Find surgical videos for
Hemorrhagic and Ischemic Stroke
online at **MediaCenter.thieme.com**!

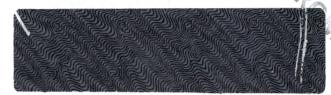
Surgical videos available online:

1. Decompressive craniectomy for stroke
2. Carotid aneurysm clip reconstruction
3. Microsurgical treatment of ruptured right posterior communicating- internal carotid artery aneurysm
4. Extracranial-Intracranial Bypass
5. Giant Thrombosed Aneurysm
6. AVM Surgery
7. ELANA bypass technique
8. Aneurysm coiling
9. Cranial AVM embolization
10. Spinal AVM and dural fistula embolization

And much more!

These videos illustrate the principles and techniques of surgical and neuroendovascular procedures used for treating stroke patients.

Total length of videos: approximately 1 hour

System requirements:

	WINDOWS	MAC	TABLET
Recommended Browser(s)**	Microsoft Internet Explorer 8.0 or later, Firefox 3.x	Firefox 3.x, Safari 4.x	HTML5 mobile browser. iPad — Safari. Opera Mobile — Tablet PCs preferred.
	** all browsers should have JavaScript enabled		
Flash Player Plug-in	Flash Player 9 or Higher* ** Mac users: ATI Rage 128 GPU does not support full-screen mode with hardware scaling*		Tablet PCs with Android OS support Flash 10.1
Minimum Hardware Configurations	Intel® Pentium® II 450 MHz, AMD Athlon™ 600 MHz or faster processor (or equivalent) 512 MB of RAM	PowerPC® G3 500 MHz or faster processor Intel Core™ Duo 1.33 GHz or faster processor 512 MB of RAM	Minimum CPU powered at 800MHz 256MB DDR2 of RAM
Recommended for optimal usage experience	Monitor resolutions: • Normal (4:3) 1024×768 or Higher • Widescreen (16:9) 1280×720 or Higher • Widescreen (16:10) 1440×900 or Higher DSL/Cable internet connection at a minimum speed of 384.0 Kbps or faster WiFi 802.11 b/g preferred.		7-inch and 10-inch tablets on maximum resolution. WiFi connection is required.

Hemorrhagic and Ischemic Stroke

Medical, Imaging, Surgical, and Interventional Approaches

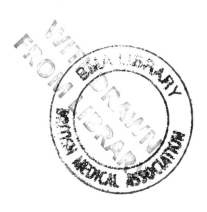

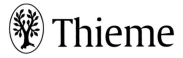

Hemorrhagic and Ischemic Stroke

Medical, Imaging, Surgical, and Interventional Approaches

Bernard R. Bendok, MD
Associate Professor
Departments of Neurological Surgery and Radiology
Northwestern University Feinberg School of Medicine
Chicago, Illinois

Andrew M. Naidech, MD, MSPH
Associate Professor
Department of Neurology, Anesthesiology, and Neurological Surgery
Northwestern University Feinberg School of Medicine
Chicago, Illinois

Matthew T. Walker, MD
Associate Professor of Radiology
Chief of Neuroradiology
Northwestern University Feinberg School of Medicine
Chicago, Illinois

H. Hunt Batjer, MD, FACS
Michael J. Marchese Professor of Neurological Surgery
Professor and Chair
Department of Neurological Surgery
Northwestern University Feinberg School of Medicine
Chicago, Illinois

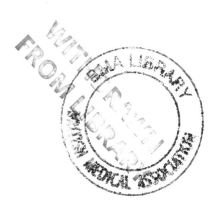

Thieme
New York • Stuttgart

Thieme Medical Publishers, Inc.
333 Seventh Ave.
New York, NY 10001

Executive Editor: Kay Conerly
Editorial Director, Clinical Reference: Michael Wachinger
Production Editor: Barbara A. Chernow
Medical Illustrator: Jennifer Pryll
International Production Director: Andreas Schabert
Senior Vice President, International Marketing and Sales: Cornelia Schulze
Vice President, Finance and Accounts: Sarah Vanderbilt
President: Brian D. Scanlan
Compositor: Agnew's, Inc.
Printer: Everbest Printing Co.

Library of Congress Cataloging-in-Publication Data

Hemorrhagic and ischemic stroke : surgical, interventional, imaging, and medical approaches / [edited by] Bernard R. Bendok . . . [et al.].
    p. ; cm.
  Includes bibliographical references and index.
  ISBN 978-1-60406-234-2
  1. Cerebrovascular disease. 2. Cerebral ischemia. 3. Diagnostic imaging. I. Bendok, Bernard R.
  [DNLM: 1. Stroke—therapy. 2. Brain Ischemia—surgery. 3. Brain Ischemia—therapy. 4. Diagnostic Imaging—methods. 5. Neurosurgical Procedures—methods. 6. Stroke—surgery. WL 356]
  RC388.5.H448   2011
  616.8'1—dc23   2011022038

Important note: Medical knowledge is ever-changing. As new research and clinical experience broaden our knowledge, changes in treatment and drug therapy may be required. The authors and editors of the material herein have consulted sources believed to be reliable in their efforts to provide information that is complete and in accord with the standards accepted at the time of publication. However, in view of the possibility of human error by the authors, editors, or publisher of the work herein or changes in medical knowledge, neither the authors, editors, nor publisher, nor any other party who has been involved in the preparation of this work, warrants that the information contained herein is in every respect accurate or complete, and they are not responsible for any errors or omissions or for the results obtained from use of such information. Readers are encouraged to confirm the information contained herein with other sources. For example, readers are advised to check the product information sheet included in the package of each drug they plan to administer to be certain that the information contained in this publication is accurate and that changes have not been made in the recommended dose or in the contraindications for administration. This recommendation is of particular importance in connection with new or infrequently used drugs.

Some of the product names, patents, and registered designs referred to in this book are in fact registered trademarks or proprietary names even though specific reference to this fact is not always made in the text. Therefore, the appearance of a name without designation as proprietary is not to be construed as a representation by the publisher that it is in the public domain.

Printed in China

5 4 3 2 1

ISBN 978-1-60406-234-2

This book is dedicated to my exceptional parents, Riad and Mima, for all their sacrifices and support; to my precious gem and wife, Karen, who makes my career possible, and my amazing children, Michael and Sarah, who are my most cherished gifts, daily joy, and inspiration; to my incomparable towering mentors and teachers, Dr. Hunt Batjer and Dr. Nick Hopkins; to all my dedicated and passionate fellows, residents, and students who make teaching worthwhile; and to my brave patients who demonstrate to me the meaning of life and the essence of human dignity every day.

—*Bernard R. Bendok*

Dedicated to the memories of Leon A. Weisberg, MD, and Charity Hospital, New Orleans. The environment sounded like jazz, smelled of cayenne pepper, and enveloped you like thick, moist air. I miss them every day.

—*Andrew M. Naidech*

I would like to acknowledge the support and mentorship of Dr. Eric J. Russell, who has been instrumental in guiding my career. I would also like to acknowledge the help and support of my diagnostic neuroradiology colleagues, neurointerventional partners, neuroradiology fellows, and radiology residents at the Feinberg School of Medicine of Northwestern University. I would also like to acknowledge the support of my family, including Karen, Grace, Owen, and, of course, Uncle Scooter!

The Neuroimaging Section is dedicated to all practicing radiologists who toil in relative obscurity while supporting and advancing the important field of high-resolution anatomical and physiological neuroimaging, which is greatly affecting the lives of stroke patients and their families. As Thomas Merton, American author, stated: "Yet it is in this loneliness that the deepest activities begin. It is here that you discover act without motion, labor that is profound repose, vision in obscurity and, beyond all desire, fulfillment whose limits extend to infinity."

—*Matthew T. Walker*

Dedicated to my great friend and mentor, Duke Samson. He taught me everything I know about cerebrovascular disease. I wish only that he had taught me all HE knows!

—*H. Hunt Batjer*

Contents

Video Contents

Foreword: Medical and Critical Care Considerations

I welcome the opprotunity to introduce the medical and critical care considerations section for this contemporary text edited by Drs. Bendok, Naidech, Walker, and Batjer. The crux of optimizing outcomes after stroke is medical management in all phases of stroke. While most centers do not have access to advanced neuroimaging and endovascular and vascular neurosurgical expertise, all clinicians who serve this patient population would benefit from reading this section, regardless of the setting of their practice. This well-written and organized section is highly appropriate for physicians training in neurology, especially those with a focus on vascular neurology and/or neurocritical care, and is an excellent resource for building concepts.

The fields of vascular neurology and neurocritical care are evolving out of a need for application of the concepts reviewed in this book. This is an exciting time for neurologists who are seeing optimism overcome the nihilistic approach that was present before demonstration of the effectiveness of IV tPA for acute ischemic stroke. I see a growing awareness of the challenges in management of this population of patients that is paralleled by the spectrum of clinical research studies in cerebrovascular disease. This text should make readers more enthusiastic about the future of the medical and critical care management of this high-risk group of patients. This book will be on my shelf adjacent to my prior gold standard stroke text.

Sheryl Martin-Schild, MD, PhD
Vascular Neurologist
Assistant Professor of Neurology
Director of the Stroke Program
Tulane University School of Medicine
New Orleans, Louisiana

Foreword: Imaging Considerations

It is a pleasure to have been asked to write the foreword to the imaging section of this comprehensive review of the imaging and treatment of stroke, edited by Drs. Bendok, Naidech, Walker, and Batjer.

Hemorrhagic and Ischemic Stroke is a user-friendly, one-stop guide for the clinical management of stroke patients. Written by renowned leaders in the stroke field, this book delivers concise, practice-oriented overviews and practical recommendations to guide decision making. *Hemorrhagic and Ischemic Stroke* includes cutting-edge information on acute stroke imaging and treatment and the latest therapies for stroke-related symptoms and disorders.

At once concise and authoritative, *Hemorrhagic and Ischemic Stroke* is the ideal reference for the clinician who wants to stay current on stroke diagnosis and therapy. This book

- answers questions that are frequently asked of neurologists, neurosurgeons and radiologists at any stage of their training;
- addresses both commonplace and rarer issues;
- covers both basic and advanced neuroimaging of stroke;
- and addresses medical, surgical, and interventional treatment of stroke.

Max Wintermark, MD
Associate Professor of Radiology, Neurology,
Neurological Surgery and Biomedical Engineering
Chief of Neuroradiology
University of Virginia
Charlottesville, Virginia

Foreword: Open Surgical Approaches

I am honored to write the foreword to the surgery section of this comprehensive text on the current multidisciplinary treatment of stroke. The editors have assembled a remarkable "cast of stars" to contribute to this book. The text is truly comprehensive dealing first with general medical, clinical, and intensive care considerations in the care of patients with both hemorrhagic and ischemic stroke. The second section, on imaging, is outstanding and deals with all the modern anatomic and physiologic imaging techniques, ending with an excellent futuristic look at upcoming technologies. The section on surgery is very comprehensive and deals not only with surgical techniques, but also with the important anesthetic considerations that are so essential to these difficult neurosurgical interventions for all common and less common vascular pathologies including aneurysms, AVMs, dural fistulas, cavernomas, and intracranial and extracranial occlusive disease. The section on interventional treatment is equally comprehensive and ends with a wonderful chapter of recent advances, innovations and the future of neurointerventional surgery.

The publication of this modern, comprehensive text is very timely given the phenomenal technological advances that we have seen over the last few years in neuro-imaging, medical and intensive care, and surgical and interventional techniques for stroke. The editors have done a remarkable job of putting it all together in a very readable, didactic and well illustrated book. I heartily congratulate them!

Roberto C. Heros, MD
Professor and Co-Chairman of Neurological Surgery
Resident Program Director
University of Miami
Miami, Florida

Foreword: Neurointerventional Approaches

I am honored to write the foreword for Section IV, Neuro-interventional Approaches, in *Hemorrhagic and Ischemic Stroke.* Having been involved in the field of interventional neuroradiology for three decades, I have had ample opportunity to witness the incredible progress that has occurred in the endovascular treatment of hemorrhagic and, more recently, ischemic stroke. More importantly, having worked in a tightly integrated multidisciplinary environment for over ten years, it became very obvious to me a long time ago that the best advances and clinical care usually result from interdisciplinary work, collaboration, and research.

In this book, Drs. Bendok, Naidech, Walker, and Batjer perfectly capture and frame this concept. They assembled a superb group of clinicians, imagers, endovascular physicians, neurosurgeons, and intensivists who, together, created a "go to" reference for every physician or trainee involved in all aspects of the diagnosis and treatment of patients with ischemic and hemorrhagic stroke.

Our daily lives are usually spent in our own subspecialty fields; even the scientific meetings we go to tend to cater to our own specialties. Reading this book gives one the opportunity to easily learn about how our other stroke colleagues contribute to patient care and become more knowledgeable team members. I hope this work strengthens the relationship that will make all of us better researchers and providers and continue to advance this very dynamic field.

Jacques Dion, MD, FRCP(C)
Professor and Head, Division of Interventional
Neuoradiology
Professor, Department of Neurosurgery
The Emory Clinic
Atlanta, Georgia

Preface

Cerebrovascular disease, both ischemic and hemorrhagic, constitutes a matter of major public health importance. These disease states are responsible for death and disability in people from infancy through late adult life. In general, hemorrhagic stroke afflicts individuals earlier in life than ischemic stroke and thus has an even higher societal cost. The past decade has seen enormous growth of endovascular strategies to treat patients with these life-threatening conditions. The diagnostic imaging field has enjoyed major advances both in the magnetic resonance domain as well as in noninvasive angiography. Modern critical care teams are armed with an enormous arsenal of drugs and devices that can maintain optimal physiologic states for protracted periods. Surgical techniques, both catheter-based and open, have also made major technologic and strategic advances.

From its inception, the goal of this project has been to produce a highly up-to-date and practical book that focuses on medical, radiologic, interventional, and surgical treatment paradigms. Conceptually, we strove to create an immediately available and user-friendly resource for trainees and those in their early postgraduate careers. As the sections of the book suggest, our audience includes neuroradiologists, neurologists, neurosurgeons, and those physicians engaged in neurologic critical care. This book can also serve as a useful reference for more experienced subspecialists in all of these areas as it reflects a state-of-the-art snapshot.

The first section of the book discusses medical and critical care issues. In this section the focus is on early diagnosis, medical decision making, and medical interventions. The second section discusses imaging in all of the facets that come into play in the diagnosis of ischemic and hemorrhagic stroke states. The third section discusses neurologic surgery. Appropriately the first chapter in this section deals with a most critical and common theme, neuroanesthesiology. Major advances have been seen in the past decade that have set the stage for an incredibly safe environment in which to perform life-threatening and lifesaving procedures. Contemporary techniques pertaining to extracranial and intracranial treatment for structural ischemic and hemorrhagic conditions are presented. The fourth section of the book discusses interventional and catheter-based techniques. Indications as well as specific technical guidance for these dramatic new procedures are put forward by the leaders in the field.

Several useful and novel features are included in this book to assist the reader in acquiring the key principles. A set of pearls is included in each chapter to highlight the key information. Almost all procedural chapters have video content that illustrates the principles of procedures, as well as the actual conduct of such a procedure both surgical and catheter-based. Artistic illustrations are provided that should enhance the readers' interpretation of the authors' description.

The editors of this book are well versed in this subject matter. Dr. Bernard Bendok is a microneurosurgeon and cranial-base surgeon who also has training and expertise in endovascular neurosurgery. Dr. Andrew Naidech is a neurologist with subspecialty expertise in neurologic critical care. Dr. Matthew Walker is the chief of neuroradiology at Northwestern University, and Dr. H. Hunt Batjer serves as chair of the Department of Neurological Surgery at Northwestern University with special interest in cerebrovascular disease. We collectively hope that this book accomplishes its purpose and provides a means of maintaining cutting-edge strategies and invasive procedures to minimize the long-term deficits that can result from these illnesses.

◆ Acknowledgments

We wish to acknowledge the tireless and creative efforts of Dr. Rudy Rahme in the creation of this book. We would also like to thank our artist, Jennifer Pryll, for the outstanding representation of often-complex concepts. We also wish to acknowledge the dedication, professionalism and constant support of Thieme editor Kay Conerly and her assistant editor Lauren Henry.

Contributors

Todd A. Abruzzo, MD
Department of Radiology
University of Cincinnati Neuroscience Institute
University of Cincinnati College of Medicine
Mayfield Clinic
Cincinnati, Ohio

Joseph G. Adel, MD
Department of Neurological Surgery
Northwestern University Feinberg School of Medicine
Chicago, Illinois

Felipe C. Albuquerque, MD
Division of Neurological Surgery
Barrow Neurological Institute
St. Joseph's Hospital and Medical Center
Phoenix, Arizona

Peter J. Amenta, MD
Department of Neurosurgery
Thomas Jefferson University Hospital
Jefferson Hospital for Neuroscience
Philadelphia, Pennsylvania

Sameer A. Ansari, MD, PhD
Department of Radiology, Neurology, and Neurosurgery
Northwestern University Feinberg School of Medicine
Chicago, Illinois

Salah G. Aoun, MD
Department of Neurological Surgery
Northwestern University Feinberg School of Medicine
Chicago, Illinois

Omar M. Arnaout, MD
Department of Neurological Surgery
Northwestern University Feinberg School of Medicine
Chicago, Illinois

Issam A. Awad, MD, MSc, FACS, MS (hon)
Professor of Surgery (Clinical Scholar)
Biological Sciences Division
Director of Neurovascular Surgery
Section of Surgery
University of Chicago Pritzker School of Medicine
Chicago, Illinois

Daniel L. Barrow, MD
Department of Neurosurgery
Emory Clinic
Department of Neurosurgery Service
Emory University Hospital
Emory MBNA Stroke Center
Atlanta, Georgia

H. Hunt Batjer, MD, FACS
Michael J. Marchese Professor of Neurological Surgery
Professor and Chair
Department of Neurological Surgery
Northwestern University Feinberg School of Medicine
Chicago, Illinois

John F. Bebawy, MD
Department of Anesthesiology
Northwestern University Feinberg School of Medicine
Chicago, Illinois

Rodney D. Bell, MD
Jefferson Hospital for the Neurosciences
Philadelphia, Pennsylvania

Bernard R. Bendok, MD
Associate Professor
Departments of Neurological Surgery and
   Radiology
Northwestern University Feinberg School of Medicine
Chicago, Illinois

Richard A. Bernstein, MD, PhD
Department of Neurology
Northwestern University Feinberg School of Medicine
Chicago, Illinois

Alan S. Boulos, MD
Division of Neurosurgery
Albany Medical Center
Albany, New York

Leonardo B.C. Brasiliense, MD
Division of Neurological Surgery
Barrow Neurological Institute
St. Joseph's Hospital and Medical Center
Phoenix, Arizona

Charles M. Cawley, MD
Department of Radiology
Emory University
Atlanta, Georgia

Neeraj Chaudhary, MD
Department of Radiology
University of Michigan Health System and Medical
  School
Ann Arbor, Michigan

Guilherme Dabus, MD
Department of Neurointerventional Surgery
Baptist Cardiac and Vascular Institute
Miami, Florida

John C. Dalfino, MD
Neurosurgery Group
Albany Medical Center
Albany, New York

Mark Dannenbaum, MD
Department of Neurosurgery
Emory Clinic
Atlanta, Georgia

Reza Dashti, MD, PhD
Department of Neurosurgery
Cerraphasa University
Istanbul, Turkey

Arthur L. Day, MD
Department of Neurosurgery
University of Texas Medical School
Houston, Texas

Valerie Dechant, MD
Department of Neurology
University of North Carolina
Chapel Hill, North Carolina

Colin P. Derdeyn, MD
Mallinckrodt Institute of Radiology
Departments of Neurology and Neurological Surgery
Center for Stroke and Cerebrovascular Disease
Washington University School of Medicine
St. Louis, Missouri

Rajat Dhar, MD
Department of Neurology
Division of Neurocritical Care
Washington University School of Medicine
St. Louis, Missouri

Andrew F. Ducruet, MD
Department of Neurological Surgery
Columbia University
New York, New York

Joshua R. Dusick, MD
Department of Neurosurgery
David Geffen School of Medicine
University of California–Los Angeles
Los Angeles, California

James D. Eastwood, MD
Department of Radiology
Duke University Medical Center
Durham, North Carolina

Christopher S. Eddleman, MD, PhD
Department of Neurological Surgery
Northwestern University Feinberg School of Medicine
Chicago, Illinois

Andrew J. Fishman, MD
Departments of Otolaryngology and Neurosurgery
Northwestern University Feinberg School of Medicine
Chicago, Illinois

John C. Flickinger, MD, FACR
Department of Radiation Oncology
University of Pittsburgh Medical Center
Shadyside Radiation Oncology
Pittsburgh, Pennsylvania

W. Christopher Fox, MD
Department of Neurosurgery
University of Michigan Health System
Ann Arbor, Michigan

Joseph J. Gemmete, MD
Division of Interventional Neuroradiology
Department of Radiology
University of Michigan Health System
Ann Arbor, Michigan

Nestor R. Gonzalez, MD
Departments of Neurosurgery and Radiology
David Geffen School of Medicine
University of California–Los Angeles
Los Angeles, California

Andrew Grande, MD
Department of Neurosurgery
University of Cincinnati Neuroscience Institute
University of Cincinnati College of Medicine
Cincinnati, Ohio

Bradley A. Gross, BS
Brigham and Women's Hospital
Boston, Massachusetts

Murat Gunel, MD
Department of Neurosurgery and Neurobiology
Section of Neurovascular Surgery
Yale University School of Medicine
New Haven, Connecticut

Dhanesh K. Gupta, MD
Departments of Anesthesiology and Neurological Surgery
Northwestern University Feinberg School of Medicine
Chicago, Illinois

Reza Hakimelahi, MD
Department of Radiology
Division of Neuroradiology
Massachusetts General Hospital
Boston, Massachusetts

Ricardo A. Hanel, MD, PhD
Department of Neurosurgery
Mayo Clinic
Jacksonville, Florida

Julie H. Harreld, MD
Diagnostic Imaging
St. Jude Children's Research Hospital
Memphis, Tennessee

Juha Hernesniemi, MD, PhD
Department of Neurosurgery
Helsinki University Central Hospital
Helsinki, Finland

L. Nelson Hopkins, MD
Departments of Neurosurgery and Radiology and Toshiba
    Stroke Research Center
School of Medicine and Biomedical Sciences
State University of New York at Buffalo
Department of Neurosurgery
Millard Fillmore Gates Hospital
Kaleida Health
Buffalo, New York

Jay U. Howington, MD
Neurological Institute of Savannah
Savannah, Georgia

Yin C. Hu, MD
Division of Neurological Surgery
Barrow Neurological Institute
St. Joseph's Hospital and Medical Center
Phoenix, Arizona

Michael C. Hurley, MD
Department of Radiology
Northwestern University Feinberg School of Medicine
Chicago, Illinois

Pascal M. Jabbour, MD
Department of Neurological Surgery
Division of Neurovascular Surgery and Endovascular
    Neurosurgery
Thomas Jefferson University Hospital
Philadelphia, Pennsylvania

Jennifer Jaffe, MPH, CCRP
Neurovascular Surgery Program and Section of
    Neurosurgery
Division of Biological Sciences and the Pritzker School of
    Medicine
University of Chicago
Chicago, Illinois

Rashid M. Janjua, MD
Department of Neurosurgery
University of South Florida
Tampa, Florida

Brian J. Jian, MD, PhD
Department of Neurosurgery
University of California, San Francisco
San Francisco, California

Jimmy Jaeyoung Kang, MD
Department of Radiology
Division of Radiology
Massachusetts General Hospital
Boston, Massachusetts

Hideyuki Kano, MD, PhD
Research Assistant Professor
Department of Neurological Surgery
University of Pittsburgh
Pittsburgh, Pennsylvania

Shah-Naz Khan, MD
Department of Neurosurgery
University of New Mexico
Albuquerque, New Mexico

Contributors

Usman Khan, MD
Department of Neurosurgery
University of Cincinnati College of Medicine
Cincinnati, Ohio

Anne Catherine Kim, MD
Department of Radiology/Imaging Services
Kaiser Permanente
Walnut Creek Medical Center
Walnut Creek, California

Antoun Koht, MD
Departments of Anesthesiology, Neurological Surgery, and
    Neurology
Northwestern University Feinberg School of Medicine
Chicago, Illinois

Douglas Kondziolka, MD, MSc, FRCS(C), FACS
Department of Neurological Surgery
University of Pittsburgh Medical Center
Pittsburgh, Pennsylvania

Peter G. Kranz, MD
Department of Radiology
Duke University Medical Center
Durham, North Carolina

Michael T. Lawton, MD
Department of Neurological Surgery
University of California, San Francisco
San Francisco, California

Martin Lehecka, MD, PhD
Department of Neurosurgery
Helsinki University Central Hospital
Helsinki, Finland

Elad I. Levy, MD
Departments of Neurosurgery and Radiology and Toshiba
    Stroke Research Center
School of Medicine and Biomedical Sciences
State University of New York at Buffalo
Department of Neurosurgery
Millard Fillmore Gates Hospital
Kaleida Health
Buffalo, New York

Richard Lochhead, MD
Division of Neurological Surgery
Barrow Neurological Institute
St. Joseph's Hospital and Medical Center
Phoenix, Arizona

L. Dade Lunsford, MD, FACS
Department of Neurological Surgery
University of Pittsburgh School of Medicine
Pittsburgh, Pennsylvania

Neil A. Martin, MD
Department of Neurosurgery
David Geffen School of Medicine
University of California–Los Angeles
Los Angeles, California

Cameron G. McDougall, MD
Division of Neurological Surgery
Barrow Neurological Institute
St. Joseph's Hospital and Medical Center
Phoenix, Arizona

Laurie McWilliams, MD
Cerebrovascular Center
Cleveland Clinic
Cleveland, Ohio

Anna G. Meader, BS
Harvard University
Massachusetts General Hospital
Boston, Massachusetts

Philip M. Meyers, MD, FAHA
Department of Neurological Surgery
Columbia University
New York, New York

Jeffery Miller, MD
Department of Radiology
Northwestern University Feinberg School of Medicine
Chicago, Illinois

Mark D. Morasch, MD
Department of Vascular Surgery
Northwestern University Feinberg School of Medicine
Chicago, Illinois

Andrew M. Naidech, MD, MSPH
Associate Professor
Department of Neurology, Anesthesiology, and Neurological
    Surgery
Northwestern University Feinberg School of Medicine
Chicago, Illinois

Sabareesh K. Natarajan, MD, MS
Department of Neurosurgery and Toshiba Stroke Research
    Center
School of Medicine and Biomedical Sciences
State University of New York at Buffalo
Department of Neurosurgery
Millard Fillmore Gates Hospital
Kaleida Health
Buffalo, New York

C. Benjamin Newman, MD
Division of Neurological Surgery
Barrow Neurological Institute
St. Joseph's Hospital and Medical Center
Phoenix, Arizona

Contributors

Christopher Nichols, MD
Department of Neurosurgery
University of Cincinnati Neuroscience Institute
University of Cincinnati College of Medicine
Cincinnati, Ohio

Mika Niemelä, MD, PhD
Department of Neurosurgery
Helsinki University Central Hospital
Helsinki, Finland

Tomi Niemi, MD, PhD
Department of Anesthesiology
Helsinki University Central Hospital
Helsinki, Finland

Anitha Nimmagadda, MD
Departments of Neurological Surgery and Radiology
Northwestern University Feinberg School of Medicine
Chicago, Illinois

Christopher S. Ogilvy, MD
Department of Neurosurgery
Massachusetts General Hospital
Boston, Massachusetts

Aditya S. Pandey, MD
Department of Neurosurgery
University of Michigan Health System and Medical
  School
Ann Arbor, Michigan

J. Javier Provencio, MD, FCCM
Cleveland Clinic
Cleveland, Ohio

Gail Pyne-Geithman, PhD
Department of Neurovascular Research
Department of Neurosurgery
University of Cincinnati
Cincinnati, Ohio

Alejandro A. Rabinstein, MD
Department of Neurology
Mayo Clinic
Rochester, Minnesota

Rudy J. Rahme, MD
Department of Neurosurgery
Northwestern University Feinberg School of Medicine
Chicago, Illinois

Andrew J. Ringer, MD
Department of Neurosurgery
University of Cincinnati Neuroscience Institute
University of Cincinnati College of Medicine and Mayfield
  Clinic
Cincinnati, Ohio

Jaakko Rinne, MD
Department of Neurosurgery
Kuopio University Hospital
Kuopio, Finland

Rossana Romani, MD
Department of Neurosurgery
Helsinki University Central Hospital
Helsinki, Finland

Javier M. Romero, MD
Department of Ultrasound
Harvard University
Massachusetts General Hospital
Boston, Massachusetts

Robert H. Rosenwasser, MD, FACS, FAHA
Department of Neurological Surgery
Jefferson Medical College
Thomas Jefferson University
Philadelphia, Pennsylvania

Howard A. Rowley, MD
Department of Neuroradiology
University of Wisconsin, Madison
Madison, Wisconsin

Eric J. Russell, MD
Department of Radiology
Northwestern University Feinberg School of Medicine
Chicago, Illinois

Pamela W. Schaefer, MD
Department of Radiology
Division of Neuroradiology
Massachusetts General Hospital
Boston, Massachusetts

Albert J. Schuette, MD
Departments of Neurosurgery and Radiology
Emory University
Atlanta, Georgia

R. Michael Scott, MD
Department of Neurosurgery
Children's Hospital Boston
Boston, Massachusetts

Ali Shaibani, MD
Department of Radiology
Northwestern University Feinberg School of Medicine
Chicago, Illinois

Sameer A. Sheth, MD, PhD
Department of Neurosurgery
Massachusetts General Hospital
Boston, Massachusetts

Sunil A. Sheth, MD
Department of Neurosurgery
Massachusetts General Hospital
Boston, Massachusetts

Adnan H. Siddiqui, MD, PhD
Departments of Neurosurgery and Radiology and Toshiba
  Stroke Research Center
School of Medicine and Biomedical Sciences
State University of New York at Buffalo
Department of Neurosurgery
Millard Fillmore Gates Hospital
Kaleida Health
Buffalo, New York

Vineeta Singh, MD
Neurology Service
San Francisco General Hospital
University of California, San Francisco
San Francisco, California

Edward R. Smith, MD
Department of Neurosurgery
Children's Hospital Boston
Boston, Massachusetts

Robert A. Solomon, MD
Department of Neurological Surgery
Neurological Institute
Columbia University College of Physicians and
  Surgeons
New York, New York

Robert F. Spetzler, MD
Barrow Neurological Institute
Phoenix, Arizona

Charles M. Strother, MD
Department of Radiology
University of Wisconsin, Madison
Madison, Wisconsin

Byron Gregory Thompson, MD
Departments of Neurosurgery, Otolaryngology, and
  Radiology
University of Michigan School of Medicine
Taubman Health Care Center
Ann Arbor, Michigan

Cornelis A.F. Tulleken, MD, PhD
Department of Neurosurgery
Rudolf Magnus Institute of Neuroscience
University Medical Center Utrecht
Utrecht, The Netherlands

Patrick A. Turski, MD
Department of Radiology
University of Wisconsin, Madison
Madison, Wisconsin

Timothy Uschold, MD
Division of Neurological Surgery
Barrow Neurological Institute
St. Joseph's Hospital and Medical Center
Phoenix, Arizona

A. van der Zwan, MD, PhD
Department of Neurosurgery
Rudolf Magnus Institute of Neuroscience
University Medical Center Utrecht
Utrecht, The Netherlands

T.P.C. van Doormaal, MD
Department of Neurosurgery
Rudolf Magnus Institute of Neuroscience
University Medical Center Utrecht
Utrecht, The Netherlands

Erol Veznedaroglu, MD, FACS, FAHA
Stroke and Cerebrovascular Center of New Jersey
Hamilton, New Jersey

Matthew Vibbert, MD
Jefferson Medical College
Philadelphia, Pennsylvania

Matthew T. Walker, MD
Associate Professor of Radiology
Chief of Neuroradiology
Northwestern University Feinberg School of Medicine
Chicago, Illinois

Huai-che Yang, MD
Department of Neurological Surgery
University of Pittsburgh School of Medicine
Pittsburgh, Pennsylvania

Carine Zeeni, MD
Department of Anesthesiology
Northwestern University Feinberg School of Medicine
Chicago, Illinois

Contributors

I

Medical and Critical Care Considerations

1

Epidemiology

Rodney D. Bell and Valerie Dechant

Pearls

◆ Stroke is the third leading cause of death and the leading cause of disability in the United States.[1]
◆ Risk factors for stroke include nonmodifiable factors such as age and gender and modifiable factors such as hypertension, diabetes, and smoking.
◆ Awareness of stroke risk factors facilitates stratification of patient stroke risk as well as therapy aimed at improving modifiable risks.

◆ Stroke Incidence

Despite the modern advances in the diagnosis and treatment of cerebrovascular disease, stroke remains an important cause of mortality and morbidity worldwide. The World Health Organization (WHO) estimates that there are 15 million cases of stroke each year. Of these, 5 million will die from the stroke and 5 million will live with long-term disability.[2] Stroke is more prevalent in industrialized nations and is a major health concern in the United States. It is estimated that 795,000 strokes occur annually in the U.S. In 2005 the American Heart Association (AHA) reported 143,579 stroke-related deaths, making stroke the third most common cause of death behind heart disease and cancer.[1]

◆ Stroke Prevalence

Although the overall stroke incidence is expected to increase with the aging population, the rate of death in stroke patients has been declining with advances in acute treatment and supportive care. Due to improved survival after stroke, there are an estimated 4,700,000 stroke survivors living in the United States; 30 to 50% of them do not regain functional independence. Recurrent stroke is common in this population. In stroke survivors of ages 40 to 69, 15% of men and 17% of women are expected to have a recurrent stroke within 5 years. For those with stroke at age 70 or older, the rate of recurrent stroke increases to 23% for men and 27% for women.[1]

◆ Frequency of Stroke Subtypes

Ischemic stroke is caused by a lack of blood flow to brain tissue. According to data derived from the Framingham Heart Study, approximately 85% of all strokes are ischemic. Sixty percent of ischemic strokes are atherothrombotic, originating from direct occlusion of either small or large vessels. Embolic strokes are caused by a piece of thrombus that migrates from a distant location, causing an occlusion of a cerebral vessel. Embolic stroke accounts for approximately 25% of ischemic strokes. Hemorrhagic stroke accounts for approximately 13% of all strokes. Eight percent of all strokes are intraparenchymal hemorrhage and 5.4% are subarachnoid hemorrhages (SAHs)[3] (**Fig. 1.1**).

◆ Stroke Risk Factors

Epidemiologic studies have shown that patients with vascular risk factors are at an increased risk of stroke. The Framingham Heart Study prospectively followed a cohort of more than 5000 subjects over several decades. Based on these data, a risk profile was created to predict the likelihood of stroke over a 10-year period. The profile includes age, systolic blood pressure, antihypertensive therapy, diabetes, cigarette smoking, cardiovascular disease, atrial fibrillation, and left ventricular hypertrophy.[4] Evaluation for risk factors is essential to assessing a patient's overall stroke risk.

Some risk factors, such as age and gender, cannot be changed. However, many vascular risk factors can be modified by appropriate medical treatment. Diligent surveillance and treatment of modifiable risk factors can significantly

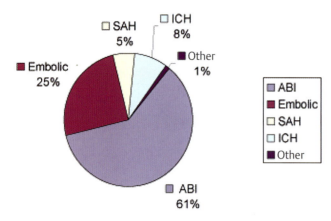

Fig. 1.1 Stroke percentages by subtype, based on data collected by the Framingham Heart Study. ABI, atherothrombotic brain infarction; ICH, intracerebral hemorrhage; SAH, subarachnoid hemorrhage. (From Mohr JP, Choi D, Grotta J, Weir B, Wolf P. Stroke: Pathophysiology, Diagnosis and Management, 4th ed. Churchill Livingstone, 2004.)

modify a patient's risk of stroke. A full list of nonmodifiable and modifiable stroke risk factors can be found in **Table 1.1**.

Nonmodifiable Risk Factors

Age

The annual incidence of stroke increases with age.[1] Data from the Framingham Heart Study's 55-year follow-up demonstrates that the stroke risk approximately doubles in each decade from ages 35 to 95 (**Fig. 1.2**).[3]

Gender

Men have a higher incidence of stroke at young ages. This gender difference narrows with advancing age (**Fig. 1.2**). For the oldest age group (≥85 years), women have a higher incidence of stroke, probably because women are more likely to live to advanced age. In 2005 women accounted for >60% of all stroke deaths.[1]

Race

Several cohort studies have assessed the effect of race on stroke risk, including the Northern Manhattan Stroke Study, the Atherosclerosis Risk in Communities Study, and the Greater Cincinnati/Northern Kentucky Stroke Study. There is a racial disparity in stroke risk in the United States, with African Americans having the highest risk, followed by Hispanics and then Caucasians. African Americans have nearly twice the stroke risk of Caucasians. This disparity is particularly prominent in patients under 55 years of age. Asian Americans have a lower risk of ischemic stroke but a higher risk of hemorrhagic stroke. Low levels of high-density lipoprotein (HDL) cholesterol are more common in Asian populations and have been linked to an increased risk of hemorrhagic stroke.[1]

Table 1.1 Modifiable and Nonmodifiable Stroke Risk Factors
Nonmodifiable Risk Factors
Age
Gender
Race/ethnicity
Genetics
Modifiable Risk Factors
Hypertension
Diabetes
Cigarette smoking
Dyslipidemia
Physical inactivity
Obesity
Excessive alcohol intake
Atrial fibrillation
Other heart disease
Drug abuse
Obstructive sleep apnea
Previous stroke/transient ischemic attack (TIA)
Hypercoagulable state
Aortic atheroma
Patent foramen ovale
Carotid artery disease

Genetics

Studies of twins and families with stroke suggest a genetic component to stroke risk. A complex interaction between multiple genetic susceptibilities and environment rather than a single gene likely conveys an individual's vulnerability to stroke. Several gene polymorphisms have been identified that may be related to increased risk of ischemic stroke, intracerebral hemorrhage, and SAH[5,6] (**Table 1.2**).

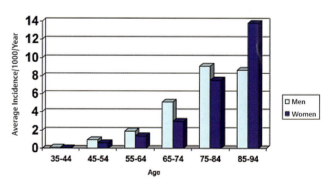

Fig. 1.2 Incidence of atherothrombotic brain infarction by age and gender. (Adapted from data from the Framingham Heart Study as presented in Mohr JP, Choi D, Grotta J, Weir B, Wolf P. Stroke: Pathophysiology, Diagnosis and Management, 4th ed. Churchill Livingstone, 2004, p. 15.)

Table 1.2 Genes with Polymorphisms Independently Associated with Stroke

Gene	Gene Function
Genes Associated with Atherothrombotic Strokes	
MTHFR	Encodes the enzyme methylenetetrahydrofolate reductase which is necessary for the breakdown of homocysteine to methionine. Defects cause homocystinuria.
IPF1	Encodes a transcriptional activator involved in the development of the pancreas and glucose regulation. Linked to early-onset diabetes.
TNFSF4	Encodes for cytokine in the tumor necrosis factor ligand family that mediates adhesion of activated T cells to vascular endothelial cells. Linked to myocardial infarction and systemic lupus erythematosus.
ITGB2	Encodes for an integrin protein involved in cell adhesion.
THBS2	Encodes a thrombospondin protein that mediates cell adhesion and migration.
IL6	Encodes a cytokine produced at sites of inflammation. Dysfunction has been linked to diabetes.
ANXA5	Encodes an anticoagulant protein involved in the coagulation cascade.
MMP12	Encodes a matrix degrading enzyme involved in inflammation. Defects are associated with accelerated atherosclerosis.
Genes Associated with Intracerebral Hemorrhage	
IL6	See above.
TNF	Encodes proinflammatory cytokine secreted by macrophages that may have a neuroprotective role.
FBN1	Encodes fibrillin-1, a protein that is part of the extracellular matrix. Dysfunction is linked to connective tissue disorders such as Marfan syndrome.
UCP1	Encodes a mitochondrial uncoupling protein. Dysfunction has been linked to obesity.
LIPC	Encodes a protein involved in lipoprotein uptake. Defects have been linked to diabetes.
CCL5	Encodes a cytokine involved chemoattraction of T cells.
Genes Associated with Subarachnoid Hemorrhage	
TNF	See above.
CCL5	See above.
MTHFR	See above.
CAPN10	Encodes a calpain protein that has been associated with non–insulin-dependent diabetes mellitus.
UCP3	Encodes a mitochondrial uncoupling protein thought to protect mitochondria against lipid-induced oxidative stress. Defects have been linked to obesity and type 2 diabetes.
OLR1	Encodes a transcription factor important in fetal development of insulin-producing β cells. Defects are linked to both insulin-dependent and non–insulin-dependent diabetes mellitus.
TGFBR2	Encodes a receptor used in cell signal transduction that influences cell growth and division. It has been implicated as a tumor suppressor. Defects have been linked to connective tissue diseases.
IL10	Encodes a cytokine produced by monocytes and lymphocytes involved in immunoregulation. Defects are linked to Crohn's disease and rheumatoid arthritis.

Source: Adapted from Yamada Y. Identification of genetic factors and development of genetic risk diagnosis systems for cardiovascular diseases and stroke. Circ J 2006;70:1240–1248. Gene functions are as described in the Online Mendelian Inheritance in Man (OMIM) genetic disorder catalog, www.ncbi.nlm.nih.gov.

Cerebral autosomal-dominant arteriopathy with subcortical infarcts and leukoencephalopathy (CADASIL) is the most common hereditary stroke related syndrome. It is caused by a mutation of the *NOTCH3* gene that phenotypically results in migraine, mood changes, and subcortical strokes in young adulthood.

Fabry's disease is an X-linked recessive condition in which deficiency of β-galactosidase A leads to accumulation of trihexosylceramide in the blood vessels, nervous system, kidneys, and skin. These patients are at an increased risk of stroke and heart attack.

Modifiable Risk Factors

Hypertension

Hypertension is the most powerful modifiable risk factor for stroke. The risk of stroke increases with increasing systolic blood pressure (SBP) above 115 mm Hg.[3,7] Effective blood pressure control can reduce stroke risk by up to one third.[8]

Diabetes

Diabetics are at an increased risk of atherosclerotic disease at multiple locations including the coronary, peripheral, and cerebral vasculature.[3] Atherosclerosis combined with an increased risk of hypertension conveys a high risk of stroke among diabetics.[9]

Patients with diabetes have strokes at a younger age than nondiabetics, possibly due to accelerated atherosclerotic disease[9]; 15 to 33% of patients with ischemic stroke have diabetes.[10]

Although glucose intolerance and elevated blood sugars have been found to increase stroke risk and may be predictors of poor outcome in patients with stroke, it is unclear whether tight glycemic control helps to ameliorate the risk of stroke in diabetic patients or improves outcome in patients who have suffered a stroke.[3,11]

Cigarette Smoking

Smokers have roughly twice the ischemic stroke risk of non-smokers after controlling for other risk factors.[1] Increased stroke risk is likely due to accelerated atherosclerosis and proinflammatory effects. Those who stop smoking can reduce their stroke risk to that of a nonsmoker after 5 years of abstinence. The AHA recommends counseling for smoking cessation for all stroke survivors.[12]

Dyslipidemia

Although elevated serum cholesterol is associated with arthrosclerosis, including carotid and coronary artery disease, a direct relationship between elevated serum cholesterol and stroke has not been consistently demonstrated.[12] The incidence of coronary artery disease is directly related to serum low-density lipoprotein (LDL) levels and inversely related to high-density lipoprotein (HDL) levels.[1,12] Based on this relationship, the AHA recommends a goal LDL of <100 mg/dL or <70 mg/dL for patients with multiple vascular risk factors.[10]

There is mounting evidence that statins, the most common medication used for the treatment of hyperlipidemia, may provide some protection against stroke. The Heart Protection Study included 3280 patients with previous stroke or transient ischemic attack (TIA) who were randomized to simvastatin or placebo. Significantly fewer recurrent strokes were seen in patients on simvastatin even in those with normal to mildly elevated cholesterol.[13] The Stroke Prevention by Aggressive Reduction in Cholesterol Levels (SPARCL) trial investigated the role of statin therapy in prevention of recurrent stroke in patients with TIA or stroke in the past 6 months. In this trial patients on statin therapy had a lower incidence of stroke.[14] The Justification for the Use of Statins in Prevention: An Intervention Trial (JUPITER) study group followed over 17,000 healthy patients without hyperlipidemia (LDL <130) but with elevated C-reactive protein. The study group found that statin use reduced the incidence of major cardiovascular events, including stroke.[15] Based on these studies, it appears that the antiatherosclerotic effects of statins extend beyond their effect on cholesterol and likely involve their antiinflammatory properties and direct antiatherosclerotic effects on the vascular wall. The AHA guidelines suggest it is reasonable to start stroke survivors on statin therapy even if they lack other indications such as elevated cholesterol or coronary artery disease.[10]

Obesity

Obesity is linked to other stroke risk factors such as diabetes mellitus, hypertension, and dyslipidemia. Associations between body mass index (BMI) and stroke risk have been reported. Although the relationship between general obesity and stroke may be mediated by the medical complications of obesity, there is evidence that abdominal obesity is an independent risk factor for ischemic stroke. Abdominal obesity has been shown to be related to prothrombotic conditions.[16]

Excessive Alcohol

Moderate consumption of alcohol may decrease ischemic stroke risk. The mechanism responsible for this is not clear. Proposed mechanisms include increased HDL, decreased platelet aggregation, and decreased fibrinogen levels. Excessive intake of alcohol is associated with an increased risk of ischemic and hemorrhagic stroke.[17] This is likely secondary to alcohol-related diseases including hypertension and cardiomyopathy.[17]

Physical Inactivity

Regular exercise may reduce stroke risk by improving risk factors such as obesity, hypertension, blood glucose control, and serum lipid ratio. Aerobic exercise may also have more direct effects such as promoting atherosclerotic plaque stability and improving endothelial functioning. Exercise may also benefit stroke survivors psychologically and improve their functional independence.[18]

Carotid Artery Disease

Atherosclerotic disease of the carotid arteries is a possible source of embolic stroke. Severe stenosis or occlusion of the carotid vessels can also lead to ischemia due to decreased perfusion of the cerebral vasculature.

The appropriate approach to treatment of carotid artery stenosis has been addressed by randomized trials. The North American Symptomatic Carotid Endarterectomy Trial (NASCET) and the European Carotid Surgery Trial (ECST) investigated the benefit of carotid endarterectomy (CEA) versus medical therapy in patients with recent nondisabling strokes or stroke-like symptoms. Both studies found a benefit for CEA over medical therapy in patients with 70 to 99% stenosis. The Asymptomatic Carotid Atherosclerosis Study (ACAS) investigated CEA versus medical management in pa-

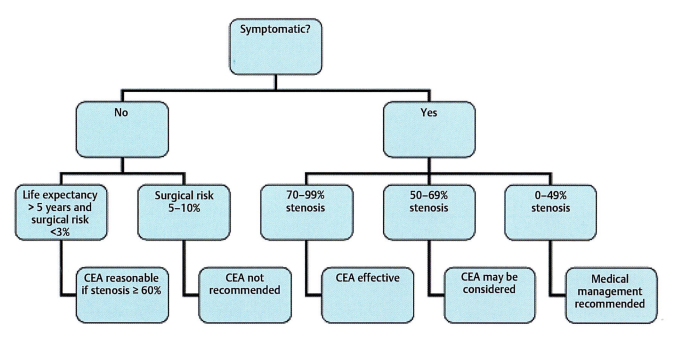

Fig. 1.3 Guidelines for carotid endarterectomy. (Adapted from recommendations in Biller J, Feinberg WM, Castaldo JE, et al. Guidelines for carotid endarterectomy: a statement for healthcare professionals from a special writing group of the Stroke Council, American Heart Association. Stroke 1998;29:554–562.)

tients with >60% carotid stenosis. The study findings suggest that CEA was beneficial over medical management in patients with >60% stenosis if procedural morbidity was minimized. The American Academy of Neurology (AAN) has published a statement regarding CEA in symptomatic and asymptomatic patients in part based on the results of NASCET[19,20] **(Fig. 1.3).**

Carotid artery stenting (CAS) is an alternative approach to the treatment of internal carotid artery (ICA) stenosis. The potential benefits, if any, of CAS over CEA are unclear, and there may be a higher risk of restenosis in patients who underwent CAS.[21] The CREST TRIAL (Carotid Revascularization Endarterectomy VS Stent Trial) showed that patients with symptomatic or asymptomatic carotid stenosis, the risk of the primary outcomes of stroke, myocardial infarction, or death did not differ between carotid endarterectomy or stenting. There was a higher risk of stroke with stenting and a higher risk of myocardial infarction in the endarterectomy group.

Atrial Fibrillation

Atrial fibrillation (AF) results in irregular and inefficient contraction of the atria of the heart. This can lead to stagnation of blood within the left atrium of the heart, which can clot and embolize to the cerebral vasculature. AF is associated with a fivefold increase in stroke risk.[22] Although the presence of AF increases stroke risk in all age groups, the independent effect of AF on stroke risk increases with advanced age.[22] Anticoagulation with warfarin decreases the risk of stroke to roughly 1% annually in patients with AF. Therefore, anticoagulation is recommended in patients without contraindications. Patients with AF who are younger than 65 and have no other vascular risk factors (lone AF) have a preanticoagulation stroke risk too low to benefit from warfarin.[23] Patients who cannot tolerate anticoagulation should be treated with antiplatelet agents. The Atrial Fibrillation Clopidogrel Trial with Irbesartan for Vascular Events (ACTIVE) study compared the use of aspirin to aspirin plus clopidogrel in patients who could not be treated with full anticoagulation. Although the combination of aspirin and clopidogrel did provide a 28% reduction in stroke versus aspirin alone, it also increased the risk of major intracerebral hemorrhage by 87%.[24]

Obstructive Sleep Apnea

Obstructive sleep apnea (OSA) is condition in which upper airway obstruction results in multiple pauses in breathing during sleep. As a result of these apneas the patient retains carbon dioxide and experiences hypoxemia. This triggers an increase in sympathetic activity resulting in vasoconstriction, which can cause extreme hypertension. OSA has been linked to endothelial dysfunction, oxidative stress, and increased platelet activation.[25] OSA has been shown to be an independent risk factor for stroke even when controlling for comorbid factors such as hypertension, diabetes, and obesity.[26]

Aortic Atheroma

Atherosclerotic disease in general is a risk factor for stroke. Atherosclerotic plaques located in the ascending aorta are of particular concern because they may directly embolize to the cerebral vasculature. A higher rate of significant ascending aortic atheroma has been identified in patients with cryptogenic stroke. The following atheroma characteristics have been found to predict higher risk of embolization leading to stroke[27]:

◆ Thicker plaques ≥4 mm
◆ Ulceration within the plaque
◆ Mobile element within the plaque

Patent Foramen Ovale

The foramen ovale is a hole in the atrial septum that facilitates blood flow during fetal circulation. Normally this communication closes at birth. When this closure is not complete a communication remains between the right and left heart. This can allow paradoxical embolism to travel from the venous system through a patent foramen ovale (PFO), into the arterial circulation, and cause cerebral infarction. Factors that may predict a high risk of recurrent stroke in patients with PFO include the following[28]:

◆ Presence of atrial septal aneurysm
◆ Large PFO
◆ High degree of right-to-left shunting
◆ Presence of a hypercoagulable state

Patent foramen ovale is found incidentally in 20 to 35% of the general population based on autopsy findings, and is seen on transesophageal echocardiography (TEE) in 10 to 25% of healthy individuals.[28] Although PFO is more common in patients with cryptogenic stroke than in the general population, there are many patients with asymptomatic PFO. There is no clear indication for treatment of asymptomatic PFO, as no prospective randomized trial has been completed at this time.

Drug Abuse

Abuse of illicit drugs is a significant cause of stroke in young patients. It is reasonable to screen young patients for drug use when they present with cryptogenic stroke. Cocaine use is associated with hemorrhagic stroke due to its tendency to induce extreme hypertension. Cocaine may also induce vasospasm, which can result in ischemic damage. Heroin use has been linked to border-zone infarctions, perhaps related to episodes of hypotension or hypoxia. Amphetamine use is associated with recurrent transient ischemic attacks, intracerebral hemorrhage, and ischemic stroke.[29]

Prothrombotic States

The coagulation system maintains a delicate balance between clotting and blood flow. Patients with abnormalities of the coagulation system may be prone to excessive bleeding or clotting. Therefore, they may be at increased risk for hemorrhagic or ischemic stroke.

Antiphospholipid antibodies include lupus anticoagulant and anticardiolipin antibodies (immunoglobulins G and M). These are associated with systemic lupus erythematosus (SLE) and other connective tissue diseases, but they may also occur independently. Patients with antiphospholipid antibodies have an increased risk of both arterial and venous thrombosis.[3,30] Although there are conflicting data, some prospective studies suggest that the risk of stroke is higher in patients with antiphospholipid antibodies.[30]

Factor V Leiden mutation is the most common hereditary cause of venous thrombosis. A mutation in factor V causing it to be resistant to breakdown by protein C leads to increased rates of venous thrombosis. The link between factor V Leiden mutation and arterial stroke is controversial.[3,30]

Protein C, protein S, and antithrombin are responsible for inactivation of the coagulation cascade. Deficiencies in these proteins are less common than factor V Leiden mutation but are more likely to cause venous thrombosis.[3] Cerebral venous thrombosis is seen in 1 to 3% of these patients.[3] The role of these mutations in arterial stroke is unclear.

Prothrombin G20210A mutation causes increased levels of prothrombin leading to a higher risk of venous thrombosis. There is some evidence to suggest that this mutation may work synergistically with other vascular risk factors to increase the risk of stroke, but existing data have not consistently confirmed this relationship.[3,30]

Elevated levels of plasma homocystine can result from defects in metabolism of methionine. High levels of homocystine are associated with premature atherosclerosis, which can lead to stroke. In the most severe form, children with homocystinuria can present with homocystine levels 20 times normal and may have a stroke at a young age. Modest elevations in homocystine (1.5 to 2 times normal) are seen in up to 30% of ischemic stroke patients.[3] High homocystine levels can be caused by insufficient intake of folate, or defects in the metabolism of methionine. Supplementation with B vitamins may lower homocystine levels but has not been shown to reduce the risk of stroke.

Web Resources

www.americanheart.org: provides links to up-to-date stroke-related statistics and information for patients and physicians

www.who.int/cardiovascular_diseases: provides links to stroke-related statistics and guidelines as well as the Atlas of Heart Disease and Stroke

www.strokecenter.org: provides links to stroke-related information for both patients and health care providers, and provides a link to the stroke trials registry

www.theheart.org: provides a summary of recent publications related to vascular disease and stroke

References

1. Goldstein LB, Adams R, Becker K, et al. Primary prevention of ischemic stroke: A statement for healthcare professionals from the Stroke Council of the American Heart Association. Stroke 2001;32:280–299. Stroke. 2001;32:280–299
2. Mackay J, Mensah G. The Atlas of Heart Disease and Stroke. Geneva: World Health Organization, 2004
3. Mohr JP, Choi D, Grotta J, Weir B, Wolf P. Stroke: Pathophysiology, Diagnosis and Management, 4th ed. New York: Churchill Livingstone, 2004
4. Wolf PA, D'Agostino RB, Belanger AJ, Kannel WB. Probability of stroke: a risk profile from the Framingham Study. Stroke 1991;22:312–318
5. Yamada Y. Identification of genetic factors and development of genetic risk diagnosis systems for cardiovascular diseases and stroke. Circ J 2006;70:1240–1248
6. Ikram MA, Seshadri S, Bis JC, et al. Genomewide association studies of stroke. N Engl J Med 2009;360:1718–1728

7. Lawes CM, Bennett DA, Feigin VL, Rodgers A. Blood pressure and stroke: an overview of published reviews. Stroke 2004;35:776–785
8. Chalmers J, Todd A, Chapman N, et al; International Society of Hypertension Writing Group. International Society of Hypertension (ISH): statement on blood pressure lowering and stroke prevention. J Hypertens 2003;21:651–663
9. Kissela BM, Khoury J, Kleindorfer D, et al. Epidemiology of ischemic stroke in patients with diabetes: the greater Cincinnati/Northern Kentucky Stroke Study. Diabetes Care 2005;28:355–359
10. Sacco RL, Adams R, Albers G, et al; American Heart Association; American Stroke Association Council on Stroke; Council on Cardiovascular Radiology and Intervention; American Academy of Neurology. Guidelines for prevention of stroke in patients with ischemic stroke or transient ischemic attack: a statement for healthcare professionals from the American Heart Association/American Stroke Association Council on Stroke: co-sponsored by the Council on Cardiovascular Radiology and Intervention: the American Academy of Neurology affirms the value of this guideline. Stroke 2006;37:577–617
11. Fuentes B, Castillo J, San José B, et al; Stroke Project of the Cerebrovascular Diseases Study Group, Spanish Society of Neurology. The prognostic value of capillary glucose levels in acute stroke: the GLycemia in Acute Stroke (GLIAS) study. Stroke 2009;40:562–568
12. Sanossian N, Ovbiagele B. Multimodality stroke prevention. Neurologist 2006;12:14–31
13. Heart Protection Study Collaborative Group. MRC/BHF Heart Protection Study of cholesterol lowering with simvastatin in 20,536 high-risk individuals: a randomised placebo-controlled trial. Lancet 2002;360:7–22
14. Amarenco P, Bogousslavsky J, Callahan A III, et al; Stroke Prevention by Aggressive Reduction in Cholesterol Levels (SPARCL) Investigators. High-dose atorvastatin after stroke or transient ischemic attack. N Engl J Med 2006;355:549–559
15. Ridker PM, Danielson E, Fonseca FA, et al; JUPITER Study Group. Rosuvastatin to prevent vascular events in men and women with elevated C-reactive protein. N Engl J Med 2008;359:2195–2207
16. Suk S-H, Sacco RL, Boden-Albala B, et al; Northern Manhattan Stroke Study. Abdominal obesity and risk of ischemic stroke: the Northern Manhattan Stroke Study. Stroke 2003;34:1586–1592
17. Sacco RL, Elkind M, Boden-Albala B, et al. The protective effect of moderate alcohol consumption on ischemic stroke. JAMA 1999;281:53–60
18. Gordon NF, Gulanick M, Costa F, et al; American Heart Association Council on Clinical Cardiology, Subcommittee on Exercise, Cardiac Rehabilitation, and Prevention; the Council on Cardiovascular Nursing; the Council on Nutrition, Physical Activity, and Metabolism; and the Stroke Council. Physical activity and exercise recommendations for stroke survivors: an American Heart Association scientific statement from the Council on Clinical Cardiology, Subcommittee on Exercise, Cardiac Rehabilitation, and Prevention; the Council on Cardiovascular Nursing; the Council on Nutrition, Physical Activity, and Metabolism; and the Stroke Council. Circulation 2004;109:2031–2041
19. Beneficial effect of carotid endarterectomy in symptomatic patients with high-grade carotid stenosis. North American Symptomatic Carotid Endarterectomy Trial Collaborators. N Engl J Med 1991;325:445–453
20. Chaturvedi S, Bruno A, Feasby T, et al; Therapeutics and Technology Assessment Subcommittee of the American Academy of Neurology. Carotid endarterectomy—an evidence-based review: report of the therapeutics and technology assessment subcommittee of the American Academy of Neurology. Neurology 2005;65:794–801
21. Bettmann MA, Katzen BT, Whisnant J, et al. Carotid stenting and angioplasty: a statement for healthcare professionals from the Councils on Cardiovascular Radiology, Stroke, Cardio-Thoracic and Vascular Surgery, Epidemiology, and Prevention, and Clinical Cardiology, American Heart Association. Circulation 1998;97:121–123
22. Wolf PA, Abbott RD, Kannel WB. Atrial fibrillation as an independent risk factor for stroke: the Framingham Study. Stroke 1991;22:983–988
23. Atrial Fibrillation Investigators. Risk factors for stroke and efficacy of antithrombotic therapy in atrial fibrillation. Analysis of pooled data from five randomized controlled trials. Arch Intern Med 1994;154:1449–1457
24. Connolly SJ, Pogue J, Hart RG, et al; ACTIVE Investigators. Effect of clopidogrel added to aspirin in patients with atrial fibrillation. N Engl J Med 2009;360:2066–2078
25. Somers VK, White DP, Amin R, et al. Sleep apnea and cardiovascular disease: an American Heart Association/American College of Cardiology Foundation Scientific Statement from the American Heart Association Council for High Blood Pressure Research Professional Education Committee, Council on Clinical Cardiology, Stroke Council, and Council on Cardiovascular Nursing. J Am Coll Cardiol 2008;52:686–717
26. Yaggi HK, Concato J, Kernan WN, Lichtman JH, Brass LM, Mohsenin V. Obstructive sleep apnea as a risk factor for stroke and death. N Engl J Med 2005;353:2034–2041
27. Fujimoto S, Yasaka M, Otsubo R, Oe H, Nagatsuka K, Minematsu K. Aortic arch atherosclerotic lesions and the recurrence of ischemic stroke. Stroke 2004;35:1426–1429
28. Thaler DE, Saver JL. Cryptogenic stroke and patent foramen ovale. Curr Opin Cardiol 2008;23:537–544
29. Neiman J, Haapaniemi HM, Hillbom M. Neurological complications of drug abuse: pathophysiological mechanisms. Eur J Neurol 2000;7:595–606
30. Rahemtullah A, Van Cott EM. Hypercoagulation testing in ischemic stroke. Arch Pathol Lab Med 2007;131:890–901

2

Clinical Evaluation

Richard A. Bernstein

Pearls

- The temporal relationship between headache and focal deficit is of major diagnostic importance in differentiating stroke from migraine and in determining the etiology of the stroke.
- Careful observation during history constitutes an important part of the physical examination.
- The presence of an enlarged pupil in a patient with altered consciousness suggests an imminent threat of irreversible brain injury or death and must prompt emergent measures to reduce cerebral edema, neuroimaging, and a neurosurgical consultation.

Acute stroke is a medical emergency requiring rapid recognition, etiologic diagnosis, and treatment. All of these steps must be performed simultaneously in an organized fashion, with clinicians keeping in mind two differential diagnoses. First, clinicians must consider the most likely diagnoses and work to rule them out. Second, and just as important, clinicians must construct a list of imminent, potentially reversible threats to the patient's safety, and either treat them empirically or rule them out rapidly, even if they are unlikely. These two parallel differential diagnoses evolve as the results of history taking, examination, and laboratory and imaging studies are synthesized. The chapter discusses an organized approach to the evaluation of patients with acute-onset neurologic deficits that could be due to stroke. It promulgates an organized approach to obtaining the key clinical information needed to determine if stroke is the cause, and if it is, the type of stroke. The approach discussed here is geared toward providing the clinician with the information needed to choose among the treatments for acute stroke that are discussed in subsequent chapters.

◆ Acute Neurologic Syndromes: General Considerations

All acute neurologic complaints should be regarded as emergencies. The brain tolerates injury poorly, and the time window during which injury can be reversed is short. Because neurology is often viewed as complex by nonneurologists and may lead to a desire to call in a specialist before routine stabilization is accomplished, it is important to remember that all acutely ill patients, including those with neurologic complaints, require attention to the basics of medical care (**Table 2.1**). These include ensuring that the patient has an open and protected airway, and establishing an artificial airway if the patient's respiratory function is compromised. The patient must have a stable, perfusing cardiac rhythm. Cardiac monitoring until the patient is stable is advised. A severe decline in blood pressure (BP) may cause central nervous system (CNS) dysfunction; determination of BP and correction of hypotension (generally defined as systolic BP <90 mm Hg with neurologic symptoms) must be accomplished. Finally, most acute neurologic syndromes including coma, stroke, and seizure, can be mimicked or caused by acute hypoglycemia. Therefore, if the blood glucose is not known at the time of first evaluation, it should be rapidly determined by bedside testing.[1] Glucose should be given intravenously if the patient is hypoglycemic or if the glucose cannot be rapidly determined. Acute thiamine deficiency may cause altered consciousness (Wernicke encephalopathy) and may be precipitated in vulnerable patients by the administration of glucose; therefore, administration of 100 mg intravenous thiamine to all patients with acute CNS dysfunction is advisable prior to the administration of glucose. Because patients with acute CNS dysfunction may have fluctuating levels of consciousness, a policy of nothing by mouth (NPO) until the patient is stable may prevent aspiration. Any patient found on the floor

Table 2.1 Emergent Management for All Stroke Patients
1. Determine if the airway is protected, and, if not, establish a stable airway
a. In general, patients with a Glasgow Coma Scale score of <9 should be considered for endotracheal intubation.
2. Establish intravenous access.
3. Oxygen if saturation <92%
4. Maintain systolic blood pressure >90 mm Hg.
5. Give thiamine 100 mg intravenously.
6. Determine serum glucose or give glucose empirically.
7. If patient found lying on the ground or floor, stabilize cervical spine until radiographically cleared.
8. Consider naloxone if opiate overdose is possible.

Table 2.2 Common Nonvascular Causes of Rapid-Onset Focal Neurologic Symptoms and Signs
1. Seizure: positive symptoms and amnesia for event
2. Migraine: slow onset of a spreading deficit followed by headache; pattern of prior similar events
3. Hypertensive encephalopathy: severe hypertension and encephalopathy out of proportion to focal findings
4. Hypoglycemia
5. Conversion disorder: lack of concern about deficit, absence of objective signs (e.g., facial weakness, abnormal reflexes)

must be presumed to have fallen and to have an unstable cervical spine injury until proven otherwise. Finally, if the overuse of sedatives or opiate analgesics is possible, a trial of naloxone should be considered

Is the Deficit Focal or Global, and Is It Likely to Be a Stroke?

The clinical hallmark of stroke is the sudden onset of a focal neurologic deficit. A focal deficit is one in which the neurologic problem can be ascribed to a lesion in a particular area of the CNS. The opposite, a global deficit, results from dysfunction of the entire cerebrum or the entire brain. The latter is less likely to be caused by acute stroke. After a patient is stabilized (**Table 2.1**), the next step in evaluation is to determine if the patient has a focal or a global deficit, because they have different etiologies and treatments. Focal deficits may be elicited by both history and examination, and this determination can take place rapidly. Focal deficits that may be rapidly identified by history and examination include aphasia (inability to speak or understand in the setting of preserved consciousness); a visual field disturbance, unilateral weakness, or weakness affecting a single limb; unilateral numbness; unilateral incoordination; truncal or gait instability; hemispatial neglect; or inability to carry out learned motor tasks despite normal motor and sensory function. Because a decline in level of consciousness (LOC) requires bihemispheric or massive brainstem dysfunction, most patients with stroke have preserved consciousness, at least initially. Global deficits are usually characterized by a decline in level of consciousness *out of proportion* to any focal symptoms or signs. A patient who is lethargic but has intact motor and brainstem function is unlikely to have a stroke (with the exception of subarachnoid hemorrhage).

Rapid-onset focal neurologic deficits should be considered to be a stroke until proven otherwise, but there are other causes of these deficits that must be considered.[1] These include the entities listed in **Table 2.2**. It is important to note

that it may not be possible to adequately rule out stroke acutely in patients with acute focal deficits purely based on clinical evaluation, even if they have features of the other conditions listed in the table. Several validated prehospital screening tools to differentiate stroke from other causes of acute brain dysfunction are available and have been shown to improve ambulance recognition of stroke.[2,3]

◆ Early Clinical Evaluation of Acute Stroke

History

Once it is determined that stroke is a likely or possible diagnosis, a focused history and physical neurologic examination may both clarify the diagnosis, guide further testing, and determine the patient's eligibility for acute treatment. It is essential to accurately determine the time of onset of the neurologic symptoms. If the patient or reliable witnesses cannot report the time of onset, the time the patient was last confirmed to be normal must be determined. In patients who are aphasic, the patient must have been heard to speak normally to establish that the deficit was not present; normal motor function without a witnessed attempt to speak does not establish the absence of a deficit, even if a motor deficit is present at the time of medical evaluation. Patients with large nondominant hemispheric lesions may not be aware of their deficit and therefore may not be able to accurately report symptom onset. Every effort must be made to contact witnesses in the home, workplace, or wherever the patient was found to determine as unambiguously as possible the time the patient was last normal.

The mode of onset of the deficit should be determined by history. Ischemic strokes often have a maximum deficit at onset, whereas deficits from intracerebral hemorrhage (ICH) may worsen over seconds to minutes due to expansion of the hematoma. Deficits that spread over contiguous parts of the body over 10 to 30 minutes suggest migraine. Deficits preceded by positive symptoms (shaking) may be due to seizure, although rarely brain ischemia may cause limb shaking. Additionally, between 2% and 10% of strokes are accompanied by a seizure at or near the time of onset.[4] Therefore, the occurrence of a seizure does not rule out the presence of a co-existing stroke.

The history should elicit the patient's handedness. The presence of stroke risk factors, such as prior stroke, prior myocardial infarction, hypertension, diabetes mellitus, smoking, atrial fibrillation, or peripheral vascular disease should be determined. A complete medication list should be obtained if possible; if not, the use of antithrombotic medications, anticoagulants, and insulin or oral hypoglycemics must be specifically queried. The use of illicit drugs should also be determined, especially sympathomimetics (cocaine, amphetamine) and herbal supplements. The presence of headache should be queried. A headache that occurred prior to or with the onset of the deficit is consistent with either ischemic or hemorrhagic stroke (including subarachnoid hemorrhage [SAH]), or may indicate arterial thrombosis or injury (dissection) or intracranial venous occlusion. A headache that comes on after a focal deficit has resolved may indicate migraine.

Finally, it is crucially important to determine if the focal complaint has resolved. If it has completely resolved and the patient feels entirely back to normal, this must be clearly documented. In some circumstances, recurrence of the deficit may then be treatable with thrombolysis even many hours later. Dramatic but incomplete improvement is also important to document. Some interventions might not be needed if the patient improves dramatically without treatment. It is usually best to describe something the patient could not do that he or she can now do (e.g., lift an arm, tie one's shoelaces, speak).

A particularly difficult situation is the recognition and evaluation of patients with in-hospital strokes.[5] These patients often have complex underlying acute medical problems and have undergone multiple medical and surgical treatments and diagnostic procedures. In this setting, the history must include an analysis of the reason for hospitalization; all medications that have been used, with a focus on antithrombotic therapies and sedatives; any recent invasive procedures, including central line placement, biopsies, surgeries, and endoscopies; and the presence of underlying infection or immune deficiencies. In addition, the occurrence of any episode of hypotension, hypoxia, hypoglycemia, or cardiac arrest or dysfunction must be determined.

Physical Examination

The importance of determining the vital signs has been discussed above. The remainder of the physical examination may be divided into a general (nonneurologic) examination, and the neurologic examination. However, it is important to note that talking with the patient while taking the history affords an invaluable chance to make observations that can focus the neurologic examination. A patient who can relate a cogent, accurate history and carry on a normal conversation is unlikely to have a clinically significant aphasia. A patient who is aware of, concerned about, and frustrated by a motor deficit

likely does not have significant anosognosia. A patient who has no recollection of a transient focal deficit that was clearly witnessed by others, and that was not accompanied by a loss of consciousness, may have had a seizure. Patients who appear to move their arms and legs normally while changing position or gesturing, despite complaints of focal weakness, may have a functional (conversion) disorder.

General Physical Examination

Cardiac examination should focus on the regularity of the pulse, looking for signs of atrial fibrillation; the presence of cardiac murmurs that could suggest endocarditis; and the presence of peripheral edema, suggesting congestive heart failure that predisposes to embolism. Pulmonary examination should search for the presence of pulmonary edema that requires treatment in its own right and suggests the presence of left ventricular dysfunction (see above). The skin should be carefully examined for stigmata of endocarditis (Osler nodes, Janeway lesions, splinter hemorrhages), and for rashes that may suggest the presence of an autoimmune disease or hypercoagulable state (e.g., livedo reticularis). Finally, signs of trauma or seizure should be sought, such as lacerations; bruises; hip, knee, or elbow pain; or a bitten tongue. The general physical examination of a stroke patient in the acute setting should take no more than 2 to 3 minutes.

Neurologic Examination

The neurologic examination is often taught as a static, detailed, tedious, and obscure collection of physical maneuvers that must be memorized and performed in its entirety. In the setting of acute stroke, the key to success is a focused neurologic examination designed to elicit focal symptoms and to grade their severity. The evaluation of a patient with an acute stroke is not the setting to test two-point discrimination over the entire body!

A focused examination facilitates an anatomic diagnosis, and provides the basis for determining if the patient merits acute interventions that carry risk. Because large artery occlusion may be treatable via endovascular therapy, it is urgent to determine if the stroke involves cortical structures fed by large arteries, or spares those structures and just affects motor and sensory white matter tracts. **Table 2.3** lists some common cortical signs that signify large vessel involvement.

The mental status should be tested, with a focus on determining the LOC, and determining if the patient is aphasic or not and if neglect is present or not. Describe the level of consciousness by relating what stimulation it takes to arouse the patient, how long the patient remains awake, and what the patient can do while awake.

Aphasia may be ruled out by the response to questioning during history taking. Formal language testing should include listening to the patient's spontaneous speech for the use of wrong words or sounds and for fluency (the number of linguistic elements per minute, or "flow" of the speech); the ability to follow one-, two-, and three-step commands;

Table 2.3 Clinical Signs of Large Artery Occlusion in Acute Stroke

1. Aphasia
2. Gaze preference with contralateral weakness
3. Unawareness of deficit (anosognosia)
4. Hemispatial neglect
5. Visual field cut
6. Neglect on the affected side to double simultaneous visual or tactile stimulation

and the ability to name some common objects rapidly and correctly. Aphasia should be graded as global (no speech, no comprehension); expressive (nonfluent, telegraphic speech with absent grammatic elements but preserved semantic content and relatively preserved comprehension); or receptive (fluent but meaningless speech, often with "jargon," and with relatively poor comprehension and insight).

Anosognosia and neglect may be examined by asking patients if they believe their arm or leg is weak when it obviously is; asking them to point to objects on their left side; and asking them to count the number of people in the room to see if they notice people on their left. A quick screen for visuospatial neglect is to enter the room and stand on the patient's left side (or right side in some left-handed patients) and see if the patient notices the examiner's presence.

Cranial nerve functions that must be tested in patients with suspected stroke include visual fields (tested in the lateral quadrants of both eyes as a screening test; each eye individually if a field deficit exists); eye movements; facial sensation, strength, and symmetry; the clarity of speech (already assessed during history taking); and tongue protrusion. Motor testing should focus on strength (the Medical Research Council [MRC] scale is a useful objective scale) and dexterity. Often the only sign of a subtle motor deficit is slow, clumsy fine finger movements in the hand with normal strength, or pronator drift without gross weakness. Sensation should be tested quickly to avoid patient boredom, which can lead to inaccurate testing. A few regions tested with a pin or cold object are sufficient in most cases. It is important to assess the response to double simultaneous stimulation; patients with subtle visual or sensory neglect may detect a stimulus on the affected side when presented in isolation, but not when presented in tandem with a stimulus on the non-affected side **(Table 2.3)**. This finding suggests a parietal lobe lesion. Coordination should be tested in all four limbs, and, if stable, the patient should be made as vertical as possible by sitting up in the gurney to assess truncal ataxia. Recording the examination, as well as the score on a standardized stroke assessment tool, such as the National Institutes of Health (NIH) stroke scale,[6] enables serial examinations to determine if the patient is stable, improving, or worsening.[1]

Testing deep tendon and plantar reflexes, muscle tone, and detailed sensory testing can often wait until other crucial diagnostic testing has been completed.

◆ Neurologic Examination Signatures of Particular Stroke Syndromes

Coma

A clinically useful model of how the brain produces consciousness makes the neurologic examination of the comatose patient straightforward. This model postulates that there are three anatomic/etiologic causes of coma (defined here as lack of normal arousal to stimulation). Coma results from a lesion in the arousal centers of the brainstem, dysfunction of both cerebral hemispheres, or a unihemispheric lesion that affects function of either the brainstem or the other hemisphere. The examination of a comatose patient should be focused on determining which of these three scenarios is present **(Table 2.4)**.

Three different patterns may be observed. First, patients may be comatose, but have intact brainstem reflexes and symmetric, often brisk withdrawal to pain in all four limbs. Such patients usually have global insults resulting in bihemispheric dysfunction (e.g., hypoglycemia, infection). The presence of this pattern of deficits is usually not due to stroke. However, a shower of small emboli to both cerebral hemispheres or emboli to both medial thalami may cause this pattern on examination. Such cases are unusual and require neuroimaging to diagnose with certainty.

The second pattern seen on examination is a comatose patient with a unilateral enlarged, unreactive pupil and contralateral hemiplegia. This may be an important sign of a mass lesion in the hemisphere (usually) ipsilateral to the enlarged pupil, with impending brainstem compression (uncal herniation). Such patients are at imminent risk of death and require emergent airway management and brain imaging; often an enlarging hematoma or ischemic stroke with mass effect is seen, and surgical decompression with or without medical therapy to reduce cerebral edema may be indicated as a lifesaving measure. On occasion, patients with uncal herniation have contralateral extension and internal rotation of the arm to pain (extensor posturing) that indicates compression of the contralateral upper brainstem. Less severe upper brainstem damage or a severe hemispheric lesion may result in flexion of the elbow and wrist and fingers to pain (flexor posturing).

The final pattern seen in comatose patients is abnormal eye movements, absent corneal reflexes (often asymmetric),

Table 2.4 Examination of the Comatose Patient

1. Level of arousal (the minimum stimulus needed to trigger a response from the patient, and the type of response)
2. Pupillary reaction to light
3. Eye movements, either spontaneous or in reaction to head movement or ice water in the ear
4. Corneal reflexes
5. Limb response to pain

Table 2.5 Clinical Characteristics of Small Artery Occlusions

1. Mental status is normal; no aphasia, neglect, gaze preference, or visual field disturbance
2. Involvement of face, arm, and leg
3. Weakness, numbness, or both may be present
4. Occasionally coexisting weakness and hemiataxia

and asymmetric motor signs. This pattern of cranial nerve and motor dysfunction in a comatose patient suggests damage to the brainstem due to either ischemic stroke or hemorrhage.

It is important to recognize these three patterns of deficits in comatose patients. The first is usually not due to stroke. The second, due to large hemispheric lesions, may be the result of either a massive intracerebral hemorrhage or a large vessel anterior circulation occlusion (internal carotid artery, middle cerebral artery). The last pattern may be due to either a brainstem hemorrhage or ischemic stroke due to basilar artery thrombosis.

Motor or Sensory Deficit Without Other Symptoms or Signs

Patients may describe severe motor or sensory deficits involving one side of their body (often including the face, arm, and leg) in the absence of aphasia, neglect, gaze preference, or visual field disturbance. These patients are usually alert and able to provide a reliable history. Examination usually shows some involvement of the face, arm, and leg, but the involvement may not be equivalently severe in all three regions. Occasional patients describe just dysarthria (as a sign of facial and lingual involvement) and clumsiness or numbness of the ipsilateral hand in the absence of other cognitive or visual symptoms. Patients may also have some combination of weakness, numbness, and incoordination on one side ("ataxic-hemiparesis") without other signs or symptoms. These "lacunar" syndromes are often due to occlusions of small penetrating arteries in the internal capsule or pons, or small hemorrhages in those regions **(Table 2.5)**. Rarely this syndrome is the result of an embolism to the motor or sensory cortex.

The importance of recognizing this constellation of symptoms and signs is that these patients rarely have a large arterial occlusion that merits endovascular therapy. Often the occluded vessel is angiographically invisible. Such patients may still respond to systemic thrombolysis, but catheter-based therapies are usually not indicated in this scenario.

Hemispheric Syndromes

The occlusion of the intracranial internal carotid artery or its branches (the middle cerebral artery [MCA] or anterior cerebral artery [ACA]) or major branches thereof usually produces symptoms and signs that indicate infarction of the cerebral cortex. In the dominant (language) hemisphere, cortical signs include either expressive or receptive aphasia or both (global aphasia). Expressive aphasia, in which the patient has slow, nonfluent, halting telegraphic speech with intact semantic content but missing grammatical words (such as "and," "but," etc.), usually signifies occlusion of the anterior division of the MCA and is usually associated with contralateral hemiparesis. Receptive aphasia, characterized by fluent but meaningless speech filled with wrong words (semantic paraphasias) or words with the wrong letter (literal paraphasias) are usually due to occlusion of the inferior division of the dominant hemisphere MCA, and is usually accompanied by a contralateral visual field disturbance. In the nondominant hemisphere, MCA occlusion may produce contralateral weakness without the patient's awareness of the deficit (anosognosia), neglect of contralateral space, and inability of the patient to recognize his or her own contralateral arm (asomatognosia) or even hatred of the weak limb (misoplegia). ACA infarction produces frontal lobe dysfunction, which may include abulia, disinhibition, executive dysfunction, and contralateral leg weakness.

Occlusion of a posterior cerebral artery produces contralateral visual field loss due to infarction of the occipital cortex, and, if extensive, may also lead to amnestic syndromes if the medial temporal lobe is involved. In the case of embolism to the basilar apex, some combination of fluctuation in consciousness, bilateral visual field loss, loss of upgaze, and an amnestic syndrome results from infarction of both occipital lobes, the medial thalami bilaterally, and the medial temporal lobes ("top of the basilar" syndrome).

Basilar artery occlusion causes infarction in the pons and/or midbrain. When extensive, infarction of the pontine base causes quadriplegia and facial paralysis and loss of all but vertical eye movements. In many cases, the patient is awake and sensate but unable to communicate except with vertical eye movements ("locked-in" syndrome). Basilar artery branch occlusions may lead to ipsilateral cranial nerve dysfunction with contralateral hemiparesis due to unilateral pontine or midbrain infarcts. One of the most distinctive brainstem syndromes is the lateral medullary syndrome of Wallenberg, in which vertigo is present along with ipsilateral facial numbness, palate weakness, and hemiataxia and contralateral body numbness to temperature and pain. This syndrome may be due to occlusion of the intracranial vertebral artery, the posterior inferior cerebellar artery, or small penetrating branches of either artery.

Transient Ischemic Attack Versus Stroke

A transient ischemic attack (TIA) should be thought of as a stroke that gets better quickly. The current definition of TIA is the occurrence of stroke symptoms that are not accompanied by acute brain infarction on neuroimaging.[7] This definition has the consequence that the use of more sensitive brain imaging techniques (e.g., magnetic resonance imaging [MRI] rather than computed tomography [CT]) will result in more diagnoses of stroke than of TIA. Any stroke syndrome may occur transiently and potentially cause TIA. Because often no health care professional is present to witness the episode and patients themselves are often poor self-observers, details of the episode may be impossible to elicit by history or by interviewing witnesses. The occurrence of isolated light-headedness, general confusion, or transient loss of consciousness is usually not due to TIA.

Patients with TIA require the same urgent evaluation as stroke patients, because the risk of stroke after TIA is as high as 5% in the following 48 hours; many of these strokes are disabling or fatal.[8] The ABCD2 score is a simple bedside scale to stratify the risk of impending stroke in patients with recent TIA (**Table 2.6**).[9] A score of zero indicates a low risk of imminent stroke. As the score increases, the risk of stroke at 48 hours and 90 days increases.[9]

Uncommon But Important Presentations of Stroke

A few rare stroke syndromes are important to recognize because they have important treatment implications. In young patients, the occurrence of severe, unusual neck pain and headache accompanied by stroke or TIA suggests the presence of a tear in the intima of a cervicocephalic artery (carotid or vertebral dissection). These injuries may be precipitated by major or minor trauma, and have been reported after chiropractic manipulation, sexual or athletic activity, vomiting, sneezing, or even in the absence of any clear trigger.[10] Diagnosis may be established by noninvasive vascular imaging (computed tomography angiography [CTA] or magnetic resonance angiography [MRA]), or in some cases cerebral angiography.[11]

Patients with hemodynamically significant carotid occlusive disease may have repeated episodes of TIA upon standing or when blood pressure falls. Typical syndromes include isolated hand or proximal arm weakness present with standing, or multiple episodes of aphasia precipitated by a drop in blood pressure. A syndrome of repeated nonepileptic contralateral shaking of the arm or leg as a result of severe carotid stenosis or occlusion has been reported (limb-shaking TIA).[12] Transient loss of vision in one eye (amaurosis fugax) has long been recognized as a potential sign of microembolism from the ipsilateral cervical internal carotid artery (ICA). The occurrence of repeated monocular visual loss in bright light with recovery in darkness is a reliable sign of retinal ischemia from carotid insufficiency.

The occurrence of systemic complaints accompanying stroke may indicate a severe underlying illness that explains both. For example, the occurrence of fever and malaise with stroke suggests the presence of bacterial endocarditis and mandates emergent echocardiography as well as brain imaging.[13] The presence of severe headache with visual loss or posterior circulation stroke suggests giant cell (temporal) arteritis. Empiric steroids and temporal artery biopsy should be considered. Finally, the combination of unexplained weight loss, venous thromboses, and ischemic stroke may indicate a hypercoagulable state due to an underlying malignancy.

Clinical Signs of Intracerebral Hemorrhage

There are a few clinical signs in stroke patients that suggest the presence of intracerebral hemorrhage (ICH) rather than ischemic stroke. Hemorrhages expand over the course of seconds to an hour or longer. The occurrence of a minor deficit that rapidly becomes more severe, especially when accompanied by a precipitous decline in consciousness, strongly suggests the presence of an expanding intracerebral hematoma. The rapid addition of blood to the intracranial vault may raise intracranial pressure or lead to shifts in brain tissue and lead to vomiting and signs of herniation (see above). Most stroke patients have increased blood pressure; patients with ICH tend to have extremely elevated blood pressure, often more than 230 mm Hg systolic. Headache is more common in ICH than in ischemic stroke, but neither its presence nor its absence is specific enough to rely upon for diagnosis.[14]

◆ Bedside Monitoring in Acute Stroke

Stroke patients face the risk of worsening neurologic deficit at any time after the onset of their stroke. Large ischemic strokes may swell and cause herniation with resultant coma. Large vessel stenoses may occlude and cause recurrent or worsening symptoms. Intracerebral hematomas may enlarge or develop perihematomal edema, leading to raised intracranial pressure (ICP) and/or herniation. Even lacunar (small vessel) strokes may fluctuate and worsen in a stepwise fashion in the first few days after occurrence. Patients with TIA are at high risk of stroke in the first 48 hours after their index event, and these strokes may be treatable with tissue-type plasminogen activator (tPA). In all cases, expectant monitoring of the patient is required to rapidly detect, and thereby act on, any worsening neurologic status.

Clinical Monitoring

In patients with an eloquent examination (e.g., not in deep coma), careful documentation of key elements of the neurologic examination is essential to detecting worsening stroke. It is important to document the level of consciousness by describing what stimulation is required to arouse the patient, and what the patient does when he or she is awake. Motor strength should be described either using standard scales (e.g., NIH stroke scale) or by describing the patient's abilities; for example, "The patient can hold his arm over the bed for 5 seconds but cannot manipulate an object with his fingers." Specific descriptions enable other observers to compare findings. The goal of this monitoring is to detect worsening cerebral edema or recurrent infarction before irreversible brain injury occurs. The most severely ill patients may be in coma with severe motor deficits; in these patients clinical monitoring may not be able to detect worsening neurologic status until herniation has occurred.

Radiographic and Invasive Monitoring

Patients with cerebral edema from hemispheric or cerebellar stroke (ischemic or hemorrhagic) are at risk for tissue shifts and herniation. In many patients, edema and shifts may worsen considerably without clinical signs. However, eventually compensatory mechanisms are exceeded and patients will then rapidly decline, often irreversibly. Serial CT scans may provide important information on the neurologic status of these patients in advance of their development of clinical signs. Most patients who experience malignant edema from a hemispheric stroke have involvement of more than half of the MCA territory.[14] Daily or twice-daily CT scans may disclose hematoma expansion (which might lead to consideration of hemostatic therapy or surgical evacuation). Serial CT scans could disclose an increase in tissue shifts from perihematomal edema or periinfarct edema that could lead to treatment with hyperosmolar therapy (mannitol) or early hemicraniectomy, or the development of obstructive hydrocephalus or brainstem compression from posterior fossa lesions. Finally, serial CT scanning may disclose hemorrhagic transformation of an ischemic infarct that could lead to a change in or discontinuation of antithrombotic therapy. The ideal frequency of serial CT scanning has not been determined. This depends upon the overall clinical status of the patient, the availability of rapid and convenient CT scanning, and the likelihood of finding changing radiographic signs in advance of clinical signs.[15,16] In general, scans once or twice per day are most useful in the first 5 days after a major stroke.

The role of invasive monitoring in patients with ischemic stroke has not been fully defined.[16] Technology exists to monitor ICP, tissue oxygenation, lactate level, and pH. However, it is unclear whether this monitoring improves outcome or changes management. Some experts suggest ICP monitoring in patients with coma due to intracerebral hemorrhage (guidelines).

References

1. Adams HP Jr, del Zoppo G, Alberts MJ, et al; American Heart Association/American Stroke Association Stroke Council; American Heart Association/American Stroke Association Clinical Cardiology Council; American Heart Association/American Stroke Association Cardiovascular Radiology and Intervention Council; Atherosclerotic Peripheral Vascular Disease Working Group; Quality of Care Outcomes in Research Interdisciplinary Working Group. Guidelines for the early management of adults with ischemic stroke: a guideline from the American Heart Association/American Stroke Association Stroke Council, Clinical Cardiology Council, Cardiovascular Radiology and Intervention Council, and the Atherosclerotic Peripheral Vascular Disease and Quality of Care Outcomes in Research Interdisciplinary Working Groups: The American Academy of Neurology affirms the value of this guideline as an educational tool for neurologists. [Erratum appears in Circulation 2007 Oct 30;116(18):e515] Circulation 2007;115:e478–e534
2. Kidwell CS, Starkman S, Eckstein M, Weems K, Saver JL. Identifying stroke in the field. Prospective validation of the Los Angeles prehospital stroke screen (LAPSS). Stroke 2000;31:71–76
3. Kothari RU, Pancioli A, Liu T, Brott T, Broderick J. Cincinnati Prehospital Stroke Scale: reproducibility and validity. [see comment] Ann Emerg Med 1999;33:373–378
4. Burn J, Dennis M, Bamford J, Sandercock P, Wade D, Warlow C. Epileptic seizures after a first stroke: the Oxfordshire Community Stroke Project. BMJ 1997;315:1582–1587
5. Alberts MJ, Brass LM, Perry A, Webb D, Dawson DV. Evaluation times for patients with in-hospital strokes. [Erratum appears in Stroke 1994 Mar;25(3):717] Stroke 1993;24:1817–1822
6. Internet Stroke Center (http://www.strokecenter.org/trials/scales/)
7. Easton JD, Saver JL, Albers GW, et al; American Heart Association; American Stroke Association Stroke Council; Council on Cardiovascular Surgery and Anesthesia; Council on Cardiovascular Radiology and Intervention; Council on Cardiovascular Nursing; Interdisciplinary Council on Peripheral Vascular Disease. Definition and evaluation of transient ischemic attack: a scientific statement for healthcare professionals from the American Heart Association/American Stroke Association Stroke Council; Council on Cardiovascular Surgery and Anesthesia; Council on Cardiovascular Radiology and Intervention; Council on Cardiovascular Nursing; and the Interdisciplinary Council on Peripheral Vascular Disease. The American Academy of Neurology affirms the value of this statement as an educational tool for neurologists. Stroke 2009;40:2276–2293
8. Johnston SC, Gress DR, Browner WS, Sidney S. Short-term prognosis after emergency department diagnosis of TIA. JAMA 2000;284:2901–2906
9. Johnston SC, Rothwell PM, Nguyen-Huynh MN, et al. Validation and refinement of scores to predict very early stroke risk after transient ischaemic attack. Lancet 2007;369:283–292
10. Debette S, Leys D. Cervical-artery dissections: predisposing factors, diagnosis, and outcome. Lancet Neurol 2009;8:668–678
11. Ansari SA, Parmar H, Ibrahim M, Gemmete JJ, Gandhi D. Cervical dissections: diagnosis, management, and endovascular treatment. Neuroimaging Clin N Am 2009;19:257–270
12. Tatemichi TK, Young WL, Prohovnik I, Gitelman DR, Correll JW, Mohr JP. Perfusion insufficiency in limb-shaking transient ischemic attacks. Stroke 1990;21:341–347
13. Baddour LM, Wilson WR, Bayer AS, et al; Committee on Rheumatic Fever, Endocarditis, and Kawasaki Disease; Council on Cardiovascular Disease in the Young; Councils on Clinical Cardiology, Stroke, and Cardiovascular Surgery and Anesthesia; American Heart Association; Infectious Diseases Society of America. Infective endocarditis: diagnosis, antimicrobial therapy, and management of complications: a statement for healthcare professionals from the Committee on Rheumatic Fever, Endocarditis, and Kawasaki Disease, Council on Cardiovascular Disease in the Young, and the Councils on Clinical Cardiology, Stroke, and Cardiovascular Surgery and Anesthesia, American Heart Association: endorsed by the Infectious Diseases Society of America. [Errata appear in Circulation 2005 Oct 11;112(15):2373; 2007 Apr 17;115(15):e408; 2007 Nov 20;116(21):e547; and 2008 Sep 16;118(12):e497] Circulation 2005;111:e394–e434
14. Broderick J, Connolly S, Feldmann E, et al; American Heart Association/American Stroke Association Stroke Council; American Heart Association/American Stroke Association High Blood Pressure Research Council; Quality of Care and Outcomes in Research Interdisciplinary Working Group. Guidelines for the management of spontaneous intracerebral hemorrhage in adults: 2007 update: a guideline from the American Heart Association/American Stroke Association Stroke Council, High Blood Pressure Research Council, and the Quality of Care and Outcomes in Research Interdisciplinary Working Group. Circulation 2007;116:e391–e413
15. Kasner SE, Demchuk AM, Berrouschot J, et al. Predictors of fatal brain edema in massive hemispheric ischemic stroke. Stroke 2001;32:2117–2123
16. Steiner T, Pilz J, Schellinger P, et al. Multimodal online monitoring in middle cerebral artery territory stroke. Stroke 2001;32:2500–2506

3

Fibrinolysis for Cerebral Ischemia

Alejandro A. Rabinstein

Pearls

- Intravenous fibrinolysis is an effective treatment for acute ischemic stroke for up to 4.5 hours after symptom onset.
- Time from symptom onset to fibrinolytic therapy is the most important determinant of the success of treatment; the chances of favorable recovery diminish with each minute lost.
- Strict adherence to the prescribed protocol for the administration of recombinant tissue-type plasminogen activator (rtPA) and postfibrinolytic care is crucial to minimize the risk of hemorrhagic complications.
- rtPA remains the only fibrinolytic agent reliably proven to improve the outcomes of stroke patients after intravenous administration.
- Selection of candidates for reperfusion therapies using penumbra imaging (diffusion- or perfusion-weighted magnetic resonance imaging or computed tomography perfusion) is a promising—albeit yet unproven—strategy to widen the therapeutic window for acute treatment of brain ischemia.
- Correction of hyperglycemia might improve the results of fibrinolysis and should be considered as part of the acute care of stroke patients undergoing reperfusion therapies.

The concept of pharmacologic fibrinolysis for the treatment of acute ischemic stroke developed from the finding that early reperfusion improved outcomes in various experimental animal models of intracranial vessel occlusion and from the recognition that the mechanisms for endogenous fibrinolysis in humans are often insufficient to prevent brain infarction in many patients.[1] The clinical application of fibrinolysis revolutionized ischemic stroke care by offering an effective treatment for a disease in which previously all medical efforts were focused on prevention of recurrent events, avoidance of secondary complications, and rehabilitation.

◆ Mechanisms of Fibrinolysis

When a clot is formed, a plasma protein called plasminogen gets trapped within it. The injured tissues and vascular endothelium then slowly release tissue-type plasminogen activator (tPA), which in turn activates and converts plasminogen to plasmin. Plasmin is a potent proteolytic enzyme that digests fibrin (the main protein component of the clot) as well as coagulation proteins, such as fibrinogen, prothrombin, factor V, factor VIII, and factor XII. This process ensures the elimination of excess clot and protects blood flow, particularly in the microcirculation, once bleeding has stopped.

Figure 3.1 offers a schematic representation of the physiologic process of fibrinolysis.

◆ Fibrinolysis for the Treatment of Ischemic Stroke

The Evidence

Early intravenous administration of recombinant tissue-type plasminogen activator (rtPA, alteplase) has been proven to improve functional outcome after acute ischemic stroke.[2] The pivotal trial leading to the international approval of intravenous rtPA for the treatment of cerebral ischemia was the National Institute of Neurological Disorders and Stroke (NINDS) rtPA Stroke Study.[3] In this trial, 624 patients were randomized to receive intravenous rtPA (0.9 mg/kg, maximum 90 mg) or a placebo within 3 hours of stroke symptom onset. Treatment with intravenous rtPA was associated with at least a 30% increase in the chances of achieving functional independence with complete or nearly complete neurologic recovery at 3 months.[3] The main risk of treatment was symptomatic intracerebral hemorrhage, which occurred in 6.4% of patients treated with rtPA versus 0.6% of patients who received placebo, but it did not result in an increase in mortality among rtPA-treated patients. Efficacy was greatest for patients treated within 90 minutes of symptom onset. For patients treated within 90 minutes, the odds ratio for complete recovery was 2.11 compared with an odds ratio of 1.69 for patients treated within 91 to 180 minutes.[4] A graphic illustration of the benefit that patients can expect when given

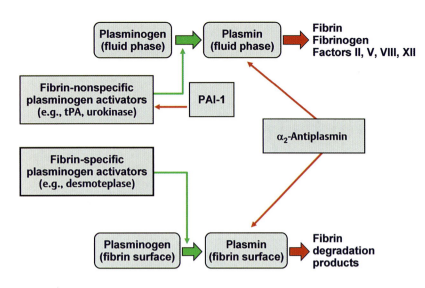

Fig. 3.1 Schematic representation of the mechanisms of fibrinolysis. Solid green arrows indicate activation, solid red arrows indicate degradation, and thin red arrows indicate inhibition. tPA, tissue-type plasminogen activator; PAI-1, plasminogen activator inhibitor-1.

intravenous rtPA within 3 hours of stroke symptom onset is presented in **Fig. 3.2**. Functional benefit was sustained at 1 year.[5] Subgroup analyses confirmed that the efficacy of intravenous rtPA extended to all patients meeting the trial inclusion and exclusion criteria, including older patients with severe strokes at presentation.[3]

Shortly after publication of the NINDS trial, rtPA was approved for intravenous use in patients with acute ischemic stroke in the United States, mostly following the patient selection criteria of the NINDS study. An additional radiologic exclusion criterion was added based on the finding that the presence of large early ischemic changes on a baseline computed tomography (CT) scan was associated with a higher risk of symptomatic intracranial hemorrhage, and results from earlier European studies that suggested poorer outcomes in patients with multilobar low-attenuation changes,[6] which had led to the exclusion of these patients from subsequent European trials. Since then, treatment with intravenous rtPA has gained acceptance worldwide, and its effectiveness has been confirmed in multiple observational studies.

The largest of these observational studies has been the Safe Implementation of Thrombolysis in Stroke–Monitoring Study (SITS-MOST),[7] which enrolled nearly 6500 patients from 14 European countries. Intravenous fibrinolysis with rtPA was at least as safe and effective in routine clinical practice as it had been in the randomized trials.[7,8] Over three quarters of treated patients had moderate to severe strokes at baseline, and 55% were independent at 3 months despite only 10.6% being treated within 90 minutes (versus half of the rtPA group in the NINDS trial). Even centers with limited experience on the administration of fibrinolysis for acute stroke achieved good results when adhering to the accepted indications and contraindications. The risk of intracranial hemorrhage, defined using various criteria, was acceptably low. Substantial neurologic decline from brain hemorrhage only occurred in 1.7% of patients.

Although intravenous fibrinolysis has become the standard of care for emergency treatment of patients with acute ischemic stroke, only a small minority of these patients receive the therapy. The main reason for the limited application of this effective intervention in clinical practice is that patients often arrive at the emergency department too late. As a consequence, there has been a lot of interest in extending the therapeutic window for acute reperfusion therapies, including intravenous rtPA.

A pooled analysis of six major trials evaluating the effectiveness of intravenous rtPA for acute ischemic stroke within 6 hours of symptom onset suggested that fibrinolysis could produce clinical benefit when administered beyond 3 hours.[9] In fact, this analysis showed that the benefit was much greater within the first 90 minutes of symptom onset, but much more similar when the time to treatment was 91 to 180 minutes and 181 to 270 minutes. These findings provided the rationale for the design of the European Cooperative Stroke Study (ECASS III) trial, a multicenter, randomized trial conducted in Europe to evaluate intravenous rtPA versus placebo administered between 3 and 4.5 hours after the onset of ischemic stroke symptoms.[10] A total of 821 patients were enrolled, nearly one-third more than in the NINDS trial. Treat-

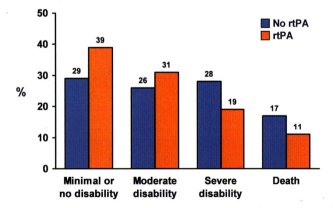

Fig. 3.2 Illustration of clinical benefit of intravenous fibrinolysis administered within 3 hours of stroke symptom onset.

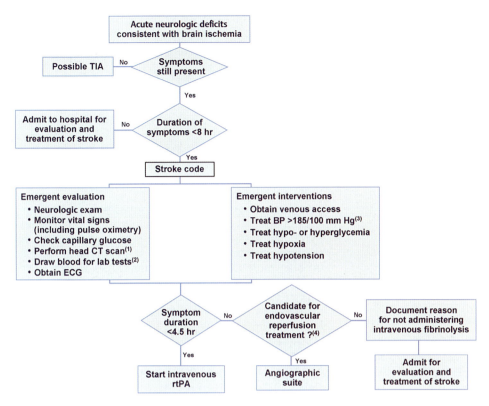

Fig. 3.3 Proposed stroke code algorithm. Annotations: (1) Multimodality computed tomography (CT) or magnetic resonance imaging (MRI) is an excellent alternative to noncontrast CT scan if these studies can be performed without delay. (2) Blood tests should include glucose, electrolytes, creatinine, cardiac enzymes, complete blood count (including platelet count), prothrombin time/international normalized ratio (INR), and activated partial thromboplastin time (aPTT). (3) Refer to **Table 3.3**. (4) Clinical deficits suspicious for large intracranial vessel occlusion or, ideally, documented penumbra on perfusion studies associated with large intracranial vessel occlusion on noninvasive angiogram; for more details, refer to the text of this chapter and to Chapter 30. BP, blood pressure; ECG, electrocardiogram; TIA, transient ischemic attack.

ment with rtPA was associated with a significant improvement in the rate of favorable functional outcome using various scales. Overall, the chances of regaining full independence were 28% higher among patients treated with rtPA, and 14 patients had to be treated for one additional patient to achieve a favorable outcome. Mortality was not significantly different between the groups, but was slightly higher in the placebo arm. The rate of symptomatic intracranial hemorrhage as defined by the NINDS criteria was 7.9% in the rtPA group (versus 6.4% in the NINDS trial), but only 2.4% of patients were considered to have worsened because of the bleeding. Intravenous fibrinolysis with rtPA within 3 and 4.5 hours was also shown to be safe in a large European observational study (Safe Implementation of Thrombolysis in Stroke–International Thrombolysis Registry (SITS-ISTR), which included over 650 patients treated in that time window.[11] Therefore, intravenous rtPA should be considered for selected patients with symptom duration of between 3 and 4.5 hours.

Patient Evaluation and Selection

Acute stroke patients must be evaluated emergently for consideration of reperfusion treatments. Hospitals need to implement a stroke code process to streamline immediate patient assessment, brain imaging, and drug administration. Development of critical care pathways (ideally starting from assessment in the field by paramedics or other first responders), easily accessible written protocols, and order sets are highly useful to ensure rapid and effective evaluation and

treatment (**Fig. 3.3**). Hospitals should monitor their performance to recognize areas for improvement and to ensure consistent compliance with the recommended time metrics (**Table 3.1**).

Strict adherence to the prescribed criteria for patient selection is crucial to avoid complications and optimize the likelihood of benefit from intravenous fibrinolysis. **Table 3.2** presents the indications and contraindications for treatment with intravenous rtPA. Note that some additional contraindications should be considered when contemplating the use of rtPA between 3 and 4.5 hours.

The importance of the careful determination of time of symptom onset cannot be overemphasized. Current guidelines on rtPA administration are based on the definition of symptom onset as the last time that the patient was symptom-free or at his/her previous baseline.[2] For patients who

Table 3.1 Target Times from Acute Stroke Presentation to Fibrinolytic Treatment

Step of care	Target time
Evaluation by physician	10 minutes
Brain imaging	25 minutes
Interpretation of brain imaging (door-to-interpretation)	45 minutes
Start of fibrinolysis (door-to-needle)	60 minutes

Table 3.2 Indications and Contraindications for Intravenous rtPA in Acute Ischemic Stroke

Indications

Diagnosis of ischemic stroke causing a measurable neurologic deficit

Onset of symptoms <4.5 hours before initiation of treatment

Contraindications

Clinical

Sustained hypertension above 180/110 mm Hg

Symptoms suggestive of subarachnoid hemorrhage

Previous history of intracranial hemorrhage

ST-elevation myocardial infarction within the previous 3 months

Major head trauma or stroke within the previous 3 months

Major surgery within the previous 14 days

Gastrointestinal or urinary tract hemorrhage within the previous 21 days

Arterial puncture at a noncompressible site within the previous 7 days

Active bleeding or acute traumatic fracture on examination

Seizure at onset with suspected postictal deficits

Minor or rapidly improving neurologic deficits

Radiologic

Head CT showing hemorrhage or multilobar infarction (i.e., hypodensity involving more than one third of the cerebral hemisphere

Laboratory

Oral anticoagulation with international normalized ratio (INR) >1.7 *

Heparin within previous 48 hours with elevated current activated partial thromboplastin time (aPTT)

Platelet count <100,000 per mm^3

Blood glucose level <50 mg/dL (2.7 mmol/L) at presentation with improving deficits following correction of hypoglycemia

Additional Contraindications for Treatment Between 3 and 4.5 hours

Age >80 years

Very severe deficits at onset (NIHSS score >25)

Combination of previous stroke and diabetes mellitus

*Oral anticoagulation regardless of current INR should be considered a contraindication for treatment at between 3 and 4.5 hours.

wake up with symptoms, the time of onset is considered the last time the patient was awake and without the symptoms. A recent transient ischemic attack similar to the current symptoms is generally not considered a contraindication for fibrinolysis; the clock can be reset to the time of onset of the new symptoms as long as there is clear knowledge that the previous symptoms resolved fully.

Some factors initially listed among the exclusion criteria for intravenous fibrinolysis in the seminal trials are no longer considered to be contraindications in practice. For instance, the report of a seizure at the onset of deficits should not preclude fibrinolysis as long as the treating physician is convinced that the persistent deficits are secondary to a stroke and not merely a postictal phenomenon.[2] Similar reasoning might be applied to hypoglycemic patients who fail to improve after administration of dextrose. One should also be careful when deciding not to treat a stroke patient with fibrinolysis because of mild or rapidly improving symptoms. All too often, these patients subsequently suffer permanent disability from these strokes.[12]

Interpretation of brain imaging in the emergency setting has the primary objective of excluding intracranial hemorrhage. Noncontrast CT scan of the head is sufficient for this objective, and emergency treatment should not be delayed to obtain more advanced imaging modalities (such as multimodality magnetic resonance imaging [MRI] and multimodality CT).[2] Apart from hemorrhage, only the presence of multilobar hypodensity (involving more than one third of the cerebral hemisphere) should be considered a radiologic contraindication for fibrinolysis **(Fig. 3.4)**. Other CT findings may have prognostic value, but they do not negate the benefit of fibrinolysis and should not preclude its use **(Fig. 3.5)**. For instance, the presence of a hyperdense middle cerebral artery sign is associated with worse prognosis[13] and higher risk of hemorrhage after fibrinolysis,[14] but intravenous rtPA can still be useful for these patients.[13] Other early signs of brain ischemia can often be seen when the CT scan is assessed in detail, such as loss of insular ribbon, obscuration of the lenticular nucleus, loss of gray-white matter differentiation, and sulcal effacement. However, these signs do not have the same implication as areas of definite hypodensity because they

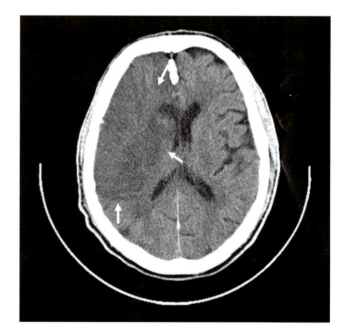

Fig. 3.4 CT scan of the head without contrast showing a multilobar hypodensity in the right hemisphere *(arrows)*.

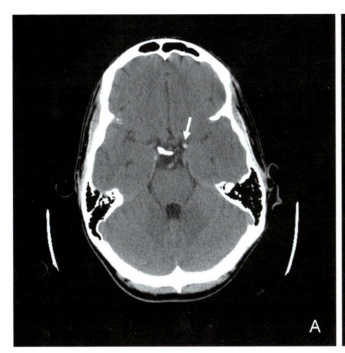 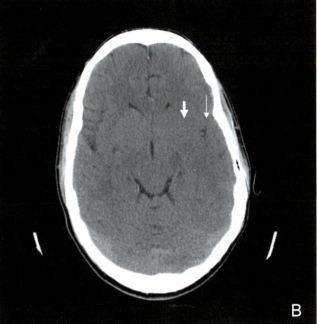

Fig. 3.5 **(A)** CT scan of the head without contrast showing a left hyperdense middle cerebral artery sign indicative of acute thrombosis *(arrow).* **(B)** CT scan of the head without contrast showing effacement of sulci and sylvian fissure *(thin arrow)* and loss of distinction of the margins of the left lenticular nucleus *(thick arrow).*

probably indicate focal tissue edema rather than established infarction.[15] Interpretation of brain imaging should be performed by a physician with expertise reading brain scans, but formal training in neuroradiology is not required.

Adequate control of blood pressure before, during, and after administration of intravenous fibrinolysis must be achieved to reduce the risk of intracranial bleeding. **Table 3.3** summarizes the recommendations for blood pressure control. Most stroke specialists deem administration of fibrinolysis unsafe for patients who require sodium nitroprusside infusion to lower the blood pressure below 185/110 mm Hg in the emergency department.

Administration of Fibrinolysis and Postfibrinolysis Care

Infusion of the fibrinolytic agent should be started in the emergency department without delay as soon as the patient is determined to be a good treatment candidate. The dose of rtPA is 0.9 mg/kg (maximum 90 mg) over 60 minutes, with 10% of the total dose given as a bolus over 1 minute. After fibrinolysis, the patient should be admitted to a stroke unit for strict neurologic monitoring by specialized nurses. Postfibrinolytic management ideally should be guided by a written protocol to ensure optimal care and avoid risks. Essential elements of postfibrinolysis care are summarized in **Table 3.4**. Patients should be kept on cardiac telemetry for at least the first 24 hours.

Bleeding complications in general and intracranial hemorrhage in particular are the most common and feared adverse

Table 3.3 Management of Arterial Hypertension in Patients with Acute Ischemic Stroke Who Are Candidates for Fibrinolysis*

Before fibrinolysis

If SBP >185 mm Hg or DBP >110 mm Hg

    Labetalol 10 to 20 mg IV over 1 to 2 minutes (may repeat once)

    or

    Nicardipine infusion at 5 to 15 mg/h

If BP controlled, administer fibrinolysis

If BP still >185/110 mm Hg, do NOT proceed with fibrinolysis

After fibrinolysis

If SBP 180 to 230 mm Hg or DBP 105 to 120 mm Hg

    Labetalol 10 to 20 mg IV over 1 to 2 minutes, may repeat every 10 to 20 minutes up to 300 mg over 24 hours

    or

    Labetalol 10 to 20 mg IV followed by infusion at 2 to 8 mg/min

    or

    Nicardipine infusion at 5 to 15 mg/h

If SBP >230 mm Hg or DBP >120 mm Hg

    Sodium nitroprusside infusion at 0.5 to 3 µg/kg/min (doses of up to 10 µg/kg/min can be safely administered for up to 10 minutes)

Abbreviations: BP, blood pressure; DBP, diastolic blood pressure; SBP, systolic blood pressure.

*This protocol also applies to other forms of reperfusion therapy apart from intravenous rtPA.

Table 3.4 Key Elements of Medical Management During and After Intravenous Fibrinolysis for Acute Ischemic Stroke

Admit to stroke unit for neurologic and cardiac monitoring

Neurologic assessments every 15 minutes during rtPA infusion, every 30 minutes thereafter for the first 6 hours, and then hourly until 24 hours after treatment

Discontinue rtPA infusion and obtain emergency CT scan if the patient develops severe headache, vomiting, or acute refractory hypertension (>180/110 mm Hg)

Measure blood pressure every 15 minutes for the first 2 hours, every 30 minutes for the next 6 hours, and then hourly to complete 24 hours

If systolic blood pressure ≥180 mm Hg or if diastolic blood pressure ≥105 mm Hg, treat with antihypertensives (see Table 3.3) and increase the frequency of blood pressure measurements

Strict monitoring of blood glucose and treatment with insulin to maintain blood sugar levels between 140 mg/dL and 180 (mg/dL)

Monitor body temperature and treat fever with antipyretics or mechanical measures

Avoid use of all antithrombotics during the first 24 hours after treatment

Delay invasive procedures (including placement of nasogastric tubes, indwelling bladder catheters, arterial catheters, and central venous catheters) until 24 hours after treatment

Obtain follow-up brain imaging at 24 hours before starting antithrombotics (antiplatelet agents or anticoagulants)

events after intravenous fibrinolysis. Yet, disabling or fatal intracranial hemorrhages after fibrinolysis typically occur in older patients with severe deficits and large areas of ischemia at presentation.[16,17] In other words, severe brain hemorrhages usually complicate fibrinolytic therapy in patients who already had very poor prognosis from presentation. As a consequence, few patients are actually harmed by intravenous rtPA (number needed to harm has been estimated to be 126 mg for a disabled or fatal outcome and 36.5 mg for worsened outcome among patients treated within 3 hours of symptom onset).[17]

Additional complications from rtPA include angioedema, which may cause partial airway obstruction, and, very rarely, myocardial rupture in patients with previous large myocardial infarctions.

Predictors of Outcome After Intravenous Fibrinolysis

Older age, worse neurologic deficits (i.e., higher National Institutes of Health Stroke Scale [NIHSS] score) and disturbances of consciousness at presentation, higher admission blood glucose level, and early ischemic changes and hyperdense middle cerebral artery sign on baseline CT scan are the main predictors of poor outcome upon initial evaluation.[3,8,13,18–20] Time to fibrinolysis has a strong inverse association with functional outcome across strokes of different severity.[4,9] Hyperglycemia and intracranial hemorrhage predict hyperacute clinical worsening after fibrinolysis.[21] Lack

of improvement at 24 hours portends a worse outcome at 3 months.[22] Hyperglycemia, time to fibrinolytic therapy, and cortical involvement have been associated with lack of improvement during the first day.[22] The detrimental effects of hyperglycemia may be at least partially explained by lower rates of recanalization, probably related to a hyperglycemia-induced decrease in fibrinolytic activity.[23]

The main predictors of symptomatic intracranial hemorrhage are older age, although intravenous rtPA can be administered to selected octogenarians with acceptable safety[24]; higher initial NIHSS; larger area of ischemia; and higher blood glucose levels.[9,16,25] Longer time to fibrinolysis has been associated with a higher risk of intracranial hemorrhage in some,[25] but not all,[9] studies. Higher systolic blood pressure may also increase the risk of intracranial hemorrhage,[8] but especially when currently recommended parameters for blood pressure control are not followed. Other protocol violations, most notably the use of antithrombotic agents during the first 24 hours, can markedly increase the risk of hemorrhage.[26]

◆ Novel Strategies for Intravenous Fibrinolysis

Selection of Candidates for Intravenous Fibrinolysis Using Penumbral Imaging

There is a strong physiologic rationale to support the concept that imaging of the ischemic penumbra with diffusion-weighted (DWI) and perfusion-weighted (PWI) MRI or with CT perfusion (CTP) can extend the therapeutic window for reperfusion therapies, including fibrinolysis. Proponents of this model argue that documentation of persistent ischemic penumbra (i.e., hypoperfused but salvageable tissue) should represent a solid indication for reperfusion treatments regardless of duration of symptoms. Assuming that brain imaging can reliably recognize penumbral tissue and discriminate patients at excessive risk for bleeding in the ischemic core, the concept should be valid. However, these assumptions remain to be proven.

The Diffusion and Perfusion Imaging Evaluation for Understanding Stroke Evolution (DEFUSE) study was a prospective observational study of 74 patients treated with intravenous rtPA between 3 and 6 hours after symptom onset.[16] All patients underwent MRI with DW-PW and MR angiogram before and a few hours after fibrinolysis, but all patients were treated regardless of the radiologic findings. The investigators found that patients with a "target mismatch profile" (i.e., large areas of hypoperfusion with much smaller areas of restricted diffusion) benefited greatly from fibrinolysis if they achieved recanalization. Conversely, patients with very large areas of restricted diffusion had unacceptably high risks of intracerebral bleeding.

The randomized Echoplanar Imaging Thrombolytic Evaluation Trial (EPITHET) assigned 101 patients to receive intravenous rtPA or placebo 3 to 6 hours after stroke onset.[27] All patients were studied with MRI with DW-PW before and a few days after treatment, but the radiologic findings did not affect treatment assignment. DW-PW was present in 86% of patients. Reperfusion occurred in 39% of the mismatch patients, and these patients had less infarct growth and better functional outcome. The rate of symptomatic intracranial hemorrhage was quite low (4%), and the risk of this complication did not correlate with baseline volume of restricted diffusion.

A recent study compared intravenous tenecteplase administered between 3 and 6 hours after symptom onset on patients with documented penumbra (defined by MRI with DW-PW or CTP) and vessel occlusion (defined by noninvasive angiogram) versus control patients treated with intravenous rtPA within 3 hours according to current guidelines.[28] Although the relatively small size of the study (n = 50, including only 15 patients treated with tenecteplase) and methodologic limitations preclude definitive conclusions, the high degrees of reperfusion (74%) and rates of recanalization (10/15 cases) among patients selected on the basis of penumbral imaging was promising. Pilot trials testing intravenous desmoteplase administered between 3 and 9 hours after symptom onset in patients with DW-PW mismatch on baseline MRI had shown encouraging results.[29,30] However, the larger Desmoteplase in Acute Ischemic Stroke (DIAS-2) study did not confirm this benefit.[31] A preponderance of mild strokes with small core lesions and mismatch volumes may have limited the power of DIAS-2 to detect some therapeutic effect.

An ongoing trial (Magnetic Resonance and Recanalization of Stroke Clots Using Embolectomy [MR RESCUE]) is assessing the value of endovascular reperfusion within 3 to 8 hours of symptom onset among patients with DW-PW mismatch on MRI. At this point, we still do not have sufficient information to recommend the use of penumbral imaging to select patients for fibrinolysis in clinical practice.

Novel Fibrinolytic Agents for Stroke

Alteplase (rtPA) is not highly fibrin-specific, needs to be cleaved by plasmin to become activated, and has been shown to produce N-methyl-D-aspartate (NMDA)- and kainite-neurotoxic effects in experimental animals. Desmoteplase, the recombinant form of a fibrinolytic agent contained in the saliva of vampire bats, does not have any of these disadvantages. It is generally only active in the presence of fibrin, it does not require the activation by plasmin, and it is not neurotoxic.[32] As described in the previous section, the initial promising results with this novel fibrinolytic agent[29,30] were not confirmed in the DIAS-2 study.[31]

Tenecteplase is a recombinant mutation of the wild-type tPA molecule that has a longer half-life and greater resistance to plasminogen activator inhibitor-1 than does rtPA.[32] It is the most commonly used fibrinolytic agent for acute myocardial infarction. There is limited information from human studies on the value of tenecteplase for acute ischemic stroke. A phase I, dose-escalation study using the same criteria currently prescribed for rtPA administration indicated that tenecteplase was safe in the doses tested (0.1 to 0.4 mg/kg).[33] Tenecteplase administration was associated with high degrees of reperfusion and high rates of recanalization in a small population of patients with symptoms for 3 to 9 hours and radiologically documented penumbra.[28]

Ultrasound-Enhanced Thrombolysis

The likelihood of intracranial vessel recanalization after intravenous fibrinolysis may be increased by combining it with ultrasound waves continuously delivered to the occlusive thrombus by means of transcranial Doppler. This concept was tested on the Combined Lysis of Thrombosis in Brain Ischemia Using Transcranial Ultrasound and tPA (CLOTBUST) study, a phase II randomized, controlled trial comparing the combination of intravenous rtPA with continuous transcranial Doppler insonation versus intravenous rtPA with placebo (i.e., no continuous insonation) within 3 hours of stroke onset.[34] The addition of continuous insonation was associated with significant improvement in the rate of complete recanalization at 2 hours (38% versus 13% without continuous ultrasound), but with only a trend toward better clinical recovery. More research in this area is being conducted.

◆ Intraarterial Fibrinolysis and Bridging Therapy

The study and application of endovascular reperfusion therapies for acute ischemic stroke has strong advocates. Unfortunately, the available evidence is highly promising but not conclusive. Therefore, endovascular interventions for acute brain ischemia cannot be considered the standard of care. Chapter 30 discusses chemical and mechanical thrombolysis in detail. Hence, this chapter only briefly reviews the most important information on intraarterial fibrinolysis and combined intravenous and intraarterial therapy (also known as bridging therapy).

The Prolyse in Acute Cerebral Thromboembolism (PROACT II) study provides the best evidence that intraarterial fibrinolysis can improve patient outcomes.[35] This was a rigorously designed, multicenter (54 centers in the U.S. and Canada), randomized, open-label study with blinded outcome assessment that enrolled 180 patients with angiographically proven middle cerebral artery occlusion and stroke symptoms for less than 6 hours to receive intraarterial pro-urokinase over 2 hours plus intravenous heparin versus intravenous heparin alone (all patients received heparin for 4 hours). Mechanical disruption of the clot was not allowed. Intraarterial fibrinolysis resulted in recanalization in 66% of cases. Favorable functional outcome at 90 days occurred in 40% of patients treated with intraarterial fibrinolysis versus 25% of patients in the control group (p = .04; number needed to treat = 7). These results were quite remarkable considering that participating patients had severe deficits at presentation (median NIHSS score 17). The rate of symptomatic intracranial hemorrhage was 10% among patients treated with the fibrinolytic agent (versus 2% among controls), but there were no differences in mortality. Following the conclusion of the study, pro-urokinase was not approved for clinical use in stroke, and its manufacturer stopped producing it. Over the subsequent years, the clinical use of intraarterial rtPA has been found to be safe.

The Middle Cerebral Artery Embolism Local Fibrinolytic Intervention Trial (MELT), a Japanese study, had a similar design to PROACT II, albeit using urokinase as the fibrinolytic agent.[36] It was prematurely aborted after enrollment of 114 patients because of the approval of intravenous rtPA treatment in Japan. Clinical outcomes were more favorable with intraarterial fibrinolysis, especially in terms of the number of patients achieving excellent function and minimal or no deficits at 90 days. Symptomatic intracranial hemorrhage occurred in 9% of fibrinolysed patients (versus 2% of controls).

The combined results of PROACT II and MELT provide strong support for the clinical use of intraarterial fibrinolysis. Yet the advent of mechanical embolectomy afforded by the introduction of clot retrieving and suctioning catheters has changed the field. Today, endovascular reperfusion procedures start with attempts to remove the clot, and fibrinolysis is usually only attempted as an adjuvant therapy when the clot cannot be mechanically retrieved or suctioned.

Bridging therapy consists of administering intravenous fibrinolysis and then proceeding to endovascular treatment if the patient fails to improve and there is persistent major intracranial vessel occlusion. The Interventional Management of Stroke (IMS II) trial tested this strategy on 81 stroke patients with severe deficits at presentation (median NIHSS score of 19).[37] Intravenous rtPA (0.6 mg/kg) was started within 3 hours and intraarterial rtPA (up to 22 mg) within 5 hours of symptom onset. Patients treated in this multicenter, open-label, single-arm pilot study had better outcomes than the rtPA-treated patients in the NINDS study despite a longer time to the start of intravenous fibrinolysis and much worse initial stroke severity. The rate of symptomatic intracranial hemorrhage was nearly 10%, but 3-month mortality was actually lower than expected (16%). IMS III is randomizing patients to standard intravenous rtPA versus a combined intravenous/intraarterial approach (including mechanical embolectomy).

References

1. Meschia JF, Miller DA, Brott TG. Thrombolytic treatment of acute ischemic stroke. Mayo Clin Proc 2002;77:542–551
2. Adams HP Jr, del Zoppo G, Alberts MJ, et al; American Heart Association; American Stroke Association Stroke Council; Clinical Cardiology Council; Cardiovascular Radiology and Intervention Council; Atherosclerotic Peripheral Vascular Disease and Quality of Care Outcomes in Research Interdisciplinary Working Groups. Guidelines for the early management of adults with ischemic stroke: a guideline from the American Heart Association/American Stroke Association Stroke Council, Clinical Cardiology Council, Cardiovascular Radiology and Intervention Council, and the Atherosclerotic Peripheral Vascular Disease and Quality of Care Outcomes in Research Interdisciplinary Working Groups: the American Academy of Neurology affirms the value of this guideline as an educational tool for neurologists. Stroke 2007;38:1655–1711
3. Tissue plasminogen activator for acute ischemic stroke. The National Institute of Neurological Disorders and Stroke rt-PA Stroke Study Group. N Engl J Med 1995;333:1581–1587
4. Marler JR, Tilley BC, Lu M, et al. Early stroke treatment associated with better outcome: the NINDS rt-PA stroke study. Neurology 2000;55:1649–1655
5. Kwiatkowski TG, Libman RB, Frankel M, et al; National Institute of Neurological Disorders and Stroke Recombinant Tissue Plasminogen Activator Stroke Study Group. Effects of tissue plasminogen activator for acute ischemic stroke at one year. N Engl J Med 1999;340:1781–1787
6. von Kummer R, Hacke W. Safety and efficacy of intravenous tissue plasminogen activator and heparin in acute middle cerebral artery stroke. Stroke 1992;23:646–652
7. Wahlgren N, Ahmed N, Dávalos A, et al; SITS-MOST investigators. Thrombolysis with alteplase for acute ischaemic stroke in the Safe Implementation of Thrombolysis in Stroke-Monitoring Study (SITS-MOST): an observational study. Lancet 2007;369:275–282
8. Wahlgren N, Ahmed N, Eriksson N, et al; Safe Implementation of Thrombolysis in Stroke-MOnitoring STudy Investigators. Multivariable analysis of outcome predictors and adjustment of main outcome results to baseline data profile in randomized controlled trials: Safe Implementation of Thrombolysis in Stroke-MOnitoring STudy (SITS-MOST). Stroke 2008;39:3316–3322
9. Hacke W, Donnan G, Fieschi C, et al; ATLANTIS Trials Investigators; ECASS Trials Investigators; NINDS rt-PA Study Group Investigators. Association of outcome with early stroke treatment: pooled analysis of ATLANTIS, ECASS, and NINDS rt-PA stroke trials. Lancet 2004;363:768–774
10. Hacke W, Kaste M, Bluhmki E, et al; ECASS Investigators. Thrombolysis with alteplase 3 to 4.5 hours after acute ischemic stroke. N Engl J Med 2008;359:1317–1329
11. Wahlgren N, Ahmed N, Dávalos A, et al; SITS investigators. Thrombolysis with alteplase 3–4.5 h after acute ischaemic stroke (SITS-ISTR): an observational study. Lancet 2008;372:1303–1309
12. Barber PA, Zhang J, Demchuk AM, Hill MD, Buchan AM. Why are stroke patients excluded from TPA therapy? An analysis of patient eligibility. Neurology 2001;56:1015–1020
13. Qureshi AI, Ezzeddine MA, Nasar A, et al. Is IV tissue plasminogen activator beneficial in patients with hyperdense artery sign? Neurology 2006;66:1171–1174
14. Derex L, Hermier M, Adeleine P, et al. Clinical and imaging predictors of intracerebral haemorrhage in stroke patients treated with intravenous tissue plasminogen activator. J Neurol Neurosurg Psychiatry 2005;76:70–75
15. Muir KW, Buchan A, von Kummer R, Rother J, Baron JC. Imaging of acute stroke. Lancet Neurol 2006;5:755–768
16. Albers GW, Thijs VN, Wechsler L, et al; DEFUSE Investigators. Magnetic resonance imaging profiles predict clinical response to early reperfusion: the Diffusion and Perfusion Imaging Evaluation for Understanding Stroke Evolution (DEFUSE) study. Ann Neurol 2006;60:508–517
17. Saver JL. Hemorrhage after thrombolytic therapy for stroke: the clinically relevant number needed to harm. Stroke 2007;38:2279–2283
18. Bruno A, Levine SR, Frankel MR, et al; NINDS rt-PA Stroke Study Group. Admission glucose level and clinical outcomes in the NINDS rt-PA Stroke Trial. Neurology 2002;59:669–674
19. Heuschmann PU, Kolominsky-Rabas PL, Roether J, et al; German Stroke Registers Study Group. Predictors of in-hospital mortality in patients with acute ischemic stroke treated with thrombolytic therapy. JAMA 2004;292:1831–1838
20. Mateen FJ, Nasser M, Spencer BR, et al. Outcomes of intravenous tissue plasminogen activator for acute ischemic stroke in patients aged 90 years or older. Mayo Clin Proc 2009;84:334–338
21. Leigh R, Zaidat OO, Suri MF, et al. Predictors of hyperacute clinical worsening in ischemic stroke patients receiving thrombolytic therapy. Stroke 2004;35:1903–1907
22. Saposnik G, Young B, Silver B, et al. Lack of improvement in patients with acute stroke after treatment with thrombolytic therapy: predictors and association with outcome. JAMA 2004;292:1839–1844
23. Ribo M, Molina C, Montaner J, et al. Acute hyperglycemia state is associated with lower tPA-induced recanalization rates in stroke patients. Stroke 2005;36:1705–1709
24. Sylaja PN, Cote R, Buchan AM, Hill MD; Canadian Alteplase for Stroke Effectiveness Study (CASES) Investigators. Thrombolysis in patients older than 80 years with acute ischaemic stroke: Canadian Alteplase for Stroke Effectiveness Study. J Neurol Neurosurg Psychiatry 2006;77:826–829
25. Kidwell CS, Saver JL, Carneado J, et al. Predictors of hemorrhagic transformation in patients receiving intra-arterial thrombolysis. Stroke 2002;33:717–724
26. Katzan IL, Furlan AJ, Lloyd LE, et al. Use of tissue-type plasminogen activator for acute ischemic stroke: the Cleveland area experience. JAMA 2000;283:1151–1158
27. Davis SM, Donnan GA, Parsons MW, et al; EPITHET investigators. Effects of alteplase beyond 3 h after stroke in the Echoplanar Imaging Thrombolytic Evaluation Trial (EPITHET): a placebo-controlled randomised trial. Lancet Neurol 2008;7:299–309
28. Parsons MW, Miteff F, Bateman GA, et al. Acute ischemic stroke: imaging-guided tenecteplase treatment in an extended time window. Neurology 2009;72:915–921
29. Furlan AJ, Eyding D, Albers GW, et al; DEDAS Investigators. Dose Escalation of Desmoteplase for Acute Ischemic Stroke (DEDAS): evidence of

safety and efficacy 3 to 9 hours after stroke onset. Stroke 2006;37:
1227–1231

30. Hacke W, Albers G, Al-Rawi Y, et al; DIAS Study Group. The Desmoteplase in Acute Ischemic Stroke Trial (DIAS): a phase II MRI-based
9-hour window acute stroke thrombolysis trial with intravenous desmoteplase. Stroke 2005;36:66–73

31. Hacke W, Furlan AJ, Al-Rawi Y, et al. Intravenous desmoteplase in patients with acute ischaemic stroke selected by MRI perfusion-diffusion
weighted imaging or perfusion CT (DIAS-2): a prospective, randomised,
double-blind, placebo-controlled study. Lancet Neurol 2009;8:141–150

32. Meretoja A, Tatlisumak T. Novel thrombolytic drugs: will they make a
difference in the treatment of ischaemic stroke? CNS Drugs 2008;22:
619–629

33. Haley EC Jr, Lyden PD, Johnston KC, Hemmen TM; TNK in Stroke Investigators. A pilot dose-escalation safety study of tenecteplase in acute
ischemic stroke. Stroke 2005;36:607–612

34. Alexandrov AV, Molina CA, Grotta JC, et al; CLOTBUST Investigators.
Ultrasound-enhanced systemic thrombolysis for acute ischemic stroke.
N Engl J Med 2004;351:2170–2178

35. Furlan A, Higashida R, Wechsler L, et al. Intra-arterial prourokinase for
acute ischemic stroke. The PROACT II study: a randomized controlled
trial. Prolyse in Acute Cerebral Thromboembolism. JAMA 1999;282:
2003–2011

36. Ogawa A, Mori E, Minematsu K, et al; MELT Japan Study Group. Randomized trial of intraarterial infusion of urokinase within 6 hours of
middle cerebral artery stroke: the Middle Cerebral Artery Embolism
Local Fibrinolytic Intervention Trial (MELT) Japan. Stroke 2007;38:
2633–2639

37. IMS II Trial Investigators. The Interventional Management of Stroke
(IMS) II Study. Stroke 2007;38:2127–2135

4

Critical Care Management

Matthew Vibbert and Andrew M. Naidech

Pearls for the Management of Intracerebral Hemorrhage

- Preventing clot growth is key to improving outcomes, especially in the first few hours after symptom onset.
- Acute hypertension should probably be controlled. A systolic blood pressure of 140 to 160 mm Hg is reasonable.
- Anticoagulation with vitamin K antagonists (e.g., warfarin) should be reversed immediately.
- Nonconvulsive seizures should be excluded, but universal anticonvulsant prophylaxis is unlikely to benefit most patients.
- Predicted poor outcome may lead to changes in goals of care and self-fulfilling prophecies.

Pearls for the Management of Subarachnoid Hemorrhage

- The risk of aneurysm rebleeding should be minimized with acute blood pressure control, early aneurysm obliteration, and potentially with hemostatic therapy.
- The incidence of vasospasm can be pharmacologically reduced.
- Symptomatic vasospasm can often be treated with hyperdynamic therapy, alone or in conjunction with endovascular therapy (covered in Section IV of this book).
- Nonconvulsive seizures should be excluded, but universal anticonvulsant prophylaxis is unlikely to benefit most patients.

Pearls for the Management of Elevated Intracranial Pressure

- Elevated intracranial pressure may be related to mass, ischemia, insufficient nutrient delivery, or other potentially reversible causes.
- A stepwise progression of therapies from short-acting (elevation of the head of the bed and titratable agents) to longer-acting (barbiturates) should be quickly employed.

◆ Critical Care Management of Intracerebral Hemorrhage

Predictors of Outcome in Acute Intracerebral Hemorrhage

Several factors on admission are associated with worse outcome after intracerebral hemorrhage (ICH). Several similar prediction scores have been developed from prognostic variables.[1]

Intracerebral Hemorrhage Volume

An acute clot is a mass in the skull. As such, it may compress adjacent structures, increase intracranial pressure (ICP), and lead to hydrocephalus, herniation, and death. Larger volumes are associated with worse outcomes.

Intracerebral hemorrhage volume frequently increases after the diagnostic computed tomography (CT) scan. Approximately one third of patients have an increase in ICH volume of one third or more. When it occurs, ICH volume growth is associated with a worse outcome. Predictors of ICH volume growth include earlier time of the diagnostic CT scan, anticoagulation, larger ICH volume on the diagnostic scan, and acute hypertension.

Location of Intracerebral Hemorrhage

Intracerebral hemorrhage in the brainstem is especially deadly because it is likely to compress brain tissue involved in respiration, bronchial hygiene, and consciousness. A moderate-sized cerebellar ICH may compress the brainstem and require neurosurgical decompression.

Age

Older age is associated with worse outcome. This is likely a combination of reduced recovery, limitations in goals of care, and reduced tolerance for cardiovascular stress if critical care is required.

Level of Consciousness and Neurologic Examination

The Glasgow Coma Scale and National Institutes of Health (NIH) Stroke Scale have both been shown to be predictors of outcome; any validated neurologic assessment is likely to be useful. A depressed level of consciousness may be related to increased ICH volume, hydrocephalus, or a seizure.

Intraventricular Hemorrhage

Hemorrhage in the basal ganglia, thalamus, or caudate nuclei more frequently extends into the third or a lateral ventricle. Intraventricular hemorrhage (IVH) leads to an increased risk of fever, hydrocephalus from obstructed flow of cerebrospinal fluid (CSF), and worse outcomes. Consultation with a neurosurgeon regarding ventricular drainage is advisable.

Blood Pressure Management for Acute Intracerebral Hemorrhage

Hypertension is a leading cause of ICH and is commonly abnormal on admission. The pathophysiology of elevated blood pressure may lead to increased ICP, a Cushing response (bradycardia with severe hypertension due to an intracranial mass), or a surge of catecholamines.

The available data generally show an association between acute hypertension and ICH volume growth. The presumed pathophysiology is that greater blood pressures lead to more acute bleeding from a small vessel and ICH volume growth. Case series of documented contrast extravasation on acute CT angiography ("spot sign") and subsequent ICH volume growth lend support to this hypothesis.[2]

The optimal timing, potency, and choice of agent for blood pressure control have not been defined, and several clinical trials are in progress. One study found that "intensive" blood pressure control (target systolic blood pressure [SBP] 140 mm Hg, medication at the discretion of the treating physician) was associated with less clot growth than standard care (target SBP 180 mm Hg)[3]; a confirmatory trial is underway. For patients with severe hypertension an SBP of 160 mm Hg should be considered, although this may be modified by elevated ICP or tailored to therapy to optimize cerebral perfusion pressure (usually targeted at 60 to 80 mm Hg).

Coagulopathy

Clotting limits the amount of bleeding into cerebral tissue. Anything that retards clotting may increase the risk of clot growth, IVH, and poor outcome. The more potent the inhibition of clotting, the more profound the risk.

Vitamin K Antagonists (Warfarin)

Warfarin (Coumadin), an antagonist of vitamin K, is commonly used for stroke prevention (especially in the setting of atrial fibrillation or artificial cardiac valves), and for the prevention of cerebrovascular and peripheral vascular disease. The intensity of anticoagulation is monitored with the international normalized ratio (INR), which corrects for variation in each laboratory's prothrombin time (PT). An INR of 1 is considered normal, with 2 to 3 being the most commonly used therapeutic range. An elevated INR is strongly associated with more and later clot growth as blood continues to ooze.

A warfarin effect should be treated emergently. The best way to correct a warfarin effect has not been clearly determined, and different institutions use different protocols. The longer the time until the INR is corrected (1.4 or less is considered desirable, although the best target has not been prospectively defined), the greater the risk of clot growth and poor outcome. Several different options are available:

◆ Fresh Frozen Plasma

Fresh frozen plasma (FFP) replaces the factors inhibited by warfarin. The greater the intensity of anticoagulation, the more units are needed. Two to four units are usually given to start with follow-up of the INR.

◆ Prothrombin Complex Concentrates

Prothrombin complex concentrates (PCCs) have relatively high concentrations of vitamin K–dependent clotting factors. A variety of PCCs are available. PCC administration may be faster and require less volume than FFP, but the cost is significantly greater; the benefit as compared with FFP is attenuated if the INR is corrected quickly.[4] One should consult in advance with a hematologist on the most appropriate PCC and dose required to avoid delay when a patient requires emergent treatment.

◆ Recombinant Factor VII

Recombinant factor VII (FVII) has been used in case series for the correction of warfarin. The INR is decreased quickly, but vitamin K–dependent clotting factors are not repleted. The effect on the INR is short-lived, so one should consider the concurrent administration of FFP or PCC.

◆ Vitamin K

Vitamin K is frequently given IV or PO. If anticoagulation is required again (such as for a mechanical cardiac valve), then the administration of vitamin K will complicate future use of warfarin, sometimes for weeks afterward. Vitamin K has a slow onset of action because clotting factors must be resynthesized by the liver, so it is not appropriate as monotherapy for warfarin-related ICH.

Heparin and Low-Molecular-Weight Heparins

Heparin is similar to warfarin in its impact on ICH, although not only the vitamin K–dependent clotting factors are involved.

The risk of ICH is related to the intensity of anticoagulation, and unintentional over-anticoagulation increases the risk of cerebral hemorrhage. Unfractionated heparin should be reversed with protamine and discontinuation of heparin. Low-molecular-weight heparins are incompletely corrected with protamine, and typically require administration of FFP or PCC.

Antiplatelet Agents (IIbIIIa Inhibitors, Aspirin, Thienopyridines [Clopidogrel])

Aspirin irreversibly acetylates a residue on platelets, which makes them less potent. Thienopyridines (of which clopidogrel is in widespread use and likely to be followed by others) inhibit platelet activation further downstream and are more potent. The classes are often combined, especially after the interventional treatment of acute coronary syndromes. Compared with monotherapy, combined antiplatelet therapy increases the risk of ICH.

Known antiplatelet medication use is generally associated with more ICH volume growth and worse outcome[5]; measurement of platelet activity may improve prediction.[6] Platelet transfusion has been used to improve platelet activity, although data from randomized trials are not yet available. The utility of other agents (desmopressin, FVII) in this setting has not been well described.

Intravenous IIbIIIa inhibitors (e.g., abciximab, etanercept) may infrequently lead to cerebral hemorrhage. The risk of cerebral hemorrhage increases with elevated blood pressure, cerebral ischemia, and reperfusion. The antiplatelet agent should be discontinued and platelets administered, with potentially repeat treatment depending on the half-agent of the offending agent.

Hemorrhage After Alteplase (Tissue-Type Plasminogen Activator) for Ischemic Stroke

Cerebral hemorrhage after alteplase (tissue-type plasminogen activator [tPA]) administration for acute ischemic stroke is infrequent (approximately 5%). Centers that follow the National Institute of Neurological Disorders and Stroke (NINDS) tPA protocol have hemorrhagic conversion rates similar to that in the original tPA trial. When it occurs, the hemorrhages tend to be severe and in ischemic or reperfused brain tissue. The risk is increased by older age, hypertension, longer time from symptom onset to treatment, greater amount of ischemic brain tissue (involvement of one third or more of the middle cerebral artery distribution increases the risk), and protocol violations (e.g., early administration of aspirin or heparin, severe hypertension).[7] Drug administration should be stopped whenever hemorrhage is suspected (change in mental status, new headache, etc.) and excluded with CT. When ICH occurs, FFP is typically given.

Acute Hemostatic Therapy

The documentation of ICH volume growth in the first hours after symptom onset implies that if clot growth could be stopped, then outcomes might be improved. There have been two randomized clinical trials with FVII as an acute hemostatic agent after ICH. In both trials, treatment led to less ICH volume growth, although functional outcomes at 90 days were improved only in the first trial.[8]

Surgical Decompression and Catheter-Based Clot Lysis

Surgical decompression and catheter-based clot lysis are covered in Section III of this book.

Seizures and Anticonvulsant Medication Use After Intracerebral Hemorrhage

There are widely varying quoted rates of seizures after ICH, from 5% to >20%. Seizures usually occur soon after ICH. A substantial number of seizures are only detected on prolonged electroencephalogram (EEG) monitoring, and such monitoring should be considered for comatose patients to exclude nonconvulsive seizures and status epilepticus. Other risk factors for seizures include cortical location, an associated subdural hematoma, and previous cerebral infarction.[9]

If a patient does not have seizures within a few days of ICH, is at low risk for seizures, or if seizures have been excluded with EEG, then the potential benefits of anticonvulsant therapy are probably low. Prophylactic anticonvulsant therapy, especially phenytoin, has been associated with more fever and worse functional outcomes.[10]

Self-Fulfilling Prophecies in Intracerebral Hemorrhage

Intracerebral hemorrhage is known to have the worst prognosis of the subtypes of stroke. Confidence in prognosis can be counterproductive, however, because clinicians who are certain of a poor outcome may direct their care away from intervention and rehabilitation toward restriction of critical care and comfort. In patients with equivalent severity of neurologic illness scores, hospitals that have higher rates of do-not-resuscitate orders have higher mortality.[11] Patients with a good outcome may, early on, be thought to have no reasonable chance of functional independence. This does not mean that intensive care is always appropriate, but rather that clinicians should be aware of their potential biases in discussions with decision makers. If you are convinced the case is hopeless, you can usually prove yourself correct.

Web Resources

Updated guidelines from the American Heart Association for the management of acute ICH are available at:

http://stroke.ahajournals.org/cgi/content/full/38/6/2001

Ongoing clinical trials in ICH can be found at:

www.stroketrials.org

◆ Critical Care Management of Subarachnoid Hemorrhage

Predictors of Outcome in Aneurysmal Subarachnoid Hemorrhage

The features that predict poor outcome in subarachnoid hemorrhage (SAH) are similar to those described for ICH. Advanced age, impaired level of consciousness, focal neurologic deficits, hemorrhage burden, and the presence of IVH are associated with poor outcome. Markers of physiologic derangement on admission, including the presence of increased A-a gradient, metabolic acidosis, hyperglycemia, hypotension, and hypertension, have been reported to predict poor outcome (**Table 4.1**).[12] Prevention of rebleeding (see below) is important to maximize the chances of good neurologic outcome.

Management of Subarachnoid Hemorrhage Prior to Aneurysm Obliteration

Early management of SAH focuses on treating elevated ICP through medical management and CSF diversion, limiting hemorrhage burden through prevention of rebleeding, and reversing physiologic derangement through aggressive resuscitation.

Airway Management

Patients with a normal level of consciousness generally do not require invasive airway control. Patients with a reduced level of consciousness are at risk for aspiration, and endotracheal intubation for poor bronchial hygiene should be considered. After intubation, effective sedation should be achieved with a short-acting sedatives and analgesics. Coughing and ventilator asynchrony may produce sharp increases in ICP and blood pressure and potentially increase the risk of aneurysm rebleeding.

Table 4.1 Predictors of Outcome in Aneurysmal Subarachnoid Hemorrhage

Grade	Hunt and Hess[31]	World Federation of Neurosurgical Societies (WFNS)[32]
1	Asymptomatic, mild headache, slight nuchal rigidity	Glasgow Coma Scale (GCS) score 15
2	Moderate to severe headache, nuchal rigidity, no neurologic deficit other than cranial nerve palsy	GCS 13–14, no motor deficit
3	Drowsiness/confusion, mild focal neurologic deficit	GCS 13–14, motor deficit
4	Stupor, moderate-severe hemiparesis	GCS 7–12
5	Coma, decerebrate posturing	GCS 3–6

Blood Pressure Management Prior to Aneurysm Obliteration

Elevated systolic blood pressure has been associated with rebleeding within 24 hours of aneurysmal SAH. Although no randomized, controlled studies have been conducted to demonstrate a reduction in rebleed rates with strict blood pressure control, a goal systolic pressure of <140 mm Hg is reasonable prior to obliteration of the aneurysm. This is generally achieved through the use of a continuous, rapidly titratable infusion of antihypertensive medications.

Although strict control of systolic blood pressure is desirable, care must be taken to avoid profound hypotension. Patients with acute SAH are commonly intravascularly volume depleted. As such, they are at risk for hypotension with initiation of antihypertensive medications, especially when given in concert with sedation. Crystalloid or colloid fluid boluses may be administered to achieve and maintain a euvolemic state; mean arterial pressures should be maintained above 70 mm Hg. Neurogenic stunned myocardium, discussed below, can make achieving this goal challenging. Central venous pressure monitoring or invasive hemodynamic monitoring may be useful.

Neurogenic Stunned Myocardium

Troponin levels are elevated following SAH in as many as 60% of patients and are associated with impaired left ventricular function and regional wall motion abnormalities.[13] Neurogenic stunned myocardium (myocardial stunning) is thought to arise from excessive catecholamine release from the cardiac sympathetic nervous system. It is associated with increased risk of arrhythmia, pulmonary edema, delayed cerebral ischemia, mortality, and disability. On pathologic examination, contraction band necrosis may be found. A correlation has been reported between adrenoreceptor polymorphisms and risk of troponin elevation and echocardiographic abnormalities, implicating autonomic function.[14]

Neurogenic stunned myocardium is an early complication of SAH and generally resolves within 5 to 7 days of the hemorrhage. Myocardial dysfunction, however, may make early resuscitation and late hyperdynamic therapy challenging. Iatrogenic support and advanced hemodynamic monitoring may be helpful in this setting.

Analgesia

Sedation should be minimized to permit frequent neurologic evaluation; however, effective analgesia must be achieved. Uncontrolled pain may contribute to hypertension and increase the risk of aneurysm rebleeding. Acetaminophen is the preferred first-line agent, but cautious use of short-acting, intravenous opiate agents is likely to be necessary.

Hydrocephalus

Subarachnoid hemorrhage extending into the third or fourth ventricle commonly causes obstructive hydrocephalus. Development of ventriculomegaly on CT should prompt emergent

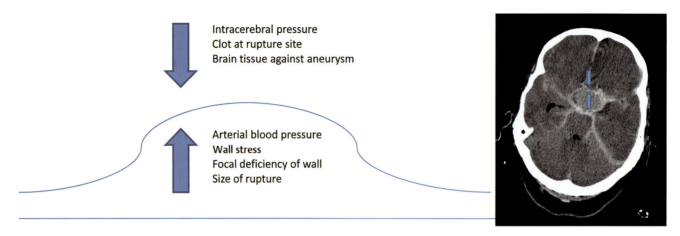

Intracerebral pressure
Clot at rupture site
Brain tissue against aneurysm

Arterial blood pressure
Wall stress
Focal deficiency of wall
Size of rupture

Fig. 4.1 Factors that influence aneurysmal rebleeding on both sides of the arterial wall. A stylized version appears on the left, and a computed tomography scan of a patient with a large aneurysm appears on the right. Arrows indicate the direction of pressure.

placement of an external ventricular drain for CSF diversion. Care should be taken not to dramatically reduce ICP at insertion, as this may favor aneurysm rebleeding as the pressure inside the aneurysm becomes greater than the pressure outside **(Fig. 4.1).**

Prevention of Rebleeding

Aneurysmal rebleeding occurs in 7 to 10% of SAH patients and is a major cause of mortality and long-term disability.[15] Rebleeding occurs within 3 days of ictus in most (73%) cases. The most important predictors of aneurysm rebleeding are neurologic grade on admission and aneurysm size.

When there is an unavoidable delay in aneurysm obliteration (patient transport, equipment malfunction, etc.), a brief course of antifibrinolytic therapy reduces the risk of aneurysm rebleeding without an increased risk of vasospasm.[16] Early surgical or endovascular obliteration of the aneurysm is preferred. Aneurysm obliteration is covered in Sections III and IV of this book.

Management of Subarachnoid Hemorrhage After Aneurysm Obliteration

Blood Pressure Management

After obliteration of the aneurysm, blood pressure parameters may be liberalized to maintain systolic blood pressures at less than 200 mm Hg as the risk of vasospasm increases from 3 to 14 days after rupture. The presence of unsecured, unruptured aneurysms should not influence blood pressure management strategies.

Vasospasm Prophylaxis

Cerebral infarction related to vasospasm is a significant source of long-term disability. Hemorrhage burden is the best predictor of vasospasm.[17] Angiographic vasospasm and elevation in transcranial Doppler (TCD) mean flow velocities occur more frequently than symptomatic vasospasm (delayed cerebral ischemia) or delayed cerebral infarction from vasospasm.[18]

Calcium channel blockers have been studied for the prevention of vasospasm. Although no agent has been demonstrated to reduce the incidence of angiographic vasospasm, improved 3-month outcomes were reported with nimodipine; a mechanism other than vasodilatation may be involved.[19] A lower dose may be considered in patients who experience significant hypotension following administration.

Several small studies have investigated the benefit of statin therapy following SAH. A recent meta-analysis described a decrease in symptomatic vasospasm, delayed ischemia, and mortality associated with statin therapy.[20]

Vasospasm Treatment

Elevated mean flow velocities and radiographic vasospasm can often be treated medically without progression to symptomatic vasospasm or cerebral infarction. Hypertension may be induced with vasopressors with the goal of reversing symptoms of cerebral ischemia or to a specified perfusion goal. Serial electrocardiogram (ECG) and measurement of troponin are advisable during the period of induced hypertension, as the increased work may lead to myocardial injury.

Patients should be maintained in a euvolemic state throughout the vasospasm period. This may be accomplished with isotonic crystalloid or colloid intravenous fluids. Hypotonic intravenous fluids should be avoided. In patients with vasospasm, central venous pressure (CVP) monitoring or advanced hemodynamic monitoring may be useful in instituting goal-directed therapy aimed at maintaining euvolemia. Inducing a hypervolemic state likely does not add significant benefit over maintenance of euvolemia.[21]

The timing and goals of packed red blood cell transfusion are controversial. Transfusion reduces oxygen extraction fraction and increases oxygen delivery after SAH.[22] Anemia increases the risk of cerebral infarction and poor outcomes,[23] but transfusion may lead to infection, volume overload, or lung injury.

Endovascular therapy (discussed in Section IV) should be considered early as an adjunct to medical therapy for vasospasm and for refractory symptoms.

Fever and Fever Control

Fever is a common medical complication of SAH and has been associated with poor outcome and prolonged intensive care unit (ICU) length of stay.[24] The use of therapeutic temperature modulation to maintain normothermia is discussed further below.

Seizure and Anticonvulsant Medication Use

Seizures commonly occur in patients with SAH, and nonconvulsive status epilepticus has been reported in as many as 20% of critically ill neurologically injured patients.[9] A period of continuous EEG monitoring is advisable for patients with abnormal mental status. The use of anticonvulsive medications, typically phenytoin, in the perioperative following SAH may be considered. In the absence of clinical or electrographic seizures, seizure prophylaxis beyond 72 hours after SAH adds little benefit.[25] Phenytoin burden has been associated with early disability and poor cognitive outcomes at 3 months following SAH.[26]

Web Resources

Updated guidelines on the management of SAH from the American Heart Association are available at:

http://www.americanheart.org/presenter.jhtml?identifier _3003999

Ongoing clinical trials are listed at:

www.stroketrials.org

◆ Critical Care Management of Acute Ischemic Stroke

This section does not discuss fibrinolysis, which is covered in Chapter 3.

Blood Pressure Management

Hypertension is the strongest risk factor for stroke, and blood pressure is frequently elevated after acute ischemic stroke. The management of blood pressure is different depending on the use of fibrinolytic therapy. Outside of the setting of fibrinolysis, there are no clear guidelines for the control of hypertension.

Hypertension in the setting of cerebral ischemia may be physiologic in that increased blood pressure may increase cerebral perfusion to ischemic tissue. If cerebral perfusion is reduced or sensitive to pressure, further decreasing blood pressure may increase ischemia and worsen the stroke. On the other hand, untreated severe hypertension may lead to hemorrhagic conversion of an ischemic stroke.

Hypotension should be avoided and volume status should be assessed on admission and at least daily. Patients with stroke may become volume depleted from reduced oral intake. Hypotonic fluids should be avoided as they may lead to cerebral edema in infarcted brain tissue. A trial of acute vasopressor therapy may be considered on a case-by-case basis for patients who are particularly pressure sensitive, although how to best select these patients is unclear.

Cardiac Monitoring

Arrhythmias and cardiac dysfunction are common causes of stroke. Atrial fibrillation leads to disorganized flow of blood and is thrombogenic. A severely depressed left ventricular ejection fraction or focal hypokinesis/akinesis (from a previous myocardial infarction) may lead to ventricular clot formation and embolism. A causative arrhythmia may not be present on admission or during the emergency evaluation, but may be intermittent. Patients admitted with acute ischemic stroke (AIS) should have telemetry monitoring for 24 to 48 hours to exclude an arrhythmic cause. An evaluation of cardiac function should be considered. Stroke is frequently associated with acute myocardial infarction; measurement of serum markers for myocardial ischemia should be performed.

Cerebral Edema After Acute Ischemic Stroke

Infarcted brain often swells, with the acme at 3 to 5 days after stroke. Larger amounts of infarcted cerebral tissue confer a greater risk of cerebral edema. Cerebral edema and the resulting mass effect are particularly likely with infarction of the middle cerebral artery territory. The evaluation and management of elevated intracranial pressure are discussed below. Patients younger than 60 years of age with complete middle cerebral artery infarction should be considered for early hemicraniectomy regardless of the side of infarction. Hemicraniectomy markedly increases the risk of survival, although some functional disability is likely.[27] Hemicraniectomy is covered in Section III.

Stroke Unit Care and the Stroke Patient in a Neuro–Intensive Care Unit

Care in specialized stroke units improves the outcomes of patients with stroke.[28] The use of best practices as a whole is more important than a specific intervention (e.g., availability of mechanical clot lysis). Accrediting organizations have developed specific guidelines (see web resources, below). Important facets of stroke unit care include improved organization, coordination of care, and protocols for routine procedures and consultations (nutrition, physical and occupational therapy, etc.). Prevention of complications is discussed below.

Stroke unit teams are composed of several disciplines including specially trained physicians, nurses, and rehabilitation personnel. A medical director oversees protocols and coordinates care among the several involved disciplines. Regular review of quality metrics ensures that best practices are enforced and new interventions are added in a timely manner. Specific training in vascular neurology is usual for some members of the team.

If a patient with stroke requires intensive care for blood pressure augmentation, ventilatory support, a medical comorbidity, or another reason, that care may be provided in the stroke unit, a neurologic intensive care unit, or a separate intensive care unit, depending on local resources. For patients who require intensive care, intensivist staffing is associated with improved outcomes. Some ICU protocols may overlap or partially conflict with protocols for stroke patients, so a clear delineation of responsibilities should be discussed ahead of time.

Web Resources for Acute Ischemic Stroke

Updated guidelines from the American Heart Association on AIS are available at:

http://stroke.ahajournals.org/cgi/content/full/38/5/1655

Accreditation criteria for a stroke center in the U.S. are available at:

http://www.jointcommission.org/CertificationPrograms/
PrimaryStrokeCenters/

◆ Management of Acute Elevated Intracranial Pressure in Ischemic and Hemorrhagic Stroke

Pathophysiology

Elevated ICP is an important treatable cause of secondary neuronal injury following ICH, SAH, and large territory ischemic stroke. Global perturbations (such as inadequate perfusion) may lead to a generalized increase in ICP. Local mass effect may lead to compression of adjacent structures. As the ICP rises, the patient may mount a compensatory systemic hypertensive response in an effort to maintain an adequate cerebral perfusion pressure (CPP). As this compensatory mechanism fails and CPP falls below a critical threshold, hypoxic and ischemic injury develops. This secondary ischemic injury produces a greater territory of edematous tissue, and ICP rises further. Left unchecked, this cycle ultimately leads to herniation and death.

Initial Management

Early recognition of elevated ICP and prompt intervention are critical to minimize neurologic injury. Early signs of elevated ICP include a decrease in the patient's level of consciousness, an increase in leg tone, and restriction of vertical gaze; an emergent CT scan should be considered. In the presence of hydrocephalus, an emergent neurosurgical consultation for the placement of an external ventricular drain is strongly advised.

Stepwise medical interventions can ameliorate or control elevated ICP in many cases.

Surgical Management

Neurosurgical consultation should be considered early. Elevated ICP due to a mass lesion (such as clot), obstructive hydrocephalus, or massive cerebral infarction is unlikely to be controllable with medical therapy alone.

Decompressive hemicraniectomy increases intracranial volume and decreases ICP, although elevated ICP may still occur. Hemicraniectomy improves mortality in patients with elevated ICP, but if there is already severe neurologic damage it does not improve the likelihood of meaningful neurologic recovery. It should be considered early, before herniation compresses the basal ganglia and brainstem.

Nonpharmacologic Interventions

Head-of-bed elevation decreases in ICP through improved venous drainage. For all patients with suspected or known elevated ICP, the head of the bed should be maintained at or above 30 degrees whenever possible. This includes during transport to and from the ICU. The head should also be maintained in a midline position to permit optimal jugular venous drainage.

Hyperventilation leads to a rapid decrease in pCO_2. This, in turn, causes cerebrovascular constriction and affects a drop in ICP. This effect persists only for hours, after which return of pCO_2 back to normal may lead to vasodilatation and rebound increased ICP. Hyperventilation should be viewed as a bridge to more definitive treatment, not maintained over days. Hyperventilation to a pCO_2 <20 to 25 mm Hg can produce severe vasoconstriction and cerebral infarction, so monitoring of pCO_2 during hyperventilation should be considered. Beware of inadvertent hyperventilation during transport by nervous or enthusiastic personnel.

Short-Acting Sedating and Analgesic Agents

Agitation and pain can contribute to elevated ICP. Patients at risk for elevated ICP should receive sedation and analgesia sufficient to produce a calm, comfortable state. A target score on a validated scale (such as the Richmond Agitation Sedation Scale) may assist in medication titration. Short-acting agents are preferred to permit brief interruptions in sedation for regularly neurologic assessments and avoid oversedation that may prolong ventilator weaning.

The short half-life of propofol makes it an attractive choice when frequent neurologic assessments are required. Prolonged use (>24 hours) in high doses (>65 µg/kg/min) in young patients with central nervous system (CNS) injury has been associated with a (usually) fatal "propofol infusion syndrome" characterized by metabolic academia, renal failure, and refractory arrhythmias. A 30-year-old woman with poor-grade subarachnoid hemorrhage and refractory status epilepticus would be at particularly high risk. There is no agreed-upon monitoring for early detection and no specific treatment, so propofol use should be minimized in this setting in favor of other agents.

Even in the absence of clinically obvious agitation or pain, sedatives and analgesics may lower ICP. These agents decrease brain metabolism and, via flow-metabolism coupling, may decrease cerebral blood volume and ICP. It is reasonable to administer IV boluses of short-acting agents in response to an acute elevation in ICP.

Hyperosmolar Therapy

Mannitol is an osmotic diuretic; a bolus of 0.5 to 1.5 g/kg may be administered through a peripheral IV with an effect starting in 15 to 30 minutes and typically persisting for several hours. Serum osmolality should be assayed following administration of mannitol, although the optimal increase in osmolality has not been clearly defined. Mannitol is a potent diuretic, so urine output and volume status should be closely monitored to avoid hypovolemia.

Hypertonic saline effectively lowers ICP and may be used alone or in conjunction with mannitol. Various concentrations have been used in this setting, including 3%, 7%, and 23.4% (compared with 0.9% "normal saline"). Administration of 30 mL of 23.4% saline (sometimes called a "bullet" because of the shape of the vial, administered over 5 to 10 minutes) through a central venous line can effectively and safely lower the ICP for several hours. More rapid administration can produce profound, transient hypotension. Serum sodium and osmolality should be monitored following administration of hypertonic saline. An infusion may be used to maintain osmolality; 3% hypertonic saline at 0.5 to 1 mL/kg/hr to maintain a serum osmolality of 315 to 325 mOsm/L is typical. If used for more than a day, either mannitol or hypertonic saline should be weaned over several days to avoid a rebound effect.

Cerebral Perfusion Pressure Optimization

Extremes of CPP may produce elevations in ICP. In response to low CPP, cerebrovascular dilatation increases cerebral blood volume and contributes to high ICP. Alternately, very high CPP may overwhelm compensatory cerebrovascular constriction, leading to an increase in cerebral blood volume and ICP.[29] The optimal target CPP for patients with elevated ICP has not been clearly established; 60 to 80 mm Hg is typical.

Therapeutic Temperature Modulation

Fever may contribute to elevated ICP. Scheduled administration of antipyretics such as acetaminophen may reduce fever and contribute to ICP control. In patients who remain febrile in spite of antipyretic administration, therapeutic temperature modulation with surface or endovascular cooling devices to achieve normothermia may be considered.

Hypothermia effectively lowers ICP, probably due to a decrease in metabolic activity. Alternately, hypothermia may favorably modulate the inflammatory response following brain injury. The optimal target temperature for ICP control has not been established. On termination of therapeutic hypothermia, slow rewarming at 0.25°C per hour or less is advisable because rapid rewarming can lead to rebound edema and elevated ICP.

Temperature modulation is frequently accompanied by shivering. Shivering increases metabolic demand, raises temperature, and increases ICP. Pharmacologic and nonpharmacologic strategies are available. Temperature modulation may not be appropriate in the presence of infection. The risk of thrombosis, infection, arrhythmia, and other complications increases after 2 to 3 days and should be weighed against the potential longer-term benefits.

Barbiturates and Long-Acting Sedative Agents

Barbiturates are effective in the management of elevated ICP but have long half-lives and significant cardiovascular side effects. Barbiturates are typically used for refractory elevated ICP. EEG monitoring may be helpful to titrate the level of sedation to a burst-suppression pattern. Once initiated, barbiturates are difficult to reverse and make a determination of brain death difficult because they confound the neurologic exam and assessment of spontaneous respiration.

◆ Minimizing Medical Complications in the Neuro–Intensive Care Unit

◆ Medical complications increase length of stay, morbidity, and potentially mortality.

◆ "Preventable" medical complications are reviewed by quality agencies, payers, and the public to determine reimbursement, ratings, and payment.

◆ The incidence of central-line–associated bloodstream infections (CLABSIs), hospital-acquired pneumonia (HAP), ventilator-acquired pneumonia (VAP), ventricular-drain–related meningitis/ventriculitis, and decubitus ulcers can be reduced in the neuro-ICU.

◆ Mechanical ventilatory support and sedation should be weaned as soon as tolerated. Early tracheostomy should be considered for patients with minimal ventilatory support who are unable to protect their airway due to coma or impaired bronchial hygiene.

Impact of Medical Complications

Treatment of patients following ischemic and hemorrhagic stroke is commonly complicated by fever, anemia, pneumonia, hyperglycemia, and venous thrombotic events (VTEs). These complications represent important sources of morbidity and prolong hospitalizations.[24] These patients are also at high risk for preventable complications such as gastric ulcers, CLABSIs, decubitus ulcers, and nutritional compromise. Prevention of these complications is considered a marker of high-quality ICU care.

Fever and Temperature Control

Fever is a common and modifiable complications following brain injury. In cases of persistent fever after administration of antipyretics, therapeutic temperature modulation may be considered to enforce normothermia, although no controlled trials have been conducted to evaluate the benefit of fever control. In general, it is reasonable to maintain normothermia throughout the period of active neuronal injury, typically 3 to 5 days for ICH and ischemic stroke and 7 to 14 days for SAH complicated by vasospasm.

Incidence of "central fever" is high following SAH, and patients may have a higher hypothalamic "set point" for body temperature. Consequently, many patients experience significant shivering even during maintenance of normothermia. Shivering may increase metabolic demand and ICP in patients with SAH. Detection and treatment of shivering is essential when therapeutic temperature modulation is employed.

Hospital-Associated Pneumonia and Ventilator-Associated Pneumonia

Patients may be at high risk for HAP or VAP from prolonged intubation, poor bronchial hygiene, aspiration, or other factors. Daily interruptions of sedation combined with spontaneous breathing trials decrease the duration of mechanical ventilation, the duration of hospital stay, and mortality. Protocols for suctioning, oral hygiene, and elevation of the head of the bed further decrease the risk. Early tracheostomy should be considered for patients likely to need prolonged airway protection even when ventilator support is not needed.

Hyperglycemia

Hyperglycemia frequently complicates neurologic injury. Untreated severe hyperglycemia (>200 mg/dL) is associated with increased myoneuropathy, prolonged ventilator weaning, and sepsis. The optimal serum glucose, however, is unclear. Glucose control, typically with a goal between 80 and 140 mg/dL, is considered reasonable.

Venous Thrombotic Events

Patients are at high risk for deep venous thrombosis (DVT) and pulmonary embolism (PE) due to immobility. Mechanical prophylaxis should be routinely instituted. Chemoprophylaxis with unfractionated heparin or low-molecular-weight heparin should be considered in patients with ICH when clot volume is stable and in patients with SAH after aneurysm obliteration.

For patients who develop DVT or PE, the optimal timing of initiation of therapeutic anticoagulation is controversial. For SAH, therapeutic anticoagulation may be initiated following obliteration. There are few data in ICH, and anticoagulation is generally avoided. After AIS, the risk for clinically significant hemorrhagic transformation is highest in the first 3 to 7 days following stroke and with increased volume of infarction. Inferior vena cava filters are often considered and seem reasonable, but there are few data.

Gastric Ulcers

Neurologically injured, critically ill patients are at high risk for clinically significant bleeding caused by gastric ulcers. This risk is increased in patients with mechanical ventilation, coagulopathy, or administration of high-dose steroids. Ulcer prophylaxis with histamine blockers or proton pump inhibitors should be routinely considered.

Central-Line–Associated Bloodstream Infections

CLABSI is considered a preventable complication in critically ill patients. Infections associated with insertion are reduced by rigid adherence to sterile technique, full barrier precautions, and handwashing protocols. Once in place, meticulous site care reduces the risk of later infections. For central venous catheters likely to be in place for more than a week, catheters coated with minocycline and rifampin have reduced colonization rates. Daily assessment of the need for central access should be performed and central lines should be removed as early as possible. In cases where peripheral access is limited or prolonged need for central access is anticipated, early placement of a peripherally inserted central catheter (PICC) may be considered.

Decubitus Ulcers

Stroke patients are at high risk for decubitus ulcers, especially when complicated by coma, immobility, or incontinence. Decubitus ulcers are considered to be preventable complications. Daily assessment for signs of pre-ulcerous skin changes, frequent patient rotation, and aggressive, early treatment of skin breakdown should be standard practice.

Nutrition

Early initiation of nutritional support should be implemented as soon as possible following initial resuscitation and within 48 hours of all forms of stroke. Enteral nutrition is preferred to parenteral nutrition because of reduced risks of infection, ease of administration and lower cost. When a feeding tube is placed, gastric and postpyloric feeds are acceptable, although postpyloric feeds may be preferred in patients at high risk for aspiration. Early placement of percutaneous gastrostomy tubes is not superior to nasogastric tube placement during the first 2 weeks following ischemic stroke.[30] A percutaneous gastrostomy tube should be considered early when the patient is unlikely to be able to take adequate nutrition by mouth for an extended period of time due to coma or aspiration. A variety of nutritional formulations are available, although none has shown particular benefit in patients with stroke.

Web Resources

Updated guidelines from the Society of Critical Care Medicine for the management and prevention of medical complications in the ICU are available at:

http://sccmwww.sccm.org/professional_resources/guide
lines/index.asp

References

1. Hemphill JC III, Farrant M, Neill TA Jr. Prospective validation of the ICH Score for 12-month functional outcome. Neurology 2009;73: 1088–1094
2. Wada R, Aviv RI, Fox AJ, et al. CT angiography "spot sign" predicts hematoma expansion in acute intracerebral hemorrhage. Stroke 2007;38: 1257–1262
3. Anderson CS, Huang Y, Wang JG, et al; INTERACT Investigators. Intensive blood pressure reduction in acute cerebral haemorrhage trial (INTERACT): a randomised pilot trial. Lancet Neurol 2008;7:391–399
4. Huttner HB, Schellinger PD, Hartmann M, et al. Hematoma growth and outcome in treated neurocritical care patients with intracerebral hemorrhage related to oral anticoagulant therapy: comparison of acute treatment strategies using vitamin K, fresh frozen plasma, and prothrombin complex concentrates. Stroke 2006;37:1465–1470
5. Saloheimo P, Ahonen M, Juvela S, Pyhtinen J, Savolainen ER, Hillbom M. Regular aspirin-use preceding the onset of primary intracerebral hemorrhage is an independent predictor for death. Stroke 2006;37: 129–133
6. Naidech AM, Jovanovic B, Liebling S, et al. Reduced platelet activity is associated with early clot growth and worse 3-month outcome after intracerebral hemorrhage. Stroke 2009;40:2398–2401
7. Tanne D, Kasner SE, Demchuk AM, et al. Markers of increased risk of intracerebral hemorrhage after intravenous recombinant tissue plasminogen activator therapy for acute ischemic stroke in clinical practice: the Multicenter rt-PA Stroke Survey. Circulation 2002;105:1679–1685
8. Mayer SA, Brun NC, Begtrup K, et al; FAST Trial Investigators. Efficacy and safety of recombinant activated factor VII for acute intracerebral hemorrhage. N Engl J Med 2008;358:2127–2137
9. Claassen J, Mayer SA, Kowalski RG, Emerson RG, Hirsch LJ. Detection of electrographic seizures with continuous EEG monitoring in critically ill patients. Neurology 2004;62:1743–1748
10. Messé SR, Sansing LH, Cucchiara BL, Herman ST, Lyden PD, Kasner SE; CHANT investigators. Prophylactic antiepileptic drug use is associated with poor outcome following ICH. Neurocrit Care 2009;11:38–44
11. Hemphill JC III, Newman J, Zhao S, Johnston SC. Hospital usage of early do-not-resuscitate orders and outcome after intracerebral hemorrhage. Stroke 2004;35:1130–1134
12. Claassen J, Vu A, Kreiter KT, et al. Effect of acute physiologic derangements on outcome after subarachnoid hemorrhage. Crit Care Med 2004;32:832–838
13. Naidech AM, Kreiter KT, Janjua N, et al. Cardiac troponin elevation, cardiovascular morbidity, and outcome after subarachnoid hemorrhage. Circulation 2005;112:2851–2856
14. Zaroff JG, Pawlikowska L, Miss JC, et al. Adrenoceptor polymorphisms and the risk of cardiac injury and dysfunction after subarachnoid hemorrhage. Stroke 2006;37:1680–1685
15. Naidech AM, Janjua N, Kreiter KT, et al. Predictors and impact of aneurysm rebleeding after subarachnoid hemorrhage. Arch Neurol 2005;62: 410–416
16. Hillman J, Fridriksson S, Nilsson O, Yu Z, Saveland H, Jakobsson KE. Immediate administration of tranexamic acid and reduced incidence of early rebleeding after aneurysmal subarachnoid hemorrhage: a prospective randomized study. J Neurosurg 2002;97:771–778
17. Hijdra A, van Gijn J, Nagelkerke NJ, Vermeulen M, van Crevel H. Prediction of delayed cerebral ischemia, rebleeding, and outcome after aneurysmal subarachnoid hemorrhage. Stroke 1988;19:1250–1256
18. Frontera JA, Fernandez A, Schmidt JM, et al. Defining vasospasm after subarachnoid hemorrhage: what is the most clinically relevant definition? Stroke 2009;40:1963–1968
19. Petruk KC, West M, Mohr G, et al. Nimodipine treatment in poor-grade aneurysm patients. Results of a multicenter double-blind placebo-controlled trial. J Neurosurg 1988;68:505–517
20. Sillberg VA, Wells GA, Perry JJ. Do statins improve outcomes and reduce the incidence of vasospasm after aneurysmal subarachnoid hemorrhage: a meta-analysis. Stroke 2008;39:2622–2626
21. Lennihan L, Mayer SA, Fink ME, et al. Effect of hypervolemic therapy on cerebral blood flow after subarachnoid hemorrhage: a randomized controlled trial. Stroke 2000;31:383–391
22. Dhar R, Zazulia AR, Videen TO, Zipfel GJ, Derdeyn CP, Diringer MN. Red blood cell transfusion increases cerebral oxygen delivery in anemic patients with subarachnoid hemorrhage. Stroke 2009;40:3039–3044
23. Naidech AM, Jovanovic B, Wartenberg KE, et al. Higher hemoglobin is associated with improved outcome after subarachnoid hemorrhage. Crit Care Med 2007;35:2383–2389
24. Wartenberg KE, Schmidt JM, Claassen J, et al. Impact of medical complications on outcome after subarachnoid hemorrhage. Crit Care Med 2006;34:617–623, quiz 624
25. Chumnanvej S, Dunn IF, Kim DH. Three-day phenytoin prophylaxis is adequate after subarachnoid hemorrhage. Neurosurgery 2007;60:99–102, discussion 102–103
26. Naidech AM, Kreiter KT, Janjua N, et al. Phenytoin exposure is associated with functional and cognitive disability after subarachnoid hemorrhage. Stroke 2005;36:583–587
27. Vahedi K, Hofmeijer J, Juettler E, et al; DECIMAL, DESTINY, and HAMLET investigators. Early decompressive surgery in malignant infarction of the middle cerebral artery: a pooled analysis of three randomised controlled trials. Lancet Neurol 2007;6:215–222
28. Stroke Unit Trialists Collaboration. How do stroke units improve patient outcomes? A collaborative systematic review of the randomized trials. Stroke 1997;28:2139–2144
29. Rose JC, Mayer SA. Optimizing blood pressure in neurological emergencies. Neurocrit Care 2004;1:287–299
30. Dennis MS, Lewis SC, Warlow C; FOOD Trial Collaboration. Effect of timing and method of enteral tube feeding for dysphagic stroke patients (FOOD): a multicentre randomised controlled trial. Lancet 2005;365: 764–772
31. Hunt WE, Hess RM. Surgical risk as related to time of intervention in the repair of intracranial aneurysms. J Neurosurg 1968;28:14–20
32. Teasdale GM, Drake CG, Hunt W, et al. A universal subarachnoid hemorrhage scale: report of a committee of the World Federation of Neurosurgical Societies. J Neurol Neurosurg Psychiatry 1988;51:1457

5

Defining Success: Basics of Measurement Scales and Clinical Research in Neurovascular Disease

Andrew M. Naidech

Pearls

- A "clinically successful outcome" should be measured with a validated scale.
- Neurologic outcome scales are typically related to function or examination.
- Bias must be carefully eliminated or minimized, or it will cloud and falsify results.
- The appropriate statistical test will highlight the hypothesized result. The wrong statistical test is more likely to be falsely negative (fails to detect a difference) or falsely positive (detects a difference where none exists).
- Running numerous statistical tests on a large data set ("data-dredging") will be apparent to sophisticated readers and reviewers.

◆ Measurement in Neurovascular Disease

Minimizing the occurrence, impact, and long-term consequences of neurovascular disease requires an ability to measure neurologic function. Not all outcomes can, or should, be measured in all patients. In general, the more accurate a scale, the more expensive (in time, equipment, and sophistication of the examiner) it is to obtain a result.

Mortality

When patients are lost to follow-up, mortality can usually be ascertained by searching publicly available vital records. Mortality is an insufficient measure in neuroscience, however, because it does not measure function or quality of life.

For many patients (and potential patients) avoiding severe disability or a vegetative state is more important than staying alive in the physiologic sense.[1]

Functional Scales

Functional scales attempt to measure what the patient can do. There are a variety of available metrics. Some are self-explanatory, have available on-line training, or can be administered with a standardized questionnaire.

Glasgow Coma Scale[2]

The Glasgow Coma Scale (GCS, **Table 5.1**) is the most widely used neurologic examination for life-threatening neurologic disease because of its simplicity and prognostic validity. There are ceiling effects (the best possible score, 15, can be associated with disability) and floor effects (the worst possible score, 3, does not mean death).

FOUR Score[3]

The Full Outline of UnResponsiveness (FOUR) score is also designed to assess comatose patients, but includes assessments of respiratory response on the ventilator and the response of pupils to light. It is more helpful for determining minimal brainstem function than the GCS.

National Institutes of Health Stroke Scale (NIHSS)[4]

The possible scores on this validated neurologic exam range from 0 (no abnormality) to 42 (the worst possible score). The

Table 5.1	Glasgow Coma Scale		
Eyes	**Motor**	**Verbal**	
	6 Follows		
	5 Localizes	5 Oriented	
4 Spontaneously open	4 Withdraws	4 Disoriented but in context	
3 Open to voice	3 Flexor posturing	3 Inappropriate words	
2 Open to pain	2 Extensor posturing	2 Unintelligible	
1 No response	1 No response	1 No response	

disadvantages of the NIHSS include its bias toward language (as opposed to visual-spatial) function,[5] and its relatively crude assessment of consciousness. Comatose patients are unable to do much of the exam.

Modified Rankin Scale

The modified Rankin Scale (mRS, **Table 5.2**)[6] is graded from 0 (no symptoms) to 6 (death). It is heavily geared toward functional independence and the ability to walk. There is a validated questionnaire that improves inter-rater reliability.[7] The score can be obtained over the phone. Serial scores can be followed over time. The mRS is not sensitive to cognitive dysfunction. An awake, interactive, but bed-bound patient scores the same as a vegetative patient.

Glasgow Outcome Scale

The Glasgow Outcome Scale (GOS) is similar to the mRS, and is graded from 1 (dead) to 5 (able to return to work or school). The major distinctions in this scale are a vegetative state, the ability to live independently, and the return to useful work. A more detailed eight-step version is the GOS-Extended (GOS-E) scale.[8]

Table 5.2	Modified Rankin Scale
0	No symptoms
1	No significant disability: despite symptoms, able to carry out all usual duties and activities
2	Slight disability: unable to perform all previous activities but able to look after own affairs without assistance
3	Moderate disability: requiring some help but able to walk without assistance
4	Moderately severe disability: unable to walk without assistance and unable to attend to own bodily needs without assistance
5	Severe disability: bedridden, incontinent and requiring constant nursing care and attention
6	Death

Barthel Index[9]

The Barthel Index focuses on the functions of daily living, including dressing, eating, and continence. Scores are from 0 (not independent in any item) to 100. It may be particularly helpful for planning rehabilitation.[10]

Sickness Impact Profile[11]

The Sickness Impact Profile (SIP) is a 136-item questionnaire that measures functioning in a variety of domains, including function, daily living, and psychosocial health. The SIP has been validated in subarachnoid hemorrhage.

Cognitive Scales

Cognitive scales are important for determining if a conscious patient can live independently or return to productive work. Unfortunately, a substantial number of patients who survive an intensive care unit (ICU) stay will not be able to complete cognitive testing. Potential barriers include the inability to present for the test, the cost of trained staff, the unavailability of clinic and testing space, and the cognitive disability itself from neurologic disease. The U.S. National Institute of Neurological Disorders and Stroke (NINDS) and the Canadian Stroke Network have proposed standards for 5-minute, 30-minute, and 60-minute batteries of complementary tests for patients with neurovascular disease.[12]

Telephone Interview for Cognitive Status (TICS)[13]

The TICS is a multistep cognitive exam for a variety of tasks including memory, attention, declarative knowledge, and orientation. It performs well compared with comprehensive batteries, and highlights patients who are likely to have abnormalities on more detailed testing.[14]

Grooved Pegboard Test

This test measures the ability of a subject to place grooved pegs in a standard board. Different results may be obtained for the dominant and nondominant hand. This test requires a cooperative patient with at least some motor skill.

Trail-Making

The primary outcome of this test is the time to connect the dots on a testing surface. Online tests are also available for remote measurement. Standard sheets are commercially available.

Mini–Mental Status Exam[15]

This popular exam measures cognitive performance in a variety of domains. It is brief and meant to be done at the patient's bedside. Brief tests of memory, cognition, visual-spatial function, and language are included.

Imaging End Points

Volume

In ischemic stroke, ischemia to large portions of the middle cerebral artery territory is associated with a higher risk for hemorrhage. The Alberta Stroke Program Early CT Score (ASPECTS) is graded from the CT scan[16] and correlates well with infarct volume by measuring whether discrete regions of brain tissue are hypodense. The intracerebral hemorrhage (ICH) volume and subsequent clot growth[17] are important predictors of outcome. The ICH volume can be calculated with dedicated software, or roughly estimated using the abc/2 method (height times width times diameter divided by 2).[18] Larger intracranial aneurysms are more difficult to obliterate and have a worse prognosis.

Cerebral Infarction

Cerebral infarction is common after a subarachnoid hemorrhage (SAH).[19] Most, but not all, infarctions can be linked to a vasospasm. Cerebral infarction should at least be recorded as present or absent. Further quantifying cerebral infarction by location (cortical, subcortical, or both) and number (single or multiple)[20] may be more accurate.

Atrophy

A variety of neural insults and cerebral infarction may lead to brain atrophy. Decreased brain volume correlates with progression of dementia[21] and a worse performance on cognitive testing.

Angiography

Angiography is a common examination for SAH and proximal ischemic stroke. Angiographic vasospasm is often scored dichotomously (present or absent), or qualitatively (none, mild, moderate, or severe). When reporting such data, the criteria should be clearly stated ("flow-limiting," based on a percentage change from baseline, diameter, etc.).

In acute ischemic stroke, important variables include the degree of stenosis, arterial occlusion, and the interventions that are performed. The faster and more completely that flow is restored, the better the radiographic and clinical outcome.

Combining Complementary End Points

Sometimes combining two scales is more helpful that using just one. For example, the NIHSS may clarify whether or not a normal GCS score is associated with a hemiparesis. A patient who is unable to live independently (mRS 4) may have a nearly normal neurologic exam but be impulsive or cognitively impaired.

◆ Key Web Resources for Neurologic Scales

- ◆ Center for Outcome Measurement in Brain Injury (www.tbims.org): provides an introduction, online training, and many commonly used outcomes scales
- ◆ Stroke Center at the University of Washington (www.strokecenter.org/trials/scales/scales-overview.htm): provides an overview of commonly used outcome scales and a registry of clinical trials in stroke
- ◆ www.NIHstrokescale.org: provides online training in the NIHSS in a variety of languages

◆ Clinical Research in Neurovascular Disease

Selection of a Condition to Study

Characteristics of potentially successful clinical projects include enrolling a sufficient number of patients (a minimum of a few per month, but they need not be enrolled at all hours of the day and night), reliable ascertainment of the patient's suitability for the study (by admission to a defined location, or enrolled by a reliable screener or by referral), clear measurement techniques, and well-trained staff working under the direction of a project leader. Examples of project topics include clinical vasospasm, severe neurotrauma, and monitoring in coma, all of which can be reasonably studied in larger medical centers. Without observational pilot data, it is difficult to judge precisely how many patients will be available. For example, ischemic stroke is common, but presentation within 3 hours is not. It is insufficient to cite an index case ("We see it") or two ("We see it over and over") as a foundation for research.

Feasibility of an Intervention

Timing

Delays in diagnosis, assessment, and administration of therapy render many treatments ineffective or dangerous. For example, intravenous (IV) tissue-type plasminogen activator (tPA) is quite effective when given within an hour of the onset of stroke symptoms, but delays of a few hours render it ineffective and increase the risk of hemorrhage.[22] In contrast, for studies on preventing vasospasm, patients can typically be enrolled within a few days of symptom onset.

Complexity

An intervention becomes less feasible if it requires more steps, more highly trained personnel, more complicated equipment, the involvement of another department (e.g., the pharmacy), or a skilled implementation (e.g., insulin infusion).

Bias

Bias is the alteration of measured outcomes by an outside factor. An unblinded examiner, exclusion of certain patients, loss to follow-up, potential gain by a third party, and other factors may lead to bias. Bias is deadly to clinical research: a study with a biased outcome may be misleading and worse than no study at all.

Minimizing Bias

The most thorough way to minimize bias is randomization, where patients are assigned by chance to one of several interventions. The larger the number randomized and the fewer the groups, the more effective randomization is likely to be. Ensuring that equal numbers of patients with certain characteristics are assigned to each intervention is known as stratification. For example, in a trial of ischemic stroke, one might stratify the side on which the stroke occurred so that each group has an equal number of left- and right-sided strokes.

Ideally, outcomes are assessed with a validated scale by an examiner who has no knowledge of the intervention. In a "double-blinded" study, neither the physician nor the patient knows which treatment has been given. This is sometimes not possible in critical care, where the intervention is obvious to the treatment team (e.g., transfusion). In that case, a separate blinded examiner who is not part of the treatment team may record the outcome ("blinded outcome ascertainment").

Informed Consent in the Patient with Altered Consciousness

The patient's right to autonomy extends to research. Many critically ill patients are not able to make their wishes known, so protocols must be carefully reviewed and approved in advance, and consent must be clearly documented.

Surrogate Consent

Prospective research often depends on the consent of a spokesperson for the patient. This person is expected to do what the patient would choose to do, not substitute his or her own beliefs for the patient's.

Presumed Consent

Some clinical scenarios make informed consent nearly impossible. This may be the case in acute, life-threatening disease where randomization must be done shortly after admission and there is no time for a surrogate to arrive. Blood cell substitutes in trauma is one example,[23] where patients present in shock, emergent treatment with presumed consent would be given anyway, and there is no time to obtain consent.

Follow-Up After Hospital Discharge

Patient status at the time of hospital discharge is important but incomplete. Improvement is often delayed for weeks or months. Patients who are disabled at 14 days often have some recovery, but predicting this is difficult. Prospective registries and trials should have some method of obtaining follow-up after discharge.

Historical studies may use outcomes from medical records or abstract outcomes after discharge. The ability to reliably extract outcomes depends on the quality of the documentation. It is difficult to abstract the mRS from clinical notes.[24]

Follow-up by telephone enables an examiner to question a patient and obtain a clearer response to a choice of outcomes. It also enables the examiner to corroborate information with another source.

Follow-up in person with an examination (preferably blinded) at a defined time is preferable for trials, but it entails the added costs of finding available space and involving the examiner and the clinic staff.

The Internet provides another potential pathway for collecting follow-up data. Major limitations include the requirement that patients be sufficiently intact to use the Internet, which is less likely in patients who survive a life-threatening neurologic event. Privacy is another concern because of the potential for identity theft (of both the patient and health care staff), insurance fraud, and informational pathogens (e.g., computer viruses). The use of codes and secure sites helps, but that often requires expertise distinct from that of the health care providers and clinical trial staff.

Registration of Clinical Trials

Charges of suppression of unfavorable trial results and selective publication[25] have led to policies that require the registration of trials. Trials must be registered at a publicly accessible Web site (see Web resources, below) to permit later consideration for publication by major medical journals. There are several advantages to examining such sites: they permit investigators to join trials in progress, and they enable investigators to see what trials others are pursuing and how trials are structured.

Key Web Resources for Neurovascular Clinical Trials

www.stroketrials.org and www.strokecenter.org/trials: stroke trials registries

www.clinicaltrials.gov: administered by the National Institutes of Health

www.icmje.org: the International Committee of Medical Journal Editors' uniform requirements for the submission of clinical trials

◆ Statistics in Neurovascular Disease, or the Tests You Need to Write Abstracts and Talk Intelligently with a Statistician

Study abstracts and reports generally include a statistical analysis to detect differences between groups. There are several excellent references on clinical trials and medical research.[26–29]

Signal/Noise Ratio

Statistical analysis shows how much variability in the data is due to factors defined by the investigator (signal), and how much is due to error or chance (noise). The greater the effect of defined variables, and the less the error, the more powerful the statistical analysis will be. Choosing the appropriate data and statistical tests are important to maximize the variability that the investigator can explain.

Investigator-Initiated Research

Define the Data of Interest

Investigators should resist the temptation to "get started now" in a haphazard fashion. Rather, they should clearly define the data they wish to collect. Narratives may be used to explain coded data that are not clear, but they should not be the primary data collection tool. Having fewer data points of high quality is more valuable than having more data points of lower quality. High-quality data are specific, have a high interrater reliability, and can be verified with source documents. The most valuable data to record prospectively are data that may need to be clarified while events are recent and are hardest to ascertain from the medical record (**Table 5.3**).

Discrete information such as laboratory values, automated times of procedures, and medications administered can often be deferred and retrieved later or with an automated query from a computer system. In general, if the data are handwritten on paper and if finding that piece of paper will require more than minimal effort later, then it is important to obtain the data now.

Research must be approved by the appropriate authority to ensure that it complies with applicable laws and ethical standards. Investigators should pay particular attention to

Table 5.3 High- and Low-Quality Data in the History of Present Illness; High Quality Data Are Specific and Use Validated Scales

High Quality	Low Quality
Time of onset: Dec. 15, 3:15 PM Time of admission: Dec. 15, 5:45 PM Glasgow Coma Scale on admit: 9 ICH Volume (abc/2), mL: 15 Glasgow Coma Scale at 24 hours: 7	Pt presented approx. 2.5 hours after lunch. Lethargic on admission, pupils equal. CT showed moderate ICH. Got worse, postured.

the identifying information (names, dates of birth, etc.) and should keep this information secure by locking hardcopies in a private office and keeping electronic data behind a firewall.

Categorical, Ordered, Normally Distributed, and Continuous Data

Neurologists ask "Where's the lesion?" because it leads to the differential diagnosis. Answering the question, "What kind of data are these?" often leads to the appropriate statistical test.

Categorical data fall into groups that are distinct and are in no particular order. Sex, ethnicity, and eye color are categorical variables. Dichotomous data are binary, such as yes/no, dead/alive, board certified/not board certified. Dichotomous data should be used only if no other information is available. For example, it is better to record GCS as a number rather than as ≤8 or >8. Ordinal data are categories with a defined sequence. The motor score of the GCS (obeys, localizes, withdraws, etc.) is ordinal.

Normally distributed data are numerical data that take the shape of a bell curve when frequency is plotted (**Fig. 5.1**). These data are appropriate for many well-known statistical tests, such as the Student's t-test.

The Meaning of P

P is the probability that the difference found is due to chance alone: $p = .05$ means there is a 5% probability that the difference is due to chance; $p = .01$ means there is a 1% probability; $p = .001$ means there is a 0.1% (or one in a thousand) probability.

$P \leq .05$ does not mean that the result is clinically significant. Many results are statistically significant but not clinically significant, such a difference of 2 mm Hg in clinical trials of blood pressure. In a population of several thousand such a difference is meaningful, but in an individual patient the error of measurement may be greater.

Chi-Squared, for Comparing Categories

Categorical variables may be compared with a chi-squared statistic. For example, one might compare a categorical variable such as the history of hypertension with another categorical variable such as coronary artery disease. A 2-by-2 table could be constructed with hypertension (presence or absence) as columns and coronary artery disease (presence or absence) as rows. The number of patients with each of four possible combinations would then be analyzed.

Student's t-Test (Two Groups) and Analysis of Variance for Groups of Normally Distributed Data

For normally distributed data (typically age, blood pressure, and most numerical characteristics) the signal is the mean value, and the noise is the variance of the data. The commonly presented standard deviation (SD) is the square root

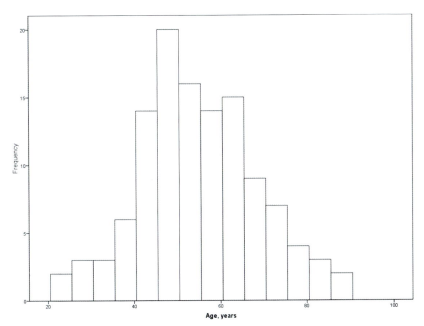

Fig. 5.1 Age is normally distributed in this data set.

of the variance. Student's *t*-test is the most commonly used test for comparing the mean value between two groups, and is a special case of the analysis of variance (ANOVA). ANOVA compares the mean between more than two groups. The statistical significance of the difference is compared with standard distribution tables. Results are expressed as mean ± SD.

Nonparametric Tests for Groups of Nonnormally Distributed Data

Sometimes data will not be normally distributed; that is, it will not be in a bell-curve distribution. In this case, one of the assumptions of the *t*-test or ANOVA does not hold. **Figure 5.1** shows normally distributed data, whereas **Fig. 5.2** shows nonnormally distributed data. Nonnormal distributions are common with measures of disease severity, pain scales, neurologic examination scales, and when there is a referral bias in a disease (if the center specializes in older patients, for example). Numerical data should always be examined for normality before deciding on the appropriate test.

If the data are not normally distributed, the appropriate test may be a nonparametric test such as the Mann-Whitney *U*. Instead of comparing the mean and error, these tests compare the ranks between groups. Numbers should be expressed

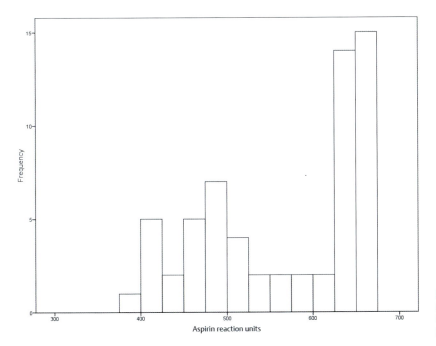

Fig. 5.2 Platelet activity (measured in aspirin reaction units) is not normally distributed in this data set. There are two normally distributed populations.

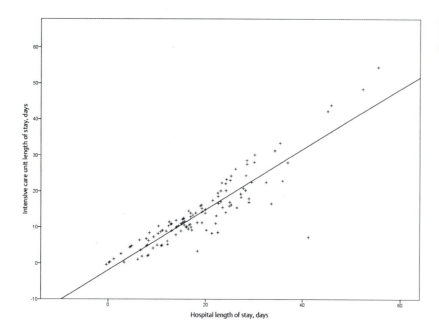

Fig. 5.3 Linear regression between intensive care unit and hospital length of stay. The two are positively correlated.

as a median (e.g., 25th percentile or 75th percentile] instead of mean ± SD.

Linear Regression, When One Number Is Associated with Another

Two numbers may move together such that a change in one is associated with a change in another. For example, hospital and ICU length of stay are often correlated, as shown in **Fig. 5.3**. A longer length of stay in the ICU corresponds to a longer length of stay in the hospital. Linear regression quantifies the relationship between the two. In this case, each day in the ICU corresponds to 0.97 days in the hospital ($p < .001$). The 95% confidence interval (CI) is 0.88 to 1.06 days. This means that we can be 95% confident that the true effect of one day longer in the ICU is between 0.88 and 1.06 days in the hospital.

Multiple linear regression uses more than one variable to predict a numerical outcome of interest. For example, ICU length of stay is not the only predictor of hospital length of stay. You might correct for other variables, such as the neurologic examination score on admission.

Logistic Regression, When One Number Is Associated with a Dichotomous Change in Another Variable

Sometimes the outcome of interest is a dichotomous one, such as mortality. For example, you might wish to predict mortality after ICH, and test the association of variables such as age. The result is not a number but rather the probability of an outcome. For example, age might increase the probability of death, but death is not certain at any particular age **(Fig. 5.4)**. Multiple logistic regression analysis is used to predict the impact of multiple variables on a dichotomous out-

come, for example, the prediction of significant disability after ICH.

Dichotomous outcomes are easy to understand, but sometimes oversimplify. Dichotomizing a good outcome as an mRS of 3 or better makes it impossible to distinguish between mRS scores of 0 and 3 and magnifies the difference between 3 and 4. A patient or surrogate, moreover, may be most interested in the chances of an excellent outcome without disability with a particular treatment (mRS 0 or 1 versus 2 to 6).

Ordinal Regression, When One Number Is Associated with a Stepwise Change in Another Variable

Sometimes the outcome of interest is a range of discrete options, such as the mRS or GOS score. Ordinal regression uses multiple, discrete, ordered categories for outcome. This strategy works best when data are present for every level of outcome. If the outcome is the mRS score at 3 months, for example, then every patient's temperature data should be recorded.

The "Right" Way

If the data are robust, then one is likely to get the same answers no matter how the data are analyzed. For example, an association between age and mortality after ICH can be shown in several ways:

- A t-test comparing the mean age of patients who die versus those who survive
- A logistic regression where death is the dependent variable and age is the independent variable

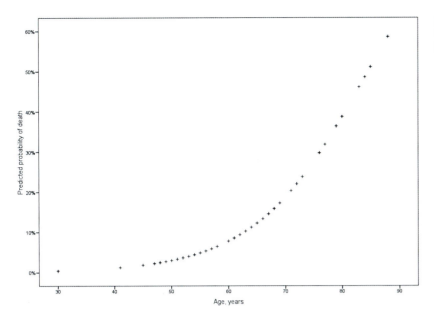

Fig. 5.4 Logistic regression between age and mortality after intracerebral hemorrhage (ICH). The greater the age, the greater the likelihood of death.

◆ A chi-squared where the category of dead versus alive is compared with the category of age greater or less than 65 years

Model Building

All statistical models are wrong in the sense that some error remains unexplained, but some are useful in that they increase understanding of the data. An interpretation should accompany the use of multiple variables to explain an outcome of interest.

Many clinical data sets have some internal confounding because sicker patients have more complications. The most statistically significant variable is not necessarily the most important, and may be confounded. Coma increases the likelihood of intubation, which increases the likelihood of pneumonia, which is associated with worse early outcomes. Thus an analysis that finds pneumonia to be the most important predictor of poor outcome might be confounded by coma.

Appropriate model building often requires teamwork between a clinician and a statistician. A statistical consultant may be necessary to determine the appropriateness of the data, the choice of model, and the statistical interpretation. The clinician must be sure to point out the variables that are clinically most appropriate to collect and are known to be associated with the outcome of interest.

Multiple Comparisons, or "Data-Dredging"

If $p = .05$ occurs 5% of the time by chance alone, then on average one must do 20 comparisons in a random data set to get one such result. With the availability of large databases for share or purchase and powerful statistical software, it is easier than ever to find "positive" results. Reviewers are well aware of this (some of them having done it themselves), and "data-dredging," making a large number of comparisons in a large data set for a few positive findings, generally looks exactly like what it is. Robust findings, as opposed to chance findings,

◆ are biologically plausible,
◆ do not become nonsignificant when controlling for obvious confounders,
◆ are associated with the outcome by more than one measure, and
◆ are significant when tested again in another, independent data set.

An abstract at a meeting is an invitation to discuss preliminary findings, and a manuscript is more a sentence in a continuing conversation than a final statement. A finding can be said not to exist until published in a peer-reviewed forum, signifying that independent investigators agree that the work is of good quality. Most medical journals require investigators to keep the data for at least several years in case questions about data integrity are raised later. Everyone expects there to be occasional false leads even when good work is done in good faith, but investigators should exercise due diligence before submission. Once their findings are published, their good name will be attached to it.

Web Resources for Statistics

The good news is that large databases for stroke research are available. The bad news is that the data are of variable quality.[30]

www.epibiostat.ucsf.edu/biostat/sites.html: the University of California at San Francisco maintains this helpful list of statistical resources

www.ahrq.gov: the Agency for Healthcare Research and Quality (AHRQ) maintains large national databases

http://wonder.cdc.gov: the Centers for Disease Control makes a wide variety of information available on this Web site through its Wonder program.

www.uhc.edu: academic medical centers may use data available from the University Hospital Consortium

References

1. Patrick DL, Pearlman RA, Starks HE, Cain KC, Cole WG, Uhlmann RF. Validation of preferences for life-sustaining treatment: implications for advance care planning. Ann Intern Med 1997;127:509–517
2. Teasdale G, Jennett B. Assessment of coma and impaired consciousness. A practical scale. Lancet 1974;2:81–84
3. Wijdicks EFM, Bamlet WR, Maramattom BV, Manno EM, McClelland RL. Validation of a new coma scale: The FOUR score. Ann Neurol 2005;58:585–593
4. Brott T, Adams HP Jr, Olinger CP, et al. Measurements of acute cerebral infarction: a clinical examination scale. Stroke 1989;20:864–870
5. Fink JN, Selim MH, Kumar S, et al. Is the association of National Institutes of Health Stroke Scale scores and acute magnetic resonance imaging stroke volume equal for patients with right- and left-hemisphere ischemic stroke? Stroke 2002;33:954–958
6. van Swieten JC, Koudstaal PJ, Visser MC, Schouten HJ, van Gijn J. Interobserver agreement for the assessment of handicap in stroke patients. Stroke 1988;19:604–607
7. Wilson JTL, Hareendran A, Grant M, et al. Improving the assessment of outcomes in stroke: use of a structured interview to assign grades on the modified Rankin Scale. Stroke 2002;33:2243–2246
8. Wilson JTL, Pettigrew LE, Teasdale GM. Structured interviews for the Glasgow Outcome Scale and the extended Glasgow Outcome Scale: guidelines for their use. J Neurotrauma 1998;15:573–585
9. Mahoney FI, Barthel DW. Functional evaluation: the Barthel Index. Md State Med J 1965;14:61–65
10. Kasner SE. Clinical interpretation and use of stroke scales. Lancet Neurol 2006;5:603–612
11. Damiano A. Sickness Impact Profile. User's Manual and Interpretation Guide. Baltimore: Johns Hopkins University Press, 1996
12. Hachinski V, Iadecola C, Petersen RC, et al. National Institute of Neurological Disorders and Stroke-Canadian Stroke Network vascular cognitive impairment harmonization standards. Stroke 2006;37:2220–2241
13. Brandt J, Spencer M, Folstein M. The telephone interview for cognitive status. Neuropsychiatry Neuropsychol Behav Neurol 1988;1:111–117
14. Mayer SA, Kreiter KT, Copeland D, et al. Global and domain-specific cognitive impairment and outcome after subarachnoid hemorrhage. Neurology 2002;59:1750–1758
15. Folstein MF, Folstein SE, McHugh PR. "Mini-mental state." A practical method for grading the cognitive state of patients for the clinician. J Psychiatr Res 1975;12:189–198
16. Barber PA, Demchuk AM, Zhang J, Buchan AM. Validity and reliability of a quantitative computed tomography score in predicting outcome of hyperacute stroke before thrombolytic therapy. ASPECTS Study Group. Alberta Stroke Programme Early CT Score. Lancet 2000;355:1670–1674
17. Flibotte JJ, Hagan N, O'Donnell J, Greenberg SM, Rosand J. Warfarin, hematoma expansion, and outcome of intracerebral hemorrhage. Neurology 2004;63:1059–1064
18. Kothari RU, Brott T, Broderick JP, et al. The ABCs of measuring intracerebral hemorrhage volumes. Stroke 1996;27:1304–1305
19. Juvela S, Siironen J, Varis J, Poussa K, Porras M. Risk factors for ischemic lesions following aneurysmal subarachnoid hemorrhage. J Neurosurg 2005;102:194–201
20. Rabinstein AA, Weigand S, Atkinson JLD, Wijdicks EFM. Patterns of cerebral infarction in aneurysmal subarachnoid hemorrhage. Stroke 2005;36:992–997
21. Brickman AM, Honig LS, Scarmeas N, et al. Measuring cerebral atrophy and white matter hyperintensity burden to predict the rate of cognitive decline in Alzheimer disease. Arch Neurol 2008;65:1202–1208
22. Clark WM, Wissman S, Albers GW, Jhamandas JH, Madden KP, Hamilton S. Recombinant tissue-type plasminogen activator (Alteplase) for ischemic stroke 3 to 5 hours after symptom onset. The ATLANTIS Study: a randomized controlled trial. Alteplase Thrombolysis for Acute Noninterventional Therapy in Ischemic Stroke. JAMA 1999;282:2019–2026
23. Chumnanvej S, Dunn IF, Kim DH. Three-day phenytoin prophylaxis is adequate after subarachnoid hemorrhage. Neurosurgery 2007;60:99–102, discussion 102–103
24. Quinn TJ, Ray G, Atula S, Walters MR, Dawson J, Lees KR. Deriving modified Rankin scores from medical case-records. Stroke 2008;39:3421–3423
25. Melander H, Ahlqvist-Rastad J, Meijer G, Beermann B. Evidence b(i)ased medicine—selective reporting from studies sponsored by pharmaceutical industry: review of studies in new drug applications. BMJ 2003;326:1171–1173
26. Friedman LM, Furberg CD, DeMets DL. Fundamentals of Clinical Trials, 3rd ed. New York: Springer, 1998
27. Gallin JI. Principles and Practice of Clinical Research. San Diego, CA: Academic Press, 2002
28. Armitage P, Berry G, Matthews J. Statistical Methods in Medical Research, 4th ed. Williston, VT: Blackwell Science, 2002
29. Guyatt G, Rennie D, Meade M, Cook D. Users Guides to the Medical Literature, 2nd ed. New York: McGraw-Hill, 2008
30. Gillum LA, Johnston SC. Analysis of large databases in stroke. Sem Cerebrovasc Dis and Stroke. 2003;3:91–99

6

Promising Developments in Critical Care

Laurie McWilliams and J. Javier Provencio

Pearls

- There are many new and old technologies currently being used in the neuro–intensive care units (NICUs) to assess brain function prior to seeing a change in the neurologic exam. Currently, these modalities have been useful in the trauma population, but need further investigation in other patient populations in the NICU prior to making conclusions regarding their efficacy.
- Many modalities for neuroprotection are being investigated, the best known and most efficacious being hypothermia.
- New medications are consistently being investigated that are useful in the NICU population. The newer antiepileptics are showing great promise. The use of conivaptan in this patient population and the clinical scenarios for its safety and efficacy are still being debated.

The near future of neurocritical care is not likely to include the large shifts that have been seen in the past two decades. The paradigm-shifting events including the development of dedicated neurologic intensive care units (NICUs) (initially in neurosurgery but more recently combined with neurology), the advent of dedicated intensive care physicians with specialization in neurocritical care, and advances in imaging and intracranial monitoring techniques have moved neurocritical care into the mainstream. In the near future, we will see refinements of existing technologies and, it is hoped, the development of fully formed treatments from the prospective treatments that have been under study for years. It is clear that the refinements in our understanding of cerebral physiology in the injured brain, control of neuroinflammation, and neuroprotection will lead the list of advances in the next decade.

Another important trend that will manifest in the years to come is not unique to neurocritical care. As we struggle to find our place in the broader field of general critical care, advances in process improvement techniques that are being implemented in many ICUs will come to the NICU as well.

In this chapter we discuss technologic advances that are and will be used more frequently, but we focus on intracranial monitoring and continuous electroencephalogram (EEG) monitoring. In addition, we discuss promising neuroprotective strategies and control of inflammation. We highlight a few medications that are likely to have a big impact on the future care of these patients. Finally, we discuss process improvement strategies that will be coming to common practice in the near future.

◆ Intracranial Monitoring and Our Understanding of Brain Physiology

Ischemic stroke, hemorrhagic stroke, and subarachnoid hemorrhage can lead to devastating neurologic deficits. In the acute setting, the goal of treatment is to protect and restore salvageable brain tissue. This goal can be accomplished by restoring blood flow to the ischemic areas and decreasing the metabolic and inflammatory mediators that potentiate further ischemic damage.

The concept of the autoregulation of the brain vasculature is critical to understanding the challenges of cerebral blood flow (CBF) in the injured brain. In normal patients, the brain and the cerebral arteries are able to maintain CBF within the cerebral perfusion pressure range of 50 to 150 mm Hg. However, in the setting of acute neurologic injury, the injured tissue loses its autoregulatory capability. The end result is a system where CBF is entirely dependent on the perfusion pressure.[1]

In these acute neurologic emergencies, blood pressure is closely monitored and adequate cerebral perfusion pressure (CPP) is tightly controlled, augmented with the use of vasopressors if needed. Unfortunately, studies have shown that altered autoregulation may include only regional areas of the brain, and global measures of systemic blood pressure may miss areas at risk.[2] To combat this problem, direct or indirect

CBF monitoring in the brain may be useful to guide management. Three specific modalities are currently in use either clinically or investigationally to measure blood flow or substrate delivery in the brain: thermodilution CBF, brain tissue oxygenation, and cerebral microdialysis.

Thermodilution Cerebral Blood Flow

Using the principles of heat dissipation, the technology includes a heating element proximal to a thermometer. The amount of energy required to maintain a temperature above the local body temperature is proportional to the washout volume, or blood flow. The technology has been tested in several neurologic conditions and is in use clinically in several centers in the United States and Europe. The major limitation of the CBF monitor is that it measures flow in a very focal area of the brain. As discussed above, there are differences in the competence of autoregulation in brain injury. There is a risk of placement errors that can either under- or overestimate the actual blood flow.[3]

Brain Tissue Oxygenation

In the setting of a primary neurologic insult (traumatic brain injury [TBI], subarachnoid hemorrhage), increased intracranial pressure or decreased CBF can result in secondary neurologic injury. Brain tissue oxygenation probes measure the partial pressure of oxygen of the interstitial space surrounding the Clark's electrode in the probe. The information obtained by this method infers oxygen delivery and so is thought to be proportional to blood flow.

Low brain tissue oxygen readings in patients with TBI are associated with worse outcome. In the trauma literature, low and prolonged brain tissue oxygenation (defined as less than 10 mm Hg for greater than 150 minutes) correlates with poor outcome in TBI patients.[4] There is still debate about whether treatment improves outcome. A review by Maloney-Wilensky and colleagues[4] reported an insertion hematoma rate of <1%, and no reported risk of infection.

There are few trials studying brain tissue oxygenation and subarachnoid hemorrhage, with no clear evidence that treatment strategies based on tissue oxygenation improve outcome.

Cerebral Microdialysis

Microdialysis exploits the movement of small molecules across a semipermeable membrane down a concentration gradient. The process entails inserting a microdialysate catheter ipsilateral to the area of damage. The catheter collects dialyzed extracellular neurochemicals that are indicators of cellular processes; lactate/pyruvate levels, glutamate, and glycerol are most common tested. Specific changes in the levels of these mediators presumably detect ischemia adjacent to the catheter.[5] This method has the advantage of measuring the output of the cell, not the delivery of substrate to determine the adequacy of substrate delivery. This minimizes the interpatient variability of substrate needs. In trauma, microdialysis has been used to detect worsening cerebral edema, allowing for interventions to take place for further interventions for reduction of elevated intercranial pressures.

In acute ischemic stroke, Schneweis et al examined potential predictors of malignant edema in large middle cerebral artery (MCA) infarcts with intracranial pressure (ICP) monitoring and microdialysis catheters.[6] The study included 10 patients and found patients who developed massive edema on computed tomography (CT) scan and elevated ICPs correlating with increased dialysate levels of lactate/pyruvate, glutamate, and glycerol. However, there was no clear pattern to elevations in dialysate levels with timing of ICP elevation. Berger et al examined the dialysate levels in 24 patients with large MCA strokes.[7] The patients were allocated to conservative management, hypothermia, or hemicraniectomy. The dialysate levels of lactate/pyruvate, glycerol, and glutamate in the conservative group were seven times higher than in the hypothermic and hemicraniectomy groups, suggesting a benefit in both hypothermia and hemicraniectomy.

Multimodal Monitoring Approaches to Patient Management

Cerebral blood flow monitoring, intraparenchymal oxygen tension monitoring, and microdialysis have all been shown to be promising therapies for the treatment of brain-injured patients. All have also been found to have limitations. In clinical practice, tissue oxygen and CBF readings are sometimes difficult to interpret in isolation. Microdialysis also has drawbacks having to do with the sampling time and rate. In the near future, it is likely that these devices will be used in combination. By having different but related data about the brain, it may be possible to develop more complete and nuanced conclusions about the brain physiology. The idea of a "bundle" of multiple brain devices has been tried in several centers in the U.S. and in Europe (**Fig. 6.1**). There is still too little evidence to suggest its use. In addition, complication risks need to be clearly evaluated along with potential benefits.

Continuous Electroencephalogram Monitoring

In addition to the intraparenchymal monitoring expansion occurring in the NICU is a resurgence in interest in the electroencephalogram (EEG), particularly continuous EEG. The standard of care for neurologic patients with worsening neurologic functioning has traditionally been CT of the head and EEG to investigate the cause of the worsening. However, continuous EEG (cEEG) may now be a better modality to assess the brain function in confused or comatose patients prior to acute clinical worsening. As stated by Vespa,[8] cEEG monitoring for the brain is like telemetry for the heart; it allows one to see changes prior to the clinical consequences. There are multiple modes of cEEG interpretation that are currently being studied.

Continuous EEG has been studied in several settings. It is illustrative to discuss the role of cEEG in ischemic stroke and

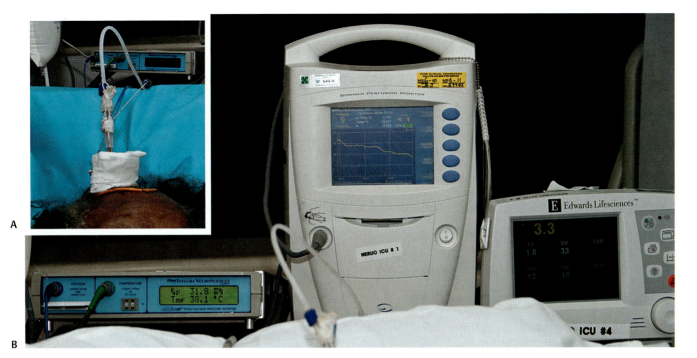

Fig. 6.1 **(A)** A patient with a subarachnoid hemorrhage and hydrocephalus, with an external ventricular catheter (EVD) and Licox and Bowman catheters inserted within the same bur hole. The tip of the EVD catheter allows monitoring of the intracranial pressures. The Licox and Bowman catheters are inserted within the brain parenchyma, specifically the white matter, near the region most susceptible to reduced blood flow from vasospasm. **(B)** In order from left to right, Licox, Bowman, and Vigileo monitors connected to the patient. The Licox catheter monitors the brain tissue oxygenation and the Bowman monitors the cerebral blood flow, on a minute-to-minute basis. The Vigileo is a cardiac output monitor used to assess the optimization of the cardiac output, to assist with vasospasm management.

intracerebral hemorrhage as it has been well studied. The frequency of clinically manifested seizures in stroke ranged from 5 to 17%, with the majority occurring from large arterial distribution and cardioembolic strokes.[8] With the use of cEEG, the actual frequency of seizures (electrographic seizures) increases to approximately 25% in some studies. Carrera et al[9] found an association of increased seizure frequency with worsening National Institutes of Health Stroke Scale (NIHSS) scores.

In addition to the detection of seizures in stroke, the pyramidal neurons of layers 3, 5, and 6 produce excitatory and inhibitory potentials that are detected by scalp electrodes and are sensitive to hypoxia. Therefore, EEG has the potential to be a sensitive, real-time detector of acute ischemia, which has been shown intraoperatively.[10] Some studies have specifically shown EEG abnormalities with changes in CBF. When CBF reaches 25 to 30 mL/100 g/min, the EEG signal changes in morphology, amplitude, and frequency, whereas when CBF decreases to less than 15 mL/100 g/min, the EEG signal becomes isoelectric.[11] Importing this real-time operating room technology to the ICU bedside has technical and logistic challenges but will likely become a standard of ICU care in the near future. More reliable means of postprocessing the EEG signal is necessary to make the analysis less time-consuming.

In primary intracerebral hemorrhage, seizure frequency is higher than in ischemic strokes, with frequencies in the high 20%. Vespa et al[8] studied seizure frequency in ischemic and hemorrhagic stroke, and noted that (1) hemorrhages with the highest seizure frequency occurred in the setting of arteriovenous malformations, and (2) seizures occurred more frequently with lobar hemorrhages but still occurred with subcortical hemorrhages. Monitoring seizures has a few intended and unintended attributes. Preventing seizures may decrease the metabolic demand incurred in partially injured neurons, allowing them to heal more effectively. From a psychological standpoint, the most common reason for death in intracerebral hemorrhage is the withdrawal of life-sustaining care. Removing the encephalopathy associated with frequent seizures makes it easier for physicians to make a clear assessment of the patient's progress before decisions of limitation of care are started.[8]

◆ Neuroprotection

The concept of neuroprotection has been studied in depth in stroke, TBI, and hemorrhages with little success. With the possible exception of nimodipine in subarachnoid hemorrhage, neuroprotectant medications are not routinely used in clinical practice. Despite this, the preclinical data for several compound classes is very promising. It is likely that some medication with neuroprotective effects will be used in the near future. Below is a brief analysis of some of the most promising classes.

Medications

Among the most promising new compounds are the spin trap compounds that derive from the parent compound α-phenyl-N-tert-butyl nitrone. They act as free radical scavengers and thereby inhibit mediators of oxidative stress. Disodium-([tert-butylimino] methyl) benzene-1,3-disulfonate N-oxide (NXY-059) was studied in two large human stroke trials, Stroke Acute Ischemic NXY-059 (SAINT) I and II. As a compound in this class, NXY-059 is unique due to its lack of polarity. This quality also confers a greater affinity for free radicals but limits its availability to the brain because poorly polar compounds do not pass through the blood–brain barrier well. This has the advantage of limiting cerebral side effects while controlling oxidative stress in the body outside the brain. The phase III stroke trial did not show improved outcome defined as disability at 90 days.[12,13] Interestingly, post hoc analysis showed a significant decreased frequency of hemorrhagic transformation (symptomatic and asymptomatic) in the patients receiving NXY-059, which may ultimately be the greatest utility of this drug.[14]

There are other spin traps that are being investigated in animal models with hopes of human trials. Stilbazunenlyl nitrone (STAZN) is an alternative spin trap molecule with increased hydrophobic properties. The rationale for this compound compared with NXY-059 is that higher concentrations are achieved in the brain, allowing for increased neuroprotective action in the brain parenchyma than in the arteries with a greater risk of neuronal side effects.[12,13]

N-methyl-D-aspartate (NMDA) antagonists have been studied for several years as neuroprotective medications. The NMDA receptor is a calcium channel found on neurons that is sensitive to glutamate (and indirectly glycine) and mediates slow calcium currents into the neuron that is important in several neuronal processes, most notably memory consolidation. The NMDA receptor has been implicated in excitotoxic secondary brain injury after acute injury. In the 1990s, several compounds were tried in clinical trials of stroke that failed to improve the outcome. Despite this, the mechanism of NMDA blockade makes sense as a therapeutic target. Currently, there are no NMDA antagonists being tried in multicenter trials in neurocritical care in the U.S.

Other Therapies

In addition to medications, there are several therapies that have been tested over the last decade that are thought to be neuroprotective. Two of these, transcranial infrared laser therapy and hypothermia, have been assessed in multicenter trials.

Transcranial Infrared Laser Therapy

In two animal models of acute stroke, rat and rabbit, it has been shown that applications of infrared laser therapy in wavelengths that are nonionizing improve neurologic function without a change in infarct volume. The proposed mechanism of infrared stimulation is activation of cytochrome oxidase C, an enzyme in the cellular respiratory chain of the mitochondria, to transfer a proton across the inner membrane, allowing phosphorylation of adenosine triphosphate (ATP), thereby generating more ATP. This leads to increased cellular metabolism. If the overall results lead to improved clinical outcome measures without decreased infarct volumes, the underlying proposed mechanism is improved neuronal recovery by increased cellular metabolism.[13]

A prospective trial, Neurothera Effectiveness and Safety Trial I (NEST-I), enrolled 120 acute ischemic stroke patients, with application of the treatment arm within 24 hours of stroke onset. The treatment application is unique in medicine and involves a fiber optic cable applied to the shaved scalp of the patient. The initial trial showed successful improvement in outcome measures at 90 days with no increase in mortality or adverse events among the treatment group. A second trial (NEST-2) included 660 patients randomized to infrared therapy applied within 24 hours of stroke onset, similar to NEST-1. The larger trial failed to show the benefit of the initial trial but continued to show no adverse events. Despite the failure of the study therapy, there was a trend for better outcome among the treated patients. More clinical trials are planned to investigate this therapy further.

Therapeutic Cooling

Hypothermia has gained increased attention in the neurologic and neurosurgical field due to its proposed neuroprotective properties. The neuroprotective mechanism of hypothermia consists of reducing excitatory mediators that lead to neurotoxic effects by inflammation and free radical production. In addition, hypothermia reduces cerebral metabolism of glucose and oxygen, leading to a decrease rate of ATP metabolism, decreasing the metabolic stress of injured tissues. Finally, glutamate release is thought to be inhibited yielding a decrease in excitatory mediators.[15] The optimal temperature for hypothermia in animal studies is between 24° and 33°C; however, at temperatures lower than 32°C in humans there are increased adverse effects including cardiac arrhythmias, coagulopathy, and infections. Methods for hypothermia consist of surface and endovascular cooling. The major impediments of effective cooling therapy are shivering and cutaneous vasoconstriction. Although counter-warming of skin and medications such as meperidine can overcome shivering, the excess sedation with meperidine makes close neurologic monitoring of patients difficult.[16]

Several trials have studied cooling in traumatic brain injury, ischemic stroke, and cardiac arrest. To date, cooling has not been shown in stroke and intracerebral hemorrhage to improve outcome. Several trials have investigated hypothermia for ischemic stroke. The Intravascular Cooling in the Treatment of Stroke (ICTuS) trial was a feasibility study including 20 awake patients with an NIHSS score >4, initiated 12 hours of stroke symptom onset.[17] The target temperature was 33°C for a duration of 12 to 24 hours. The ICTuS trial showed hypothermia could be performed via endovascular cooling, but with several side effects including deep venous thrombosis at a rate of 22% and bradycardia.

The Cooling for Acute Ischemic Brain Damage (COOL AID) trial attempted to show feasibility in endovascular cooling post–ischemic stroke. The study was not powered to show an efficacy difference. The authors concluded that there was no significant difference in complication rate between the hypothermic and normothermic groups, but there was clearly an increased incidence of both pulmonary edema and pneumonia in the cooled group.[18]

A German study by Schwab and colleagues[19] enrolled 23 patients with large MCA strokes and evidence of edema on CT scan of the head. Patients with elevated ICPs were cooled to a target temperature of 33°C for 48 to 72 hours. Despite the fact that many patients developed refractory edema upon rewarming, the mortality rate was 44% (less than reported in the literature).

In general, there is a potential role for hypothermia in the management of acute ischemic stroke; however, we currently do not have the ideal method for cooling patients due to potential side effects. It is expected that we will see more advances in this area in the near future.

◆ Restorative Treatment

When all attempts to save brain tissues have failed, restoring function may be a matter of replacing neurons. Animal studies have explored restorative treatments in acute stroke, including those that are cell and pharmacology based. The main idea with restorative treatment is to be able to stimulate growth of cells within the infracted tissue, and allow for maturation to improve functional outcome. Within the brain, there are two populations of neural stem cells: the subventricular zone and the dentate gyrus of the hippocampus. In addition, there are many populations of stem cells outside the brain that have been studied in animal models. Bone marrow mesenchymal cells, embryonic stem cells, fetal neural stem cells, and human umbilical cord blood all hold promise for future therapies to restore brain function after cell loss.[20] None of these therapies is in multicenter human trials for acute stroke or intracerebral hemorrhage.

Closer on the horizon than stem cell therapies may be medical therapies that exploit the brain's own restorative function to improve brain recovery. The two processes most targeted experimentally are neurogenesis and angiogenesis. There are many molecular pathways involved that have striking similarity.

Potential targets for therapies in this field are still under study. A few promising molecular pathways include the phosphatidylinositol 3-kinase Akt signaling pathway in the neuroprogenitor cells, vascular endothelial growth factor (VEGF) and its receptor (VEGF receptor 2), and angiopoietin-1.[20] Overall, the area of neurorestorative therapies in acute and subacute stroke is promising. We look forward to seeing advancements in this area to add to the modalities for stroke treatment.

◆ Inflammation in Vascular Brain Injury

There is a robust literature based on the inflammatory mediators and pathways involved in the response of the brain to trauma. Less work has been devoted to the study of stroke and intracerebral injury syndromes. Although it is tempting to lump all of these categories together, there are clear differences among injury mechanisms. Inflammation causing cerebral edema occurs immediately in the setting of traumatic brain injury and increases over the first 24 to 48 hours, whereas cerebral edema in ischemic stroke and intracerebral hemorrhage takes a noticeably different course, with the edema developing over the first 3 to 4 days.

Study of inflammatory mediators in ischemic stroke has led to a better understanding of cytokine signals that rev up the inflammation. Multiple proinflammatory cytokines including interleukin-1β (IL-1β), IL-6, and tumor necrosis factor-α (TNF-α) have been implicated in the development of cerebral edema. In addition, aquaporin-4 (although not classically associated with inflammation) seems to play a critical role in the passage of water across the blood–brain barrier in the development of edema.

In subarachnoid hemorrhage, the study of inflammation has revolved around the development of delayed cerebral vasospasm (deficits incurred by patients 3 days to a week after the initial hemorrhage presumably due to spasm of the arteries around the circle of Willis). Although the initial work in this area focused on the typical proinflammatory cell signals, work now is focused on interactions between the endothelium and the glial cells. In addition, there is new evidence that the innate immune system (the part of the immune system that is hard wired and does not adapt to bacteria and viruses) may be critically important in the process.[21]

Future therapies for the cerebral edema associated with stroke and primary intracerebral hemorrhage and the delayed effects of subarachnoid hemorrhage will depend largely on where the research takes us. The mechanisms of these interactions are not yet well enough understood to point to any one medication that may help.

◆ New Medications Coming into the Practice of Neurocritical Care

There are several medications that are new to the treatment of NICU patients and will undoubtedly have longstanding impact. We focus here on Food and Drug Administration (FDA)-approved medications. Three in particular are likely to have an impact on the care of neurovascular patients: conivaptan, lacosamide, and dexmedetomidine.

Conivaptan

Hyponatremia is encountered in the NICU setting. Hyponatremia is commonly seen in subarachnoid patients, traumatic brain injury, and intracerebral hemorrhage. In the setting of subarachnoid hemorrhage, the differential diagnosis of hyponatremia includes the syndrome of inappropriate antidiuretic hormone (SIADH) (euvolemic hyponatremia), water intoxication (hypervolemic hyponatremia), and cerebral salt wasting (hypovolemic hyponatremia). (Water intoxication is uncommon and is not discussed here, and a discussion of the differences between the remaining two is beyond the scope of this chapter.) This distinction is important due to the consequences of the treatments, which are diametrically opposed.

Conivaptan is the first drug to be FDA approved for hyponatremia in the setting of SIADH, though it is also thought to be safe in the setting of hypervolemic hyponatremia. It is unclear if it is safe in hypovolemic patients such as those with cerebral salt wasting. Conivaptan is a V1A and V2 vasopressin antagonist, allowing free water excretion (aquaresis) without electrolyte excretion. The approved dosing of conivaptan is a 20-mg bolus followed by infusion of 20 to 40 mg over 24 hours. Common adverse effects include overcorrection of hyponatremia, infusion-site reactions, phlebitis, and hypotension.

There are two trials of conivaptan in the neurocritical care patient population. The first study included 22 patients with euvolemic hyponatremia who were given conivaptan as an initial bolus followed by infusion 20 to 40 mg over 1 to 4 days.[22] The primary goal was to increase serum sodium >6 mEq/L from baseline sodium, and the secondary goal was to maintain a serum sodium greater than 135 mEq over a 24-hour period after the medication was discontinued. In their study 86% of the patients achieved the primary goal within an average time frame of 13 hours, whereas 50% of the patients required conivaptan in addition to other traditional therapies for hyponatremia (normal saline, 3% normal saline, salt tabs, or fludrocortisone). Of the 86% who attained a sodium level greater than 135 mEq, 47% reached the goal 24 hours after discontinuation of treatment, 32% where non-responders during treatment, and 21% had recurring hyponatremia posttreatment. There were no sodium overcorrections in the study group, although 31% of participants experienced infusion-site reactions and one patient experienced hypotension.

Murphy and colleagues[23] investigated the use of bolus doses of conivaptan without the infusion. The primary goal was to analyze the response of conivaptan over a 12-hour period postadministration. They observed that 40% of the patient population had an increase in serum sodium in 8 hours, 25% reached peak sodium 72 hours after the administration of one dose, and 69% patients sustained the correction after a single dose within 72 hours of drug administration. When comparing the change in serum sodium with the concurrent use of intravenous fluids, normal saline and conivaptan increased sodium by 5.3 ± 3.1 mEq/L, and 3% normal saline by 7.2 ± 3.4 mEq/L. When comparing the doses of conivaptan used, 20 mg increased sodium by 5.6 ± 3.4 mEq/L and 40 mg by 6.2 ± mEq/L. There were no incidences of phlebitis or significant hypotension.

Based on these two studies, it appears that conivaptan is safe to use in neurologic patients with euvolemic hyponatremia, without serious adverse effects. There is still no consensus about the treatment of hypovolemic patients, and

caution should be used in subarachnoid patients at risk of vasospasm.

Lacosamide

Lacosamide is a new antiepileptic drug that has been studied in phase II and III trials as an adjunctive agent to other antiepileptic drugs for partial-onset seizures with or without secondary generalization. It is a modified amino acid with the mechanism of enhancing slow inactivation of sodium channels without altering fast inactivation. In addition, it binds to collapsing-response mediator protein-2 (CRMP2), which is involved with neuroplasticity. Orally, lacosamide absorption is not affected by coadministration with food. It is excreted by the kidneys, 40% unchanged in the urine. Protein binding is less than 15%, and there are no pharmacokinetic interactions with carbamazepine, valproic acid, metformin, digoxin, oral contraceptives, or omeprazole. Its metabolite has no activity.[24]

Phase II and III trials studied its efficacy as an adjunctive antiepileptic drug at doses of 200, 400, and 600 mg per day. The 400 mg/day dose was the most efficacious, with a 50% responder rate and minimal adverse effects. It was well tolerated in the clinical trials, with typical adverse effects for an antiepileptic medication including dizziness, nausea, diplopia, abnormal coordination, ataxia, vomiting, and nystagmus.[24]

Intravenous administration is safe and well tolerated. The safety profile is comparable for IV and oral administration. There was no reported QTc prolongation, but a minimal PR prolongation.[24]

Dexmedetomidine

Sedation in the NICU is always a difficult proposition. On the one hand, the neurologic examination is the foundation of monitoring patients. In fact, many of the most important changes in our patients are manifest first in the neurologic exam. So administering any medication that inhibits the sensorium can significantly impair the physical exam. On the other hand, patients with neurologic disease often are confused and anxious. Interventions such as mechanical ventilation, invasive intracranial monitors, and vascular catheters are important, and if removed incorrectly, can be dangerous. The introduction of propofol to the NICU setting in the 1990s was an improvement because it allowed rapid lightening and evaluation of patients. The drawback to propofol is that during therapy patients cannot participate in an examination, and some patients wake up from propofol very agitated, putting themselves at additional risk for self-harm.

Dexmedetomidine is an analogue of clonidine, an antihypertensive used commonly. It is a central-acting α-adrenergic receptor blocker that can be administered intravenously. The advantage over propofol is that although the patient is sedated with this medication, he or she can still respond to commands and participate in the examination. The effect is akin to being in a sleep state from which one can be wakened while still on the medication. In addition, because it has no respiratory depression, it can be used in patients who are not mechanically ventilated. Although it has been extensively studied in the operating room and in the surgical and medical ICU, there is less evidence of safety and efficacy in the neurologically critically ill patient.[25] The major side effects include hypotension and bradycardia, which are typically experienced with the administration of boluses and during initiation of therapy. In the near future, it is likely that this drug, or another from its class, may play a large role in the treatment of NICU patients.

◆ Process Improvement in the Intensive Care Unit

Intensive care unit management is extremely complicated. It requires coordination of multiple practitioners with different training working in an individual but highly coordinated fashion. This is similar in complexity to launching a rocket or flying military missions, but with the additional responsibility of addressing the patient's and family's emotional issues. In this environment, it is very easy to forget aspects of the care plan or to be less diligent about the small details.

There was recently a hallmark study done in Michigan that showed that the small details make a difference.[26] The investigators showed that in multiple ICUs across the entire state, they were able to decrease mortality by adopting a checklist approach to make sure that they adhere to the small details **(Table 6.1)**. Considering that the administration of recombinant tissue-type plasminogen activator (rtPA) for acute stroke has not been shown to improve mortality, it suggests that the most profound and important aspect of neurocritical care is presence in the ICU of nurses, physicians, respiratory therapists, pharmacists, and technicians so that the details are not missed.

In the near future, there will be increased interest in and vigilance about getting the small things correct: preventing pneumonia and line infections, making sure patients are fed as soon as possible, getting them out of bed and starting physical therapy as soon possible, evaluating mechanically ventilated patients so that they can be extubated as soon as possible. The new NICU will be a busier place with systems and backup systems in place to make sure that even the smallest of jobs is done in a timely manner. The coalescence of these small matters will become the driver that will likely have the largest effect on patient mortality and morbidity. The challenge will be to have enough physicians, nurses, and other staff in the ICU to do this correctly. It is very clear that the days when physicians could do rounds in the ICU first thing in the morning and then go about their day in the clinic or operating room are coming to an end. *Presence* is a buzzword that is going to become commonplace in the ICU vernacular.

◆ Conclusion

The future for neurocritical care looks exciting. We have come from fighting for respect and equality with the other ICU

Table 6.1 Example of a Neuro–ICU Checklist

History and physical exam completed within 24 hours of admission?

Medication reconciliation done at admission?

Verbal orders signed?

Are restraints necessary? Is the order written?

Deep vein thrombosis prophylaxis administered?

Stress ulcer prophylaxis?

Head of bed elevated >30 degrees?

Skin check completed?

Nasal devices? Contraindicated?

Is central line or arterial line essential?

Wound checks/dressings checked and changed?

Can sedation be reduced?

Plan discussed with assigned nurse?

Is patient on ventilator support?

Plan discussed with assigned respiratory therapist?

Is enteral nutrition at target level?

Family updated within last 24 hours?

Plan of care discussed with on-call resident?

If patient is on insulin, is the blood glucose level 70 to 115 more than 50% of time?

Can patient activity level be increased?

Staphylococcus aureus screening completed? Are the test results positive?

Dysphagia screen completed before anything given PO?

specialties to a place where the care of NICU patients is seen as unique and important. Small strides have been made in the care of critically ill neurological patients. The next era will bring to fruition many of the monitoring techniques and therapies that have been in development.

References

1. Rose JC, Mayer SA. Optimizing blood pressure in neurological emergencies. Neurocrit Care 2004;1:287–299
2. Diringer MN, Axelrod Y. Hemodynamic manipulation in the neuro-intensive care unit: cerebral perfusion pressure therapy in head injury and hemodynamic augmentation for cerebral vasospasm. Curr Opin Crit Care 2007;13:156–162
3. Vajkoczy P, Roth H, Horn P, et al. Continuous monitoring of regional cerebral blood flow: experimental and clinical validation of a novel thermal diffusion microprobe. J Neurosurg 2000;93:265–274
4. Maloney-Wilensky E, Gracias V, Itkin A, et al. Brain tissue oxygen and outcome after severe traumatic brain injury: a systematic review. Crit Care Med 2009;37:2057–2063
5. Johnston AJ, Gupta AK. Advanced monitoring in the neurology intensive care unit: microdialysis. Curr Opin Crit Care 2002;8:121–127
6. Schneweis, S; Grond, M; Staub, F; Brinker, G; Neveling, M; Dohmen, C; Graf, R; Heis, WD; Shuaib, A. Predictive Value of Neurochemical Monitoring in Large Middle Cerebral Artery Infarction. Stroke. 2001; 32: 1863–1867.

7. Berger C, Annecke A, Aschoff A, Spranger M, Schwab S. Neurochemical monitoring of fatal middle cerebral artery infarction. Stroke. 1999;30: 460–463.

8. Vespa P. Continuous EEG monitoring for the detection of seizures in traumatic brain injury, infarction, and intracerebral hemorrhage: "to detect and protect". J Clin Neurophysiol 2005;22:99–106

9. Carrera E, Michel P, Despland PA, et al. Continuous assessment of electrical epileptic activity in acute stroke. Neurology 2006;67:99–104

10. Suzuki A, Nishimura H, Yoshioka K, et al. New display methods of combined topographic EEG and cerebral blood flow images in the evaluation of cerebral ischemia. Brain Topogr 1996;8:275–278

11. Jordan KG. Emergency EEG and continuous EEG monitoring in acute ischemic stroke. J Clin Neurophysiol 2004;21:341–352

12. Lapchak PA, Araujo DM. Advances in ischemic stroke treatment: neuroprotective and combination therapies. Expert Opin Emerg Drugs 2007; 12:97–112

13. Lampl, Y; Zivin, JA; Fisher, M; Lew, R; Welin, L; Dahlof, B; Borenstein, P; Anderson, B; Perez, J; Caparo, C; Ilic, S; Oron, U. Infrared Laser Therapy for Ishcemic Stroke: A New Treatment Strategy. Stroke. 2007; 38: 1843–1849.

14. Lees KR, Zivin JA, Ashwood T, et al; Stroke-Acute Ischemic NXY Treatment (SAINT I) Trial Investigators. NXY-059 for acute ischemic stroke. N Engl J Med 2006;354:588–600

15. Lyden PD, Krieger D, Yenari M, Dietrich WD. Therapeutic hypothermia for acute stroke. Int J Stroke 2006;1:9–19

16. Hemmen TM, Lyden PD. Hypothermia after acute ischemic stroke. J Neurotrauma 2009;26:387–391

17. Lyden PD, Allgren RL, Ng K, et al. Intravascular Cooling in the Treatment of Stroke (ICTuS): early clinical experience. J Stroke Cerebrovasc Dis 2005;14:107–114

18. De Georgia MA, Krieger DW, Abou-Chebl A, et al. Cooling for Acute Ischemic Brain Damage (COOL AID): a feasibility trial of endovascular cooling. Neurology 2004;63:312–317

19. Schwab S, Georgiadis D, Berrouschot J, Schellinger PD, Graffagnino C, Mayer SA. Feasibility and safety of moderate hypothermia after massive hemispheric infarction. Stroke 2001;32:2033–2035

20. Zhang ZG, Chopp M. Neurorestorative therapies for stroke: underlying mechanisms and translation to the clinic. Lancet Neurol 2009;8: 491–500

21. Provencio JJ, Vora N. Subarachnoid hemorrhage and inflammation: bench to bedside and back. Semin Neurol 2005;25:435–444

22. Wright WL, Asbury WH, Gilmore JL, Samuels OB. Conivaptan for hyponatremia in the neurocritical care unit. Neurocrit Care 2009;11:6–13

23. Murphy T, Dhar R, Diringer M. Conivaptan bolus dosing for the correction of hyponatremia in the neurointensive care unit. Neurocrit Care 2009;11:14–19

24. Halford JJ, Lapointe M. Clinical perspectives on lacosamide. Epilepsy Curr 2009;9:1–9

25. Venn RM, Karol MD, Grounds RM. Pharmacokinetics of dexmedetomidine infusions for sedation of postoperative patients requiring intensive caret. Br J Anaesth 2002;88:669–675

26. Pronovost PJ, Berenholtz SM, Goeschel C, et al. Improving patient safety in intensive care units in Michigan. J Crit Care 2008;23:207–221

II

Imaging Considerations

7

Computed Tomography in Hemorrhagic and Ischemic Stroke

Julie H. Harreld, Peter G. Kranz, and James D. Eastwood

Pearls

- Because hyperacute or subacute hemorrhage can be of similar attenuation to that of brain, recognition can be difficult. Clues to the presence of isodense hemorrhage include subtle mass effect; displacement of sulci from the calvaria (in the case of subdural or epidural hemorrhage); obscuration of the basal cisterns or sulci (in subarachnoid hemorrhage); or subtle alterations in ventricular contour (intraventricular hemorrhage or periventricular parenchymal hemorrhage).
- Acute hemorrhage in anemic patients (hematocrit <30%) may be of lower density, and possibly isodense in the acute phase, making it more difficult to recognize.
- The presence of a hematocrit "layering" effect, with graded increase in density from antidependent to dependent, is suggestive of coagulopathy or anticoagulation, though it is not specific.[1]
- The appearance of hyperdensity within a previously isodense or low-density hemorrhage is evidence of acute-on-chronic (i.e., repeat) hemorrhage.
- Subacute hemorrhage may enhance peripherally, mimicking neoplasm.

Potential Pitfall

- A congenitally hypoplastic or absent transverse venous sinus can mimic thrombosis. The caliber of the ipsilateral jugular vein can provide a clue: if it is small, the sinus is likely hypoplastic or aplastic; if normal in caliber, thrombosis is likely. Partial recanalization of a thrombosed vein or sinus can occur in subacute or chronic thrombosis, resulting in irregularity and decreased caliber.

◆ Role of Computed Tomography Imaging in Stroke

Computed tomography (CT) imaging has been, for nearly 35 years, the most often used imaging modality for the initial assessment of stroke patients. Modern CT scanning equipment and techniques permit a detailed study of the brain tissue and blood vessels and can even provide physiologic information about perfusion and vascular permeability. Each of these techniques can provide information helpful for the care of patients with ischemic and hemorrhagic stroke.

Noncontrast CT (NCT) remains the first-line imaging modality of choice at most institutions for evaluation of patients with acute stroke. The reasons for this include the wide availability, sensitivity to hemorrhage, and lower cost of CT compared with magnetic resonance imaging (MRI). Although MRI provides valuable information, it is often performed as a second imaging test after CT. The first diagnostic assessment is whether or not intracranial hemorrhage is present, as intracranial hemorrhage changes both the diagnosis and the management. This assessment is typically determined from the nonenhanced CT scan. If hemorrhage is present, a CT angiogram is often helpful to determine if the cause of hemorrhage is a vascular lesion (e.g., arteriovenous malformation [AVM], aneurysm). Finally, brain hemodynamic measurements with CT (or CT perfusion [CTP]) can provide increased physiologic information in patients with stroke. Such measurements include blood flow, blood volume, transit time, and even blood–brain barrier permeability.

◆ Acquisition and Display Techniques

Nonenhanced Computed Tomography

A typical adult noncontrast head CT protocol consists of 5-mm axial images every 5 mm from skull to vertex, parallel to the orbitomeatal line at 120 kVp and 120 mA for a 2-second scan. A typical display field of view (DFOV) of 25 cm with a matrix size of 512 × 512 results in a pixel size of 0.5 mm (FOV/matrix size).

Computed Tomography Angiography

In CT angiography (CTA) of the head, thin axial images acquired in the arterial phase of the infused contrast bolus are reconstructed in two-dimensional (2D) and three-dimensional (3D) fashion for diagnosis of arterial stenosis or occlusion in the setting of stroke. Optimal arterial enhancement is essential, but variable due to both technical and patient-related hemodynamic factors such as decreased cardiac output or severe arterial stenosis. In a patient with normal cardiac output, optimal arterial enhancement can be achieved with an iodine injection rate of 2.2 g/s, which translates to 6 mL/s for 370 mg/mL contrast, or a total volume of 120 mL during a 20-second scan.[3] Because of this short acquisition time and wide variability in hemodynamics between patients, a bolus-triggering technique for timing the scan following contrast administration is preferable to a fixed delay, which in some patients can result in missing the arterial phase of the bolus altogether.[3] For the bolus triggering technique, the scan is scheduled to begin a certain number of seconds after the attenuation in the chosen reference vessel (i.e., the aorta) reaches a certain value. Typical acquisition parameters are slice thickness of 0.625 mm acquired at a 0.625-mm interval with a helical CT pitch ratio of 0.56 to 1, 5.625 mm table speed, 120 kVp and auto mA (80–220) with 0.7-second scans. Images should be transferred to a 3D workstation and multiplanar 2D and 3D reconstructions evaluated.

A CTA of the neck may be appropriate in the setting of suspected arterial dissection, carotid or vertebral occlusive disease of the neck, or trauma. Scanning parameters and reconstruction/viewing guidelines are similar to the above.

Computed Tomography Venography

Computed tomography venography (CTV) involves the acquisition of thin axial images of the head in venous phase, which may then be transferred to a workstation for 3D and multiplanar reconstruction. A typical protocol would be acquisition of 0.625-mm images from vertex to skull base with a 0.625-mm interval, pitch of 0.56 to 1, table speed of 5.625 per revolution, 0.7 second scans with 120 kVp, and auto mA with noise index 8.0 (minimum 80, maximum 220) with an FOV of 22. As with CTA, scan timing may be with a simple delay (typically 30 to 40 seconds) following power injection of approximately 100 mL of 350 to 370 mg/mL iodinated contrast at 3 to 4 mL/s. Alternatively, the scan may be performed with a bolus-triggering technique to allow for variability in patient hemodynamics. Images should be processed and viewed as 3D and multiplanar 2D reconstructions. Although rendering of maximum intensity projection (MIP) images of the venous sinuses in isolation may be performed, this requires subtraction of osseous structures from the images (usually manually) and can be very time consuming without adding diagnostic information. For this reason, we usually favor multiplanar assessment of the venous system.

Computed Tomography Perfusion

Computed tomography perfusion is used in stroke imaging to try to define the ischemic penumbra, to follow perfusion after therapy for embolic stroke, and to predict ischemia due to vasospasm following subarachnoid hemorrhage. Dynamic first-pass CTP estimates capillary-level tissue perfusion via serial imaging of a slab of brain following the administration of intravenous contrast, taking advantage of the relationship between contrast concentration and attenuation (in Hounsfield units [HU]) to measure regional cerebral blood flow (rCBF), regional cerebral blood volume (rCBV), and mean transit time (MTT). CTP is performed at 80 kVp to reduce the dose and to exploit the k-edge of iodinated contrast.[4] Following administration of 35 to 50 mL of contrast (350–370 mg/mL) at 4 to 6 mL/s followed by a 20- to 40-mL saline "chaser," a 20- to 40-mm slab of supraorbital brain (proximal middle cerebral artery [MCA]/anterior cerebral artery [ACA] territory) is scanned in two phases: (1) one image per second for approximately 45 seconds, and then (2) one image every 2 to 3 seconds for approximately 45 seconds, for a total imaging time of 90 seconds (100 mAs, FOV = 24 cm).[5] Permeability measurements can also be performed but require a third phase in which an image is acquired every 10 to 15 seconds for 2 minutes.[4] An additional slab may also be chosen; CTP can be performed before or after CTA. Perfusion parameters are calculated by dedicated software according to user-defined regions of interest (ROIs).

◆ Ischemic Stroke

Acute Stroke: Nonenhanced Computed Tomography

The expected findings on noncontrast CT will depend on the duration of time from onset of the ictus to the time of imaging, as well as the severity and location of ischemia. Within the first 6 hours, CT of the brain may appear normal.[6] The use of newer generation CT scanners and stroke-specific window/level review settings has increased the sensitivity for early ischemic changes in the <6-hour time period.[7] After 6 to 12 hours, most patients with ongoing cortical ischemia develop fairly clear-cut findings on CT. Presently, the primary role of CT imaging is to exclude hemorrhage, and a secondary role is to confirm the diagnosis of ischemic stroke. In general, the imaging findings related to acute ischemia can be classified as (1) intravascular thrombus and (2) brain edema. Intravascular thrombus is hyperattenuating on CT, whereas the CT findings associated with edema (in order of most subtle to most obvious) are sulcal effacement, loss of the normal gray matter–white matter attenuation difference, and parenchymal hypodensity.

Hyperdense Vessels

The presence of acute thrombus within a segment of the intracranial vasculature may result in increased density of that vessel on CT compared with other cerebral vessels of similar caliber. This sign is most commonly encountered in the M1 segment of the MCA ("hyperdense MCA" sign; **Fig. 7.1A**), but can be observed in any vessel, including the internal carotid arteries, anterior cerebral arteries, posterior cerebral arteries, and basilar artery. Typically, normal vessels measure 30 to 40 HU, whereas arteries containing acute thrombus may measure higher, on the order of approximately 80 HU. The reported specificity of the sign is high, but the sensitivity is low, and the absence of the finding should not be used to exclude intravascular thrombus.[8] When present, recognizing the presence of the hyperdense artery is important, as it portends a worse clinical outcome. Confirmation of vessel occlusion and evaluation of the extent of the thrombus can be obtained with CT angiography (**Fig. 7.1B**) or MR angiography in equivocal cases, especially if catheter directed intra-arterial therapy is considered. The hyperdense appearance of the artery may resolve following spontaneous vessel recanalization or treatment with thrombolytics.

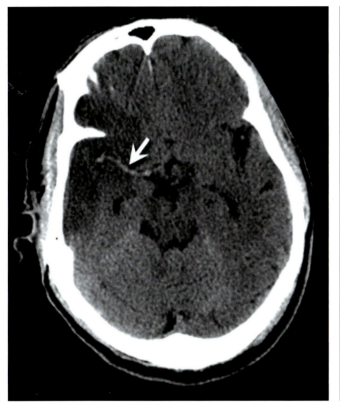

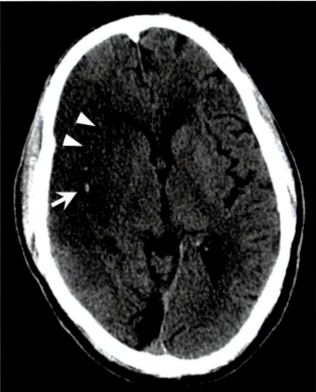

A

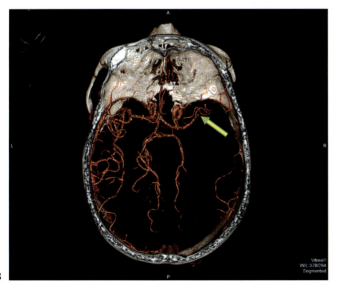

B

Fig. 7.1 **(A)** Axial computed tomography (CT) images in a patient with acute right middle cerebral artery (MCA) infarct demonstrate hyperdense appearance of the right MCA and its insular branches *(white arrows)*, loss of the insular ribbon *(white arrowheads)*, parenchymal hypodensity, effacement of sulci, and mild mass effect. **(B)** Computed tomography angiography (CTA) performed in the same patient demonstrates abrupt cutoff of the right MCA *(yellow arrow)* due to intravascular thrombus. By convention, three-dimensional (3D) reconstructed CTA images are viewed as if from the top of the patient.

Ischemic Brain Edema

Loss of normal gray-white attenuation difference is an important early ischemic change on CT. In nonischemic brain, the gray matter of the cortex and basal ganglia is normally of greater attenuation than the white matter, causing it to appear brighter on CT images. Because gray matter is preferentially subject to edema in early ischemia, ischemic gray matter often shows a decrease in density (and thus decreased brightness). As a result, the visual contrast between the gray and white matter becomes less pronounced, resulting in obscuration of the normal gray-white differentiation. There are two well-described signs that reflect loss of gray-white contrast in the MCA territory. First, when thrombus in the M1 segment of the MCA occludes blood flow in the lateral lenticulostriate branches, developing edema leads to obscuration of the lentiform nucleus, called the "loss of basal ganglia" sign **(Fig. 7.2)**. Second, if blood flow to the insular branches of the MCA is reduced, there is obscuration of the normal gray-white attenuation difference of the insular cortex, leading to the so-called "loss of insular ribbon" sign. Although these are commonly described signs specific to MCA ischemia, the general principle that the loss of gray-white attenuation difference can be a sign of early ischemia is applicable to all vascular territories.

As the water content of the ischemic brain increases, hypodensity also develops in the affected parenchyma on CT. The degree of hypodensity at a given time is influenced by both the duration and degree of ischemia, which on the anatomic level are determined by both the location and extent of proximal vascular occlusion and the degree of collateral blood flow. Early hypoattenuation (within the first 6 hours of stroke) has been shown to correlate with irreversible ischemia, greater severity of symptoms, and worse clinical outcome.[9,10]

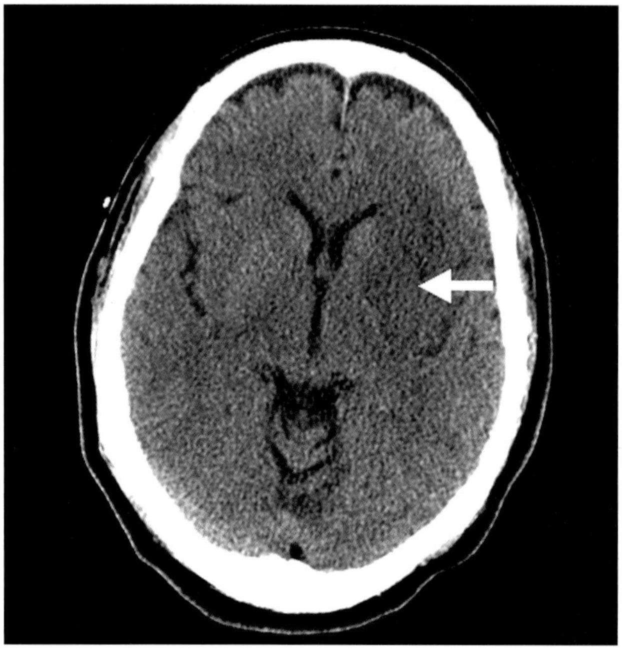

The presence of hypodensity alone is not sufficient to make the diagnosis of ischemia. A wide variety of other pathologic processes that affect the brain, such as neoplasms, infections, metabolic disorders, and trauma, can result in hypodensity. To distinguish stroke from these other etiologies, the hypodensity should conform to a known vascular territory. Knowledge of the geographic areas of the brain supplied by the major branches of the anterior and posterior circulation is therefore useful in making a successful interpretation. If CT hypodensity crosses major vascular territories, an etiology other than stroke should be considered first. Moreover, in stroke, the hypodensity frequently involves both gray and white matter; hypodensity that spares the cortex suggests vasogenic edema, such as due to tumor or infection, or venous ischemia.

Extent of Acute Computed Tomography Abnormality

Whether or not the size of the observed hypodensity can be used to influence therapeutic decision making remains controversial. Post hoc evaluation of the data from the European Cooperative Acute Stroke Study (ECASS-I) demonstrated a higher risk of fatal hemorrhage in patients with hypodensity in greater than one third of the expected MCA territory who were treated with recombinant tissue-type plasminogen activator (rtPA).[10] This and other similar observations led to reservations about treating patients with intravenous thrombolytic therapy when large areas of hypodensity were present on initial CT. This finding was not replicated, however, in the data analysis from the National Institute of Neurological Disorders and Stroke (NINDS) rtPA trial, in which patients with hypodensity in greater than one third of the territory of the MCA who were treated with rtPA demonstrated clinical benefit, without significantly higher rates of symptomatic hemorrhage.[11] The American Heart Association/American Stroke Association consensus guidelines from 2007 conclude that "data are insufficient to state that, with the exception of hemorrhage, any specific CT finding (including evidence of ischemia affecting more than one third of a cerebral hemisphere) should preclude treatment with rtPA within 3 hours of onset of stroke (class IIb, level of evidence A)."[12] Nevertheless, this remains a controversial topic and the subject of ongoing investigation.

The Alberta Stroke Program Early CT Score (ASPECTS) was developed in 2000 as a standardized method for quantifying early ischemic changes on CT.[13] This system, which divides the MCA territory into 10 subregions, each of which is assigned one point if normal and zero points if abnormal on CT, was created in response to the observation that even among those experienced in stroke diagnosis and care, there was poor reproducibility in identifying and classifying the extent of early ischemic change.[14] The authors reported that the ASPECTS score demonstrated good reproducibility, correlated

Fig. 7.2 "Loss of the basal ganglia" sign. Decreased conspicuity of the left lentiform nucleus *(arrow)* compared with the right due to early left MCA infarct.

inversely with National Institutes of Health Stroke Scale (NIHSS), and predicted functional outcome and risk of hemorrhage. Subsequent evaluations of ASPECTS have demonstrated mixed results in its ability to predict outcomes and help plan therapy.[15-17]

Potential Pitfalls: Acute Ischemic Stroke

Early Mass Effect

A potential pitfall in evaluating early mass effect may be seen in the setting of diffuse cerebral volume loss. Cerebral volume loss can be the result of normal aging, a variety of medical therapies (including steroids and chemotherapeutic agents), atherosclerotic disease, or toxins (including alcohol and illicit drugs). In these patients, the sulci are abnormally wide at baseline due to the volume loss. In the situation of ischemia, there may be a pseudonormalization of the sulcal width within the region of ischemia, thereby making the changes less apparent than in a patient without baseline global volume loss, and leading to a false-negative interpretation. For this reason, an assessment of overall brain volume and comparison of sulci with the contralateral hemisphere to evaluate for asymmetry can be performed.

Hyperdense Vessel

Not all hyperattenuating arteries contain thrombus. Increased hematocrit may result in diffuse increased density of the intracerebral vessels. Atherosclerotic disease with diffuse calcification in the vessel wall, and beam hardening artifact, particularly affecting the basilar artery, can all result in apparent high attenuation within the vessel. Knowledge of the presenting clinical symptoms, pretest probability for acute stroke, and evaluation of the contralateral vasculature for density and atherosclerotic disease can be helpful in avoiding false-positive results.

Tissue Hypodensity

A pitfall to the use of the "obscuration of basal ganglia" sign is that patients are frequently asymmetrically positioned such that the appearance of the right-sided basal nuclei on a given slice may be different from that of the left-sided basal nuclei. In practice, we have found this a difficult sign to use, especially when other signs are not present. Interpretation of such a finding should be carefully correlated with the side of symptoms.

Sometimes more than one major vascular territory can be involved in stroke at the same time. For example, MCA stroke can be accompanied by ACA stroke or even posterior cerebral artery (PCA) stroke. Also, lacunar infarcts, infarcts due to occlusion of small penetrating arteries that are usually <1.5 mm in size, often produce focal hypodensities in the deep gray matter or the white matter, and typically do not involve the cortex.

Watershed infarcts, caused by focal or global decreased perfusion pressure (e.g., hemodynamic stroke; stroke due to hypotension) often cause decreased blood flow to the boundary zones between major vascular distributions, and involve regions of brain between, rather than within, the major arterial territories. Furthermore, watershed strokes may involve a disproportionally larger amount of white matter than gray matter and, in fact, can affect solely white matter in some cases. Finally, in ischemia due to venous occlusion, cortical gray matter may or may not be involved, and the pattern of hypodensity depends on the patterns of venous drainage, and therefore is not confined to normal arterial distributions.

Venous ischemia should be suspected particularly in patients with risk factors for venous thrombosis (hypercoagulable states, dehydration, oral contraceptive use, peripartum patients), with bilateral or midline distributions of hypodensity, with primarily subcortical hypodensity, and when hypodensity crosses normal arterial boundaries. Hemorrhage is commonly associated with venous infarcts, very commonly at the gray matter–white matter junction.

Subacute and Chronic Stroke

Beyond the acute phase, the appearance of ischemic stroke on noncontrast CT continues to evolve. Wedge-shaped, cortically based hypodensity becomes more pronounced over the first week, with progressively sharper definition of the affected area. Mass effect increases initially, usually peaking around 3 to 5 days, then progressively decreases. At approximately 2 to 3 weeks, the infarcts may become isodense to the adjacent brain, the so-called fogging effect. This is hypothesized to be due to the influx of macrophages and the proliferation of astrocytes, endothelial cells, and new blood vessels.[18] During this period, the infarct may be inapparent, and could be overlooked if prior imaging is not available for comparison. Contrast enhancement can be seen in the subacute phase as the result of breakdown of the blood–brain barrier, which usually peaks at 2 to 3 weeks, although uncommonly can be seen earlier.[19] Patterns of enhancement may be patchy, cortical, ring enhancement, or homogeneous.[20]

After approximately 1 month, the affected brain once again becomes hypodense as the parenchyma is replaced by gliotic tissue. In the chronic stage, encephalomalacia results in volume loss of the affected brain, with corresponding atrophy of gyri, widening of sulci, and *ex vacuo* dilation of the adjacent ventricular system. Injury to neurons may result in degeneration of the axon distal to the site of injury, known as wallerian degeneration. This can result in volume loss and hypodensity along white matter tracts remote from the original ischemic insult. A frequently observed manifestation of this phenomenon is atrophy of the cerebral peduncle ipsilateral to a chronic MCA infarct, due to injury of the corticospinal tracts.

Use of Computed Tomography Angiography in Stroke Imaging

Computed tomography angiography, as an adjunct to nonenhanced CT, has become a very helpful clinical tool for assessment of patients with acute ischemic stroke. CTA can help to locate or exclude arterial stenoses and occlusions, and often can provide the specific cause of stroke (e.g., arterial dissection or carotid atherosclerosis). In the special case of ischemia due to post–subarachnoid hemorrhage (SAH) vasospasm, the extent and severity of vasospasm can be documented. Occasionally, CTA can help to make an unusual diagnosis such as cerebral vasculitis.

Computed Tomography Perfusion in Ischemic Stroke

Ischemic stroke is likely the most important potential clinical application for cerebral blood flow (CBF) imaging. CTP is a highly sensitive method for detecting hemodynamic alteration. Thus, detection of perfusion abnormality, especially if it corresponds well to an expected arterial territory, can be helpful for confirming ischemia in a patient with acute symptoms.

Computed tomography perfusion imaging also provides access to knowledge of the pathophysiologic pattern of a lesion. For example, nearly all ischemic lesions are characterized by prolonged MTT but often have variable measurements of CBF and cerebral blood volume (CBV). It has been proposed that different patterns may be present for viable and nonviable ischemic tissue. For example, it has been proposed that viable tissue may be characterized by increased MTT, decreased CBF, and normal-to-increased CBV, whereas nonviable tissue may be characterized by increased MTT, decreased CBF, and decreased CBV.[21] Characterizing tissue by prognosis and developing treatment protocols related to tissue prognosis is an area of very active research.[22,23] At the present time, the available evidence does not support treatment based on CT perfusion imaging.

Evaluation of the axial CTA source images has also been proposed to be helpful as a marker for hypoperfusion. Although partly dependent on technique and individual hemodynamics, underperfused regions of brain can have decreased uptake of iodinated contrast material and so the apparent attenuation difference between hypoperfused regions and adjacent normal regions can be accentuated, making them easier to recognize.[24] It is not clear at the time of this writing that the evidence supports the general use of CTA source images to make treatment decisions.

◆ Hemorrhagic Stroke

Intracerebral hemorrhage (ICH) accounts for between 10% and 30% of all strokes and has a mortality rate greater than that of ischemic stroke, up to 50% in the first month; half of these deaths occur within the first 48 hours.[25] Hemorrhagic stroke is most often primary (80%) and seen in the setting of hypertension. Secondary causes (20%) include vascular anomalies, neoplasm, coagulopathy, infection, drugs, venous thrombosis, cerebral hypoperfusion syndrome, amyloid, and trauma.

Nonenhanced Computed Tomography

In the hyperacute stage (within minutes) blood measures 30 to 60 HU on CT, similar to the cerebral cortex (**Table 7.1**). In

Table 7.1 Attenuation Values in Hounsfield Units (HU) for Blood and Cranial Structures on CT

Tissue	HU
Air	−1000
Fat	−50 to −100
Water	0
Cerebrospinal fluid	15
White matter	20 to 30
Gray matter	40 to 45
Subacute blood	30 to 50
Acute blood	40 to 90
Muscle	40
Calcification	120 to 200
Bone	1000

the acute stage (minutes to hours, up to 3 days), clot formation results in increasing density, with attenuation ranging from 60 to 80 HU. Subsequent retraction of clot and resorption of serum increases the attenuation of the hematoma to 80 to 100 HU. In the subacute phase (approximately 3 days to 2 weeks), clot breakdown, beginning at the periphery, results in attenuation decrease to 30 to 50 HU (similar to gray matter and white matter; see **Table 7.1**).[1] Peripheral contrast enhancement is common in the subacute phase, and should not be confused with abscess or tumor. Over time, continued decrease in hematoma volume and attenuation eventually result in a small residual low density within the brain parenchyma.

Once hemorrhage is identified on noncontrast head CT, the hemorrhage should next be localized to compartment and anatomic location, as the location provides insight into the cause and therefore the next step in determining the diagnosis and management (**Table 7.2**). Hematoma volume should next be assessed, as it has been found to be a strong predictor of 30-day mortality, regardless of location; hematoma volume greater than 30 mL^3 at baseline is associated with poor outcome, and patients with hematoma volume >60 mL^3 with a Glasgow Coma Scale (GCS) score of 8 or less had a 91% mortality in a study by Broderick et al.[26] Hematoma growth and intraventricular hemorrhage are associated with poor outcome.[27] Posterior fossa hematoma can be a surgical emergency, as space limitations may result in rapid basal cistern effacement, herniation, impingement of the brainstem, and associated potentially life-threatening neurologic deficits; early involvement of the neurosurgery service can help to limit morbidity. Midline shift, hydrocephalus, and degree of associated edema should also be evaluated. Though hemorrhage into a neoplasm often cannot be confirmed until resolution of the hematoma, such lesions may demonstrate associated vasogenic edema to a greater degree than expected with simple ICH (**Fig. 7.3**). Contrast-enhanced imaging at the time of hemorrhage can sometimes show evidence of a mass. In studies initially negative for tumor, repeat scanning (in 6

Table 7.2 Causes of Hemorrhage by Location

Location	Underlying Cause	Comment
Basal ganglia	Hypertension	Most common, particularly in older patients with elevated blood pressure
	Vascular lesion (AVM, aneurysm, cavernoma)	In up to 30% of all basal ganglia hemorrhage, and in approximately 13% of hypertensive patients[28]
Posterior fossa/cerebellum	Hypertension	
	Vascular lesion (AVM, aneurysm, cavernoma)	Approximately 20%
	Tumor	
	Amyloid	Rare
Brainstem	Hypertension	Highest mortality for hemorrhage in this location[1]
	Cavernoma	
	AVM	
	Neoplasm	
Lobar (cortical or subcortical)	Amyloid	Particularly in the parietal lobes; look for microbleeds on MR
		Rare in patients <55 years of age
	Aneurysm	Hemorrhage may dissect into adjacent brain, such as medial frontal lobes in anterior Cerebral/anterior communicating artery aneurysm, or temporal lobe in MCA aneurysm
Subarachnoid	Aneurysm	
	Extension of parenchymal Hemorrhage	
Intraventricular	Aneurysm	Particularly ACA
	Choroidal vascular Malformation	
	Extension of parenchymal Hemorrhage	
	Moyamoya	
	Hypertension	
	Neoplasm	
Subdural	Trauma	
	Coagulopathy	
Epidural	Trauma	
Nonarterial distribution, bilateral	Hemorrhagic venous Infarction	

to 8 weeks) with contrast following resolution of hematoma may confirm underlying enhancing tumor, with the caveat that peripheral enhancement of prior parenchymal hemorrhage may also occur.

Computed tomography angiography or catheter angiography should be performed in the setting of spontaneous ICH if an underlying vascular lesion is suspected, such as in patients younger than 45, in patients without preexisting hypertension, and in lobar hemorrhage. In a study by Zhu et al,[27] 34% of 206 patients with isolated spontaneous parenchymal hemorrhage had a vascular lesion as demonstrated by angiography. Angiography was positive in 45% of normotensive patients and in 9% of patients with preexisting hypertension; angiography was more likely to be positive in patients under 45 years of age. In patients with a history of hypertension presenting with thalamic, putaminal, or posterior fossa hemorrhage, an underlying vascular lesion on angiography was extremely unlikely (0%); however, 48% of hypertensive patients 45 or younger had angiographically evident lesions underlying bleeds in the same locations. Of patients with isolated intraventricular hemorrhage, 67% of those 45 and over and 63% of those under 45 had findings at angiography.

Halpin et al[28] found similar results, with 12.8% of hypertensive patients having an underlying AVM or aneurysm. Hino et al[29] found that in patients with initially negative angiography in the acute phase of subcortical hemorrhage, those who underwent subsequent repeat angiography had positive findings 18% of the time. Thus, if initial angiography is negative, a repeat angiogram or CTA should be strongly

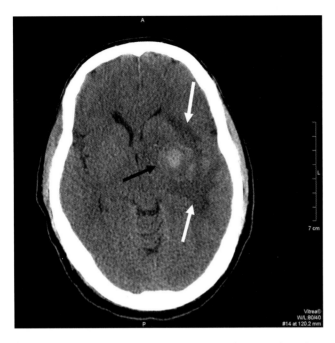

Fig. 7.3 Glioblastoma multiforme centered in the left basal ganglia *(black arrow)* mimics hypertensive hemorrhage, but the significant associated vasogenic edema is suggestive of underlying neoplasm *(white arrows).*

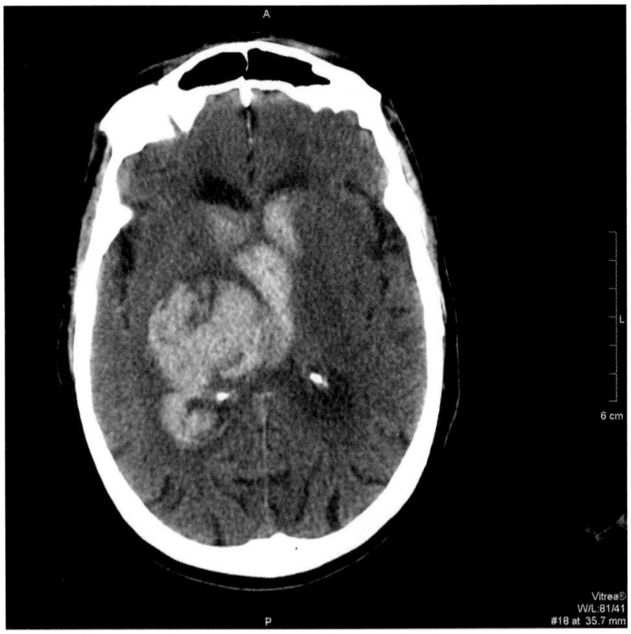

Fig. 7.4 Hypertensive hemorrhage. A large right basal ganglia hemorrhage in a patient with a history of hypertension, accompanied by hydrocephalus, intraventricular hemorrhage, and midline shift, all poor prognostic indicators.

considered, particularly if the location of the hemorrhage and the clinical picture are suspicious. CTA may reveal extravasation of contrast into the hematoma as evidenced by focal high density, which correlates with active bleeding and poor prognosis.[1]

The role of CT perfusion in hemorrhagic stroke continues to be investigated. Though it has been proposed that aggressive blood pressure reduction measures targeted toward decreasing expansion of hematoma may result in perihemorrhage or global decreases in CBF leading to ischemia,[30] there is conflicting evidence.[31] Recent work suggests that altered permeability of the blood–brain barrier as measured by CT perfusion may predict hemorrhagic transformation of ischemic infarct.[32]

Primary Intracerebral Hemorrhage

Primary, hypertensive hemorrhage is responsible for approximately 80% of hemorrhagic strokes **(Fig. 7.4)**. Long-standing hypertension results in lipohyalinosis and Charcot-Bouchard microaneurysms involving small penetrating arteries/arterioles, predominantly lenticulostriates and thalamic, brainstem, and cerebellar perforators. As a result, the most common areas for primary hemorrhagic infarction are the basal ganglia (40–50%), cerebrum (20–50%), thalamus (10–15%), cerebellum (15%), and brainstem (<10%).[31] Suspicion for an underlying vascular lesion should be increased and prompt CTA or other angiographic interrogation for aneurysm or AVM in normotensive or young patients, or in patients with lobar hemorrhage. However, a significant number of hypertensive

and older patients may have underlying vascular abnormalities such as AVM or aneurysm, and one should not assume that the presence of hypertension excludes the presence of such a lesion. Indeed, hypertension can be a secondary condition due to intracranial hemorrhage and associated increased intracranial pressure itself, with resultant Cushing response. Drug-induced hypertension due to sympathomimetics (amphetamine, pseudoephedrine, phenylpropanolamine) or cocaine can present with similar hemorrhage, with the same caveat regarding underlying vascular lesions.

Secondary Intracerebral Hemorrhage

Even in hypertensive patients, up to 34% of hemorrhagic stroke may be associated with an underlying cause or lesion, such as aneurysm, AVM, cavernoma, coagulopathy, venous thrombosis, vasculitis, and vasculopathy.[27,28] Ischemic stroke may undergo hemorrhagic transformation. Certain primary and secondary brain neoplasms have a propensity for hemorrhage as well.

Although primary ICH occurs more commonly in the deep gray matter or posterior fossa, lobar hemorrhage is more frequently secondary[1] **(Table 7.2)**. When both deep and lobar/subcortical hemorrhage are present, the origin is more likely to be deep.[1] Whenever patient history, age, or location of hemorrhage is suspicious for an etiology other than simple hypertensive hemorrhage, further investigation is warranted. Even in cases of traumatic intracranial hemorrhage such as in motor vehicle collision, if the hemorrhage is not in a typical or expected location for traumatic injury the patient's

Table 7.3 Localization of Aneurysm by Distribution of Hemorrhage

Aneurysm	Hemorrhage
MCA	Sylvian fissure, temporal lobe
ACoA	Interhemispheric fissure, lateral ventricle
PICA	4th ventricle
Pericallosal artery	Anterior falx

Abbreviations: MCA, middle cerebral artery; ACoA, anterior communicating artery; PICA, posterior inferior communicating artery.

history should be carefully culled for clues that hemorrhage secondary to underlying lesion may have been the initial incident, rather than the reverse.

Aneurysmal Hemorrhage

Although aneurysmal hemorrhage is usually into the subarachnoid space, there may be intraparenchymal hemorrhage in approximately 15% of cases.[33] The location of parenchymal hemorrhage or the preponderance of subarachnoid hemorrhage on a noncontrast head CT can often suggest the location of the aneurysm **(Table 7.3).** CTA is a rapid, noninvasive, and effective tool to screen for aneurysm in the acute setting. The vast majority of cerebral aneurysms occur at branch points of the circle of Willis; in descending frequency, ACA/anterior communicating artery (ACoA), MCA/posterior communicating artery (PCoA), MCA bifurcation, basilar tip,

and posterior inferior cerebellar artery (PICA). Though the majority of aneurysms are located in the anterior circulation **(Fig. 7.5),** posterior circulation aneurysms are believed more likely to rupture and to be associated with increased morbidity and mortality. Aneurysms in unusual locations, distal to the circle of Willis, are suspicious for underlying or associated abnormality such as mycotic aneurysm, moyamoya, AVM, or atrial myxoma. In the absence of such an associated abnormality, peripheral aneurysms tend to be large, fusiform, and not at arterial branch points.[34] Fusiform aneurysms can occur in other locations, as well, and careful attention should be paid to vessel caliber, as not all aneurysms are saccular. In general, aneurysms greater than 10 mm are believed to be at higher risk of rupture. Increased rupture risk is also associated with apical bleb, multilobed configuration, and length/neck ratio >1.6.[35] Aneurysms >2.5 cm are termed "giant."

Traumatic aneurysms are most commonly pseudoaneurysms, the result of disruption of all layers of the vessel wall with contained, localized rupture. The location should be consistent with the trauma, for example, cortical aneurysms developing subjacent to a calvarial fracture or in a region of penetrating injury.

Coagulopathy

A hematocrit layering effect within a hematoma is suggestive of an underlying coagulopathy, but it is not pathognomonic, as it may be found in other types of hemorrhage if the time to CT is short, and it is likely due to incomplete clotting.[1] Elements of the coagulation cascade, thrombin and fibrinogen in particular, have been linked to the development of perihematoma edema, which results in increased intracranial

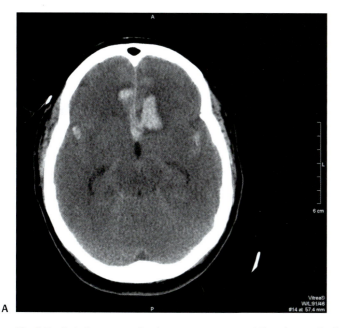

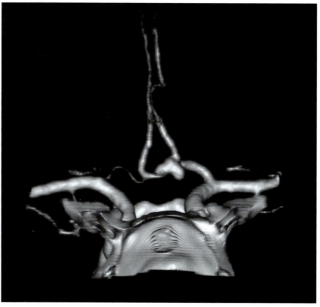

Fig. 7.5 Anterior communicating artery aneurysm. **(A)** Widespread subarachnoid hemorrhage with parafalcine predominance and bifrontal parenchymal hemorrhage is suggestive of the location of this bilobed anterior communicating artery aneurysm **(B).**

pressure and subsequent poor outcome; this may explain why ICH related to thrombolysis or coagulopathy tends to result in less perihematoma edema than hemorrhage from other causes.[36] Such hemorrhage tends to be solitary and lobar.

Vascular Malformations

Arteriovenous malformations (AVMs) consist of abnormal connections of arteries and veins without an intervening capillary bed. Brain tissue is generally present between the vessels. Larger AVMs are more likely to present with symptoms related to mass effect, such as seizures, whereas smaller AVMs are more likely to hemorrhage, possibly related to hemodynamic factors. The majority of AVMs are supratentorial, and approximately 7% have an associated aneurysm.[37] Factors associated with increased risk of hemorrhage include periventricular location, deep venous drainage, deep location, and associated aneurysm.[2] Surgical risk is assessed by the Spetzler-Martin grading scale, which grades AVMs from I to VI according to size, pattern of venous drainage, and location with respect to eloquent cortex. Grade I AVMs are small, have superficial drainage, and are located in non-eloquent cortex; at the other end of the spectrum, grade VI AVMs are large, have deep venous drainage, and are located in eloquent cortex, making them essentially inoperable.[38] The appearance on noncontrast CT is variable, ranging from occult small lesions to visualization of serpentine vessels; approximately 30% show evidence of calcification. CTA demonstrates serpentine dilated arteries and veins to good advantage.

Cavernous hemangiomas (cavernomas) are composed of abnormal vascular sinusoids/"caverns" without intervening brain. These lesions are generally considered to be angiographically occult, though a faint blush of enhancement may be seen on CTA or angiography. On noncontrast CT, they may appear as an iso- or hyperattenuating mass, and may demonstrate the classic "popcorn" calcification centrally. The characteristic appearance is best appreciated on MRI, which demonstrates internal stippled T1 hyperintensity from calcification/blood products, often with peripheral hemosiderin susceptibility from prior hemorrhage. The majority of cavernomas are supratentorial and asymptomatic. They are commonly associated with venous angiomas (24% in one series), in which case they have been found to have a higher incidence of hemorrhage and posterior fossa location.[39]

Capillary telangiectasias and venous angiomas/developmental venous anomalies (DVAs) are fairly common, and are not associated with a high risk of intracranial hemorrhage. Capillary telangiectasias are most commonly seen in the pons on postcontrast T1-weighted MRI, but typically demonstrate no abnormal density on pre- or postcontrast CT. Calcification may rarely be seen on noncontrast CT. Developmental venous anomalies or venous angiomas are the most common cerebral vascular malformation, and are generally asymptomatic. However, they are associated with cavernomas, in which case there is a higher incidence of cavernoma-related intracranial hemorrhage.[39] Less common presentations include venous congestion and draining vein thrombosis. Rarely, supratentorial hemorrhage can occur due to the DVA itself

when arteriovenous connections are present.[40] On contrast-enhanced CT, DVAs appear as a "caput medusae" of veins draining normal intervening brain parenchyma, converging to a dilated draining vein. Dural arteriovenous fistulas are likely the sequela of chronic venous thrombosis, and present more often with objective pulsatile tinnitus and headache than with intracranial hemorrhage.

Cerebral Amyloid Angiopathy

Cerebral amyloid angiopathy (CAA) is the result of deposition of amyloid protein in the walls of cortical, subcortical, and leptomeningeal vessels, resulting in weakening of the vessel walls and predisposition to hemorrhage in the event of alterations of blood pressure or minor trauma.[1,36,37,41] Though the disorder may rarely be sporadic and present in younger patients, it is most common in those over 60 years of age, with the incidence increasing with age, and is a common, if not the most common, cause of lobar hemorrhage in the elderly.[1,37,41] Noncontrast head CT is the initial imaging study of choice and demonstrates cortical/subcortical hemorrhage, most commonly parieto-occipital but also possible in the brainstem, basal ganglia, or cerebellum.[36] Subarachnoid extension is common, with subdural or rarely intraventricular hemorrhage possible.[1,36,41] Leukoencephalopathy (white matter low density) and atrophy are common. The typical chronic microhemorrhages at the gray-white junction seen on MR susceptibility sequences are not visualizable on CT.

Venous Thrombosis

Cerebral venous thrombosis (**Fig. 7.6**) is an imaging emergency, as prompt recognition and treatment can result in reversal, thereby averting significant morbidity and mortality. Noncontrast head CT and CT venography are effective and rapid diagnostic tools. The sigmoid and transverse sinuses are most often involved, with cortical vein involvement in approximately 6%.[42] Gyral enhancement, possibly extending to the adjacent white matter, can occur in up to 29% due to breakdown of the blood–brain barrier in the setting of edema.[42]

Reperfusion Injury/Hemorrhagic Transformation/Cerebral Hyperperfusion Syndrome

Reperfusion of ischemic brain tissue, in which the blood–brain barrier is compromised due to ischemic damage, may result in hemorrhagic transformation in up to 40% of patients with ischemic stroke and may occur within several hours to up to 1 week from onset.[43] Such reperfusion injury can occur in the setting of intravenous, intraarterial or mechanical thrombolysis, or due to natural recanalization of occlusion. Severity of hemorrhage may range from subtle, gyriform petechial hemorrhage to large parenchymal hematoma with mass effect. The type of hemorrhage and the size of the parenchymal hematoma with respect to the infarct size should be noted, as large hematomas have a poorer prognosis. Recent

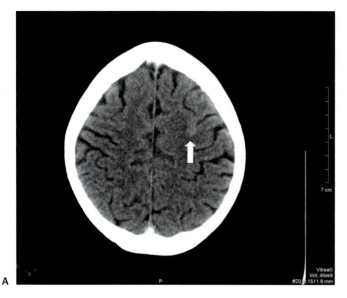

A

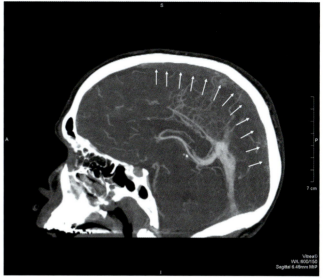

B

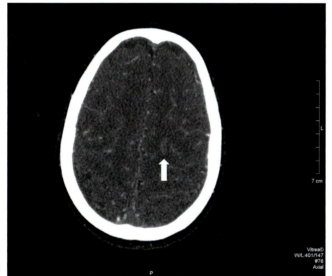

C

Fig. 7.6 Venous sinus thrombosis. **(A)** Noncontrast CT shows subtle left frontal hemorrhage *(arrow)* in this 40-year-old woman on oral contraceptives with decreased consciousness, due to sagittal sinus thrombosis as seen on CT venogram **(B)** *(small arrows)*. **(C)** The parenchymal hemorrhage *(arrow)* is less conspicuous on the contrasted study (scanned at a different angle), emphasizing the importance of a noncontrast head CT in evaluating intracranial hemorrhage.

work suggests that altered permeability of the blood–brain barrier as measured by CT perfusion may predict hemorrhagic transformation.[32] Cerebral hemorrhage following carotid endarterectomy, known as cerebral hyperperfusion syndrome, may occur in hyperperfused healthy brain tissue (as opposed to infarcted tissue) following carotid endarterectomy or carotid stenting.[31,44] Patients with hypertension, recent stroke, and anticoagulation are at increased risk.

Vasculitis/Vasculopathy

Though ischemia is the most common presentation in central nervous system (CNS) vasculitis, parenchymal or subarachnoid hemorrhage may be present. Such findings on a noncontrast or contrast head CT, particularly if multifocal, should raise the question of vasculitis. Multiple focal vascular stenoses are suggestive of the diagnosis, but may not be seen in every case. Vasculitis less frequently manifests as multiple microaneurysms.

Central nervous system vasculitis may be seen as a nonspecific response to numerous inflammatory or infectious disorders, and can involve large, medium, or small vessels. Though the size of the vessel that is involved may provide clues as to the etiology, the findings are nonspecific, and definitive diagnosis is through a biopsy. Potential etiologies include primary systemic vasculitides, primary angiitis of the CNS (PACNS), benign angiopathy of the CNS (BACNS), or secondary vasculitis due to infection, inflammation, or drugs. Radiation vasculopathy, Behçet's, fibromuscular dysplasia, HIV vasculitis, and neurosyphilis should be considered in the appropriate clinical setting. The differential diagnosis also includes vasospasm, cerebral autosomal-dominant arteriopathy with subcortical infarcts and leukoencephalopathy (CADASIL), and migraine.

Moyamoya

Moyamoya disease is characterized by progressive occlusion of the distal intracranial internal carotid arteries, as well as of the unilateral or bilateral MCAs and sometimes ACAs, with formation of numerous small vessel collaterals. Resultant weakening of the vascular walls and abnormal hemodynamic stress predisposes to cerebral hemorrhage. Intracranial hemorrhage is the most common presentation of moyamoya disease in adults, whereas ischemia is more common in children. Patients may also develop aneurysms or pseudoaneurysms in collateralized lenticulostriates, thalamoperforators, or other small arterial branches (moyamoya vessels) distal to the circle of Willis. Idiopathic moyamoya disease may be sporadic or genetic.[45] A moyamoya vascular pattern may also be seen in patients with sickle cell disease, neurofibromatosis, and Down syndrome, among others. Noncontrast head CT to evaluate for hemorrhage and CTA of the entire head to evaluate for the typical moyamoya vascular pattern and potential aneurysm formation are useful for initial evaluation.

Neoplasm

Hemorrhage into a preexisting primary or secondary neoplasm can obscure the underlying lesion and mimic primary, or other secondary, causes of intracranial hemorrhage (**Fig. 7.3**). In cases where there is suspicion for underlying neoplasm, follow-up imaging to search for tumor enhancement should be performed following resolution of the hematoma. Though subacute hematoma may demonstrate peripheral enhancement, the presence of additional foci of enhancement consistent with metastatic disease confirms the diagnosis of metastasis if present. Metastases are more likely to hemorrhage than primary brain neoplasms. Primary and secondary neoplasms with a propensity for hemorrhage are listed in **Table 7.4**.

Drugs

Patients on anticoagulants and undergoing treatment with thrombolytic drugs have an increased risk of intracranial hemorrhage. Sympathomimetic drugs such as cocaine and amphetamine may cause intracranial hemorrhage by either inducing vasculitic changes with subsequent hemorrhage or transiently increasing blood pressure with resultant hypertensive-like hemorrhage.

◆ Future Directions

Penumbra Imaging

There is substantial interest in the neuroimaging community to try to develop ways of using imaging to select stroke patients for treatment. Imaging of the so-called ischemic penumbra remains an area of very active research. In animal models, the MR diffusion–MR perfusion model has been studied extensively as an approach to imaging nonviable (ischemic core) and viable (penumbra) tissue.[46] However, in humans validation of core and penumbra imaging as a clinically useful tool has been more problematic, and simple extrapolation does not seem to account for differences between human and experimental stroke. Substantial effort has been made in recent years to determine if dynamic CT perfusion imaging with intravenous contrast can help to depict the sizes of the core and penumbra.[23] Two strategies that have been considered for assessing the core and penumbra with CT are CBF threshold measurement and comparison of two or more perfusion parameters. The idea behind CBF threshold measurement is based on work previously published using the xenon (Xe)-CT method of measuring CBF.[47] In theory, if the CBF values obtained by CT perfusion are comparable to those obtained by Xe-CT perfusion, then the threshold values for the core (approximately 0 to 8 cc/100 g/min) and penumbra (approximately 9 to 18 cc/100 g/min) established previously could be used. Previously published validation work in humans and animals has supported the idea that accurate, reproducible CBF values can be obtained using dynamic CT perfusion imaging.[48] However, in our practical experience, we have found thresholds difficult to use reliably because of image noise and the relatively small volume of tissue typically measuring in the "penumbral" range (9 to 18 cc/100 g/min). A second issue involves published reports of CBF value variability arising from the use of arterial and venous (input function) regions of interest (ROIs). Arterial and venous input functions are widely used in a type of CBF computation called deconvolution analysis. The user must choose or affirm the computer's choice of an appropriate artery and vein to use for analysis. Small variations in placement of these input function ROIs can produce substantial variation in CBF.[49] For these reasons, we do not use quantitative CBF threshold analysis at our institution.

Multiparameter analysis compares two or more perfusion parameters to try to assess the extent of core and penumbra. The two formulations that have received the most attention are comparison of CBF and CBV (**Fig. 7.7**) and comparison of MTT and CBV. In both scenarios, low CBV values are believed to be the marker for irreversibly infarcted tissue (core) whereas the larger regions of MTT or CBF abnormality (**Fig. 7.8**) are thought to be viable tissue at risk.[23] Previously published work has emphasized correlations based on retro-

Table 7.4 Tumors with a Propensity for Hemorrhage[1,2]	
Primary	Glioblastoma multiforme
	High-grade glioma
	Oligodendroglioma
Secondary/metastatic	Bronchogenic carcinoma
	Renal cell carcinoma
	Choriocarcinoma
	Melanoma
	Thyroid carcinoma

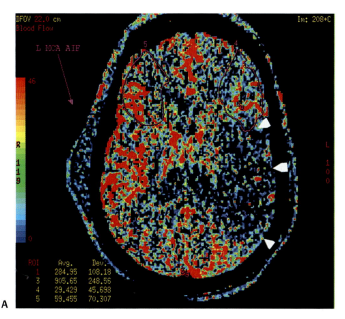

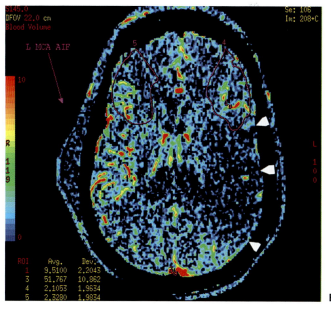

Fig. 7.7 Matched abnormalities of cerebral blood flow **(A)** and cerebral blood volume **(B)** in the left hemisphere in the territory of the middle cerebral artery *(arrowheads)*. One hypothesis that has been of interest is that the use of multiparameter imaging differentiates reversible ischemia from irreversible ischemia. Decreases in observed blood volume are thought to represent irreversible ischemia, though this is an area of active research.

spective analysis. Furthermore, there has not been a systematic control for early reperfusion, which likely plays an important role in tissue outcomes. Thus, at present, there is not a universally accepted and validated formula for assessment of core and penumbra imaging using CT. It remains an area of very active research because the clinical potential is very enticing.

Permeability/Risk of Hemorrhage

Computed tomography perfusion imaging has been studied as a possible predictor of hemorrhage following ischemic stroke. The major hypothesis is that blood–brain barrier insufficiency can be measured related to the extravasated iodine within a lesion. Preliminary investigations support the

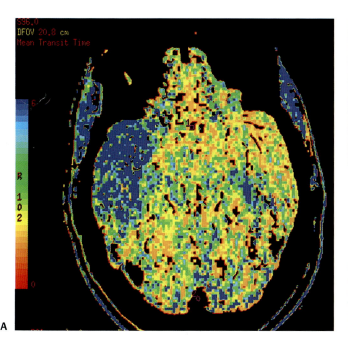

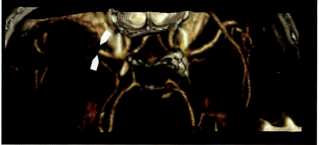

Fig. 7.8 **(A)** Dynamic CT perfusion imaging shows a well-defined region of prolonged mean transit time (MTT) in the right hemisphere, depicted as blue. Prolonged transit time is a sensitive indicator of hemodynamic alteration and is related to reduced cerebral perfusion pressure such as in stroke. **(B)** CTA image in the same patient depicts right MCA occlusion *(arrows)*.

notion that such alterations are measurable and may be related to the risk of hemorrhage.[32] Work in this field is ongoing.

Collateral/Miscellaneous

One variable that likely influences tissue outcome following stroke is the presence and sufficiency of collateral blood flow. This variable has been inconsistently studied in the past, but previously published work suggests that tissue and clinical outcomes are better when collateral flow is present. This is a very commonsensical idea and is appealing for this reason. Assessment of collaterals includes circle-of-Willis collaterals and pial-to-pial collaterals. The former lend themselves readily to study with CTA, whereas the latter are more difficult to assess. One possible marker for pial collaterals may actually be an increase in the perfusion parameter CBV. There is a physiologic reason that CBV may depict pial collateral flow: as perfusion pressure drops (such as in arterial occlusion), autoregulatory vasodilation attempts to increase flow locally. Arteriolar vasodilation increases local blood volume. Thus, when CBV is increased, presumably this provides information about the status of pial collateralization. This also is an area of ongoing research.

References

1. Smith EE, Rosand J, Greenberg SM. Hemorrhagic stroke. Neuroimaging Clin N Am 2005;15:259–272, ix
2. Aygun N, Masaryk TJ. Diagnostic imaging for intracerebral hemorrhage. Neurosurg Clin N Am 2002;13:313–334, vi
3. Konstas AA, Goldmakher GV, Lee TY, Lev MH. Theoretic basis and technical implementations of CT perfusion in acute ischemic stroke, part 2: technical implementations. AJNR Am J Neuroradiol 2009;30:885–892
4. Wintermark M, Albers GW, Alexandrov AV, et al. Acute stroke imaging research roadmap. AJNR Am J Neuroradiol 2008;29:e23–e30
5. Nguyen-Huynh MN, Wintermark M, English J, et al. How accurate is CT angiography in evaluating intracranial atherosclerotic disease? Stroke 2008;39:1184–1188
6. Inoue Y, Takemoto K, Miyamoto T, et al. Sequential computed tomography scans in acute cerebral infarction. Radiology 1980;135:655–662
7. Tomura N, Uemura K, Inugami A, Fujita H, Higano S, Shishido F. Early CT finding in cerebral infarction: obscuration of the lentiform nucleus. Radiology 1988;168:463–467
8. Tomsick T, Brott T, Barsan W, et al. Prognostic value of the hyperdense middle cerebral artery sign and stroke scale score before ultraearly thrombolytic therapy. AJNR Am J Neuroradiol 1996;17:79–85
9. Wardlaw JM, Mielke O. Early signs of brain infarction at CT: observer reliability and outcome after thrombolytic treatment—systematic review. Radiology 2005;235:444–453
10. von Kummer R, Allen KL, Holle R, et al. Acute stroke: usefulness of early CT findings before thrombolytic therapy. Radiology 1997;205:327–333
11. Patel SC, Levine SR, Tilley BC, et al; National Institute of Neurological Disorders and Stroke rt-PA Stroke Study Group. Lack of clinical significance of early ischemic changes on computed tomography in acute stroke. JAMA 2001;286:2830–2838
12. Adams HP Jr, del Zoppo G, Alberts MJ, et al; American Heart Association; American Stroke Association Stroke Council; Clinical Cardiology Council; Cardiovascular Radiology and Intervention Council; Atherosclerotic Peripheral Vascular Disease and Quality of Care Outcomes in Research Interdisciplinary Working Groups. Guidelines for the early management of adults with ischemic stroke: a guideline from the American Heart Association/American Stroke Association Stroke Council, Clinical Cardiology Council, Cardiovascular Radiology and Intervention Council, and the Atherosclerotic Peripheral Vascular Disease and Quality of Care Outcomes in Research Interdisciplinary Working Groups: the American Academy of Neurology affirms the value of this guideline as an educational tool for neurologists. Stroke 2007;38:1655–1711
13. Barber PA, Demchuk AM, Zhang J, Buchan AM. Validity and reliability of a quantitative computed tomography score in predicting outcome of hyperacute stroke before thrombolytic therapy. ASPECTS Study Group. Alberta Stroke Programme Early CT Score. Lancet 2000;355:1670–1674
14. Grotta JC, Chiu D, Lu M, et al. Agreement and variability in the interpretation of early CT changes in stroke patients qualifying for intravenous rtPA therapy. Stroke 1999;30:1528–1533
15. Hill MD, Rowley HA, Adler F, et al; PROACT-II Investigators. Selection of acute ischemic stroke patients for intra-arterial thrombolysis with pro-urokinase by using ASPECTS. Stroke 2003;34:1925–1931
16. Demchuk AM, Hill MD, Barber PA, Silver B, Patel SC, Levine SR; NINDS rtPA Stroke Study Group, NIH. Importance of early ischemic computed tomography changes using ASPECTS in NINDS rtPA Stroke Study. Stroke 2005;36:2110–2115
17. Weir NU, Pexman JH, Hill MD, Buchan AM; CASES investigators. How well does ASPECTS predict the outcome of acute stroke treated with IV tPA? Neurology 2006;67:516–518
18. Scuotto A, Cappabianca S, Melone MB, Puoti G. MRI "fogging" in cerebellar ischaemia: case report. Neuroradiology 1997;39:785–787
19. Ito U, Tomita H, Kito K, Ueki Y, Inaba Y. CT enhancement after prolonged high-dose contrast infusion in the early stage of cerebral infarction. Stroke 1986;17:424–430
20. Hornig CR, Busse O, Buettner T, Dorndorf W, Agnoli A, Akengin Z. CT contrast enhancement on brain scans and blood-CSF barrier disturbances in cerebral ischemic infarction. Stroke 1985;16:268–273
21. Eastwood JD, Lev MH, Wintermark M, et al. Correlation of early dynamic CT perfusion imaging with whole-brain MR diffusion and perfusion imaging in acute hemispheric stroke. AJNR Am J Neuroradiol 2003;24:1869–1875
22. Murphy BD, Fox AJ, Lee DH, et al. White matter thresholds for ischemic penumbra and infarct core in patients with acute stroke: CT perfusion study. Radiology 2008;247:818–825
23. Wintermark M, Flanders AE, Velthuis B, et al. Perfusion-CT assessment of infarct core and penumbra: receiver operating characteristic curve analysis in 130 patients suspected of acute hemispheric stroke. Stroke 2006;37:979–985
24. Hunter GJ, Hamberg LM, Ponzo JA, et al. Assessment of cerebral perfusion and arterial anatomy in hyperacute stroke with three-dimensional functional CT: early clinical results. AJNR Am J Neuroradiol 1998;19:29–37
25. Santalucia P. Intracerebral hemorrhage: medical treatment. Neurol Sci 2008;29(Suppl 2):S271–S273
26. Broderick JP, Brott TG, Duldner JE, Tomsick T, Huster G. Volume of intracerebral hemorrhage. A powerful and easy-to-use predictor of 30-day mortality. Stroke 1993;24:987–993
27. Zhu XL, Chan MS, Poon WS. Spontaneous intracranial hemorrhage: which patients need diagnostic cerebral angiography? A prospective study of 206 cases and review of the literature. Stroke 1997;28:1406–1409
28. Halpin SF, Britton JA, Byrne JV, Clifton A, Hart G, Moore A. Prospective evaluation of cerebral angiography and computed tomography in cerebral haematoma. J Neurol Neurosurg Psychiatry 1994;57:1180–1186
29. Hino A, Fujimoto M, Yamaki T, Iwamoto Y, Katsumori T. Value of repeat angiography in patients with spontaneous subcortical hemorrhage. Stroke 1998;29:2517–2521
30. Qureshi AI, Bliwise DL, Bliwise NG, Akbar MS, Uzen G, Frankel MR. Rate of 24-hour blood pressure decline and mortality after spontaneous intracerebral hemorrhage: a retrospective analysis with a random effects regression model. Crit Care Med 1999;27:480–485
31. Wang DZ, Talkad AV. Treatment of intracerebral hemorrhage: what should we do now? Curr Neurol Neurosci Rep 2009;9:13–18
32. Aviv RI, d'Esterre CD, Murphy BD, et al. Hemorrhagic transformation of ischemic stroke: prediction with CT perfusion. Radiology 2009;250:867–877
33. van der Jagt M, Hasan D, Bijvoet HW, et al. Validity of prediction of the site of ruptured intracranial aneurysms with CT. Neurology 1999;52:34–39
34. Nussbaum ES, Madison MT, Goddard JK, Lassig JP, Nussbaum LA. Peripheral intracranial aneurysms: management challenges in 60 consecutive cases. J Neurosurg 2009;110:7–13
35. Osborn AG, Salzman KL, Katzman GL, et al. Diagnostic Imaging: Brain, 1st ed. Salt Lake City: Amirsys, 2004
36. Woo D, Broderick JP. Spontaneous intracerebral hemorrhage: epidemiology and clinical presentation. Neurosurg Clin N Am 2002;13:265–279, v
37. Barnes B, Cawley CM, Barrow DL. Intracerebral hemorrhage secondary to vascular lesions. Neurosurg Clin N Am 2002;13:289–297, v
38. Spetzler RF, Martin NA. A proposed grading system for arteriovenous malformations. J Neurosurg 1986;65:476–483

39. Abdulrauf SI, Kaynar MY, Awad IA. A comparison of the clinical profile of cavernous malformations with and without associated venous malformations. Neurosurgery 1999;44:41–46, discussion 46–47
40. Oran I, Kiroglu Y, Yurt A, et al. Developmental venous anomaly (DVA) with arterial component: a rare cause of intracranial haemorrhage. Neuroradiology 2009;51:25–32
41. Chao CP, Kotsenas AL, Broderick DF. Cerebral amyloid angiopathy: CT and MR imaging findings. Radiographics 2006;26:1517–1531
42. Leach JL, Fortuna RB, Jones BV, Gaskill-Shipley MF. Imaging of cerebral venous thrombosis: current techniques, spectrum of findings, and diagnostic pitfalls. Radiographics. 2006;26(Suppl 1):S19–41; discussion S2–3
43. Mullins ME, Lev MH, Schellingerhout D, Gonzalez RG, Schaefer PW. Intracranial hemorrhage complicating acute stroke: how common is hemorrhagic stroke on initial head CT scan and how often is initial clinical diagnosis of acute stroke eventually confirmed? AJNR Am J Neuroradiol 2005;26:2207–2212
44. Lapsiwala S, Moftakhar R, Badie B. Drug-induced iatrogenic intraparenchymal hemorrhage. Neurosurg Clin N Am 2002;13:299–312, v–vi v–vi.
45. Burke GM, Burke AM, Sherma AK, Hurley MC, Batjer HH, Bendok BR. Moyamoya disease: a summary. Neurosurg Focus 2009;26:E11
46. Shen Q, Meng X, Fisher M, Sotak CH, Duong TQ. Pixel-by-pixel spatio-temporal progression of focal ischemia derived using quantitative perfusion and diffusion imaging. J Cereb Blood Flow Metab 2003;23: 1479–1488
47. Rubin G, Firlik AD, Levy EI, Pindzola RR, Yonas H. Xenon-enhanced computed tomography cerebral blood flow measurements in acute cerebral ischemia: Review of 56 cases. J Stroke Cerebrovasc Dis 1999;8: 404–411
48. Wintermark M, Thiran JP, Maeder P, Schnyder P, Meuli R. Simultaneous measurement of regional cerebral blood flow by perfusion CT and stable xenon CT: a validation study. AJNR Am J Neuroradiol 2001;22: 905–914
49. Kealey SM, Loving VA, Delong DM, Eastwood JD. User-defined vascular input function curves: influence on mean perfusion parameter values and signal-to-noise ratio. Radiology 2004;231:587–593

8

Magnetic Resonance Imaging in Hemorrhagic and Ischemic Stroke

Anne Catherine Kim, Jimmy Jaeyoung Kang, Reza Hakimelahi, and Pamela W. Schaefer

---

Pearls

- Susceptibility weighted imaging differs from conventional echo planar imaging (EPI) or gradient echo (GRE) T2*-weighted imaging in that both phase and magnitude information are incorporated.
- Susceptibility weighted imaging has greater sensitivity for detection of microbleeds, diffuse axonal injury hemorrhages, intratumoral hemorrhage, and cerebral cavernous malformations.
- Susceptibility weighted imaging may depict slow-flow lesions such as capillary telangiectasias.
- Susceptibility weighted imaging may distinguish calcium from hemorrhage.
- See also **Table 8.13.**

◆ Acute Ischemic Stroke

The introduction of magnetic resonance imaging (MRI) for acute ischemic stroke imaging has greatly improved our ability to identify stroke, understand the underlying pathophysiology, triage patients, and select appropriate treatments. Of the multiple parameters, diffusion weighted imaging is the most reliable for detecting acute ischemic stroke, and it can do so with high sensitivity and specificity, within 30 minutes of symptom onset. Perfusion MRI depicts hemodynamic conditions at the microvascular level, and can therefore identify regions of brain tissue that are viable, but at risk of infarction if timely reperfusion does not occur. This chapter discusses how diffusion and perfusion MRI can help identify infarct core, penumbra, benign oligemia, and the risk of hemorrhagic transformation, and how diffusion and perfusion MRI can be used to predict patient outcome and select appropriate therapy. This chapter also discusses magnetic resonance angiography (MRA) and its uses and applications.

Conventional Magnetic Resonance Imaging

Acute Stroke

Conventional MRI sequences (fluid-attenuated inversion recovery [FLAIR] and T2) are most useful for assessing extent and age of subacute and chronic infarctions **(Figs. 8.1 and 8.2; Table 8.1).** Their utility rests on detection of edema-related changes after an occlusive event. In the acute setting (first 6 hours), tissue changes are primarily due to shifts of water from the extra- to intracellular space, with relatively little increase in total tissue water. Consequently, the sensitivity of FLAIR and T2-weighted images for detecting the parenchymal changes associated with acute stroke are very low, ranging from 8.3 to 26% in the first 6 hours after symptom onset.[1–3]

The FLAIR and T2-weighted images are therefore most useful as adjuncts to diffusion-weighted imaging (DWI) and vessel imaging. When a patient presents with stroke symptoms of unknown duration, with a DWI-hyperintense lesion but little or no associated FLAIR hyperintensity, it is generally accepted that the stroke is less than 6 hours old. FLAIR can also show a thrombus or slow flow, demonstrated as high signal in the affected vessel, and present in up to 65% of cases.[4,5] On T2-weighted images, thrombus and slow flow can be detected by the absence of normal flow voids.[6]

Gradient echo T2* images are typically included in acute stroke protocols, as they are highly sensitive to the detection of paramagnetic blood products, and are at least as sensitive as computed tomography (CT) for the detection of hemorrhage.[7] They also have relatively high sensitivity (86% sensitivity in one large study[8]) for the detection of acute thrombus. Gadolinium-enhanced T1-weighted sequences can also be obtained; in the acute period, arterial vessels in the affected region may enhance due to slow flow in collateral vessels.[6] During this period, the parenchyma usually does not

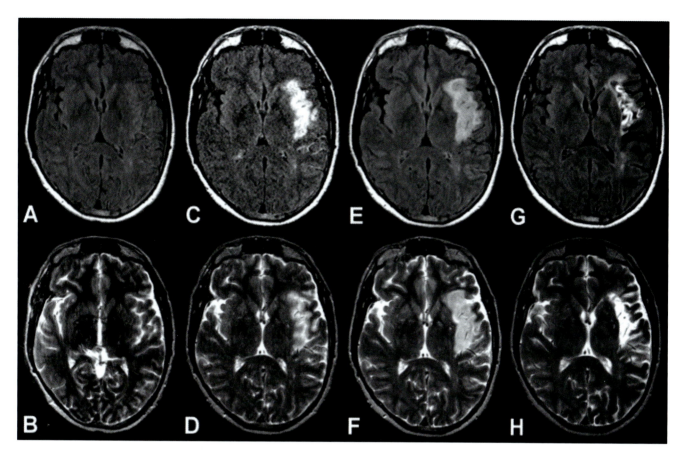

Fig. 8.1 Stroke evolution on conventional magnetic resonance imaging (MRI). A 53-year-old man with right hemiparesis and aphasia. Fluid-attenuated inversion recovery FLAIR **(A)** and T2-weighted images **(B)** demonstrate minimal hyperintensity in the left insula and subinsular lesion. Left middle cerebral artery (MCA) branches are hyperintense, due to slow flow. At 31 hours, the infarction has become markedly hyperintense [FLAIR **(C)** and T2 **(D)**], with persistence of the vascular hyperintensity. By 5 days [FLAIR **(E)** and T2 **(F)**], the infarct has increased in size due to vasogenic edema and swelling. The vascular hyperintensity has resolved. At 5 months [FLAIR **(G)** and T2 **(H)**], there is tissue loss with some cavitation (low signal on FLAIR images).

enhance. However, in rare cases, early parenchymal enhancement may occur when there is early reperfusion or good collateralization.[9]

Subacute and Chronic Stroke

In the early subacute period (1 to 7 days), vasogenic edema predominates, resulting in increased T2 and FLAIR hyperintensity, T1 hypointensity, and brain swelling. The brain swelling peaks at 3 to 5 days and usually resolves by 7 to 10 days. Vascular enhancement can persist for 1 week, and arterial FLAIR hyperintensity can persist for up to 2 weeks.[10]

During this period, parenchymal, gyral, and meningeal enhancement can also be seen. Parenchymal enhancement (usually gyral) is due to collateral circulation, or recanalization and breakdown of the blood–brain barrier. It is consistently present by 6 days after stroke, and usually persists for 6 to 8 weeks. Gyral enhancement without mass effect is unusual in other settings, and therefore is almost pathognomonic for late subacute infarction. Meningeal enhancement, thought to represent reactive hyperemia, usually occurs within 1 to 3 days and disappears within 1 week.[11]

By 6 weeks, the chronic stage of infarction is well established: the inflammatory response is complete, edema has resorbed, and the blood–brain barrier and reperfusion have been established. Enhancement of parenchyma, meninges, or vessels has resolved. This stage is characterized by encephalomalacia, with cystic cavitation and increased water content causing T2 hyperintensity and T1 hypointensity. Peripheral gyriform T1 shortening, due to laminar necrosis, can also occur. Large middle cerebral artery (MCA) territory infarcts usually have associated wallerian degeneration, with T2 hyperintensity and tissue loss of the ipsilateral cortical spinal tract.[11–13]

Diffusion Magnetic Resonance Imaging of Acute Stroke

Basic Physics

For detailed descriptions of the physics of diffusion weighted imaging, several reviews are available.[14,15] Briefly, DWI is based on a spin-echo echo planar imaging sequence, with a large magnetic field gradient applied before a radiofrequency (RF)

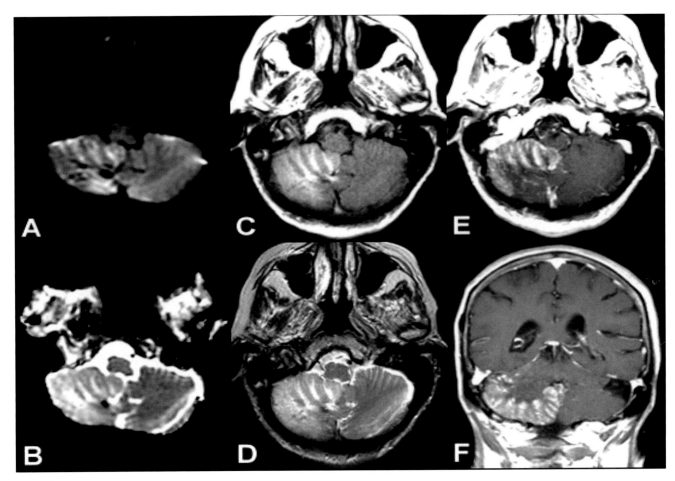

Fig. 8.2 Subacute stroke. A 53-year-old woman with dizziness and ataxia for 2 weeks. The right cerebellar stroke is isointense on diffusion-weighted imaging (DWI) **(A)** and hyperintense on apparent diffusion coefficient (ADC) **(B)** images, consistent with a late subacute stroke. The lesion is hyperintense on FLAIR **(C)** and T2 **(D)** due predominantly to vasogenic edema. Gadolinium-enhanced axial **(E)** and coronal **(F)** T1-weighted images demonstrate gyriform enhancement.

pulse, followed by application of equal and opposite gradient pulses. The first gradient de-phases protons, and the second gradient re-phases them. Within any given voxel, if there is no net movement of water protons, the two balanced gradients negate each other. However, if there is net movement of water molecules due to diffusion, the protons experience the first gradient pulse at one location and the second gradient pulse at a different location; the two gradients are no longer experienced as equal in magnitude, and therefore do not cancel each other out. Faster-moving water protons undergo a larger net dephasing. The resultant signal intensity of a voxel of tissue containing moving protons is equal to its signal intensity on a T2-weighted image, decreased by an amount related to the rate of diffusion. Therefore, tissue with the most restricted protons (e.g., in acute ischemic tissue) has the highest signal.[14,15]

It is important to note that in addition to contrast due to differences in diffusion, DWI images also have T2-weighted contrast. Signal intensity is linearly related to T2 signal, and exponentially related to diffusion. To remove the T2 contrast,

a map of apparent diffusion coefficient (ADC) values is created by obtaining two image sets, one with a very low b value and one with $b = 1000$ second/mm^2. By plotting the natural logarithm of the signal intensity versus b for these two b values, the ADC can be determined from the slope of this line. Alternatively, the DWI can be divided by the echoplanar spin echo (SE) T2 image (or low b value image), to give an "exponential image," the signal intensity of which is exponentially related to the ADC.[14]

Regions with abnormally restricted diffusion are hyperintense on DWI. However, regions with normal or increased diffusion may be hypo-, iso-, or hyperintense, depending on the strength of the diffusion and T2 components (T2 shine-through effect). For this reason, review of the ADC maps or the exponential images is essential; a DWI-hyperintense lesion with truly restricted diffusion is dark on ADC maps and bright on exponential images. These images are also useful for detecting areas of increased diffusion that may be masked by T2 effects on the DWI images.[14]

Table 8.1 Appearance of Arterial Infarcts on Conventional Magnetic Resonance Imaging

Stage	T1	T2	FLAIR	GRE T2*
Hyperacute (0–6 h)	Postcontrast may show vessel enhancement No parenchymal enhancement	Absence of flow void Little to no parenchymal abnormality	Hyperintense vessels Little to no parenchymal abnormality	Susceptibility in region of clot
Acute (6–24 h)	Postcontrast vessel enhancement No parenchymal enhancement	Gyriform high signal, sulcal effacement Persistent vascular findings from hyperacute stage	Gyriform high signal, sulcal effacement Persistent vascular findings from hyperacute stage	Can show gyriform susceptibility from petechial hemorrhage
Subacute (1 day to 2 weeks)	Gyriform high signal due to petechial blood, Arterial meningeal, parenchymal enhancement	Gyriform high signal, sulcal effacement	Gyriform high signal, sulcal effacement	Susceptibility from petechial hemorrhage
Chronic	Low signal from cavitation	High signal from gliosis and wallerian degeneration	High signal from gliosis and wallerian degeneration	Susceptibility from petechial hemorrhage

Theory for Restricted Diffusion in Acute Stroke

The physiologic basis for the restricted diffusion associated with acute stroke is still under investigation **(Table 8.2)**. The predominant theory is that acute ischemia causes adenosine triphosphate (ATP) concentrations to fall, and Na^+/K^+ adenosine triphosphatase (ATPase) and other ionic pumps to fail. This leads to net translocation of water from the extracellular into the intracellular compartment where water movement is relatively more restricted. Resultant cell swelling causes a decrease in the size of the extracellular space, leading to more restricted movement of protons in that space as well. Degradation of intracellular components, leading to increased intracellular viscosity, may also play a role. Temperature decreases and cell membrane permeability have also been proposed as minor contributing factors.[15]

Time Course of Acute Stroke in Diffusion-Weighted Imaging

Restricted diffusion in the setting of acute stroke, manifest as high signal on diffusion-weighted images and low signal on ADC maps, has been reported in as early as 11 minutes,[16] and is reliably visible 30 minutes after symptom onset[15] **(Fig. 8.3; Table 8.3)**. Diffusion continues to decrease, reaching a nadir at 1 to 4 days. Several hours after stroke onset, the release of inflammatory mediators from ischemic brain tissue results in increasing vasogenic edema and increasing numbers of more mobile water molecules. Cell membrane breakdown and degradation result in the further removal of obstacles to water diffusion. Consequently, after 1 to 4 days, the ADC begins to rise, returning to baseline ("pseudo-normalizing") at 1 to 2 weeks. At this point, the infarct is isointense on ADC and exponential images but remains hyperintense on DWI images due to the T2 component. As the infarct cavitates and

fluid or gliosis replace the dead tissues, the ADC continues to rise; in the chronic stage, ADC maps demonstrate increased signal, whereas exponential images demonstrate decreased signal. DWI images may vary from slight hypointensity to slight hyperintensity, due to the varying contributions of diffusion and T2-weighting.

The time course is influenced by several factors including infarct type and patient age.[17] For example, in lacunar infarcts, ADC reaches its nadir more slowly, and increases later than in other stroke types. In non-lacunes, younger patients demonstrate faster increases in ADC.[18] Early reperfusion may also alter the time course: in acute stroke patients who

Table 8.2 Theory of Decreased Diffusion in Stroke

Theory

Failure of Na^+/K^+ ATPase and other ionic pumps; loss of ionic gradients and net transfer of water from the extracellular to the intracellular compartment; intracellular organelles, cytoskeletal macromolecules, and other structures provide barriers to random motion of water molecules

Reduced extracellular space volume and increased extracellular space pathway tortuosity due to cell swelling

Increased intracellular space viscosity and tortuosity from fragmentation of cellular components such as microtubules

Decreased cytoplasmic mobility

Increased cell membrane permeability

Temperature decrease

Abbreviation: ATPase, adenosinetriphosphatase.

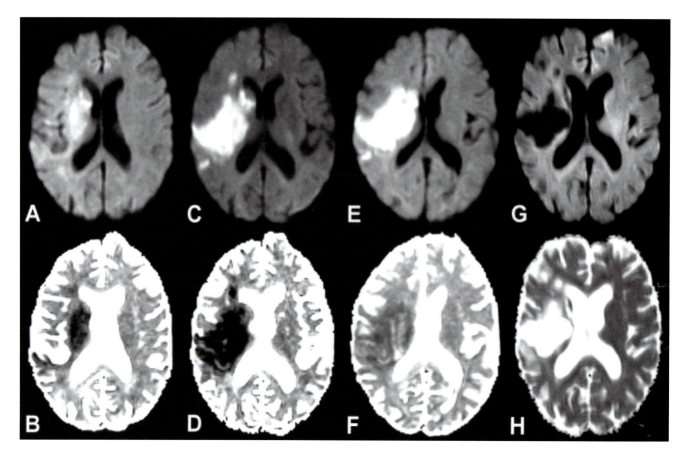

Fig. 8.3 Time course of a DWI lesion. Acute right MCA stroke. Top row, DWI images. Bottom row, ADC images. At 6 hours **(A,B),** the acute right MCA infarction is clearly visualized and is hyperintense on DWI and hypointense on ADC images due to cytotoxic edema. By 30 hours **(C,D),** the infarction has reached maximal hyperintensity on DWI images and hypointensity on ADC images due to cytotoxic edema. By 5 days **(E,F),** the ADC has pseudo-normalized or returned to baseline due to the development of cell lysis and vasogenic edema. The infarction is still hyperintense on DWI images due to the T2 component. By 3 months **(G,H),** the infarction is markedly hypointense on DWI and hyperintense on ADC images, due to tissue cavitation and gliosis.

Table 8.3 Appearance of Stroke on Diffusion-Weighted Imaging

	Hyperacute (0–6 h)	**Acute (6–24 hr)**	**Early Subacute (1–7 d)**	**Late Subacute (7–14 d)**	**Chronic**
(6–24 hour)	Early Subacute (1–7 days)	Late subacute (7–14 days)	Chronic		
Reason for changes	Cytotoxic edema	Cytotoxic edema	Cytotoxic edema with small amount of vasogenic edema	Cytotoxic and vasogenic edema	Gliosis and neuronal loss
DWI	Hyperintense	Hyperintense	Hyperintense, gyral hypo-intensity from petechial hemorrhage	Hyperintense (due to T2 shine through)	Iso- to hypointense
ADC	Hypointense	Hypointense	Hypointense	Isointense	Hyperintense
EXP	Hyperintense	Hyperintense	Hyperintense	Isointense	Hypointense
Echoplanar T2	Isointense	Hyperintense	Hyperintense, gyral hypo-intensity from petechial hemorrhage	Hyperintense	Hyperintense

Abbreviation: ADC, apparent diffusion coefficient; DWI, diffusion-weighted imaging; EXP, exponential images.

receive intravenous recombinant tissue-type plasminogen activator (rTPA) within 3 hours of symptom onset, pseudo-normalization can occur as early as 1 to 2 days.[19] Furthermore, there can be different rates of tissue evolution within the same lesion. One study demonstrated that while the average ADC of an ischemic lesion is depressed within 10 hours, different zones within an ischemic lesion may demonstrate low, pseudo-normal, or elevated ADCs.[20] In spite of these variations, in the absence of thrombolysis, tissue with reduced ADC nearly always progresses to infarction.

Accuracy of Diffusion-Weighted Imaging in Acute Stroke

Diffusion-weighted imaging is highly sensitive and specific for the detection of hyperacute and acute infarction. Reported sensitivities range from 88 to 100% and reported specificities range from 86 to 100%.[3,21] Infarctions not identified on DWI are usually very small and located in the brainstem, deep gray nuclei, or cortex[22] **(Fig. 8.4)**. False-positive acute infarctions can occur in patients with subacute or early chronic infarcts that appear bright on DWI due to T2 shine-through. This error is easily avoided by interpreting the DWI images in combination with ADC maps or exponential images. False-positive DWI images can also occur with restricted diffusion due to several other entities, as outlined in **Table 8.4**. When reviewed in conjunction with conventional MRI images, these lesions can usually be easily distinguished from acute infarc-

tions.[15] Certain entities, including hypoglycemia **(Fig. 8.5)**, acute demyelinative lesions, and hemiplegic migraine, can present with an acute neurologic deficit and a single FLAIR hyperintense, nonenhancing lesion with restricted diffusion. Because of this, they are at times misdiagnosed as acute strokes.[15]

Diffusion-Weighted Imaging Reversibility

It is commonly accepted that DWI represents tissue that is destined to infarct. The ultimate volume of an infarct is usually larger than that seen on initial DWI images, encompassing both the initial DWI abnormality and other tissue into which the infarct extends. Indeed, reversibility (abnormal on initial DWI but normal on follow-up images) of DWI hyperintense lesions is very rare except in the setting of early reperfusion, usually following intravenous or intraarterial thrombolysis **(Fig. 8.6; Table 8.5)**.

In fact, more recent studies have suggested that partial DWI reversal following thrombolysis with early reperfusion is relatively common. For example, of the 32 of 74 patients enrolled in the Diffusion and Perfusion Imaging Evaluation for Understanding Stroke Evolution (DEFUSE) trial who had early recanalization following administration of intravenous tissue-type plasminogen activator (rTPA), 23 had partial reversal of the initial DWI lesion, with an average 47% reversal of the original DWI lesion size to the follow-up 3-month T2

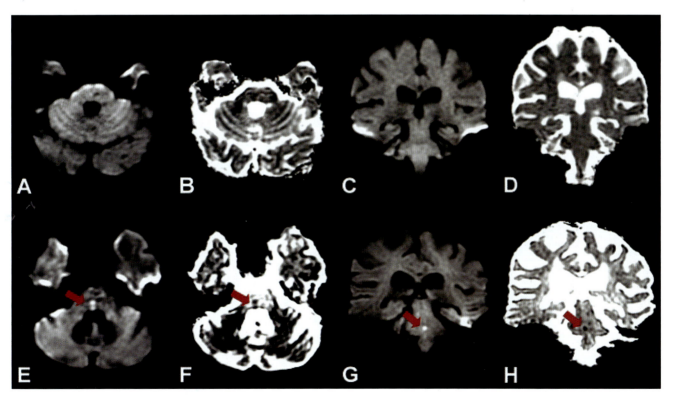

Fig. 8.4 False-negative DWI lesion. A 69-year-old woman with visual disturbance. Initial axial and coronal DWI **(A,C)** and ADC **(B,D)** images obtained at 12 hours after symptom onset show no definite acute infarction. Follow-up DWI **(E,G)** images obtained at 3 days demonstrate a hyperintense lesion *(arrow)*, consistent with a punctate acute infarction, in the dorsal pons. The lesion is hypointense on ADC **(F,H)** images.

Table 8.4 False Positives and Negatives on Diffusion-Weighted Imaging

DWI False-Negative Lesions	DWI False-Positive Lesions	Mechanism for Decreased Diffusion in False-Positive Lesions
Brainstem or deep gray nuclei lacunes	T2 shine-through	Predominance of T2 effect
	Abscess	Viscous pus
	Lymphoma and medulloblastoma	Dense tumor cellularity
	Actively demyelinating lesions	Inflammatory infiltrate, tissue vacuolization
	Hemorrhage—oxyhemoglobin, extracellular methemoglobin	Cell membranes intact for oxyhemoglobin, high protein content for both oxyhemoglobin and extracellular methemoglobin
	Herpes encephalitis	Cytotoxic edema
	Seizures	Cytotoxic edema
	Hypoglycemia	Cytotoxic edema
	Diffuse axonal injury	Cytotoxic edema or axonal retraction balls
	Creutzfeldt-Jakob disease	Spongiform change
	Heroin leukoencephalopathy	Tissue vacuolization
	Hemiplegic migraine	Cytotoxic edema or spreading depression
	Transient global amnesia	Cytotoxic edema or spreading depression
	Metronidazole toxicity (dentate nuclei)	Cytotoxic edema
	Venous sinus thrombosis	Cytotoxic edema

lesion size.[23] However, it should be noted that judging whether tissue with a diffusion abnormality is normal at follow-up can be difficult. Kidwell et al[24] reported a decrease in size from the initial to the follow-up DWI abnormality immediately after intraarterial thrombolysis in eight of 18 patients, with a mean decrease in lesion volume of 52%. However, despite the initial apparent recovery, a subsequent increase in DWI lesion volume was observed in five of the eight patients. Additionally, because tissue loss is a feature of chronic infarction, diminished infarct volumes on 1-month follow-up could be due to tissue loss rather than to reversal of the initial DWI lesion.

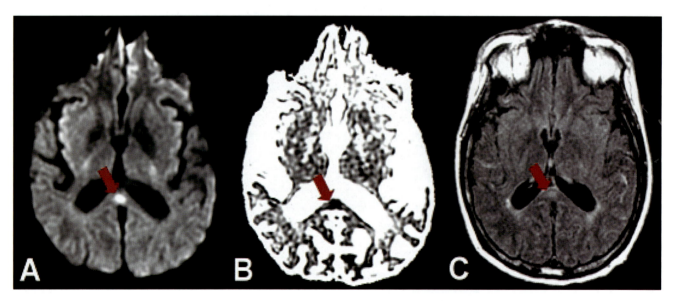

Fig. 8.5 False-positive DWI lesion due to hypoglycemia. A 56-year-old man presented with ophthalmoplegia, abnormal speech, and hypoglycemia. DWI **(A)** and ADC **(B)** images demonstrate restricted diffusion in the splenium *(arrow)* of the corpus callosum. The lesion is FLAIR hyperintense **(C)**. The patient's hypoglycemia was corrected and the diffusion abnormality resolved.

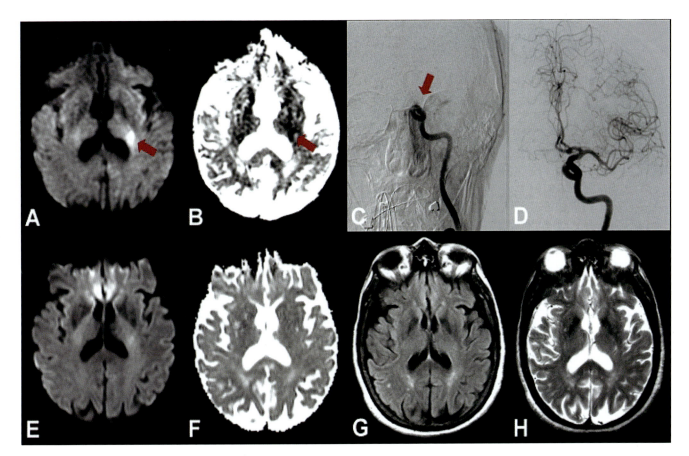

Fig. 8.6 DWI reversibility. A 79-year-old woman with acute right hemiparesis imaged at 8 hours after stroke onset with an initial National Institutes of Health Stroke Scale (NIHSS) score of 22. Initial DWI **(A)** and ADC **(B)** images demonstrate restricted diffusion in the posterior limb of the left internal capsule *(arrow),* consistent with acute infarction. The initial anteroposterior (AP) cerebral angiogram **(C)** shows no opacification of the distal left internal carotid artery or of the proximal left internal carotid artery (ICA) or MCA. The patient underwent successful intravascular recanalization therapy at 10:20, and the ICA, MCA, and ACA appear normal on the follow-up digital subtraction angiographic images **(D)**. Follow-up DWI **(E)**, ADC **(F)**, FLAIR **(G)**, and T2-weighted **(H)** images at 41 hours show no definite abnormality in the left internal capsule. The patient's follow up NIHSS score was 2.

Table 8.5 Diffusion-Weighted Imaging Reversibility

Definition	DWI abnormal tissue that appears normal at follow-up imaging
Entities with DWI reversibility	Acute stroke—usually following thrombolysis and/or recanalization procedures, with early reperfusion
	Venous infarction
	Hemiplegic migraine
	Transient global amnesia
	Hypoglycemia
	Seizures
Lesion location	White matter more than gray matter
Amount of DWI reversible tissue in arterial strokes following tissue-type plasminogen activator (rTPA)	Variable, 47% mean reduction in size from initial DWI to follow-up lesion for recanalizers in the DEFUSE study
Apparent diffusion coefficient (ADC) values	Higher in DWI-reversible versus nonreversible tissue
	663 to 732 × 10⁻⁶ mm²/sec in DWI reversible regions compared with 608 to 650 × 10⁻⁶ mm²/sec in DWI abnormal regions that progress to infarction
	49% of tissue with relative ADC of 70 to 80% reverses

Although an absolute ADC threshold for tissue infarction has not been defined, a number of studies have demonstrated that ADC values are significantly higher in DWI-reversible tissue compared with DWI-abnormal tissue that progresses to infarction. Mean ADCs range from 663 to 732×10^{-6} mm^2/sec in DWI reversible regions compared with 608 to 650×10^{-6} mm^2/sec in DWI abnormal regions that progress to infarction.[24,25] Fiehler et al[26] also showed that 49% of acute ischemic tissue with a relative ADC of 70 to 80% demonstrated DWI reversal, whereas only 6% of acute ischemic tissue with a relative ADC of less than 50% demonstrated reversal.

Perfusion Magnetic Resonance Imaging of Acute Stroke

Perfusion-weighted imaging (PWI) describes techniques that visually depict hemodynamic conditions that occur in capillaries and other microscopic blood vessels. Because impairment at the microvascular level most directly causes ischemic damage to brain tissue, PWI can guide acute stroke therapy by identifying regions of brain tissue that are underperfused but not yet infarcted, and can thus be rescued by timely initiation of appropriate treatment.

Dynamic Susceptibility Contrast: Principles

In the acute stroke setting, perfusion imaging is generally performed with a bolus tracking technique, dynamic susceptibility contrast (DSC) imaging. DSC relies on the decrease in signal due to magnetic susceptibility effects of gadolinium as it passes through the intracranial vasculature. Because blood passes through the brain parenchyma rapidly, the most commonly used sequence is a single-shot gradient echo echo planar imaging (EPI) sequence capable of multiple slice acquisitions from a single repetition time (TR). Typically, gadolinium is injected rapidly (5 to 7 cc/s) into a peripheral intravenous catheter, and then images are obtained repeatedly as the contrast agent passes through the brain. The technique takes approximately 1 to 2 minutes, and is performed so as to track the first pass of the contrast bolus through the intracranial vasculature, without recirculation effects. Approximately 60 images are obtained for each 5-mm brain slice, covering the entire brain.[27]

Perfusion Maps and Technical Considerations

The images obtained in the examination are converted by a computer to a contrast agent concentration-versus-time curve. The cerebral blood volume (CBV), the fraction of tissue that is occupied by blood within a given voxel, is proportional to the area under the curve. The cerebral blood flow (CBF), cubic centimeter of blood per minute per cubic centimeter of tissue, and mean transit time (MTT), the average time it takes a tracer to pass through the tissue, are typically computed with an arterial input function (AIF) and deconvolution methodology. These three cerebral perfusion parameters are related according to the central volume theorem: MTT = CBV/CBF. Other transit time measures that are commonly obtained are time to peak (TTP), the time it takes to reach maximal susceptibility effect; and T_{max}, the time-to-peak of the deconvolved residue function.

Singular value decomposition (SVD) is the standard deconvolution algorithm used to create perfusion maps. However, maps created with this algorithm are susceptible to error introduced by a delay in the bolus arrival, and dispersion or dilution of the bolus.[28] Selecting an ipsilateral AIF proximal to the region of interest minimizes delay but increases dispersion, whereas selecting a contralateral AIF increases delay and minimizes dispersion.[29] In general, delay and dispersion cause underestimation of the CBF and overestimation of the tissue at risk. To reduce this error, automated, bolus-delay corrected, and tracer arrival time-insensitive AIF selection have been proposed as solutions.[30,31]

Other Types of Perfusion-Weighted Imaging

In arterial spin labeling (ASL), an additional MRI coil is placed over the patient's neck and used to excite hydrogen nuclei ("spins") as they pass through one of the major cervical arteries en route to the brain. The spins themselves serve as an endogenous contrast agent. Passage of these spins through the brain can be used to measure cerebral blood flow. This method is attractive because it is completely noninvasive and can be used safely in patients with contrast allergies. In addition, individual cervical arteries can be selectively labeled, so that the vascular territory of each cervical artery can be individually imaged. However, current ASL pulse sequences are more time-consuming than DSC and thus more susceptible to patient motion. In addition, the maps generated are far noisier, with poorer spatial resolution than DSC maps. They require further validation as a tool in acute stroke.[32]

Diffusion and Perfusion in Acute Stroke Treatment

Correlation of Diffusion-Weighted Imaging and Perfusion-Weighted Imaging with Clinical and Tissue Outcome

A number of studies have shown that DWI can be used to predict clinical and radiologic outcomes. Initial DWI lesion volume correlates well with final infarct volume on T2 and FLAIR images, and slightly underestimates it, with correlation coefficients ranging from 0.72 to 0.9.[3,21,25,31,33] Initial DWI lesion volume also correlates well with clinical outcome, as measured by multiple neurologic assessment tests, including the National Institutes of Health Stroke Scale (NIHSS) score, Canadian Neurological Scale, Glasgow Outcome Scale, Barthel index, and modified Rankin Scale.[3,34] Correlation coefficients between DWI lesion volume and clinical outcome range from 0.65 to 0.78. In general, correlations are stronger for cortical strokes than for penetrator artery strokes and for left-sided versus right-sided strokes.[34] Recent work in early reperfusion trials shows that DWI correlates best with final infarct and with clinical outcome scales when there is complete reperfusion.[35] Furthermore, large initial DWI volumes predict poor outcome. For example, one study demonstrated that for internal carotid artery (ICA) and MCA strokes treated with various therapies including thrombolytic agents, a DWI volume greater than 89 cc was highly predictive of early neurologic deterioration (receiver operating characteristics [ROC] curve with 85.7% sensitivity and 95.7% specificity).[36] Another study, performed in patients with proximal MCA emboli, who received intravascular thrombolytic agents, demonstrated that patients with an initial DWI lesion volume of greater than 70 cc had a much worse outcome compared with those patients with an initial DWI lesion volume of less than 70 cc (71.5% vs. 0% 90-day mortality).[37] A third study, investigating anterior circulation strokes treated with intraarterial therapy, showed that 100% of patients with an initial DWI lesion volume greater than 70 cc did poorly (defined as a modified Rankin Scale score of 3 to 6).[31] Because patients with an initial large DWI

stroke volume have poor outcomes and an increased risk of intracranial hemorrhage, those with an initial DWI lesion volume of greater than one third of the MCA territory or greater than 100 cc are typically excluded from acute stroke trials.[33] The CBV abnormality (depicting changes due to capillary collapse) also represents infarct core; however, it is not as accurate as DWI and is only used if the DWI images are technically inadequate.

In general, perfusion parameters such as CBF, MTT, TTP, and T_{max} lesion volumes are generally much larger than the DWI lesions, correlate less well with final infarct volume, and on average greatly overestimate final infarct volume[23,38] **(Table 8.6)**. Tissue that appears normal on DWI but abnormal on the perfusion images is thought to represent the ischemic penumbra. The ischemic penumbra usually surrounds the core, where collateral vessels supply some residual perfu-

Table 8.6 Common Perfusion-Weighted Imaging (PWI) Parameters

Parameter	Comments
DWI	Represents ischemic infarct "core," is usually irreversible in the absence of early reperfusion
	Highly predictive of final infarct volume with strokes on average growing 20%
	With thrombolysis, a portion of the DWI abnormality may be reversible, especially in white matter
	Lower ADC ratios and values trend toward irreversibility; threshold difficult to define
	Best parameter for predicting patient outcome; patients with DWI lesion volume greater than 70–100 cc do poorly
CBV	Less reliable than DWI to evaluate infarct core
	Low CBV is predictive of infarction
	Markedly elevated CBV is unstable; may or may not infarct
CBF	Measures operational penumbra; in general overestimates final infarct size
	With proximal occlusions, is usually larger than DWI
	? Best parameter for distinguishing between penumbra likely to infarct from penumbra likely to survive in spite of intervention; relative threshold for tissue viability—0.27 in early recanalizers and 0.41 in late recanalizers and nonrecanalizers
MTT	With proximal occlusions, is usually larger than DWI and yields the largest operational penumbra
	Usually overestimates final infarct size
	Controversy as to whether or not MTT is useful for distinguishing between penumbra likely to infarct and that likely to survive; one large study suggests a relative threshold of 1.78
TTP	Measures operational penumbra and in general overestimates final infarct size
	With proximal occlusions is usually larger than DWI
	TTP of 6 to 8 seconds correlates well with final infarct size
T_{max}	Measures operational penumbra and in general overestimates final infarct size
	With proximal occlusions is usually larger than DWI
	T_{max} of 4 to 6 seconds and relative T_{max} of 1.45 correlate well with final infarct size
Factors affecting calculations of thresholds for tissue viability	Timing of reperfusion
	Gray versus white matter
	Timing of initial and follow-up scans
	Variability in post ischemic tissue responses

Abbreviations: CBF, cerebral blood flow; CBV, cerebral blood volume; DWI, diffusion-weighted imaging; MTT, mean transit time; T_{max}, the time-to-peak of the deconvolved residue function; TTP, time to peak.

sion. The penumbra represents tissue that may progress to infarction or may recover depending on the timing of reperfusion and the degree of collateralization.[39]

The number of patients who have an ischemic penumbra is estimated to be at least 80% within the first 3 hours.[40] Additionally, a penumbra is much more likely to occur with proximal arterial occlusions than with lacunar or distal infarcts. In fact, a recent study showed that 80% of patients with untreated proximal artery occlusions can have mismatches that last for more than 9 hours.[41] Volumes of perfusion lesions also correlate with clinical outcome. The correlations are highest when there is no reperfusion and the infarction eventually extends into the penumbra.

The best perfusion parameter for determining the penumbra has been a subject of much investigation; a recent study comparing different PWI parameters within the same cohort found large variances in penumbral estimates, within the same patient.[42] There is no current consensus on which PWI lesion to measure, how to measure it, and which postprocessing software to use. Earlier studies suggested that deconvolved MTT maps best predicted follow-up tissue outcome. However, more recent studies have found no benefit of MTT over other transit time measures.[43] In general, MTT, TTP or T_{max} are chosen to represent the penumbra because contrast-to-noise ratios are higher on these maps compared with others.

Furthermore, the PWI defect may contain regions with benign oligemia, that is, tissue that will survive whether or not there is early reperfusion. To separate true mismatch from benign oligemia, some investigators have compared thresholded blood flow and transit time map lesion volumes with follow-up lesion volumes in patients who did not reperfuse. A T_{max} of 4 to 6 seconds provided the best estimate of final infarct volume in a subset of patients from the DEFUSE trial.[44] Christensen et al[43] demonstrated that a relative T_{max} of 1.45 seconds, a relative MTT of 1.78 seconds, and a relative first moment of 3.51 seconds were the optimal operating points on ROC curves comparing initial transit time abnormalities to follow-up infarct, on a voxel by voxel basis.

In patients who reperfuse, a threshold for tissue infarction is more difficult to define because the thresholds are dependent on the timing of reperfusion. In a seminal primate study, the CBF threshold for tissue infarction was 17 to 18 mL/100 g/min if the subject experienced permanent occlusion. However, if perfusion was reestablished in 2 to 3 hours, the subject could tolerate a much lower CBF, 10 to 12 mL/100 g/min, before infarction occurred.[45] Similarly, Schaefer et al,[46] comparing initial CBF with follow-up infarction on a voxel by voxel basis, demonstrated optimal relative CBF thresholds of 0.27 (i.e., relative CBF 27% of normal) for tissue reperfused at less than 6 hours, versus 0.41 for tissue that is reperfused at greater than or equal to 6 hours. Better models to predict tissue at risk are under development. For example, Wu et al[47] developed a voxel-based generalized linear threshold model utilizing DWI and multiple perfusion maps that improved predictive value of tissue outcome compared with models based on a single parameter.

Mismatch and Patient Selection

After a patient presents with an acute stroke syndrome, the current standard of care is to perform noncontrast head CT, which if negative for a hemorrhage or for a >100 cc hypodensity in an MCA territory, allows for administration of IV rTPA. This is based on well-accepted clinical data dating back to the National Institute of Neurological Disorders and Stroke (NINDS) study in 1995.[48] A recent large phase 3 thrombolysis trial suggested that administration of IV rTPA up to 4.5 hours after the onset of the stroke is efficacious.[49,50] If a patient presents with acute stroke but is outside the 3- to 4.5-hour window for IV therapy, delayed IV therapy, or intraarterial recanalization, currently recommended up to 6 hours after onset of symptoms, may be attempted.[49] In either case, to ensure best application of an aggressive treatment with inherent risks, proper patient selection is crucial. This is where PWI in conjunction with DWI is most useful.

There are five possible scenarios when obtaining DWI and PWI, as outlined in **Table 8.7** and **Figs. 8.7, 8.8,** and **8.9.** A DWI lesion without a PWI lesion or larger than the PWI lesion implies early spontaneous reperfusion. If the DWI lesion is equal to the PWI lesion, it is generally accepted that the infarct has completed. Patients with these patterns usually do not receive thrombolytic therapy or recanalization because

Table 8.7 Mismatch Patterns

Pattern	Cause	Comment
PWI, no DWI	Proximal occlusion or critical stenosis with ischemic tissue perfused via collaterals	DWI abnormalities may develop depending on collateralization and timing of reperfusion; good candidate for reperfusion therapy
PWI > DWI	Proximal occlusion or critical stenosis with penumbra partially perfused via collaterals	DWI may expand into part or all of the PWI abnormality depending on collateralization and timing of reperfusion; good candidate for reperfusion therapy
PWI = DWI	Usually occurs with lacunes or distal occlusions	Entire territory has infarcted; no tissue at risk
PWI < DWI	Proximal, distal, or lacunar infarct	Ischemic tissue has reperfused; no tissue at risk
DWI but no PWI	Proximal, distal, or lacunar infarct	Ischemic tissue has reperfused; no tissue at risk; also, tiny infarctions not seen on PWI due to lower resolution

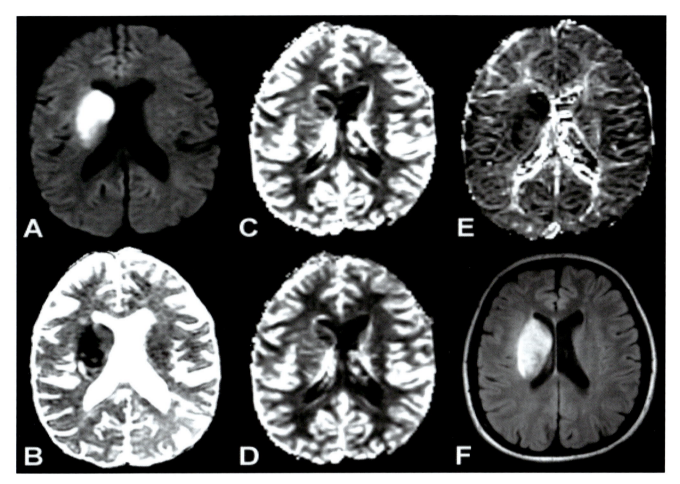

Fig. 8.7 A DWI lesion larger than a mean transit time (MTT) lesion. A 37-year-old woman with left hemiparesis, imaged 1 day following recanalization therapy. There is a DWI-hyperintense **(A)** and ADC-hypointense **(B)** lesion in the right corona radiata, consistent with an early subacute acute infarction. There is mildly elevated cerebral blood volume (CBV) **(C)** and cerebral blood flow (CBF) **(D)** and decreased MTT **(E)** within the lesion, consistent with reperfusion. Follow-up FLAIR image **(F)** shows no evidence of infarct extension.

the infarction is not expected to extend.[51,52] Aggressive therapies generally concentrate on two groups, a DWI lesion smaller than the PWI lesion, or a PWI lesion without a DWI lesion, because those are the patients with tissue at risk of further infarction.

Several clinical trials addressing the use of intravenous thrombolytic agents beyond the 3-hour time window have validated the mismatch concept. The Desmoteplase in Acute Ischemic Stroke (DIAS) trial[51] and the Dose Escalation of Desmoteplase for Acute Ischemic Stroke (DEDAS) trial[53] utilized a 20% mismatch between the PWI and DWI lesions as a trial entry criterion; patients were given intravenous desmoteplase (a thrombolytic agent derived from bat venom) or placebo at between 3 and 9 hours after symptom onset. These trials demonstrated that administration of desmoteplase was associated with dose-dependent rates of higher reperfusion and better clinical outcomes compared with placebo. In the DEFUSE study, 74 patients recruited on the basis of CT findings received IV rTPA within 3 to 6 hours after stroke onset. Early reperfusion was associated with a significantly increased chance of a favorable clinical response in patients with at least a 20% DWI-PWI mismatch, whereas patients without a mismatch did not benefit from early reperfusion.[52] In the Echoplanar Imaging Thrombolytic Evaluation Trial (EPITHET), 101 patients were recruited on the basis of CT selection criteria and received IV rTPA or placebo within 3 to 6 hours after stroke onset; of these, 86% had a mismatch. Although there was no significant difference in infarct growth between patients who received placebo and those who received IV rTPA, there was increased reperfusion in those with a mismatch; additionally, reperfusion was associated with less infarct growth and improved clinical outcomes.[54] When mismatch as a target for therapy was first introduced, it was arbitrarily defined as PWI lesion 20% larger than the baseline DWI lesion volume. However, some investigators have suggested using a larger mismatch. For example, the DEFUSE investigators retrospectively determined an optimum PWI/DWI ratio of 2.6 (i.e., a PWI lesion 2.6 times larger than the DWI lesion) for the best chance of a favorable outcome after early reperfusion.[55] The EPITHET investigators suggest a 2.0 ratio.[56] The MRA-DWI mismatch is a possible alternative model. THE DEFUSE investigators found that patients with a

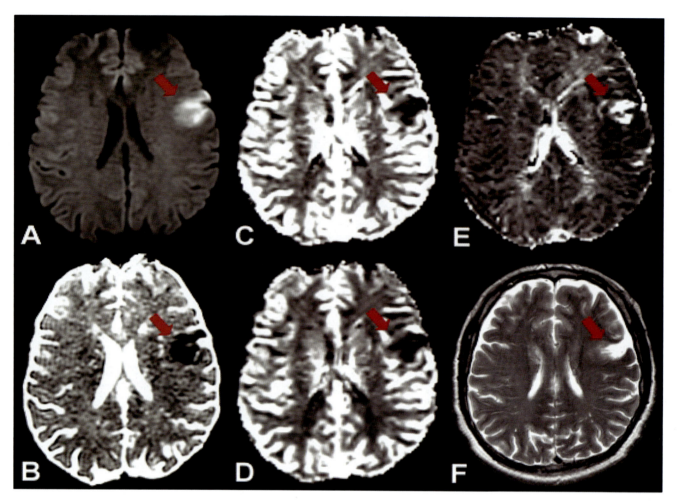

Fig. 8.8 A matched DWI-MTT lesion. A 54-year-old man with acute aphasia who was imaged initially at 5 hours following symptom onset. The initial DWI **(A)** and ADC **(B)** maps demonstrate an acute infarction in the left inferior frontal region. The lesion is of similar size on the CBV **(C)**, CBF **(D)**, and MTT **(E)** maps, indicating no tissue at risk. Follow-up T2-weighted image **(F)** obtained at 7 days demonstrates no infarct extension.

MRA-DWI mismatch (defined as a DWI lesion less than 25 cc with a proximal vessel occlusion, or a DWI lesion less than 15 cc with a proximal vessel stenosis or distal abnormal vessel) had an increased rate of favorable clinical response when reperfused compared with those without a mismatch.[57]

Most patients do not receive MRI prior to intraarterial therapy due to the relative inaccessibility of MRI and the consequent delay in treatment. However, one recent study demonstrated that in patients with proximal occlusions, large diffusion-perfusion mismatches and initial infarct volumes greater than 70 cc had significantly better clinical outcomes if they recanalized early, versus those who recanalized late or not at all.[58] Another study, showed that patients with a clinical-diffusion mismatch (NIHSS scale >8 and DWI lesion volume <25 cc) and presentation beyond 8 hours of symptom onset could be successfully revascularized without intracranial hemorrhage or early neurologic deterioration.[59]

For patients for whom the stroke onset time is unknown, early MRI may also be helpful. One study assessed 32 pa-

tients with unclear onset time, little to no FLAIR changes, a DWI abnormality, and a PWI-DWI mismatch who were treated with IV rTPA within 3 hours and/or intraarterial urokinase within 6 hours of symptom detection. There was no difference in recanalization rates, early neurologic improvement, symptomatic intra cranial hemorrhage, or 3-month clinical outcome in these patients compared with 223 patients with known stroke onset time.[60]

Predicting Risk of Hemorrhage

Hemorrhagic transformation of an acute ischemic stroke occurs because of recirculation into severely ischemic tissue with an abnormally permeable vascular bed.[61] Severe ischemia compromises the basal lamina of the blood vessels comprising the blood–brain barrier. Then, extravasation of blood allows inflammatory markers and mediators into the compromised region, further increasing capillary permeability.[62]

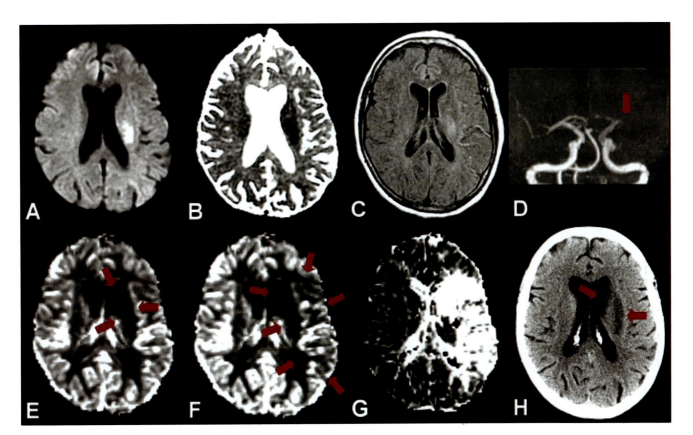

Fig. 8.9 Small initial infarction with a large diffusion perfusion mismatch. An 85-year-old woman with right hemiplegia and dysarthria, imaged at 4.75 hours from stroke onset. There is hyperintensity on the DWI image **(A)**, hypointensity on the ADC map **(B)**, and hypointensity on the CBV map **(E)** in the left corona radiata, consistent with a small infarct core. The infarct is only slightly hyperintense on the FLAIR image **(C)**, consistent with an infarct that is less than 6 hours old. **(D)** The three-dimensional (3D) time-of-flight (TOF) MR angiogram demonstrates no flow-related enhancement distal to the proximal left MCA stem, consistent with acute thrombus. There is low CBF (hypointense, **F**) and prolonged MTT (hyperintense, **G**) throughout much of the left MCA territory. The DWI-normal but CBF- and MTT-abnormal tissue is thought to represent the ischemic penumbra. The patient underwent aggressive hypertensive therapy. Follow-up computed tomography (CT) **(H)** at 5 days demonstrates hypodensity, consistent with infarction, of the left basal ganglia and corona radiata (regions initially characterized by DWI hyperintensity). None of the penumbra has progressed to infarction.

Hemorrhagic transformation (HT) has an incidence of 15 to 26% during the first 2 weeks, and up to 43% after the first month.

Hemorrhagic transformation can be classified into four categories as seen in **Table 8.8**.[63] It should be noted that these classifications do not take into account the clinical impact of such findings and that an increased risk of hemorrhage does not necessarily imply poor patient outcome. For example, a study of 32 patients with proximal MCA occlusion treated with rTPA found that the nine patients with HI-type hemorrhages had a statistically significant higher rate of improvement, compared with patients with both parenchymal hemorrhage and those with no intracranial hemorrhage.[9] The term "symptomatic intracranial hemorrhage" generally refers to deterioration of the patient's clinical condition in the judgment of the clinician.[48] In both European Cooperative Acute Stroke Study (ECASS) trials, only hemorrhages of the PH-2 type impacted long-term outcome; therefore, PH-2 has been suggested as a standardized safety point for future trials.[64] However, there is still controversy with regard to whether less severe forms of hemorrhage are important.

Many factors contribute to HT. Thrombolytic therapy increases the risk of hemorrhage, with an odds ratio of 3.37 according to one review.[65] Clinical risk factors include greater severity of baseline stroke symptoms, elevated blood glucose,

Table 8.8 Types of Hemorrhagic Transformation

Type of hemorrhage	Description
HI-1	Small petechiae along margins of infarct
HI-2	More confluent petechiae without mass effect
PH-1	Hematoma involving 30% or less of infarct, with mild mass effect
PH-2	Dense hematoma greater than 30% of infarct; any hemorrhage outside infarct

advanced age, increased time to treatment, low platelets, hypertension, prior history of congestive heart failure (CHF), and cardioembolic etiology of stroke.[66] Imaging risk factors demonstrated on angiography or CT in early stroke studies include hypodensity on noncontrast CT in greater than one third of the MCA territory, good collateral circulation, and early reperfusion.[67]

More recently, a number of investigators have reported MRI parameters that are predictive of HT (**Fig. 8.10; Table 8.9**): (1) a DWI lesion greater than one third of the MCA territory, (2) a PWI lesion greater than 100 cc with T_{max} >8, (3) low ADC values in the infarct core (ranging from 300×10^{-6} mm²/s to $\leq 550 \times 10^{-6}$ mm²/s), (4) abnormal visibility of transcerebral veins on T2*-weighted images, (5) moderate to severe deep white matter lesions, (6) early parenchymal enhancement, (7) CBF ratio of less than 0.18 on MR perfusion imaging, (8) and increased permeability on dynamic contrast-enhanced T1-weighted images.[68–72]

Several recent large studies have demonstrated that microhemorrhages on T2* images are not associated with an increased risk of symptomatic HT of acute ischemic stroke. For example, in a study of 65 patients for anterior circulation strokes treated with thrombolytic agents, the presence of microbleeds was not an independent risk factor for early HT or symptomatic hemorrhage.[73] A 2007 prospective study of 152 patients suggested that microbleeds are a clinically irrelevant phenomenon related to reperfusion after ischemia with or without the use of thrombolytics, whereas parenchymal hemorrhage appears to be mediated by a separate pathophysiologic pathway related to the presence of rTPA.[74] More clarification is needed.

Magnetic Resonance Angiography in Acute Stroke

Magnetic resonance angiography can be useful in the acute stroke setting to assess the presence and degree of stenosis or occlusion and the presence of collateral flow (**Table 8.10**). In the setting of acute stroke, a typical protocol is a three-dimensional (3D) time-of-flight (TOF) sequence through the

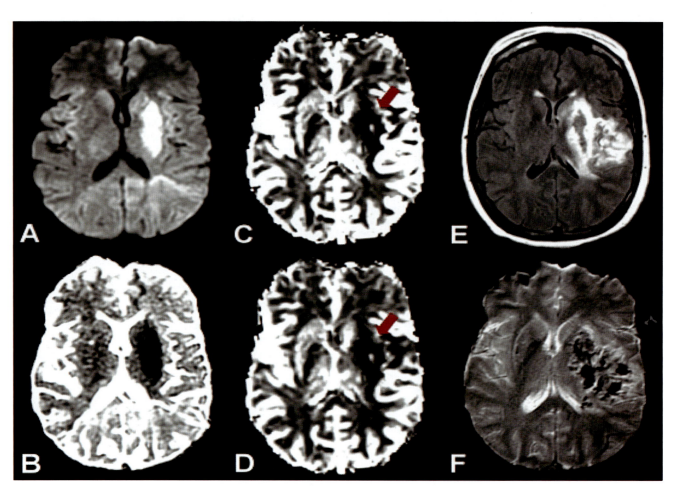

Fig. 8.10 Hemorrhagic transformation. A 58-year-old woman with right hemiparesis, who received IV tissue-type plasminogen activator (rTPA) and was imaged at 5 hours after stroke onset. DWI **(A)** and ADC **(B)** images demonstrate an acute infarction in the left basal ganglia. The lesion is markedly hypointense on ADC images, consistent with very low ADC values. There is also marked hypointensity on the CBV **(C)** and CBF **(D)** maps in the left basal ganglia and inferior frontal lobe, consistent with very low blood volume and flow, respectively. Follow-up FLAIR **(E)** image at 19 days shows extension of the infarction into the inferior frontal lobe and hemorrhagic transformation, characterized by low signal on gradient echo T2* sequences **(F).**

Table 8.9 Factors Predictive for Hemorrhagic Transformation

Imaging findings	DWI greater than one third of the MCA territory
	Severely decreased ADC values in the infarct core
	Abnormal visibility of transcerebral veins on T2* images
	Moderate to severe deep white matter lesions
	Early parenchymal enhancement
	CBF ratio <0.18
	PWI greater than 100 cc, with T_{max} >8
	Increased permeability
Clinical findings	High National Institutes of Health Stroke Scale (NIHSS) score
	Elevated blood glucose
	Advanced age
	Low platelets
	Hypertension
	History of congestive heart failure (CHF)
Vascular variables	Embolic stroke etiology
	Good collaterals
	Early reperfusion
Therapies undertaken	Anticoagulation
	Thrombolytic therapy
	Increased time to treatment

circle of Willis, and a contrast-enhanced sequence through the neck. For patients who cannot receive a gadolinium injection, a two-dimensional (2D) or 3D TOF sequence through the neck is performed. To determine the presence of arterial dissection, an axial fat-saturated T1-weighted image can be performed as well.

Neck

For patients who cannot receive gadolinium, TOF MRA is typically performed. TOF is a gradient echo technique that images vascular flow by repeatedly applying an RF pulse to a given volume of tissue and subsequently obtaining images; because their spins have been saturated, the stationary tissues give little or no signal, whereas protons carried into the block of tissue within a blood vessel and unexposed to the saturating pulses remain bright. To avoid imaging of venous structures, a saturation pulse is placed superior to the block.

In the neck, TOF can be performed in a 2D technique utilizing multiple contiguous axial thin sections.[75] However, several limitations exist. If flowing blood does not exit a slice before the next RF pulse, it is subject to saturation and signal loss; signal loss is frequently seen in horizontal portions of arteries, such as the vertebral arteries where they turn around C1, and the petrous internal carotid arteries.[76] Vessel

stenoses can also be overestimated due to slow flow in the periphery of vessels, or turbulent flow leading to intravoxel phase dispersion and signal loss. In general, 2D TOF images overestimate stenoses, and do not reliably assess the arch and great vessel origins.

Three-dimensional TOF imaging of the neck can also be performed by exciting a volume of tissue and using an extra phase-encoding step to divide it into multiple contiguous thin sections. Compared with 2D TOF MRA, 3D TOF offers higher spatial resolution and less signal loss due to intravoxel dephasing. However, it is limited by increased saturation effects and can only cover a small area of interest such as the carotid bifurcation.

For patients who can receive gadolinium, contrast-enhanced MRA of the neck is the protocol of choice. Images are typically acquired in the coronal plane and the peak of the contrast bolus is mapped to the center of k-space. It has several advantages over 2D TOF imaging. Contrast-enhanced MRA can cover a larger area of anatomy (the arch, great vessel origins, and whole neck) in a shorter time with less susceptibility to patient motion. It has a higher signal-to-noise ratio, and does not overestimate stenoses as much as TOF because it is less susceptible to turbulence-related dephasing and loss of signal due to saturation effects. However, it requires imaging during a narrow window of time to avoid venous contamination; if the bolus is missed, it cannot be repeated until the gadolinium has cleared. The edge of the imaged slab often has a poor signal-to-noise ratio, and respiratory motion can particularly affect imaging of the aorta and major cervical arterial origins.[76]

Head

Because the head is a smaller area to cover, routine MRA is typically performed with 3D TOF, which offers better spatial resolution, signal-to-noise ratio, and less intravoxel dephasing compared with 2D TOF. However, its longer acquisition time renders it more susceptible to saturation artifact. Because it typically utilizes a small flip angle, background tissues with intrinsically high T1-weighted signal such as fat or hemorrhage may also appear as foci of high signal and may be mistaken for flow-related enhancement.

Contrast-enhanced MRA is not typically used in the head because it requires an extra dose of gadolinium, has inferior spatial resolution, and can often be compromised by venous contamination. However, recent studies have used contrast-enhanced MRA of the head to improve sensitivity for distal stenoses or occlusions, mostly in the setting of transient ischemic attack. A prospective study utilizing both 3 Tesla noncontrast and contrast MRAs in conjunction with MRI for patients with transient ischemic attacks showed that those patients with a DWI lesion were 2.6 times more likely to have a new stroke, and those with a lesion and an intracranial occlusion were 8.9 times more likely.[77]

Other Magnetic Resonance Angiography Techniques

Phase-contrast MRA is another noncontrast technique based on the principle that inflowing blood causes a phase shift.

Table 8.10 Magnetic Resonance Angiography (MRA) Techniques and Applications

	Advantages	Disadvantages	Clinical Applications
2D time of flight (2DTOF)	• Noninvasive • Can image slow flow • Can image large volume of tissue • Can repeat if suboptimal	• Overestimates vessel stenosis • In-plane signal loss • Signal loss from turbulence • Low spatial resolution • Artifact from T1 hyperintense lesions	• Back up neck MRA if ceMRA not optimal • Routine for MR venography • Physiologic—can suggest subclavian steal if combined with ceMRA
3D time of flight (3D TOF)	• Noninvasive • High spatial resolution • Shows complex vascular flow • Less susceptible to intravoxel dephasing • Can be repeated if suboptimal • Can be obtained after contrast	• Only small volumes due to marked saturation effects • Cannot image slow flow because of saturation effects • Time consuming, susceptible to patient motion • Artifact from T1 hyperintense lesions	• Routine to evaluate circle of Willis for large vessel stenoses/ occlusions • Can estimate carotid bifurcation stenoses
2D phase contrast (2D PC MRA)	• Can show direction and magnitude of flow • No artifact from T1 hyperintense lesions • Can show very slow moving blood. • Can be obtained after contrast • Can be repeated if suboptimal	• Low spatial resolution • More susceptible to turbulent dephasing than TOF MRA • Can have aliasing artifact • 2D PC of neck is longer than 2D TOF of neck	• Can determine collateral flow around circle of Willis (COW) • Can detect subclavian steal and abnormal flow direction in neck • Can detect slow flow if near-occlusion is suspected
3D phase contrast (3D PC MRA)	• High spatial resolution • Does not show high signal artifact from T1 hyperintense lesions	• Time consuming; 3D TOF MRA is faster, with similar resolution	• Rarely used • Used if intravascular clot will confuse 3D TOF MRA interpretation
Contrast-enhanced MRA (ceMRA)	• Fast, minimizing patient motion artifact • Less susceptible to signal loss from flow turbulence • No saturation artifact • Good signal-to-noise ratio • Images large volume of tissue • No high signal artifact from T1 hyperintense lesions • Accurate in estimating stenoses • Helps differentiate occlusion from near-occlusion	• Lower spatial resolution than 3D TOF MRA • Occasionally underestimates stenosis • must be obtained in arterial phase • Cannot be repeated until IV contrast has cleared • Requires rapid power injection of contrast	• Routinely used to evaluate stenoses and occlusions of neck vessels and origins

Two sets of images are obtained after an initial RF pulse; the first is obtained after a gradient and the second after an equal and opposite gradient. The two sets of images are subtracted. Stationary tissue has little to no signal because the equal and opposite gradient pulses result in zero phase shift. For moving spins there is a net phase shift, resulting in signal that is proportional to their velocity. Phase-contrast MRA is useful in that it can demonstrate flow direction; it can also show very slow flow that is typically saturated out on TOF images. Because background tissues are completely subtracted, it is not subject to the T1-hyperintense background artifacts that limit 3D TOF MRA. However, because of longer acquisition time, it is more subject to motion artifact; because of a longer echo time (TE), it is more prone to signal loss due to intravoxel dephasing. For these reasons, it is usually only used in a problem-solving manner to determine the presence and/ or direction of flow in the anterior or posterior communicating arteries, basilar artery, or severely stenotic internal carotid arteries.

Accuracy

In the acute setting, detection of severely stenotic or occlusive lesions is especially important if catheter-based therapies are being considered. However, MRA is generally used less frequently than computed tomography angiography (CTA) because its accuracy is inferior to that of CTA, it is less readily available, and is more time consuming.

Magnetic resonance angiography of the head in acute stroke is useful mostly for identifying acute proximal large vessel occlusions, and is less useful for detecting distal occlusions. Its overall sensitivity and specificity for detecting acute proximal large vessel occlusions range from 70 to 100%.[49] As mentioned above, a MRA-DWI mismatch (defined as a DWI lesion less than 25 cc with a proximal vessel occlusion, or a DWI lesion volume less than 15 cc with proximal vessel stenosis or an abnormal finding of a distal vessel) has been reported as a possible marker of patients with stroke who are likely to benefit from reperfusion therapy.[57,78]

Magnetic resonance angiography of the neck is quite accurate for identifying severe (greater than 70%) ICA stenosis and occlusion **(Fig. 8.11)**. A recent meta-analysis comparing 2D and 3D TOF MRA to diagnostic catheter angiography demonstrated sensitivity and specificity of 91% and 88% for TOF MRA, and 95% and 92% for contrast-enhanced (CE) MRA, in identifying severe (70–99%) ICA stenosis. For identifying ICA occlusions, TOF sensitivity and specificity were 95% and 99%, and CE MRA sensitivity and specificity were 99% and 100%. For less severe stenoses, TOF performed poorly, with a sensitivity and specificity of 38% and 92%, whereas CE MRA demonstrated a sensitivity and specificity of 66% and 94%.[79]

Magnetic Resonance Angiography for Dissection

Cervical artery dissections are a relatively common cause of ischemic stroke in younger populations[80] **(Fig. 8.12)**. They can be spontaneous or posttraumatic, or can occur in an underlying disease state affecting the connective tissues, such

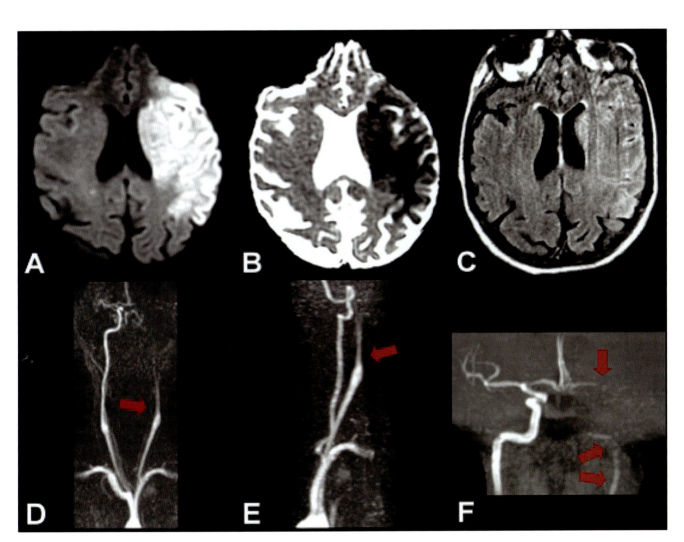

Fig. 8.11 Magnetic resonance angiography (MRA) demonstrating string sign and acute ICA embolus. A 51-year-old woman with acute left hemiparesis, imaged at 7 hours. DWI **(A)** and ADC **(B)** images demonstrate a large acute infarction involving most of the left MCA territory. The infarction is mildly hyperintense on FLAIR images **(C)**. Contrast-enhanced MRA of the neck **(D,E)** and 3D time-of-flight MRA of the circle of Willis **(F)** demonstrate a left ICA string sign extending from the origin to the precavernous ICA. There is no flow-related enhancement in the distal left internal carotid artery or in the proximal left middle or anterior cerebral arteries.

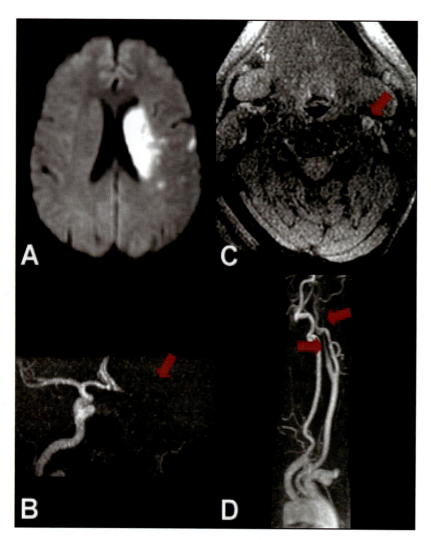

Fig. 8.12 An MRI and MRA demonstrating dissection. A 50-year-old man with right hemiparesis. **(A)** DWI demonstrates a left MCA territory infarction involving predominantly the left caudate body and corona radiata. Fat-saturated T1-weighted axial images **(B)** demonstrate T1 hyperintensity (methemoglobin) within the left ICA wall, consistent with dissection. Contrast-enhanced MRA of the neck **(C)** demonstrates tapering of the left ICA *(arrow)* from its origin into a string sign. 3D TOF MRA of the circle of Willis **(D)** demonstrates minimal flow-related enhancement in the vertical petrous left ICA, but no flow-related enhancement in the more distal ICA or in the proximal ACA or MCA, consistent with slow flow and occlusion.

as fibromuscular dysplasia or Marfan disease. Most often dissection occurs in the carotid arteries as they enter the skull base, and in the vertebral arteries from C2 to the foramen magnum. Conventional MRI has relatively high sensitivity (84%) and specificity (99%) for detecting ICA dissection, typically showing eccentric T1 hyperintensity representing subacute hemorrhage in the false lumen **(Fig. 8.12).** Three-dimensional TOF MRA also has excellent sensitivity (95%) and specificity (99%) for detecting ICA dissection, compared with conventional angiography. For vertebral artery dissection, MRI/MRA is less useful; conventional MRI has a sensitivity of 60% and specificity of 58%, and 3D TOF MRA has a sensitivity of 20%, with a specificity of 100%.[80,81]

◆ Hemorrhagic Stroke

Hemorrhagic stroke encompasses both nontraumatic intraparenchymal hemorrhage and subarachnoid hemorrhage, has an incidence of roughly 30 to 75/100,000 persons per year and comprises approximately 9 to 18% of strokes in adults of ages 45 to 84.[82] Risk factors for intraparenchymal

hemorrhage include male sex, advanced age, hypertension, and high alcohol intake, with weaker associations with concurrent smoking and diabetes.[83] Risk factors for subarachnoid hemorrhage include hypertension, smoking, and high alcohol intake.[84]

Primary intraparenchymal hemorrhage in adults results from rupture of small deep or cortical penetrating arteries within the brain parenchyma, which is most often the result of hypertension or amyloid angiopathy and accounts for 78 to 88% of cases.[85] Secondary intraparenchymal hemorrhage accounts for the remainder of cases and occurs as a result of vascular lesions (such as arteriovenous malformations, aneurysms, arteriovenous fistulas, and cavernous malformations), venous sinus thrombosis, primary or metastatic tumors, coagulopathy, trauma, or drug abuse **(Table 8.11).** Relatively less common causes include moyamoya disease, posterior reversible encephalopathy syndrome (PRES), reversible vasoconstriction syndrome, and vasculitis. Subarachnoid hemorrhage most commonly results from ruptured aneurysm (85%) followed by nonaneurysmal perimesencephalic hemorrhage (10%), with other uncommon etiologies accounting for the remaining cases.[84,86]

Table 8.11 Etiologies of Hemorrhagic Stroke

Hypertension*

Amyloid angiopathy*

Coagulopathy*

Vascular lesions*

Cavernous malformation

Arteriovenous malformation

Aneurysm

Dural arteriovenous fistula

Tumor*

Cerebral venous sinus thrombosis*

Moyamoya

Posterior reversible encephalopathy syndrome

Reversible vasoconstriction syndrome

Vasculitis

Infection

Septic emboli

Toxoplasmosis

Aspergillus

Mucormycosis

Herpes simplex virus

Drug abuse

*Most common causes in adults with hypertension and amyloid angiopathy accounting for 78 to 88%.

In the pediatric population, hemorrhagic stroke accounts for approximately one half of all strokes with an incidence of 1.1 to 1.4/100,000 person-years, with roughly two thirds classified as intraparenchymal and one third as subarachnoid hemorrhage.[87] In this population, the most common etiologies of intraparenchymal hemorrhage include arteriovenous malformations accounting for 14 to 57%, hematologic abnormalities (including thrombocytopenia, hemophilia, and coagulopathy) accounting for 10 to 30%, brain tumors accounting for 2 to 22%, and cavernous malformations accounting for 3 to 27%.[88]

Imaging Approach

Imaging typically begins with a noncontrast head CT scan that serves to identify and localize the hemorrhage. Further imaging with a CT angiogram is then indicated to search for an underlying vascular lesion. Predictors of underlying vascular etiology include age 45 years or younger, absence of known hypertension or coagulopathy, female sex, lobar or infratentorial location of hemorrhage, and lobar intraparenchymal hemorrhage with associated intraventricular hemorrhage.[86] Intraarterial digital subtraction angiography is typically performed when further characterization of a vascular lesion demonstrated on CTA is required or when CTA does not show an underlying vascular lesion but the patient is age 45 years or younger, does not have risk factors for hypertension and is not anticoagulated, or has hemorrhage in unusual locations. MRI may be performed to further characterize a vascular lesion for surgical planning. In cases where no vascular lesion is detected by CTA, MRI is performed to search for other underlying etiologies. Typically gadolinium is administered to improve detection of an underlying mass lesion, and susceptibility sensitive images are obtained to detect additional hemorrhages that may suggest a specific diagnosis, as described in more detail below.

Conventional Magnetic Resonance Imaging of Hemorrhage

Computed tomography has traditionally been the first-line imaging modality in the workup of acute stroke largely to determine the presence of hyperacute/acute blood products. This stems in part from the belief that MRI is relatively insensitive to their detection. However, MRI with T2*-weighted gradient echo images has comparable sensitivity to CT for the detection of hyperacute hemorrhage[89] and is more sensitive than CT for the detection of subacute and chronic hemorrhage.[89] High sensitivity has also been reported for the detection of hyperacute subarachnoid hemorrhage with proton density and FLAIR images.[90]

The signal characteristics of hemorrhage are dependent on the chemical state of hemoglobin or the presence of its breakdown products, red blood cell membrane integrity, the pulse sequence, and magnetic field strength.[91] Intraparenchymal hematoma undergoes a predictable pattern of evolution with time on T1 and FLAIR/T2-weighted images (**Table 8.12**).

In the hyperacute phase (up to 12 to 24 hours), the hematoma contains primarily diamagnetic oxyhemoglobin, which is isointense on T1- and hyperintense on T2-weighted images.[91] In the acute phase (1 to 3 days), paramagnetic deoxyhemoglobin within intact red blood cells, which exhibits isointensity on T1- and hypointensity on T2-weighted images, predominates. This is followed by the oxidation of deoxyhemoglobin to paramagnetic methemoglobin within intact red blood cells in the early subacute phase (4 to 7 days), which demonstrates hyperintensity on T1- and hypointensity on T2-weighted images. As red blood cell lysis occurs, extracellular methemoglobin appears during the late subacute phase (1 week to several months); it is hyperintense on both T1- and T2-weighted images. In the chronic phase (after several months), macrophages containing paramagnetic ferritin and hemosiderin lead to hypointensity on both T1- and T2-weighted images.[91]

Subdural and epidural hematomas and subarachnoid hemorrhage undergo temporal evolution that is relatively slower than intraparenchymal hematomas due to higher oxygen tension within their respective compartments.[91] The MRI pattern is similar to parenchymal hematomas, with the exception of the chronic stage in which hemosiderin is less likely to be present.[91,92]

T2*-weighted images performed with the gradient echo or echo planar technique accentuate susceptibility effects. They demonstrate signal hypointensity in the setting of the para-

Table 8.12 MRI Appearance of Intraparenchymal Hemorrhage

	Hemoglobin State	T1	T2	FLAIR	T2*/SWI	DWI
Hyperacute (up to 12–24 hour)	Oxyhemoglobin core, peripheral Deoxyhemoglobin	Isointense	Hyperintense	Hyperintense	Central hyperintensity, hypointense rim	Hyperintense
Acute (1–3 days)	Deoxyhemoglobin	Hypo- or isointense	Hypointense	Hypointense	Hypointense	Hypointense
Early subacute (4–7 days)	Intracellular methemoglobin	Hyperintense	Hypointense	Hypointense	Hyperintense, no susceptibility	Hypointense
Late subacute (1 week to several months)	Extracellular methemoglobin	Hyperintense	Hyperintense	Hyperintense	Hyperintense	Hyperintense
Chronic (after several months)	Hemosiderin, ferritin	Hypointense	Hypointense	Hypointense	Hypointense	Hypointense

magnetic hemoglobin products deoxyhemoglobin, intracellular methemoglobin, ferritin, and hemosiderin secondary to spin dephasing that occurs due to local magnetic field nonuniformity.[91]

Diffusion-Weighted Imaging of Hemorrhage

Intraparenchymal hematomas are hyperintense on diffusion-weighted images in the hyperacute (oxyhemoglobin) and late subacute (extracellular methemoglobin) phases and hypointense in the acute (deoxyhemoglobin), early subacute (intracellular methemoglobin), and chronic (hemosiderin) phases.[93] High signal intensity of oxyhemoglobin may be due to restricted diffusion within intact red blood cells or high protein content. High signal on diffusion-weighted images of extracellular methemoglobin is likely due to high protein content. Low signal on DWI of deoxyhemoglobin, intracellular methemoglobin, and hemosiderin/ferritin is due to susceptibility effects, and calculation of actual ADC values in this setting is problematic.[94]

Susceptibility-Weighted Imaging

Susceptibility-weighted imaging (SWI) is a relatively new technique that utilizes both phase and magnitude information obtained from high-resolution 3D gradient echo–based sequences to create images that accentuate differences in magnetic susceptibilities of tissues. Raw phase images are converted into high-pass filtered phase images and then into a "phase mask" that is subsequently multiplied into the magnitude images to create a final susceptibility-weighted magnitude image set.[95]

Susceptibility-weighted imaging is superior to conventional T2*-weighted gradient echo imaging for the evaluation of intracranial hemorrhage. It is superior in detecting cerebral microbleeds, diffuse axonal injury hemorrhages, cerebral cavernous malformations, and intratumoral hemorrhage.[96] Pre- and postcontrast SWI can also differentiate

between intratumoral hemorrhage and neovascularity. Furthermore, normal vessels and vascular abnormalities including slow-flow lesions such as capillary telangiectasias are well demonstrated with SWI because of the accentuation of intravascular deoxyhemoglobin. In addition, SWI is highly sensitive for the detection of acute venous sinus thrombosis due to the presence of deoxyhemoglobin within the clot. SWI may also detect secondary signs of sinus thrombosis such as venous engorgement.[96]

Susceptibility-weighted imaging can differentiate calcium from hemorrhage (deoxyhemoglobin, methemoglobin, hemosiderin, ferritin). Although both calcium and hemorrhage appear hypointense on conventional T2*-weighted gradient echo images and on SWI magnitude images, calcium appears hyperintense and hemorrhage hypointense on SWI filtered phase images in a right-handed system. Because calcium is diamagnetic and hemorrhage (deoxyhemoglobin, methemoglobin, hemosiderin, ferritin) is paramagnetic, calcium has a positive phase and hemorrhage has a negative phase.[97]

Perihematomal Region

Edema in the region surrounding an intraparenchymal hematoma, as demarcated by hyperintense signal on T2-weighted and FLAIR images increases by approximately 75% during the first 24 hours.[98] Subsequently, it slowly increases up to day 14 and decreases thereafter.[99] Increased diffusion in the perihematoma region, consistent with vasogenic edema, and hypoperfusion (prolonged mean transit time) with spontaneous normalization within 3 to 5 days have been reported.[100,101] These findings correlate with a ^{15}O positron emission tomography (PET) study demonstrating decreased CBF and a disproportionately greater decrease in the cerebral metabolic rate of oxygen ($CMRO_2$), resulting in a decrease in oxygen extraction fraction in the perihematomal region; these findings suggest that perihematomal hypoperfusion reflects reduced metabolic demand or diaschisis rather than ischemia.[102]

Etiologies of Hemorrhagic Stroke

Imaging pearls and pitfalls for the following entities are outlined in **Table 8.13**.

Hypertensive Hemorrhage

Hypertension is a major risk factor for the development of intraparenchymal hemorrhage.[83] Perforating vessels such as the lenticulostriates, thalamoperforators, and pontine perforators are the most susceptible to hypertension-induced changes such as intimal thickening, atherosclerosis, lipohyalinosis, smooth muscle medial degeneration, and occasional miliary aneurysms. Consequently hypertension-associated hemorrhage most commonly occurs in deep structures such as the basal ganglia, thalamus, brainstem, and cerebellum, and less commonly in the lobar regions.[103]

Cerebral Amyloid Angiopathy

Cerebral amyloid angiopathy describes the pathologic process in which amyloid deposition occurs predominantly in small and medium-sized cerebral blood vessels including cortical and leptomeningeal arteries, arterioles, capillaries, and less commonly veins.[104] Luminal duplication, intimal obliteration, hyaline degeneration, microaneurysm formation, and fibrinoid necrosis are the pathologic hallmarks.[105] Affected vessels are most commonly located in the parietal and occipital cortices, less commonly in the cerebellum, and uncommonly in the subcortical white matter, hippocampi, basal ganglia, thalami, and brainstem.[105] Cerebral amyloid angiopathy is common in the elderly, found in 57% of patients 60 years of age and older in an autopsy series.[106]

Clinical diagnosis according to the Boston Criteria for probable cerebral amyloid angiopathy may be made with demonstration of multiple lobar, cortical, subcortical, or cerebellar hemorrhages in a patient older than 55 without other causes of hemorrhage.[107] In one study, 73% of patients presenting with an acute neurologic deficit and lobar hemorrhage on MRI had additional microhemorrhages on gradient echo T2* images (**Fig. 8.13**).[107] Additional imaging findings are hemosiderosis, and edema and leptomeningeal enhancement associated with a more recently recognized inflammatory form of amyloid angiopathy.

Microhemorrhage

Cerebral microhemorrhages are small foci of signal loss measuring less than 5 mm, best demonstrated on T2*-weighted gradient echo or SWI sequences, that represent foci of hemosiderin-containing macrophages due to prior small vessel hemorrhage.[108] Microhemorrhages associated with hypertension are commonly found in the basal ganglia, thalamus, brainstem, and cerebellum (**Fig. 8.14A**). Microhemorrhages associated with cerebral amyloid angiopathy are more common in the lobar regions, at gray white matter junctions with a posterior predominance (temporal and occipital lobes) (**Fig. 8.14B**).[109] In patients with primary lobar hemorrhage due to amyloid angiopathy, the number of concurrent microhemorrhages has been shown to be predictive of a higher risk of future symptomatic intracerebral hemorrhage.[110]

Microhemorrhages are also seen in the setting of cerebral autosomal-dominant arteriopathy with subcortical infarcts and leukoencephalopathy (CADASIL). The radiologic differential diagnosis of numerous small foci of signal hypointensity on T2*-weighted images also includes diffuse axonal injury,

Table 8.13 Imaging Pearls and Pitfalls

	Pearls	Pitfalls
Hypertension	Most common in deep gray nuclei and cerebellum	Location in cerebellum overlaps with amyloid angiopathy related hemorrhage
Amyloid angiopathy	Posterior lobar predominance and cerebellum	May occasionally present as a peripherally located enhancing mass lesion ("inflammatory form")
Coagulopathy	Fluid-blood levels	
Tumor	Solid enhancement associated with hematoma	Intrinsic T1 hyperintensity of subacute blood products may obscure gadolinium enhancement
Cavernous malformation	Complete low signal hemosiderin rim classically described	
Cerebral venous sinus thrombosis	Susceptibility effect aids in detection of thrombosed sinuses and cortical veins	Thrombus with intrinsic T1 hyperintensity simulates flow-related signal on time of flight MRV
Arteriovenous malformation	Time-resolved MRA allows more dynamic evaluation	
Aneurysm	Rupture may present with intraparenchymal hematoma (anterior temporal lobe for middle cerebral artery bifurcation aneurysm, inferior frontal lobe for anterior communicating artery aneurysm)	

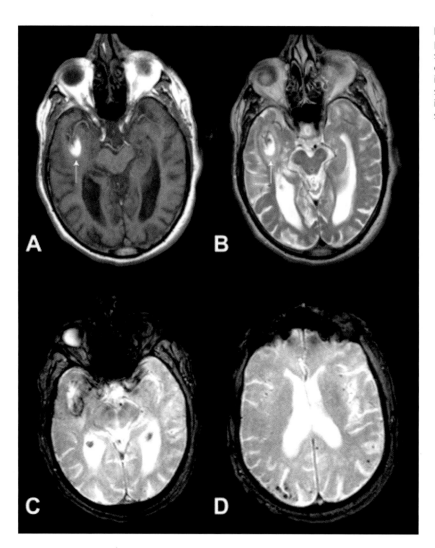

Fig. 8.13 Amyloid angiopathy. An 80-year-old patient who initially presented with acute mental status change. T1- **(A)** and T2- **(B)** weighted images demonstrate a hyperintense hematoma *(arrow)* in the right temporal lobe consistent with late subacute blood products. Selected T2*-weighted images **(C,D)** demonstrate multiple other cortical/subcortical foci of chronic microhemorrhage.

vasculitis, multiple cavernous malformations, hemorrhagic micrometastasis, and postradiation change.[111]

Coagulopathy

Oral anticoagulation therapy is associated with a 7- to 10-fold increase in the risk of intracranial hemorrhages, the majority of which are intraparenchymal hematomas (70%).[112] Risk factors include age greater than 75 years, hypertension, history of cerebrovascular disease, and concomitant aspirin use.[113] The presence of microhemorrhage is independently associated with intraparenchymal hemorrhage associated with oral anticoagulant use.[114] Leukoaraiosis is also an independent risk factor for oral anticoagulant–related hemorrhage in the setting of prior ischemic stroke. Intraparenchymal hemorrhages associated with oral anticoagulation therapy occur in the lobar regions (30%), deep cerebral structures (46%), cerebellum (17%), and brainstem (6%) with a notable relative greater cerebellar predilection compared with noncoagulopathic controls (8 to 14%).[115] On MRI, fluid-blood levels demonstrated a 98% specificity for coagulopathy[116] **(Fig. 8.15).**

Hemorrhage Secondary to Brain Tumor

Many vascular central nervous system (CNS) tumors can present with intracranial hemorrhage. In one large series, the most common tumors were glioblastoma **(Fig. 8.16)** and metastases. Other primary tumors such as anaplastic astrocytomas, low-grade gliomas, meningiomas, pituitary adenomas, hemangioblastomas, and pineoblastomas can present with intracranial hemorrhage. The most common hemorrhagic metastases are melanoma, bronchogenic carcinoma, breast carcinoma, thyroid carcinoma, choriocarcinoma, and renal cell carcinoma.[117]

Hemorrhagic brain tumors may be distinguished from primary intracerebral hemorrhage by the presence of solid enhancing elements, delay in the temporal pattern of evolution of hemorrhage, and a greater extent of or longer persistence of the "edematous" T2 hyperintense region surrounding the hematoma.[118] The hemosiderin rim surrounding the hematoma in the chronic phase may also be incomplete or less pronounced[118] **(Table 8.14).** Furthermore, small metastases are best detected on T2*-weighted images. In one study, 7% of melanoma metastases were only detected on these images.[119]

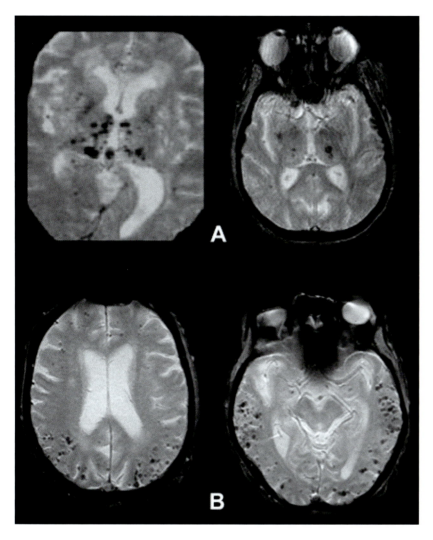

Fig. 8.14 Microhemorrhages. **(A)** T2*-weighted images in two patients with hypertension demonstrating multiple foci of microhemorrhage, predominantly located in the deep gray nuclei. **(B)** An 82-year-old woman with dementia with numerous cortical and subcortical microhemorrhages with a posterior predominance, consistent with amyloid angiopathy.

Cavernous Malformations

Cavernous malformations are multilobulated, well-circumscribed lesions that consist of thin-walled vascular spaces containing blood products of various durations, with surrounding gliotic, hemosiderin-stained tissue. They are usually supratentorial, can be associated with developmental venous anomalies, have a 0.5% prevalence, and have a 3.1% hemorrhage rate per patient-year.[120]

Cavernous malformations are heterogeneous on T1- and T2-weighted images due to the presence of blood products in various stages of evolution **(Fig. 8.17)**. They frequently have fluid-fluid levels on T2-weighted images and a complete low signal hemosiderin rim. T2*-weighted images demonstrate blooming low signal due to the susceptibility effect from blood products. Hyperintensity surrounding the lesion may be present on FLAIR images, reflecting gliosis or edema, and patchy enhancement may be present. Recently, T1 hyperintensity within the perilesional edema has been described as being a specific sign associated with cavernous malformations.[121]

Table 8.14 Characteristics of Benign Versus Malignant Hemorrhage

Benign	Malignant
Edema resolves in 1–2 months	More edema than benign etiologies, persists >1–2 months
Complete hemosiderin ring	Incomplete, less pronounced hemosiderin ring
Normal temporal evolution of blood products	Delayed temporal evolution of blood products
No underlying enhancement	Underlying enhancement (not all)
Smooth margins	Irregular margins
No corpus callosum involvement	Corpus callosum involvement

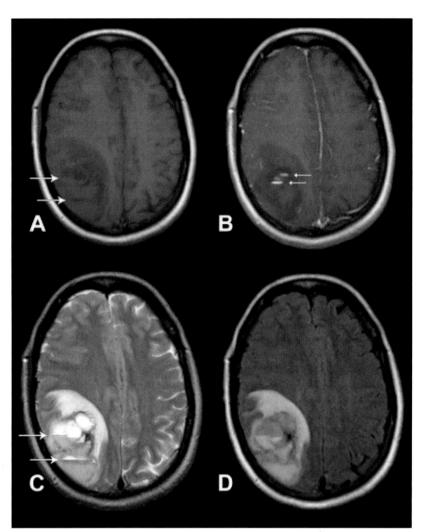

Fig. 8.15 Coagulopathy. A 46-year-old woman with lung adenocarcinoma, on Lovenox. **(A)** T1-weighted image demonstrates a heterogeneous hematoma in the right parietal lobe with fluid-blood levels *(arrows)*. **(B)** T1-weighted postgadolinium image demonstrates active extravasation of contrast *(arrows)*. **(C)** T2-weighted image demonstrates fluid-blood levels *(arrows)* within the hematoma. **(D)** FLAIR image demonstrates hyperintense signal consistent with vasogenic edema surrounding the hematoma.

Cerebral Venous Sinus Thrombosis

Both gross and petechial hemorrhages may occur in the setting of cerebral venous sinus thrombosis. Subcortical or cortical T2 hyperintense lesions reflecting vasogenic edema or infarction can also occur **(Fig. 8.18)**. Parenchymal signal changes and associated hemorrhage are often present near the midline in the frontal, parietal, or occipital lobes in the case of superior sagittal sinus thrombus; posterior temporal lobe in the setting of transverse sinus/vein of Labbé thrombus; and in the basal ganglia, thalamus, periventricular white matter, or superior cerebellum in the case of internal cerebral vein or straight sinus thrombosis.[122]

Magnetic resonance imaging characteristics of the thrombosed venous sinuses have been described in three stages.[123] In the acute stage (0 to 7 days), thrombus is composed of predominantly deoxyhemoglobin and is isointense on T1-weighted images and hypointense on T2-weighted images. Thrombus in the subacute stage (7 to 14 days) is hyperintense on both T1- and T2-weighted images due to the presence of extracellular methemoglobin. In the chronic phase (greater than 15 days), the affected sinus is isointense on T1- and hyperintense on T2-weighted images secondary to vascularized connective tissue within chronic thrombus. An intermediate phase demonstrating hyperintensity on T1- and hypointensity on T2-weighted images secondary to intracellular methemoglobin can also be observed. The susceptibility effect due to the presence of paramagnetic hemoglobin breakdown products is most pronounced in the acute phase and less prominent in the subacute and chronic phases.[123] The susceptibility effect also aids in the detection of isolated cortical vein thrombus in both the acute and chronic stages.

Magnetic resonance venography (MRV) demonstrates the absence of flow-related signal in the thrombosed veins on 2D TOF and phase contrast sequences and a filling defect on 3D gadolinium-enhanced sequences. Thrombus demonstrating T1 hyperintensity simulating flow-related signal on 2D TOF MRV exams is a potential pitfall. In one recent study directly comparing MRV with CT venography, CT showed thrombosis in a total of 81 sinuses/veins compared with 77 for MRI.[124]

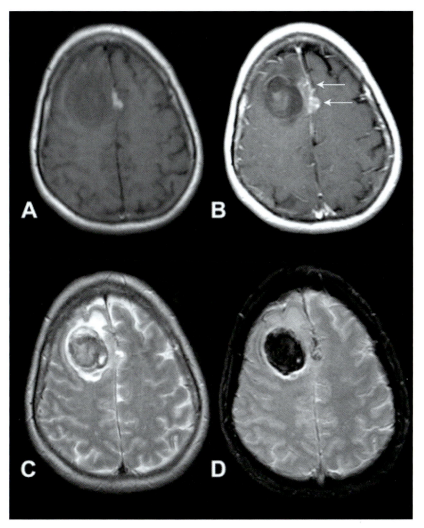

Fig. 8.16 Hemorrhagic glioblastoma multiforme. A 55-year-old woman, found unresponsive. **(A)** T1-weighted image demonstrates an isointense acute hematoma in the right frontal lobe with a small associated focus of T1-hyperintense hemorrhage adjacent to the falx. **(B)** T1-weighted postgadolinium image demonstrates an enhancing solid component adjacent to the hematoma *(arrows)*. **(C)** T2-weighted image demonstrates heterogeneous hypointensity consistent with an acute hematoma. **(D)** T2*-weighted gradient echo (GRE) image demonstrates low signal within the hematoma secondary to the presence of paramagnetic deoxyhemoglobin.

Arteriovenous Malformations

Arteriovenous malformations (AVMs) are defined by the presence of abnormal arterial to venous shunting via a nidus of abnormal vessels without an interposed normal capillary bed. AVM rupture may result in both intraparenchymal and subarachnoid hemorrhage.

Imaging evaluation of AVMs must include the accurate delineation of feeding arteries, draining veins, and the nidus itself. Although intraarterial digital subtraction angiography remains the gold standard, noninvasive imaging with CTA and/or MRA plays an important role in pre- and postoperative evaluation **(Fig. 8.19)**. MRI of AVMs may be undertaken with 3D TOF MRA, contrast-enhanced MRA, and dynamic time-resolved techniques; 3D TOF MRA provides a static delineation of the angioarchitecture of the AVM. Limitations of the TOF technique include spin saturation due to slow flow, spin dephasing due to turbulent flow, and the proximity of vessels to substances with intrinsic T1 hyperintensity.[125] The improved signal-to-noise ratio afforded by 3.0-tesla imaging has increased the sensitivity for detection of feeding arteries as well as superficial and deep draining veins versus 1.5-tesla, with the trade-off of increased susceptibility effects.[126]

Contrast-enhanced MRA possesses inherent advantages compared with TOF MRA; these include a higher signal-to-noise ratio, shorter acquisition time, and relative insensitivity to slow or turbulent flow effects.[125] The relatively narrow window for optimal contrast bolus timing is a primary limitation.[125] Improved depiction of the AVM nidus and draining veins has been reported with contrast-enhanced MRA compared with TOF MRA at 1.0 tesla.[127]

Time-resolved contrast-enhanced MRA or MR digital subtraction angiography (DSA) facilitates a more dynamic evaluation of AVMs by obtaining contrast-enhanced images at multiple time points. Although early applications were hampered by relatively limited spatial resolution, section thickness of the imaging slab, and temporal resolution,[128] more recent improvements of the technique have been developed taking advantage of parallel imaging and selective k-space sampling strategies.[129]

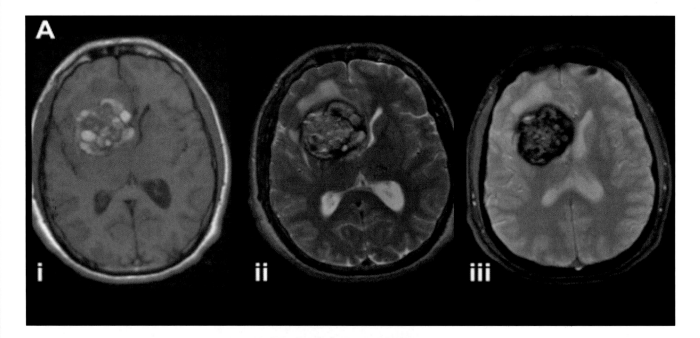

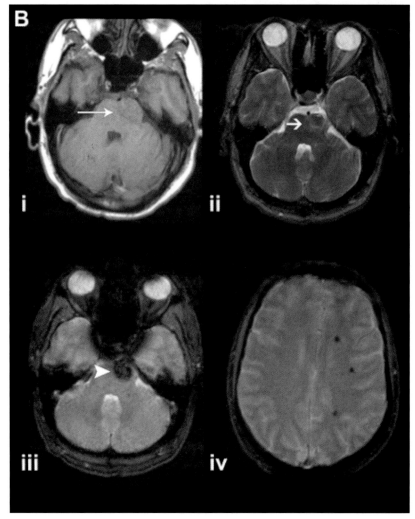

Fig. 8.17 Cavernous malformations. **(A)** A 50-year-old patient with left-sided weakness. T1-weighted (i), T2-weighted (ii), and T2*-weighted images (iii) demonstrate a mass with heterogeneous signal characteristics consistent with blood products of various durations typical of a cavernous malformation. Complete hemosiderin rim and surrounding T2 hyperintensity consistent with gliosis and/or edema are present. **(B)** A 40-year-old patient with multiple cavernous malformations including one lesion in the left pons with acute hemorrhage. T1-weighted (i) and T2-weighted (ii) images demonstrate isointensity *(long arrow)* and mild hypointensity *(short arrow)* consistent with acute blood products. T2*-weighted images (iii, iv) demonstrate hypointensity *(arrowhead)* in the region of hemorrhage in the left pons and multiple other supratentorial foci of susceptibility, consistent with additional cavernous malformations.

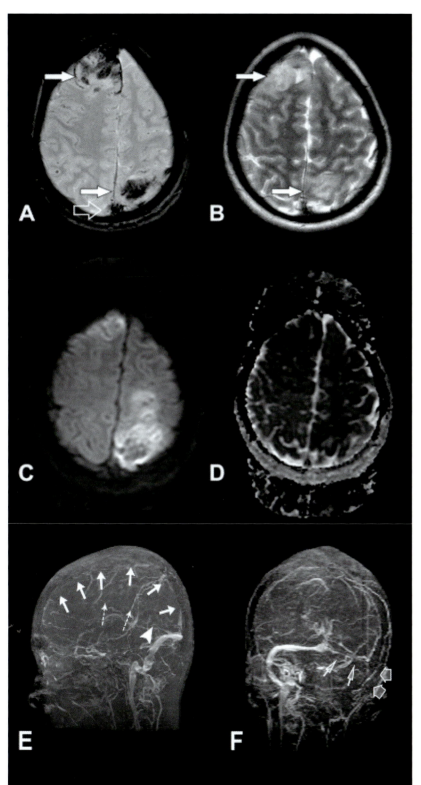

Fig. 8.18 Venous sinus thrombosis. A 26-year-old woman with a history of ulcerative colitis with headache. **(A)** T2* GRE image demonstrates hemorrhages *(solid arrows)* in the right anterior frontal lobe and paramedian left frontal and parietal lobes as well as susceptibility effect in the superior sagittal sinus *(open arrow)*. **(B)** T2-weighted images demonstrate gyriform hyperintensity and cortical swelling associated within the regions of hemorrhage *(arrows)*. Diffusion-weighted image **(C)** and ADC map **(D)** demonstrate restricted diffusion in these regions, consistent with venous infarction. **(E,F)** Selected maximum intensity projection (MIP) images from a 2D TOF MRV demonstrate absence of flow-related signal in the superior sagittal sinus *(arrows)*, inferior sagittal sinus *(dashed arrows)*, straight sinus *(arrowhead)*, left transverse sinus *(thin open arrows)*, and sigmoid sinus *(thick open arrows)* consistent with thrombosis.

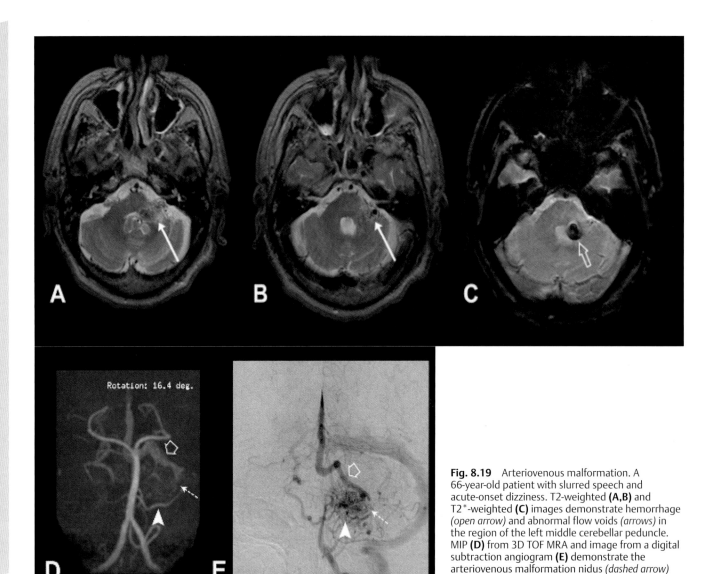

Fig. 8.19 Arteriovenous malformation. A 66-year-old patient with slurred speech and acute-onset dizziness. T2-weighted **(A,B)** and T2*-weighted **(C)** images demonstrate hemorrhage *(open arrow)* and abnormal flow voids *(arrows)* in the region of the left middle cerebellar peduncle. MIP **(D)** from 3D TOF MRA and image from a digital subtraction angiogram **(E)** demonstrate the arteriovenous malformation nidus *(dashed arrow)* with left anterior inferior cerebellar feeding artery *(arrowhead)* and perimesencephalic draining vein *(open arrowhead).*

Aneurysms

Aneurysm rupture most commonly results in subarachnoid hemorrhage, with intraparenchymal or subdural hemorrhage occurring less commonly. Common intraparenchymal locations are the anterior temporal lobe due to MCA bifurcation aneurysm rupture and the inferior frontal lobe due to anterior communicating artery aneurysm rupture. Initial imaging typically includes noncontrast CT followed by CTA. However, recent studies have demonstrated that MRA is similar to CTA in the detection of aneurysms. In one study using intraarterial DSA as the reference standard, 3D TOF MRA at 3 tesla achieved a sensitivity of 89% and specificity of 76% for the detection of aneurysms, with multidetector 64 slice CT angiography (MDCTA) achieving a sensitivity of 87% and specificity of 79%.[130] Although intraarterial DSA is accepted as the gold standard for aneurysm detection, Jager et al[131]

reported five aneurysms in five patients presenting with acute subarachnoid hemorrhage detected by 3D TOF MRA at 1.5 tesla that were thought not to be present on initial DSA, and five aneurysms in four patients detected by DSA that were thought not to be present on MRA, suggesting, that the two modalities should be viewed as complementary.

Other Conditions

◆ Moyamoya

Moyamoya manifests as progressive narrowing of the intracranial internal carotid arteries and its proximal branches, with *moyamoya syndrome* referring to patients with known risk factors such as prior radiation therapy, neurofibromatosis type 1, sickle cell disease, or Down syndrome, and *moyamoya disease* referring to the condition in which no known predisposing risk factor exists.[132] Hemorrhage complicates moyamoya in 20% of adults and 2.8% of children, and may be intraparenchymal, subarachnoid, or intraventricular in location.[132]

◆ Posterior Reversible Encephalopathy Syndrome

Posterior reversible encephalopathy syndrome is complicated by hemorrhage in 15% of cases.[133] Small parenchymal hemorrhages, focal intraparenchymal hematomas, or sulcal subarachnoid hemorrhages occur with roughly equal frequency. Hemorrhage in the setting of PRES is most common in patients who have undergone allogenic bone marrow transplantation and patients who are therapeutically anticoagulated at the time of onset.

◆ Reversible Vasoconstriction Syndrome

Reversible vasoconstriction syndrome presents clinically with a thunderclap headache either with or without associated neurologic deficits and angiographically with multifocal areas of stenosis and dilatation of the cerebral arteries. In one series, subarachnoid hemorrhage was present in 22% of cases and intraparenchymal hematoma in 6%.[134]

◆ Vasculitis

Intraparenchymal and subarachnoid hemorrhage is also seen in the setting of primary CNS angiitis and secondary CNS vasculitides due to viral causes, autoimmune disease, and illicit drug use.

◆ Conclusion

In the past 15 years, new advances in MR technology have greatly increased the role of neuroimaging of acute ischemic stroke. MR angiography can identify the precise location of vascular occlusion. Diffusion-weighted imaging can identify acute ischemic infarction with high sensitivity and specificity and can approximate infarct core. Perfusion MRI can estimate the ischemic penumbra or area of tissue at risk of infarction. Diffusion and perfusion parameters appear to be useful in predicting tissue viability, HT, and clinical outcome. Furthermore, these new imaging modalities have become an integral component to guide treatment decisions. Clot location on MRA, initial DWI lesion size, and ischemic penumbra size are already being used to select patients for thrombolysis.

Advances in MR technology have also greatly increased the role of neuroimaging in the workup of hemorrhagic stroke. T2* and SWI are more sensitive than CT for the detection of intracranial hemorrhage. Their detection of microhemorrhages in association with a primary hemorrhage can confirm specific diagnoses. SWI and gadolinium enhancement can identify vascular lesions with slow flow. Gadolinium-enhanced images can also detect the presence of an underlying mass lesion. Advanced MR angiography techniques can identify and delineate the presence of underlying vascular lesions.

Further advances in MRI will undoubtedly improve our understanding of stroke, improve our treatment strategies, and improve patient outcome.

References

1. Perkins CJ, Kahya E, Roque CT, Roche PE, Newman GC. Fluid-attenuated inversion recovery and diffusion- and perfusion-weighted MRI abnormalities in 117 consecutive patients with stroke symptoms. Stroke 2001;32:2774–2781
2. Sunshine JL, Tarr RW, Lanzieri CF, Landis DM, Selman WR, Lewin JS. Hyperacute stroke: ultrafast MR imaging to triage patients prior to therapy. Radiology 1999;212:325–332
3. González RG, Schaefer PW, Buonanno FS, et al. Diffusion-weighted MR imaging: diagnostic accuracy in patients imaged within 6 hours of stroke symptom onset. Radiology 1999;210:155–162
4. Cosnard G, Duprez T, Grandin C, Smith AM, Munier T, Peeters A. Fast FLAIR sequence for detecting major vascular abnormalities during the hyperacute phase of stroke: a comparison with MR angiography. Neuroradiology 1999;41:342–346
5. Noguchi K, Ogawa T, Inugami A, et al. MRI of acute cerebral infarction: a comparison of FLAIR and T2-weighted fast spin-echo imaging. Neuroradiology 1997;39:406–410
6. Provenzale JM, Jahan R, Naidich TP, Fox AJ. Assessment of the patient with hyperacute stroke: imaging and therapy. Radiology 2003;229:347–359
7. Arnould MC, Grandin CB, Peeters A, Cosnard G, Duprez TP. Comparison of CT and three MR sequences for detecting and categorizing early (48 hours) hemorrhagic transformation in hyperacute ischemic stroke. AJNR Am J Neuroradiol 2004;25:939–944
8. Flacke S, Urbach H, Keller E, et al. Middle cerebral artery (MCA) susceptibility sign at susceptibility-based perfusion MR imaging: clinical importance and comparison with hyperdense MCA sign at CT. Radiology 2000;215:476–482
9. Molina CA, Alvarez-Sabín J, Montaner J, et al. Thrombolysis-related hemorrhagic infarction: a marker of early reperfusion, reduced infarct size, and improved outcome in patients with proximal middle cerebral artery occlusion. Stroke 2002;33:1551–1556
10. Ricci PE, Burdette JH, Elster AD, Reboussin DM. A comparison of fast spin-echo, fluid-attenuated inversion-recovery, and diffusion-weighted MR imaging in the first 10 days after cerebral infarction. AJNR Am J Neuroradiol 1999;20:1535–1542
11. Crain MR, Yuh WT, Greene GM, et al. Cerebral ischemia: evaluation with contrast-enhanced MR imaging. AJNR Am J Neuroradiol 1991;12:631–639
12. Kuhn MJ, Mikulis DJ, Ayoub DM, Kosofsky BE, Davis KR, Taveras JM. Wallerian degeneration after cerebral infarction: evaluation with sequential MR imaging. Radiology 1989;172:179–182
13. Boyko OB, Burger PC, Shelburne JD, Ingram P. Non-heme mechanisms for T1 shortening: pathologic, CT, and MR elucidation. AJNR Am J Neuroradiol 1992;13:1439–1445
14. Schaefer PW, Copen WA, Lev MH, Gonzalez RG. Diffusion-weighted imaging in acute stroke. Neuroimaging Clin N Am 2005;15:503–530, ix–x
15. Schaefer PW, Grant PE, Gonzalez RG. Diffusion-weighted MR imaging of the brain. Radiology 2000;217:331–345
16. Hjort N, Christensen S, Sølling C, et al. Ischemic injury detected by diffusion imaging 11 minutes after stroke. Ann Neurol 2005;58:462–465
17. Schwamm LH, Koroshetz WJ, Sorensen AG, et al. Time course of lesion development in patients with acute stroke: serial diffusion- and hemodynamic-weighted magnetic resonance imaging. Stroke 1998;29:2268–2276
18. Copen WA, Schwamm LH, González RG, et al. Ischemic stroke: effects of etiology and patient age on the time course of the core apparent diffusion coefficient. Radiology 2001;221:27–34
19. Marks MP, Tong DC, Beaulieu C, Albers GW, de Crespigny A, Moseley ME. Evaluation of early reperfusion and i.v. tPA therapy using diffusion- and perfusion-weighted MRI. Neurology 1999;52:1792–1798
20. Nagesh V, Welch KM, Windham JP, et al. Time course of ADCw changes in ischemic stroke: beyond the human eye! Stroke 1998;29:1778–1782
21. Lövblad KO, Laubach HJ, Baird AE, et al. Clinical experience with diffusion-weighted MR in patients with acute stroke. AJNR Am J Neuroradiol 1998;19:1061–1066
22. Engelter ST, Wetzel SG, Bonati LH, Fluri F, Lyrer PA. The clinical significance of diffusion-weighted MR imaging in stroke and TIA patients. Swiss Med Wkly 2008;138:729–740
23. Olivot JM, Mlynash M, Thijs VN, et al. Relationships between cerebral perfusion and reversibility of acute diffusion lesions in DEFUSE: insights from RADAR. Stroke 2009;40:1692–1697

24. Kidwell CS, Saver JL, Starkman S, et al. Late secondary ischemic injury in patients receiving intraarterial thrombolysis. Ann Neurol 2002;52: 698–703
25. Schaefer PW, Hunter GJ, He J, et al. Predicting cerebral ischemic infarct volume with diffusion and perfusion MR imaging. AJNR Am J Neuroradiol 2002;23:1785–1794
26. Fiehler J, Knudsen K, Kucinski T, et al. Predictors of apparent diffusion coefficient normalization in stroke patients. Stroke 2004;35:514–519
27. Wu O, Ostergaard L, Sorensen AG. Technical aspects of perfusion-weighted imaging. Neuroimaging Clin N Am 2005;15:623–637, xi
28. Calamante F, Gadian DG, Connelly A. Quantification of perfusion using bolus tracking magnetic resonance imaging in stroke: assumptions, limitations, and potential implications for clinical use. Stroke 2002; 33:1146–1151
29. Lythgoe DJ, Ostergaard L, William SC, et al. Quantitative perfusion imaging in carotid artery stenosis using dynamic susceptibility contrast-enhanced magnetic resonance imaging. Magn Reson Imaging 2000;18: 1–11
30. Wu O, Østergaard L, Koroshetz WJ, et al. Effects of tracer arrival time on flow estimates in MR perfusion-weighted imaging. Magn Reson Med 2003;50:856–864
31. Rose SE, Janke AL, Griffin M, Finnigan S, Chalk JB. Improved prediction of final infarct volume using bolus delay-corrected perfusion-weighted MRI: implications for the ischemic penumbra. Stroke 2004;35:2466–2471
32. Petersen ET, Zimine I, Ho YC, Golay X. Non-invasive measurement of perfusion: a critical review of arterial spin labelling techniques. Br J Radiol 2006;79:688–701
33. Sibon I, Ménégon P, Orgogozo JM, et al. Inter- and intraobserver reliability of five MRI sequences in the evaluation of the final volume of cerebral infarct. J Magn Reson Imaging 2009;29:1280–1284
34. Lövblad KO, Baird AE, Schlaug G, et al. Ischemic lesion volumes in acute stroke by diffusion-weighted magnetic resonance imaging correlate with clinical outcome. Ann Neurol 1997;42:164–170
35. Olivot JM, Mlynash M, Thijs VN, et al. Relationships between infarct growth, clinical outcome, and early recanalization in diffusion and perfusion imaging for understanding stroke evolution (DEFUSE). Stroke 2008;39:2257–2263
36. Arenillas JF, Rovira A, Molina CA, Grivé E, Montaner J, Alvarez-Sabín J. Prediction of early neurological deterioration using diffusion- and perfusion-weighted imaging in hyperacute middle cerebral artery ischemic stroke. Stroke 2002;33:2197–2203
37. Sanák D, Nosál' V, Horák D, et al. Impact of diffusion-weighted MRI-measured initial cerebral infarction volume on clinical outcome in acute stroke patients with middle cerebral artery occlusion treated by thrombolysis. Neuroradiology 2006;48:632–639
38. Grant PE, He J, Halpern EF, et al. Frequency and clinical context of decreased apparent diffusion coefficient reversal in the human brain. Radiology 2001;221:43–50
39. Kidwell CS, Alger JR, Saver JL. Beyond mismatch: evolving paradigms in imaging the ischemic penumbra with multimodal magnetic resonance imaging. Stroke 2003;34:2729–2735
40. Darby DG, Barber PA, Gerraty RP, et al. Pathophysiological topography of acute ischemia by combined diffusion-weighted and perfusion MRI. Stroke 1999;30:2043–2052
41. Copen WA, Rezai Gharai L, Barak ER, et al. Existence of the diffusion-perfusion mismatch within 24 hours after onset of acute stroke: dependence on proximal arterial occlusion. Radiology 2009;250:878–886
42. Kane I, Carpenter T, Chappell F, et al. Comparison of 10 different magnetic resonance perfusion imaging processing methods in acute ischemic stroke: effect on lesion size, proportion of patients with diffusion/perfusion mismatch, clinical scores, and radiologic outcomes. Stroke 2007;38:3158–3164
43. Christensen S, Mouridsen K, Wu O, et al. Comparison of 10 perfusion MRI parameters in 97 sub-6-hour stroke patients using voxel-based receiver operating characteristics analysis. Stroke 2009;40:2055–2061
44. Olivot JM, Mlynash M, Thijs VN, et al. Optimal Tmax threshold for predicting penumbral tissue in acute stroke. Stroke 2009;40:469–475
45. Jones TH, Morawetz RB, Crowell RM, et al. Thresholds of focal cerebral ischemia in awake monkeys. J Neurosurg 1981;54:773–782
46. Mui K, Yoo AJ, Verduzco L, et al. Cerebral blood flow thresholds for tissue viability in acute ischemic stroke patients treated with intra-arterial thrombolysis depend on timing of reperfusion. 46th Annual Meeting of the American Society of Neuroradiology, New Orleans, 2008
47. Wu O, Christensen S, Hjort N, et al. Characterizing physiological heterogeneity of infarction risk in acute human ischaemic stroke using MRI. Brain 2006;129(Pt 9):2384–2393
48. Tissue plasminogen activator for acute ischemic stroke. The National Institute of Neurological Disorders and Stroke rt-PA Stroke Study Group. N Engl J Med 1995;333:1581–1587
49. Adams HP Jr, del Zoppo G, Alberts MJ, et al; American Heart Association; American Stroke Association Stroke Council; Clinical Cardiology Council; Cardiovascular Radiology and Intervention Council; Atherosclerotic Peripheral Vascular Disease and Quality of Care Outcomes in Research Interdisciplinary Working Groups. Guidelines for the early management of adults with ischemic stroke: a guideline from the American Heart Association/American Stroke Association Stroke Council, Clinical Cardiology Council, Cardiovascular Radiology and Intervention Council, and the Atherosclerotic Peripheral Vascular Disease and Quality of Care Outcomes in Research Interdisciplinary Working Groups: the American Academy of Neurology affirms the value of this guideline as an educational tool for neurologists. Stroke 2007;38: 1655–1711
50. Hacke W, Kaste M, Bluhmki E, et al; ECASS Investigators. Thrombolysis with alteplase 3 to 4.5 hours after acute ischemic stroke. N Engl J Med 2008;359:1317–1329
51. Hacke W, Albers G, Al-Rawi Y, et al; DIAS Study Group. The Desmoteplase in Acute Ischemic Stroke Trial (DIAS): a phase II MRI-based 9-hour window acute stroke thrombolysis trial with intravenous desmoteplase. Stroke 2005;36:66–73
52. Albers GW, Thijs VN, Wechsler L, et al; DEFUSE Investigators. Magnetic resonance imaging profiles predict clinical response to early reperfusion: the diffusion and perfusion imaging evaluation for understanding stroke evolution (DEFUSE) study. Ann Neurol 2006;60:508–517
53. Furlan AJ, Eyding D, Albers GW, et al; DEDAS Investigators. Dose Escalation of Desmoteplase for Acute Ischemic Stroke (DEDAS): evidence of safety and efficacy 3 to 9 hours after stroke onset. Stroke 2006;37: 1227–1231
54. Davis SM, Donnan GA, Parsons MW, et al; EPITHET investigators. Effects of alteplase beyond 3 h after stroke in the Echoplanar Imaging Thrombolytic Evaluation Trial (EPITHET): a placebo-controlled randomised trial. Lancet Neurol 2008;7:299–309
55. Kakuda W, Lansberg MG, Thijs VN, et al; DEFUSE Investigators. Optimal definition for PWI/DWI mismatch in acute ischemic stroke patients. J Cereb Blood Flow Metab 2008;28:887–891
56. Donnan GA, Baron JC, Ma H, Davis SM. Penumbral selection of patients for trials of acute stroke therapy. Lancet Neurol 2009;8:261–269
57. Lansberg MG, Thijs VN, Bammer R, et al. The MRA-DWI mismatch identifies patients with stroke who are likely to benefit from reperfusion. Stroke 2008;39:2491–2496
58. Yoo AJ, Verduzco LA, Schaefer PW, Hirsch JA, Rabinov JD, González RG. MRI-based selection for intra-arterial stroke therapy: value of pretreatment diffusion-weighted imaging lesion volume in selecting patients with acute stroke who will benefit from early recanalization. Stroke 2009;40:2046–2054
59. Janjua N, El-Gengaihy A, Pile-Spellman J, Qureshi AI. Late endovascular revascularization in acute ischemic stroke based on clinical-diffusion mismatch. AJNR Am J Neuroradiol 2009;30:1024–1027
60. Cho AH, Sohn SI, Han MK, et al. Safety and efficacy of MRI-based thrombolysis in unclear-onset stroke. A preliminary report. Cerebrovasc Dis 2008;25:572–579
61. Fisher M, Adams RD. Observations on brain embolism with special reference to the mechanism of hemorrhagic infarction. J Neuropathol Exp Neurol 1951;10:92–94
62. Derex L, Nighoghossian N. Intracerebral haemorrhage after thrombolysis for acute ischaemic stroke: an update. J Neurol Neurosurg Psychiatry 2008;79:1093–1099
63. Hacke W, Kaste M, Fieschi C, et al; The European Cooperative Acute Stroke Study (ECASS). Intravenous thrombolysis with recombinant tissue plasminogen activator for acute hemispheric stroke. JAMA 1995; 274:1017–1025
64. Khatri P, Wechsler LR, Broderick JP. Intracranial hemorrhage associated with revascularization therapies. Stroke 2007;38:431–440
65. Wardlaw JM, Zoppo G, Yamaguchi T, Berge E. Thrombolysis for acute ischaemic stroke. Cochrane Database Syst Rev 2003:CD000213
66. Kidwell CS, Saver JL, Carneado J, et al. Predictors of hemorrhagic transformation in patients receiving intra-arterial thrombolysis. Stroke 2002;33:717–724
67. von Kummer R, Allen KL, Holle R, et al. Acute stroke: usefulness of early CT findings before thrombolytic therapy. Radiology 1997;205:327–333
68. Neumann-Haefelin T, Hoelig S, Berkefeld J, et al; MR Stroke Group. Leukoaraiosis is a risk factor for symptomatic intracerebral hemorrhage after thrombolysis for acute stroke. Stroke 2006;37:2463–2466
69. Hermier M, Nighoghossian N, Derex L, et al. Hypointense transcerebral veins at T2*-weighted MRI: a marker of hemorrhagic transformation risk in patients treated with intravenous tissue plasminogen activator. J Cereb Blood Flow Metab 2003;23:1362–1370
70. Vo KD, Santiago F, Lin W, Hsu CY, Lee Y, Lee JM. MR imaging enhancement patterns as predictors of hemorrhagic transformation in acute ischemic stroke. AJNR Am J Neuroradiol 2003;24:674–679

71. Kassner A, Roberts T, Taylor K, Silver F, Mikulis D. Prediction of hemorrhage in acute ischemic stroke using permeability MR imaging. AJNR Am J Neuroradiol 2005;26:2213–2217
72. Schaefer PW, Roccatagliata L, Schwamm L, et al. Assessing hemorrhagic transformation with diffusion and perfusion MR imaging. 41st Annual Meeting of the American Society of Neuroradiology, Washington, DC, 2003
73. Kim HS, Lee DH, Ryu CW, et al. Multiple cerebral microbleeds in hyperacute ischemic stroke: impact on prevalence and severity of early hemorrhagic transformation after thrombolytic treatment. AJR Am J Roentgenol 2006;186:1443–1449
74. Thomalla G, Schwark C, Sobesky J, et al; MRI in Acute Stroke Study Group of the German Competence Network Stroke. Outcome and symptomatic bleeding complications of intravenous thrombolysis within 6 hours in MRI-selected stroke patients: comparison of a German multicenter study with the pooled data of ATLANTIS, ECASS, and NINDS tPA trials. Stroke 2006;37:852–858
75. Sellar RJ. Imaging blood vessels of the head and neck. J Neurol Neurosurg Psychiatry 1995;59:225–237
76. Green D, Parker D. CTA and MRA: visualization without catheterization. Semin Ultrasound CT MR 2003;24:185–191
77. Coutts SB, Simon JE, Eliasziw M, et al. Triaging transient ischemic attack and minor stroke patients using acute magnetic resonance imaging. Ann Neurol 2005;57:848–854
78. Ma L, Gao PY, Lin Y, et al. Can baseline magnetic resonance angiography (MRA) status become a foremost factor in selecting optimal acute stroke patients for recombinant tissue plasminogen activator (rt-PA) thrombolysis beyond 3 hours? Neurol Res 2009;31:355–361
79. Debrey SM, Yu H, Lynch JK, et al. Diagnostic accuracy of magnetic resonance angiography for internal carotid artery disease: a systematic review and meta-analysis. Stroke 2008;39:2237–2248
80. Rodallec MH, Marteau V, Gerber S, Desmottes L, Zins M. Craniocervical arterial dissection: spectrum of imaging findings and differential diagnosis. Radiographics 2008;28:1711–1728
81. Lévy C, Laissy JP, Raveau V, et al. Carotid and vertebral artery dissections: three-dimensional time-of-flight MR angiography and MR imaging versus conventional angiography. Radiology 1994;190:97–103
82. Sudlow CL, Warlow CP; International Stroke Incidence Collaboration. Comparable studies of the incidence of stroke and its pathological types: results from an international collaboration. Stroke 1997;28:491–499
83. Ariesen MJ, Claus SP, Rinkel GJE, Algra A. Risk factors for intracerebral hemorrhage in the general population: a systematic review. Stroke 2003;34:2060–2065
84. van Gijn J, Kerr RS, Rinkel GJE. Subarachnoid haemorrhage. Lancet 2007;369:306–318
85. Qureshi AI, Tuhrim S, Broderick JP, Batjer HH, Hondo H, Hanley DF. Spontaneous intracerebral hemorrhage. N Engl J Med 2001;344: 1450–1460
86. Delgado Almandoz JE, Schaefer PW, Forero NP, Falla JR, Gonzalez RG, Romero JM. Diagnostic accuracy and yield of multidetector CT angiography in the evaluation of spontaneous intraparenchymal cerebral hemorrhage. AJNR Am J Neuroradiol 2009;30:1213–1221
87. Fullerton HJ, Wu YW, Zhao S, Johnston SC. Risk of stroke in children: ethnic and gender disparities. Neurology 2003;61:189–194
88. Jordan LC, Hillis AE. Hemorrhagic stroke in children. Pediatr Neurol 2007;36:73–80
89. Kidwell CS, Chalela JA, Saver JL, et al. Comparison of MRI and CT for detection of acute intracerebral hemorrhage. JAMA 2004;292:1823–1830
90. Wiesmann M, Mayer TE, Yousry I, Medele R, Hamann GF, Brückmann H. Detection of hyperacute subarachnoid hemorrhage of the brain by using magnetic resonance imaging. J Neurosurg 2002;96:684–689
91. Bradley WG Jr. MR appearance of hemorrhage in the brain. Radiology 1993;189:15–26
92. Fobben ES, Grossman RI, Atlas SW, et al. MR characteristics of subdural hematomas and hygromas at 1.5 T. AJR Am J Roentgenol 1989;153:589–595
93. Kang BK, Na DG, Ryoo JW, Byun HS, Roh HG, Pyeun YS. Diffusion-weighted MR imaging of intracerebral hemorrhage. Korean J Radiol 2001;2:183–191
94. Maldjian JA, Listerud J, Moonis G, Siddiqi F. Computing diffusion rates in T2-dark hematomas and areas of low T2 signal. AJNR Am J Neuroradiol 2001;22:112–118
95. Haacke EM, Mittal S, Wu Z, Neelavalli J, Cheng YC. Susceptibility-weighted imaging: technical aspects and clinical applications, part 1. AJNR Am J Neuroradiol 2009;30:19–30
96. Haacke EM, Mittal S, Wu Z, Neelavalli J, Cheng YC. Susceptibility-weighted imaging: technical aspects and clinical applications, part 1. AJNR Am J Neuroradiol 2009;30:19–30
97. Wu Z, Mittal S, Kish K, Yu Y, Hu J, Haacke EM. Identification of calcification with MRI using susceptibility-weighted imaging: a case study. J Magn Reson Imaging 2009;29:177–182
98. Gebel JM Jr, Jauch EC, Brott TG, et al. Natural history of perihematomal edema in patients with hyperacute spontaneous intracerebral hemorrhage. Stroke 2002;33:2631–2635
99. Inaji M, Tomita H, Tone O, Tamaki M, Suzuki R, Ohno K. Chronological changes of perihematomal edema of human intracerebral hematoma. Acta Neurochir Suppl (Wien) 2003;86:445–448
100. Carhuapoma JR, Wang PY, Beauchamp NJ, Keyl PM, Hanley DF, Barker PB. Diffusion-weighted MRI and proton MR spectroscopic imaging in the study of secondary neuronal injury after intracerebral hemorrhage. Stroke 2000;31:726–732
101. Butcher KS, Baird T, MacGregor L, Desmond P, Tress B, Davis S. Perihematomal edema in primary intracerebral hemorrhage is plasma derived. Stroke 2004;35:1879–1885
102. Zazulia AR, Diringer MN, Videen TO, et al. Hypoperfusion without ischemia surrounding acute intracerebral hemorrhage. J Cereb Blood Flow Metab 2001;21:804–810
103. Takebayashi S, Kaneko M. Electron microscopic studies of ruptured arteries in hypertensive intracerebral hemorrhage. Stroke 1983;14: 28–36
104. Pezzini A, Padovani A. Cerebral amyloid angiopathy-related hemorrhages. Neurol Sci 2008;29(Suppl 2):S260–S263
105. Yamada M. Cerebral amyloid angiopathy: an overview. Neuropathology 2000;20:8–22
106. Yamada M, Tsukagoshi H, Otomo E, Hayakawa M. Cerebral amyloid angiopathy in the aged. J Neurol 1987;234:371–376
107. Knudsen KA, Rosand J, Karluk D, Greenberg SM. Clinical diagnosis of cerebral amyloid angiopathy: validation of the Boston criteria. Neurology 2001;56:537–539
108. Fazekas F, Kleinert R, Roob G, et al. Histopathologic analysis of foci of signal loss on gradient-echo T2*-weighted MR images in patients with spontaneous intracerebral hemorrhage: evidence of microangiopathy-related microbleeds. AJNR Am J Neuroradiol 1999;20:637–642
109. Rosand J, Muzikansky A, Kumar A, et al. Spatial clustering of hemorrhages in probable cerebral amyloid angiopathy. Ann Neurol 2005; 58:459–462
110. Greenberg SM, Eng JA, Ning M, Smith EE, Rosand J. Hemorrhage burden predicts recurrent intracerebral hemorrhage after lobar hemorrhage. Stroke 2004;35:1415–1420
111. Blitstein MK, Tung GA. MRI of cerebral microhemorrhages. AJR Am J Roentgenol 2007;189:720–725
112. Hart RG, Boop BS, Anderson DC. Oral anticoagulants and intracranial hemorrhage. Facts and hypotheses. Stroke 1995;26:1471–1477
113. Cavallini A, Fanucchi S, Persico A. Warfarin-associated intracerebral hemorrhage. Neurol Sci 2008;29(Suppl 2):S266–S268
114. Lee S-H, Ryu W-S, Roh J-K. Cerebral microbleeds are a risk factor for warfarin-related intracerebral hemorrhage. Neurology 2009;72: 171–176
115. Flaherty ML, Haverbusch M, Sekar P, et al. Location and outcome of anticoagulant-associated intracerebral hemorrhage. Neurocrit Care 2006;5:197–201
116. Pfleger MJ, Hardee EP, Contant CF Jr, Hayman LA. Sensitivity and specificity of fluid-blood levels for coagulopathy in acute intracerebral hematomas. AJNR Am J Neuroradiol 1994;15:217–223
117. Licata B, Turazzi S. Bleeding cerebral neoplasms with symptomatic hematoma. J Neurosurg Sci 2003;47:201–210, discussion 210
118. Atlas SW, Grossman RI, Gomori JM. Hemorrhagic intracranial malignant neoplasms: spin-echo MR imaging. Radiology 1987;164:71–77
119. Gaviani P, Mullins ME, Braga TA, et al. Improved detection of metastatic melanoma by T2*-weighted imaging. AJNR Am J Neuroradiol 2006;27:605–608
120. Moriarity JL, Wetzel M, Clatterbuck RE, et al. The natural history of cavernous malformations: a prospective study of 68 patients. Neurosurgery 1999;44:1166–1171, discussion 1172–1173
121. Yun TJ, Na DG, Kwon BJ, et al. A T1 hyperintense perilesional signal aids in the differentiation of a cavernous angioma from other hemorrhagic masses. AJNR Am J Neuroradiol 2008;29:494–500
122. Connor SEJ, Jarosz JM. Magnetic resonance imaging of cerebral venous sinus thrombosis. Clin Radiol 2002;57:449–461
123. Leach JL, Strub WM, Gaskill-Shipley MF. Cerebral venous thrombus signal intensity and susceptibility effects on gradient recalled-echo MR imaging. AJNR Am J Neuroradiol 2007;28:940–945
124. Khandelwal N, Agarwal A, Kochhar R, et al. Comparison of CT venography with MR venography in cerebral sinovenous thrombosis. AJR Am J Roentgenol 2006;187:1637–1643
125. Ozsarlak O, Van Goethem JW, Maes M, Parizel PM. MR angiography of the intracranial vessels: technical aspects and clinical applications. Neuroradiology 2004;46:955–972

126. Heidenreich JO, Schilling AM, Unterharnscheidt F, et al. Assessment of 3D-TOF-MRA at 3.0 Tesla in the characterization of the angioarchitecture of cerebral arteriovenous malformations: a preliminary study. Acta Radiol 2007;48:678–686

127. Unlu E, Temizoz O, Albayram S, et al. Contrast-enhanced MR 3D angiography in the assessment of brain AVMs. Eur J Radiol 2006;60: 367–378

128. Tsuchiya K, Katase S, Yoshino A, Hachiya J. MR digital subtraction angiography of cerebral arteriovenous malformations. AJNR Am J Neuroradiol 2000;21:707–711

129. Taschner CA, Gieseke J, Le Thuc V, et al. Intracranial arteriovenous malformation: time-resolved contrast-enhanced MR angiography with combination of parallel imaging, keyhole acquisition, and k-space sampling techniques at 1.5 T. Radiology 2008;246:871–879

130. Hiratsuka Y, Miki H, Kiriyama I, et al. Diagnosis of unruptured intracranial aneurysms: 3T MR angiography versus 64-channel multidetector row CT angiography. Magn Reson Med Sci 2008;7:169–178

131. Jäger HR, Mansmann U, Hausmann O, Partzsch U, Moseley IF, Taylor WJ. MRA versus digital subtraction angiography in acute subarachnoid haemorrhage: a blinded multireader study of prospectively recruited patients. Neuroradiology 2000;42:313–326

132. Scott RM, Smith ER. Moyamoya disease and moyamoya syndrome. N Engl J Med 2009;360:1226–1237

133. Hefzy HM, Bartynski WS, Boardman JF, Lacomis D. Hemorrhage in posterior reversible encephalopathy syndrome: imaging and clinical features. AJNR Am J Neuroradiol 2009;30:1371–1379

134. Ducros A, Boukobza M, Porcher R, Sarov M, Valade D, Bousser MG. The clinical and radiological spectrum of reversible cerebral vasoconstriction syndrome. A prospective series of 67 patients. Brain 2007;130(Pt 12):3091–3101

9

Positron Emission Tomography in Ischemic and Hemorrhagic Stroke

Colin P. Derdeyn and Rajat Dhar

Pearls

- Positron emission tomography (PET) measurements of hemo-dynamic parameters, including cerebral blood flow and oxygen extraction fraction, are not Food and Drug Administration (FDA)-approved for diagnostic use and are presently used for research purposes only. PET studies have yielded important knowledge regarding human cerebrovascular disease, including the following pearls.
- The best indicator of viable penumbral tissue in acute ischemic stroke is preserved oxygen metabolism. Flow parameters are not specific for whether tissue is alive or dead.
- Autoregulation is intact in tissue around an acute ischemic infarction.
- There is no evidence that intracranial hemorrhage causes ischemic changes in adjacent brain.
- Autoregulation is frequently impaired in patients with aneurysmal–subarachnoid hemorrhage (SAH)-induced vasospasm.

Positron emission tomography (PET) remains an important research tool for in vivo investigations of human cerebrovascular pathophysiology. PET imaging provides regional, quantitative measurements of important parameters such as cerebral blood flow (CBF) and oxygen metabolism, as well as molecular imaging using specific physiologic and pathologic chemical compounds (molecular imaging). The measurements are also useful in the assessment of therapeutic interventions, such as red cell transfusion in cerebral vasospasm, for example, on different physiologic parameters. The ability to measure oxygen metabolism, in addition to CBF, facilitates the comprehensive assessment of the impact of therapeutic interventions on the ischemic vulnerability of brain tissue. Many of these applications are unique to PET imaging. This chapter reviews the knowledge gained from PET studies regarding the pathophysiology and treatment of acute ischemic and hemorrhagic stroke, as well as chronic oligemia from arterial occlusive disease. The first section is a review of the basic principles and important limitations of PET. The second section is a review of normal cerebral hemodynamics and metabolism. The third section is a discussion of the responses of the brain and its vasculature to reductions in perfusion pressure, primarily autoregulatory vasodilation and increased oxygen extraction fraction. The remaining sections briefly review the contributions of PET studies to our understanding of pathophysiology and treatment in the settings of chronic arterial occlusive disease, acute ischemic stroke, acute intracerebral hemorrhage, and subarachnoid hemorrhage.

◆ Positron Emission Tomography Imaging Physics

Positron emission tomography imaging requires two or three components: a positron-emitting isotope (radiotracer), a tomographic imaging system to detect the location and to measure the quantity of radiation, and often a mathematical model relating the physiologic process under study to the detected radiation.[1] For example, the method used in our laboratory for the measurement of cerebral blood flow uses a bolus injection of O-15 labeled water ($H_2^{15}O$, the radiotracer).[1] The PET camera system records the location and number of counts during the circulation of the water through the brain. Finally, the tomographic PET images of raw counts are converted into maps of regional quantitative CBF using computer algorithms. This processing requires measurement of arterial blood counts and incorporates models and assumptions regarding the transit of water through the cerebral circulation.

Radiotracers are radioactive molecules administered in such small quantities that they do not affect the physiologic process under study. PET radiotracers decay by positron emission and may be separated into two broad categories: normal biologic molecules, such as ^{15}O-labeled water, or nonbiologic elements attached to organic molecules as radiolabels, such as ^{18}F-labeled deoxyglucose.

Positron emission tomography imaging detection systems use the phenomenon of annihilation radiation both to localize and to measure physiologic processes in the brain. In the body, the positron (a positively charged electron emitted by the radionuclide) travels up to a few millimeters before encountering an electron. This encounter results in the annihilation of both the positron and electron and the consequent generation of two gamma photons of equal energy. These two photons are emitted in characteristic 180-degree opposite directions. A pair of detectors positioned on either side of the source of the annihilation photons detects them simultaneously. This allows localization of the point source of the radiation.

The most important limitations of PET imaging of physiologic processes relate to the phenomenon of full-width, half-maximum (FWHM) and a related phenomenon of partial-volume averaging. Detected radiation is observed over a larger area than the actual source. The spread or distribution of activity is approximately gaussian for a point source of radiation, with the maximum located at the original point. The FWHM describes the degree of smearing of radioactivity in a reconstructed image. The ability of a PET scanner to discriminate between two small adjacent structures or accurately measure the activity in a small region depends on the FWHM of the system as well as on the amount and distribution of activity within the region of interest and the surrounding areas. Because of the smearing or redistribution of detected radioactivity, any given region in the reconstructed image does not contain all the activity actually within the region. Some of the activity spills over into adjacent areas. This phenomenon is known as the partial-volume effect. An important consequence of this principle is that PET always measures a gradual change in activity where an abrupt change actually exists, such as in an infarct, hemorrhage, or at the border of different structures such as the brain and cerebrospinal fluid (CSF) or gray and white matter.[2]

Finally, the externally measured tissue concentration of the positron-emitting radiotracer (PET counts) is quantitatively related to the physiologic variable under study by a mathematical model. The PET scanner measures the total counts in a volume of tissue over time. The model then calculates how that measured activity reflects the physiologic parameter under study. These calculations account for several factors related to the tracer biomechanics and metabolism. These factors include the mode of tracer delivery to the tissue, the distribution and metabolism of the tracer within the tissue, the egress of the tracer and metabolites from the tissue, the recirculation of both the tracer and its labeled metabolites, and the amount of tracer and metabolites remaining in the blood.

◆ Normal Cerebral Hemodynamics and Metabolism

A brief introduction and definition of the common physiologic parameters measured with PET is useful prior to the discussion of normal hemodynamics and metabolism. *Cerebral blood flow* (CBF) is the volume of blood delivered to a defined mass of tissue per unit time, generally in milliliters of blood per 100 g of brain per minute (mL/(100 g · min)) **(Fig. 9.1)**. ^{15}O-labeled water is the most commonly used tracer for measurements of CBF and the method used in our laboratory.[1] Other methods are in common use as well, including O-15 labeled butanol.[3]

Cerebral blood volume (CBV) is the volume of blood within a given mass of tissue and is expressed as milliliters of blood per 100 g of brain tissue. Regional CBV measurements may serve as an indicator of the degree of cerebrovascular vasodilatation, as discussed below. CBV can be measured by PET with either trace amounts of ^{15}O-labeled carbon monoxide or ^{11}CO[1] **(Fig. 9.1)**. Both carbon monoxide tracers label the red blood cells. Blood volume is then calculated using a correction factor for the difference between peripheral vessel and cerebral vessel hematocrit. *Mean transit time* (MTT) is usually calculated as the ratio of CBV/CBF. By the central volume theorem, this ratio yields mean transit time, the hypothetical mean time for a particle to pass through the cerebral circulation. Increased MTT is used as an indicator of autoregulatory vasodilation. Some PET groups have advocated the use of the inverse of this ratio instead.[4]

Oxygen extraction fraction (OEF) is the proportion of oxygen delivered that is extracted by tissue for metabolism. In the brain OEF normally varies between 0.25 and 0.5, with values over 0.5 signifying increased extraction. It is measured in our laboratory by an O^{15}O inhalation scan and independent measurements of CBF and CBV[1] **(Fig. 9.1)**. The CBF accounts for the amount of oxygen delivered to the brain. The CBV corrects for oxygen in the blood that is not extracted. An alternative count based method uses the ratio of the counts after an O^{15}O inhalation scan to the counts from an O^{15}O water scan, without CBV correction.[5] Other similar methods are also in common use. *Cerebral metabolic rate of oxygen* (CMRO$_2$) is the amount of oxygen consumed by tissue metabolism, measured in milliliters of oxygen per 100 g of brain tissue per minute[1] **(Fig. 9.1)**. CMRO$_2$ is equal to the CBF multiplied by OEF and the CaO$_2$ (delivery of oxygen times the fraction extracted times the amount of available oxygen).

Molecular imaging studies in ischemic and hemorrhagic stroke patients have used several different labeled substances,[6] including 11-C-labeled FK506 (tacrolimus) copper-60, ^{11}C-flumazenil (FMZ), ^{18}F-fluoromisonidazole (^{18}F-FMISO), and a host of other labeled neurotransmitters. *Glucose metabolism* (CMRGlu) is most frequently measured using the glucose analogue ^{18}F-fluorodeoxyglucose (FDG). CMRGlu measurements are limited in pathologic conditions such as ischemia, however, because the ratio of tissue uptake of glucose and its analogue, DG, varies with the severity of ischemia. Glucose metabolism can be measured directly with 1-^{11}C-D–glucose.[7]

Whole-brain mean CBF of the adult human brain is approximately 50 mL per 100 g per minute. Functional activation increases local or regional CBF, but global CBF generally remains unchanged. CBF for any brain region is determined by the ratio of cerebral perfusion pressure (CPP) and cerebral vascular resistance (CVR) in that region. Cerebral perfusion

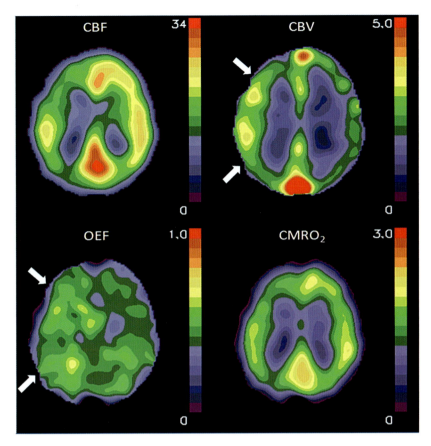

Fig. 9.1 Severe hemodynamic impairment. These images show a unilateral reduction in cerebral blood flow (CBF) distal to a carotid occlusion in a patient with a complete atherosclerotic carotid occlusion. Cerebral blood volume (CBV) is elevated owing to autoregulatory vasodilation *(arrows)*. Cerebral metabolic rate of oxygen (CMRO₂) is relatively preserved owing to the increase in oxygen extraction fraction (OEF) *(arrows)*.

pressure is the difference between the arterial pressure forcing blood into the cerebral circulation and the intracranial pressure or the pressure in the venous system. The venous pressure is negligible under most conditions, so the CPP is generally equal to the systemic arterial pressure. Several different pathologic processes result in reduced perfusion pressure secondary to venous disease, however. These include venous sinus thrombosis, dural arteriovenous fistulas, and possibly other conditions such as jugular foraminal narrowing. The venous pressure also increases with increased intracranial pressure.

Under normal conditions any change in regional CBF (rCBF) must be caused by a change in regional CVR. Vascular resistance is mediated by alterations in the diameter of small arteries or arterioles. In the resting brain with normal CPP, CBF is also closely matched to the metabolic rate of the tissue. Regions with higher metabolic rates have higher levels of CBF. For example, gray matter has a higher CBF than white matter. Although there is wide variation in levels of flow and metabolism, the ratio between rCBF and metabolism is nearly constant in all areas of the brain. Consequently, the maps of OEF and glucose extraction (not metabolism) from the blood show little regional variation.[8] One exception to this is seen with physiologic activation, where blood flow increases well beyond the metabolic needs of the tissue. This leads to a relative decrease of OEF and a reduction in local venous deoxyhemoglobin.[9] This phenomenon is the basis for the use of magnetic resonance imaging (MRI) as a means to map brain function.

◆ Responses to Reductions in Cerebral Perfusion Pressure: Oligemia and Ischemia

An arterial stenosis or occlusion may cause a reduction in perfusion pressure if collateral sources of flow are not adequate.[10] The presence of arterial stenosis or occlusion does not equate with hemodynamic impairment: up to 50% of patients with complete carotid artery occlusion and prior ischemic symptoms have no evidence of reduced CPP.[11] The adequacy of collateral sources of flow determines whether an occlusive lesion will cause a reduction in perfusion pressure. When perfusion pressure falls owing to an occlusive lesion and an inadequate collateral system, the brain and its vasculature maintain the normal delivery of oxygen and glucose through two mechanisms: autoregulatory vasodilation and increased oxygen extraction fraction.[12] The presence of these mechanisms has been extensively studied, primarily in animal models employing acute reductions in perfusion pressure. The extent to which these models are applicable to humans with chronic regional reductions in perfusion pressure is not completely known. Autoregulatory vasodilation and increased OEF may also occur in response to reduced CPP owing to increases in venous back pressure.[13]

Changes in perfusion pressure have little effect on CBF over a wide range of pressure owing to vascular autoregulation. Increases in mean arterial pressure produce vasocon-

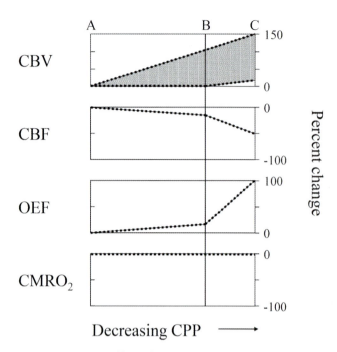

Fig. 9.2 Schematic of hemodynamic and metabolic responses to reductions in cerebral perfusion pressure (CPP). The x-axis represents progressive reduction in perfusion pressure. The region between points A and B is the autoregulatory range. The region between points B and C is the region of autoregulatory failure where CBF falls passively as a function of pressure. Point C represents the exhaustion of compensatory mechanisms to maintain normal oxygen metabolism and the onset of true ischemia. CBV either remains unchanged or increases with autoregulatory vasodilation, depending largely on the methods used to measure CBV. With autoregulatory failure, most investigations have found further increases in CBV. CBF falls slightly through the autoregulatory range. Once autoregulatory capacity is exceeded, CBF falls passively as a function of pressure down to 50% of baseline values. OEF increases slightly with the reductions in CBF through the autoregulatory range. After autoregulatory capacity is exceeded and flow falls up to 50% of baseline, OEF may increase up to 100% from baseline. CMRO$_2$ remains unchanged throughout this range of CPP reduction owing to both autoregulatory vasodilation and increased OEF. (From Derdeyn CP, Videen TO, Yundt KD, et al. Variability of cerebral blood volume and oxygen extraction: stages of cerebral haemodynamic impairment revisited. Brain 2002;125(Pt 3): 595–607. Reprinted by permission.)

striction of the pial arterioles, serving to increase vascular resistance and maintain CBF at a constant level.[14] Conversely, when the pressure falls, reflex vasodilation maintains CBF at near-normal levels.[15] Two measurable parameters that indicate autoregulatory vasodilation are increases in MTT and CBV (**Fig. 9.2**). Despite vasodilation, there is some slight reduction in CBF through the autoregulatory range as perfusion falls, leading to a slight increase in oxygen extraction to compensate for the reduced delivery of oxygen.[12]

At some point the capacity for autoregulatory vasodilation can be exceeded. The threshold value for autoregulatory failure is variable between patients and can be shifted higher or lower by prior ischemic injury or long-standing hypertension. Beyond this point, CBF falls linearly as a function of pressure. Direct measurements of arteriovenous oxygen differences (CaO$_2$ × OEF) using jugular venous oximetry have

demonstrated the brain's capacity to increase oxygen extraction (OEF) and maintain normal cerebral oxygen metabolism (CMRO$_2$) in circumstances where oxygen delivery diminishes due to decreasing CBF[16] (**Figs. 9.1 and 9.2**). The precise mechanism by which OEF increases is not completely understood. Oxygen passively diffuses from the blood to the tissue. The best current hypothesis is that more of the oxygen that diffuses into the tissue is used for oxidative metabolism, thus reducing the amount of oxygen available to diffuse back to the capillaries.[17]

If the perfusion pressure of the brain continues to fall beyond the capacity for increases in OEF to compensate for the reduced delivery of oxygen, oxygen extraction becomes insufficient to meet the energy requirements of the brain.[18] CMRO$_2$ begins to fall and neurologic dysfunction occurs. This may be reversible if oxygen delivery is rapidly restored. Persistent or further declines in flow can lead to permanent tissue damage, depending on the duration and degree of ischemia.[19] Below approximately 20 mL per 100 g per minute, normal brain electrical activity ceases and neurologic symptoms may appear. The energy supply becomes insufficient owing to the inadequate supply of oxygen, preventing normal aerobic glycolysis. The high-energy phosphate stores of adenosine triphosphate (ATP) and phosphocreatine (PCr) become depleted. Anaerobic metabolism of the small amount of glucose remaining in the intracellular stores or from the diminished blood flow leads to a lactic acidosis. Once CBF has fallen to 10 to 12 mL per 100 g per minute, the integrity of cell membranes is lost and intracellular K$^+$ leaks out of the cells whereas extracellular Ca$^+$ leaks in. Cell death ultimately follows unless reperfusion occurs quickly.

Once tissue damage has occurred, the normal mechanisms of cerebrovascular control may no longer operate.[20] Therefore, in some patients who have had transient ischemic attacks (TIA) or mild ischemic strokes with subsequent recanalization, autoregulation or the normal cerebrovascular response to PaCO$_2$ may be abnormal for up to several weeks.[21] Over time, flow falls to match the metabolic needs of the tissue, and autoregulatory capacity is regained. Following reperfusion, the biochemical and ionic abnormalities resolve to a degree dependent on the severity of the initial ischemic insult. The acidosis of anaerobic glycolysis may be replaced by alkalosis.

Chronic oligemia may lead to other compensatory mechanisms, in addition to autoregulatory vasodilation and increased OEF. These include possible reversible metabolic downregulation, accompanied by a reversible cognitive impairment.[22] This phenomenon remains an unproven hypothesis and is being evaluated in ongoing trials.

◆ Positron Emission Tomography PET Studies in Chronic Arterial Occlusive Disease (Oligemia)

The identification of compensatory responses to reduced perfusion pressure, or hemodynamic impairment as it is frequently called, may play an important role in medical decision making in several subacute or chronic arterial occlusive disorders. These conditions include atherosclerotic carotid occlusion, arterial dissection, moyamoya disease, and possibly asymptomatic atherosclerotic carotid stenosis. PET and other hemodynamic studies in these patient populations have been aimed primarily at establishing if the presence of these compensatory mechanisms is associated with future stroke risk (natural history studies), and if particular medical or surgical interventions can improve cerebral hemodynamics (i.e., using imaging as a secondary end point). Pivotal intervention studies of efficacy based on hemodynamic criteria have also been done. This section reviews PET methods for identification of autoregulatory vasodilation and increased OEF, and reviews clinical studies in different patient populations.

Identification of Compensatory Reponses to Reduced Perfusion Pressure with Positron Emission Tomography

As discussed above, the hemodynamic effect of an arterial stenosis or occlusion depends on the adequacy of collateral circulation as well as the degree of stenosis. An occluded carotid artery, for example, often has no measurable effect on the distal CPP because the collateral flow through the circle of Willis is adequate. Many imaging techniques, such as arteriography, MRI, computed tomography angiography, and Doppler ultrasound, can identify the presence of these collaterals. These tools show us the highways for blood flow, but not the traffic on them.

It is important to recognize that a single measurement of flow is meaningless when investigating the effects of an arterial lesion. Normal values of CBF do not exclude the presence of autoregulatory vasodilation, and reduced CBF may be present with normal perfusion pressure. This second situation may occur with prior stroke in the region of interest or in a remote area. Prior lacunar stroke in the basal ganglia may lead to profound reduction in metabolic demand of the overlying cortex and secondary reduction in flow. This phenomenon has been termed diaschisis (**Fig. 9.3**).

Three basic PET strategies for defining the degree of hemodynamic compromise caused by arterial occlusive disease have emerged, based on the known compensatory responses of the brain to reduction in CPP as discussed above. Two approaches are used to identify autoregulatory vasodilation and the third identifies increased OEF. The first method relies on resting measurements of CBV and CBF. When CPP is reduced, autoregulatory vasodilatation causes an increase in CBV. The CBV/CBF ratio (MTT) increases. The second strategy employs paired measurements of rCBF at rest and during some

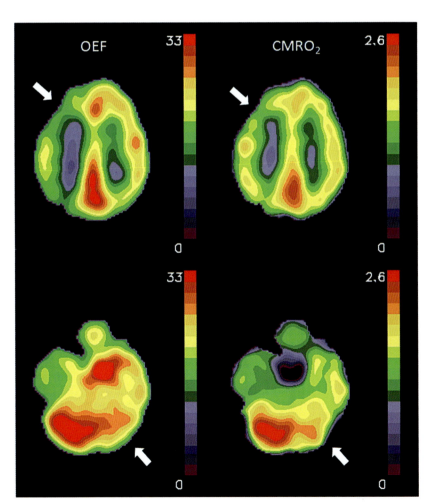

Fig. 9.3 Diaschisis. This patient has a complete atherosclerotic occlusion of the right internal carotid artery and previous stroke in this territory. Consequently, the CMRO₂ image demonstrates reduced oxygen metabolism relative to the contralateral hemisphere *(arrow)*. The reduced metabolic activity in the right frontal area has caused reduced metabolic activity in the structurally normal left cerebellar hemisphere. This phenomenon is known as diaschisis. The primary reduction in metabolism in the cerebellum leads to a reduction in CBF in both the frontal lobe and the cerebellum *(arrows)*.

form of vasodilatory stimulus, such as with acetazolamide (Diamox) or CO_2 inhalation. Reduction of the normal increase in CBF seen in response to these stimuli is taken as evidence of preexisting autoregulatory vasodilatation, which would mute such an increase.

Atherosclerotic Carotid Occlusion

The condition that has been the focus of the most investigations has been atherosclerotic carotid artery occlusion. The presence of increased OEF as measured by PET has been established as a powerful and independent risk factor for future stroke in these patients.[11] Based on this information, a clinical trial of surgical revascularization is underway—the Carotid Occlusion Surgery Study (COSS).[23] The details of these natural history studies and the design and rationale for the current trial are described in this section.

Patients with complete atherosclerotic occlusion of the carotid artery are at high risk for future stroke. A randomized trial of extracranial (EC) to intracranial (IC) arterial bypass (the EC/IC Bypass Trial) failed to show a benefit of surgical revascularization in over 800 patients randomized to surgery or aspirin.[24] One possible reason for the failure of this study to show a benefit was the lack of an effective tool to establish whether flow was normal or impaired. A procedure intended to improve flow is unlikely to provide any benefit if flow at baseline is normal. It is possible that a benefit of bypass was missed for a subgroup at particularly high risk due to hemodynamic impairment.

The St. Louis Carotid Occlusion Study was designed to determine if such a subgroup existed.[11] This was a blinded, prospective study of stroke risk designed to test the hypothesis that increased OEF in patients with symptomatic atherosclerotic carotid occlusion predicted future stroke risk. Eighty-one patients with complete carotid occlusion and ipsilateral ischemic symptoms were enrolled. At baseline, 17 clinical, epidemiologic, and laboratory stroke risk factors were recorded. PET measurements of oxygen extraction were obtained.[25] Thirty-nine of the 81 patients had increased OEF. All 81 patients were followed for a mean duration of 3.1 years. Fifteen total and 13 ipsilateral ischemic strokes occurred during this period. Eleven of the 13 ipsilateral strokes occurred in the 39 patients with increased OEF. Multivariate analysis found only age and OEF as predictors of stroke risk. Log-rank analysis demonstrated increased OEF to be a powerful predictor of subsequent stroke ($p = .004$) (**Fig. 9.4**). Similar results were found by Yamauchi and coworkers.[26]

Prior studies with PET have shown that the superficial temporal artery to middle cerebral artery bypass procedure is capable of reversing the OEF abnormality.[20,27] Based on these facts, the COSS was funded by the National Institutes of Health and is underway.[23] Patients with complete atherosclerotic carotid artery occlusion and recent (120 days) ipsilateral cerebral ischemic symptoms are eligible for enrollment. PET studies are obtained on enrollment to identify patients with increased OEF for randomization to surgery or best medical therapy. The primary hypothesis is that bypass surgery will prevent stroke in this high-risk group.

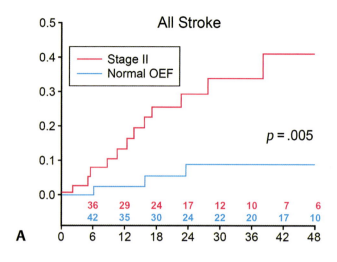

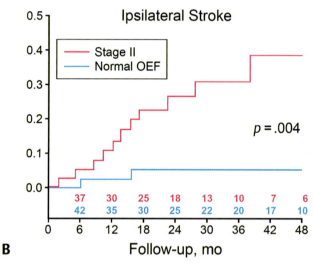

Fig. 9.4 Carotid Occlusion Surgery Study (COSS) outcome. Kaplan-Meier cumulative failure curves for the primary end point of all stroke **(A)** and the secondary end point of ipsilateral ischemic stroke **(B)**. Data for stage II subjects (increased OEF) are shown in red and data for subjects with normal OEF are shown in blue. The number of patients who remained event free and available for follow-up evaluation at each 6-month interval is shown in the appropriate color for each group at the bottom of the graph. (From Grubb RL Jr, Derdeyn CP, Fritsch SM, et al. Importance of hemodynamic factors in the prognosis of symptomatic carotid occlusion. JAMA 1998;280:1055–1060. Copyright © 1998, American Medical Association. All rights reserved. Reprinted by permission.)

Border-Zone Hemodynamics

Acute reductions in perfusion pressure can cause ischemic infarction of the cortex and adjacent subcortical white matter located at the border zones between major cerebral arterial territories, such as the middle and anterior cerebral arteries.[28] Severe systemic hypotension is a well-recognized cause of multiple bilateral discrete cortical border-zone infarctions.[28] However, the mechanism of cortical border-zone infarction in most patients with carotid atherosclerotic disease is likely embolic and not purely hemodynamic.[29,30]

In addition to this cortical arterial border zone, there is good evidence for an arterial border zone within the white matter of the centrum semiovale and corona radiata.[31] This has been called the internal arterial border zone (between lenticulostriate perforators and deep penetrating branches of the distal middle cerebral artery).[31] There is a strong association between hemodynamic impairment of the hemisphere and prior stroke in the white matter, but not in the cortical border zone.[29] Interestingly, the degree of oligemia as indicated by increased OEF is not higher in noninfarcted white matter regions than in the overlying cortex in patients with chronic carotid disease.[32] This suggest that these white matter infarctions may occur at the time of occlusion or soon after (when some selective increase in OEF is present) and not in the chronic situation.

Improvement in Hemodynamics Over Time

In some patients with atherosclerotic carotid occlusion, hemodynamic impairment can improve over time, as collateral flow increases.[33] We repeated PET measurements in 10 patients with complete atherosclerotic carotid artery occlusion who exhibited increased OEF by PET and had no interval stroke 12 to 59 months after the initial examination. Quantitative regional measurements of CBF, CBV, $CMRO_2$, and OEF were obtained. Regional measurements of the cerebral rate of glucose metabolism (CMRGlu) were also made on followup in five patients. As a group, the ratio of ipsilateral to contralateral OEF declined from a mean of 1.16 to 1.08 ($p = .022$). Greater reductions were seen with longer duration of followup ($p = .023$, r = 0.707). The CBF ratio improved from 0.81 to 0.85 ($p = .021$). No change in CBV or $CMRO_2$ was observed. CMRGlu was reduced in the ipsilateral hemisphere ($p = .001$ compared with normal), but the $CMRO_2$/CMRGlu ratio was normal. These findings allowed us to conclude that increased glucose transport was not a compensatory response to chronic hemodynamic impairment.

This improvement in collateral sources of flow over time may be a factor that accounts for the reduction in stroke risk over time in all the major cerebral revascularization trials. The greatest risk for stroke in medically treated patients in the symptomatic carotid stenosis trials, the EC/IC Bypass Trial, and the St. Louis Carotid Occlusion Study was in the first 2 years after stroke.[24]

Moyamoya Disease

Moyamoya disease is an obliterative vasculopathy of unknown etiology affecting the anterior circulation at the circle of Willis. In North America, it most frequently affects women in their third and fourth decades. Ischemic symptoms of stroke or transient ischemic attacks are the most common presentation.[34] It is highly likely that hemodynamic mechanisms play a role in the pathogenesis of stroke in these patients. Hemodynamic assessment may be able to provide prognostic information regarding stroke risk in this patient population, analogous to the atherosclerotic carotid occlusion.

We have used PET to study 42 patients with moyamoya disease and found the frequency of hemodynamic impairment to be quite variable despite uniformly severe vasculopathy: 29 had normal OEF, eight had elevated unilateral OEF, and five had elevated bilateral OEF. Interval improvement in CBF and OEF was observed in one patient with increased OEF at baseline who underwent surgical revascularization. Whether increased OEF predicts stroke risk in this patient population (as it does in atherosclerotic carotid occlusion) is an area of ongoing study.[35]

◆ Positron Emission Tomography Studies in Acute Ischemic Stroke

Human and animal PET studies have provided a detailed description of the time course of changes in CBF and metabolism that occur during and after transient and permanent interruption of normal CBF. Pappata et al[36] have shown in a baboon model of middle cerebral artery (MCA) occlusion that a zone of increased OEF first develops centrally and then moves progressively more peripherally over time. OEF reflects the mismatch between oxygen deliver (CBF) and metabolism. OEF was elevated in the MCA territory both at 1 hour and at 3 hours after occlusion. At 3 hours the regional $CMRO_2$ ($rCMRO_2$) had fallen in the central or deep MCA territory, consistent with infarction. In peripheral, cortical regions, however, $CMRO_2$ was only moderately reduced, suggesting viability. These peripheral regions usually go on to infarction within hours even without further reduction in CBF. This gradual movement of reduced oxygen metabolism from central to peripheral has been termed the dynamic penumbra by Heiss and coworkers,[37] who have described this phenomenon in cats as lasting up to 24 hours.

A brief period of hyperperfusion often occurs immediately after the arterial occlusion ceases. This phenomenon where CBF becomes elevated in a region of infarction is called luxury perfusion. A prolonged period of depressed CBF, reduced below normal values, then follows. During this period of postischemic hypoperfusion, metabolism may recover or even rise above normal levels. Consequently, OEF may be increased during postischemic hypoperfusion. In one patient with persistently increased OEF 4 days after acute stroke, Wise and coworkers[38] raised the systemic blood pressure via angiotensin infusion. Flow to the infarcted region increased, OEF fell, but $CMRO_2$ remained unchanged and no neurologic improvement was observed. Later, CBF may rise above normal while metabolism falls. These changes are typically observed over a period of several days. CBF eventually returns to a level that matches that of the reduced metabolic rate of the infarcted tissue.

Positron emission tomography studies performed in the setting of acute ischemia (less than 24 or 48 hours) have demonstrated regions of both decreased and increased blood flow.[36,37] The regions of decreased CBF are thought to be due to persisting ischemia or postischemic hypoperfusion. Regions with increased CBF are attributed to early postischemic hyperperfusion, caused by either clot lysis or collateral reperfusion. In acute ischemic stroke, focal reduction of CBF is accompanied by a reduction in rCMRO$_2$. The OEF is often elevated due to a greater reduction in CBF than in CMRO$_2$.[20]

Marchal et al[39] studied regional blood flow and oxygen metabolism in 18 patients with acute MCA stroke between 5 and 18 hours after onset of symptoms and correlated their findings with neurologic outcome at 2 months. They categorized their patients into three groups based on the PET scan results. The first group had reduced blood flow and metabolism, suggesting irreversible damage; these patients had a poor outcome. The second group demonstrated reduced flow and metabolism but to a lesser extent than did the first group; this pattern was associated with a variable recovery of function. The third group showed increased perfusion and largely unchanged oxygen metabolism; this group had excellent return of function, suggesting early spontaneous reperfusion and collaterals that were able to maintain the minimum necessary flow during the period of occlusion. Further work from these authors and others has confirmed the observation that early postischemic hyperperfusion is likely a harmless phenomenon.[40,41]

Investigators have also used PET to measure central benzodiazepine receptor binding sites after acute ischemia. Sette and coworkers[42] measured ^{11}C-labeled flumazenil, an antagonist of central benzodiazepine receptors and ^{11}C-labeled PK 11195, a peripheral benzodiazepine receptor antagonist, as well as CBF, CBV, and OEF in a baboon model of stroke. They demonstrated a delayed (20 to 40 days to peak binding) increase of the uptake of the peripheral antagonist, likely reflecting glial and macrophage reaction at this time point. More importantly, they noted a marked early and prolonged reduction in the uptake of the central receptor antagonist, ^{11}C-flumazenil, within the area of infarction that was unchanged after day 2 postinfarction. This reduction was time and perfusion independent. The authors concluded that this method would be useful for the identification of completed infarction in the subacute setting.

Read et al[43] reported the use of ^{18}F-FMISO in patients after ischemic stroke to identify hypoxic but viable peri-infarct tissue. Uptake was identified in peri-infarct regions up to 6 days after stroke onset. The temporal and regional patterns of uptake suggest that this tracer may allow identification of ischemic but viable tissue. Subsequent animal studies using a rat model have validated this tracer as a reliable marker of the ischemic penumbra, although the technique is sensitive to the timing of tracer injection.[44]

More recent studies have investigated the effects of rapid reductions of blood pressure in hypertensive patients after recent ischemic stroke.[45] Investigators at our institution recently performed a PET study to investigate whether aggressive reductions in blood pressure affected peri-infarct CBF in hypertensive patients with recent ischemic stroke.[45] Nine patients with systolic blood pressure of more than 145 mm Hg were studied 1 to 11 days after symptom onset of stroke. Mean arterial pressure was rapidly reduced using intravenous nicardipine infusion. CBF measurements were obtained before and after blood pressure reduction. No regional or peri-infarct reductions in CBF were observed. Two patients had global CBF reductions of greater than 19% in both hemi-

spheres, likely due to an upward shift of the autoregulatory curve as a consequence of chronic hypertension.

Diaschisis

A common finding in PET studies of both acute and chronic stroke has been areas of reduced flow and metabolism at sites distant from the site of infarction (**Fig. 9.3**). The remote reductions in flow and metabolism generally occur in areas linked by afferent or efferent pathways from the primary lesion. This phenomenon has been termed diaschisis.[46] The degree of reduction of CBF is slightly greater than that of CMRO$_2$.[47] The classic and most common example is seen in the contralateral cerebellar hemispheres after frontal infarction (**Fig. 9.2**). Diaschisis has been observed in the visual cortex with local reduction in CMRGlu after infarction involving the optic radiations. Similar findings have been reported in other cortical sites, particularly those overlying subcortical infarctions. Decreased metabolism of the ipsilateral thalamus after cortical or subcortical infarction has been reported as well as the converse condition of decreased cortical metabolism after ipsilateral thalamic infarction.

◆ Acute Intracerebral Hemorrhage

The mechanisms by which spontaneous intracerebral hemorrhage (ICH) causes brain injury remain unclear. The initial hemorrhage causes a direct mechanical injury to the brain parenchyma. There is good evidence that there is also a secondary injury that follows, owing to factors including hematoma enlargement, edema, inflammation, toxic effects of blood products, apoptosis, and local ischemia from compression.[48]

Zazulia et al,[49] from our group, studied 19 subjects within 24 hours of ICH to determine whether ischemia exists in the region around the clot. Peri-clot measurements of CBF, OEF, and CMRO$_2$ were determined by drawing a 1-cm-wide area around the hyperdense clot on each computed tomography (CT) slice containing clot and then superimposing this area on the PET images.[2] Although CBF and CMRO$_2$ were both significantly reduced, OEF was reduced less than in other brain regions. Thus, despite hypoperfusion, there was no evidence for peri-clot ischemia in acute ICH. These findings are consistent with a study by Hirano et al[50] using ^{18}F-fluoromisonidazole PET, a marker of hypoxia, which also found no area of reduced uptake around the clot. The reduced CBF appears to match a primary reduction in metabolism that may be related to mitochondrial dysfunction.[51]

In a subsequent study of 13 subjects with ICH, Zazulia et al[52] found evidence of a transient focal increase in FDG uptake in perihematoma regions occurring 2 to 4 days after ICH. The underlying pathophysiology of this finding remains unclear. They also studied the effects of lowering blood pressure in hypertensive patients with acute ICH. Using PET to study 14 patients within 24 hours of ICH, they reduced the mean arterial pressure (MAP) by 16% and found no drop in global or perihematomal CBF.[53] Therefore, it appears that autoregulation is preserved in patients with acute ICH (at least for mild to moderate-sized clots).

◆ Aneurysmal Subarachnoid Hemorrhage

Positron emission tomography studies in subarachnoid hemorrhage (SAH) have provided valuable data regarding the initial brain injury, as well as the mechanisms and treatment of delayed ischemic deficits (DIDs). Regarding the latter, there is good evidence that autoregulatory dysfunction is a major factor in the development of DID **(Fig. 9.5).** PET has consistently shown that oxidative metabolism and CBF is depressed after SAH.[54] The majority of studies report normal measurements of OEF in this early period, suggesting that ischemia is not a major factor.[55] In contrast, a study by Frykholm et al[56] involving PET measurements of CBF and OEF in 11 patients soon after SAH (22 to 53 hours after onset) identified several brain regions with apparent ischemia (increased OEF), in contrast to the prior reports. The mechanism and significance of this possible early ischemia is unclear.

With the onset of arteriographic vasospasm and DID, CBF falls further and OEF increases as a compensatory mechanism to maintain metabolism (CMRO$_2$).[54] Clinical deficits have been associated with a regional CBF less than 20 mL per 100 g per minute in patients with SAH-induced vasospasm,[57] similar to the values reported with other arterial occlusive

conditions.[58] The causes of reduced CBF in patients with DID can be primarily related to three key factors: (1) narrowing of large intracranial arteries (leading to reduced downstream perfusion), (2) intravascular volume depletion often related to cerebral salt wasting and associated with hyponatremia,[59] and (3) a loss of normal autoregulatory function in the distal circulation.[60] Increased intracranial pressure (related to cerebral edema or hydrocephalus) may play a role in a minority of patients.

Studies have shown that patients with SAH have an abnormal autoregulatory response to changes in systemic blood pressure.[61] The presence of abnormal autoregulation has been associated with the degree of arteriographic vasospasm. Heilbrun et al[62] measured regional CBF in 10 patients after SAH. Measurements were made at the time of cerebral arteriography using direct intracarotid injections of 133 xenon. After baseline CBF measurements, blood pressure was briefly lowered and raised with trimethaphan and angiotensin, respectively, and CBF measurements were repeated. All patients with arterial vasospasm ($n = 5$) had regional or global impairment of autoregulation. Voldby and colleagues[57] studied 26 patients after aneurysmal SAH using the same method. CBF responses to hypotension were measured between days 3 and 13 after SAH. Mean MAP reductions were 13.4% ± 5.8%. They categorized the patients based on arteriographic findings. One of the 10 patients with a normal angiogram had global impairment of autoregulation as compared with six of the eight patients with mild vasospasm. Autoregulatory

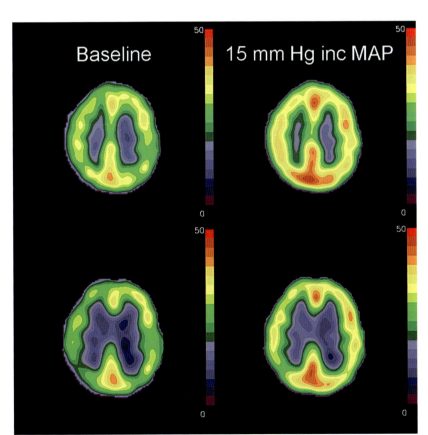

Fig. 9.5 Increased CBF with increased mean arterial pressure (MAP) consistent with a loss of normal autoregulatory function after subarachnoid hemorrhage (SAH)-induced vasospasm. Baseline CBF images are on the left. After an increase (inc) in MAP of 15 mm Hg (using a phenylephrine infusion), a repeat CBF study demonstrates a global increase in CBF. In normal subjects, a mild increase in MAP does not increase CBF owing to autoregulatory vasoconstriction.

dysfunction was regional in five and global in one. Of the eight patients with severe vasospasm all showed autoregulatory dysfunction (regional in three and global in three). Failure of autoregulation is important in SAH as it undermines the normal ability of the brain to respond to a drop in perfusion (related to vasospasm or hypovolemia) and maintain normal levels of CBF.

The inability to regulate constant levels of CBF in response to increased MAP in the study by Manno et al[61] and in response to decreased MAP in the studies of Heilbrun et al[62] and Voldby et al[57] could arise from either of two factors or a combination of both: (1) autoregulatory capacity of distal vessels is normal but the proximal large vessel spasm has reduced distal CPP to the extent that maximal vasodilation has occurred and any fall in CPP now leads to a fall in CBF (downward slope of the autoregulation curve); or (2) autoregulatory capacity of distal vessels to dilate in response to CPP is impaired.

Prior work at our institution has demonstrated that normal autoregulatory vasodilation is absent in patients with SAH.[60] Hemodynamic PET data from 29 patients with aneurysmal SAH were compared with data from 19 normal volunteers and five patients with carotid artery occlusion. SAH patients with vasospasm and controls with carotid occlusion both showed comparable reductions in rCBF (28.3 ± 7.9 versus 30.1 ± 4.4 mL per 100 g per minute) and elevations in rOEF (0.51 ± 0.09 versus 0.54 ± 0.08). The rCBV findings were very different, however. In patients with vasospasm, rCBV (3.81 ± 0.94 mL per 100 mg) was significantly lower than normal (4.62 ± 1.1), whereas in patients with carotid occlusion, rCBV (5.60 ± 1.4) was significantly higher than normal. CBV is an index of vasodilation and normally increases in situations of hemodynamic compromise, including chronic atherosclerotic disease, acute ischemic stroke, and experi-

mental animal studies of global hemorrhagic hypotension.[10] These data show that CBV is reduced in patients with vasospasm under conditions of tissue hypoxia (reduced CBF, increased OEF) that produce increased CBV in patients with carotid occlusion. These observations provide evidence that distal parenchymal vessels do not exhibit normal autoregulatory vasodilation in patients with angiographic large-vessel vasospasm and reduced perfusion after SAH.

The management of DID related to vasospasm centers around reversing the reduction in flow and oxygen delivery, as well as increased OEF, which leads to delayed cerebral ischemia. Traditional strategies have employed "triple-H" therapy (hypertension, hypervolemia, hemodilution) in an attempt to improve cerebral perfusion and CBF. The physiologic response of the cerebral circulation to these interventions is incompletely understood; we have undertaken a series of clinical experiments to examine whether CBF, DO_2 (oxygen delivery), and OEF are positively impacted by these commonly used treatments.

We studied the effect of volume expansion on CBF in six patients with arteriographic and clinical evidence of vasospasm.[63] Patients received a normal saline bolus of 15 mL/kg administered over 1 hour after baseline PET measurement of CBF. A second CBF measurement was performed after the bolus was completed. Regional CBF in territories with baseline flows below the threshold of 25 mL per 100 g per minute increased significantly with volume expansion, whereas volume expansion did not elevate CBF in regions with preserved flow or improve global CBF. The improvement in flow observed was sustained when measurements were repeated 2 to 3 hours later. Interestingly, rCBF did not improve within regions of arteriographic vasospasm (not all of which had CBF <25 mL/100 g/min). There was a weak relationship between low flow and regions with vasospasm, an observation

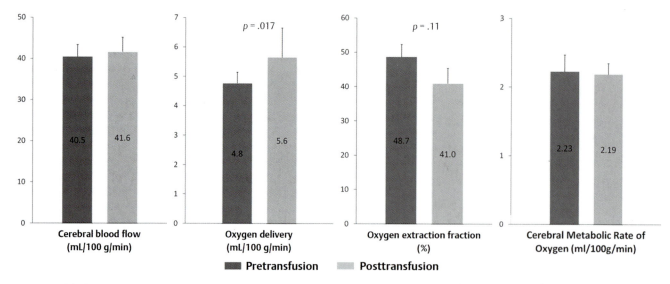

Fig. 9.6 Global CBF, oxygen delivery (DO_2), OEF, and $CMRO_2$ before and after transfusion in patients with subarachnoid hemorrhage–induced vasospasm. Mean global CBF was unchanged after transfusion, resulting in DO_2 rising by almost 20% on average. This increase in DO_2 was associated with a fall in OEF and a stable $CMRO_2$. (From Dhar R,

Zazulia AR, Videen TO, Zipfel GJ, Derdeyn CP, Diringer MN. Red blood cell transfusion increases cerebral oxygen delivery in anemic patients with subarachnoid hemorrhage. Stroke 2009;40:3039–3044. Reprinted by permission.)

we have consistently observed in other PET studies. Low flow in regions not affected by large vessel vasospasm may be related to distal vasospasm.

We have also investigated the role of red blood cell transfusion to augment cerebral oxygen delivery after SAH.[64] Anemia is a common problem in patients with SAH and may exacerbate the reduction in DO_2 (related to low CBF) underlying delayed cerebral ischemia. Lower hemoglobin levels have been associated with worse outcome, including more cerebral infarcts. However, blood transfusion is controversial in this setting because higher hemoglobin may increase viscosity and further impair CBF in the setting of vasospasm. As mentioned above, hemodilution (essentially the opposite of transfusion) has been employed by many in the management of vasospasm. Although hemodilution reduces viscosity and may improve flow, by reducing CaO_2, it may actually be detrimental to DO_2 ($CBF \times CaO_2$). How transfusion will impact DO_2 and ultimately OEF and metabolism had not been previously evaluated. To answer this question, we studied eight patients with aneurysmal SAH and hemoglobin <10 g/dL with ^{15}O-PET before and after transfusion of 1 unit of red blood cells. Transfusion resulted in a significant rise in cerebral DO_2 without lowering global CBF (**Fig. 9.6**). This response was associated with a fall in OEF but no rise in oxygen metabolism. The rise in DO_2 and fall in OEF was greater in regions with oligemia (low DO_2 and OEF ≥0.5) at baseline but the rise in DO_2 was attenuated within territories exhibiting angiographic vasospasm, where CBF actually fell 7%. Transfusion may be a novel therapy to augment DO_2 in the face of reduced perfusion and anemia. By reducing OEF it may provide vulnerable brain tissue at risk for cerebral ischemia a greater buffer before compensatory reserve is exhausted. However, further studies are needed to confirm the clinical benefit of transfusion on delayed cerebral ischemia and balance its ability to raise DO_2 and lower OEF against potential systemic and cerebral risks.

◆ Conclusion

Positron emission tomography imaging is a unique and critical tool for the investigation of cerebrovascular pathophysiology and the physiologic effects of therapies in living humans. We have gained a deeper understanding of the responses of the brain and brain vasculature to acute and chronic ischemia, spontaneous intracerebral hemorrhage, and subarachnoid hemorrhage-induced vasospasm.

References

1. Derdeyn CP. Positron emission tomography imaging of cerebral ischemia. Neuroimaging Clin N Am 2005;15:341–350, x–xi
2. Videen TO, Dunford-Shore JE, Diringer MN, Powers WJ. Correction for partial volume effects in regional blood flow measurements adjacent to hematomas in humans with intracerebral hemorrhage: implementation and validation. J Comput Assist Tomogr 1999;23:248–256
3. Quarles RP, Mintun MA, Larson KB, Markham J, MacLeod AM, Raichle ME. Measurement of regional cerebral blood flow with positron emission tomography: a comparison of [15O]water to [11C]butanol with distributed-parameter and compartmental models. J Cereb Blood Flow Metab 1993;13:733–747
4. Sette G, Baron JC, Mazoyer B, Levasseur M, Pappata S, Crouzel C. Local brain haemodynamics and oxygen metabolism in cerebrovascular disease. Positron emission tomography. Brain 1989;112(Pt 4):931–951
5. Derdeyn CP, Videen TO, Simmons NR, et al. Count-based PET method for predicting ischemic stroke in patients with symptomatic carotid arterial occlusion. Radiology 1999;212:499–506
6. Davies JR, Rudd JH, Weissberg PL. Molecular and metabolic imaging of atherosclerosis. J Nucl Med 2004;45:1898–1907
7. Baron JC, Frackowiak RS, Herholz K, et al. Use of PET methods for measurement of cerebral energy metabolism and hemodynamics in cerebrovascular disease. J Cereb Blood Flow Metab 1989;9:723–742
8. Baron JC, Rougemont D, Soussaline F, et al. Local interrelationships of cerebral oxygen consumption and glucose utilization in normal subjects and in ischemic stroke patients: a positron tomography study. J Cereb Blood Flow Metab 1984;4:140–149
9. Fox PT, Raichle ME. Focal physiological uncoupling of cerebral blood flow and oxidative metabolism during somatosensory stimulation in human subjects. Proc Natl Acad Sci U S A 1986;83:1140–1144
10. Powers WJ, Tempel LW, Grubb RL Jr, et al. Clinical correlates of cerebral hemodynamics. Stroke 1987;18:284
11. Grubb RL Jr, Derdeyn CP, Fritsch SM, et al. Importance of hemodynamic factors in the prognosis of symptomatic carotid occlusion. JAMA 1998; 280:1055–1060
12. Derdeyn CP, Videen TO, Yundt KD, et al. Variability of cerebral blood volume and oxygen extraction: stages of cerebral haemodynamic impairment revisited. Brain 2002;125(Pt 3):595–607
13. Wei EP, Kontos HA. Increased venous pressure causes myogenic constriction of cerebral arterioles during local hyperoxia. Circ Res 1984;55: 249–252
14. Forbes HS. The cerebral circulation, I: observation and measurement of pial vessels. Arch Neurol Psychiatry 1928;19:751–761
15. Fog M. Cerebral circulation. The reaction of the pial arteries to a fall in blood pressure. Arch Neurol Psychiatry 1937;24:351–364
16. McHenry LC Jr, Fazekas JF, Sullivan JF. Cerebral hemodynamics of syncope. Am J Med Sci 1961;241:173–178
17. Mintun MA, Lundstrom BN, Snyder AZ, Vlassenko AG, Shulman GL, Raichle ME. Blood flow and oxygen delivery to human brain during functional activity: theoretical modeling and experimental data. Proc Natl Acad Sci U S A 2001;98:6859–6864
18. Marshall RS, Lazar RM, Mohr JP, et al. Higher cerebral function and hemispheric blood flow during awake carotid artery balloon test occlusions. J Neurol Neurosurg Psychiatry 1999;66:734–738
19. Heiss WD, Rosner G. Functional recovery of cortical neurons as related to degree and duration of ischemia. Ann Neurol 1983;14:294–301
20. Powers WJ, Martin WR, Herscovitch P, Raichle ME, Grubb RL Jr. Extracranial-intracranial bypass surgery: hemodynamic and metabolic effects. Neurology 1984;34:1168–1174
21. Powers WJ. Cerebral hemodynamics in ischemic cerebrovascular disease. Ann Neurol 1991;29:231–240
22. Chmayssani M, Festa JR, Marshall RS. Chronic ischemia and neurocognition. Neuroimaging Clin N Am 2007;17:313–324, viii
23. Grubb RL Jr, Powers WJ, Derdeyn CP, Adams HP Jr, Clarke WR. The carotid occlusion surgery study. Neurosurg Focus 2003;14:e9
24. The EC/IC Bypass Study Group. Failure of extracranial-intracranial arterial bypass to reduce the risk of ischemic stroke. Results of an international randomized trial. N Engl J Med 1985;313:1191–1200
25. Derdeyn CP, Yundt KD, Videen TO, Carpenter DA, Grubb RL Jr, Powers WJ. Increased oxygen extraction fraction is associated with prior ischemic events in patients with carotid occlusion. Stroke 1998;29: 754–758
26. Yamauchi H, Fukuyama H, Nagahama Y, et al. Significance of increased oxygen extraction fraction in five-year prognosis of major cerebral arterial occlusive diseases. J Nucl Med 1999;40:1992–1998
27. Baron JC, Bousser MG, Rey A, Guillard A, Comar D, Castaigne P. Reversal of focal "misery-perfusion syndrome" by extra-intracranial arterial bypass in hemodynamic cerebral ischemia. A case study with 15O positron emission tomography. Stroke 1981;12:454–459
28. Adams JH, Brierley JB, Connor RC, Treip CS. The effects of systemic hypotension upon the human brain. Clinical and neuropathological observations in 11 cases. Brain 1966;89:235–268
29. Derdeyn CP, Khosla A, Videen TO, et al. Severe hemodynamic impairment and border zone—region infarction. Radiology 2001;220:195–201
30. Torvik A. The pathogenesis of watershed infarcts in the brain. Stroke 1984;15:221–223
31. Zuelch KJ. On the pathogenesis and localization of cerebral infarction. Zentralbl Neurochir 1961;21:158–178
32. Derdeyn CP, Simmons NR, Videen TO, et al. Absence of selective deep white matter ischemia in chronic carotid disease: a positron emission tomographic study of regional oxygen extraction. AJNR Am J Neuroradiol 2000;21:631–638

33. Derdeyn CP, Videen TO, Fritsch SM, Carpenter DA, Grubb RL Jr, Powers WJ. Compensatory mechanisms for chronic cerebral hypoperfusion in patients with carotid occlusion. Stroke 1999;30:1019–1024

34. Chiu D, Shedden P, Bratina P, Grotta JC. Clinical features of moyamoya disease in the United States. Stroke 1998;29:1347–1351

35. Zipfel GJ, Sagar J, Miller JP, et al. Cerebral hemodynamics as a predictor of stroke in adult patients with moyamoya disease: a prospective observational study. Neurosurg Focus 2009;26:E6

36. Pappata S, Fiorelli M, Rommel T, et al. PET study of changes in local brain hemodynamics and oxygen metabolism after unilateral middle cerebral artery occlusion in baboons. J Cereb Blood Flow Metab 1993; 13:416–424

37. Heiss W-D, Graf R, Wienhard K, et al. Dynamic penumbra demonstrated by sequential multitracer PET after middle cerebral artery occlusion in cats. J Cereb Blood Flow Metab 1994;14:892–902

38. Wise RJS, Bernardi S, Frackowiak RS, Legg NJ, Jones T. Serial observations on the pathophysiology of acute stroke. The transition from ischaemia to infarction as reflected in regional oxygen extraction. Brain 1983;106(Pt 1):197–222

39. Marchal G, Serrati C, Rioux P, et al. PET imaging of cerebral perfusion and oxygen consumption in acute ischaemic stroke: relation to outcome. Lancet 1993;341:925–927

40. Marchal G, Young AR, Baron JC. Early postischemic hyperperfusion: pathophysiologic insights from positron emission tomography. J Cereb Blood Flow Metab 1999;19:467–482

41. Heiss WD, Graf R, Löttgen J, et al. Repeat positron emission tomographic studies in transient middle cerebral artery occlusion in cats: residual perfusion and efficacy of postischemic reperfusion. J Cereb Blood Flow Metab 1997;17:388–400

42. Sette G, Baron JC, Young AR, et al. In vivo mapping of brain benzodiazepine receptor changes by positron emission tomography after focal ischemia in the anesthetized baboon. Stroke 1993;24(12):2046–2057, discussion 2057–2058

43. Read SJ, Hirano T, Abbott DF, et al. Identifying hypoxic tissue after acute ischemic stroke using PET and 18F-fluoromisonidazole. Neurology 1998; 51:1617–1621

44. Spratt NJ, Donnan GA, Howells DW. Characterisation of the timing of binding of the hypoxia tracer FMISO after stroke. Brain Res 2009;1288: 135–142

45. Powers WJ, Videen TO, Diringer MN, Aiyagari V, Zazulia AR. Autoregulation after ischaemic stroke. J Hypertens 2009;27:2218–2222

46. Feeney DM, Baron JC. Diaschisis. Stroke 1986;17:817–830

47. Yamauchi H, Fukuyama H, Kimura J. Hemodynamic and metabolic changes in crossed cerebellar hypoperfusion. Stroke 1992;23:855–860

48. Qureshi AI, Suri MF, Ostrow PT, et al. Apoptosis as a form of cell death in intracerebral hemorrhage. Neurosurgery 2003;52:1041–1047, discussion 1047–1048

49. Zazulia AR, Diringer MN, Videen TO, et al. Hypoperfusion without ischemia surrounding acute intracerebral hemorrhage. J Cereb Blood Flow Metab 2001;21:804–810

50. Hirano T, Read SJ, Abbott DF, et al. No evidence of hypoxic tissue on 18F-fluoromisonidazole PET after intracerebral hemorrhage. Neurology 1999;53:2179–2182

51. Kim-Han JS, Kopp SJ, Dugan LL, Diringer MN. Perihematomal mitochondrial dysfunction after intracerebral hemorrhage. Stroke 2006;37: 2457–2462

52. Zazulia AR, Videen TO, Powers WJ. Transient focal increase in perihematomal glucose metabolism after acute human intracerebral hemorrhage. Stroke 2009;40:1638–1643

53. Powers WJ, Zazulia AR, Videen TO, et al. Autoregulation of cerebral blood flow surrounding acute (6 to 22 hours) intracerebral hemorrhage. Neurology 2001;57:18–24

54. Carpenter DA, Grubb RL Jr, Tempel LW, Powers WJ. Cerebral oxygen metabolism after aneurysmal subarachnoid hemorrhage. J Cereb Blood Flow Metab 1991;11:837–844

55. Hayashi T, Suzuki A, Hatazawa J, et al. Cerebral circulation and metabolism in the acute stage of subarachnoid hemorrhage. J Neurosurg 2000; 93:1014–1018

56. Frykholm P, Andersson JL, Långström B, Persson L, Enblad P. Haemodynamic and metabolic disturbances in the acute stage of subarachnoid haemorrhage demonstrated by PET. Acta Neurol Scand 2004;109:25–32

57. Voldby B, Enevoldsen EM, Jensen FT. Regional CBF, intraventricular pressure, and cerebral metabolism in patients with ruptured intracranial aneurysms. J Neurosurg 1985;62:48–58

58. Marshall RS, Lazar RM, Pile-Spellman J, et al. Recovery of brain function during induced cerebral hypoperfusion. Brain 2001;124(Pt 6):1208–1217

59. Solomon RA, Post KD, McMurtry JG III. Depression of circulating blood volume in patients after subarachnoid hemorrhage: implications for the management of symptomatic vasospasm. Neurosurgery 1984;15: 354–361

60. Yundt KD, Grubb RL Jr, Diringer MN, Powers WJ. Autoregulatory vasodilation of parenchymal vessels is impaired during cerebral vasospasm. J Cereb Blood Flow Metab 1998;18:419–424

61. Manno EM, Gress DR, Schwamm LH, Diringer MN, Ogilvy CS. Effects of induced hypertension on transcranial Doppler ultrasound velocities in patients after subarachnoid hemorrhage. Stroke 1998;29:422–428

62. Heilbrun MP, Olesen J, Lassen NA. Regional cerebral blood flow studies in subarachnoid hemorrhage. J Neurosurg 1972;37:36–44

63. Jost SC, Diringer MN, Zazulia AR, et al. Effect of normal saline bolus on cerebral blood flow in regions with low baseline flow in patients with vasospasm following subarachnoid hemorrhage. J Neurosurg 2005;103: 25–30

64. Dhar R, Zazulia AR, Videen TO, Zipfel GJ, Derdeyn CP, Diringer MN. Red blood cell transfusion increases cerebral oxygen delivery in anemic patients with subarachnoid hemorrhage. Stroke 2009;40:3039–3044

10

Ultrasound Assessment in Ischemic and Hemorrhagic Stroke

Javier M. Romero and Anna G. Meader

Pitfall

◆ Although peak systolic velocity is the most common criterion for grading stenosis in duplex ultrasonography (DUS), it is not always entirely reliable in its estimation. Cases in point are the differentiation between occlusion and pseudo-occlusion of the carotid artery and subclavian steal physiology, as well as pseudo-normalization, otherwise known as "velocities falling off."

◆ Carotid Duplex Ultrasonography

Justification for Use

Although many causes of anterior circulation stroke exist, emboli from carotid occlusive disease account for a significant percentage as well as for the majority of stroke morbidity and mortality.[1] The North American Carotid Endarterectomy Trial (NASCET) (1991) demonstrated strong evidence that, for symptomatic patients with greater than 70% stenosis, surgical intervention provides a greater reduction in ischemic stroke risk than medical treatment alone.[2] Furthermore, the Asymptomatic Carotid Atherosclerosis Studies (ACAS) as well as the Asymptomatic Carotid Surgery Trial (ACST) showed a clear benefit, albeit less dramatic than the NASCET, for intervention in asymptomatic patients with greater than 60% stenosis.[3,4] In addition to carotid endarterectomy (CEA), surgical options for carotid revascularization include carotid angioplasty and stent placement.[5,6] Because the efficacy of intervention in reducing ischemic events directly relates to the severity of stenosis of the internal carotid artery (ICA) in symptomatic patients, noninvasive imaging determining the degree of stenosis plays a pivotal role in defining which patients may benefit from carotid artery revascularization.

Noninvasive imaging of the ICAs is indicated in several clinical settings **(Table 10.1),** including as a preoperative eval-

uation prior to coronary artery bypass graft (CABG) surgery,[7] in patients who have experienced transient ischemic attacks (TIAs), patients with ischemic stroke, and asymptomatic patients who have carotid bruits. Carotid bruits are neither a specific nor a sensitive indicator for severe carotid disease, however, as many as one third of patients with bruits do have severe ICA stenosis.[8] Patients with cervical bruits should undergo evaluation for carotid disease. All patients who have TIAs should be evaluated for carotid stenosis as soon as possible due to a significantly increased risk of stroke in the months following a TIA.[6] Patients undergoing evaluation for acute stroke should undergo carotid imaging due to the large proportion of embolic strokes originating from the carotid artery.[1] Although carotid screening is not recommended for every CABG candidate, all patients over the age of 60 years or presenting with a minimum of two risk factors, such as elevated cholesterol or known coronary artery disease, should undergo carotid evaluation to reduce the risk of perioperative stroke.[9,10] Sequential follow-up status post–carotid revascularization should also be performed to search for restenosis and intimal hyperplasia.[2] Intimal hyperplasia results secondary to operative trauma and is characterized by redundant granulation or scar tissue. Intimal hyperplasia with smooth muscle cell and matrix accumulation is the prominent feature in all of these situations, with evidence of intense cell proliferation and cell death.[11] Intimal hyperplasia usually peaks at 9 months postsurgery and generally does not progress after the first year.

Technique

In a standard carotid duplex ultrasonography (DUS), a bilateral examination of the common carotid arteries (CCAs), ICA, external carotid arteries (ECAs), and vertebral arteries (VAs) is performed. Gray-scale images in both transverse and longitudinal planes are obtained throughout the course of

Table 10.1 Clinical Indications for Carotid Duplex Examination
Carotid bruit
Transient ischemic attack
Ischemic stroke
Preoperative coronary artery bypass graft
Post–carotid endarterectomy or poststenting follow-up

Table 10.2 Standard Spectral Carotid Duplex Ultrasound Technique
1. Obtain waveforms from a longitudinal axis view of the artery, using a small sample volume placed in the center stream of flow or center to the flow "jet"
2. Align the cursor parallel to the vessel wall/flow jet
3. Standardize the Doppler angle, with the recommended Doppler angle being 40–60 degrees; if the angle is correct, the cursor will be parallel to the vessel wall; a correct Doppler angle is required to calculate the peak systolic velocity (PSV)

the CCA and ICA, whereas in the ECA and VA, longitudinal images only are obtained. B-mode imaging is conducted as a separate segment of the exam from the spectral Doppler evaluation. Utilizing gray-scale B-mode imaging, color and Doppler flow provide the necessary imaging tools to determine the severity of ICA stenosis. The presence of hemodynamically significant disease in the ICA is determined by an increase in the Doppler-derived blood flow velocity, B-mode findings, and color flow images. Spectral Doppler waveforms are obtained from eight standardized sites, with a defined technique **(Table 10.2)**: the proximal, middle, and distal CCA; the proximal, middle, and distal ICA; the proximal ECA; and the proximal/middle VA. Although many guidelines have been published for the detection of significant stenosis (>70%), we favor the internal correlation with angiograms (computed tomography [CT] or conventional catheter) for a practice-oriented guideline **(Table 10.3)**.

Each vessel has a characteristic normal waveform pattern based on the vascular bed distal to the artery **(Table 10.4)**.

Occlusion Versus Pseudo-Occlusion

Vessel occlusion, for instance in the ICA, is typically indicated by a lack of signal or Doppler shift within the vessel. How-

ever, even with a critical stenosis very slow flow may be present, and routine ultrasonography may be insensitive to such low velocities. Therefore, the possibility of a pseudo-occlusion, otherwise known as a hairline residual lumen, must be considered. The technique should be optimized by placing the Doppler signal in the ghost vessel while increasing the color gain to the maximum level and decreasing filters and pulse repetition frequency (PRF). With these parameters carotid ultrasound shows an 80 to 90% sensitivity in detecting hairline lumina.[12]

When clinical suspicion is high for pseudo-occlusion, meaning a lack of flow with ultrasound or magnetic resonance angiography (MRA) two-dimensional (2D) time of flight (TOF), CT angiography may be required for a definitive diagnosis.[13] Perhaps the most definitive technique may be conventional catheter arteriography, still considered the standard of reference for distinguishing between pseudo- and true occlusions.[14]

Velocities Falling Off

Typically, as the percent stenosis in a vessel increases, peak systolic velocities increase correspondingly due to the increase of the pressure gradient. However, when stenosis ap-

Table 10.3 Carotid Noninvasive Ultrasound

Degree of Stenosis	Peak Systolic Velocity (cm/s)	Approx. % Degree of Stenosis	Luminal Diameter (mm)	Other Indirect Signs (Periorbital Doppler TCD, Assumes NL ECAs)
NL	<150		>3	
Mild	150–200	50–60%	2.5–3	
Mod	200–300	60–70%	2–2.5	
Severe	300–400	70–80%	1–2 mm	Reversal flow ipsilateral ACA (TCD) Supraorbital Doppler reversal
Critical	>400	80–90%	0.7–1	Reversal flow Ophthalmic artery (TCD) Supratrochlear Doppler reversal
	Falling off	>90%	<0.7	MRA shows absent distal ICA signal (slow flow versus occlusion), consider CTA

Abbreviations: ACA, anterior cerebral artery; CTA, computed tomography angiography; ECA, external carotid artery; ICA, internal carotid artery; MRA, magnetic resonance angiography; NL, normal; TCD, Transcranial Doppler ultrasonography.
Source: Velocity guidelines for determining degree of vessel stenosis in carotid DUS adapted from the Neurovascular Laboratory, Massachusetts General Hospital, Boston.

Fig. 10.1 Carotid duplex ultrasound demonstrating dampened waveforms and low peak systolic velocities in the left internal carotid artery, a result of a hairline lumen. (Courtesy of Massachusetts General Hospital Imaging.)

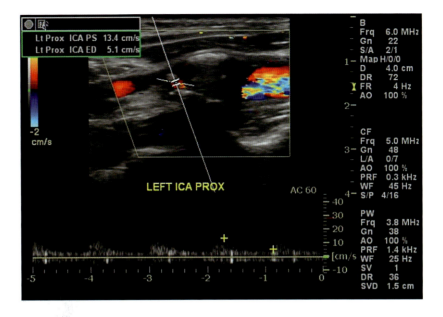

Table 10.4 Typical Vascular Waveform Characteristics for Carotid Duplex Ultrasonography

Vessel	Normal Carotid DUS Waveform Patterns
ICA	Low resistance waveform with continuous forward flow throughout the diastole
ECA	High-resistance waveform with a rapid sharp systolic upstroke and diminished diastolic flow
CCA	A mixture of the ICA and ECA waveforms with a low resistance waveform and continuous flow throughout the diastole
VA	Low-resistance waveform with continuous forward flow throughout the diastole

Abbreviations: CCA, common carotid arteries; DUS, duplex ultrasonography; ECA, external carotid artery; ICA, internal carotid artery; VA, vertebral artery.

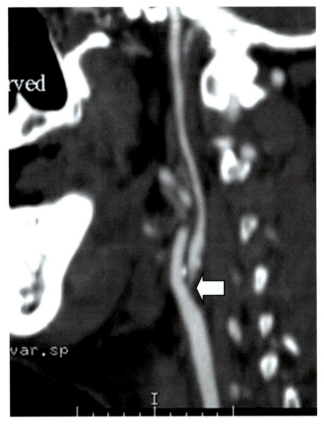

Fig. 10.2 Computed tomography angiogram: curved reformat centered in the left internal carotid artery demonstrating a hairline lumen of the proximal segment *(arrow).* (Courtesy of Massachusetts General Hospital Imaging.)

proaches 100%, leaving only a residual hairline lumen open, velocities may suddenly decrease in a process referred to as pseudonormalization (**Fig. 10.1**). This phenomenon, otherwise known as "velocities falling off," results in a downward recapitulation of the velocity values into ranges associated with less severe stenosis or absence of stenosis.[2] Pseudonormalization is problematic due to the fact that it may lead to an inaccurate description of vessel stenosis, whereas in fact the vasculature may be critically stenotic (**Fig. 10.2**), and peak systolic velocities indicate a low degree of stenosis (**Fig. 10.1**), if any, with the result that severe carotid disease may be overlooked.

Fortunately, turbulent flow (**Fig. 10.3**), decreases in the resistance index, spectral broadening (**Fig. 10.4**), dampening of the distal vessel waveform (curved waveforms **Fig. 10.5**), and a pinpoint residual lumen on color flow images in either the longitudinal or transverse plane may be used to correctly identify a "velocities falling off" situation. Additionally, a ret-

rograde flow direction in the ophthalmic artery detected via transcranial Doppler ultrasonography may be used to identify pseudonormalization. Evidence of reversal of flow begins at approximately the same time velocities start to fall off as

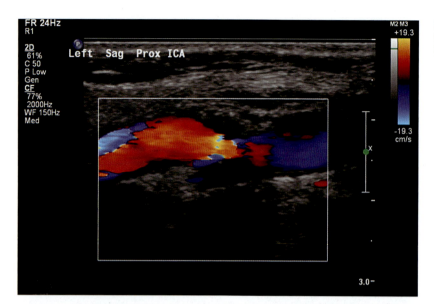

Fig. 10.3 Turbulent color flow demonstrated in the left internal carotid artery. (Courtesy of Massachusetts General Hospital Imaging.)

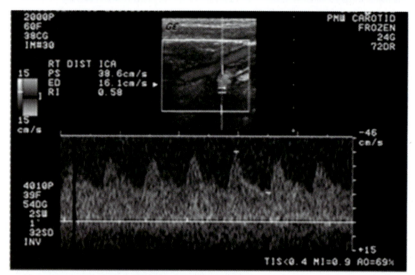

Fig. 10.4 Spectral broadening and decreased resistance index, demonstrated in the waveform of the distal right internal carotid artery. (Courtesy of Massachusetts General Hospital Imaging.)

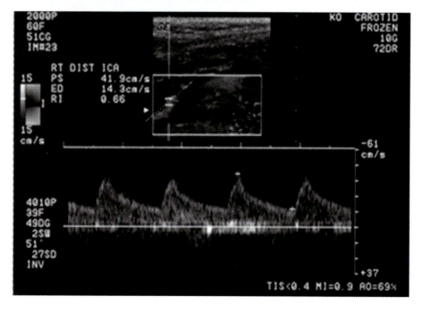

Fig. 10.5 A curved waveform demonstrated in the right distal internal carotid artery. (Courtesy of Massachusetts General Hospital Imaging.)

the internal carotid artery narrows. Also a dissociation among the degree of stenosis being evaluated in b-mode, the color flow, and the measured velocities should always be interrogated and further investigated.

Tandem Lesions

A tandem lesion in the carotid artery is defined as two separate stenoses at least 3 cm apart that result in severe stenosis along the carotid artery. In such cases, the second lesion, located downstream from the insonated lesion, causes dampening of the peak systolic velocity between the two lesions. It is the stenosis with the greatest narrowing that determines the hemodynamic compromise.[13,15] In this situation, despite evidence of severe stenosis as indicated by B-mode imaging, peak systolic velocities and spectral configuration of flow of

the poststenotic segment remain within normal or slightly abnormal limits **(Fig. 10.6)**.[13] When tandem lesions are suspected due to a discrepancy between B-mode images and Doppler velocities, CT angiography, gadolinium-enhanced magnetic resonance imaging (MRI), or conventional angiography should be used for a definitive diagnosis **(Fig. 10.6C)**.

Subclavian Steal

A subclavian steal phenomenon is clinically characterized by vertigo during arm exertion, as well as by hand or arm pain due to hypoperfusion. Moreover, patients typically exhibit marked differences in blood pressure between the left and right arms. The incidence of subclavian steal is rare, approximately 2%, and the relevance of a steal in asymptomatic patients remains small or unknown.[16]

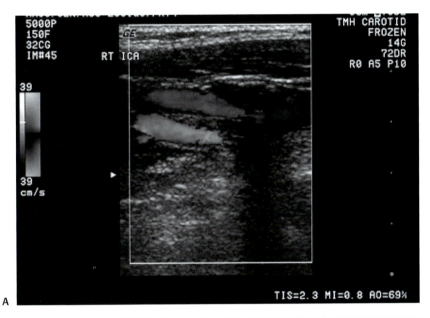

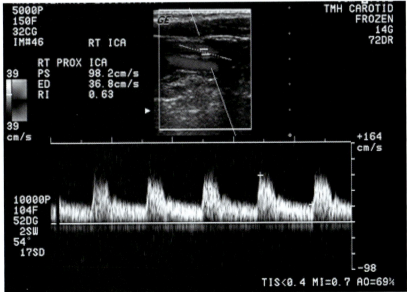

Fig. 10.6 Carotid duplex ultrasound images demonstrating tandem lesions in the right internal carotid artery. **(A)** Gray-scale imaging. **(B)** Waveforms. (Courtesy of Massachusetts General Hospital Imaging.) *(continued on next page)*

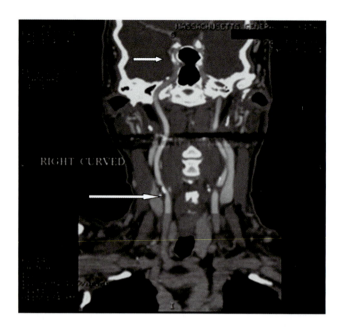

Fig. 10.6 *(continued)* **(C)** Tandem lesion: coronal curved reformat of the right carotid artery. Severe stenosis of the proximal right internal carotid artery *(long arrow);* severe stenosis of the cavernous segment of the right internal carotid artery *(short arrow).* (Courtesy of Massachusetts General Hospital Imaging.)

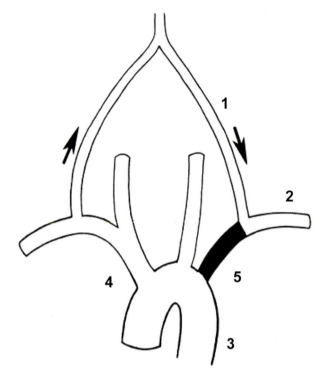

Fig. 10.7 Depiction of a left subclavian steal phenomenon. The vessel diagram depicts the left vertebral artery (1), the left subclavian artery (2), the aortic arch (3), the brachiocephalic arch (4), and the subclavian region of stenosis (5). (Adapted from Horrow MM, Stassi J. Sonography of the vertebral arteries: a window to disease of the proximal great vessels. AJR Am J Roentgenol 2001;177:53–59.)

Retrograde flow evident in the VA is the classic hallmark of an advanced subclavian steal phenomenon (**Fig. 10.7**); however, subtle waveform changes are evident even in the early stages of steal development. In a 957-subject trial, Kliewer et al[10] demonstrated four distinctly identifiable waveform changes indicative of advancing subclavian steal physiology. Although all four waveforms share an abrupt decline in flow velocity in early systolic upstroke, each characteristic waveform is defined by the ratio of the flow velocity at the midsystolic notch to the flow velocity at end diastole. The greater the ratio, the more advanced the steal phenomenon, with the class IV steal displaying the greatest degree of retrograde flow (**Fig. 10.8**). Angiographic correlation supports the conclusion that increasing hemodynamic changes evident in the VA are associated with disease severity.[10]

◆ Vulnerable Plaque Characterization

Many recent trials have concentrated on the characterization of vulnerable plaque morphology. Seminal papers regarding plaque characterization were based on ultrasound technology; the Cardiovascular Health Physicians Trial in particular demonstrated a close relationship between hypoechoic carotid plaque and neurologic symptoms.[17] This was one of the largest trials to date demonstrating a relationship of symptoms different from the one risk based on significant stenosis. In contrast, more recent trials have indicated that a hyperechoic state may represent calcification of the plaque,[18] and therefore may confer or represent a certain degree of protec-

tion, probably secondary to a more mature stage of this plaque and lack of inflammatory component; in other words, a hyperechoic plaque may represent a stable plaque.

Detection of the lipid core as a defined characteristic of vulnerable plaque has also been demonstrated with multiple modalities such as MRI, CT, and ultrasound; a few studies have demonstrated a good correlation of hypoechoic plaque with the presence of a lipid core.[19–21] Although other plaque characteristics such as a thin fibrous cap and plaque enhancement have been shown to possess a strong relationship with symptoms, these findings are difficult to evaluate with ultrasound due to the small dimension of the fibrous capsule, particularly as it is apparently more prone to rupture when the capsule reaches a very thin diameter.[22]

Recent ultrasound trials have additionally demonstrated the possibility of detecting vasa vasorum with contrast agents.[23,24] This finding has been investigated with computed tomographic angiography (CTA) and demonstrated a larger proportion of vessels with increased vasa vasorum enhancement, hence neovascularization in symptomatic patients compared with asymptomatic patients.[25] Neovascularization of the vasa vasorum within the adventitia is a hallmark of inflammation not only of the carotid plaque (**Fig. 10.9**) but also within the iliac and coronary arteries.[26]

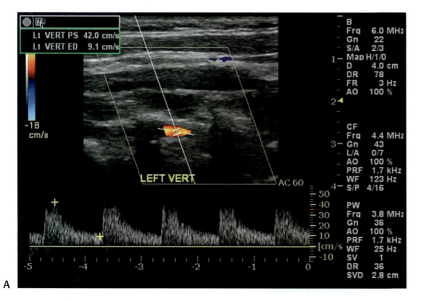

A

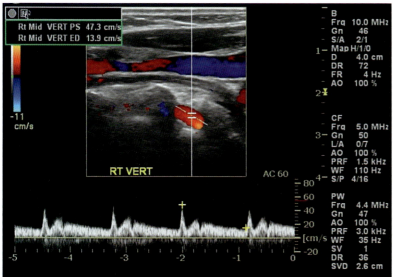

B

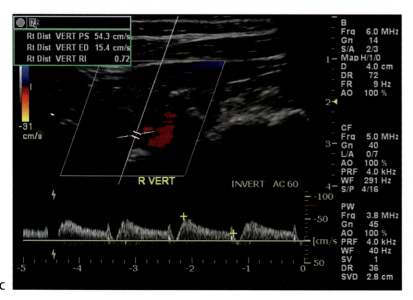

C

Fig. 10.8 The four categories of subclavian steal waveform in order of increasing severity. **(A)** Type I subclavian steal waveform, characterized by a mild notch between two systolic peaks. **(B)** Type II subclavian steal waveform, characterized by a more pronounced notch between the two systolic peaks, with the second peak shorter than the first; note also the mild diastolic notch. **(C)** Type III subclavian steal waveform, characterized by a systolic notch falling at or slightly below baseline, but with resumption of forward flow prior to diastole. (*continued on next page*)

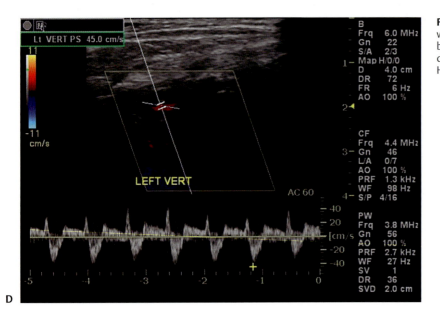

Fig. 10.8 (*continued*) **(D)** Type IV subclavian steal waveform, characterized by a systolic notch falling below baseline and the recovery of forward flow during diastole. (Courtesy of Massachusetts General Hospital Imaging.)

◆ Intima-Media Thickness

Multiple noninvasive imaging trials have assessed the carotid artery for characteristics that may be related to increased cardiovascular risk.[27–29] Of the multiple characteristics evaluated, intima–media thickness (IMT) as measured with ultrasound has the benefit of being a very accessible measure, as well as a reproducible and economical method with strong correlation to increased cardiovascular risk.[30] The carotid intima media is a layer of the arterial wall, constituted by endothelium (tunica intima) and a layer of multiple elastic lamellae alternating with thin layers of circularly oriented smooth muscle (tunica media) (**Fig. 10.10**). B-mode imaging is used to determine both the carotid intimal and medial thickness. Because of its strong correlation with increased cardiovascular risk, carotid IMT may be used as a surrogate marker and intermediate phenotype for early atherosclerosis.[31]

Patients with increased thickness of the intima media layer of the carotid artery present not only a higher incidence of myocardial infarction but also a higher incidence of stroke.[32,33] The normal measurements of the intima media at different age ranges are shown in **Table 10.5**. According to Juonala et al,[34] when adjustments for risk factors and carotid diameter are taken into account, there is no significant difference between the IMT of healthy men and that of healthy women. A 2007 meta-analysis by Lorenz et al[32] has pooled many studies of carotid IMT as measured by ultrasound, including a total of 37,197 patients. The analysis found that for an absolute carotid IMT difference of 0.1 mm, the future risk of myocardial infarction increases by 10 to 15%, and the stroke risk increases by 13 to 18%. However, the study also highlighted the difficulties comparing the different trial protocols measuring IMT. Additionally, multiple recent studies have demonstrated the reduction of IMT via the administration of statins, with clinical impact in reduction of stroke risk.[35–37]

◆ Transcranial Doppler Ultrasonography

Technique

Transcranial Doppler (TCD) ultrasonography technology is based on pulsed-wave Doppler measurements of blood flow velocity, and it combines two-dimensional gray-scale imag-

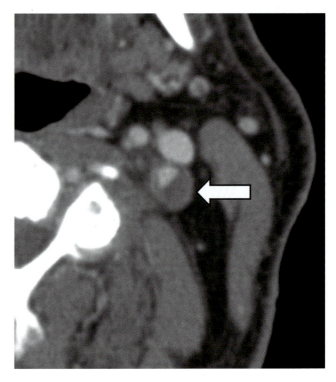

Fig. 10.9 Axial computed tomography angiogram of the neck at the level of proximal left internal carotid artery demonstrating enhancement of the carotid wall (vasa vasorum; *arrow*). (Courtesy of Massachusetts General Hospital Imaging.)

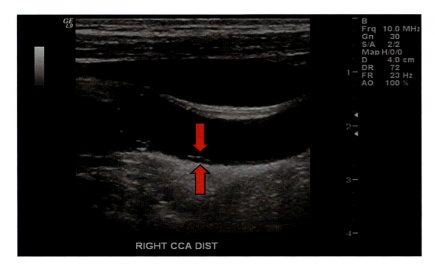

Fig. 10.10 Intimal medial thickening demonstrated in the right distal common carotid artery. (Courtesy of Massachusetts General Hospital Imaging.)

ing with real-time Doppler, providing a color-coded representation of blood flow velocity.[38] Advantages of the method include its noninvasive nature, enabling bedside examination, as well as its reproducibility.

In a full TCD examination, a bilateral examination of the anterior cerebral arteries (ACAs), middle cerebral arteries (MCAs), and posterior cerebral arteries (PCAs), as well as the intracranial and extracranial VAs, proximal basilar artery, ophthalmic arteries (OphAs), and carotid siphon region is performed (**Table 10.6**).

Table 10.5 Reference Limits for Ultrasound Measurements of Intima-Media Thickness (IMT) in Healthy Patients

Age/Sex	Carotid IMT (mm)	
	Lower Limit	Upper Limit
Women		
24 years	0.411	0.698
27 years	0.420	0.719
30 years	0.430	0.742
33 years	0.440	0.765
36 years	0.451	0.789
39 years	0.462	0.814
Men		
24 years	0.411	0.734
27 years	0.422	0.760
30 years	0.433	0.787
33 years	0.444	0.816
36 years	0.456	0.846
39 years	0.469	0.878

Source: Adapted from Juonala M, Kähönen M, Laitinen T, et al. Effect of age and sex on carotid intima-media thickness, elasticity and brachial endothelial function in healthy adults: the cardiovascular risk in Young Finns Study. Eur Heart J 2008;29:1198–1206.

The presence and degree of hemodynamically significant vessel stenosis is determined by the velocities (**Table 10.7**) as well as direction of flow and waveform characteristics. Flow should be oriented toward the probe when insonating the MCA and ophthalmic arteries, and oriented away from the probe when insonating the ACA and PCA. The direction of flow may vary when insonating the carotid siphon region, basilar artery, and VAs. Waveforms of high resistance are typically found in the ophthalmic arteries, whereas low-resistance waveforms may be found throughout the rest of the intracranial vasculature.

Utility in Subarachnoid Hemorrhage Vasospasm

Vasospasm, defined as the delayed narrowing of large capacitance intracranial arteries, is the greatest source of mortality and morbidity in subarachnoid hemorrhage (SAH) patients who survive symptom onset.[39] Vasospasm is characterized by an increase in mean blood flow velocity above the upper limit for a patient's age; see **Table 10.8** for information regarding normal mean blood flow velocity. As severe vasospasm has a hemodynamic effect similar to that of stenosis, both producing an increase in blood flow velocity, transcranial Doppler ultrasound has been shown to be a sensitive method of diagnosing and monitoring SAH vasospasm.[40] Although conventional angiography may be considered the "gold standard" in vasospasm diagnosis, unfortunately it should not be used in frequent monitoring due to its invasive nature, radiation exposure, and increased risk of cerebral ischemia.[38,41] The ability to perform repeated noninvasive studies with easily reproducible results makes TCD a popular method of SAH vasospasm patient monitoring. It must be remembered, however, that TCD provides a measurement of vessel flow velocity, and therefore does not provide any direct indication of decreased tissue perfusion.[39] Additionally, recording Doppler signals from spastic arteries with a small diameter or beyond the reach of the TCD bone window may be technically difficult.[40]

Transcranial Doppler ultrasonography is most reliable in diagnosing vasospasm of the M1 segment, followed by the basilar and vertebral arteries; currently TCD is not considered

Table 10.6 Guidelines for Transcranial Doppler Vessel Insonation

Vessel	Depths (mm)	Flow Direction in Reference to Probe	Window	Optimal Boost Setting
MCA	65 to 45	Toward	Temporal	Medium
ACA	65 to 75	Away	Temporal	Medium
PCA	65 to 75	Away	Temporal	Medium
OphA	45 to approximately 65	Toward	Orbital	Low
Siphon	Approximately 65 to 75	Either	Orbital	Medium
Vertebral				
Extracranial	45 to 55	Away	Mastoid	Low
Intracranial	60 to 75	Away	Foraminal	Medium
Basilar	80 to 120	Away	Foraminal	Medium

Abbreviations: ACA, anterior cerebral artery; MCA, middle cerebral artery; OphA, ophthalmic artery; PCA, posterior cerebral artery.

Source: Standard guidelines for vascular insonation by transcranial Doppler ultrasound, adapted from the guidelines of the Neurovascular Laboratory of Massachusetts General Hospital, Boston.

reliable for diagnosis of ACA (A2) vasospasm.[38] Typically, MCA velocities above 120 cm/s are considered suggestive of vasospasm, with velocities above 200 cm/s considered a critical vasospasm.[38,41] A mean blood flow velocity may also be considered indicative of critical vasospasm when it is approximately five times greater than a typical blood flow velocity for the patient's age.[41] Transcranial Doppler results should always be compared with baseline values obtained early (during the first 3 days postictus) to evaluate progression of disease. In addition to increased intracranial velocities, the Lindegaard ratio may be used to determine the presence of vasospasm; if the ratio of MCA flow velocity to extracranial ICA flow velocity (Lindegaard ratio) is greater than 3, vasospasm is the likely diagnosis, whereas if the mean MCA velocity is greater than 120 cm/s and the Lindegaard ratio is less than 3, hyperemia is the likely diagnosis.[42,43]

Use in Pediatric Sickle Cell Disease

Children with sickle cell disease (SCD) carry an increased risk of stroke when a critical low level of hemoglobin is reached; the incidence of stroke is highest during the first decade of life.[44] These low levels of hemoglobin may require polytransfusions to decrease stroke risk; however, polytransfusions carry the risk of secondary effects such as iron overload and alloimmunization.[45] Adams et al[46] first demonstrated the effectiveness of Doppler in screening for cerebrovascular disease in pediatric patients with SCD. Since then, TCD has been repeatedly demonstrated to be an accurate tool for detecting a high risk for stroke and identifying those patients who would benefit most from transfusion therapy.[47–49]

Table 10.7 A Concise Guide to Determining Vessel Stenosis Based on Insonated Vessel Velocity

Degree of Stenosis	Velocity of Pulse Wave (cm/s)	
	Anterior	Vertebral and Basilar
"Gray zone"		80–100
Mild	120–160	101–150
Moderate	161–200	150–180
Severe	>200	>180

Table 10.8 Normal Reference for Carotid Blood Flow Velocities (cm/s) in Different Age Groups

	20–40 Years	41–60 Years	>60 Years
Common carotid artery			
Peak systolic	96	75	61
End diastolic	23	21	16
Internal carotid artery			
Peak systolic	65	61	51
End diastolic	27	25	18
Vertebral artery			
Peak systolic	49	48	45
End diastolic	17	17	14

Source: Adapted from Babikian VL, Wechsler LR, Higashida RT. Ultrasound images of cerebrovascular disease. In: Babikian VL, Wechsler LR, Higashida RT, eds. Imaging Cerebrovascular Disease. Philadelphia: Butterworth Heinemann, 2003:3–35.

Table 10.9 Indicators of Cerebrovascular Disease in Sickle Cell Disease Patients

1	Maximum ophthalmic artery velocity greater than 35 cm/s
2	Time-averaged mean maximum velocity of greater than 170 cm/s in the MCA
3	RI ophthalmic artery less than 60 cm/s
4	Ophthalmic artery velocity greater than that of the ipsilateral MCA
5	Maximum PCA, vertebral, or basilar velocity greater than the maximum MCA velocity
6	Turbulent flow
7	PCA visualized without the MCA
8	Any RI less than 30 cm/s
9	Peak systolic MCA velocity greater than 200 cm/s

Abbreviations: MCA, middle cerebral artery; PCA, posterior cerebral artery; RI, resistance index.

Source: Adapted from Seibert JJ, Glasier CM, Kirby RS, et al. Transcranial Doppler, MRA, and MRI as a screening examination for cerebrovascular disease in patients with sickle cell anemia: an 8-year study. Pediatr Radiol 1998;28:138–142.

Transcranial Doppler Ultrasonography Criteria for Sickle Cell Disease in Children for Increased Risk of Stroke

The Stroke Prevention Trial in Sickle Cell Anemia (STOP)[48] determined that children who demonstrated a time-averaged mean maximum velocity of ≥200 cm/s in the intracranial vasculature are at an increased risk for stroke. Time-averaged mean maximum velocity differs from peak systolic velocity (PSV); the time-averaged mean refers to the time mean of the peak velocity envelope, with the envelope considered to be the trace of the peak flow velocity as a function of time.[45] More specifically, children with velocities ≥200 cm/s in the distal ICA or proximal MCA have a stroke risk 10 to 20 times greater than that of the general sickle cell population of the same age. Subsequently, using TCD, MRA, and MRI, Seibert et al[50] identified nine TCD indicators for an increased risk of stroke (**Table 10.9**).

◆ Cerebrovascular Reserve

Cerebrovascular reserve (CVR), also known as cerebral vascular reactivity, is a measure of the ability of the cerebral vasculature to dilate when there is an increase of partial pressure of blood CO_2 (PCO_2). This vascular reactivity has been postulated to be the mechanism by which patients regulate sudden changes of local metabolism to changes in blood pressure, hydration, and pulse pressure to maintain an adequate blood flow to all areas of the brain. When this mechanism fails to sustain the required blood flow levels in the border-zone areas of the brain, ischemic changes may result secondary to unmet requirements of metabolic demand.

When there is an exhausted cerebral vascular reserve the patient is at risk for a border-zone ischemia (**Fig. 10.11**). Many conditions may be related to a decreased vascular reserve or reactivity; the most common of these is the presence of a long-standing stenosis of the ICA, MCA, or a cardiac

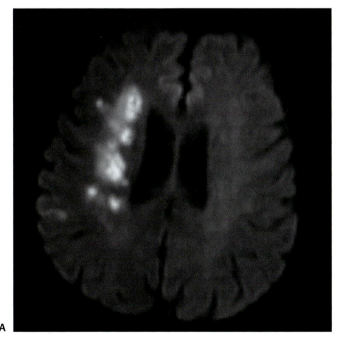
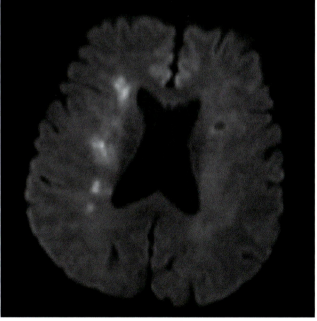

Fig. 10.11 **(A,B)** Axial diffusion-weighted images of the brain demonstrate multiple foci of restricted diffusion within the right corona radiata, likely border-zone infarctions given the patient's critical right internal carotid artery stenosis. (Courtesy of Massachusetts General Hospital Imaging.)

condition.[5] Other less frequent causes of decreased vascular reactivity are medications, and pathologies such as amyloid angiopathy and diabetes mellitus.[51] Impaired vascular reserve has been related to the increased risk of border-zone infarcts, in the setting of severe carotid stenosis or occlusion, with an odds ratio of 14.4.[52]

Many modalities have been used to measure vascular reactivity, including positron emission tomography (PET), CT perfusion, single photon emission computed tomography (SPECT), CT xenon, and TCD. The discussion here is limited to cerebrovascular reactivity as measured with TCD and as compared with other modalities.[8,53]

The MCA stem (M1) has a constant diameter during increase of PCO_2, which facilitates accurate measurement of any changes of blood velocity. With an increase of PCO_2 there is a reactive vasodilatation of the arterioles distal to the M1 segment of the MCA stem that decreases the intraluminal pressure within this vasculature. This change or increase of pressure gradient facilitates the increase of blood flow through the MCA, which consequently has to increase its flow velocity, reflected in the increase of peak systolic velocity (PSV) of the MCA as measured by the TCD. Numerous trials have measured the normal values for vascular reactivity of the MCA during the administration of CO_2 at 6%, 8%, or 10%, with breath hold or Valsalva maneuver.[1,6,9]

◆ Emboli Detection in Asymptomatic Patients: High-Intensity Transient Signal

Carotid artery atheromatous disease promoting clot formation is the culprit behind many anterior circulation ischemic strokes. The pathophysiology of this event was first described by C. Miller Fisher in his landmark paper, *Occlusion of the Carotid Arteries*.[54] Based on this premise, the detection of emboli during their course to the intracranial circulation has been the aim of many techniques. Doppler ultrasound is valuable in that it has the capacity to detect emboli originating from the heart or surrounding vessels via the continuous monitoring of the Doppler spectrum of the intracranial arteries, most often the MCA. Detection of these events with TCD is possible because these emboli particles emit a high-intensity transient signal (HITS) during their course through

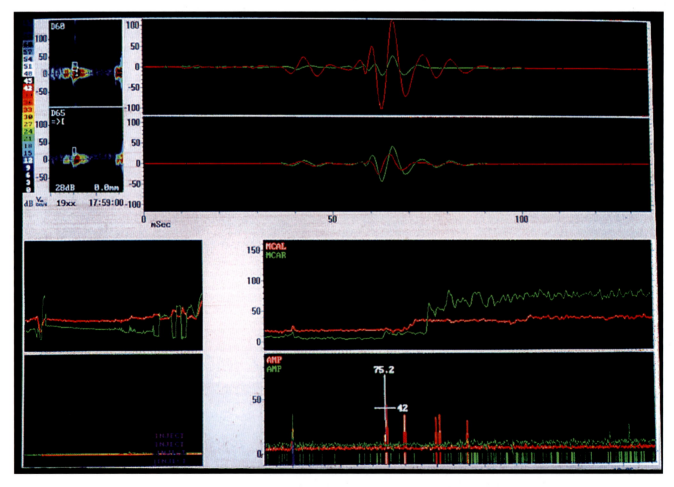

Fig. 10.12 Transcranial Doppler ultrasonography detection of a high-intensity transient signal (HITS) in the left middle cerebral artery, likely secondary to emboli in a patient with auricular fibrillation. (Courtesy of Massachusetts General Hospital Imaging.)

the MCA.[55,56] HITS detection is most often undertaken over the period of approximately 1 hour, as intraindividual variations increase when monitored over long periods of time.[57,58] The detection of HITS and its relation to symptomatic patients has been evaluated in multiple trials including some multicentric trials.[59,60]

The HITS is caused by an increased reflection of sound by the embolus surface. Signal intensity is dependent on embolus size and composition; however, because intensity is dependent upon multiple factors, no conclusions about embolus nature may be drawn from signal intensity alone. Signals are unidirectional and occur at random throughout the cardiac cycle, in addition to sounding a specific note known as a "chirp" or "blip" (**Fig. 10.12**).[61]

References

1. Aaslid R, Markwalder TM, Nornes H. Noninvasive transcranial Doppler ultrasound recording of flow velocity in basal cerebral arteries. J Neurosurg 1982;57:769–774
2. Barnett HJM; North American Symptomatic Carotid Endarterectomy Trial Collaborators. Beneficial effect of carotid endarterectomy in symptomatic patients with high-grade carotid stenosis. N Engl J Med 1991;325:445–453
3. Rothwell PM, Goldstein LB. Carotid endarterectomy for asymptomatic carotid stenosis: asymptomatic carotid surgery trial. Stroke 2004;35:2425–2427
4. Young B, Moore WS, Robertson JT, et al. An analysis of perioperative surgical mortality and morbidity in the asymptomatic carotid atherosclerosis study. ACAS Investigators. Asymptomatic Carotid Atherosclerosis Study. Stroke 1996;27:2216–2224
5. Ringelstein EB, Sievers C, Ecker S, Schneider PA, Otis SM. Noninvasive assessment of CO2-induced cerebral vasomotor response in normal individuals and patients with internal carotid artery occlusions. Stroke 1988;19:963–969
6. Aaslid R, Lindegaard KF, Sorteberg W, Nornes H. Cerebral autoregulation dynamics in humans. Stroke 1989;20:45–52
7. Cirillo F, Leonardo G, Renzulli A, et al. Carotid Atherosclerosis is Associated with In-hospital Mortality After CABG Surgery. Int J Angiol 2002;11:210–215
8. Aaslid R, Markwalder TM, Nornes H. Noninvasive transcranial Doppler ultrasound recording of flow velocity in basal cerebral arteries. J Neurosurg 1982;57:769–774
9. Bishop CCR, Powell S, Rutt D, Browse NL. Transcranial Doppler measurement of middle cerebral artery blood flow velocity: a validation study. Stroke 1986;17:913–915
10. Kliewer MA, Hertzberg BS, Kim DH, Bowie JD, Courneya DL, Carroll BA. Vertebral artery Doppler waveform changes indicating subclavian steal physiology. AJR Am J Roentgenol 2000;174:815–819
11. Zubilewicz T, Wronski J, Bourriez A, et al. Injury in vascular surgery—the intimal hyperplastic response. Med Sci Monit 2001;7:316–324
12. Fürst G, Saleh A, Wenserski F, et al. Reliability and validity of noninvasive imaging of internal carotid artery pseudo-occlusion. Stroke 1999;30:1444–1449
13. Romero JM, Lev MH, Chan S-T, et al. US of neurovascular occlusive disease: interpretive pearls and pitfalls. Radiographics 2002;22:1165–1176
14. Thiele BL, Young JV, Chikos PM, Hirsch JH, Strandness DE Jr. Correlation of arteriographic findings and symptoms in cerebrovascular disease. Neurology 1980;30:1041–1046
15. Rouleau PA, Huston J III, Gilbertson J, Brown RD Jr, Meyer FB, Bower TC. Carotid artery tandem lesions: frequency of angiographic detection and consequences for endarterectomy. AJNR Am J Neuroradiol 1999;20:621–625
16. Ackermann H, Diener HC, Seboldt H, Huth C. Ultrasonographic follow-up of subclavian stenosis and occlusion: natural history and surgical treatment. Stroke 1988;19:431–435
17. Polak JF, Shemanski L, O'Leary DH, et al. Hypoechoic plaque at US of the carotid artery: an independent risk factor for incident stroke in adults aged 65 years or older. Cardiovascular Health Study. Radiology 1998;208:649–654
18. Tegos TJ, Sohail M, Sabetai MM, et al. Echomorphologic and histopathologic characteristics of unstable carotid plaques. AJNR Am J Neuroradiol 2000;21:1937–1944
19. Grønholdt MLM, Wiebe BM, Laursen H, Nielsen TG, Schroeder TV, Sillesen H. Lipid-rich carotid artery plaques appear echolucent on ultrasound B-mode images and may be associated with intraplaque haemorrhage. Eur J Vasc Endovasc Surg 1997;14:439–445
20. Kagawa R, Moritake K, Shima T, Okada Y. Validity of B-mode ultrasonographic findings in patients undergoing carotid endarterectomy in comparison with angiographic and clinicopathologic features. Stroke 1996;27:700–705
21. Grønholdt MLM, Nordestgaard BG, Wiebe BM, Wilhjelm JE, Sillesen H. Echo-lucency of computerized ultrasound images of carotid atherosclerotic plaques are associated with increased levels of triglyceride-rich lipoproteins as well as increased plaque lipid content. Circulation 1998;97:34–40
22. Carr S, Farb A, Pearce WH, Virmani R, Yao JST. Atherosclerotic plaque rupture in symptomatic carotid artery stenosis. J Vasc Surg 1996;23:755–765, discussion 765–766
23. Feinstein SB. Contrast ultrasound imaging of the carotid artery vasa vasorum and atherosclerotic plaque neovascularization. J Am Coll Cardiol 2006;48:236–243
24. Goertz DE, Frijlink ME, Tempel D, et al. Contrast harmonic intravascular ultrasound: a feasibility study for vasa vasorum imaging. Invest Radiol 2006;41:631–638
25. Romero JM, Babiarz LS, Forero NP, et al. Arterial wall enhancement overlying carotid plaque on CT angiography correlates with symptoms in patients with high grade stenosis. Stroke 2009;40:1894–1896
26. Fleiner M, Kummer M, Mirlacher M, et al. Arterial neovascularization and inflammation in vulnerable patients: early and late signs of symptomatic atherosclerosis. Circulation 2004;110:2843–2850
27. Finn AV, Kolodgie FD, Virmani R. Correlation between carotid intimal/medial thickness and atherosclerosis: a point of view from pathology. Arterioscler Thromb Vasc Biol 2010;30:177–181
28. Griffin M, Nicolaides A, Tyllis T, et al. Carotid and femoral arterial wall changes and the prevalence of clinical cardiovascular disease. Vasc Med 2009;14:227–232
29. Mauriello A, Sangiorgi GM, Virmani R, et al. A pathobiologic link between risk factors profile and morphological markers of carotid instability. Atherosclerosis 2010;208:572–580
30. Pignoli P, Tremoli E, Poli A, Oreste P, Paoletti R. Intimal plus medial thickness of the arterial wall: a direct measurement with ultrasound imaging. Circulation 1986;74:1399–1406
31. Verçoza AM, Baldisserotto M, de Los Santos CA, Poli-de-Figueiredo CE, d'Avila DO. Cardiovascular risk factors and carotid intima-media thickness in asymptomatic children. Pediatr Cardiol 2009;30:1055–1060
32. Lorenz MW, Markus HS, Bots ML, Rosvall M, Sitzer M. Prediction of clinical cardiovascular events with carotid intima-media thickness: a systematic review and meta-analysis. Circulation 2007;115:459–467
33. Bots ML, Hoes AW, Koudstaal PJ, Hofman A, Grobbee DE. Common carotid intima-media thickness and risk of stroke and myocardial infarction: the Rotterdam Study. Circulation 1997;96:1432–1437
34. Juonala M, Kähönen M, Laitinen T, et al. Effect of age and sex on carotid intima-media thickness, elasticity and brachial endothelial function in healthy adults: the cardiovascular risk in Young Finns Study. Eur Heart J 2008;29:1198–1206
35. Crouse JR III, Grobbee DE, O'Leary DH, et al; Measuring Effects on intima media Thickness: an Evalution Of Rosuvastatin study group. Measuring effects on intima media thickness: an evaluation of rosuvastatin in subclinical atherosclerosis—the rationale and methodology of the METEOR study. Cardiovasc Drugs Ther 2004;18:231–238
36. Meaney A, Ceballos G, Asbun J, et al. The VYtorin on Carotid intima-media Thickness and Overall arterial Rigidity (VYCTOR) study. J Clin Pharmacol 2009;49:838–847
37. Forst T, Wilhelm B, Pfützner A, et al. Investigation of the vascular and pleiotropic effects of atorvastatin and pioglitazone in a population at high cardiovascular risk. Diab Vasc Dis Res 2008;5:298–303
38. Babikian VL, Wechsler LR, Higashida RT. Ultrasound images of cerebrovascular disease. In: Babikian VL, Wechsler LR, Higashida RT, eds. Imaging Cerebrovascular Disease. Philadelphia: Butterworth Heinemann, 2003:3–35
39. Babikian VL, Wechsler LR, Higashida RT. Subarachnoid hemorrhage. In: Babikian VL, Wechsler LR, Higashida RT, eds. Imaging Cerebrovascular Disease. Philadelphia: Butterworth Heinemann, 2003:241–269
40. Seiler RW, Newell DW. Subarachnoid hemorrhage and vasospasm. In: Seiler RW, Newell DW, eds. Transcranial Doppler. New York: Raven Press, 1992:101–107
41. Aaslid R, Huber P, Nornes H. Evaluation of cerebrovascular spasm with transcranial Doppler ultrasound. J Neurosurg 1984;60:37–41
42. Lindegaard KF, Nornes H, Bakke SJ, Sorteberg W, Nakstad P. Cerebral vasospasm after subarachnoid haemorrhage investigated by means of transcranial Doppler ultrasound. Acta Neurochir Suppl (Wien) 1988;42:81–84

43. Gupta AK. Monitoring the injured brain in the intensive care unit. J Postgrad Med 2002;48:218–225
44. Ohene-Frempong K. Stroke in sickle cell disease: demographic, clinical, and therapeutic considerations. Semin Hematol 1991;28:213–219
45. Bulas D. Screening children for sickle cell vasculopathy: guidelines for transcranial Doppler evaluation. Pediatr Radiol 2005;35:235–241
46. Adams R, McKie V, Nichols F, et al. The use of transcranial ultrasonography to predict stroke in sickle cell disease. N Engl J Med 1992;326:605–610
47. Adams RJ, McKie VC, Carl EM, et al. Long-term stroke risk in children with sickle cell disease screened with transcranial Doppler. Ann Neurol 1997;42:699–704
48. Adams RJ, McKie VC, Brambilla D, et al. Stroke prevention trial in sickle cell anemia. Control Clin Trials 1998;19:110–129
49. Armstrong-Wells J, Grimes B, Sidney S, et al. Utilization of TCD screening for primary stroke prevention in children with sickle cell disease. Neurology 2009;72:1316–1321
50. Seibert JJ, Glasier CM, Kirby RS, et al. Transcranial Doppler, MRA, and MRI as a screening examination for cerebrovascular disease in patients with sickle cell anemia: an 8-year study. Pediatr Radiol 1998;28:138–142
51. Fülesdi B, Limburg M, Bereczki D, et al. Impairment of cerebrovascular reactivity in long-term type 1 diabetes. Diabetes 1997;46:1840–1845
52. Markus H, Cullinane M. Severely impaired cerebrovascular reactivity predicts stroke and TIA risk in patients with carotid artery stenosis and occlusion. Brain 2001;124(Pt 3):457–467
53. Maeda H, Etani H, Handa N, et al. A validation study on the reproducibility of transcranial Doppler velocimetry. Ultrasound Med Biol 1990;16:9–14
54. Fisher M. Occlusion of the carotid arteries: further experiences. AMA Arch Neurol Psychiatry 1954;72:187–204
55. Sliwka U, Job FP, Wissuwa D, et al. Occurrence of transcranial Doppler high-intensity transient signals in patients with potential cardiac sources of embolism. A prospective study. Stroke 1995;26:2067–2070
56. Mackinnon AD, Aaslid R, Markus HS. Ambulatory transcranial Doppler cerebral embolic signal detection in symptomatic and asymptomatic carotid stenosis. Stroke 2005;36:1726–1730
57. Droste DW, Decker W, Siemens HJ, Kaps M, Schulte-Altedorneburg G. Variability in occurrence of embolic signals in long term transcranial Doppler recordings. Neurol Res 1996;18:25–30
58. Droste DW, Ringelstein EB. Detection of high intensity transient signals (HITS): how and why? Eur J Ultrasound 1998;7:23–29
59. Daffertshofer M, Ries S, Schminke U, Hennerici M. High-intensity transient signals in patients with cerebral ischemia. Stroke 1996;27:1844–1849
60. Babikian VL, Hyde C, Pochay V, Winter MR. Clinical correlates of high-intensity transient signals detected on transcranial Doppler sonography in patients with cerebrovascular disease. Stroke 1994;25:1570–1573
61. van Zuilen EV, Moll FL, Vermeulen FEE, Mauser HW, van Gijn J, Ackerstaff RGA. Detection of cerebral microemboli by means of transcranial Doppler monitoring before and after carotid endarterectomy. Stroke 1995;26:210–213

11

Neuroangiography in Hemorrhagic and Ischemic Stroke

Guilherme Dabus, Michael C. Hurley, and Eric J. Russell

Pearls

- Neuroangiography remains the gold standard for the evaluation of cerebrovascular diseases, and it is the foundation for neurointervention and neuroendovascular surgery.
- The mastery of the techniques necessary for safe and effective neuroangiography is essential for anyone who is venturing into the area of neurointervention and neuroendovascular surgery.
- Before starting the procedure, it is important to have a plan based on the disease being evaluated (which vessels to inject, which anatomic segment to image, need for three-dimensional imaging, etc.).
- As with any other procedure, it is important to be familiar with the devices and other equipment.
- Although very uncommon, severe complications may occur; it is important to be prepared to recognize and deal with them.

Neuroangiography is the dynamic study of the cerebral and spinal vasculature performed by means of an endovascular arterial catheter that is used to inject radiopaque contrast media. Imaging is then performed during the injection of contrast, and a series of arterial, capillary/parenchymal, and venous phase frames are acquired using the digital subtraction technique. Usually, repeat injections in multiple planes are necessary for an adequate cerebral study. More recently, three-dimensional (3D) rotational angiography has become an important tool in the angiographic evaluation of vascular lesions, particularly intracranial aneurysms, and may reduce the need for additional angulated series.

Despite the constant advances in and improvement of less invasive techniques such as magnetic resonance angiography (MRA) and computed tomography angiography (CTA), cerebral catheter angiography (CA) remains the gold standard for the evaluation of cerebrovascular diseases. Moreover, CA is the foundation for neurointervention, enabling the creation of a functional angiographic map that facilitates intelligent planning of targeted neuroendovascular surgical procedures. The mastery of the techniques necessary for safe and effective neuroangiography is essential for anyone who is venturing into the area of neurointervention and neuroendovascular surgery.

◆ Historical Facts

- Wilhelm Conrad Roentgen produced and detected electromagnetic radiation (x-ray) in November 1895.[1]
- An angiographic study of an amputated arm was performed in Vienna using a mixture of quicklime, petroleum, and mercuric sulfide in 1896.[2]
- Antonio Egas Moniz, a Portuguese neurologist who attended the Treaty of Versailles following World War I, and who received the Nobel Prize for developing frontal leucotomy as a treatment for psychiatric diseases, performed the first cerebral angiograms in cadavers. In 1927, he performed the first cerebral angiogram in a living human, assisted by his colleagues Almeida Lima and Almeida Dias; the patients had diagnoses of paralysis of the insane, parkinsonism, and brain tumors. Interestingly, the first patient with a successful series of angiographic images suffered thromboembolic complications and died soon after the procedure. In Moniz's series, strontium bromide and then sodium iodide were used as contrast media.[2-4]
- In 1931, Thorotrast, a colloidal solution of thorium, was used for cerebral angiography. Due to high rates of carcinogenesis, the use of this agent was discontinued in the early 1950s. Additional follow-up studies also showed a significantly increased incidence of malignancies (hepatobiliary, leukemia, and others) in patients who had received this agent.[2,4]

◆ Cerebral angiography gained popularity and was established as an important tool for evaluation of intracranial diseases in the late 1950s; at that time it was performed by direct puncture of the cervical arteries.[5]

◆ In the late 1960s cerebral angiography through femoral access was introduced.[6]

◆ Until the 1970s, cerebral angiography was performed for evaluation of all kinds of intracranial processes; the development of computed tomography (CT) in 1973 resulted in a shift toward cerebral angiography being reserved predominantly for evaluation of neurovascular diseases.[4]

◆ In the 1980s digital subtraction angiography (DSA) replaced film-screen techniques, and became the angiographic technique of choice, providing good resolution and image contrast with much more efficient workflow.

◆ More recent technologies, including 3D rotational angiography and flat-panel detectors capable of acquiring data that can be reconstructed into computed tomography (CT)-like images, are rapidly becoming an essential component for diagnostic or therapeutic procedures in neurointerventional departments around the world.

◆ Performing a Neuroangiography

A physician who performs cervicocerebral or spinal angiography must have received adequate training based on published accepted standards, and must demonstrate high success and low complication rates.[7,8] The procedure can be effective and safely performed using several different techniques depending on physician preference. It is important to mention that there is no "right" way to perform the procedure; however, safety thresholds need to be respected. Patient selection and preparation, meticulous technique executing the procedure, and postprocedural care are key steps to avoid complications.

Plan

Patient History and Review of Previous Studies

As in any other interventional procedure, the patient's clinical history is extremely important. The rationale and the risks and benefits of performing the procedure need to be determined individually. It is important to ask if the patient's clinical issue could be just as well assessed using a less invasive imaging modality such as magnetic resonance imaging (MRI), CT, MRA, or CTA. All prior procedures and imaging studies relevant to the case at hand need to be reviewed prior to the procedure during the decision-making process.

Allergies, Medical Problems, and Medications

Other important questions need to be addressed: Does the patient have an allergy to any medication or contrast agent that will be used during the procedure? Has the patient been exposed to iodine in the past (CT with IV contrast or intravenous urogram)? Does the patient need to be premedicated before

the procedure? In our institution we use premedication when a prior reaction to iodine is reported, and if there is a history of a severe reaction, the procedure is performed with anesthesia standby, monitored anesthesia care (MAC), or, in the worst-case scenario, under general anesthesia (GA). Our premedication protocol includes 50 mg of prednisone administered 13 hours, 7 hours, and 1 hour before the procedure, and 50 mg of diphenhydramine given 1 hour before the procedure.

Coexistent medical problems such as high blood pressure, diabetes, decreased renal function or renal failure, and diseases that result in a prothrombotic state and require anticoagulation can also potentially increase the risks of the procedure and need to be factored in to the plan prior to the procedure. Certain medications that require special attention include heparin, warfarin, and metformin; any decision made to discontinue these medications before the procedure need to be discussed with the referring physician. In patients on heparin therapy, it is our practice to hold the heparin 2 hours before the puncture and restart it immediately after the procedure if a closure device is successfully deployed, or to restart it after 2 to 4 hours if manual compression of the puncture site is performed. Warfarin is usually stopped 5 days prior to the procedure and the international normalized ratio (INR) is rechecked the day before the procedure. It can then be restarted the same day after the procedure. It is important to discuss with the referring physician the need for heparin bridging therapy during the period when the INR is subtherapeutic, depending on the primary reason for anticoagulation. Metformin, an oral antihyperglycemic medication that is excreted predominantly by the kidneys, increases the risk of lactic acidosis, a rare but serious complication, when associated with contrast administration. It is recommended to hold the Metformin until 48 hours after contrast administration and restart it after making sure that renal function is normal.[9]

Another category of patients that requires special attention are those with decreased renal function. Because there is an increased chance of worsening renal function due to contrast-induced nephrotoxicity, pretreatment of this patient population is recommended. It is our routine to give two 1200-mg doses of *N*-acetylcysteine 12 hours prior to contrast exposure and two doses after the procedure. On the day of the procedure we hydrate these patients with an intravenous solution of sodium bicarbonate (150 mEq/L in 1000 mL of D5W), 3 mL/kg for the first hour before contrast administration and 1 mL/kg/h for 6 hours after the procedure. The use of low- or iso-osmolar contrast media is also important.[10]

Neurologic Examination

A baseline neurologic examination prior to the procedure is extremely important. Knowing the patient's neurologic status also makes the clinical diagnosis of neurologic complications during the procedure fairly straightforward.

Laboratory Workup

The preprocedural laboratorial workup should include, at least, complete blood count, chemistry panel, and coagulation panel. Women should also have a pregnancy test done prior to the procedure to avoid radiation to the fetus, if possible. The most important questions to ask in regard to laboratory workup are the following: Is the patient severely anemic? Is the platelet count acceptable for the procedure? Is there an infection? What is the renal function? Are the prothrombin time (PT), INR, and partial thromboplastin time (PTT) acceptable for the procedure?

Type of Contrast to Be Used

Most contrast agents used for cerebral angiography are nonionic. Examples of nonionic low-osmolarity agents include iopamidol (Isovue; Bracco Diagnostics, Princeton, NJ), iohexol (Omnipaque; GE Healthcare, Princeton, NJ), ioversol (Optiray; Mallinckrodt, Hazelwood, MO), and iopromide (Ultravist; Bayer Vital, Leverkusen, Germany). The iodine content of the contrast media is included in the label for nonionic agents (e.g., Isovue-370 has 370 mgI/mL of solution; Omnipaque-300 has 300 mgI/mL of solution). For most nonionic agents, the osmolality depends on the concentration. Recently, a new nonionic contrast agent has been introduced; iodixanol (Visipaque; GE Healthcare, Princeton, NJ). A nonionic dimeric contrast agent that is iso-osmolar to blood, Visipaque 320, has 320 mgI/mL of solution with an osmolality of 290 mOsm/kg H_2O.[11] At our institution we reserve the use of iso-osmolar contrast agents for patients with decreased renal function or difficult spinal angiograms where increased volume of contrast might be necessary.

Sedation Assessment

Sedation assessment is another important issue. Does the patient have breathing problems? Are there airway/facial abnormalities? Does the patient have sleep apnea? Is there a history of airway problems or difficult intubation? Is the patient's mental status depressed? Does the patient respond appropriately and follow commands? What is the American Society of Anesthesiologists (ASA) status? The vast majority of cases can be performed under moderate sedation (conscious sedation) as long as the patient responds purposefully to verbal commands or light tactile stimulation. In these cases spontaneous ventilation is adequate and no intervention is required to maintain a patent airway or cardiovascular function.[12] Usually adequate moderate sedation can be achieved with the careful use of a sedative agent (commonly a benzodiazepine) associated with an analgesic drug (opioids). During the moderate sedation period the patient's vital signs and responsiveness should be carefully monitored by an independent observer, to guard against respiratory depression. If oversedation occurs, the benzodiazepine should be reversed using flumazenil; for opioid reversal, naloxone is the agent of choice.[13,14] Patients who are combative, who are not following commands, or who have delicate cardiovascular or respiratory stability may need anesthesia support (MAC or GA). In those cases an anesthesia consult is appropriate.

Arterial Access

Gaining access through a successful arterial puncture is the first step in cerebral angiography. Several different sites and arteries have been used for this particular purpose.[2,4,6,15–18]

The femoral artery puncture became the standard for access in the early 1970s. It was introduced in the late 1960s when most of the procedures were performed by direct puncture of the carotid or vertebral arteries.[6] The common femoral artery should be punctured below the inguinal ligament. A high puncture can result in difficulty obtaining hemostasis at the end of the procedure and increases the risk of retroperitoneal hematoma. The femoral head can be used as a landmark for puncture. The skin incision should be performed over the inferior third of the femoral head after application of local anesthesia (**Fig. 11.1**). This usually corresponds to 2 to 3 cm below the inguinal ligament. The puncture needle is then advanced in a 45-degree cephalad angle until the artery is punctured. Note that because the needle is angled superiorly, the artery will be punctured approximately 1 to 2 cm above the skin incision (**Fig. 11.2**).

A variety of puncture techniques can be used, including single wall, double wall, and micropuncture depending on the physician's preference. At our institution we routinely perform the arterial puncture using a micropuncture kit (**Fig. 11.3**). In this technique a 21-gauge needle is used to puncture the artery. An 0.018-inch micro-guidewire is passed into the arterial lumen to the level of the common iliac artery or proximal abdominal aorta. The needle is then removed and

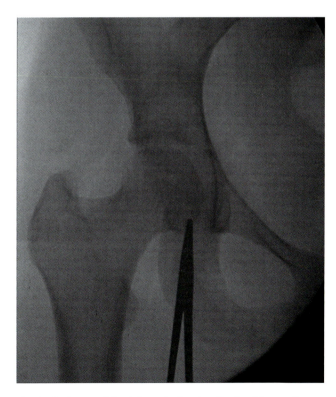

Fig. 11.1 Image of the right groin showing the tip of the needle driver positioned over the inferior third of the femoral head.

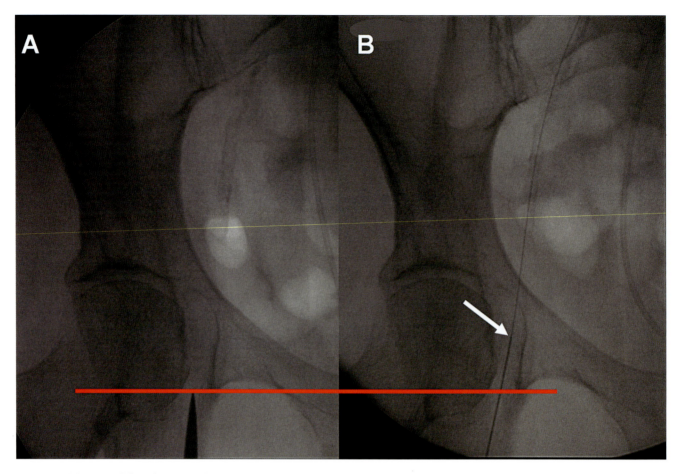

Fig. 11.2 **(A)** Image of the right groin with the marker over the skin incision site at the inferior third of the femoral head. **(B)** Right groin after the common femoral artery was punctured. Note that the exact puncture site is approximately 1 to 2 cm over the skin incision *(red line)*.

the wire is kept in the vessel lumen. A 4- or 5-French (F) introducer is then advanced over the wire. Subsequently, the inner part of the introducer and the micro-guidewire are removed together and a 0.035-inch J-wire or Bentson wire is advanced into the abdominal aorta and the outer piece of the introducer is removed. After that, a 4F or 5F arterial sheath is inserted in the common femoral artery over the wire. Finally, the wire and the sheath's inner portion are removed, leaving the outer canula in place. Axillary, brachial, and radial artery puncture follow the same principles.

It is our practice to always use arterial sheaths. It has been demonstrated in a randomized controlled trial that they decrease the incidence of intraprocedural bleeding at the femoral puncture site and increase the ease of catheter manipulation without increasing the number of groin complications.[19]

Cerebral angiography using the radial or ulnar artery approach has been shown to be feasible and safe, with limited complications.[15–17,20] In these cases the patient is examined using the modified Allen test to ensure adequate collateral circulation from the ulnar artery.[16,17,20] The artery is then punctured using the micropuncture technique described above. Due to the small size of these vessels, some authors recommend infusion of a mixture of medications including heparin, verapamil, lidocaine, and nitroglycerin through the

introducer sheath for vasospasm prevention or treatment.[16,20] The main advantages of these approaches over the conventional transfemoral approach are easier hemostasis and greater comfort for the patient (the patient is not required to lie flat for several hours after the procedure).[16,17,21]

When extreme tortuosity of the aortic arch and proximal supraaortic trunks makes selective catheterization impossible via the transfemoral approach or through one of the upper extremities approaches, the cervical arteries can be punctured directly. In a recent series of patients who underwent endovascular treatment of intracranial diseases, direct puncture of the cervical arteries, predominantly the common carotid artery followed by the vertebral artery, was felt to be effective and relatively safe.[18]

Catheters

Many different catheter shapes have been used successfully in performing selective catheterization of the cervical arteries. In more than 90% of cases, all cervical vessels can be successfully selected using all-purpose catheters such as the angled taper, vertebral, Berenstein, Davis, and Headhunter types. If the aortic arch is elongated and very tortuous, or in

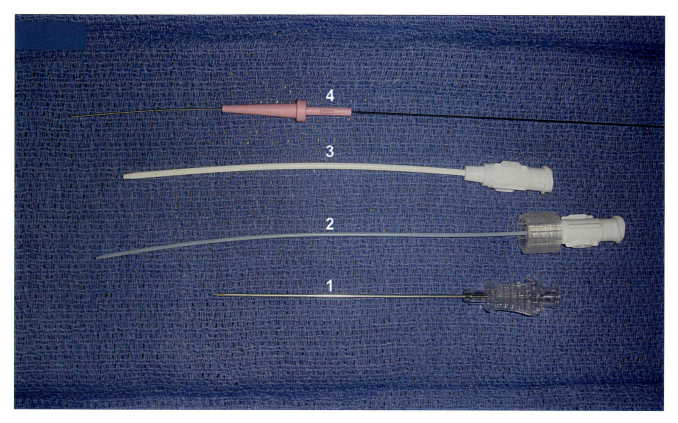

Fig. 11.3 Micropuncture kit. 1, a 21-gauge micropuncture needle; 2 and 3, inner and outer pieces of the introducer, respectively; 4, an 0.018-inch microwire.

cases of bovine arch, catheters such as the Simmons-II, Vitek, and HN-4 might be necessary to perform selective catheterization of the supraaortic arteries.

For spinal angiography, useful catheters include the Cobra-2, HS-1, Simmons-I, and Headhunter (useful for upper thoracic segmental arteries).

Continuous Flush Versus Double Flush

Here is another choice that is dependent on the operator's experience and preference. Both techniques are effective and safe if used carefully. Using a continuous flush system, a solution of heparinized saline (3000 to 5000 U/L) is infused in a drip fashion under pressure through the catheter. This allows for the catheter lumen to be filled by clean heparinized saline at all times, preventing blood stagnation and clot from forming within the catheter. At our institution, continuous flush is almost always used. **Figure 11.4** shows our setup when a mechanical injector is connected and when hand injections are used.

Double flushing the catheter is also very safe and effective as long as a meticulous technique is used. This technique consists of the aspiration of the catheter with one syringe to clear all bubbles and possible clots from the catheter lumen. This syringe is then disconnected and another syringe with clean heparinized saline is subsequently connected to the catheter. A small aspiration with subsequent flush of the catheter with heparinized saline is then performed. This maneuver should be repeated every time a wire is used and every time a new vessel is selected, or every 2 minutes, to prevent clots from forming in the catheter lumen.

Selecting Cervicocranial Vessels

After selecting the catheter of choice, the cervicocranial vessels are selected using standard over-the-wire technique. In this technique, a hydrophilic wire is advanced carefully under fluoroscopic guidance to select the target vessel. Subsequently, the wire is pinned and the catheter is advanced over the wire into the target vessel. Depending on vessel tortuosity, the presence of atherosclerotic disease, or operator preference, techniques such as roadmap or fluoro-fade guidance can be of significant help during this task (**Fig. 11.5**).

Another technique frequently used is the puff-and-push technique. Using this technique the operator connects a syringe of contrast directly to the catheter or flush system. The operator then repeatedly puffs small amounts of contrast and pushes the catheter into the target vessel without a guidewire in place. In this technique it is very important that the sequence of tasks is respected. Puffing first displaces the tip of the catheter away from the vessel wall, allowing the catheter to be pushed safely into the target vessel. This technique should be used in young patients with fairly straight anatomy and no significant atherosclerotic disease. In older patients

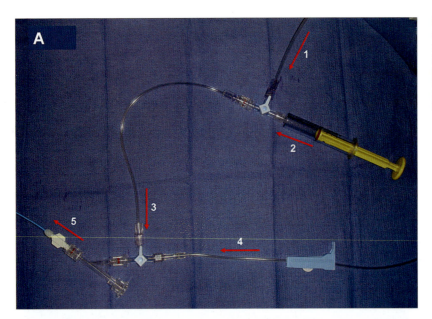

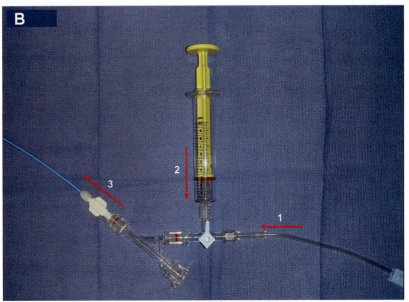

Fig. 11.4 Setup with continuous flush and the mechanical power injector connected. **(A)** 1, mechanical power injector tubing; 2, syringe for roadmap/flush; 3, connecting tubing; 4, heparinized pressurized saline infusion; 5, catheter. **(B)** Setup for hand injection with continuous flush: 1, heparinized pressurized saline infusion; 2, syringe for contrast injection; 3, catheter.

with tortuous vessels and significant atherosclerotic disease, the over-the-wire technique is safer and should always be used.

Catheter-Induced Vasospasm

It is important that when advancing the wire or catheter that the vessel anatomy and its curves be respected to avoid complications such as dissection or severe vasospasm (**Fig. 11.6**). Catheter-induced spasm is usually a self-limited condition and requires no treatment in most cases (**Fig. 11.7**). If severe catheter-induced vasospasm is noted, slow infusion of 1 to 5 mg of verapamil or 100 to 200 μg of nitroglycerin can be used to treat it.[22]

For spinal angiography the selective catheterization of the thoracic and lumbar segmental arteries are performed using anatomic landmarks with sequential catheterization of the levels above or below on each side.

Contrast Injection Rates (Mechanical Power Injection Versus Hand Injection)

The suggested rates and volumes of contrast for mechanical power injections are as follows:

◆ Aortic arch: 20 to 30 mL/s for 25 to 40 mL of contrast
◆ Common carotid artery: 7 to 10 mL/s for 10 to 14 mL of contrast

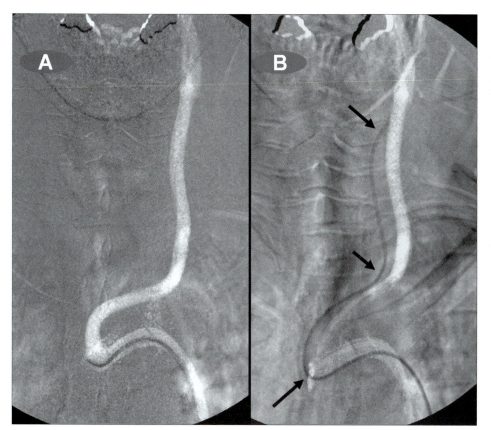

Fig. 11.5 **(A)** Roadmap image showing a tortuous left common carotid artery with an unfavorable angle from the arch. **(B)** Roadmap image after the left common carotid artery was catheterized; *arrows* point to the catheter.

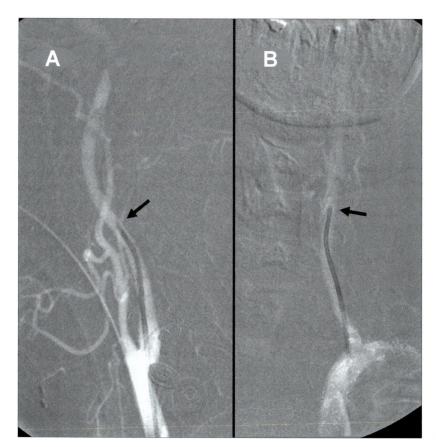

Fig. 11.6 Roadmap images after selective catheterization demonstrating the correct position of the tip of the catheters *(arrows)*, respecting the curvature of the arteries. **(A)** Internal carotid artery. **(B)** Left vertebral artery.

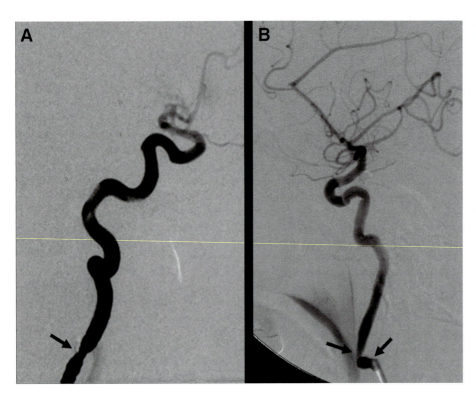

Fig. 11.7 (A,B) Examples of catheter-induced vasospasm.

- Internal carotid artery: 4 to 6 mL/s for 6 to 10 mL of contrast
- External carotid artery: 1 to 3 mL/s for 4 to 6 mL of contrast
- Vertebral artery: 3 to 6 mL/s for 6 to 8 mL of contrast
- Subclavian artery with pressure cuff inflated on the ipsilateral proximal upper extremity: 7 to 9 mL/s for 15 to 20 mL of contrast
- Segmental arteries (intercostal or lumbar): 1 to 2 mL/s for 4 to 6 mL of contrast

A randomized study demonstrated no statistically significant difference between these methods when evaluated for image quality and contralateral vessel reflux. The radiation exposure to the operator's hand and body, however, was reduced by up to 70% by using a mechanical injector during selective digital subtraction cerebral angiography. There was also a tendency of increased safety favoring mechanical injection, as all complications in the study were related to hand injection.[23] **Figure 11.4** shows our setup when a mechanical injector is connected and when hand injections are used.

No matter which technique is used, the operator needs to be attentive when setting up the mechanical power injector or when hooking up the contrast syringe for hand injection, so that no air is introduced into the system and subsequently injected into the patient's intracranial circulation. Air embolism is known to cause neurologic deficits in humans.[24] Interestingly, in a study where transcranial Doppler ultrasonography was used to monitor the presence of air emboli in the middle cerebral arteries of seven patients undergoing cerebral angiography, air embolism was noted in all cases, but none of the patients developed a focal neurologic deficit, suggesting that, in most cases, small degrees of air embolism do not result in focal neurologic deficit.[25]

Standard Imaging and Projections

Every cervicocerebral angiogram should start with a postero-anterior (PA) and lateral view of the anterior circulation (**Fig. 11.8**) and a Towne and lateral view of the posterior circulation (**Fig. 11.9**). At our institution we also perform a set of bilateral obliques for each internal carotid or vertebral artery injected. Depending on the pathology being evaluated, special techniques such as 3D rotational angiography for aneurysms or increased frame rate (6 frames/second) for documenting arteriovenous malformations and fistulas may be helpful.

Manual Pressure

Manual compression at the site of arterial puncture is a feasible, very safe, and effective method to achieve hemostasis for most patients undergoing a diagnostic neuroangiogram where a 4F or 5F sheath is used. The major disadvantages of this method are patient discomfort during the compression period and the necessity of bedrest with the patient lying flat for 2 to 6 hours afterward.[26–28] Patients on oral antiplatelet agents such as aspirin and clopidogrel may require slightly prolonged compression times. Anticoagulation (heparin) should be stopped 2 hours before the procedure and restarted 2 to 4 hours after hemostasis is achieved with manual compression.

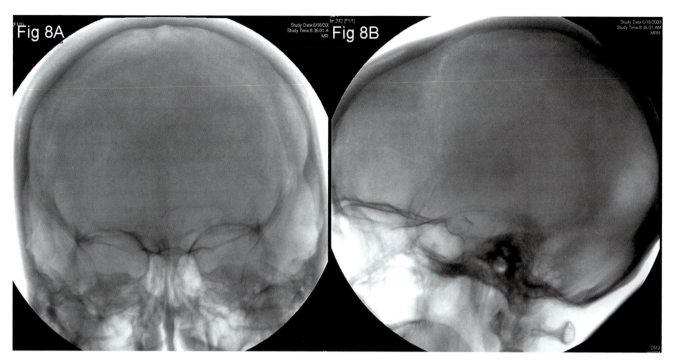

Fig. 11.8 Posteroanterior (PA) **(A)** and lateral **(B)** views for anterior circulation imaging. Note on the PA view the petrous ridges projecting in the middle of the orbits. Note on the lateral view that the internal auditory canals are aligned, allowing a straight lateral projection.

Manual compression should be performed with three fingers immediately above the skin incision. This technique ensures that the compression is being made exactly at the arterial puncture site (usually 2 cm above the skin incision).

The amount of pressure held should be enough to avoid subcutaneous collections or external oozing, but the femoral pulse should always be felt. Extreme compression can result in vessel occlusion. Manual compression is usually held for

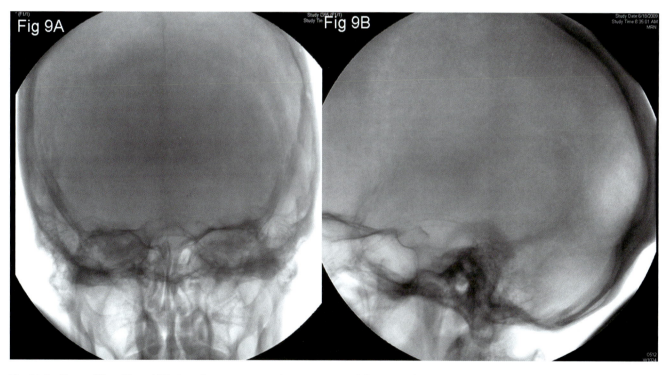

Fig. 11.9 Towne **(A)** and lateral **(B)** views for posterior circulation angiography. In the Towne view the petrous ridges project above the orbits. It is important that the superior two thirds of the nasal cavity and the occipital suture are fully included in the field of view. In the lateral projection the upper aspect of C1 needs to be included in the field of view.

10 to 20 minutes depending on the case. After this period the physician should inspect the groin, making sure that no hematoma has formed or is actively forming, even in the absence of external oozing. The lower extremity pulses are again re-evaluated to ensure adequate lower extremity blood supply. The patient is then kept in an observation unit with orders for bedrest with the patient lying flat for 4 hours. After the initial 4 hours the patient can sit, and after another 2 hours the patient is allowed to ambulate. The punctured groin and lower extremity pulses, along with the patient's vital signs, are monitored every 15 minutes during the first hour, every 30 minutes during the next 2 hours, and every hour for the last 3 hours.

Closure Devices

Several femoral arteriotomy closure devices are available. They have been observed to reduce the time to hemostasis, result in less bruising, achieve earlier ambulation, and improve patient satisfaction when compared with manual compression. They have also demonstrated a very safe profile, although complications such as device failure, infection, vessel occlusion, and embolization to the distal lower extremity are of concern.[26–28]

Devices with different mechanisms of action are currently available:

◆ Collagen plugs: with devices that employ collagen plugs, hemostasis is augmented by the exposure of the collagen to the blood. The swelling of the collagen mass mechanically seals the arteriotomy site.[29] Angio-Seal has been demonstrated to be safe and effective for arteriotomy management after neuroangiography and neurointerventional procedures.[28] Biodegradation of the collagen is expected to occur within 4 to 6 weeks, and complete dissolution by chemical analysis occurs by 90 days.[29,30] Reaccessing the same femoral artery should be avoided within that period, although there is suggestion that this may be safe.[31]

  • Angio-Seal (St. Jude Medical, Secaucus, NJ)
  • VasoSeal (Datascope, Fairfield, NJ)
  • Duett Pro (Vascular Solutions, Minneapolis, MN)

◆ Sutures: devices that use sutures employ small needles to deploy the sutures through the arteriotomy site. With this method repuncturing the artery is not a problem.[29] These devices demonstrated high success rates and low complications in a neurointerventional patient population in one study.[32]

  • Perclose (Abbott Vascular, Abbott Park, IL)
  • X Site (Datascope, Fairfield, NJ)
  • SuperStitch (Sutura Inc., Fountain Valley, CA)

◆ Staples/clips: these devices deploy an extravascular clip promoting occlusion of the arteriotomy site and hemostasis.[29] Reaccess is usually not a problem with these devices.

  • EVS (Medtronic, Minneapolis, MN)
  • StarClose (Abbott Vascular, Abbott Park, IL)

Multiple studies have been performed to compare different closure devices and manual compression.[26,27,33,34] A prospective study that evaluated the acute and chronic arterial blood flow and vascular pathology after vessel closure using Angio-Seal and StarClose in a porcine model showed that the StarClose device is associated with less short-term vessel injury compared with Angio-Seal.[34] In the StarClose and Angio-Seal Trial (SCOAST) study, a randomized controlled trial comparing Angio-Seal to StarClose, hemostasis, complication rates, patient pain perception, and patient satisfaction were similar in both groups. StarClose, however, resulted in significantly less bruising 1 week postprocedure.[33] A study that compared Angio-Seal, StarClose, and manual compression concluded that all three methods were similarly safe. The StarClose was associated with oozing postdeployment more often than Angio-Seal. Patient comfort was better with closure devices when compared with manual compression.[27] Another randomized controlled trial that compared the routine use of the Angio-Seal closure device with manual compression demonstrated that the group treated with the closure device had earlier mobilization, less bruising, and increased patient satisfaction, with no increase in other complications in comparison to manual pressure.[26]

At our institution we have extensive expertise deploying Angio-Seal and StarClose closure devices. No matter the device used, our protocol is as follows:

◆ Angiography of the puncture site: we consider the puncture site amenable for a closure device if the puncture is in the common femoral artery, no branch or bifurcation lies within 1 cm of the puncture site, and there is no evidence of intimal injury.

◆ The area is re-prepped and draped using clean sterile towels.

◆ All operators involved change their gloves for new, clean ones.

◆ After the device is deployed, gentle compression is applied for an extra 1 to 2 minutes.

◆ The femoral and pedal pulses are rechecked.

◆ Ambulation is allowed after 2 hours.

◆ Although controversial, we routinely administer antibiotics in cases where closure device use is anticipated (cefazolin 1 to 2 g; clindamycin 600 to 900 mg).

◆ Cerebral Angiography: Specific Indications, Tips, and Protocols

Atherosclerotic and Ischemic Disease

If the patient has not had a good-quality CTA or MRA of the neck, angiographic images of the aortic arch can be obtained to check for occlusive disease and stenosis of the supraaortic vessels, as well as the general anatomy of the arch (which vertebral artery is dominant, and anatomic variants, such as the presence of a bovine arch, a left vertebral artery from the arch, the presence of stenosis or occlusion of the origin of the

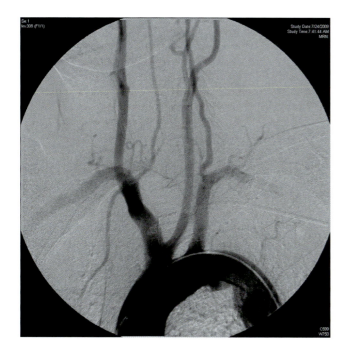

Fig. 11.10 Aortic arch angiography in a patient referred for evaluation of embolic strokes and atherosclerotic disease. Information such as the presence of plaque in the arch, common origin of the left common carotid artery (LCCA) and brachiocephalic trunk, and dominance of the left vertebral artery can be obtained from this image.

vertebral arteries, the direction of blood flow, antegrade versus retrograde filling, and subclavian steal) **(Fig. 11.10)**.

For selective catheterization of the common carotid arteries, we routinely perform angiography of the carotid bi-

furcation in the PA and lateral views. Oblique views should be performed to profile the narrowest degree of stenosis when appropriate. The angiographer should evaluate the presence of stenosis/occlusive disease, and the blood flow through the internal carotid artery (slow with delayed washout versus normal). A 3D rotational angiogram may be performed providing, an accurate estimation of the degree of stenosis[35] **(Fig. 11.11)**.

If there is mild bifurcation stenosis and intracranial disease is suspected, selective internal carotid artery (ICA) catheterization can be performed. If selective catheterization of the ICA is thought not to be safe (moderate or severe stenosis; ulcerated plaque), then common carotid injections and imaging of the intracranial circulation are performed. Intracranially, the presence of stenosis, occlusions, or incidental findings such as an aneurysm or an arteriovenous malformation is investigated on PA, lateral, and bilateral oblique views. Depending on the findings, additional views might be necessary **(Fig. 11.12)**.

When cervical, petrous, or cavernous ICA occlusion or severe stenosis is demonstrated, evaluation of the external carotid artery should be performed to determine the presence of external carotid artery (ECA) to ICA collateral anastomosis.

If atherosclerotic disease of the posterior circulation is suspected, the evaluation should start with subclavian artery angiography demonstrating adequately the origin and cervical portions of the vertebral arteries **(Fig. 11.13)**. If no significant stenosis is noted, selective catheterization of the vertebral artery is performed. If selective catheterization of the vertebral artery is thought not to be safe (moderate or severe stenosis; severe tortuosity), injection of the subclavian artery with the pressure cuff inflated on the ipsilateral proximal upper extremity is performed, and images of the

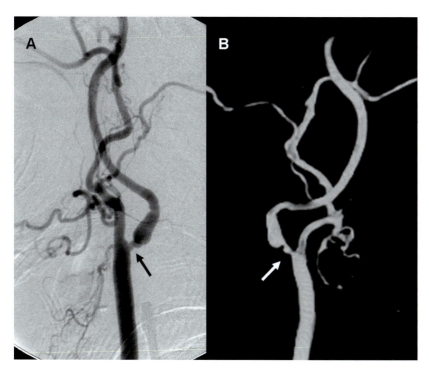

Fig. 11.11 **(A)** Stenosis of the origin of the left internal carotid artery that is better assessed with 3D rotational angiography **(B)**.

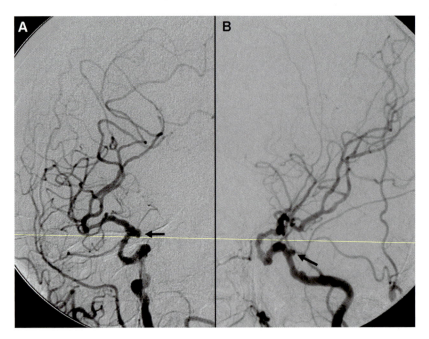

Fig. 11.12 Patient being evaluated for diffuse cervical and intracranial atherosclerotic disease. **(A,B)** Images confirm the presence of diffuse intracranial atherosclerotic disease with no significant stenosis. Incidentally, an anterior choroidal and a proximal cavernous internal carotid artery (ICA) aneurysm is seen *(arrow)*.

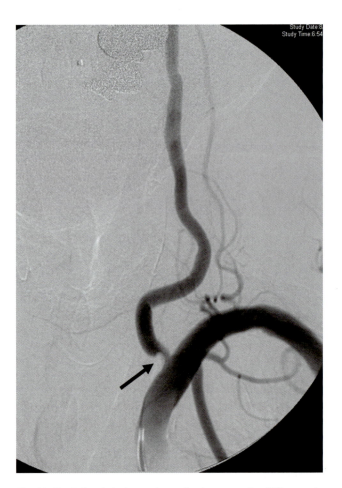

Fig. 11.13 Left subclavian angiography demonstrating 60% stenosis of the origin of the left vertebral artery *(arrow)*.

intracranial vasculature are obtained. As with the anterior circulation, the presence of stenosis, occlusions, or incidental findings such as an aneurysm or an arteriovenous malformation is investigated on PA, lateral, and bilateral oblique views. Depending on the findings, additional views might be necessary.

The patency and anatomic variations of the circle of Willis should always be assessed, as it often provides robust collateral flow in cases of cervicocerebral occlusive/stenotic disease.

Intracranial Aneurysms

Although still a matter of passionate debate, practice in recent years has seen a shift from catheter cerebral angiography to CTA in the workup of intracranial aneurysms.[36–39] Several studies have demonstrated that CTA has good reproducibility and high accuracy for detection and morphologic evaluation of intracranial aneurysms; it is also useful in the triage of patients for either coiling or clipping.[40–45]

Cerebral angiography, however, remains an important tool in the detection and evaluation of intracranial aneurysms. It should always be performed in cases of CTA-negative subarachnoid hemorrhage or when CTA results are equivocal.[42] Cerebral angiography also may better demonstrate vessels arising close to or from the neck or dome of the aneurysm.[43] The sensitivity of the CTA decreases significantly for aneurysms of less than 3 mm[40] **(Fig. 11.14).**

Three-dimensional rotational catheter angiography became available in the 1990s. It is a true technical revolution and a major step in the detection and evaluation of intracranial aneurysms.[35,46] It is less operator dependent; the image can be manipulated in any angle and direction, depicting even

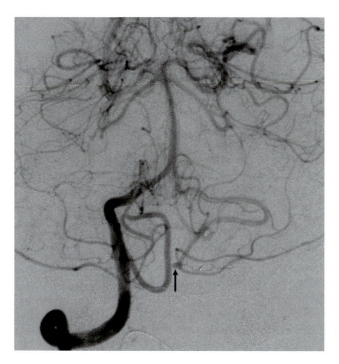

Fig. 11.14 Patient presenting with diffuse subarachnoid hemorrhage with predominance around the foramen magno. Computed tomography angiography (CTA) was negative. Patient was referred for cerebral angiography, which revealed a 1.5 mm distal left posterior inferior cerebellar artery (PICA) aneurysm *(arrow)*.

complex anatomic relationships; and measurements can be performed directly from the reconstructed 3D images.[35,46] Studies have shown that 3D rotational angiography is superior to conventional cerebral angiography (DSA) in the detection of small aneurysms. In one series, nearly 30% of small aneurysms detected on 3D rotational angiography were missed on the DSA by two experienced observers.[46]

Cerebral angiography for the detection and evaluation of intracranial aneurysms should include a four-vessel study with PA and lateral views. We routinely also perform bilateral oblique views for each vessel injected. If an aneurysm is identified, additional views to better demonstrate the neck are obtained. If 3D rotational angiography is available, it should be performed after the initial PA and lateral views, because it may reduce the number of off-angle views required for aneurysm definition. Subsequently, using the reconstructed 3D images, the best projection to demonstrate the neck and the aneurysm relationships can be obtained.

Factors to consider when evaluating an aneurysm include location, size, neck size and dome-to-neck ratio, shape, the presence of lobulations or daughter sac, the presence of vessels incorporated in the aneurysm neck or dome, and which way the aneurysm projects (**Fig. 11.15**).

When the cerebral angiogram is performed for evaluation of CTA-negative subarachnoid hemorrhage, it is our protocol to perform a six-vessel angiogram with selective catheterization of both vertebral internal and external carotid arteries. If the cerebral angiogram is also initially negative and

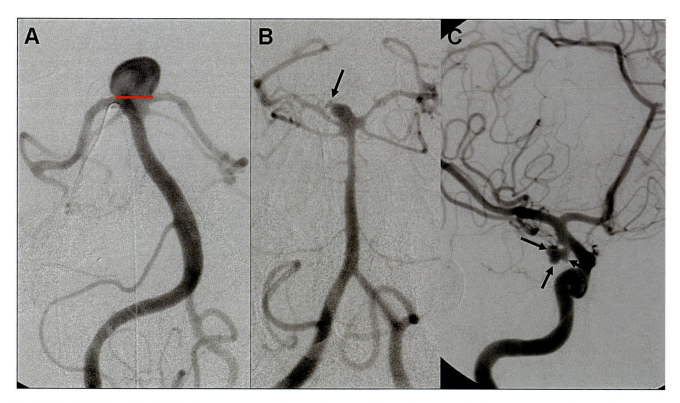

Fig. 11.15 **(A)** Wide neck *(red line)* basilar tip aneurysm with smooth contour. **(B)** Irregular ruptured basilar tip aneurysm with a daughter sac *(arrow)*, presumably the site of rupture. **(C)** Tri-lobulated narrow neck posterior communicating region aneurysm *(arrows)*.

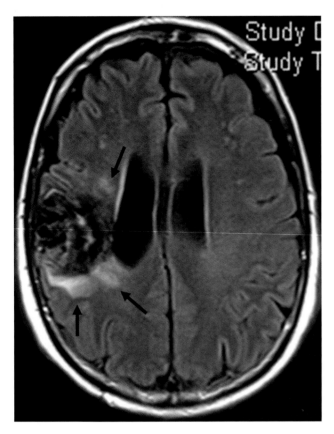

Fig. 11.16 Magnetic resonance imaging (MRI) fluid-attenuated inversion recovery (FLAIR) sequence demonstrating a right frontoparietal arteriovenous malformation (AVM) associated with adjacent encephalomalacia *(arrows)* and ex-vacuo dilatation on the right lateral ventricle due to an old hemorrhage.

there is predominance of blood in a specific location on cross-sectional imaging, 3D rotational angiography should be performed in the respective vascular tree.[47]

Cerebral Arteriovenous Malformations

Cross-sectional imaging is usually the first step in the evaluation of brain arteriovenous malformations (AVMs). CT and MRI usually provide useful information regarding the location and estimated size of the AVM, the presence of hemorrhage or calcifications, as well as changes in the adjacent brain parenchyma[48] (**Fig. 11.16**). Most recently, functional MRI has been used in the evaluation of the functionality of the parenchyma adjacent to the lesion.

The angiographic evaluation of cerebral AVMs should include all vasculature that could potentially supply the vascular territory where the lesion is located, including external carotid angiography (for evaluation of dural supply). Multiple views with an increased frame rate (usually six frames per second) are necessary for adequate evaluation of the angioarchitecture of the AVM and for the detection of intranidal aneurysms (**Fig. 11.17**).

An adequate angiographic evaluation of a cerebral AVM should demonstrate the hemodynamic balance of the brain (watershed zone transfer, pial collateralization, angiomatous changes, venous drainage of the normal parenchyma), individual feeding arteries, the size of the nidus, and the number of draining veins and the pattern of venous drainage (superficial or deep). The Spetzler and Martin classification takes into consideration the size, drainage pattern (superficial versus deep), and the eloquence of the parenchyma where the AVM is located. This system was designed to predict the surgical morbidity and mortality, and is frequently used in the decision-making process when microsurgical resection of an AVM is being considered.[49]

Other important architectural features that need to be demonstrated in the angiogram include changes related to high-flow angiopathy, including arterial stenosis and ectasia, flow-related arterial aneurysms (which are located on the feeding vessel), intranidal aneurysms, venous ectasia, (pseudo)aneurysms, and varices and venous thrombosis/occlusion[48] (**Figs. 11.17 and 11.18**).

It is important to mention that the angiographic evaluation of an AVM may be limited by the large number of overlapping structures that might make the evaluation of small intranidal aneurysms very difficult.[48] In such cases, superselective angiography may be more definitive.

Dural Arteriovenous Fistulas

Dural arteriovenous fistulas (DAVFs) are acquired abnormal arteriovenous connections located anywhere within the dura.[50] To adequately define the lesion, the angiographic evaluation of a DAVF should include selective angiography of both internal and external carotids and bilateral vertebral arteries. Exception can be made for anterior cranial fossa DAVFs where vertebral artery injection would not provide any useful information.

Important angiographic features include identification of the individual dural feeders, the presence of any pial supply, the presence of a sinus thrombosis, and, most important, the venous drainage pattern (drainage through the dural sinus antegrade or retrograde and the presence of cortical venous reflux/drainage)[51,52] (**Fig. 11.19**). The presence of cortical venous reflux/drainage is associated with an aggressive presentation (approximately 10% annual mortality rate and 15% annual rate of hemorrhagic or nonhemorrhagic neurologic deficit), and usually requires prompt identification and treatment.[53] It is also important to determine if the drainage occurs through an accessory sinus or through a septated compartment within the dural sinus, as this might have implications when treatment is planned.[54]

Carotid-Cavernous Fistula

A carotid-cavernous fistula (CCF) may be direct (spontaneous or traumatic) or indirect (dural fistula). They are classified into four types: type A, direct high-flow shunts between the internal carotid artery and the cavernous sinus; type B, shunts between dural branches of the internal carotid artery and

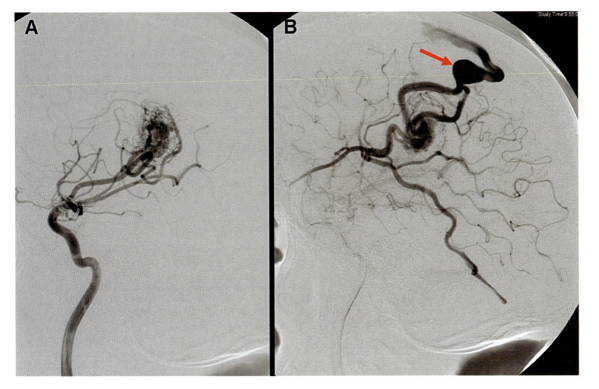

Fig. 11.17 **(A)** Arterial phase of the right ICA injection demonstrating the nidus of a right frontoparietal AVM. **(B)** Cortical (superficial) early venous drainage. Focal venous ectasia is demonstrated in the major draining vein *(arrow)*.

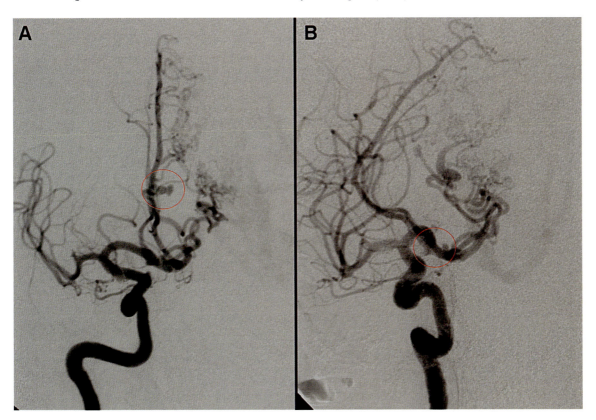

Fig. 11.18 Patient with known basal ganglia AVM was referred for angiographic evaluation after suffering intraventricular hemorrhage. **(A)** Irregular lobulated lenticulostriate flow-related aneurysm *(red circle)*, presumably the hemorrhage culprit. **(B)** Another two small flow-related aneurysms are seen.

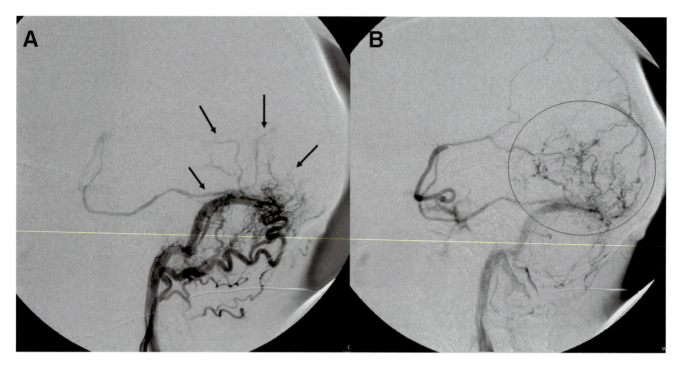

Fig. 11.19 **(A,B)** Injection of the left occipital artery demonstrates a transverse-sigmoid dural arteriovenous fistula with retrograde cortical venous reflux *(arrows)*.

the cavernous sinus; type C, shunts between dural branches of the external carotid artery and the cavernous sinus; and type D, shunts between dural branches of both the internal and external carotid arteries and the cavernous sinus[55] **(Fig. 11.20)**. Type A (spontaneous or traumatic) is also known as direct CCF and types B, C, and D (dural) are called indirect.

The angiographic evaluation of the indirect types (B, C, and D) follows the same principles described above for the evalu-

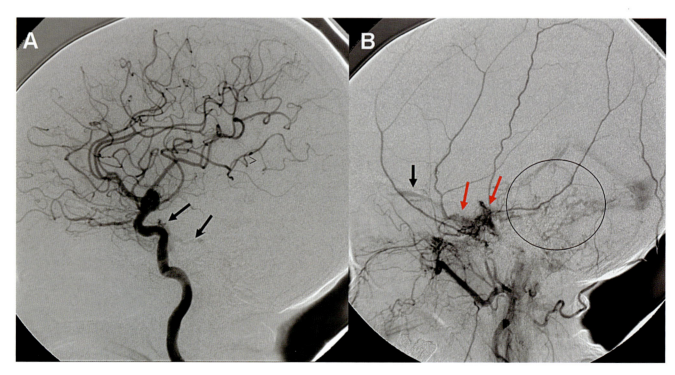

Fig. 11.20 Indirect (dural) carotid-cavernous fistula Barrow type D. **(A)** Supply from the meningohypophyseal trunk off the ICA *(arrows)*. **(B)** Supply from multiple external carotid branches. Black arrow points to drainage through the superior ophthalmic vein. Also note the cortical venous drainage *(circle)*. *Red arrows* indicate the cavernous sinus.

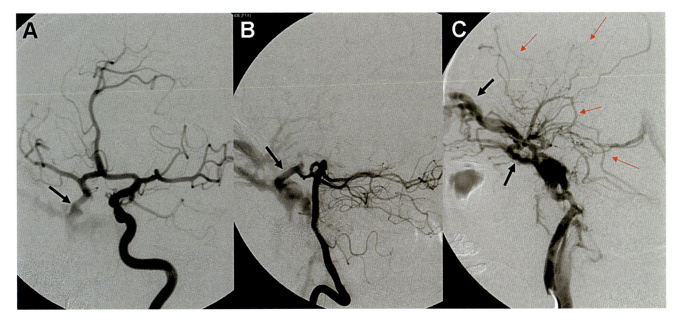

Fig. 11.21 Patient with a history of trauma presenting with proptosis, chemosis, and decreased visual acuity. **(A)** Left internal carotid injection demonstrates cross-filling with retrograde opacification of the supraclinoid right ICA *(arrow),* feeding a direct right-sided carotid-cavernous fistula. **(B)** Vertebral injection shows retrograde opacification of the right supraclinoid ICA via the posterior communicating artery to the level of the fistula *(arrow).* **(C)** Right internal carotid injection confirms the right carotid-cavernous fistula (CCF) and demonstrates no opacification distal to the fistula. Note the retrograde cortical venous reflux/drainage *(red arrows)* as well as the anterior retrograde drainage through the superior and inferior ophthalmic veins *(black arrows).*

ation of DAVF. Both internal and external carotid arteries need to be selected, and, depending on the case, one or both vertebral arteries. It is important to determine the type of venous drainage **(Fig. 11.20).** Retrograde drainage through the superior ophthalmic vein may be present, increasing the intraorbital and in some cases the intraocular pressure, posing a risk for vision loss. The presence of retrograde cortical venous drainage increases the chances of cerebral hemorrhage and nonhemorrhagic neurologic deficits (venous infarction). Drainage toward the contralateral cavernous sinus through the basilar and intercavernous venous plexus may be seen. Another reason why it is important to identify the venous drainage is that frequently, for this kind of lesion, the transvenous endovascular route is the preferred way to access and treat the lesion. For example, identification of a patent inferior petrosal sinus makes this approach quite straightforward.

Direct CCF is the result of a large communication between the cavernous carotid artery and the cavernous sinus. When the history and physical exam are clear, a three-vessel angiogram (bilateral ICA and the dominant vertebral artery) should be performed. These lesions may have such high flow that adequate visualization of the supraclinoid carotid artery and its branches might be difficult with ipsilateral angiography. Therefore, angiography of the other territory (contralateral carotid or vertebral circulations) may opacify the affected ICA to the level of the fistula in a retrograde fashion, providing important information about the exact fistula location and size. Moreover, it is important to determine how the blood supply to the ipsilateral distal territory is being provided, as, in some cases, carotid sacrifice may be necessary **(Fig. 11.21).**

The venous drainage pattern is again important, as detailed above for indirect CCF **(Fig. 11.21).**

Vasculopathy

Vasculopathy is a nonspecific term used to describe several different situations and different pathologic processes that may involve the cervicocranial vasculature. These include primary central nervous system (CNS) angiitis, vasospasm, vasoconstriction syndromes, vasculitis secondary to specific processes (infection, drugs, malignancy), systemic vasculitis with CNS involvement (giant cell arteritis, Takayasu's arteritis, Wegner's granulomatosis, polyarteritis nodosa), and other nonvasculitic processes and connective tissue disorders (fibromuscular dysplasia, systemic lupus erythematosus, scleroderma, Marfan's and Ehlers-Danlos syndromes, neurofibromatosis, sickle cell disease)[56–58] **(Fig. 11.22).**

The protocol for angiographic evaluation of cervicocerebral vasculopathy should include a three- or four-vessel angiography with selection of both internal carotid arteries and one or both vertebral arteries if the suspected disease process is intracranial. Magnified views of the intracranial circulation are highly recommended, as sometimes the findings such as vessel wall irregularity can be quite subtle. When systemic vasculitis, nonvasculitic processes, or connective tissue disorders are suspected, aortic arch, common carotid, and external carotid artery (particularly in case of giant cell arteritis) angiography should be performed.

Angiographic findings associated with vasculopathy include focal narrowing and irregularity of the vessels **(Fig. 11.23);**

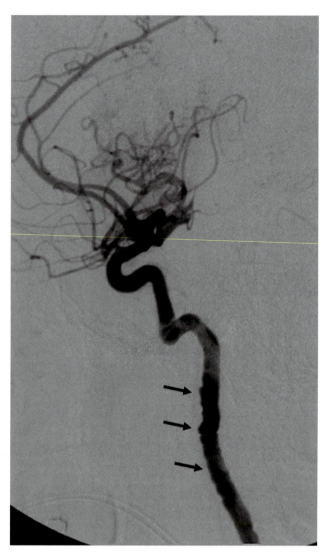

Fig. 11.22 Lateral images of an ICA injection demonstrating multiple irregularities in the distal cervical ICA with no significant stenosis typical for fibromuscular dysplasia *(arrows)*.

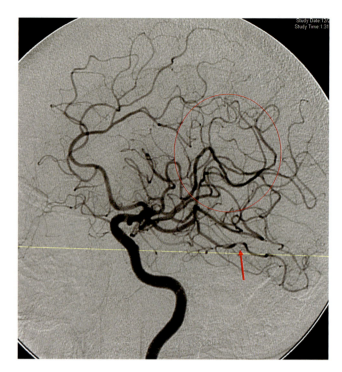

Fig. 11.23 Patient referred for cerebral angiography for workup of vasculitis, demonstrating multiple focal areas of narrowing and irregularity in distal anterior cerebral artery (ACA), middle cerebral artery (MCA), and posterior cerebral artery (PCA) branches *(arrow and circle)*.

Spinal Angiography

The indications for spinal angiography include evaluation of spinal arteriovenous malformations, myelopathy, spinal canal and spinal cord hemorrhage, vertebral lesions, and identifying the origins of the spinal radiculomedullary arteries prior to surgical procedures such as aortic dissection repair.

The evaluation of spinal arteriovenous malformation and its consequences (hemorrhage, myelopathy) has evolved over the years. Currently, time-resolved MRA provides accurate information for diagnosis and the general localization of the lesion, facilitating a more focused catheter spinal angiogram.[62] At our institution, when a vascular lesion is localized with time-resolved MRA, a focused spinal angiography usually extending two to three levels above and two to three levels below is performed. There are, however, cases where the patients' myelopathy or hemorrhage cannot be explained with current noninvasive imaging studies. In these cases, a full catheter spinal angiogram needs to be performed. Because these are usually lengthy procedures, and even a small degree of patient motion can degrade the images significantly, all complete spinal angiograms in our institution are performed under general anesthesia.

A full spinal angiogram requires study of the vertebral arteries, external carotid arteries, costocervical and thyrocervical trunks, all thoracic and lumbar segmental arteries, the median sacral artery (which arises at the aortic bifurcation),

alternating areas of dilatation and stenosis; mycotic and oncotic aneurysms (in cases of infectious and malignant vasculitis) **(Fig. 11.24)**; vessel occlusions; string of beads, pseudoaneurysm, dissection, and arteriovenous fistula (particularly in cases of fibromuscular dysplasia); proximal supraaortic arterial stenosis and occlusion (Takayasu's disease); and irregularity, narrowing, or occlusion in the external carotid branches, most importantly in the superficial temporal artery (giant cell arteritis).[56,57]

The angiographic findings are usually nonspecific and may be the same for several different underlying pathologic processes; correlation with clinical and laboratory data as well as available imaging studies is extremely important.[59] Cerebral angiography may be negative in cases of biopsy-proven primary CNS angiitis in more than 50% of cases[60]; angiography has also been shown to have low specificity and positive predictive value (PPV) in these cases.[19,61]

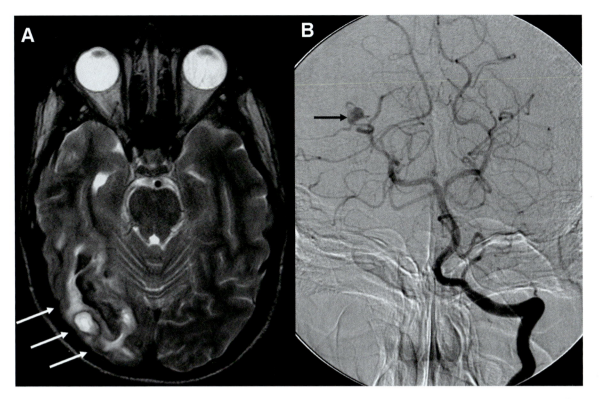

Fig. 11.24 **(A)** Patient with endocarditis and septic emboli presenting with a right temporo-occipital hemorrhage *(arrows)*. **(B)** Angiography of the posterior circulation reveals a mycotic aneurysm in the posterior temporal branch of the right posterior cerebral artery *(arrow)*.

and the lateral sacral arteries (which arise from the internal iliac arteries).

It is important to identify the levels that will give origin to radiculomedullary arteries that supply the anterior spinal artery and the radiculopial arteries that will supply the posterior spinal arteries. The number and level of origin of these vessels is variable.[63] Radiculopial arteries are more numerous compared with radiculomedullary arteries, ranging from 11 to 16 throughout the spinal axis.[64] The number of radiculomedullary arteries averages six, and the most common levels of origin include the V4 segment of the vertebral artery close to the vertebrobasilar junction (**Figs. 11.25 and 11.26**), the V2 segment of the vertebral artery or the ascending cervical artery (artery of the cervical enlargement) (**Fig. 11.26**), and the segmental arteries from T8 down to L2, more often on the left (artery of Adamkiewicz)[63,64] (**Fig. 11.27**). Both radiculomedullary and radiculopial arteries have a typical hairpin appearance angiographically. It is very important to make sure that the spinous processes are aligned in the midline of the vertebral bodies when acquiring frontal images during the spinal angiogram. Ensuring adequate technique makes the differentiation between anterior and posterior spinal arteries possible. Anterior spinal arteries are midline in location, whereas posterior spinal arteries are parasagittal (off midline).

Because spinal angiography requires multiple vessel injections (far more than for a cerebral angiography), it is important to be careful when considering the total amount of contrast used during a complete study.

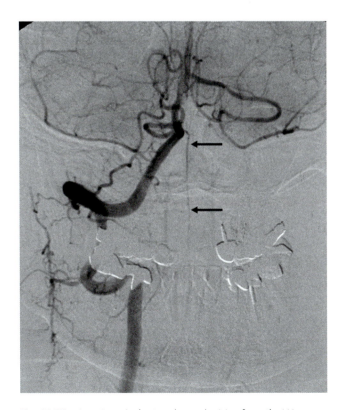

Fig. 11.25 Anterior spinal artery *(arrows)* arising from the V4 segment of the right vertebral artery close to the vertebrobasilar junction.

147

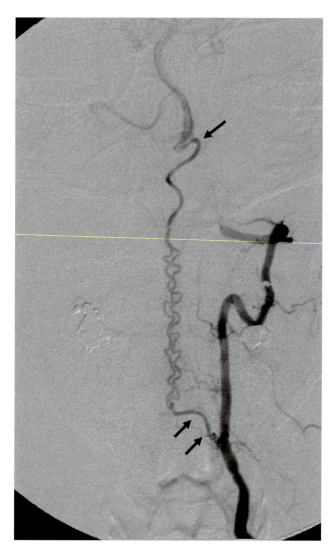

Fig. 11.26 Left vertebral injection demonstrates occlusion of the distal left vertebral artery (V3/4). This patient's right vertebral artery is also occluded, and blood supply to the basilar artery is provided by the artery of the cervical enlargement *(double arrows)* of the V2 segment of the left vertebral artery, which retrogradely fills the basilar artery through the anterior spinal artery *(single arrow)*.

◆ **Complications**

Neuroangiography is an invasive procedure, and therefore complications ranging from asymptomatic or clinically not significant to disabling or fatal may occur.[8,65–71] Cervicocerebral angiography in now performed by practitioners from several different medical specialties with different background and training. Radiologists, neurologists, neurosurgeons, vascular surgeons, and cardiologists are performing cervicocranial angiography, sometimes in the same clinical facility.[8,65,69] Independent of what specialty is performing the procedure, it is extremely important that the physician who does so has received appropriate training and has adequate experience, as suggested by published guidelines.[8] Clinical and technical knowledge as well as appropriate under-

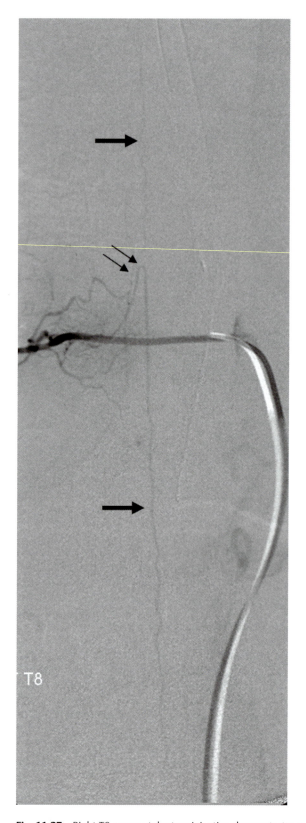

Fig. 11.27 Right T8 segmental artery injection demonstrates a radiculomedullary artery (artery of Adamkiewicz) opacifying the anterior spinal artery *(single arrows)*. Note the typical hairpin appearance of the radiculomedullary artery supplying the anterior spinal artery *(double arrows)*.

standing of the neurovascular anatomy and physiology along with excellent catheter skills are key to performing a successful and safe procedure. Physicians who practice neuroangiography or neurointervention must make sure that the risks of the procedure are minimized to ensure patient safety.

Complications can happen during any portion of the procedure as well as after it; therefore, constant continuous care is necessary. The following complications have been reported: vessel dissection and occlusion, pseudoaneurysm or arteriovenous fistula, infection, hematoma (superficial or retroperitoneal), contrast or medication allergies or reaction, contrast nephropathy, transient and permanent (stroke) neurologic deficits, myocardial infarct, and death.[65–71] Headache, whether or not accompanied by nausea and vomiting, is one of the most common problems following cerebral angiography, with a frequency of approximately 30%.[72,73] One of the proposed mechanisms is the release of vasoactive mediators during the procedure.[72] A variety of neurologic conditions such as transient global amnesia, cortical blindness, and mental status changes may occur infrequently as a complication of cerebral angiography related to contrast media neurotoxicity or microembolism.[72,74]

Quality guidelines have been issued for neuroangiography, suggesting complication-specific thresholds for neurologic and nonneurologic major complications[7] (Table 11.1). Recent published series have demonstrated that neuroangiography is a safe procedure even in pediatric patients.[65–71,75] Table 11.2 outlines the data of major series.

Several factors have been associated in the literature with increased risk during neuroangiography[65–67,69–71]:

◆ Symptomatic cerebrovascular disease
◆ Atherosclerotic disease
◆ Age older than 55
◆ Vascular comorbidities
◆ Length of the procedure
◆ Use of multiple catheters
◆ Experience of the operator

Table 11.2 Data from Major Series Demonstrating Safety of Neuroangiography

Study	Number of Patients	Permanent Neurologic Deficit	Transient and Reversible Neurologic Deficit
Dawkins et al[66]	2924	0	0.0034
Hussain et al[69]	661	0.002	0.002
Willinsky et al[71]	2899	0.005	0.009
Kaufmann et al[70]	19826	0.0014	0.025
Dion et al[67]	1002	0.004	0.027
Fifi et al[68]	3636	0	0

Another important consideration is silent embolism as demonstrated by MR diffusion-weighted imaging (MR-DWI); it has been reported following cerebral angiography and neurointerventional procedures.[76–78] These lesions have been reported in 10 to 20% of patients and are often asymptomatic. Risk factors include atherosclerosis, vasculitis, hypercoagulable state, amount of contrast medium used, fluoroscopy time, the number of vessels difficult to probe, multiple catheters, and operator experience.[77,78] A randomized prospective trial showed that the use of systemic heparin and air filters may reduce the incidence of silent ischemic events detected by MR-DWI after cerebral angiography.[76] Although the clinical significance of this phenomenon is unclear, it is recommended that all measures should be taken to reduce the occurrence of these silent lesions, and it is our belief that meticulous technique can minimize or eliminate the incidence of these events.

◆ Conclusion

Despite clear advances in noninvasive neurovascular imaging techniques such as MRA and CTA, catheter neuroangiography is still an extremely important tool in the evaluation of cerebrovascular diseases. It is the gold standard for several indications and can provide superior information about neurovascular anatomic details and hemodynamics. Moreover, mastering the technique necessary to perform an effective and safe neuroangiogram is the foundation for all neurointerventional and neuroendovascular procedures.

Table 11.1 Complication-Specific Thresholds for Neurologic and Nonneurologic Major Complications

Permanent neurologic deficit 1.0%
Reversible neurologic deficit 2.5%
Renal failure 0.2%
Arterial occlusion 0.2%
Arteriovenous fistula/pseudoaneurysm 0.2%
Hematoma requiring transfusion or surgical evacuation 0.5%

Source: Modified from American Society of Neuroradiology. American Society of Interventional and Therapeutic Neuroradiology. Society of Cardiovascular and Interventional Radiology. Quality improvement guidelines for adult diagnostic neuroangiography. Cooperative study between the ASNR, ASITN, and the SCVIR. AJNR Am J Neuroradiol 2000;21:146–150.

References

1. Mould RF. The early history of x-ray diagnosis with emphasis on the contributions of physics 1895-1915. Phys Med Biol 1995;40:1741–1787
2. Morris P. Introduction. In: Morris P, ed. Practical Neuroangiography, 1st ed. Baltimore: Lippincott Williams & Wilkins, 1997:3–6
3. Moniz E. Subsidies for the history of angiography. Med Contemp 1955;73:329–346
4. Huber P. History of cerebral angiography. In: Huber P, ed. Krayenbuhl/Yasargil Cerebral Angiography, 2nd ed. New York: Thieme Medical Publishers, 1982:2–4
5. Dagi TF. Neurosurgery and the introduction of cerebral angiography. Neurosurg Clin N Am 2001;12:145–153, ix

6. Hinck VC, Judkins MP, Paxton HD. Simplified selective femorocerebral angiography. Radiology 1967;89:1048–1052
7. American Society of Neuroradiology. American Society of Interventional and Therapeutic Neuroradiology. Society of Cardiovascular and Interventional Radiology. Quality improvement guidelines for adult diagnostic neuroangiography. Cooperative study between the ASNR, ASITN, and the SCVIR. AJNR Am J Neuroradiol 2000;21:146–150
8. Connors JJ III, Sacks D, Furlan AJ, et al; American Academy of Neurology; American Association of Neurological Surgeons; American Society of Interventional and Therapeutic Neuroradiology; American Society of Neuroradiology; Congress of Neurological Surgeons; AANS/CNS Cerebrovascular Section; Society of Interventional Radiology; NeuroVascular Coalition Writing Group. Training, competency, and credentialing standards for diagnostic cervicocerebral angiography, carotid stenting, and cerebrovascular intervention: a joint statement from the American Academy of Neurology, the American Association of Neurological Surgeons, the American Society of Interventional and Therapeutic Neuroradiology, the American Society of Neuroradiology, the Congress of Neurological Surgeons, the AANS/CNS Cerebrovascular Section, and the Society of Interventional Radiology. Neurology 2005;64:190–198
9. Widmark JM. Imaging-related medications: a class overview. Proc Bayl Univ Med Cent 2007;20:408–417
10. Goldfarb S, McCullough PA, McDermott J, Gay SB. Contrast-induced acute kidney injury: specialty-specific protocols for interventional radiology, diagnostic computed tomography radiology, and interventional cardiology. Mayo Clin Proc 2009;84:170–179
11. Singh J, Daftary A. Iodinated contrast media and their adverse reactions. J Nucl Med Technol 2008;36:69–74, quiz 76–77
12. American Society of Anesthesiologists Task Force on Sedation and Analgesia by Non-Anesthesiologists. Practice guidelines for sedation and analgesia by non-anesthesiologists. Anesthesiology 2002;96:1004–1017
13. Olkkola KT, Ahonen J. Midazolam and other benzodiazepines. Handb Exp Pharmacol 2008;182:335–360
14. Goodman AJ, Le Bourdonnec B, Dolle RE. Mu opioid receptor antagonists: recent developments. ChemMedChem 2007;2:1552–1570
15. Layton KF, Kallmes DF, Kaufmann TJ. Use of the ulnar artery as an alternative access site for cerebral angiography. AJNR Am J Neuroradiol 2006;27:2073–2074
16. Levy EI, Boulos AS, Fessler RD, et al. Transradial cerebral angiography: an alternative route. Neurosurgery 2002;51:335–340, discussion 340–342
17. Matsumoto Y, Hongo K, Toriyama T, Nagashima H, Kobayashi S. Transradial approach for diagnostic selective cerebral angiography: results of a consecutive series of 166 cases. AJNR Am J Neuroradiol 2001;22:704–708
18. Blanc R, Piotin M, Mounayer C, Spelle L, Moret J. Direct cervical arterial access for intracranial endovascular treatment. Neuroradiology 2006;48:925–929
19. Moran CJ, Milburn JM, Cross DT III, Derdeyn CP, Dobbie TK, Littenberg B. Randomized controlled trial of sheaths in diagnostic neuroangiography. Radiology 2001;218:183–187
20. Nohara AM, Kallmes DF. Transradial cerebral angiography: technique and outcomes. AJNR Am J Neuroradiol 2003;24:1247–1250
21. Layton KF, Kallmes DF, Cloft HJ. The radial artery access site for interventional neuroradiology procedures. AJNR Am J Neuroradiol 2006;27:1151–1154
22. Feng L, Fitzsimmons BF, Young WL, et al. Intraarterially administered verapamil as adjunct therapy for cerebral vasospasm: safety and 2-year experience. AJNR Am J Neuroradiol 2002;23:1284–1290
23. Hughes DG, Patel U, Forbes WS, Jones AP. Comparison of hand injection with mechanical injection for digital subtraction selective cerebral angiography. Br J Radiol 1994;67:786–789
24. Menkin M, Schwartzman RJ. Cerebral air embolism. Report of five cases and review of the literature. Arch Neurol 1977;34:168–170
25. Markus H, Loh A, Israel D, Buckenham T, Clifton A, Brown MM. Microscopic air embolism during cerebral angiography and strategies for its avoidance. Lancet 1993;341:784–787
26. Behan MW, Large JK, Patel NR, Lloyd GW, Sulke AN. A randomised controlled trial comparing the routine use of an Angio-Seal STS device strategy with conventional femoral haemostasis methods in a district general hospital. Int J Clin Pract 2007;61:367–372
27. Deuling JH, Vermeulen RP, Anthonio RA, et al. Closure of the femoral artery after cardiac catheterization: a comparison of Angio-Seal, StarClose, and manual compression. Catheter Cardiovasc Interv 2008;71:518–523
28. Geyik S, Yavuz K, Akgoz A, et al. The safety and efficacy of the Angio-Seal closure device in diagnostic and interventional neuroangiography setting: a single-center experience with 1,443 closures. Neuroradiology 2007;49:739–746
29. Hon LQ, Ganeshan A, Thomas SM, Warakaulle D, Jagdish J, Uberoi R. An overview of vascular closure devices: what every radiologist should know. Eur J Radiol 2010;73:181–190
30. Nash JE, Evans DG. The Angio-Seal hemostatic puncture closure device. Concept and experimental results. Herz 1999;24:597–606
31. Applegate RJ, Rankin KM, Little WC, Kahl FR, Kutcher MA. Restick following initial Angioseal use. Catheter Cardiovasc Interv 2003;58:181–184
32. Morris PP, Braden G. Neurointerventional experience with an arteriotomy suture device. AJNR Am J Neuroradiol 1999;20:1706–1709
33. Veasey RA, Large JK, Silberbauer J, et al. A randomised controlled trial comparing StarClose and AngioSeal vascular closure devices in a district general hospital—the SCOAST study. Int J Clin Pract 2008;62:912–918
34. Sanghi P, Virmani R, Do D, et al. A comparative evaluation of arterial blood flow and the healing response after femoral artery closure using Angio-Seal STS Plus and StarClose in a porcine model. J Interv Cardiol 2008;21:329–336
35. Anxionnat R, Bracard S, Macho J, et al. 3D angiography. Clinical interest. First applications in interventional neuroradiology. J Neuroradiol 1998;25:251–262
36. Agid R, Willinsky RA, Farb RI, Terbrugge KG. Life at the end of the tunnel: why emergent CT angiography should be done for patients with acute subarachnoid hemorrhage. AJNR Am J Neuroradiol 2008;29:e45, author reply e46–e47
37. Fox AJ, Symons SP, Aviv RI. CT angiography is state-of-the-art first vascular imaging for subarachnoid hemorrhage. AJNR Am J Neuroradiol 2008;29:e41–e42, author reply e46–e47
38. Westerlaan HE, Eshghi S, Oudkerk M, et al. Re: Death by nondiagnosis: why emergent CT angiography should not be done for patients with subarachnoid hemorrhage. AJNR Am J Neuroradiol 2008;29:e43, author reply e46–e47
39. Kallmes DF, Layton K, Marx WF, Tong F. Death by nondiagnosis: why emergent CT angiography should not be done for patients with subarachnoid hemorrhage. AJNR Am J Neuroradiol 2007;28:1837–1838
40. Lubicz B, Levivier M, François O, et al. Sixty-four-row multisection CT angiography for detection and evaluation of ruptured intracranial aneurysms: interobserver and intertechnique reproducibility. AJNR Am J Neuroradiol 2007;28:1949–1955
41. Agid R, Lee SK, Willinsky RA, Farb RI, terBrugge KG. Acute subarachnoid hemorrhage: using 64-slice multidetector CT angiography to "triage" patients' treatment. Neuroradiology 2006;48:787–794
42. Westerlaan HE, Gravendeel J, Fiore D, et al. Multislice CT angiography in the selection of patients with ruptured intracranial aneurysms suitable for clipping or coiling. Neuroradiology 2007;49:997–1007
43. Taschner CA, Thines L, Lernout M, Lejeune JP, Leclerc X. Treatment decision in ruptured intracranial aneurysms: comparison between multi-detector row CT angiography and digital subtraction angiography. J Neuroradiol 2007;34:243–249
44. Jayaraman MV, Mayo-Smith WW, Tung GA, et al. Detection of intracranial aneurysms: multi-detector row CT angiography compared with DSA. Radiology 2004;230:510–518
45. Uysal E, Oztora F, Ozel A, Erturk SM, Yildirim H, Basak M. Detection and evaluation of intracranial aneurysms with 16-row multislice CT angiography: comparison with conventional angiography. Emerg Radiol 2008;15:311–316
46. van Rooij WJ, Sprengers ME, de Gast AN, Peluso JP, Sluzewski M. 3D rotational angiography: the new gold standard in the detection of additional intracranial aneurysms. AJNR Am J Neuroradiol 2008;29:976–979
47. van Rooij WJ, Peluso JP, Sluzewski M, Beute GN. Additional value of 3D rotational angiography in angiographically negative aneurysmal subarachnoid hemorrhage: how negative is negative? AJNR Am J Neuroradiol 2008;29:962–966
48. Valavanis A. The role of angiography in the evaluation of cerebral vascular malformations. Neuroimaging Clin N Am 1996;6:679–704
49. Spetzler RF, Martin NA. A proposed grading system for arteriovenous malformations. J Neurosurg 1986;65:476–483
50. Nogueira RG, Dabus G, Rabinov JD, et al. Preliminary experience with onyx embolization for the treatment of intracranial dural arteriovenous fistulas. AJNR Am J Neuroradiol 2008;29:91–97
51. Borden JA, Wu JK, Shucart WA. A proposed classification for spinal and cranial dural arteriovenous fistulous malformations and implications for treatment. J Neurosurg 1995;82:166–179
52. Cognard C, Gobin YP, Pierot L, et al. Cerebral dural arteriovenous fistulas: clinical and angiographic correlation with a revised classification of venous drainage. Radiology 1995;194:671–680
53. van Dijk JM, terBrugge KG, Willinsky RA, Wallace MC. Clinical course of cranial dural arteriovenous fistulas with long-term persistent cortical venous reflux. Stroke 2002;33:1233–1236
54. Piske RL, Campos CM, Chaves JB, et al. Dural sinus compartment in dural arteriovenous shunts: a new angioarchitectural feature allowing superselective transvenous dural sinus occlusion treatment. AJNR Am J Neuroradiol 2005;26:1715–1722

55. Barrow DL, Spector RH, Braun IF, Landman JA, Tindall SC, Tindall GT. Classification and treatment of spontaneous carotid-cavernous sinus fistulas. J Neurosurg 1985;62:248–256
56. Greenan TJ, Grossman RI, Goldberg HI. Cerebral vasculitis: MR imaging and angiographic correlation. Radiology 1992;182:65–72
57. Hurst RW. Angiography of non-atherosclerotic occlusive cerebrovascular disease. Neuroimaging Clin N Am 1996;6:651–678
58. Kadkhodayan Y, Alreshaid A, Moran CJ, Cross DT III, Powers WJ, Derdeyn CP. Primary angiitis of the central nervous system at conventional angiography. Radiology 2004;233:878–882
59. Chu CT, Gray L, Goldstein LB, Hulette CM. Diagnosis of intracranial vasculitis: a multi-disciplinary approach. J Neuropathol Exp Neurol 1998; 57:30–38
60. Younger DS, Hays AP, Brust JC, Rowland LP. Granulomatous angiitis of the brain. An inflammatory reaction of diverse etiology. Arch Neurol 1988;45:514–518
61. Duna GF, Calabrese LH. Limitations of invasive modalities in the diagnosis of primary angiitis of the central nervous system. J Rheumatol 1995;22:662–667
62. Mull M, Nijenhuis RJ, Backes WH, Krings T, Wilmink JT, Thron A. Value and limitations of contrast-enhanced MR angiography in spinal arteriovenous malformations and dural arteriovenous fistulas. AJNR Am J Neuroradiol 2007;28:1249–1258
63. Nelson PK, Setton A, Berenstein A. Vertebrospinal angiography in the evaluation of vertebral and spinal cord disease. Neuroimaging Clin N Am 1996;6:589–605
64. Thron AK. Vascular anatomy of the spine and spinal cord. In: Hurst RW, Rosenwasser RH, eds. Interventional Neuroradiology, 1st ed. New York: Informa Healthcare USA, 2008:39–56
65. Al-Ameri H, Thomas ML, Yoon A, et al. Complication rate of diagnostic carotid angiography performed by interventional cardiologists. Catheter Cardiovasc Interv 2009;73:661–665
66. Dawkins AA, Evans AL, Wattam J, et al. Complications of cerebral angiography: a prospective analysis of 2,924 consecutive procedures. Neuroradiology 2007;49:753–759
67. Dion JE, Gates PC, Fox AJ, Barnett HJ, Blom RJ. Clinical events following neuroangiography: a prospective study. Stroke 1987;18:997–1004
68. Fifi JT, Meyers PM, Lavine SD, et al. Complications of modern diagnostic cerebral angiography in an academic medical center. J Vasc Interv Radiol 2009;20:442–447
69. Hussain SI, Wolfe TJ, Lynch JR, Fitzsimmons BF, Zaidat OO. Diagnostic cerebral angiography: the interventional neurology perspective. J Neuroimaging 2010;20:251–254
70. Kaufmann TJ, Huston J III, Mandrekar JN, Schleck CD, Thielen KR, Kallmes DF. Complications of diagnostic cerebral angiography: evaluation of 19,826 consecutive patients. Radiology 2007;243:812–819
71. Willinsky RA, Taylor SM, TerBrugge K, Farb RI, Tomlinson G, Montanera W. Neurologic complications of cerebral angiography: prospective analysis of 2,899 procedures and review of the literature. Radiology 2003;227:522–528
72. Pryor JC, Setton A, Nelson PK, Berenstein A. Complications of diagnostic cerebral angiography and tips on avoidance. Neuroimaging Clin N Am 1996;6:751–758
73. Ramadan NM, Gilkey SJ, Mitchell M, Sawaya KL, Mitsias P. Postangiography headache. Headache 1995;35:21–24
74. Saigal G, Bhatia R, Bhatia S, Wakhloo AK. MR findings of cortical blindness following cerebral angiography: is this entity related to posterior reversible leukoencephalopathy? AJNR Am J Neuroradiol 2004;25: 252–256
75. Burger IM, Murphy KJ, Jordan LC, Tamargo RJ, Gailloud P. Safety of cerebral digital subtraction angiography in children: complication rate analysis in 241 consecutive diagnostic angiograms. Stroke 2006;37: 2535–2539
76. Bendszus M, Koltzenburg M, Bartsch AJ, et al. Heparin and air filters reduce embolic events caused by intra-arterial cerebral angiography: a prospective, randomized trial. Circulation 2004;110:2210–2215
77. Bendszus M, Koltzenburg M, Burger R, Warmuth-Metz M, Hofmann E, Solymosi L. Silent embolism in diagnostic cerebral angiography and neurointerventional procedures: a prospective study. Lancet 1999;354: 1594–1597
78. Krings T, Willmes K, Becker R, et al. Silent microemboli related to diagnostic cerebral angiography: a matter of operator's experience and patient's disease. Neuroradiology 2006;48:387–393

12

Promising Developments in Stroke Imaging

Howard A. Rowley, Patrick A. Turski, and Charles M. Strother

Pearls

- Stroke triage requires rapid yet comprehensive neurovascular imaging.
- Computed tomography (CT) protocols should provide time-resolved CT angiography of the head and neck and CT perfusion of the brain to facilitate diagnosis and treatment selection.
- Magnetic resonance (MR) approaches now produce noninvasive, multidimensional, time-resolved vascular imaging data to assess anatomy, flow patterns, velocities, and pressure gradients.
- Angiography systems now offer a unified technical platform to image brain parenchyma and vessels, thereby facilitating combined diagnosis and intervention.

◆ Overview of Future Imaging

The future of stroke imaging is bright, multifaceted, and central to the diagnosis and management of patients with neurovascular disease. This chapter outlines some of the logical extensions of current computed tomography (CT), magnetic resonance (MR), and angiographic techniques. We cover both the state of the art in current practice as well as our "blue-sky" vision of future imaging developments related to ischemia and hemorrhage in the brain. Undoubtedly, other technologies, including targeted molecular imaging, will be incorporated as these methods mature. As with any scientific development, advancement in the field requires not only technical improvements but also a mindset and willingness to evaluate and embrace new work flow, diagnostic approaches, and treatment algorithms. Growth in this area is a synergistic parallel development process because new imaging methods promote and enable new treatment possibilities, and vice versa. Imaging advances are crucial to improved patient outcomes both today and tomorrow.

Neurovascular Computed Tomography

From the perspective of acute stroke triage based on CT, the future is here already. A 10-minute protocol can already screen brain parenchyma, blood vessels of the head and neck, and brain perfusion. In some ways, advanced technical abilities of current and emerging modalities already produce more information than we know what to do with in practice. Such a rich data set provides a solid basis for patient triage and management of either ischemic or hemorrhagic stroke. The next major advances in this area will include new scanner hardware such as flat panel machines with extended z-axis coverage. Here we will see a technical convergence with angiographic platforms. New CT scanners will be deployed with multi-energy, undersampled data acquisition protocols and advanced noise-reduction reconstruction algorithms to produce low-dose, multidimensional data sets. Such an approach will yield time-resolved computed tomography angiography (CTA) and CT perfusion data from the heart to the top of the head in a 1-minute examination. Fully automated postprocessing will be done at the scanner console for immediate review.

Clinical implementation of any new advanced technology must consider not only the diagnostic performance of the technique itself but how and when to deploy it. This is particularly true with respect to the timing of acute stroke imaging; it is not just the question of what test to do, but of when to do it. It can be argued that comprehensive CT and magnetic resonance imaging (MRI) neurovascular protocols should be done immediately on first presentation with suspected neurovascular disease. Patients with either acute ischemic or hemorrhagic conditions in the brain benefit from immediate, rapidly performed, and fully comprehensive stroke protocols to address the brain parenchymal patterns of injury, relevant vascular lesions of both the head and neck, and perfusion characteristics. Such comprehensive imaging data can

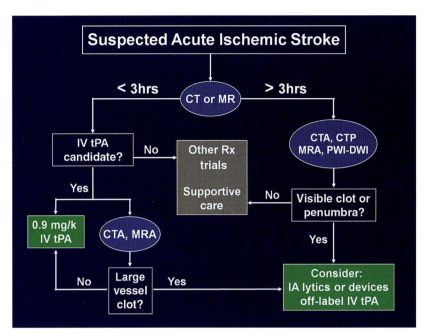

Fig. 12.1 Imaging triage for patients with acute ischemic stroke. The first priority is to identify and treat patients who are good intravenous (IV) tissue-type plasminogen activator (tPA) candidates. Comprehensive vascular and perfusion imaging tests are simultaneously performed to identify treatable vascular lesions and to assess current physiologic status. Imaging findings are used to rationally choose the best therapies on an individual basis. CT, computed tomography; CTA, computed tomography angiography; CTP, computed tomography perfusion; DWI, diffusion-weighted imaging; IA, intraarterial; MR, magnetic resonance; MRA, magnetic resonance angiography; PWI, perfusion-weighted imaging.

be useful in acute triage and in the selection of therapy based on the individual patient's physiology and anatomy rather than on the clinical features or arbitrary time windows.[1] In stroke or transient ischemic attack (TIA), it has been shown that rapid referral for treatment of underlying vascular lesions also leads to improved outcome with reduction in secondary strokes. If an examination is ultimately appropriate for a patient with acute stroke, why not perform it immediately from the emergency room, rather than a few days later, and have the information available for definitive management from that point forward?

A suggested acute stroke triage algorithm using advanced CT and MR protocols is shown in **Fig. 12.1**. This incorporates current therapies including intravenous tissue-type plasminogen activator (tPA) as well as approved endovascular devices and other intraarterial interventional strategies. Current and future efforts must streamline the work flow from the moment the patient reaches the emergency room until the definitive treatment is administered. With the realization that up to 2 million neurons die per minute in a typical middle cerebral artery occlusion, every second counts in both data acquisition and postprocessing.[2] Quality data must be rapidly produced and conveyed to the treatment team to facilitate fast yet fully informed decisions.

In our hospital, automated software running at the MR scanner console has been quickly providing multiparametric perfusion data for the past 10 years (**Fig. 12.2**). Postprocessing of color maps requires no physician input or specialized training, takes about 1 minute per scan, and maps are sent to the picture archiving and communication system (PACS) before the patient is rolled out of the MR suite. Such approaches, when combined with diffusion data, form the basis for treatment based on mismatch, or so-called penumbral imaging.[3] Treatment decisions are refined by knowledge of the vascular occlusion anatomy and filling patterns provided through fast time-resolved CTA or magnetic resonance angiography (MRA).

Innovations in Magnetic Resonance Angiography Stroke Evaluation

Imaging of the cerebrovascular system is a critical step in the evaluation of patients presenting with symptoms of stroke. A clinically desirable MRA stroke protocol would include features such as short examination time, four-dimensional (4D) temporal resolution, high spatial resolution, volumetric whole brain coverage, no or minimal risk to the patient, robustness, insensitivity to patient motion, and the ability to assess hemodynamic changes in vivo. In this section we present techniques in development that will improve the performance of MRA in stroke patients. In addition, we discuss HYPRFlow angiography as a comprehensive MRA method to evaluate stroke patients.

The MR systems of the future must be able to match the speed, ease of access, and reliability of CT if MR is to continue to play a major role in the evaluation of patients with stroke. MR systems will be increasing sited in the emergency department and staffed 24 hours a day, 7 days a week. The examinations will be transmitted to members of the stroke team simultaneously and contemporaneously with the imaging. The images will be viewed on hand-held devices that resemble small netbooks and will activate when an acute stroke patient has been identified. The hand-held devices will also permit voice and text communication among the members of the stroke team and instantaneous access to online tools.

Barriers to using MR in the emergency department (ED) are eliminated in the future through the use of revolutionary new procedures and technologies developed to quickly screen

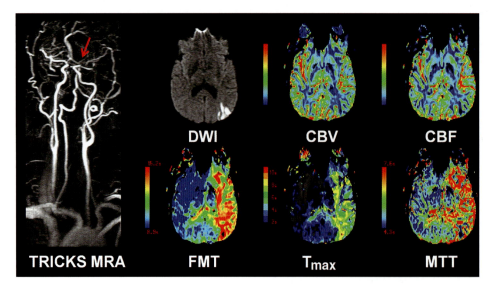

Fig. 12.2 Fast magnetic resonance imaging (MRI) triage of acute left hemisphere stroke at 4½ hours. Oblique maximum intensity projection (MIP) of time-resolved imaging of contrast kinetics (TRICKS) MRA (54 seconds) shows an occlusion of the supraclinoid left internal carotid artery. Diffusion (40 seconds) and perfusion maps (1 minute 13 seconds, automatically reconstructed at the scanner in 1 minute) show a small diffusion lesion with an extensive area of hypoperfusion in the left hemisphere. This perfusion-diffusion mismatch suggested a large ischemic penumbra. The patient was emergently treated with endovascular techniques and made a full clinical recovery. CBF, cerebral blood flow; CBV, cerebral blood volume; FMT, fluorescence molecular tomography; MTT, mean transit time; T$_{max}$, the time-to-peak of the deconvolved residue function.

patients. This technology will be adapted from new methods to screen passengers prior to boarding airline flights. The screening process will be further enhanced by the widespread use of MR-compatible clips, pacemakers, and stimulators. The screening will be completed during patient transport to the hospital and will be confirmed by a physician member of the stroke team. Thus the patients will quickly be made eligible for the MR examination.

Following clinical evaluation, the patient is prepared to be placed into the ultra-wide-bore, 3-tesla magnet. The patient is placed on a detachable ED/MR table that has intravenous pumps, anesthesia equipment, oxygen, electrocardiogram (ECG), and other support systems integrated into the table. The interior of the magnet has been modified to greatly increase the bore size and decrease the length of the bore. This has been accomplished by creating a gradient system that is only a few millimeters in thickness. The gradients enable echo times of less than 1 millisecond and repetition times of less than 2 milliseconds, roughly twice as fast as today's gradient systems. The dB/dT and SAR concerns are minimized though innovative coil and pulse sequence design. There is no sound produced by the scanner. Remote patient monitoring is easy to achieve via wireless telemetry.

The ED/MR table is constructed with a comfortable and conformable coil system. The global array has 128 channels and covers the heart, aortic arch, neck, and head in one coil system. The coils are divided into a 32-channel cardiopulmonary subgroup, a 32-channel aortic arch subgroup, a 32-channel neck subgroup, and a 32-channel head subgroup. The coil system is designed to provide high-resolution images from the heart to the brain. Cardiac imaging is routinely included to search for sources of emboli, eliminating the need for additional testing such as echocardiography. The multiple arrays generate images with high spatial resolution over a large anatomic region.

After placing the patient into the coil system and connecting the appropriate support systems, the patient is moved into the magnet room for a 15-minute comprehensive stroke evaluation. One might wonder how so much data can be acquired in only 15 minutes. There are several acceleration methods that can accomplish this. These include short repetition times, parallel imaging, radial undersampling, compressed sensing, random k-space sampling, and other methods to acquire the minimum data necessary to provide the image quality needed for diagnosis.

These cutting edge developments have their genesis in observations made decades ago. When Harry Nyquist was an engineer at AT&T, he wrote 12 articles on signal transmission. His publications led to the development of the Nyquist theorem, which states that the highest frequency in a transmission that can be accurately represented is less than one half of the sampling rate. If the sampling rate is too low, aliasing will occur and the signal (audio waves in Nyquist's day) will be distorted. Thus, for over two decades MR scientists assumed that a MR scan needed to be nearly fully sampled to prevent aliasing and suppress image artifacts. What the MR community did not realize is that meaningful images can be created with very little data and that artifacts can be minimized if the structures of interest within the imaging volume are sparse. The Nyquist theorem provides a sufficient condition, but not a necessary one, for perfect reconstruction. Vascular structures are sparse within the brain, and thus MRA lends itself to acceleration techniques such as undersampled radial imaging and compressed sensing.

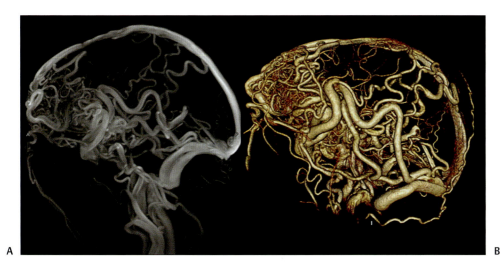

Fig. 12.3 Phase-contrast MRA using parallel imaging. The superficial venous drainage from the right frontal lobe AVM can be easily appreciated on the MIP **(A)** and surface-rendered **(B)** displays.

The first innovation to dramatically accelerate stroke imaging is related to the 128-channel coil array.[4,5] Signal from each coil is used to provide additional spatial encoding. Acceleration is achieved by reducing the number of phase-encoding steps (k-space lines) and substituting the spatial information acquired from the coil array. Pruessmann et al[6] introduced sensitivity encoding (SENSE), a parallel imaging method in which the data are first Fourier transformed, resulting in aliased images. The images are then unwrapped by using the spatial information from the coil sensitivity profiles. The SENSE calculations are conducted in image space, and a coil-sensitivity calibration (coil map) is required to carry out the calculations. **Figure 12.3** demonstrates the excellent spatial resolution than can be obtained using three-dimensional (3D) phase-contrast MRA and parallel imaging.

An alternate approach includes the coil-sensitivity calibration during the scan, and the calculations are performed in k-space. There are some advantages to this approach; it has a slightly better signal-to-noise ratio (SNR) and can cover a larger field of view.[7] Using very short repetition times (TRs) and parallel imaging techniques, one can predict at least a four- to eight-fold acceleration in MRA.

When parallel imaging is used, the coil performance must also be considered. The geometry factor (g factor) will impact the noise in the images. Currently coils are constructed out of conventional materials (such as copper wire). Future coils will use superconducting receivers with two to four times the performance of current systems.

Even higher levels of acceleration can be achieved through undersampling. In the brain, the vessels are relatively sparse within the imaging volume. Sparsity is a feature that we can exploit to our advantage. Because the vessels are sparse within the imaging volume, we can generate images of the vessels by acquiring only a small amount of signal from the volume of interest. A strategy developed by Mistretta's group[8] uses radial acquisition and projection reconstruction to acquire signal from vascular structures in a fraction of the imaging time required for Cartesian imaging.

Radial readout trajectories have several advantages over the rectilinear Cartesian approach that has dominated MRI for decades. The most compelling advantage is that the time-consuming phase-encoding stepping process is eliminated in 3D radial acquisition. For 3D radial imaging the spatial resolution is defined by the field of view and the readout gradient. For example, a 256 readout at a 25.6-cm field of view (FOV) produces isotropic 1 mm^3 voxels, and a 512 readout using the same FOV provides isotropic $0.5 \times 0.5 \times 0.5$ mm voxels. In both instances there is no phase encoding. In fact, by adjusting the readout bandwidth, both acquisitions can be obtained in the same imaging time! The elimination of phase encoding removes a fundamental barrier to image acceleration. A logical question is why was radial acquisition not pursued earlier. The answer is that fully sampled radial acquisition is slightly less efficient than fully sampled Cartesian imaging. However, when radial readout trajectories are used, the acquisition can be vastly undersampled with minimal loss of image quality. The huge advantage of radial imaging is that the undersampling artifacts are either propagated outside of the region of interest or the artifacts contribute to a slight increase in noise in the image. Vastly undersampled radial imaging can be used to obtain gated phase-contrast MR examinations of the entire head with $0.7 \times 0.7 \times 0.7$ mm resolution in less than 5 minutes. A similar examination using Cartesian rectilinear readout and phase encoding would take over an hour.

Radial 3D phase-contrast MRA[9] is similar to previous implementations in that stationary background tissue is subtracted from the angiographic images, and quantitative measurements of velocity are obtained from the velocity-induced phase shift. The velocity measurements are used to display hemodynamic conditions such as wall shear stress, relative pressure gradients, flow streamlines, and particle paths. Examples of 3D radial phase-contrast MRA examinations are shown in **Figs. 12.4** and **12.5**.

Radial undersampling is only one novel angiographic approach. Undersampling acquisition methods that are under

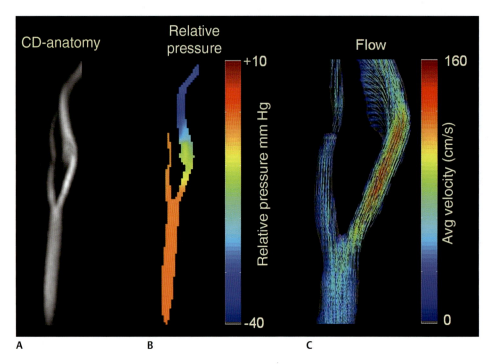

Fig. 12.4 Hemodynamic parameters obtained using highly acceler-ated radial undersampled phase-contrast MRA (PC VIPR). **(A)** The speed image reveals a stenosis of the proximal internal carotid artery. **(B)** Using the Navier-Stokes equations, a pressure gradient was calculated from the velocity data. There is approximately a 30 mm Hg drop in mean pressure across the stenosis. **(C)** The velocity vector plot shows velocities greater than 125 cm/s in the region of the stenosis. CD, complex difference. (Courtesy of Aquilla Turk, MD.)

investigation are compressed sensing and variable density sampling. Compressed sensing, also known as compressive sensing, compressive sampling, and sparse sampling, is a tech-nique for acquiring and reconstructing a signal utilizing the prior knowledge that it is sparse or compressible. The con-cept has existed for at least four decades, but recently the field has exploded.

If we think of another compression method, JPEG, a format commonly used for photographic images, the image data are routinely compressed by a factor of 10 with minimal loss of diagnostic information. So the question is how much infor-mation is really necessary to create the MRA image. For com-pressed sensing to work, the structures of interest must be sparse in the imaging or temporal domain. In addition the sampling method should produce incoherent artifacts when undersampled, and a reconstruction is needed to suppress noise-like artifacts and isolate the sparse vessel signal. For brain MRA the vessels are sparse in the imaging domain and

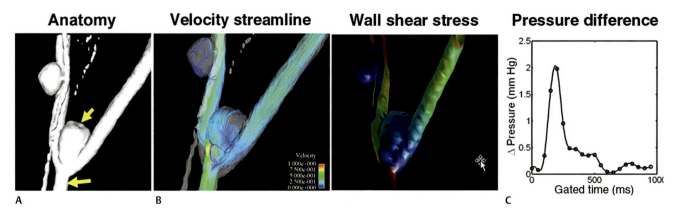

Fig. 12.5 Hemodynamic parameters obtained using highly acceler-ated radial undersampled phase-contrast MRA (PC VIPR). **(A)** The speed image shows two experimental canine aneurysms, a proximal bifurcation aneurysm, and a side wall aneurysm distally. **(B)** Velocity streamlines indicated greater flow in the bifurcation aneurysms compared with the side wall aneurysm. **(C)** The pressure gradient was measured from the parent artery (**A,** *lower arrow*) to the dome of the bifurcation aneurysm (**A,** *upper arrow*). Note the pressure difference of 2 mm Hg during the systolic phase of the cardiac cycle.

can be completely reconstructed from a highly undersampled examination. Acceleration factors of over 50 are possible. When combined with parallel imaging and ultrashort TRs, a high-resolution MRA of the head can be acquired in less than 1 second.[10,11]

Variable-density k-space sampling is a method to reduce aliasing artifacts in MR images. Because most of the energy of an image is concentrated around the k-space center, aliasing artifacts contain mostly low-frequency components if the k-space is uniformly undersampled. On the other hand, because the outer k-space region contains little energy, undersampling that region does not contribute severe aliasing artifacts. Therefore, a variable-density trajectory may sufficiently sample the central k-space region to reduce low-frequency aliasing artifacts and may undersample the outer k-space region to reduce scan time and to increase resolution. Variable-density sampling methods have been implemented for spiral imaging and 2D and 3D Fourier transform imaging. This method can significantly reduce the total energy of aliasing artifacts. In general, this method can be applied to all types of k-space sampling trajectories.[12]

Time-Resolved Magnetic Resonance Angiography Using HYPR Reconstruction

Contrast-enhanced, time-resolved MRA using HighlY constrained backPRojection (HYPR reconstruction) takes advantage of information sparsity in the time domain. The introduction of a smaller convolution kernel applied to local regions (HYPR LR) enabled more accurate waveforms and reduced signal contamination between neighboring structures. Iterative HYPR algorithms are also available that provide improved results in situations involving images of limited sparsity or complex temporal behavior.

In HYPR reconstruction, individual images are obtained by multiplying an averaged constraining image, also known as a composite image, by an appropriately produced weighting image. In HYPR LR the weighting images are given by the ratio of low-resolution versions of the undersampled time frame and composite images. The weighting images typically have poor spatial resolution but preserve temporal information. This situation is reversed for the composite image, which contains little information about temporal behavior but engenders high spatial resolution and SNR. Such approach yields high-quality time-resolved images with much higher accelerations.

Another benefit of HYPR algorithms is that the SNR and spatial resolution of individual time frames is largely determined by those of the composite image. Usually, in HYPR a composite image is formed from all of, or a subset of, the data acquired during a time-resolved examination. However, it can also be obtained in a separate, non–time-resolved scan or even from another imaging modality, thereby splitting the task of providing temporal and spatial resolution/SNR between two examinations.[13]

When a phase-contrast MRA (PC VIPR) is used as the composite image the resulting examination includes a time-resolved dynamic phase that shows the inflow and outflow

of contrast and a velocity field the encompasses the entire brain. This is called HYPRFlow, a synergistic technique that provides multidimensional physiologic and anatomic information (**Fig. 12.6**).

Beyond the blood vessels, imaging of the brain parenchyma will also be accelerated, predominantly through the use of parallel imaging technologies and high-performance coils. Two scans will be used to identify a hemorrhage on MR. The first is an isotropic whole-brain 3D fluid-attenuated inversion recovery (FLAIR) that is modified specifically to detect subarachnoid hemorrhage. The second scan produces a high-resolution isotropic 3D whole-brain susceptibility-weighted data set highly sensitive to parenchymal hemorrhage. These methods are supplemented by motion-suppressed T2 and diffusion-weighted images obtained using radial methods such as PROPELLER.[14] Quantitative perfusion studies are evaluated by a computer-assisted diagnostic (CAD) program, by which an analysis of the perfusion/diffusion mismatch is displayed as well as measurements of infarct size, volume, and location. The data are downloaded into a structured reporting macro.

Image Analysis and Display

The volume of images and data require new approaches to review. Data must be presented in an efficient way to facilitate both visual recognition and cognitive assimilation of key diagnostic features. Initially, maps of speed, velocity, estimated shear stress, and pressure differentials are displayed in axial, coronal, and sagittal projections. If a significant abnormality is identified, a small region of interest is placed over the vessel of interest, and physiologic information from that location is displayed. In this fashion, the radiologist can focus on regions of pathology and avoid distraction from large amounts of normal data. Pressure maps quickly identify hemodynamically significant stenoses. The estimated shear stress maps stratify aneurysms based on the location of inflow jets and points of high shear stress. Arteriovenous malformation (AVM) classification is expanded to include size, location, venous drainage, volume flow, pressure within the feeding arteries, and venous drainage.

Reporting and Quality

Structured reporting will be widely used for patients with stroke. Fields will be populated by data downloaded from imaging workstations. The imaging protocol and physiologic data are embedded in macros or templates. Key quality metrics such as radiation dose, SAR data, contrast type, and dose will all autopopulate to the report template from the scanner data fields. Important decision points such as permeability changes are highlighted and placed in the impression. The approved report is simultaneously transmitted to all members of the stroke team. The information is automatically downloaded into a stroke registry. To facilitate continuous quality improvement, work-flow data such as the time from examination completion to final report signature will be embedded and tracked.

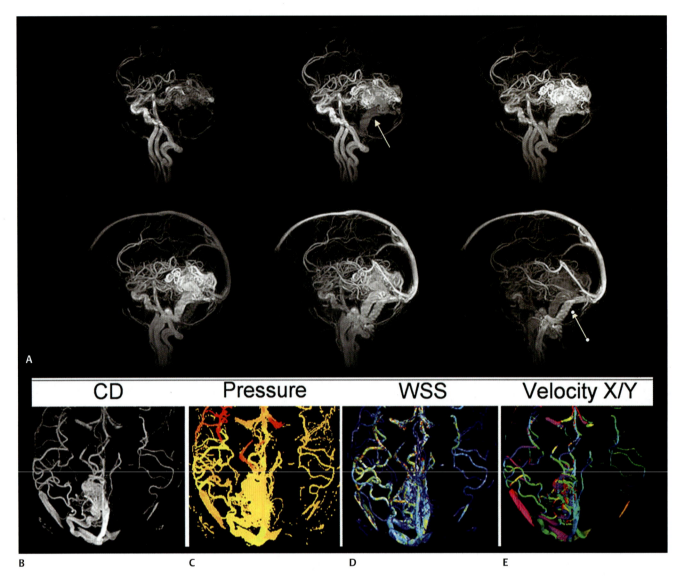

Fig. 12.6 Time-resolved MRA using highly constrained projection reconstruction (HYPR). A PC VIPR examination was used to constrain the time series. The combination of HYPR reconstruction and PC VIPR acquisition has been termed HYPRFlow. **(A)** Six images from a 64-image time series. There is excellent separation of arterial and venous structures. The right transverse *(arrow)* sinus fills rapidly due to the shunt through the arteriovenous malformation (AVM). The left transverse sinus *(arrow with circles)* fills during the venous phase of the acquisition. **(B–E)** Hemodynamic information from the PC VIPR scan is displayed. Complex difference (CD) speed image of the arterial and venous anatomy **(B)**, pressure gradient map **(C)**, estimated wall shear stress (WSS) **(D)**, and velocity vector plot **(E)**.

◆ Digital Subtraction Angiography, C-Arm Computed Tomography, and Computational Flow Studies in the Diagnosis and Management of Hemorrhagic and Ischemic Stroke

Over the last two decades 3D digital subtraction angiography (DSA) has become an integral component in the diagnosis and management of people with a large variety of central nervous system vascular diseases. The availability of flat panel detectors on C-arm configured angiographic systems has further expanded the capability of this technique, so that now high-quality tomographic image volumes can be quickly acquired and displayed. When acquired in conjunction with an injection of contrast medium over a 5- to 20-second acquisition, these images provide the opportunity to obtain detailed vascular and soft tissue information that had not previously been possible using x-ray angiographic systems. They also seem to offer some advantages over currently available CTA in that (1) there is no limitation in vascular visualization associated with the bone of the skull base, (2) there is some reduction in the amount of contrast medium required, and (3) there are some advantages in spatial resolution. The following section discusses and illustrates the current and evolving techniques using DSA and C-arm CT as they relate to

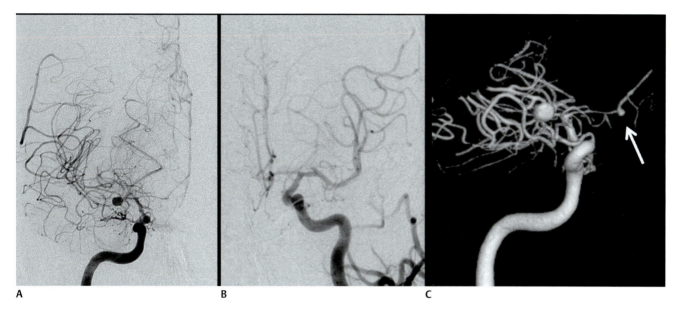

Fig. 12.7 Left **(A)** and right **(B)** internal carotid artery angiograms showing severe vasospasm and a right middle cerebral artery aneurysm. No abnormality is seen in the anterior communicating artery complex. **(C)** Three-dimensional digital subtraction angiography (3D-DSA) shows a small aneurysm at the junction between the A1 and A2 segments of the right anterior cerebral artery *(arrow)*.

the diagnosis and management of patients with hemorrhagic and ischemic strokes.

Digital Subtraction Angiography in the Diagnosis and Endovascular Therapy of Aneurysms and Arteriovenous Malformations

Aneurysmal subarachnoid hemorrhage (SAH) is a common and often lethal disease. Accurate diagnosis and recognition of the bleeding site, at the time of an initial hemorrhage, is essential if further morbidity and mortality are to be limited. Although current CTA is an excellent method for the initial screening of individuals with an aneurysmal SAH, it has been shown to be inferior to combinations of 2D and 3D DSA for aneurysm recognition. This is especially true in regard to aneurysms measuring less than 3 mm in size or ones that are located in regions where the vasculature is obscured by bones of the skull base.[15] More recently 3D-DSA has also been shown to be superior to standard multiprojection 2D-DSA for recognition of both asymptomatic and ruptured aneurysms.[16,17] **Figure 12.7** illustrates left and right internal carotid artery 2D-DSA angiograms and a left internal carotid 3D-DSA volume reconstruction from a patient seen 5 days after rupture of an aneurysm. The 2D-DSA images show a 4- to 5-mm right middle cerebral artery aneurysm, severe vasospasm, and what seems to be a normal anterior communicating artery complex. The 3D-DSA clearly shows a small, but potentially lethal, anterior communicating artery aneurysm. Both aneurysms were coiled successfully.

When done in conjunction with the injection of contrast medium and processed with appropriate algorithms, 3D acquisitions also provide a means to display both vascular and soft tissue structures. This results in interactive images that

are excellent tools for diagnostic analysis of anatomic relationships and also for treatment planning in both endovascular and open surgical interventions. In our practice, these images have proven to be especially helpful in understanding key anatomic relationships in circumstances where aneurysms are located at the skull base, and in defining the arterial and venous anatomy of complex vascular malformations. **Figure 12.8** shows a series of images taken from a 3D-DSA reconstruction acquired during injection of contrast medium into the left internal carotid artery of a patient with a large unruptured paraclinoid aneurysm. The volume was then reconstructed and unsubstracted, and viewed at a threshold appropriate for viewing both bone and vascular structures. By use of a region-of-interest cut-out tool on the angiographic workstation, a large section of the skull was removed, leaving a "model" with which structures are viewed from multiple projections. **Figure 12.9** shows a series of images taken from a 3D-DSA reconstruction acquired during injection of contrast medium into the left vertebral artery. As with the paraclinoid aneurysm discussed previously, the volume was reconstructed and unsubstracted, and viewed at a threshold appropriate for viewing both bone and vascular structures. Using the region-of-interest cut-out tool to perform a "virtual craniotomy," these images allow one to clearly visualize the location of the AVM nidus, its arterial supply, the venous drainage, and the presence of two small pseudoaneurysms that were likely responsible for the patient's hemorrhage. Although all of these structures could be seen on the 2D-DSA images, doing so requires one to obtain multiple projections, and even with these, important relationships are much more difficult to define than is the case with the 3D images.

It has long been recognized that color sharpens one's ability in visual tasks involving a search, that is, for identification and recognition. Recently a temporal and intensity color-coded

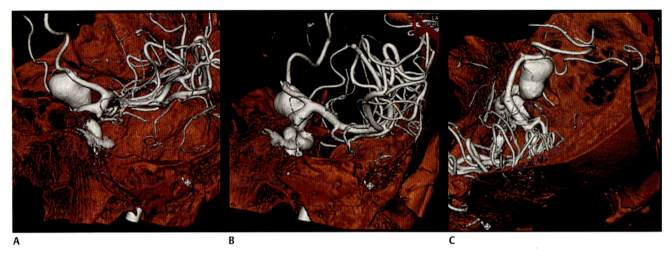

Fig. 12.8 **(A–C)** Series of views from a 3D-DSA showing the relationships of a large paraclinoid aneurysm to the skull base.

algorithm has become available that, when applied to a standard 2D-DSA sequence, provides a color-coded composite image of the entire acquisition. In preliminary studies, use of this algorithm improves the conspicuity of complex vascular structures and flow patterns; as a parametric image, it also allows one to extract functional information about circulation that cannot be gained from viewing either a single 2D-DSA image or a complete 2D-DSA acquisition.[4] About 30% of those patients who suffer an aneurysmal SAH develop symptomatic vasospasm. Many of them will be treated with a variety of endovascular techniques, such as balloon angioplasty and infusion of vasodilator drugs. Although the impact of these treatments on the large arteries at the base of the brain is often readily visualized on standard 2D-DSA images, it is usually very difficult to estimate angiographically the impact of these treatments on brain perfusion. **Figure 12.10** shows images from a 2D-DSA performed before and after treatment of vasospasm in a patient with aneurysmal SAH. Application of the color-coded algorithm to extract the time-to-half-maximum parameter and contrast concentration to the pre- and posttreatment standard DSA image series pro-

vides composite images that clearly demonstrate an increase in the speed of blood flow to the parenchyma; although this is not a quantitative measure, it seems very likely that, as is the case with the time-to-peak parameter that is frequently used in CT perfusion studies, it provides useful information about brain perfusion. **Figure 12.11** is another example of the application of this algorithm to a 2D-DSA acquisition. The 2D-DSA images show a large, complex arteriovenous malformation that receives supply from the right internal carotid artery. The composite color-coded images, displaying the time-to-half-maximum contrast concentration, allow one to more easily visualize the sequence of nidal filling and emptying and also to easily identify and separate venous structures that are arterialized from ones that are not involved with flow from the AVM. Preliminary studies indicate that information such as that shown in **Figs. 12.10** and **12.11** is helpful to physicians both in planning and in assessing therapeutic interventions.[18]

There is solid evidence that aneurysm development, growth, and rupture are all closely tied to hemodynamic factors.[19] Because the characteristics of blood flow in a particu-

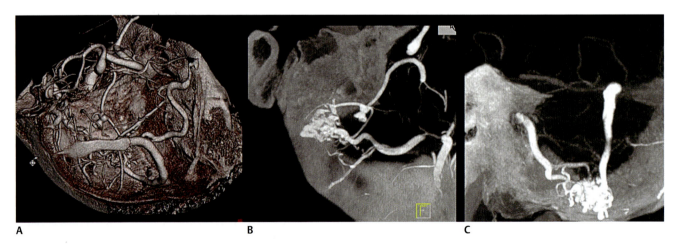

Fig. 12.9 **(A–C)** A series of views from a 3D-DSA reconstruction unsubtracted to show the relationships of a small arteriovenous malformation (AVM) with two pseudoaneurysms to the skull base. **(B,C)** Views of this volume as CT-like slices.

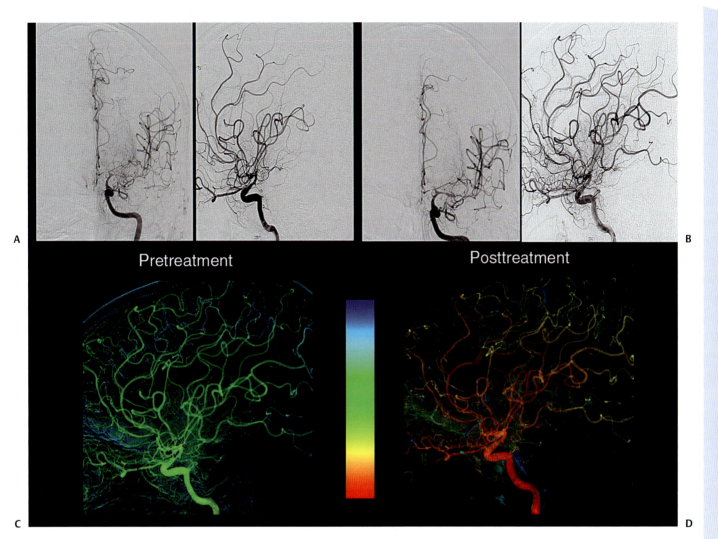

Fig. 12.10 Pre- **(A)** and post- **(B)** DSA images following treatment of vasospasm. The increased caliber of the middle and anterior cerebral arteries is evident. It is difficult to assess the degree to which this has improved tissue perfusion. **(C,D)** Composite color images of the DSA sequences done before **(C)** and after **(D)** treatment. The increase in blood flow to the parenchyma is more easily appreciated on these images than on standard DSA sequences.

lar aneurysm are primarily governed by the geometries of the aneurysm, its parent artery, and adjacent branches, there is increasing interest in evaluating the value of specific geometric factors such as the aspect ratio (AR) and the ratio of ostium area to aneurysm volume (VOR) as predictors for the risk of aneurysm rupture. Spatial resolution of images acquired with current flat detector angiographic equipment is superior to that of either CT or MR, and 3D-DSA studies can be used to display and calculate these and other geometric parameters, with greater accuracy than has been previously possible. The mortality and morbidity associated with aneurysm rupture and the lack of a reliable method to estimate rupture risk make it worthwhile to further explore the use of these tools to identify and analyze geometric characteristics that may be predictive of aneurysm natural history.

Geometric features are also key elements in determining whether or not a particular aneurysm is suitable for endovascular treatment. One such feature is the ratio between the neck width of an aneurysm and the height of its dome (the dome to neck [D/N] ratio). Aneurysms with a D/N ratio of >1.5, in general, can be treated with coiling without the need for using an adjunct device, such as balloon neck protection or coil-assisted stenting. The use of 3D-DSA reconstructions, however, provides a means for a more complete analysis of geometric features important in predicting the success of endovascular treatment, such as the percentage of parent artery circumference incorporated into the aneurysm ostium, than does an assessment based on 2D images.[20]

Digital Subtraction Angiography in the Diagnosis and Endovascular Therapy of Ischemic Stroke

There is a clinical imperative to quickly triage and treat patients presenting with TIA or stroke. Evidence is accumulating that symptoms of different etiologies, such as carotid stenosis and atrial fibrillation, are associated with different incidences of stroke risk, and that these risks may respond

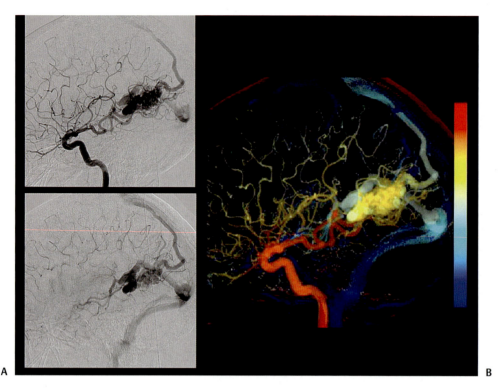

Fig. 12.11 **(A)** Lateral projections from a right internal carotid angiogram showing a large temporal arteriovenous malformation. **(B)** Composite color-coded images of the DSA sequence. Nidal filling and venous outflow are easier to appreciate on the color-coded images.

differently to different types of therapy, such as anticoagulation or antiplatelet therapy.[21] These data serve to point up the need for techniques that enable rapid and accurate diagnostic assessments and, when indicated, intervention with minimal delay. Up until now, imaging evaluation has proceeded from an initial CT or MRI to angiography for appropriate candidates. The availability of flat detector angiographic equipment capable of providing CT-like images of the brain as well as high spatial resolution 2D and 3D vascular images has significantly enhanced the resources of the angiographic suite in which diagnostic and therapeutic procedures are performed on patients with cerebrovascular disease. These techniques can now be used to obtain key physiologic measurements of brain perfusion, such as cerebral blood volume (CBV). The comprehensive diagnostic capabilities of such angiographic suites will allow more rapid diagnosis and revascularization in stroke patients.

Evolving Imaging Strategies in the Evaluation of Patients with Suspected Occlusive or Embolic Cerebrovascular Disease

Work is already underway to assess the potential of DSA to replace CTA or MRA as the initial vascular diagnostic test performed in the acute setting. Recently, a pilot study comparing images obtained with state-of-the-art equipment (dual-source CT and 3-tesla MR) indicated that the two modalities were comparable, except that for visualization of small intracranial arteries, MRA was somewhat better than CTA.[22]

Another recent study comparing CTA with DSA in the evaluation of intracranial atherosclerotic disease concluded that CTA had a high sensitivity and specificity for detecting 50% or greater stenosis of large intracranial arterial segments, and that it could be used as a screening tool for detection of intracranial arterial disease and stenosis. The authors of this study commented, however, that because of the techniques used for measurement and the special training that was given to the physicians who evaluated the images, "CTA may not be as accurate in clinical practice as reported here."[23] To our knowledge, no significant data are available comparing the advantages, if any, of 3D-DSA over 2D-DSA, CTA, or MRA for lesion detection in this patient population. Three potential advantages of using DSA instead of CTA or MRA for the initial evaluation of patients presenting with signs or symptoms suggestive of cervical or intracranial vascular disease bear consideration. First, 3D-DSA, done with flat detector angiographic equipment, has superior spatial and contrast resolution compared with both CTA and MRA. Second, preliminary experience indicates that a screening examination can be performed with a lower x-ray dose and a lower volume of contrast medium than can be done with CT. Third, from a single rotational acquisition using less than 100 cc of contrast medium injected into a peripheral vein, one can obtain not only a high spatial resolution 3D vascular volume and a noncontrast CT of the brain, but also a map of CBV **(Fig. 12.12).**

Currently, the C-arm CT images of the brain are not adequate for recognition of small amounts of blood or the early, but important, signs of acute ischemic injury. However, ongoing efforts to reduce scatter radiation and to minimize

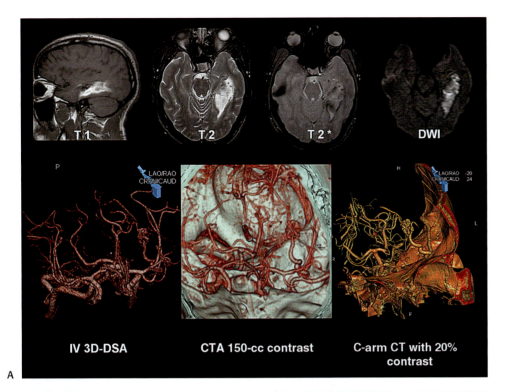

A

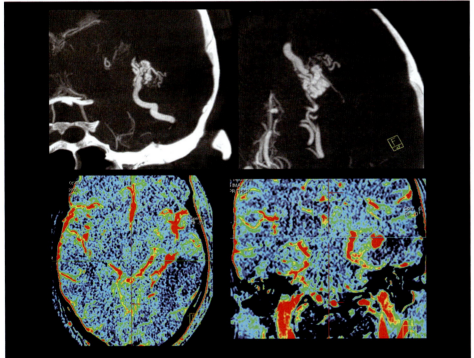

B

Fig. 12.12 **(A)** Upper panel: Series of MR images showing a left temporal lobe and ventricular hematoma. This was secondary to rupture of a small AVM. Lower panel: IV 3D-DSA done with 80 cc of contrast; CTA done with 150 cc of contrast; intraarterial (IA) C-arm CT done with 20% contrast injected throughout a 20-second acquisition. The IV 3D-DSA has equal or better spatial resolution than does the CTA.

There is no artifact caused by bone at the skull base on the IV 3D-DSA. **(B)** Upper panel: Sagittal and axial views of the IV 3D-DSA reconstructed native fill rather than subtracted. These views show excellent definition of the AVM nidus. Lower panel: Axial and coronal CBV maps generated from the IV 3D-DSA acquisition. The area of the hematoma is clearly seen as an area with reduced CBV.

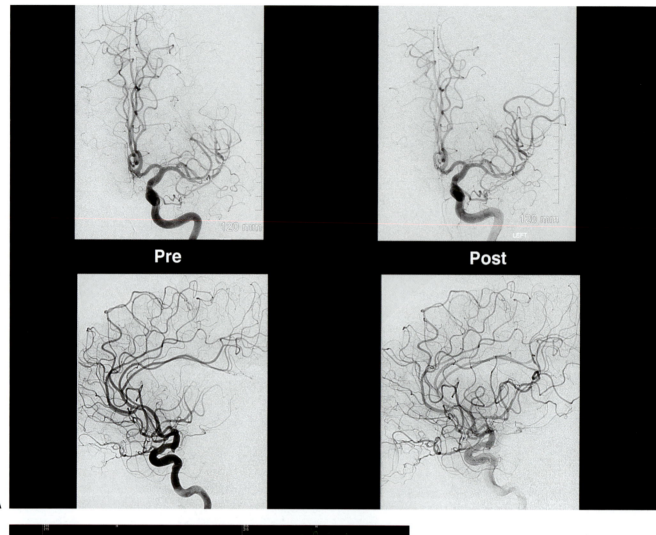

Pre

Post

A

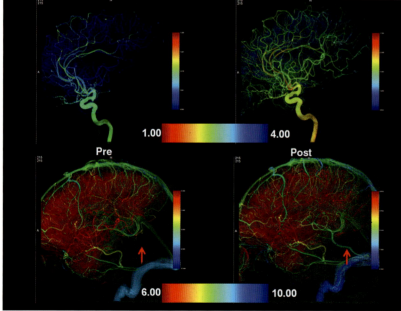

Pre

Post

1.00

4.00

6.00

10.00

B

Fig. 12.13 **(A)** Anteroposterior and lateral DSA images done pre- *(left)* and post- *(right)* balloon angioplasty of an in-stent stenosis of the left middle cerebral artery (MCA). Improved flow through the cortical branches of the MCA is evident. It is difficult to assess how or if this has improved parenchymal perfusion. **(B)** Upper panel: Color-coded lateral images pre- *(left)* and post- *(right)* angioplasty of the MCA stenosis. These composite images obtained at 1 to 4 seconds of acquisition clearly show the improved speed of flow throughout the MCA distribution. Lower panel: Composite color-coded images depicting flow between 6 and 10 seconds clearly show improved parenchymal opacification. Note filling of the vein of Labbé *(red arrow)* on the post angioplasty image.

artifacts due to patient motion are likely to improve image quality to a point that these deficiencies are eliminated. When this occurs it should prove feasible to perform in the angiographic suite both the initial assessment and triage of patients suspected of having an acute ischemic stroke. Ultimate clinical outcomes and the incidence of complications related to revascularization are both closely linked to the duration and the severity of ischemia. Initial evaluation and triage of patients with an acute ischemic stroke in an environment where both diagnosis and treatment can be performed, such as the angiography suite, should add value, both in safety and efficacy, to the care of these patients by reducing the interval between the time that a patient arrives at a hospital and the time that an accurate diagnosis is made and appropriate treatment instituted. Finally, use of the temporal and intensity color-coded algorithm already discussed in conjunction with 2D-DSA acquisitions done for evaluation of patients with cerebrovascular occlusive disease seems to improve the ability to use these images both to assess qualitatively the impact of a stenosis on brain perfusion as well as to then determine changes in perfusion that occur following angioplasty and stenting (**Fig. 12.13**).

Assessing the impact of an ischemic insult on brain viability can best be accomplished using physiologic rather than morphologic criteria, especially in the acute interval when anatomic changes are minimal and the options for revascularization are greater and most effective. Until recently, the measurement of cerebral perfusion parameters has required imaging either with CT or with MRI. Limitations in the speed of angiographic C-arm gantry rotation prohibit acquisition of rotational angiographic data sets of sufficient temporal resolution to determine either cerebral blood flow (CBF) or mean transit time (MTT). As mentioned briefly above, it is possible using currently available flat detector angiographic equipment to collect data that is suitable for determination of the CBV, a key perfusion parameter indicative of the state of autoregulation.

In studies of both normal canines and in animals in which an ischemic injury had been induced, we have demonstrated

that CBV maps obtained using C-arm CT compare well with ones obtained using standard perfusion CT (PCT). Preliminary studies in humans also indicate that the results of CBV measurements with the two modalities compare equally well. Because of limitations in the speed of the C-arm gantry rotation, it is necessary that the contrast medium be injected using an injection technique designed such that there is a steady state of contrast within the brain parenchyma during data acquisition. The details of this technique as well as a description of the algorithm used for calculation and display of the CBV maps are provided in our recent reports on this topic[24,25] (**Fig. 12.14**).

Computational Flow Studies/Simulations

Advances in computational techniques and computer hardware now make it possible to perform blood flow simulations using patient-specific geometric models at times that, in many cases, allow them to be used as adjuncts to decisions regarding the choice of optimal therapy. Although a majority of the research has addressed the use of these simulations for evaluation of intracranial aneurysms, they are also increasingly relevant to the study of stenotic lesions.

Solid evidence closely links aneurysm growth, thrombosis, and rupture to hemodynamic factors. As these are, in turn, largely governed by the geometric relationships among an aneurysm, its parent artery, and adjacent branches, accurate determination of these anatomic and geometric features is critical in creation of the models that are used for flow simulations. 3D-DSA provides the highest spatial resolution data available for this purpose. Combining such patient-specific geometric data with patient-specific waveforms and boundary conditions obtained from either ultrasound or phase-contrast MR studies, simulations closely mimic measured velocities and patterns of blood flow obtained using advanced phase-contrast MRI techniques.[26] Very significant advances have been made over the last few years in measuring patterns of flow and velocities using these advanced phase-contrast

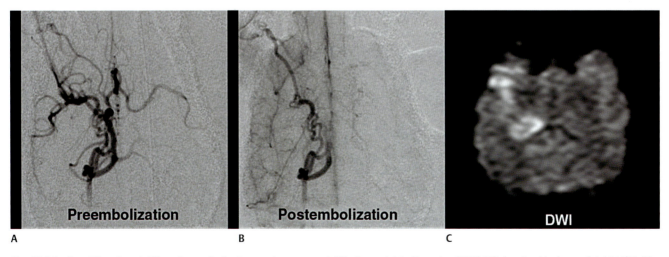

A   B   C

Fig. 12.14 Pre- **(A)** and post- **(B)** canine embolization angiograms and diffusion-weighted imaging (DWI) **(C)** showing blockage of right MCA. The DWI done at 4 hours confirms early right MCA infarction. (*continued on next page*)

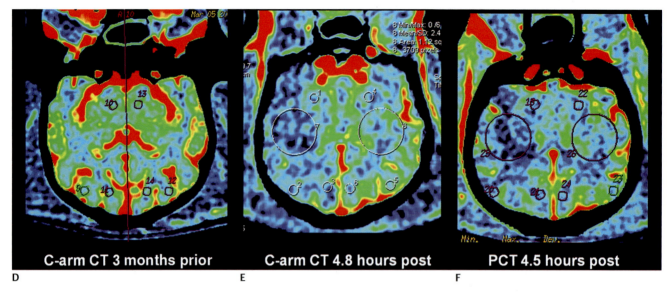

C-arm CT 3 months prior   **C-arm CT 4.8 hours post**   **PCT 4.5 hours post**

D   E   F

Fig. 12.14 (*continued*)   The DWI done at 4 hours confirms early right MCA infarction. C-arm CT CBV map **(D)** done 3 months prior to creation of stroke; C-arm CT CBV map **(E)** done 4.8 hours after embolization; conventional perfusion CT (PCT) CBV map **(F)** done just prior to the C-arm CBV study. There is excellent correlation between the area of reduced CBV shown on C-arm CT and conventional CT CBV perfusion maps.

MRI techniques.[27] One significant potential value of simulations over actual measurements of blood flow is that, with computational studies, a variety of physiologic states can be simulated and analyzed; with techniques that measure directly flow characteristics, it is challenging, if not impossible, to accurately vary and maintain altered physiologic states. As an example, we have recently performed simulations looking at changes in blood flow characteristics at three different heart rates in human aneurysms. These studies indicate, as would be expected, that hemodynamic parameters are much different, and perhaps more likely to cause vascular injury, at higher cardiac frequencies than at lower frequencies.[28] Evidence is accumulating that certain predisposing hemodynamic patterns are related to the natural history, such as the rupture risk of intracranial aneurysms. For example, Cebral and colleagues,[29] in a large series of anterior circulation aneurysms, have shown a correlation between aneurysm rupture and the pattern of inflow into an aneurysm; aneurysms with high-velocity inflow jets that impact a small area of the aneurysm wall were more likely to have ruptured than those where this pattern was not present. Although it is not yet possible for simulations such as these to be performed outside of facilities with specialized capabilities and personnel, there is evidence that simple geometric features alone may be predictive of certain hemodynamic phenotypes.[30] These geometric features are easily available from routine 3D-DSA, CTA, and MRA studies.

References

1. Latchaw RE, Alberts MJ, Lev MH, et al; American Heart Association Council on Cardiovascular Radiology and Intervention, Stroke Council, and the Interdisciplinary Council on Peripheral Vascular Disease. Recommendations for imaging of acute ischemic stroke: a scientific statement from the American Heart Association. Stroke 2009;40:3646–3678
2. Saver JL. Time is brain—quantified. Stroke 2006;37:263–266
3. Rowley HA. Extending the time window for thrombolysis: evidence from acute stroke trials. Neuroimaging Clin N Am 2005;15:575–587, x
4. McDougall MP, Wright SM. 64-channel array coil for single echo acquisition magnetic resonance imaging. Magn Reson Med 2005;54:386–392
5. Wiggins GC, Triantafyllou C, Potthast A, Reykowski A, Nittka M, Wald LL. 32-channel 3 tesla receive-only phased-array head coil with soccerball element geometry. Magn Reson Med 2006;56:216–223
6. Pruessmann KP, Weiger M, Scheidegger MB, Boesiger P. SENSE: sensitivity encoding for fast MRI. Magn Reson Med 1999;42:952–962
7. Griswold MA, Jakob PM, Heidemann RM, et al. Generalized autocalibrating partially parallel acquisitions (GRAPPA). Magn Reson Med 2002;47:1202–1210
8. Barger AV, Block WF, Toropov Y, Grist TM, Mistretta CA. Time-resolved contrast-enhanced imaging with isotropic resolution and broad coverage using an undersampled 3D projection trajectory. Magn Reson Med 2002;48:297–305
9. Gu T, Korosec FR, Block WF, et al. PC VIPR: a high-speed 3D phase-contrast method for flow quantification and high-resolution angiography. AJNR Am J Neuroradiol 2005;26:743–749
10. Gamper U, Boesiger P, Kozerke S. Compressed sensing in dynamic MRI. Magn Reson Med 2008;59:365–373
11. Lustig M, Donoho D, Pauly JM. Sparse MRI: the application of compressed sensing for rapid MR imaging. Magn Reson Med 2007;58:1182–1195
12. Lee J, Nishimura D, Osgood B. Optimal variable-density k-space sampling in MRI. Paper presented at International Symposium of Biomedical Imaging (ISBI), 2004
13. Mistretta CA. Undersampled radial MR acquisition and highly constrained back projection (HYPR) reconstruction: potential medical imaging applications in the post-Nyquist era. J Magn Reson Imaging 2009;29:501–516
14. Pipe JG. Motion correction with PROPELLER MRI: application to head motion and free-breathing cardiac imaging. Magn Reson Med 1999;42:963–969
15. Romijn M, Gratama van Andel HA, van Walderveen MA, et al. Diagnostic accuracy of CT angiography with matched mask bone elimination for detection of intracranial aneurysms: comparison with digital subtraction angiography and 3D rotational angiography. AJNR Am J Neuroradiol 2008;29:134–139
16. van Rooij WJ, Peluso JP, Sluzewski M, Beute GN. Additional value of 3D rotational angiography in angiographically negative aneurysmal subarachnoid hemorrhage: how negative is negative? AJNR Am J Neuroradiol 2008;29:962–966
17. van Rooij WJ, Sprengers ME, de Gast AN, Peluso JP, Sluzewski M. 3D rotational angiography: the new gold standard in the detection of additional intracranial aneurysms. AJNR Am J Neuroradiol 2008;29:976–979

18. Strother CM, Bender F, Deuerling-Zheng Y, et al. Parametric color coding of digital subtraction angiography. AJNR Am J Neuroradiol 2010;31:919–924

19. Stehbens WE. Etiology of intracranial berry aneurysms. J Neurosurg 1989;70:823–831

20. Karmonik C, Arat A, Benndorf G, et al. A technique for improved quantitative characterization of intracranial aneurysms. AJNR Am J Neuroradiol 2004;25:1158–1161

21. Famakin BM, Chimowitz MI, Lynn MJ, Stern BJ, George MG; WASID Trial Investigators. Causes and severity of ischemic stroke in patients with symptomatic intracranial arterial stenosis. Stroke 2009;40:1999–2003

22. Mühlenbruch G, Das M, Mommertz G, et al. Comparison of dual-source CT angiography and MR angiography in preoperative evaluation of intra- and extracranial vessels: a pilot study. Eur Radiol 2010;20:469–476

23. Nguyen-Huynh MN, Wintermark M, English J, et al. How accurate is CT angiography in evaluating intracranial atherosclerotic disease? Stroke 2008;39:1184–1188

24. Ahmed AS, Zellerhoff M, Strother CM, et al. C-arm CT measurement of cerebral blood volume: an experimental study in canines. AJNR Am J Neuroradiol 2009;30:917–922

25. Bley T, Strother CM, Pulfer K, et al. C-arm CT measurement of cerebral blood volume in ischemic stroke: an experimental study in canines. AJNR Am J Neuroradiol 2010;31:536–540

26. Boussel L, Rayz V, Martin A, et al. Phase-contrast magnetic resonance imaging measurements in intracranial aneurysms in vivo of flow patterns, velocity fields, and wall shear stress: comparison with computational fluid dynamics. Magn Reson Med 2009;61:409–417

27. Markl M, Harloff A, Bley TA, et al. Time-resolved 3D MR velocity mapping at 3T: improved navigator-gated assessment of vascular anatomy and blood flow. J Magn Reson Imaging 2007;25:824–831

28. Jiang J, Strother C. Computational fluid dynamics simulations of intracranial aneurysms at varying heart rates: a "patient-specific" study. J Biomech Eng 2009;131:091001

29. Cebral JR, Castro MA, Burgess JE, Pergolizzi RS, Sheridan MJ, Putman CM. Characterization of cerebral aneurysms for assessing risk of rupture by using patient-specific computational hemodynamics models. AJNR Am J Neuroradiol 2005;26:2550–2559

30. Ford MD, Lee SW, Lownie SP, Holdsworth DW, Steinman DA. On the effect of parent-aneurysm angle on flow patterns in basilar tip aneurysms: towards a surrogate geometric marker of intra-aneurismal hemodynamics. J Biomech 2008;41:241–248

Open Surgical Approaches

13

Anesthesia Considerations for Neurovascular Surgery

Carine Zeeni, John F. Bebawy, Dhanesh K. Gupta, and Antoun Koht

Pearls

- Plasma biomarkers of cardiac dysfunction (e.g., troponin-I, serum B-type natriuretic peptide) are predictive of cardiovascular dysfunction after subarachnoid hemorrhage (SAH) and should be measured in all SAH patients. In the presence of elevated levels, or clinical symptoms of cardiac dysfunction (e.g., pulmonary edema, hemodynamic instability), a transthoracic echocardiogram should be performed and central venous or pulmonary artery monitoring should be considered for perioperative management.
- Maintaining global and local cerebral perfusion pressure to avoid focal ischemia due to vasospasm or inadequate watershed blood flow is just as important as avoiding cerebral hypertension, which can cause aneurysm rupture or cerebral hyperemia.
- Brain relaxation not only facilitates surgical dissection, but also may avert neurologic injury due to a local decrease in cerebral perfusion pressure. Hyperosmotic therapy with mannitol and/or hypertonic saline along with maneuvers that optimize cerebral venous drainage (e.g., reverse Trendelenburg position, limited intrathoracic pressure, avoidance of excessive jugular vein torsion) are simple methods that may achieve and maintain adequate brain relaxation long after the effects of hypocapnia have waned.
- Intraoperative maintenance of normoglycemia (80–120 mg/dL) during aneurysm clip ligation is associated with improved neuropsychiatric and Glasgow Outcome Scale outcomes at 3 and 12 months. Intensive insulin therapy with bolus and infusions of insulin can rapidly achieve normoglycemia; however, to avoid hypoglycemia, frequent monitoring of serum glucose is required (i.e., every 15 to 30 minutes).
- Anatomically directed neurophysiologic monitoring may serve as an early warning sign of impending neurologic injury. Systematic investigation of the etiology of a change in neurophysiologic monitoring may allow early intervention to circumvent surgical or physiologic insults that produce intraoperative neuronal damage and postoperative neurologic morbidity.

The fundamental goal of general anesthesia is to produce a patient state in which surgical procedures can be safely performed. Besides maintaining an unaware patient who is oblivious to noxious stimulation, much time and effort is spent in maintaining homeostasis by frequently monitoring hemodynamic parameters and titrating and adding pharmacologic agents to maintain adequate perfusion to all organs. As more and more complex neurosurgical procedures are performed in patients with more severe acute and chronic coexisting diseases, the anesthesiologist also spends a significant amount of time monitoring and treating abnormalities in oxygen delivery and coagulation while employing more sophisticated monitors of neurologic well-being (e.g., processed electroencephalograms, evoked neurologic electrophysiologic responses) to maintain adequate blood flow to the neuronal tissue at risk. This chapter focuses on the physiologic and pharmacologic concepts that form the foundation for providing perioperative care of the complex neurovascular patient.

◆ Preoperative Management

Close collaboration and communication between the surgical and anesthesia teams allows formulation of the most appropriate perioperative plan for the patient. The preoperative laboratory tests that should be obtained prior to even urgent neurovascular surgery are presented in **Table 13.1**. When time permits, it is essential that all patients with complex intracranial lesions undergo preoperative cardiac testing. The goal of this evaluation is not to identify candidates in need of cardiac revascularization, but rather to identify patients who may require more invasive hemodynamic monitoring to allow the safe administration of vasoactive agents to maintain intraoperative cerebral perfusion. Patients who have poorly controlled hypertension, metabolic syndrome,

Table 13.1 Preoperative Laboratory Tests Prior to Neurovascular Surgery

Electrocardiogram

Hemoglobin, hematocrit, and platelet count

Prothrombin time (PT), international normalized ratio (INR), activated partial thromboplastin time (aPTT), and fibrinogen

Sodium, potassium, and glucose

Blood urea nitrogen (BUN) and creatinine

Platelet function assay

Type and crossmatch for two packed red blood cells[1]

[1]Depending on the surgical approach, likelihood of intraoperative blood loss, and the presence of antibodies on the crossmatch, additional units of packed red blood cells should be crossmatched and available in the operating room.

known coronary artery disease, or congestive heart failure should undergo, at a minimum, preoperative resting echocardiography. When clinical signs of angina are present, and to minimize the chances of a hypertension-induced aneurysmal rupture, adenosine sestamibi or thallium nuclear stress testing should be considered in place of treadmill or dobutamine-induced stress tests. The data from these tests will identify those patients with either a decreased ejection fraction (<25%) or significant coronary artery disease who may require perioperative pulmonary artery catheterization.

Patients presenting with subarachnoid hemorrhage (SAH) usually represent a more complex group to evaluate preoperatively because of the high incidence of electrocardiographic abnormalities, the presence of major clinical risk factors for concomitant coronary artery and systemic arterial atherosclerosis, and the real phenomenon of SAH-induced cardiac dysfunction.[1,2] Electrical disturbances as well as possible myocardial lesions are summarized in **Table 13.2**, in increasing order of severity. Despite the association between post-SAH electrocardiogram (ECG) abnormalities and post-SAH 3-month mortality, there is no association between SAH-induced ECG abnormalities and myocardial function.[2] In fact, myocardial wall motion abnormalities, which are well documented by echocardiogram or nucleotide venticulography,

Table 13.2 Cardiac Findings in Patients with Subarachnoid Hemorrhage

Electrocardiogram	• ST segment abnormalities
	• T wave abnormalities
	• QT segment prolongations
	• Ventricular tachycardia
	• Ventricular fibrillation
Myocardial lesions	• Diastolic dysfunction
	• Ventricular hypokinesis and reduced ejection fraction (including clinical heart failure)

are not related to coronary artery disease.[3] These transient wall motion abnormalities (<14 days) are caused by the catecholamine surge that occurs with SAH and follow a noncoronary artery distribution. Because of the strong association between plasma biomarkers of myocardial injury (e.g., cardiac troponin I [cTI], and serum B-type natriuretic peptide [BNP]) and clinically significant left ventricular dysfunction, all patients with SAH should have a baseline cTI and BNP measured on admission.[4,5] Subsequent preoperative workup is based on these levels and the presence or absence of clinical signs of heart failure (**Fig. 13.1**). Those patients with clinically significant ventricular dysfunction are more likely to require perioperative vasoactive agents to maintain cerebral perfusion pressure that may necessitate the placement of a cardiac output monitors (e.g., pulmonary artery catheter, transesophageal echocardiography).

◆ Intraoperative Management

Perioperative management of a patient undergoing neurovascular intervention should focus on the following goals:

1. Maintaining adequate cerebral perfusion pressure and avoiding secondary cerebral ischemia due to hypoperfusion

2. Optimizing working conditions for the neurosurgeon, including providing adequate brain relaxation throughout surgery to minimize the risk of retractor injury

3. Monitoring for impending neurologic injury and performing corrective maneuvers to undo surgical and physiologic induced changes that may be associated with neurologic injury

Hemodynamic Management

One of the most important goals of intraoperative management of neurovascular patients is to maintain adequate cerebral perfusion pressure, thereby preventing secondary cerebral injury due to hypoperfusion (ischemia). In addition, it is important to avoid unnecessary hypertension, which can lead to aneurysmal rupture or perfusion pressure breakthrough (e.g., perilesion edema, resection bed hemorrhage). All anesthetic regimens that maintain patient amnesia/sedation, prevent patient movement in response to noxious stimulation, and provide hemodynamic stability have demonstrated equal safety and efficacy in intracranial surgery.[6] The following perioperative events may be associated with transient noxious stimulation that can lead to rapid increases in blood pressure:

1. Laryngoscopy and tracheal intubation

2. Placement in Mayfield head fixation

3. Surgical incision

4. Dural traction

5. Brainstem manipulation

6. Placement of brain retractors during posterior fossa and middle fossa surgery

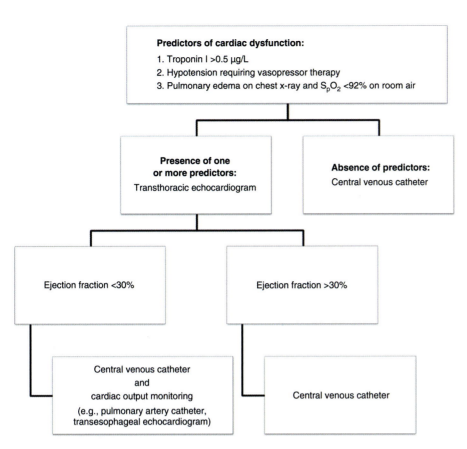

Overly aggressive prophylaxis for treatment of hypertension may lead to unintended hypotension and inadequate cerebral perfusion. Therefore, with the use of ultrarapid offset opioids (e.g., remifentanil or alfentanil) and short-acting vasoactive agents (e.g., esmolol, nicardipine, or nitroprusside), hypertension from these brief, noxious stimuli can be prevented or treated, whereas unintended hypotension is limited in duration and easily corrected. Special consideration should be given to hemodynamic management at the time of temporary occlusion of feeding vessels to facilitate permanent clip placement. To ensure adequate distal cerebral perfusion through collateral vessels, it is necessary to increase mean arterial pressure (MAP) at this time by approximately 20% from baseline values. Once temporary clips are removed and neuromonitoring signals are confirmed to be unchanged, MAP can be returned to its original level.

When temporary clipping of parent vessels is not an option for anatomic/morphologic reasons, adenosine-induced flow arrest offers a unique method of transiently and profoundly reducing systolic blood pressure so as to facilitate clip ligation of the aneurysm.[7] Other techniques to reduce aneurysm neck turgor that have been described include deep hypothermic circulatory arrest, temporary occlusion of the extracranial common carotid artery, and endovascular balloon catheter retrograde suction deflation.[8] These methods, however, are logistically more difficult to carry out. Brief periods of profound hypotension can also be produced by infusions and boluses of sodium nitroprusside or esmolol, although both of these drugs are less predictable in their dose–response relationships. Adenosine has proven to be a safe, predictable agent for achieving the brief flow arrest often needed to apply a permanent clip, and can be used repeatedly. Compared with deep hypothermic circulatory arrest, adenosine offers the advantage of avoiding the coagulopathy associated with deep hypothermia, as well as the hyperglycemia and rebound hyperthermia that occur after cardiopulmonary bypass.[9] Based on our observational series, in patients receiving a background anesthetic consisting of remifentanil, 0.5 minimum alveolar concentration (MAC) of volatile anesthetic, and a propofol infusion achieving a burst suppression ratio of 0.7, there is a significant linear relationship between the dose of adenosine, the duration of asystole, and the duration of profound hypotension **(Fig. 13.2).** An adenosine dose of 0.35 mg per kilogram of ideal body weight (preferably delivered via a central venous catheter) is the recommended starting dose to achieve approximately 45 seconds of profound systemic hypotension.[10] Timing of adenosine administration, whether planned or after inadvertent intraoperative rupture of an aneurysm, must be carefully coordinated with the neurosurgeon so that adequate working time is available for the successful placement of each clip or series of clips.

Patient Positioning

Neurovascular surgical procedures can often last anywhere from 5 to 24 hours. Careful attention by the entire operative

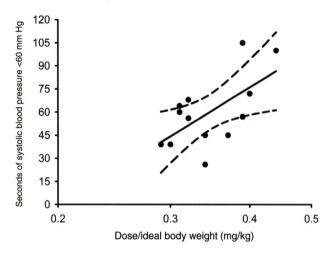

Fig. 13.2 Scattergram of the adenosine dose (normalized to ideal body weight) and the resulting duration of systolic blood pressure <60 mm Hg from the first dose administered to 13 patients in this series (raw data). The solid lines depict the log-linear dose–response curves, and the dashed lines depict the 95% confidence intervals of the models. Note that the x-axis is a log_{10} scale.

team should be paid to the positioning of the patient. Prolonged pressure or stretch of peripheral nerves (e.g., brachial plexus, ulnar nerve) may result in peripheral neuropathy. This risk may be minimized by using sufficient padding to vulnerable pressure points, adjusting all joints so that there is not extreme stretch on any neural plexus, and utilizing neurophysiologic monitors to warn of the development of peripheral nerve injury and adjusting the affected limb to correct the problem.[11] Positioning may also impact the surgical field if the patient's trunk and limbs are not adequately secured to allow sufficient manipulation or rotation of the operating table without shifting the body. Finally, ignoring the effects of a patient's position on jugular venous drainage or the pressure on the abdomen and chest may result in inadequate cerebral venous drainage that may impede adequate brain relaxation despite aggressive therapeutic maneuvers (e.g., excessive hyperosmotic therapy or cerebrospinal fluid [CSF] drainage). In addition, excessive neck flexion or rotation may impede venous drainage from the tongue, which, in the extremes of circumstances, could result in tongue edema and even necrosis, requiring prolonged endotracheal intubation due to airway obstruction.

Brain Bulk Management

Actively managing brain bulk, even in those patients with a normal starting intracranial pressure, may reduce direct pressure exerted by retractors in the field, thereby minimizing the risk of retractor-induced brain ischemia and injury.[12] Aside from acute short-term hyperventilation, hyperosmolar therapy has long been the cornerstone of brain bulk and intracranial pressure treatment. Mannitol and hypertonic saline are the osmotic agents of choice (**Table 13.3**).[13–15] Both agents decrease brain bulk and intracranial pressure by two different mechanisms. The initial mechanism is a decrease in blood viscosity that improves flow and increases oxygen delivery to brain tissue. This results in a compensatory vasoconstriction that reduces cerebral blood volume and therefore intracranial pressure. The delayed but major mechanism of reduced brain bulk is an osmotically mediated decrease in brain water content. Mannitol is renally excreted and produces a strong osmotic diuretic effect. Hypertonic saline, on the other hand, has a relatively small natriuretic effect, making it an attractive alternative to mannitol in certain circumstances (e.g., when cerebral perfusion pressure is difficult to maintain otherwise). Prospective, randomized, double-blind studies comparing the effects of hypertonic saline and mannitol on brain relaxation and serum electrolyte balance showed that both modalities were efficacious, though hypertonic saline may be more efficacious in achieving brain relaxation in supratentorial brain tumor patients. In addition, the mannitol group had decreased serum sodium, a greater fluid deficit, and increased plasma lactate levels compared with the hypertonic saline group.[14,15] Depending on the extent of initial brain bulk, 0.25 to 1 g/kg of mannitol is usually infused intravenously over 10 to 20 minutes. Alternatively, a dose of 1 to 2 mL/kg of 3% saline can be given as an intravenous bolus, followed by an infusion of 1 to 2 mL/kg/h with a plasma sodium goal of 145 to 155 mEq/dL. If repeated doses of mannitol, or long-term infusions of hypertonic saline, are needed, plasma osmolality should be closely monitored and kept under 320 mOsm/L. In addition, care should be taken to monitor for rebound cerebral edema that may occur with the abrupt discontinuation of any infusions of a hyperosmotic agent.[16]

There are other effective ways of decreasing brain bulk (**Table 13.4**). Perhaps the simplest, and often most effective, way to manage brain bulk is to pay close attention to head and neck positioning. During fixation of the Mayfield device to the operating room table, care must be taken to avoid excessive flexion or rotation of the neck that may obstruct ce-

Table 13.3	Hyperosmolar Therapy—Doses, Goals, and Major Adverse Effects			
Agent	**Bolus Dose**	**Infusion Dose**	**Goal**	**Major Adverse Effects**
Mannitol	0.25 to 1 g/kg	—	Plasma osmolarity <320 mOsm/L	• Hyponatremia • Hypovolemia
3% saline	1 to 2 mL/kg	0.5 to 1 mL/kg/h	Plasma sodium 145 to 155 mEq/dL	• Rebound intracranial hypertension • Centropontine myelinolysis

Table 13.4 Methods of Brain Bulk Management

Speed of Effect	Maneuver	Mechanism
Fast	Elevate head of bed Neutral head position	Decreased cerebral blood volume
	Hyperventilation	Decreased cerebral blood volume
	Hypnotic bolus/infusion	Decreased cerebral blood volume
	Cerebral spinal fluid drainage	Decreased cerebral spinal fluid volume
Intermediate	Hyperosmolar therapy	Decreased brain water content
	Loop diuretics	Decreased brain water content
Slow	Hypothermia	Decreased cerebral blood volume
	Corticosteroids	Decreased brain water content

rebral venous outflow. Placing the patient in 10 to 30 degrees of reverse Trendelenburg position facilitates venous outflow as well as CSF drainage and lowers intracranial pressure (ICP). However, if orthostatic hypotension occurs it should be treated with volume replacement or vasoconstrictors to maintain adequate cerebral perfusion pressure.

As mentioned above, hyperventilation-induced hypocapnia, with a goal $PaCO_2$ of 30 mm Hg, rapidly and effectively reduces ICP; more aggressive hyperventilation can aggravate cerebral ischemia through excessive vasoconstriction. This effect on cerebral arterial resistance is short lived because the brain compensates for CSF respiratory alkalosis by increasing bicarbonate elimination from the CSF.

Decreasing the cerebral metabolic rate (CMR) effectively reduces brain bulk by decreasing cerebral blood flow requirements. There are two methods of decreasing CMR. The administration of a bolus or infusion of a hypnotic such as thiopental or propofol is the most rapid and controllable method. Hypothermia, on the other hand, is more difficult to achieve rapidly without overshoot. Moreover, hypothermia is not only difficult to reverse due to the lack of efficient rewarming devices, but also, if the core temperature is <33.5°C, it may produce a coagulopathy and hypokalemia that not only cause surgical and hemodynamic disturbances, respectively, but also may result in delayed awakening secondary to decreased metabolic clearance of anesthetics (e.g., propofol, neuromuscular junction blocking agents). Although volatile agents decrease CMR, they are direct cerebral arterial dilators. Therefore, when other modalities have failed to provide adequate brain relaxation, their discontinuation can also be considered, and a total intravenous anesthesia technique, utilizing an opioid and 100 to 200 µg/kg/min of propofol, can be used instead.[6]

Cerebral Protection

A variety of pharmacologic and physiologic tools have been proposed experimentally to decrease the vulnerability of the brain to injury by prolonging tolerance to temporary ischemia. Proposed mechanisms for cerebral protection are reduction of the CMR, prevention of activation of the apoptotic pathways, and prevention of excessive influx of glucose and calcium into ischemic cells. Unfortunately, anesthetic neuroprotective techniques have not been shown to be effective in humans with clear and unequivocal success (**Table 13.5**).[17]

Glucose Control

Hyperglycemia at the cellular level together with the absence of oxygen leads to anaerobic glycolysis and the production of lactate, resulting in intracellular acidosis. This acidosis is capable of further neuronal injury, and may increase the size of cerebral infarcts. Human data demonstrate that tight glucose control improves neurologic outcomes after SAH, stroke, and traumatic brain injury.[18] Blood sugar levels should be obtained

Table 13.5 Anesthetics and Cerebral Protection

Drug	Mechanism(s)	Advantage	Disadvantage
Barbiturates	CMR decrease	Human evidence	Long duration of action
Propofol	CMR decrease	Short duration of action	Propofol infusion syndrome
Etomidate	CMR decrease	Hemodynamic stability	Cerebral tissue acidosis
			Adrenocortical suppression
Ketamine	NMDA receptor blockade	Hemodynamic stability	Dysphoria
			Possible direct neurotoxicity
Volatile agents	CMR decrease	Short duration of action	Systemic vasodilatation
			Direct cerebral arterial vasodilation
Lidocaine	Sodium channel blockade	Hemodynamic stability	Possible direct neurotoxicity

Abbreviations: CMR: cerebral metabolic rate; NMDA, N-methyl-D-aspartate.

in all neurosurgical patients undergoing any kind of surgery, and insulin therapy, utilizing a combination of boluses and a titratable infusion, should be instituted if hyperglycemia (>150 mg/dL) occurs. However, frequent glucose monitoring should be performed during insulin therapy to avoid hypoglycemia, which is also detrimental.

Corticosteroids

Corticosteroids are used most frequently in neurosurgery to decrease peritumoral vasogenic edema. There are no sufficient data to show any beneficial effect of steroids on focal or global cerebral ischemia or in cases of brain trauma; in fact, some animal evidence shows that they may exacerbate ischemic injury by increasing plasma glucose levels.

Hypothermia

Since the 1950s, mild hypothermia has been thought to provide some degree of cerebral protection, although extensive research done recently has found little benefit in neurologic outcomes. Recently, reports of the usefulness of mild hypothermia in out-of-hospital cardiac arrests, as well as slightly older studies postulating its utility in cases of severe adult traumatic brain injury, have brought back interest in the possible use of this modality in the operating room. The neuroprotective effects of hypothermia are thought to be due most probably to the reduction in the CMR. It is believed that because the energy requirements of neuronal tissue are decreased during mild hypothermia, this tissue is able to withstand ischemia for a longer period of time, thereby affording the neurosurgeon more operative ischemic time.[19] This theoretical benefit, however, should be weighed against the detrimental effects of hypothermia, including inhibition of platelet activation and coagulation factor activation, as well as increased susceptibility to cardiac dysrhythmias and the frequency of postoperative wound infections. Mild hypothermia may also be associated with hyperglycemia, and rewarming poses an added risk to neuronal tissue both because of the risk of hyperglycemia at this time and the risk of hyperthermia, which is certainly detrimental because of its effect on the CMR.

Mild systemic hypothermia has been shown to definitively decrease neurologic morbidity after ventricular fibrillation arrest.[20] There are data suggesting a clinical benefit of hypothermia in traumatic brain injury. The Intraoperative Hypothermia for Aneurysm Surgery Trial (IHAST) was conducted to compare the effects of intraoperative mild hypothermia (33.5°C) to normothermia (36.5°C) on neurologic outcome in patients with SAH undergoing surgical treatment of aneurysms.[21] This trial prospectively enrolled 1001 study subjects with World Federation of Neurosurgical Societies (WFNS) scores <3, and mild systemic hypothermia showed no benefit in terms of neurologic outcomes. Furthermore, length of hospital stay, discharge destination, and mortality were the same in both the hypothermia and the normothermia groups. The only significant difference seen between the two groups was an increased incidence of bacteremia in the hypothermia group. Based on these data, the routine use of mild hypother-

mia for cerebral protection in aneurysm surgery has been abandoned by some practitioners.

There is general consensus that deep hypothermia (18–25°C), especially when specifically targeting the brain temperature, is a useful technique for providing neuroprotection against ischemia. This has been borne out in clinical experience and animal studies; patients cooled systemically to temperatures of 18° to 25°C may be able to tolerate up to 60 minutes of ischemic brain time without major neurologic sequelae. Serious cardiac arrhythmias may occur with body temperatures of less than 32°C, and deep hypothermic circulatory arrest (DHCA) with cardiopulmonary bypass is usually used when profound levels of hypothermia are desired.[9]

Monitoring for Impending Neurologic Injury

Monitors of patients' cerebral well-being while in the anesthetized state may be extremely useful in detecting cerebral ischemia prior to irreversible neuronal damage. An ideal monitor would react rapidly and reliably to even small changes in regional cerebral blood flow. Unfortunately, methods that measure cerebral blood flow either directly (xenon washout, transcranial Doppler) or indirectly (brain tissue oxygen tension, cerebral oximetry) are limited by their inability to monitor multiple cerebral regions simultaneously, their impracticality of continuous use during craniotomy, or the fact that they are imperfect surrogate markers of cerebral blood flow.[22] Although electrophysiologic measurements of the brain do not directly measure regional or global cerebral blood flow, they are exquisitely related to disruptions of their respective pathways by ischemic events or surgical maneuvers. Thus, electrophysiologic monitoring has become a commonly accepted method of monitoring potential neuronal injury in neurovascular surgery.

Electrophysiologic monitoring of the brain with standard electroencephalography (EEG) is generally of limited use in the intraoperative setting, in part due to the difficulty of interpreting real-time EEG, and because of the inability to place surface electrodes in their precise locations when they overlap with the surgical incision. On the other hand, having access to EEG monitoring in the operating room can be useful to even the novice for the purpose of ensuring that the patient is in a burst-suppression or isoelectric state when these electrophysiologic states are desired.

Brainstem auditory evoked potentials (BAEPs) and somatosensory evoked potentials (SSEPs) have been utilized in neurovascular surgery for many years to assess the integrity of neural pathways and to detect impending neurologic injury. In up to 25% of operations using these modalities, however, SSEP signals may remain unchanged despite the appearance of a new motor deficit upon awakening. In contrast, utilizing transcranial or transcortical motor evoked potentials (MEPs) to monitor the integrity of the motor pathways decreases this lack of specificity. A comparison of the clinical characteristics of SSEPs and MEPs is outlined in **Table 13.6**.[23]

Evoked potential neuromonitoring signals are modified by several different factors, including technical, physiologic, anesthetic, and surgical factors. Good-quality signals may also be difficult to obtain in myelopathic patients or patients

Table 13.6 Characteristics of Somatosensory and Motor Evoked Potentials

	Somatosensory and Evoked Potential	Motor Evoked Potential
Speed of acquisition	2 minutes (averaged signal)	<5 seconds
Anatomic region monitored	• Dorsal columns • Subcortical tracts • Cortex	• Anterior columns • Cortex and subcortical tracts (lumped)
Parameters monitored	• Amplitude • Latency • Central conduction time	• Amplitude • Latency
Induced patient movement	• If muscle relaxants used, none • If no muscle relaxants, moderate	Moderate
Potential for spontaneous patient movement	• If muscle relaxants used, none • If no muscle relaxants, moderate	High (also potential shivering)
Muscle relaxants	Improve signal acquisition	Diminish/abolish signal
Volatile anesthetics	Dose dependent reduction (>0.5 MAC)	Dose dependent reduction (>0.5 MAC)
Opioids	Minimal	Minimal
Propofol	Minimal	Minimal
Temperature	Dose dependent reduction	Dose dependent reduction
Limiting patient factors	Sensory neuropathy	• Motor neuron disease • Primary muscle disease

who otherwise have preexisting neurologic deficits. Although there is no specific anesthesia regimen that is required for neurovascular procedures that employ neuromonitoring, strategies to obtain the best possible evoked potential signals are listed in **Table 13.7**.[24]

Sudden decrements in neuromonitoring signals, defined as an increase in latency of >10% or a decrease in amplitude of >50% for SSEPs, and a decrease in amplitude of >50% or an increase in threshold voltage needed to generate a signal for MEPs, should be considered signs of real or impending cerebral ischemia until proven otherwise. However, there are many other factors of a technical, physiologic, or pharmacologic nature that can severely affect signal quality, causing false-positive signal loss or decrement.[25] When faced with sudden neuromonitoring signal changes, it is imperative to follow a stepwise algorithm to identify the true cause(s) of these changes, as described in **Table 13.8**.

Once false-positive causes of signal change/loss have been eliminated and it is determined that cerebral ischemia is the most likely origin of these changes, a stepwise series of actions should be undertaken to minimize or reverse that ischemia, as shown in **Table 13.9**. Recovering neuromonitoring signals at a higher stimulation intensity or following an anesthetic change to enhance the signals seems to be associated with better outcomes than if signals are not recovered at all after maximum stimulation. Recovery of signals under these conditions, however, does not indicate correction of the ischemic insult.

Intraoperative Anatomic Monitoring

Clip misplacement with impingement of parent or perforating arteries can result in potentially disastrous outcomes. Intraoperative vascular imaging can be valuable in reducing

Table 13.7 Signal Enhancement Techniques

Technical aspect	Ensure correct anatomic location of stimulating and recording needles and pads
	Deliver adequate amount of stimulation intensity
Anesthetic aspect	Avoid nitrous oxide
	Keep volatile agents at ≤0.5 MAC; if signals still weak, consider total intravenous anesthesia
	Avoid abrupt anesthetic depth changes
	Avoid abrupt hemodynamic changes
	Avoid muscle relaxants when monitoring motor evoked potentials
	Augment signals by using etomidate or ketamine
Environmental aspect	Avoid hypothermia
	Check arm and leg position (avoid excessive nerve compression/stretch)

Table 13.8 Eliminating False-Positive Signal Changes/ Troubleshooting Signal Changes

Technical origin	Make sure that the signal loss is reproducible
	Make sure that stimulating/recording leads are still in place
	Make sure that adequate stimulation is being delivered by checking impedances
Pharmacologic origin	Check for any administered anesthetic boluses (propofol, thiopental, muscle relaxants) or increases in volatile agents or nitrous oxide
Physiologic origin	Check blood pressure, ensure that no sudden hypotension has occurred
	Check blood loss, ensure no acute blood loss has occurred

Table 13.9 Management of Ischemic (Surgical) Loss of Neuromonitoring Signals

Reverse the last surgical maneuver (remove the temporary or permanent clip, remove the retractor)

Increase the blood pressure to awake baseline or higher (a lighter plane of anesthesia can be considered)

Correct any hypovolemia

Consider transfusing the patient to a hemoglobin level of >10 mg dL

Increase stimulation intensity (so as to recover any signal after complete loss)

Consider computed tomography scan, angiogram, or aborting the procedure and waking the patient for a neurologic examination

the morbidity of intracranial vascular surgery; it provides real-time information in detecting the patency of the parent vessel, the branching and perforating arteries, and the presence of residual aneurysm filling. Intraoperative angiography remains the gold standard for assessment of intracranial vascular structures; however, it is logistically complex and carries some risk for vessel injury and embolic stroke. Indocyanine green (ICG) angiography is a simpler method of anatomic visualization that has shown clinical value in intracranial vascular surgery.[26] Routine doses for ICG are 0.2 to 0.5 mg/kg administered as a bolus, preferably through a central venous catheter, with a maximum daily dose of 5 mg/kg. ICG is hepatically eliminated, with a plasma half-life of 3 minutes. Repeat imaging can be performed after the background signal of the previous injection disappears—approximately 10 minutes later.

◆ Anesthesia Considerations for Carotid Surgery

Carotid endarterectomy can be conducted under general or local/regional anesthesia. The current literature does not support the superiority of one anesthesia technique over the other; both methods are safe with no obvious difference in short- or long-term outcomes.[27]

General anesthesia has the advantage of offering complete patient insensibility to discomfort due to anxiety, surgical manipulation, and positioning; definitive control of the patient airway; and the possible added benefit of anesthesia-induced neuroprotection. A distinct disadvantage of general anesthesia is the inability to obtain a neurologic exam to directly assess the adequacy of cerebral perfusion, especially following carotid cross-clamping. To mitigate this problem, some surgeons systematically insert shunts to bypass the cross-clamped carotid, whereas others rely on one or multiple neuromonitoring techniques such as stump pressure measurement, transcranial Doppler measurement of blood flow in the middle cerebral artery (MCA), near-infrared spectroscopy, EEG, and/or SSEP monitoring to help guide selective shunting.[28]

Although continuous neurologic assessment of the patient undergoing a carotid endarterectomy under local/regional anesthesia may offer the most reliable method of monitoring the adequacy of cerebral blood flow after carotid cross-clamp, the use of a local/regional anesthesia technique does not prevent patient anxiety or patient discomfort from positioning. In addition, administration of more than a modicum of sedatives or analgesics may result in significant airway obstruction or ventilatory depression. Even though the detrimental effects of moderate hypoxemia (e.g., myocardial ischemia, cerebral ischemia) or moderate to severe hypoventilation (e.g., carbon dioxide narcosis, sympathetic stimulation with resultant hypertension and tachycardia) can be prevented, the neurologic examination is most likely compromised by excessive patient sedation. Therefore, careful selection of the patient who is not overly anxious, is extremely motivated about the potential benefits of local/regional anesthesia-based surgery, and does not have coexisting disease that would preclude the administration of any anxiolytic or analgesic (e.g., obstructive sleep apnea) is essential for the successful performance of this technique. In addition, in patients who have a high likelihood of either developing significant cerebral ischemia during carotid cross-clamp without shunting or in patients who have a priori anatomic characteristics that predict difficulty in tracheal intubation, it may be preferable to electively intubate the patient and perform the surgery under general anesthesia to avoid the need to urgently/emergently intubate the patient under the surgical drapes with the carotid artery exposed and possibly cross-clamped and/or shunted.

Successful performance of carotid surgery under locoregional anesthesia is also dependent on the administration of adequate local anesthesia. Although anesthetizing both the deep and superficial cervical plexus is the definitive method of providing complete anesthesia to the surgical field, the preoperative use of anticoagulants increases the risks of performing a blind deep cervical block and adds hematoma formation to the list of complications that are related to inadvertent injection of a local anesthetic into the epidural space, the CSF, or the vertebral artery. Therefore, many anesthesiologists perform a superficial cervical plexus block and rely on the surgeon to infiltrate a local anesthetic into the deeper structures under direct vision and with small needles. However, if the deep structures require local anesthesia injection by the surgeon, it is important to wait an adequate period of time for the local anesthetic to adequately establish a field block (e.g., 5 minutes for 1% lidocaine and 10 to 15 minutes for 0.25% bupivacaine) to avoid pain that may make the patient more anxious with anticipation of further discomfort.

◆ Anesthesia Considerations for Neuroendovascular Procedures

An increasing proportion of neurovascular patients are being managed endovascularly, and neuroanesthesiologists are increasingly providing anesthesia care outside of the operating room and in the neuroendovascular suite. Although many of the considerations and techniques for safe anesthesia patient care remain the same as those that apply to the operating room, management of complications specific to endovascular surgery are worth mentioning.[29]

Hemorrhagic Complications

Aneurysm, arteriovenous malformation (AVM), or normal vessel perforation is usually recognized by dye extravasation during angiography. Moderate to severe hemorrhage is usually accompanied by a rise in ICP that may produce systemic hypertension and bradycardia. In most cases, immediate reversal of heparin with protamine is indicated. However, in patients who have previously been exposed to protamine (e.g., prior endovascular procedures, prior cardiac surgery, diabetics having taken protamine complexed insulin), idiopathic pulmonary hypertension or anaphylaxis may occur. For patients who have been taking antiplatelet medications (e.g., GIIbIIIa antagonists after cardiac stent placement or for intracranial stent placement), transfusion of 12.5 units of platelets (e.g., approximately two adult doses) should be administered to provide functional platelets for hemostasis. Additional transfusion of platelets or the administration of coagulation factors (e.g., fresh frozen plasma, cryoprecipitate, recombinant factor VIIa) should be guided by platelet function assays and specific coagulation tests. Depending on the degree of intracerebral hemorrhage, hyperventilation should be instituted, and a bolus of thiopental or propofol in a dose capable of causing a burst-suppression ratio of >0.7 should be considered. Hyperosmolar therapy with mannitol or hypertonic saline should also be instituted while preparations are made for possible emergent transfer to the operating room for craniotomy if interventional methods of achieving hemostasis are not successful. Emergent placement of an external ventricular drain may be warranted in select circumstances where immediate drainage of CSF to prevent cerebral or cerebellar herniation is necessary. Reducing systemic blood pressure can help control bleeding; however, maintaining adequate cerebral perfusion pressure (CPP) is of paramount importance. When an ICP monitor is available, systemic mean arterial pressure should be adjusted to maintain a CPP >60 mm Hg.

Thromboembolic Complications

Thromboses can form around catheters and coils placed intravascularly, or catheters and coils can themselves inadvertently migrate and embolize into the distal circulation. In these cases, anticoagulation is usually instituted while the interventionalist attempts to chemically or mechanically remove or lyse the thrombus. Cerebral perfusion pressure should be maintained or increased in the meantime to reduce the amount of ischemia (via augmentation of collateral circulation). Other methods of cerebral protection, such as reduction of the CMR with anesthetic agents, should also be considered.

To reduce the probability of inadvertently embolizing vessels responsible for perfusion of eloquent areas of the brain, superselective anesthesia functional examination (SAFE; e.g., a superselective Wada test) is conducted on awake patients prior to therapeutic embolization of each vessel of interest. During the test, a small dose of anesthetic (e.g., amobarbital, methohexital, propofol, thiopental, or etomidate) is injected into the artery of interest via a superselective endovascular microcatheter held in the position from which permanent embolic material is potentially going to be administered. If the patient develops a transient neurologic deficit after intraarterial anesthesia administration, permanent embolic material is not administered from that location. The microcatheter is either repositioned further downstream, if a branch of the feeding artery can be further isolated, and the SAFE is reperformed, or embolism of the artery is abandoned. Because of the trend toward performing endovascular procedures under general anesthesia, which promotes a completely still patient for long procedures, some investigators have started to utilize anatomically directed neurophysiologic monitoring (EEG and SSEPs) in patients undergoing neuroendovascular treatment of AVMs and aneurysms under general anesthesia. Although these results are clinically promising and intellectually appealing, controlled studies are needed to confirm their benefit.

◆ Postoperative Care

Emergence from anesthesia can be associated with intracranial and systemic hypertension and subsequent perfusion pressure breakthrough. Therefore, emergence from anesthesia should focus on minimizing noxious stimulation associated with intracranial and systemic hypertension.

Systemic Hypertension on Emergence

The main cause of systemic hypertension on emergence from anesthesia after intracranial surgery is usually untreated pain. Despite the previous belief that intracranial surgery is associated with minimal postoperative pain, a growing body of evidence suggests the contrary: postcraniotomy patients often experience moderate to severe pain, especially in the first 48 hours after surgery. Moreover, that pain is often undertreated because of a reluctance to give opioids that might cause respiratory depression and an increase in ICP. Opioids cause nausea and vomiting that can be mistaken for signs of increasing ICP and neurologic deterioration; they also cause miosis and sedation that can interfere with neurologic examination. It is important, however, to bear in mind that apart from causing patient discomfort, untreated postoperative pain can result in major cardiac morbidity due to increased myocardial strain and can be responsible for hypertension-induced cerebral hyperemia and intracranial hemorrhage (e.g., normal perfusion pressure breakthrough [NPPB]). A recent prospective randomized-controlled trial demonstrated the superiority of intravenous fentanyl delivered by patient-controlled analgesia (PCA) compared with conventional as-needed (PRN) therapy for treating postoperative craniotomy pain, without any major side effects or alterations in the neurologic examination.[30] Alternative pain control regimens could include preincisional infiltration of the operative site with a long-acting local anesthetic such as bupivacaine to help reduce postoperative pain and subsequent opioid requirements. Infratentorial surgery is associated with significantly more postoperative pain compared with supratentorial surgery; anesthesiologists as well as neurosurgeons should be aware of the possible increased requirement for analgesia in this patient population. Once postoperative pain has been treated adequately and is no longer thought to be the primary cause of hypertension, short-acting antihypertensive agents, including nicardipine, labetalol, and hydralazine, can be used to establish a normal systemic blood pressure.

In contrast to intracranial surgery, systemic hypertension after carotid endarterectomy is often not due to pain, but rather due to surgical disruption of the carotid baroreceptors. In light of the possible vasoparalysis of the previously chronically ischemic cerebrovasculature, it is imperative to maintain normotension or even mild hypotension to avoid cerebral hyperperfusion syndrome. However, this needs to be balanced with the possible contralateral perfusion requirements in the presence of untreated contralateral carotid arterial stenosis.

Intracranial Hypertension on Emergence

The main cause of intracranial hypertension during emergence is coughing. The strongest stimulus for coughing during emergence is the endotracheal tube. Early (deep) extubation would be ideal to avoid any kind of irritation. However, careful clinical judgment is warranted at the time of extubation due to the concern for airway protection, especially following posterior fossa surgery. In addition, aspiration and hypoxemia are possible complications of early extubation. The use of an infusion of short-acting opioids such as remifentanil may help blunt the cough reflex during emergence.[31] Other techniques that may be beneficial in this regard include the administration of intravenous lidocaine, or lidocaine instilled directly into the endotracheal tube cuff.

Postoperative nausea and vomiting (PONV) can cause cerebral venous hypertension. Besides increasing ICP, this can also lead to resection bed disruption and hematoma formation. PONV prophylaxis can be achieved by several medications, including 5-hydroxytryptamine receptor inhibitors (e.g., ondansetron), low-dose dexamethasone, subhypnotic propofol infusions, and dopamine antagonists (e.g., metoclopramide).[32] Droperidol is an effective antiemetic but has recently fallen out of favor due to the rare but significant incidence of prolongation of the QT interval corrected for heart rate (QT_C). On the horizon are even less sedating drugs with different mechanisms of action, such as the neurokinin-1 receptor antagonists.

◆ Conclusion

The anesthesia care of neurovascular patients requires careful planning and communication between the surgeon and anesthesiologist to meet basic anesthesia goals while also providing optimal surgical conditions. Communication should include preoperative coexisting diseases, intraoperative changes in neurologic monitoring, and postoperative hemodynamic goals. Communication is also essential in critical situations in which the operative team as a whole must rapidly perform multiple resuscitative or salvage maneuvers (e.g., intraoperative aneurysmal rupture, malignant cerebral edema, massive blood loss, thromboembolic events, venous air embolism). Relying on and returning to the fundamental physiologic and pharmacologic principles of cerebrovascular disease can rapidly guide the neuroanesthesiologist, neurologic surgeon, and neurointensivist toward the appropriate plan of action for the best care of these patients.

References

1. Tung P, Kopelnik A, Banki N, et al. Predictors of neurocardiogenic injury after subarachnoid hemorrhage. Stroke 2004;35:548–551
2. Coghlan LA, Hindman BJ, Bayman EO, et al; IHAST Investigators. Independent associations between electrocardiographic abnormalities and outcomes in patients with aneurysmal subarachnoid hemorrhage: findings from the intraoperative hypothermia aneurysm surgery trial. Stroke 2009;40:412–418
3. Kothavale A, Banki NM, Kopelnik A, et al. Predictors of left ventricular regional wall motion abnormalities after subarachnoid hemorrhage. Neurocrit Care 2006;4:199–205
4. Naidech AM, Kreiter KT, Janjua N, et al. Cardiac troponin elevation, cardiovascular morbidity, and outcome after subarachnoid hemorrhage. Circulation 2005;112:2851–2856
5. Tung PP, Olmsted E, Kopelnik A, et al. Plasma B-type natriuretic peptide levels are associated with early cardiac dysfunction after subarachnoid hemorrhage. Stroke 2005;36:1567–1569
6. Cole CD, Gottfried ON, Gupta DK, Couldwell WT. Total intravenous anesthesia: advantages for intracranial surgery. Neurosurgery 2007;61(5, Suppl 2)369–377, discussion 377–378
7. Hashimoto T, Young WL, Aagaard BD, Joshi S, Ostapkovich ND, Pile-Spellman J. Adenosine-induced ventricular asystole to induce transient profound systemic hypotension in patients undergoing endovascular therapy. Dose-response characteristics. Anesthesiology 2000;93:998–1001
8. Parkinson RJ, Bendok BR, Getch CC, et al. Retrograde suction decompression of giant paraclinoid aneurysms using a No. 7 French balloon-containing guide catheter. Technical note. J Neurosurg 2006;105:479–481
9. Young WL, Lawton MT, Gupta DK, Hashimoto T. Anesthetic management of deep hypothermic circulatory arrest for cerebral aneurysm clipping. Anesthesiology 2002;96:497–503

10. Bebawy JF, Gupta DK, Bendok BR, et al. Adenosine-induced flow arrest to facilitate intracranial aneurysm clip ligation: dose-response data and safety profile. Anesth Analg 2010;110:1406–1411

11. Anastasian ZH, Ramnath B, Komotar RJ, et al. Evoked potential monitoring identifies possible neurological injury during positioning for craniotomy. Anesth Analg 2009;109:817–821

12. Grände PO, Asgeirsson B, Nordström CH. Volume-targeted therapy of increased intracranial pressure: the Lund concept unifies surgical and non-surgical treatments. Acta Anaesthesiol Scand 2002;46:929–941

13. McDonagh DL, Warner DS. Hypertonic saline for craniotomy? Anesthesiology 2007;107:689–691

14. Rozet I, Tontisirin N, Muangman S, et al. Effect of equiosmolar solutions of mannitol versus hypertonic saline on intraoperative brain relaxation and electrolyte balance. Anesthesiology 2007;107:697–704

15. Wu C-T, Chen L-C, Kuo C-P, et al. A comparison of 3% hypertonic saline and mannitol for brain relaxation during elective supratentorial brain tumor surgery. Anesth Analg 2010;110:903–907

16. Kofke WA. Mannitol: potential for rebound intracranial hypertension? J Neurosurg Anesthesiol 1993;5:1–3

17. Warner DS. Perioperative neuroprotection: are we asking the right questions? Anesth Analg 2004;98:563–565

18. Lanier WL, Pasternak JJ. Refining perioperative glucose management in patients experiencing, or at risk for, ischemic brain injury. Anesthesiology 2009;110:456–458

19. Todd MM, Warner DS. A comfortable hypothesis reevaluated. Cerebral metabolic depression and brain protection during ischemia. Anesthesiology 1992;76:161–164

20. Bernard SA, Gray TW, Buist MD, et al. Treatment of comatose survivors of out-of-hospital cardiac arrest with induced hypothermia. N Engl J Med 2002;346:557–563

21. Todd MM, Hindman BJ, Clarke WR, Torner JC; Intraoperative Hypothermia for Aneurysm Surgery Trial (IHAST) Investigators. Mild intraoperative hypothermia during surgery for intracranial aneurysm. N Engl J Med 2005;352:135–145

22. Neuloh G, Schramm J. What the surgeon wins, and what the surgeon loses from intraoperative neurophysiologic monitoring? Acta Neurochir (Wien) 2005;147:811–813

23. Neuloh G, Schramm J. Monitoring of motor evoked potentials compared with somatosensory evoked potentials and microvascular Doppler ultrasonography in cerebral aneurysm surgery. J Neurosurg 2004;100:389–399

24. Sloan TB, Janik D, Jameson L. Multimodality monitoring of the central nervous system using motor-evoked potentials. Curr Opin Anaesthesiol 2008;21:560–564

25. Banoub M, Tetzlaff JE, Schubert A. Pharmacologic and physiologic influences affecting sensory evoked potentials: implications for perioperative monitoring. Anesthesiology 2003;99:716–737

26. Killory BD, Nakaji P, Gonzales LF, Ponce FA, Wait SD, Spetzler RF. Prospective evaluation of surgical microscope-integrated intraoperative near-infrared indocyanine green angiography during cerebral arteriovenous malformation surgery. Neurosurgery 2009;65:456–462, discussion 462

27. Lewis SC, Warlow CP, Bodenham AR, et al; GALA Trial Collaborative Group. General anaesthesia versus local anaesthesia for carotid surgery (GALA): a multicentre, randomised controlled trial. Lancet 2008;372:2132–2142

28. Kalkman CJ. Con: Routine shunting is not the optimal management of the patient undergoing carotid endarterectomy, but neither is neuromonitoring. J Cardiothorac Vasc Anesth 2004;18:381–383

29. Hashimoto T, Gupta DK, Young WL. Interventional neuroradiology—anesthetic considerations. Anesthesiol Clin North America 2002;20:347–359, vi vi

30. Morad AH, Winters BD, Yaster M, et al. Efficacy of intravenous patient-controlled analgesia after supratentorial intracranial surgery: a prospective randomized controlled trial. Clinical article. J Neurosurg 2009;111:343–350

31. Aouad MT, Al-Alami AA, Nasr VG, Souki FG, Zbeidy RA, Siddik-Sayyid SM. The effect of low-dose remifentanil on responses to the endotracheal tube during emergence from general anesthesia. Anesth Analg 2009;108:1157–1160

32. Gan TJ, Meyer TA, Apfel CC, et al; Society for Ambulatory Anesthesia. Society for Ambulatory Anesthesia guidelines for the management of postoperative nausea and vomiting. Anesth Analg 2007;105:1615–1628 table of contents

14

Bypass for Acute and Chronic Ischemic States

Joshua R. Dusick, Nestor R. Gonzalez, and Neil A. Martin

Pearls

- Do not treat embolic stroke with a bypass!
- Do not base treatment solely on the presence of anatomic occlusion. Instead, focus on treating defined hemodynamic abnormalities in symptomatic individuals.
- Careful planning of the incision is critical to allow adequate vessel dissection and reduce the risk of superficial temporal artery (STA) injury. The Doppler probe is used to map and mark the course of the STA. Very gentle handling of the donor artery is critical. Overly aggressive maneuvers can either damage the artery or lead to vasospasm of the graft. Adventitial irrigation with papaverine solution can help to reduce spasm of the artery. Care should also be taken in planning the anastomosis to avoid kinking or twisting of the graft.
- Improper orientation or twisting of vein grafts is an important pitfall in executing a vein graft bypass. Orientation should ensure that the vein valves are aligned to allow the flow of blood in the intended direction. Every effort should be made to ensure that the graft does not twist or kink as it is passed through the subcutaneous tunnel from the cervical to cranial incision, as twisting and kinking have been shown to be common reasons for graft thrombosis and failure.

◆ Indications

The Extracranial-to-Intracranial Bypass Trial

After the introduction of extracranial-to-intracranial (EC-IC) arterial bypass in 1967 by Donaghy and Yasargil,[1] the techniques were further developed and refined by numerous surgeons over the following years. Initially envisioned as a strategy to prevent ischemic stroke in patients with cerebrovascular arterial occlusion, bypass later found utility as flow replacement in the treatment of complex cerebral aneurysms and skull base tumors as well. However, following the publication of the results of the international EC-IC bypass trial in 1985, the utility of bypass for cerebrovascular ischemic disease was cast into serious doubt.[2] The study demonstrated that patients randomized to surgical treatment did no better than patients with medical treatment in terms of subsequent risk for stroke. However, subsequent evaluations of the study design have pointed to serious flaws that may compromise the validity of the study findings.[3,4] Most significantly, beyond demonstration of anatomic cerebrovascular occlusive disease, there was no hemodynamic evaluation performed in these patients, principally because the study preceded effective cerebral blood flow testing methods. Therefore, patients with embolic strokes and otherwise relatively normal cerebral blood flow may have been treated by bypass, which is not the preferred management in this setting.

Other factors also compromise the findings of the study. The study group was quite heterogeneous, enrolling patients with various types of cerebrovascular lesions including internal carotid artery (ICA) occlusion, ICA siphon stenosis, middle cerebral artery (MCA) stenosis, and MCA occlusion. Only anterior circulation disease was treated. There also appeared to be a selection bias in that some patients were treated by bypass without randomization and not included in the study, suggesting that those patients who were perceived to be most in need of bypass, and therefore most likely to benefit, were not enrolled.[4] Interestingly, both medical and surgical treatment groups, had a low rate of major ipsilateral stroke following enrollment, suggesting that most patients had adequate collateral circulation and probably did not need surgery. Although some of these patients may have been symptomatic briefly when the acute occlusion occurred, due to acute embolization or infarction of areas with inadequate circulation, the remaining circulation following occlusion had or developed adequate native collateral flow.

The subsequent St. Louis Carotid Occlusion Study assessed risk factors for stroke in patients with asymptomatic and symptomatic carotid occlusion.[5–7] Patients were studied with oxygen-15 positron emission tomography (PET) for evidence of hemodynamic failure **(Fig. 14.1).** Elevated oxygen extraction fraction (OEF) as measured by this method (so-

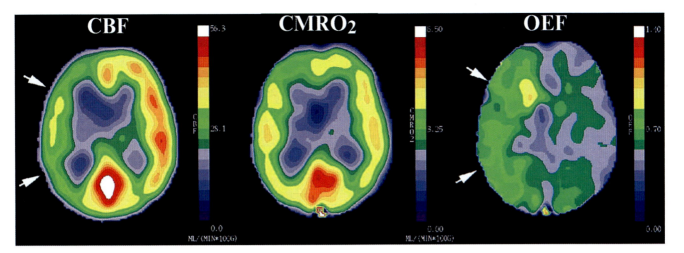

Fig. 14.1 Oxygen-15 positron emission tomography (PET) allows the measurement of cerebral blood flow (with $^{15}O\text{-}H_2O$), cerebral blood volume (with $^{15}O\text{-}CO$), and the cerebral metabolic rate of oxygen (with $^{15}O\text{-}O_2$). These values can be used to calculate the oxygen extraction fraction (OEF). Increased OEF (stage II hemodynamic failure) is an indicator of misery perfusion and maximum vasodilatory compensation. This patient demonstrates a holohemispheric hypoperfusion (low cerebral blood flow [CBF]) correlated with an elevated OEF. CMRO$_2$, cerebral metabolic rate of oxygen.

called stage II hemodynamic failure) is a marker of hemodynamic failure, indicating increased extraction of oxygen by ischemic brain tissue. It was found in this study that not all patients with carotid occlusion have hemodynamic failure. Over 50% of patients with carotid occlusion had normal OEF. It was also shown that patients with carotid occlusion and ipsilateral elevation in OEF had a significantly higher risk for subsequent stroke than patients without elevated OEF (2-year ipsilateral stroke rates of 26.5% and 5.3%, respectively). This stroke rate in patients with hemodynamic failure as demonstrated by O-15 PET was much higher than the overall stroke rate of patients in the EC-IC bypass trial, suggesting that many patients in the prior study did not have hemodynamic failure. In fact, the stroke rate in the EC-IC trial was close to those who had carotid occlusion without hemodynamic failure.

Despite its shortcomings, the EC-IC bypass trial remains the only large prospective randomized trial to assess cerebrovascular bypass for the prevention of stroke. Therefore, bypass cannot be generally recommended as a routine treatment for stroke prevention in patients with ICA or MCA occlusion or stenosis. However, because of these shortcomings of the EC-IC bypass trial, the use of bypass in the treatment of cerebrovascular ischemic disease has continued, albeit with stricter attention paid to patient selection to avoid the problems with the trial. Most notably, cerebrovascular bypass is currently being reevaluated by both the Carotid Occlusion Surgery Study (COSS)[6] and the Japanese EC-IC Bypass Trial (JET).[8] These studies are utilizing modern techniques to evaluate hemodynamic parameters indicative of cerebrovascular insufficiency and only randomizing patients with hemodynamic failure thought to be at highest risk for subsequent stroke. At present, COSS has randomized close to 200 patients to bypass or medical treatment, with an ultimate target of 372 randomized patients. The results of this study are not likely to be available for several years.

Patient Selection

Embolic Stroke Versus Hemodynamic Compromise

Although we do not yet have the results of these ongoing studies to establish guidelines that support current treatment, with the information we already have we can begin to plan a patient selection and treatment algorithm to determine the suitability of bypass in the treatment of these diseases for individual patients. One of the first considerations when evaluating a patient with ischemic symptomatology, including strokes, transient ischemic attacks (TIAs), cognitive decline, and other manifestations of focal or widespread ischemia, is to determine whether the underlying pathology is related to embolism or hypoperfusion. Embolic stroke, due to embolism from an extracranial source such as cervical internal carotid atherosclerotic stenosis, valvular or intracardiac thrombus, or MCA stenosis, does not represent an ongoing failure of cerebrovascular blood flow but rather a discrete blockage of blood flow in one distribution due to a clot. Therefore, bypass for these patients does not treat the underlying problem and does not prevent subsequent embolic stroke, as was seen in the EC-IC bypass trial. Once identified, embolic sources of cerebral infarction are best treated by removal of the embolic source (e.g., carotid endarterectomy, endovascular angioplasty and stenting, treatment of atrial fibrillation) or medical management (antiplatelet medications or anticoagulation). Transcranial Doppler may be useful to directly document spontaneous microemboli.

Alternatively, if a patient with ischemic symptomatology does not have findings consistent with embolic disease but has anatomic evidence of cerebrovascular occlusive disease (either cervical or intracranial), a workup for hemodynamic compromise and consideration of a bypass are warranted. The decision to treat these patients by bypass should be based on these blood flow considerations and not entirely based on the demonstration of stenotic or occlusive disease. For example, even patients with complete carotid occlusion may not be at significant risk for stroke if their collateral circulation is adequately supplying the needs of that hemisphere.[7] Asymptomatic patients and those with adequate cerebral blood flow and without markers of hemodynamic compromise are not likely to benefit from bypass. As stated previously, the St. Louis Carotid Occlusion Study demonstrated a low annual risk for stroke in patients with occlusion but adequate perfusion (by O-15 PET parameters).[5–7] Less than 50% of patients with carotid occlusion were found to have stage II hemodynamic failure (elevated ipsilateral OEF).

With stenosis or occlusion, if there is a mild to moderate decrease in blood flow, autoregulatory compensation occurs, in which vasodilation maintains a normal cerebral blood flow (CBF). These patients have a reduced cerebrovascular reserve capacity. At more severe levels of compromise, blood flow drops below the level that can be regulated by vasodilation, and CBF will begin to decrease, marked by an increased extraction of oxygen from the blood, often termed "misery" perfusion or stage II hemodynamic failure. It has been shown that this subgroup of patients with a severe compromise in cerebrovascular reserve capacity or frank misery perfusion are at significantly higher risk of stroke.[9–11] Demonstration of misery perfusion by PET has been associated with a 2-year stroke risk of approximately 30%.[5] This subgroup has been chosen for randomization to bypass in the COSS trial.

There are a couple of clinical situations that warrant special mention when considering bypass for patients with an occlusive lesion. Some patients with occlusion may present with episodic symptoms related to orthostatic hypotension despite adequate baseline collateral circulation. Some patients treated for hypertension are on excessive doses of antihypertensive medications, which result in severe postural hypotension. A careful history and physical can usually identify this as the cause of a patient's symptoms. In these cases, medication adjustments may be adequate to prevent hypotension, and the resulting ischemic episodes as their blood flow may be adequate under normal blood pressure parameters.

A minor stroke or TIA at the time of acute ICA or MCA occlusion may occur due to transient embolization or obstruction of small perforator branches. However, some of these patients stabilize after the acute occlusion if collateral circulation is adequate. Despite the initial symptoms, these patients do not necessarily require a bypass if they do not have ongoing TIAs and their hemodynamic assessment does not reveal hemodynamic failure.

Hemodynamic Assessment

There are several current methods to assess the hemodynamic status of a patient with cerebrovascular occlusive disease, including O-15 PET, xenon computed tomography (CT), single photon emission computed tomography (SPECT), transcranial Doppler (TCD), and magnetic resonance imaging (MRI) perfusion protocols.[12] Currently, O-15 PET is considered the gold standard because of its ability to demonstrate both misery perfusion, as indicated by an increased oxygen extraction

fraction (OEF), and reduced cerebrovascular reserve capacity, as indicated by increased cerebral blood volume (CBV) or CBV/CBF ratio, which reflect autoregulatory vasodilation. Although patients with misery perfusion (stage II hemodynamic failure) are at the highest risk of stroke, patients with reduced reserve may also be at risk of stroke, particularly if the causative occlusive lesion is not stable and progresses.

Because O-15 PET imaging is not always readily available, other indicators of hemodynamic compromise have been used. In cases of severely reduced perfusion, CT- and MRI-based perfusion studies can be useful to demonstrate ischemia. However, these studies do not demonstrate reduced reserve capacity while autoregulatory vasodilation is compensating for reduced blood flow directly. If PET is not available to assess CBV, provocative testing along with SPECT, xenon CT, or MRI perfusion can be used to measure the degree of reduction in reserve. Blood flow measurements are taken at baseline and then following a vasodilatory stimulus (acetazolamide [Diamox] administration, hypercapnia, or physiologic tasks such as hand movement).[12] Currently, xenon CT is not readily available and rarely used due to problems with Food and Drug Administration (FDA) approval. Therefore, currently MRI perfusion with and without Diamox is often used to assess hemodynamic failure. In patients with severe hemodynamic compromise, no improvement in hypoperfusion is seen with Diamox. Likewise, TCD can be used in cases of ICA occlusion to evaluate flow before and after carbon dioxide inhalation. TCD has the added advantage of allowing for detection of spontaneous microembolization. Several small studies have suggested that assessing cerebrovascular reserve vasoreactivity by SPECT, xenon CT, MRI, or TCD with Diamox or hypercapnea challenge can predict patients at highest risk for subsequent stroke.[9–11,13,14]

A relatively new technique for measuring flow velocities in individual intracranial arteries is available—quantitative magnetic resonance angiography (MRA). This software (noninvasive optimal vessel analysis [NOVA], VasSol, Inc., Chicago, IL) allows the measurement of absolute blood flow velocities along with flow direction for all major intracranial arteries and has been validated in both in vitro and in vivo studies.[15,16] This emerging technology can play an important role both in assessing preoperative blood flow volume to identify patients for whom bypass may be beneficial as well as in following bypasses postoperatively in a noninvasive manner. Additionally, because it has the capability to show the direction of flow, it can help elucidate very complex flow patterns and suggest the most efficient way to improve that patient's perfusion. For example, it has been used to demonstrate subclavian steal and reverse vertebral flow as the offender in a patient with anterior circulation hypoperfusion.[17] This finding suggested correctly that treatment of the subclavian stenosis was the best management, not bypass to the MCA. It may also, along with PET or other perfusion techniques, help to demonstrate normal flow that does not require a bypass. It therefore suggests the correct treatment target and can help avoid unnecessary bypasses.

Hemodynamic studies can also be used to follow patients post-bypass. Some small studies have already demonstrated

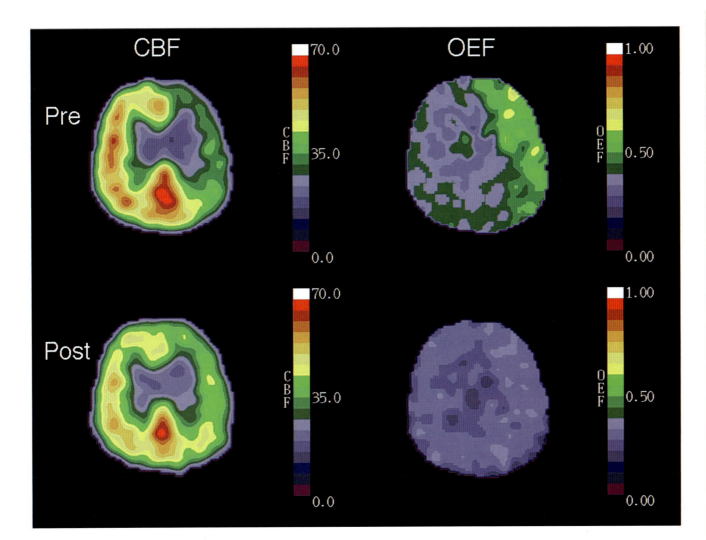

Fig. 14.2 Hemodynamic studies such as ^{15}O PET can be used both to identify patients with stage II hemodynamic failure as well as to follow patients after bypass. Preoperatively (top row), this patient's middle cerebral artery (MCA) territory had depressed CBF correlating with an elevated OEF. Post-bypass (bottom row), the CBF improved and the OEF returned to normal.

improvement in misery perfusion as measured by PET following bypass[18,19] and we have observed this in patients of our own (**Fig. 14.2**).

Indications for Bypass

Considering both patient-specific factors and the hemodynamic assessment of cerebral blood flow, the following general indications for bypass have been suggested[20]:

1. Poor cerebrovascular reserve or misery perfusion as demonstrated by hemodynamic imaging (xenon CT, PET, SPECT, MRI perfusion, TCD, quantitative MRA, etc.)
2. Failure of maximal medical treatment
3. Symptomatic patient with radiographic findings demonstrating an occlusive lesion consistent with symptoms
4. Lack of other major medical comorbidity that would be a contraindication to bypass surgery

Chronic States

The most common ischemic indications for bypass are chronic conditions that result in decreased cerebral blood flow. The most common underlying pathologies include cervical carotid occlusion without adequate distal collateral circulation and intracranial atherosclerosis. As mentioned previously, occlusion alone is not indication enough for bypass. If adequate collateral circulation exists, stenosis or occlusion of cervical or intracranial blood vessels does not in and of itself warrant bypass. Moyamoya disease can be another less common cause of decreased cerebral blood flow chronically.

Anterior Circulation Ischemia

Occlusive disease of the carotid circulation, either cervical or intracranial, can be a cause of hemodynamic failure and cerebral ischemia. Although the COSS trial is still underway and there is no evidence to support it, the finding that hemodynamic failure, as measured by increased OEF on PET or vasodilatory challenge with TCD or MRI perfusion, is highly associated with subsequent stroke risk supports the aggressive treatment of these patients. The COSS trial is randomizing patients to superficial temporal artery (STA)-MCA bypass if they have symptomatic carotid disease with hemodynamic failure.

Patients with chronic ICA or MCA occlusion should be considered for bypass only if they have a documented occlusive lesion with impaired hemodynamic reserve and continue to have refractory ischemic symptoms (TIAs or strokes) despite maximal medical therapy with antiplatelet or anticoagulant medications and correction of hypotension. Currently, we assess hemodynamic failure in these patients by MRI perfusion with and without Diamox or with TCD with carbon dioxide reactivity.

◆ Treating Stenosis

It should be noted that there is even more controversy in regard to treating intracranial atherosclerotic stenotic disease by bypass. Some patients with intracranial occlusive lesions, particularly if they have complete intracranial occlusion with hemodynamic failure, may benefit from bypass. The ongoing JET trial is testing the safety and efficacy of bypass in these patients with intracranial arterial occlusive disease.

However, the EC-IC bypass trial suggested that patients with stenosis actually fared worse after bypass. The competitive flow from the bypass changes the flow dynamics such that it can precipitate flow stasis and thrombosis at the location of the stenosis. In some cases this may cause a thrombus that can occlude the lenticulostriate arteries, propagate, or embolize, resulting in infarction. Therefore, stenosis without occlusion is a contraindication for bypass and should be treated with antiplatelet or anticoagulant therapy and endovascular techniques (angioplasty and stenting) when possible. In rare cases, symptomatic stenoses not amenable to endovascular and medical treatment can be considered for indirect revascularization procedures. These procedures provide additional collateral without the sudden hemodynamic change associated with a direct bypass that may result in acute occlusion.

◆ Moyamoya Disease

Moyamoya disease represents a unique case of intracranial stenosis or occlusion, and the indications for revascularization have not been definitively established by a randomized trial. We consider revascularization in any patient with significant, symptomatic moyamoya disease because it is usually progressive. In the case of ICA or MCA stenosis, we strongly prefer the use of indirect revascularization (encephaloduroarteriosynangiosis with or without bur holes) to avoid competing flows precipitating occlusion and stroke. In the case of complete obstructive lesions, bypass or indirect revascularization has been shown to be of benefit in preventing future ischemic events.

Posterior Circulation Ischemia

Symptomatic vertebrobasilar occlusive disease carries a high stroke risk, estimated at 10 to 15% per year despite maximal medical management.[21,22] Patients with stenosis are generally treated by anticoagulation with or without endovascular angioplasty or stenting.[23] Most patients who present with complete occlusion of bilateral vertebral arteries or the basilar artery have acute, severe, and often life-threatening, strokes at the time of occlusion. However, some patients survive with chronic bilateral vertebral artery occlusion because they develop collaterals through posterior communicating arteries that are present but inadequate or through other unusual collateral pathways such as the anterior spinal artery. These patients may be disabled by recurrent, frequent TIAs or strokes. In the case of complete bilateral occlusion, there are no endovascular options for treatment. In these patients with medically refractory TIAs or recurrent strokes and demonstrated occlusive lesions (by MRA, computed tomography angiography [CTA] or angiography), posterior circulation bypass may be a treatment option to consider. However, because of the higher rate of complications, morbidity, and mortality associated with the more technically demanding posterior circulation bypasses, caution must be used in considering these treatments. Of note, cerebrovascular reactivity and perfusion studies are technically ineffective and therefore are rarely performed. However, quantitative MRA (NOVA) demonstrating low distal flow has shown some utility in predicting those patients at highest risk for subsequent stroke in preliminary studies.[24]

Acute States

There is only rarely an indication for surgical revascularization in the setting of acute ischemic disease. The large majority of cerebral infarctions that present acutely, within hours of the onset of symptoms, are best treated by rapid interventions including IV administration of recombinant tissue-type plasminogen activator (rtPA), intraarterial chemical thrombolysis, or mechanical clot retrieval. Those that present outside of the 3- to 6-hour window will generally only be treated with anticoagulation and treatment of the embolic source (carotid disease, cardiac disease, etc.), if applicable. These patients may also benefit from treatment with partial aortic occlusion as evaluated in the Safety and Efficacy of NeuroFlo Technology in Ischemic Stroke (SENTIS) trial.[25,26] The results of this trial are promising, but the mechanism of action has not been completely elucidated. Bypass performed acutely after an occlusion with a large acute infarction is contraindicated as it can induce hyperperfusion and cerebral swelling or hemorrhagic transformation or intracerebral hemorrhage in the area of the infarction.

Occasionally, patients with underlying chronic atherosclerosis may present acutely with a rapidly progressive deterioration in perfusion, resulting in an unstable pattern of symptoms such as crescendo TIAs, waxing and waning neurologic deficit, or gradually progressive "stuttering" neurologic deficits. In these clinical circumstances, if hemodynamic assessment determines that hypoperfusion, and not embolic occlusion, is the culprit, and symptoms are not stabilized rapidly with anticoagulation or induced arterial hypertension in the intensive care unit (ICU), acute bypass may be an appropriate line of action.

◆ Types of Bypass

How Much Blood Volume Do You Need and Where to Put It?

Flow Augmentation Versus Flow Replacement

When considering a bypass for any pathology, planning of the appropriate bypass graft should first take into consideration the flow needs of the patient. In patients with some native flow, *flow augmentation* aims to supplement the existing blood flow to a vascular territory. In other words, it adds blood flow to a territory that has blood flow but not enough to fully supply the demands of that tissue territory. Because less flow is needed, flow-augmentation procedures do not require bypasses with high flow rates. Native scalp arteries, the superficial temporal artery and occipital artery, almost always supply enough supplemental flow in these cases. *Flow replacement*, on the other hand, aims to completely replace the blood flow to a particular vascular territory. Because a large amount of blood flow is needed immediately following bypass, larger, high-flow grafts are sometimes required in this setting. What type of graft is needed to supply this flow depends on the size and normal flow of the artery in question. Although in smaller terminal branches (distal MCA, posterior inferior communicating artery [PICA], etc.) flow can be replaced by an STA or occipital artery graft, larger arteries (complete vertebrobasilar system with atretic posterior communicating arteries, entire internal carotid artery, etc.) may require higher-flow grafts such as a saphenous vein graft or radial artery graft.

True flow replacement is generally only required when there is a planned, intentional occlusion of a blood vessel without adequate collateral circulation to supply the area irrigated by that artery. This most commonly occurs in cases of complex or giant aneurysms or invasive tumor surgery with planned blood vessel sacrifice.[27] Some large or complex aneurysms, including fusiform aneurysms, cannot be treated by standard clipping or coiling techniques. Occlusion of the artery may require proximal hunterian ligation or completely trapping the aneurysm, occluding it and the parent artery from the circulation. In some cases there will still be distal blood flow through collateral circulation. However, if distal collateral circulation is very poor or absent (determined by angiogram or balloon test occlusion), a flow replacement bypass may be required. In the treatment of ischemic disease, flow replacement is rarely required.

Patients with ischemic disease due to hemodynamic compromise have some level of basal blood flow hovering near the ischemic threshold (otherwise they would have infarcted the entire territory already) and supplementing that blood flow is generally all that is required to prevent further ischemic injury. In fact, a high-flow bypass in a patient with some native flow may create a hyperperfusion syndrome or precipitate hemorrhage into an infarcted area of brain.[28] A high-flow graft is almost never required to treat ischemia because if patients have such a profound decrease in blood flow, far below the ischemic threshold, they generally have a large stroke quickly and are not candidates for bypass. After bypass, if the patient's underlying collateral flow continues to become progressively worse, this generally occurs chronically and the flow through the bypass can increase over time to accommodate it. Therefore, flow augmentation is almost always sufficient for the treatment of cerebrovascular ischemic disease.

Superficial Temporal Artery to Middle Cerebral Artery Bypass

The STA to MCA bypass is one of the most widely used bypass grafts for anterior circulation ischemic disease. Although the superficial temporal artery is capable of delivering less blood flow immediately than a saphenous vein or radial artery graft, it is generally sufficient in these clinical circumstances given that flow augmentation, not flow replacement, is required. The STA-MCA bypass has the following advantages:

1. It is a native arterial graft, which has been shown to have better long-term patency rates than vein grafts.[2,29,30]

2. It is easily accessible in the scalp directly adjacent to the MCA territory, making it ideal for anterior circulation revascularization.

3. It is a pedicled arterial graft so only one anastomosis is required, making the procedure faster and less complex, with decreased temporary occlusion times.

4. The "cut flow" blood flow rate is higher than the native STA flow (due to lower distal vascular resistance), and flow volume can increase over time as the graft matures and as hemodynamic demand increases.[31,32]

The native STA in the scalp has a low flow, approximately 5 to 15 mL/min, because the peripheral resistance of the scalp is relatively high. Once the distal vascular resistance decreases, as is demonstrated by the "cut flow," the flow rate of the cut artery (measured with a flow monitor intraoperatively) increases considerably with bypass flows reported from approximately 15 to 154 mL/min.[31,33–35] Patients with cerebral hypoperfusion have very low vascular resistance because autoregulation leads to maximal vasodilation in the affected cerebral territory. Therefore, after anastomosis of the graft, the final flow approaches that of the cut flow in most patients.[31] Additionally, over time, the STA graft can increase in size and provide even greater blood flow, an advantage for pathologies that may become progressively worse over time (atherosclerotic stenosis or moyamoya disease, for example).[32]

Of note, two techniques utilizing the STA have been shown to immediately result in greater flow volumes than the standard STA-MCA graft. In one, using a short vein graft from the proximal STA trunk to an MCA branch supplies greater flow than a direct STA-MCA bypass.[36–38] The other is a STA-MCA bypass in which the sylvian fissure is opened so that a larger, more proximal MCA branch in the fissure can be used as the recipient artery.[39] Both of these have the advantage of increased flow immediately and can be useful in those circumstances when a higher flow rate is thought to be advantageous. The short vein graft can also be used in circumstances where the distal STA is too small or discontinuous to use directly.

Vein and Arterial Free Grafts

Saphenous vein and radial artery grafts supply considerably more blood flow immediately than do pedicled arterial grafts (STA or occipital). A saphenous vein graft, bypassed from the external carotid artery (ECA) or cervical ICA stump, supplies approximately 70 to 140 mL/min of blood flow, and may exceed 250 mL/min.[34,40] A radial artery graft supplies moderately less flow, approximately 40 to 70 mL/min, but still more than an STA graft.[27,34]

These free grafts have the advantage of supplying a large amount of flow immediately. However, in the setting of cerebral hypoperfusion, this level of flow may actually be too much and unnecessary. In fact, delivering too much flow can sometimes be detrimental, resulting in a hyperperfusion state.[28] Although these large grafts may be beneficial or even imperative in the setting of complete flow replacement (as with hunterian ligation of the ICA for treatment of a complex or giant aneurysm or carotid resection for the treatment of a skull base or head and neck cancer, as examples), they are rarely recommended simply for flow augmentation. In fact, the primary bypass types used for the EC-IC bypass trial as well as the current COSS and JET studies are exclusively STA-MCA bypasses.

Posterior Circulation

There are various ways to revascularize the posterior circulation in the setting of ischemia. The specific anatomy and hemodynamic features of each patient will help to determine which best addresses their needs. The occipital artery can be harvested as a pedicle graft from the scalp, although it is somewhat more technically demanding than an STA graft. Through a posterior fossa craniectomy the occipital artery (OA) can be used to bypass to the PICA.[41,42] The OA-PICA bypass is the most commonly employed posterior circulation bypass. More rarely, the occipital artery can be used to bypass to the anterior inferior cerebellar artery (AICA) as well.

If proximal posterior circulation revascularization to the PICA or AICA does not address the perfusion problems, as in patients with basilar artery atherosclerotic stenosis or occlusion, a more distal bypass may be warranted. Although the occipital artery cannot reach the distal posterior circulation, the STA can be used to bypass to either the posterior cerebral artery (PCA) or superior cerebellar artery (SCA), through a low temporal craniotomy and passing under the temporal lobe to reach these arteries adjacent to the midbrain at the tentorial incisura. When more robust flow is needed, a saphenous vein graft can be used for the same recipient arteries.

Indirect Revascularization

Indirect revascularization involves giving native vessels in the scalp and dura more direct access to the brain, allowing neovascularization to develop as is needed for a hypoperfused brain without performing a direct bypass. Various techniques of indirect revascularization have been developed. Some of the most common currently include variations of encephaloduroarteriosynangiosis, in which the STA vessel, left in continuity, is isolated and laid on the surface of the brain, and bur holes. Over time, the brain has been shown to recruit new blood vessel growth from the STA and its branches in the scalp, the middle meningeal artery and its branches in the dura, and temporalis muscle vessels. The advantages of indirect revascularization are that it is less technically demanding than a bypass, does not require a period of temporary occlusion of cerebral vessels to complete an anastomosis, and can allow revascularization of multiple vascular territories, guided by the hemodynamic demands of the underlying brain. However, it has the disadvantage that the new blood supply takes some time to develop, and therefore there is a window after surgery during which the patient is still at risk for ischemic injury.

Indirect revascularization techniques have seen their greatest application in patients with Moyamoya disease, progressive idiopathic stenosis, and occlusion of intracranial arteries at the base of the brain. Many studies have shown benefit for these patients, reducing the risk for subsequent stroke. However, it has been suggested that indirect techniques could be used to treat patients with other causes of cerebral hemodynamic failure. In particular, because they appear to be less suited to direct bypass, patients with intracranial atherosclerotic stenosis and occlusion may benefit from indirect revascularization. However, there is scarce literature to support its use at present. In fact, one small study concluded that these treatments do not reduce the rate of postoperative TIAs and cerebral infarctions.[43] However, this study only compared patients to medically managed patients from previous reports, not to a control group. Additionally, most patients had complete ICA or MCA occlusion. It remains to be seen if indirect revascularization could benefit patients with symptomatic intracranial stenosis not amenable to endovascular treatments.

◆ Techniques

Preoperative Planning and Preparation for Bypass

Although the determination of reduce perfusion is generally made by less anatomic studies, such as PET or MRI perfusion, angiographic studies to define the cerebral vascular anatomy are critical to planning the bypass procedure. Most importantly, the donor and recipient vessels should be clearly visualized and assessed to determine the optimal site of bypass.

Most patients are given preoperative anticonvulsants if the cerebral hemisphere is expected to be exposed or retracted. Steroid administration is not necessary. Hyperglycemia is monitored and treated as appropriate pre- and intraoperatively. Before surgery, all patients are administered aspirin (325 mg daily) to prevent thrombosis and occlusion of the bypass graft.

Intraoperative Management and Monitoring

Evoked potentials and electroencephalographic activity are monitored continuously in every case. When administering metabolic suppressive agents for brain protection (e.g., barbiturates, etomidate, or propofol), the electroencephalogram (EEG) is used to monitor burst suppression. Evoked potential give an indication of sensory cortex and subcortical and brainstem activity during the procedure.

Throughout the procedure, anesthesia is instructed to keep strict management of the blood pressure to avoid episodes of hypotension, which could put the ischemic brain at further risk, particularly during temporary occlusion of intracranial arteries. The systolic blood pressure is generally kept above 120 mm Hg and below 140 mm Hg, throughout the procedure. In patients who are typically hypertensive preoperatively, higher limits may be set to ensure adequate collateral circulation. The anesthetist is also instructed to avoid hyperventilation to preclude the vasoconstriction associated with hypocapnia. Additionally, adequate analgesia is important to avoid postoperative pain and hyperventilation.

We most commonly administer thiopental as a metabolic suppressive agent for cerebral protection during the period of temporary cerebral artery occlusion while the bypass is being performed.[44] Barbiturates such as thiopental as protection against transient focal ischemia is well supported by the literature.[44,45] The barbiturates are administered to induce EEG burst suppression until the bypass anastomosis is complete and the cerebral recipient artery temporary clips are removed. Although hypothermia is not actively induced, the patient is allowed to become mildly hypothermic (34–36°C).[44]

Systemic heparinization is not used during bypass procedures because the combination of aspirin, mild hypothermia, and systemic heparin administration can cause a problematic degree of coagulopathy, increasing the risk of the surgical procedure. Instead, all patients are premedicated with 325 mg aspirin PO for at least 3 days, including the day of surgery. Local intraluminal anticoagulant irrigation (heparinized saline) is also employed. Both the donor and recipient vessels are flushed prior to anastomosis, and the anastomosis is irrigated after completion with heparinized saline. All patients are kept on daily aspirin postoperatively.

The Superficial Temporal Artery to Middle Cerebral Artery Bypass

The most commonly employed graft for anterior circulation revascularization is the STA-MCA bypass **(Fig. 14.3).** Prior to surgery, an angiogram should be performed to clearly demonstrate the course, patency, and caliber of the STA branches on the side the bypass will be performed. Although a four-vessel angiogram is typically performed, CTA with three-dimensional (3D) reconstruction can also demonstrate the anatomy clearly. The course and location of the recipient artery should also be assessed preoperatively.

At surgery, prior to opening, a Doppler probe is used to identify the STA, and its course is marked on the scalp. The largest STA branch as identified on the preoperative angiogram is selected as the donor vessel. A linear incision is made over the artery distally. Gentle spreading of the scalp with a small curved hemostat helps to identify the STA, which is located just superficial to the galea. In this manner the artery is followed and slowly exposed down to the level of the zygomatic arch in front of the ear. It is carefully separated from the adjacent subcutaneous tissue, leaving a cuff of adventitia. The artery should be left in continuity until detached for anastomosis.

Once the donor artery has been exposed and protected, an underlying craniotomy centered 6 cm above the external auditory meatus (Chater's point) is made. This location is typically chosen because several large MCA branches emerge from the distal sylvian fissure at this point. If the parietal branch of the STA is used, the same cut-down incision used to identify the artery can be used for the craniotomy. If the frontal branch of the STA is selected, a second vertically oriented incision is required over Chater's point. If the two incisions are unconnected, the STA can be tunneled to the other in the subgaleal plane.

The temporalis muscle is split, and anterior and posterior flaps are developed to allow for a small oval craniotomy. After the dura is opened, an appropriate recipient artery branch of the MCA (at least 1.0 mm in diameter) is selected and the arachnoid membrane over this vessel is opened. A 10-mm length of the vessel should be prepared. As the distal end of the STA is prepared for bypass, the anesthesiologist is now instructed to begin the administration of barbiturates. The STA donor should be occluded with a temporary clip and is then divided distally and flushed with heparinized saline. The distal end of the vessel is prepared by removing the adventitial and beveling the orifice to fit a 3 to 4 mm arteriotomy. It is important to leave the STA segment sufficiently long to avoid any tension on the anastomosis or kinking of the graft and to easily allow rotation of the artery so that the front and back walls of the anastomosis can be sutured easily.

Once the distal end of the donor vessel is prepared, the MCA branch is occluded proximally and distally with small, low-pressure temporary clips. A 3- to 4-mm linear arteriotomy is made in the middle of the occluded segment. The proximal and distal ends of the oval STA orifice are sutured into place to the ends of the MCA arteriotomy using 9-0 or 10-0 monofilament nylon sutures. The anastomosis is then completed with approximately six interrupted 10-0 sutures on each of the front and back walls. After the anastomosis is complete, the distal MCA temporary clip is removed first to allow backfilling of the anastomosis, which enables inspection for major leaks prior to opening the proximal MCA, and then the STA clips. Any leaks are treated by mild pressure with Surgifoam on the anastomotic site, or, if this maneuver is insufficient, by the addition of sutures at the bleeding site. The dura is

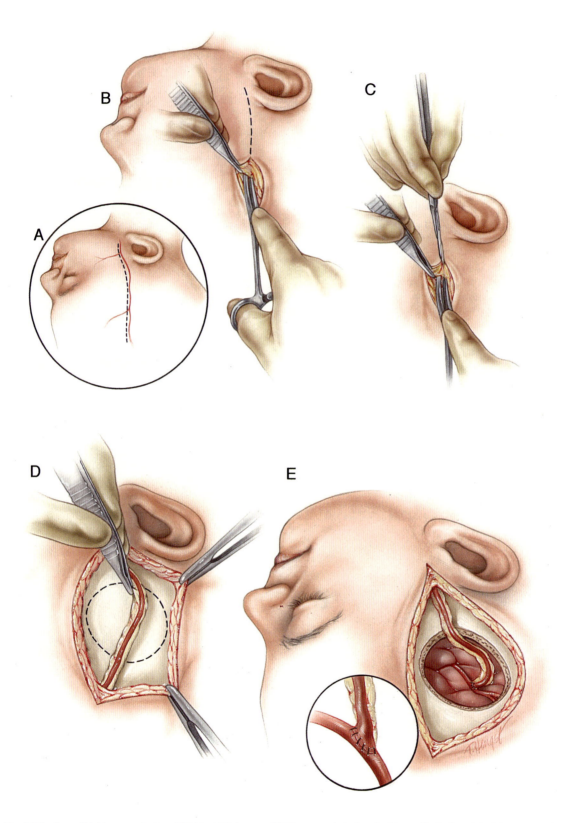

Fig. 14.3 Superficial temporal artery (STA) to MCA bypass. **(A)** The STA in the scalp is first identified with a Doppler probe and marked. **(B)** A cut-down incision over the artery is performed, and it is carefully identified. **(C)** The incision is extended to slowly reveal the full course of the STA down to the root of the zygoma. **(D)** Once the donor artery is isolated with a cuff of adventitia, it is protected and a circular craniotomy *(dotted line)* over Chater's point is opened. **(E)**. The STA is cut and anastomosed to a branch of the MCA emerging from the sylvian fissure in an end-to-side fashion.

reapproximated loosely, allowing room for the donor vessel to pass through unobstructed. The bone flap should also be trimmed to allow a smooth opening for the bypass vessel to pass through without kinking prior to securing it in place. Finally, the temporalis muscle is closed loosely. The scalp is then closed in a watertight fashion. A sterile Doppler probe can be utilized periodically to confirm that bypass flow remains uncompromised during each step of the closure.

Occipital Artery to Posterior Inferior Cerebellar Artery Bypass

The lateral position, with the operative side up, is the preferred positioning for OA-PICA bypass. With the head fixed in moderate flexion, the course of the occipital artery is identified with the Doppler probe and marked. Unlike the STA bypass, in which a cut-down incision is made directly over the artery, a hockey-stick incision, with the transverse limb located 1 cm above the superior nuchal line, is made. The occipital artery is first identified and exposed at the nuchal line, after which it is carefully dissected proximally from the subcutaneous tissue and suboccipital musculature. It is dissected from the undersurface of the myocutaneous suboccipital flap as it is slowly retracted laterally. Unlike the STA, the occipital artery does not travel in only one tissue plane and must be slowly, and painstakingly, dissected out of the scalp and muscle planes it traverses. The vessel should be left in continuity until just before the anastomosis is to be made.

At the bottom of the exposure, the occiput, the arch of C1, and the laminae of C2 are exposed. To allow access to the caudal loop of the PICA where the anastomosis will be placed, the craniotomy is extended from just beyond the midline almost to the region of the occipital condyle. The dura can then be opened and the PICA loop identified, which may require elevation of the cerebellar tonsil. The loop rarely has any branches in that area and therefore can usually be mobilized by carefully dividing the small arachnoid fibers that fix it to the dorsal surface of the medulla. After the loop is fully exposed and prepared, the distal end of the occipital artery is divided and prepared in a fashion similar to that of the STA in the STA-MCA bypass, and the patient is given barbiturates to induce burst-suppression. The PICA is then occluded proximally and distally and the anastomosis is completed in a fashion similar to that for the STA-MCA bypass. Because the dura must be left open slightly to allow unobstructed passage of the occipital artery and because the risk of cerebrospinal fluid leak is higher with posterior fossa craniotomies, the muscle closure should be performed in multiple layers in a meticulous fashion to form a completely watertight seal. Care should be taken to avoid kinking or compressing the occipital artery during this closure, and a Doppler probe may be used to check its flow at each stage of the muscle closure.

Superficial Temporal Artery to Superior Cerebellar Artery or Posterior Cerebral Artery Bypasses

The STA-to-SCA or STA-to-PCA bypass can be used as flow augmentation to the distal posterior circulation. A lumbar drain is typically placed to allow cerebrospinal fluid (CSF) drainage. The STA is first isolated in a manner similar to an STA-to-MCA bypass. However, the incision should be extended posteriorly above and behind the ear to allow for a temporal craniotomy. The lumbar drain is opened to drain approximately 10 cc of CSF, allowing easier elevation of the temporal lobe. The area of the tentorial incisura is exposed and the arachnoid in the area is opened widely to expose the SCA or PCA artery lateral to the midbrain. After administration of barbiturates, an unbranching length of the recipient vessel is isolated and occluded proximally and distally. A 3- to 4-mm arteriotomy is made along its lateral surface, and a sufficient length of STA is isolated and brought down to the recipient artery. The STA graft should have as much slack as possible to allow easy manipulation for access to the front and back walls of the anastomosis. The anastomosis is completed in the same fashion as the STA-to-MCA anastomosis.

Extracranial Carotid Artery to Middle Cerebral Artery Saphenous Vein Graft

A saphenous vein graft is typically connected end-to-end to the proximal stump of the ICA or end-to-side to the ECA. For the distal intracranial anastomosis, more proximal MCA branches in the sylvian fissure are typically a better size match to the size of the saphenous vein.

The carotid bifurcation is exposed in the neck and a pterional craniotomy is opened. The sylvian fissure should be opened widely. The MCA recipient site, usually an M2 or M3 branch free of perforating vessels, is exposed and dissected free of any arachnoid bands. The saphenous vein is exposed and isolated in the leg but left in situ and in continuity until just before it is to be used for the bypass. In our institution, we have a cardiac surgery fellow or physician's assistant who is very experienced at harvesting vein grafts harvest the graft using endoscopic technique. Meticulous care is used while exposing the vein to avoid any trauma that can cause the bypass to thrombose.[29,46,47] The alignment of the vein should be marked with a 6-0 Prolene suture through the adventitia to help define the proper orientation of the vein, to avoid twisting the vein as it is tunneled and positioned for the bypass. The vein is ligated, excised, and then immediately flushed, without overdistending it, with cool, heparinized saline.

A large clamp is used to tunnel from the cranial incision behind the zygomatic arch root to the cervical incision. The vein is aligned such that the end that was proximal in the leg is used for the cranial distal anastomosis so that the vein valves allow passage of blood in the intended direction. The vein graft is gently pulled through a large chest tube, the orientation of the vein being very carefully observed to ensure it does not twist as it passes through the tube. The chest tube is then pulled from the cervical incision to the cranial incision with the long clamp. The tube is then gently removed from the subcutaneous tunnel, leaving the vein in place. The graft is filled with cool, heparinized saline and occluded both distally and proximally with temporary aneurysm clips.

Sundt et al[37] suggested that the intracranial anastomosis be performed first, allowing the surgeon to take advantage of slack in the graft, which can be manipulated freely to suture the front and back walls of the anastomosis. The distal 5- to 6-mm of the graft are cleaned of adventitia and the end is cut on a bevel to create an orifice of approximately 5- to 6-mm in diameter. Barbiturates are administered, and a 10- to 15-mm length of the MCA is occluded proximally and distally with temporary clips. A linear arteriotomy matching the diameter of the vein graft orifice is made in the MCA. The vein graft is then fixed to the MCA at the ends using 8–0 monofilament nylon sutures and a running suture is completed. After completion of the anastomosis, the temporary clips are removed and the barbiturates can be stopped.

Slack or redundancy of the vein graft is removed by gently pulling it into the cervical incision, again being careful not to twist or kink the graft. The vein-carotid anastomosis is performed with 6-0 Prolene sutures. The temporary occluding clips are then removed and if widely patent a bounding pulse should be visible and palpable in the graft. The Doppler can also be used to confirm a normal signal flow. If there is any doubt about the graft flow or if there is concern that the graft is twisted or kinked in the subcutaneous tunnel, an intraoperative angiogram can be considered to inspect the graft and ensure that it has a smooth, normal contour with good flow.

The craniotomy is closed, allowing room in the bone flap, dura, and muscle layers for the graft to traverse without kinking or compression. The cervical incision can then be closed in standard fashion.

The ELANA Bypass Technique

Developed by Tulleken and colleagues, the excimer laser-assisted nonocclusive anastomosis (ELANA) is a technique to create anastomoses to intracranial arteries without the need for suturing or occluding the recipient artery.[48] To date, it is only applicable to saphenous vein graft bypass grafts and generally only applies to the distal intracranial anastomosis. Although both anastomoses can theoretically be performed with ELANA through a linear incision in the middle of the vein graft, the cervical anastomosis is generally still performed by hand. However, the advantage of the technology lies in its shortening of surgery time and in avoiding completely temporary occlusion of intracranial vessels, thus theoretically preventing operative ischemic morbidity.

◆ Complications

One of the most important acute complications of bypass is early graft occlusion. In the majority of cases, thrombosis and occlusion of the graft can be avoided by gentle and meticulous surgical technique and the use of heparinized saline for flushing of the graft and recipient artery. As mentioned previously, twisting, kinking, stretching, or tension of the graft can all contribute to thrombosis or stenosis of the graft. In arterial grafts, administration of adventitial papaverine irrigation can help prevent vasospasm. Perioperative antiplatelet also helps to decrease the risk of thrombosis of the bypass.

If there is any question intraoperatively about the patency of a bypass, intraoperative angiography should be performed. If a problem with stenosis or occlusion of the bypass vessel is found, it can often be revised immediately. Sometimes simply repositioning the bypass vessel is adequate, but some cases require undoing at least one of the anastomoses, removing the thrombus, and then resuturing.

A small number of graft occlusions may occur in a graft that is technically perfect but in which preoperative evaluation was not complete. If a bypass is performed to a blood vessel that has adequate blood flow already, the graft flow may be very low and will quickly become stagnant and thrombose. In most of these cases, had the flow and perfusion been carefully investigated prior to surgery, the normal flow could have been identified and it would be clear that a bypass was not necessary. This supports the rule that the decision to perform a bypass should primarily be based on flow dynamics and perfusion, not solely on demonstration of an anatomic occlusion.

Ischemic neurologic deficits can become evident postoperatively. In some cases they reflect the prolonged period of temporary arterial occlusion during anastomosis superimposed on an already hypoperfused brain. However, cerebral protection with administration of barbiturates, moderate hypothermia, and maintenance of normal or slightly hypertensive blood pressure usually minimize the risk. There has also been the suggestion that bypass in a patient with a tight MCA stenosis can precipitate thrombosis of the proximal stenotic segment.[2] Although the distal circulation in that territory is protected by the bypass, if that proximal segment supplies some perforator arteries, they may become occluded, leading to small, deep infarctions.

In the past, when systemic heparinization was used for bypass procedures, the rate of postoperative subdural or epidural hemorrhage was higher. Now, patients are given only aspirin and local anticoagulation, with heparinized saline for flushing the bypass grafts. However, because the dura is left partially open to allow the passage of the bypass graft, meticulous attention should be paid to hemostasis prior to and during closure. Any small amount of oozing from the dura, bone edges, muscle, or scalp can accumulate and cause an intracranial hematoma.

One final complication that should be noted is postoperative hyperemia. In some patients, the additional blood flow supplied by a bypass can lead to excessive cerebral blood flow, particularly with high-flow grafts such as a saphenous vein graft. Excessive flow into an already vasodilated vascular bed can lead to an acute hyperperfusion state that is generally transient but can present with transient or permanent neurologic symptoms.[28,49] This phenomenon reinforces two points: (1) preoperative assessment should assess native blood flow to avoid bypassing to a territory that already has adequate flow; and (2) flow replacement, high-flow grafts are rarely if ever needed in the setting of hypoperfusion.

◆ Outcomes

The results of the EC-IC bypass trial, published in 1985, have led to significantly decreased numbers of bypasses being performed for cerebral ischemic disease.[2] The results of that study of 1377 patients showed stroke occurred both more often and earlier in those patients who were treated with bypass. Notably, patients with severe middle cerebral artery stenosis fared much worse than those treated medically. Because of these poor results with bypass, there has been less interest in bypass for ischemic disease. However, because of the shortcomings of this trial, discussed previously, many surgeons have continued to perform bypasses for select patients with demonstration of hemodynamic failure.

The COSS trial and JET study are both prospectively studying these treatments for patients with demonstrated hemodynamic insufficiency. Because both are ongoing, no outcome data are yet available. However, some small studies have reported findings that are suggestive that bypass may be advantageous in select clinical circumstances. For example, improvements in PET parameters of hypoperfusion have been shown to improve following bypass.[18,19] Some of these studies have shown evidence of clinical improvement in many of these patients as well.[50]

◆ Case Illustrations

Case 1: Anterior Circulation, Chronic Ischemia

This patient is a 49-year-old woman with a history of diabetes mellitus, hypertension, hyperlipidemia, and three previous ischemic strokes (**Fig. 14.4**). Most recently, she presented with an episode of right leg weakness and transient dizziness. Workup at that time revealed small, acute mesial left frontal lobe and caudate infarctions as well as evidence of older left frontoparietal infarctions. She was found to have a left ICA occlusion with poor filling of the anterior cerebral artery (ACA) and MCA and almost no flow from the anterior communicating artery (ACoA) and posterior communicating artery (PCoA) to that side. The only significant collateral flow seen on angiogram was from leptomeningeal collaterals from the left PCA. Xenon CT with Diamox challenge revealed left frontal hypoperfusion with practically no effect of Diamox, demonstrating exhausted cerebrovascular reserve. ^{15}O PET was also performed which revealed an elevated OEF in the left hemisphere. During the workup she again had an episode of transient right-sided weakness without any new ischemic lesions on MRI. This patient was treated with a STA-to-MCA bypass and has had no new ischemic symptomatology since treatment.

Case 2: Anterior Circulation, Chronic Ischemia

This 81-year-old man had a history of coronary artery disease, aortic valve disease, peripheral valve disease, and a distant history of a right-sided transient ischemic attack consisting of a mild left-sided weakness. More recent "spells" of confusion and weakness were also suggestive of TIA. The patient was being treated medically with anticoagulation with Coumadin. During workup for aortic valve repair surgery, CT perfusion with Diamox challenge and transcranial

Doppler with CO_2 reactivity were both performed and demonstrated severe hemodynamic failure in the right hemisphere. Because of his high risk for stroke during a prolonged cardiac procedure, it was recommended that he undergo cerebral revascularization prior to open-heart surgery. He underwent STA-to-MCA bypass and subsequent aortic valve replacement without complications.

Case 3: Anterior Circulation, Acute Ischemia

A 73-year-old woman with a history of diabetes and hypertension presented with a rapid onset of left hemiparesis, confusion, and dysarthria (**Fig. 14.5**). Workup revealed a small MCA territory stroke but with a large MCA perfusion deficit on MRI secondary to a complete right ICA occlusion. The ACoA and PCoA on that side were very small. During her acute hospitalization, she experienced a worsening of her upper-extremity weakness and MRI revealed an expanding infarct. She was treated with an urgent STA-to-MCA bypass, which halted the progression of her infarctions and reversed the MRI perfusion defect.

Case 4: Posterior Circulation

This 71-year-old man with a history of hypertension and hyperlipidemia presented complaining of transient episodes of numbness, dizziness, and ataxia, lasting approximately 6 minutes each (**Fig. 14.6**). He was found to have bilateral vertebral artery occlusions proximal to the PICA origins. The only collateral to the posterior circulation was from tiny vessels from the dura and anterior spinal artery. The upper basilar territory was supplied by a very small PCoA on one side. He continued to have frequent episodes despite maximal medical treatment with aspirin and Coumadin and was felt to be at high risk for catastrophic posterior circulation infarction. He underwent a STA-to-SCA bypass to augment flow to the posterior circulation. Following bypass, the patient has been TIA and stroke free on Coumadin.

Case 5: Posterior Circulation

This patient is a 61-year-old man with a history of hypertension who developed acute nausea, dizziness, dysarthria, and ataxia. He was found to have bilateral upper cervical vertebral artery occlusions with a very small right PCoA. MRI revealed acute cerebellar infarctions in the PICA and AICA territories. Despite maximal antithrombotic therapy and blood pressure support, the patient's symptoms progressed while in the hospital, and it was felt that flow augmentation was warranted. Although a bypass to the superior cerebellar artery or PCA was considered, it was felt that simultaneous decompression of the posterior fossa would be beneficial given a considerable amount of cerebellar swelling due to the acute infarctions. Therefore, the patient was treated with an occipital artery-to-PICA bypass and made a slow recovery in rehabilitation without further evolution of his ischemic lesions.

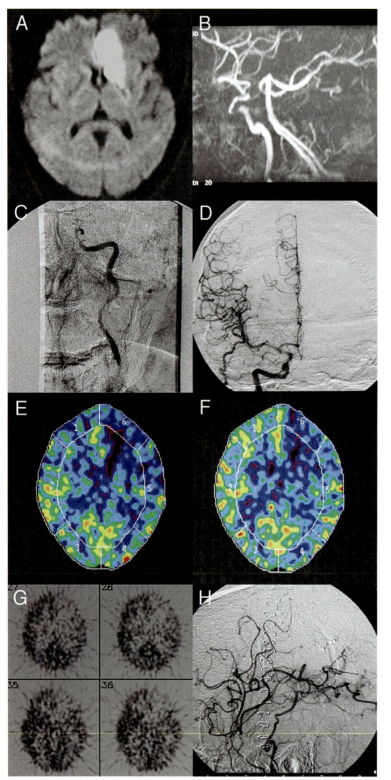

Fig. 14.4 Case 1: This 49-year-old woman with a history of prior strokes presented with right-sided weakness and transient dizziness. **(A)** Diffusion-weighted magnetic resonance imaging (MRI) revealed an acute mesial frontal lobe and caudate infarction. Magnetic resonance angiography (MRA) **(B)** and cerebral angiography **(C)** revealed a complete internal carotid artery (ICA) occlusion at the cavernous segment, with poor collateral circulation from the contralateral side **(D).** Xenon computed tomography (CT) **(E)** revealed hypoperfusion in the left frontal MCA and anterior cerebral artery (ACA) distributions that did not improve significantly after administration of Diamox **(F).** **(G)** Oxygen-15 PET was also performed, which revealed decreased cerebral blood flow and elevated oxygen extraction in the same region. The patient underwent an STA-to-MCA bypass, which provided good revascularization of the left hemisphere, as seen on a postoperative angiogram **(H).**

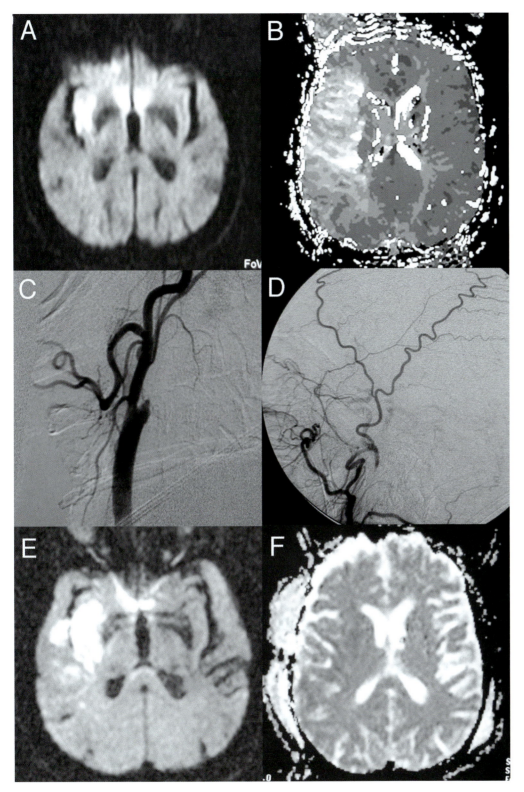

Fig. 14.5 Case 3: This 73-year-old woman experienced an acute progression of left hemiparesis, confusion, and dysarthria. Diffusion-weighted MRI revealed only a small right insular infarction **(A)** but with a large MCA perfusion deficit on MRI perfusion **(B).** Angiography revealed complete ICA occlusion **(C)** and poor collateral reconstitution of the intracranial ICA **(D).** Her clinical exam deteriorated in the hospital, and follow-up MRI demonstrated a progression of the insular and temporal infarction **(E).** Following STA-to-MCA bypass, the MRI perfusion defect was reversed **(F).**

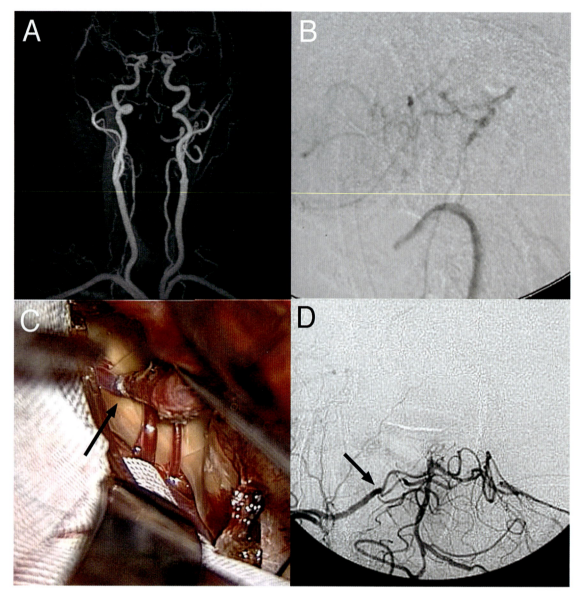

Fig. 14.6 Case 4: A 71-year-old man presented with transient episodes of numbness, dizziness, and ataxia refractory to anticoagulation. MRA **(A)** and angiography **(B)** diagnosed bilateral vertebral artery occlusion proximal to the posterior inferior cerebellar artery (PICA) with small amounts of collateral reconstituting the vertebrobasilar territory through the anterior spinal artery and a small posterior communicating artery PCoA. He underwent STA-to-SCA bypass **(C,D;** arrows indicate the site of the anastomosis).

References

1. Donaghy R, Yasargil MG. Microvascular Surgery. St. Louis: CV Mosby, 1967
2. The EC/IC Bypass Study Group. Failure of extracranial-intracranial arterial bypass to reduce the risk of ischemic stroke. Results of an international randomized trial. N Engl J Med 1985;313:1191–1200
3. Goldring S, Zervas N, Langfitt T. The Extracranial-Intracranial Bypass Study. A report of the committee appointed by the American Association of Neurological Surgeons to examine the study. N Engl J Med 1987; 316:817–820
4. Sundt TM Jr. Was the international randomized trial of extracranial-intracranial arterial bypass representative of the population at risk? N Engl J Med 1987;316:814–816
5. Grubb RL Jr, Derdeyn CP, Fritsch SM, et al. Importance of hemodynamic factors in the prognosis of symptomatic carotid occlusion. JAMA 1998; 280:1055–1060
6. Grubb RL Jr, Powers WJ, Derdeyn CP, Adams HP Jr, Clarke WR. The Carotid Occlusion Surgery Study. Neurosurg Focus 2003;14:e9
7. Powers WJ, Derdeyn CP, Fritsch SM, et al. Benign prognosis of never-symptomatic carotid occlusion. Neurology 2000;54:878–882
8. Mizumura S, Nakagawara J, Takahashi M, et al. Three-dimensional display in staging hemodynamic brain ischemia for JET study: objective evaluation using SEE analysis and 3D-SSP display. Ann Nucl Med 2004; 18:13–21
9. Kuroda S, Houkin K, Kamiyama H, Mitsumori K, Iwasaki Y, Abe H. Long-term prognosis of medically treated patients with internal carotid or middle cerebral artery occlusion: can acetazolamide test predict it? Stroke 2001;32:2110–2116
10. Ogasawara K, Ogawa A, Yoshimoto T. Cerebrovascular reactivity to acetazolamide and outcome in patients with symptomatic internal carotid or middle cerebral artery occlusion: a xenon-133 single-photon emission computed tomography study. Stroke 2002;33:1857–1862

11. Webster MW, Makaroun MS, Steed DL, Smith HA, Johnson DW, Yonas H. Compromised cerebral blood flow reactivity is a predictor of stroke in patients with symptomatic carotid artery occlusive disease. J Vasc Surg 1995;21:338–344, discussion 344–345

12. Derdeyn CP, Grubb RL Jr, Powers WJ. Cerebral hemodynamic impairment: methods of measurement and association with stroke risk. Neurology 1999;53:251–259

13. Kleiser B, Widder B. Course of carotid artery occlusions with impaired cerebrovascular reactivity. Stroke 1992;23:171–174

14. Vernieri F, Pasqualetti P, Passarelli F, Rossini PM, Silvestrini M. Outcome of carotid artery occlusion is predicted by cerebrovascular reactivity. Stroke 1999;30:593–598

15. Amin-Hanjani S, Shin JH, Zhao M, Du X, Charbel FT. Evaluation of extracranial-intracranial bypass using quantitative magnetic resonance angiography. J Neurosurg 2007;106:291–298

16. Zhao M, Charbel FT, Alperin N, Loth F, Clark ME. Improved phase-contrast flow quantification by three-dimensional vessel localization. Magn Reson Imaging 2000;18:697–706

17. Langer DJ, Lefton DR, Ostergren L, et al. Hemispheric revascularization in the setting of carotid occlusion and subclavian steal: a diagnostic and management role for quantitative magnetic resonance angiography? Neurosurgery 2006;58:528–533, discussion 528–533

18. Muraishi K, Kameyama M, Sato K, et al. Cerebral circulatory and metabolic changes following EC/IC bypass surgery in cerebral occlusive diseases. Neurol Res 1993;15:97–103

19. Nagata S, Fujii K, Matsushima T, et al. Evaluation of EC-IC bypass for patients with atherosclerotic occlusive cerebrovascular disease: clinical and positron emission tomographic studies. Neurol Res 1991;13:209–216

20. Amin-Hanjani S, Charbel FT. Is extracranial-intracranial bypass surgery effective in certain patients? Neurosurg Clin N Am 2008;19:477–487, vi–vii

21. The Warfarin-Aspirin Symptomatic Intracranial Disease WASID) Study Group. Prognosis of patients with symptomatic vertebral or basilar artery stenosis. Stroke 1998;29:1389–1392

22. Qureshi AI, Ziai WC, Yahia AM, et al. Stroke-free survival and its determinants in patients with symptomatic vertebrobasilar stenosis: a multicenter study. Neurosurgery 2003;52:1033–1039, discussion 1039–1040

23. Coward LJ, McCabe DJ, Ederle J, Featherstone RL, Clifton A, Brown MM; CAVATAS Investigators. Long-term outcome after angioplasty and stenting for symptomatic vertebral artery stenosis compared with medical treatment in the Carotid and Vertebral Artery Transluminal Angioplasty Study (CAVATAS): a randomized trial. Stroke 2007;38:1526–1530

24. Amin-Hanjani S, Du X, Zhao M, Walsh K, Malisch TW, Charbel FT. Use of quantitative magnetic resonance angiography to stratify stroke risk in symptomatic vertebrobasilar disease. Stroke 2005;36:1140–1145

25. Hussain MS, Bhagat YA, Liu S, et al. DWI lesion volume reduction following acute stroke treatment with transient partial aortic obstruction. J Neuroimaging 2010;20:379–381

26. Uflacker R, Schönholz C, Papamitisakis N; SENTIS trial. Interim report of the SENTIS trial: cerebral perfusion augmentation via partial aortic occlusion in acute ischemic stroke. J Cardiovasc Surg (Torino) 2008;49:715–721

27. Sekhar LN, Bucur SD, Bank WO, Wright DC. Venous and arterial bypass grafts for difficult tumors, aneurysms, and occlusive vascular lesions: evolution of surgical treatment and improved graft results. Neurosurgery 1999;44:1207–1223, discussion 1223–1224

28. Kim JE, Oh CW, Kwon OK, Park SQ, Kim SE, Kim YK. Transient hyperperfusion after superficial temporal artery/middle cerebral artery bypass surgery as a possible cause of postoperative transient neurological deterioration. Cerebrovasc Dis 2008;25:580–586

29. Regli L, Piepgras DG, Hansen KK. Late patency of long saphenous vein bypass grafts to the anterior and posterior cerebral circulation. J Neurosurg 1995;83:806–811

30. Schick U, Zimmermann M, Stolke D. Long-term evaluation of EC-IC bypass patency. Acta Neurochir (Wien) 1996;138:938–942, discussion 942–943

31. Amin-Hanjani S, Du X, Mlinarevich N, Meglio G, Zhao M, Charbel FT. The cut flow index: an intraoperative predictor of the success of extracranial-intracranial bypass for occlusive cerebrovascular disease. Neurosurgery 2005;56(1, Suppl)75–85, discussion 75–85

32. Chang SD, Steinberg GK. Superficial temporal artery to middle cerebral artery anastomosis. Tech Neurosurg 2000;6:86–100

33. Bendok BR, Murad A, Getch CC, Batjer HH. Failure of a saphenous vein extracranial-intracranial bypass graft to protect against bilateral middle cerebral artery ischemia after carotid artery occlusion: case report. Neurosurgery 1999;45:367–370, discussion 370–371

34. Liu JK, Kan P, Karwande SV, Couldwell WT. Conduits for cerebrovascular bypass and lessons learned from the cardiovascular experience. Neurosurg Focus 2003;14:e3

35. Mohit AA, Sekhar LN, Natarajan SK, Britz GW, Ghodke B. High-flow bypass grafts in the management of complex intracranial aneurysms. Neurosurgery 2007;60(2, Suppl 1)ONS105–ONS122, discussion ONS122–ONS123

36. Eguchi T. Results of EC-IC bypass with and without long vein graft. In: Spetzler RF, Carter LP, Selman WR, Martin N, eds. Cerebral Revascularization for Stroke. New York: Thieme-Stratton, 1985:584–590

37. Sundt TM Jr, Piepgras DG, Marsh WR, Fode NC. Saphenous vein bypass grafts for giant aneurysms and intracranial occlusive disease. J Neurosurg 1986;65:439–450

38. Little JR, Furlan AJ, Bryerton B. Short vein grafts for cerebral revascularization. J Neurosurg 1983;59:384–388

39. Diaz FG, Umansky F, Mehta B, et al. Cerebral revascularization to a main limb of the middle cerebral artery in the sylvian fissure. An alternative approach to conventional anastomosis. J Neurosurg 1985;63:21–29

40. Jafar JJ, Russell SM, Woo HH. Treatment of giant intracranial aneurysms with saphenous vein extracranial-to-intracranial bypass grafting: indications, operative technique, and results in 29 patients. Neurosurgery 2002;51:138–144, discussion 144–146

41. Ausman JI, Diaz FG, Vacca DF, Sadasivan B. Superficial temporal and occipital artery bypass pedicles to superior, anterior inferior, and posterior inferior cerebellar arteries for vertebrobasilar insufficiency. J Neurosurg 1990;72:554–558

42. Sundt TM Jr, Piepgras DG. Occipital to posterior inferior cerebellar artery bypass surgery. J Neurosurg 1978;48:916–928

43. Komotar RJ, Starke RM, Otten ML, et al. The role of indirect extracranial-intracranial bypass in the treatment of symptomatic intracranial atherooclusive disease. J Neurosurg 2009;110:896–904

44. Solomon RA. Principles of aneurysm surgery: cerebral ischemic protection, hypothermia, and circulatory arrest. Clin Neurosurg 1994;41:351–363

45. Lawton MT, Hamilton MG, Morcos JJ, Spetzler RF. Revascularization and aneurysm surgery: current techniques, indications, and outcome. Neurosurgery 1996;38:83–92, discussion 92–94

46. Sundt TM III, Sundt TM Jr. Principles of preparation of vein bypass grafts to maximize patency. J Neurosurg 1987;66:172–180

47. Sundt TMr. Sundt TM, Jr. Maximizing patency and saphenous vein bypass grafts: principles of preparation learned from coronary and peripheral vascular surgery. In: Meyer FB, ed. Sundt's Occlusive Cerebrovascular Disease. Philadelphia: WB Saunders, 1994:479–488

48. Langer DJ, Vajkoczy P. ELANA: Excimer Laser-Assisted Nonocclusive Anastomosis for extracranial-to-intracranial and intracranial-to-intracranial bypass: a review. Skull Base 2005;15:191–205

49. Fujimura M, Mugikura S, Kaneta T, Shimizu H, Tominaga T. Incidence and risk factors for symptomatic cerebral hyperperfusion after superficial temporal artery-middle cerebral artery anastomosis in patients with moyamoya disease. Surg Neurol 2009;71:442–447

50. Nussbaum ES, Erickson DL. Extracranial-intracranial bypass for ischemic cerebrovascular disease refractory to maximal medical therapy. Neurosurgery 2000;46:37–42, discussion 42–43

15

Moyamoya: Surgical Indications and Strategies

Bradley A. Gross, Mark Dannenbaum, Edward R. Smith, Arthur L. Day, and R. Michael Scott

Pearls

- Early diagnosis of moyamoya is critical to good outcome
- Fluid-attenuated inversion recovery (FLAIR) magnetic resonance imaging (MRI) can document slow flow and corroborate angiography findings.
- Preoperative planning is helped by an angiogram that includes external carotid artery (ECA) injections to identify and preserve transdural collaterals and to assist with mapping of the graft vessel.
- Maintaining aspirin treatment right up to the day of surgery and immediately postoperatively can reduce the perioperative stroke risk.
- Wide arachnoid opening on both direct and indirect operations can improve collateral development.
- Preoperative admission the night before surgery with intravenous hydration and continuation of postoperative intravenous hydration can minimize perioperative ischemic events.

Moyamoya is an arteriopathy defined by progressive stenosis of intracranial arteries, usually involving the internal carotid artery and proximal portions of its major branches—the anterior and middle cerebral arteries. This stenotic process is accompanied by concomitant formation of fragile collateral vessels, which leads to successive ischemic and hemorrhagic events (the latter more common in adults). Takeuchi and Shimizu[1] first described the phenomenon of bilateral hypoplasia of the internal carotid arteries in 1957, and the term *moyamoya,* meaning "puff of smoke," in reference to the collaterals, was later coined by Suzuki and Takaku.[2] Subsequently, the international classification of diseases has distinguished between moyamoya *disease,* which is idiopathic and bilateral, and moyamoya *syndrome,* which pertains to patients with unilateral findings or patients with bilateral angiographic findings in the setting of associated medical conditions. Such conditions include neurofibromatosis, sickle cell disease, Down syndrome, prior cranial irradiation, congenital cardiac anomalies, renal artery stenosis, giant cervicofacial hemangiomas, and hyperthyroidism, among others.[3]

◆ Epidemiology (Table 15.1)

Although first described in Japan,[1,4,5] subsequent studies have reported on the epidemiology of moyamoya in the United States, Korea, Taiwan, and Europe.[6–10] Across the Japanese studies, the female-to-male ratio has ranged from 1.8 to 2.2:1 and the incidence from 0.35 to 0.94 per 100,000.[4,5,11] The reported incidence has increased in recent years, paralleling improvements in imaging technology. Although studies of other ethnicities also show a female predilection,[8–10] the incidence of the disease is notably lower: 0.048 per 100,000 in a Taiwanese study,[7] 0.052 and 0.086 per 100,000 in American studies,[8,9] and one-tenth the incidence in Japan in a European study.[10] Interestingly, the American study of Uchino et al[9] demonstrated ethnicity-specific incidence rate ratios of 4.6 for Asian-Americans, 2.2 for African Americans, and 0.5 for Hispanics as compared with Caucasians. The incidence of moyamoya among Asian-Americans—0.28 per 100,000—approaches that reported among Japanese studies. Taken together with a 10% prevalence of familial cases among Japanese studies,[5,11] a genetic component to the idiopathic form of moyamoya is implicated. Supporting this premise, abnormalities on chromosomes 3, 6, and 17 have been identified in association with moyamoya disease.

Epidemiologic studies have demonstrated a bimodal age distribution with one peak involving children under 10 years of age and another involving adults approximately in their fourth decade.[4,6–11] This dichotomous age distribution parallels the differing clinical presentations between age groups.

Table 15.1 Moyamoya Epidemiology

Study	Pts	Location	F:M	Prevalence*	Incidence*	Age Peaks	Familial
Baba et al, 2008[4]	267	Japan	2.2	10.5	0.94	Highest 45–49 Second 5–9	
Han et al, 2000[6]	334	Korea	1.4			6–15 31–40	1.5%
Hung et al, 1997[7]	92	Taiwan	1.3	0.44	0.048	31–40	
Kuriyama et al, 2008[5]	1269	Japan	1.8	6.03	0.54	**	12%
Uchino et al, 2005[9]	298	USA	2.1		0.086	5–9 55–59	
Wakai et al, 1997[11]	1176	Japan	1.8	3.16	0.35	Highest 10–14 40–49	10%
Wetjen et al, 1998[8]	30	USA	2.4	1.2	0.052	30–50 Less than 16	
Yonekawa et al,19 97[10]	168	Europe	1.4		"1/10" that of Japan" 0.3 pt/center/yr	0–9 20–29	

Abbreviations: F:M, female-to-male ratio; Pts, patients.

*Prevalence and incidence are per 100,000 people.

**Three male peaks: ages 10–14, 35–39, 55–59; and two female peaks: ages 20–24 and 50–54 were noted.

◆ Natural History and Clinical Presentation

The majority of pediatric cases of moyamoya disease present with ischemic symptoms secondary to progressive occlusion of vessels of the circle of Willis **(Table 15.2)**. This is closely paralleled in pediatric series of moyamoya syndrome in association with sickle cell disease and Down syndrome with 67 to 100% of patients presenting with transient ischemic attack (TIAs) or strokes.[12] Symptoms are commonly precipitated by events that reduce blood flow to the brain in the setting of a tenuous vascular supply such as dehydration or hyperventilation. Reductions in $PaCO_2$—as in hyperventilation (particularly pertinent in crying children)—induce constriction of already maximally dilated cerebral vessels. Dehydration can reduce blood pressure and promote hypercoagulable states,

Table 15.2 Larger Series Depicting Clinical Presentation Among Pediatric Cases

Study	Pts	Location	Ischemic Presentation	Hemorrhagic Presentation	Other Presentation
Fung et al, 2005[33]	1448		80%	2.5%	5% seizure
Han et al, 2000[6]	334*	Korea	61%	9%	23% seizure
Karasawa et al, 1992[16]	104		55% TIA 42% CVA		3% other
Kurokawa et al, 1985[13]	27	Japan	70%		30% "non-TIA"—includes hemorrhagic
Kim et al, 2002[39]	67	Japan	58% TIA + CVA 28% TIA 8% CVA	6%	
Scott et al, 2004[3]	143	USA	68% CVA 43% TIA	3%	6% seizure 6% HA 4% choreiform mvmt 4% ASx
Suzuki et al, 1997[15]	38	Japan	82% TIA/seizures		11% choreiform mvmt 3% HA

Abbreviations: ASx, asymptomatic; CVA, cerebrovascular accident, referring to ischemic stroke; HA, headache; mvmt, movements; Pts, patients; TIA, transient ischemic attack.

*Total of 334 pediatric and adult patients.

Table 15.3 Natural History of Hemorrhagic Moyamoya

Study	Pts	Bleed Type	Outcome After Initial Bleed	Follow-Up (Years)	Rebleeds	Outcome After Rebleed
Ikezaki et al, 1997[20]	232			3.9	16% of patients*	
Kawaguchi et al, 2000[31]	11	39% IVH 39% IPH 27% IVH + IPH	12% mortality	8.7	18% of patients	100% worse
Kobayashi et al, 2000[21]	42	38% IVH + IPH 31% IVH 21% IPH 5% SAH	46% good outcome 7% mortality	6.7	7% annual rate All had IVH	21% good outcome 29% mortality
Saeki et al, 1997[23]	20		60% good outcome 5% mortality	6.2	35% of patients	40% good outcome 25% mortality
Yoshida et al, 1999[22]	28	36% IVH 25% IPH 21% IVH + IPH 18% SAH	18% mortality	14.2	38% of patients	67% mortality

Abbreviations: IVH, intraventricular hemorrhage; IPH, intraparenchymal hemorrhage; Pts, patients; SAH, subarachnoid hemorrhage.
*Regardless of whether intervention was performed.

both of which can adversely affect blood flow through stenotic parent vessels and small collaterals.

In pediatric patients, recurrent TIAs or those that alternate sides can suggest the diagnosis of moyamoya. Up to 25% of previously healthy moyamoya patients become dependent on full-time care or die within 3 years.[13] In the study of Olds et al,[14] nearly 90% of untreated patients continued to have ischemic symptoms during an average follow-up period of 3.5 years. This relentless course is also seen in patients with moyamoya syndrome and sickle cell disease, with 58% of children having new strokes despite optimal medical therapy.[12]

Other clinical presentations include seizures (up to 23% of pediatric cases)[3,6] and choreiform movements in up to 11% of cases.[3,15] These movements may result from ischemia in the basal ganglia or mass effect on these areas from dilated collaterals. Dilation of meningeal and leptomeningeal collaterals may explain headache as a presenting symptom in 3 to 6% of cases.[3,15,16] Rupture of these collaterals resulting in hemorrhage occurs relatively infrequently in the pediatric population (2.5 to 9%)[3,6,17] and may portend a worse prognosis.

In contrast, hemorrhage is typically one of the most common presentations among the adult moyamoya population, occurring in up to two thirds of cases[18–20] **(Table 15.3).** Most hemorrhages are intraventricular (IVH) or intraparenchymal (IPH). Of those with IPH, approximately three fourths are in the basal ganglia or thalamus. Mortality rates after hemorrhage have been reported to be as high as 18%. Approximately one third of patients rebleed, with a reported annual rate of 7%.[21] After a second hemorrhage, mortality is as high as 67%. Rehemorrhage can occur in a delayed fashion, with reports of bleeding at 20 years following the initial ictus.[22] In the study of Kobayashi et al,[21] five patients rebled at least 10 years after their first bleed, with a mean time of 6.5 years between hemorrhages. The authors also noted that the second bleed often occurred in a different location, suggesting diffuse vulnerability of moyamoya vessels. Saeki et al[23] noted that females were at higher risk factor of rebleeding.

The female sex was also found to be a significant risk factor for radiographic progression. In the general adult moyamoya natural history study of Kuroda et al,[24] 63 adults were followed prospectively for a mean of 6.1 years, and progression was seen in 17.4% of hemispheres (23.8% of patients) over a mean interval of 5 years. The odds ratio for disease progression in males was 0.2. More impressive are the clinical consequences of untreated moyamoya. An American study reported a 65% risk of recurrent stroke within 5 years of initial symptomatic presentation; this risk increased to 82% among patients with bilateral moyamoya and ischemic symptomatic presentation.[25] Even for the limited number of patients without any evident clinical symptoms—that is, only radiographic disease—there remains a 27% risk of symptomatic stroke over 5 years. A recent Japanese study of asymptomatic radiographic moyamoya reported a 3.2% annual risk of ischemic or hemorrhagic events.[26] In this population, radiographic studies portended the progressive nature of this disease; 20% of hemispheres showed evidence of completed strokes and 40% exhibited disturbed cerebral hemodynamics.

◆ Diagnosis

Radiographic investigation of children and adults presenting with ischemic or hemorrhagic symptoms often begins with computed tomography (CT). Among those with ischemic symptoms, small hypodense areas are often seen in the basal ganglia, deep white matter, periventricular regions, or watershed zones. Hemorrhagic presentation is often seen in the ventricular system, basal ganglia, thalamus, or medial temporal lobes.

Table 15.4	Suzuki Stages of Moyamoya Disease
Stage	**Appearance**
1	Bilateral internal carotid artery stenosis
2	Collateral vessels begin to form
3	Prominence of collateral vessels
4	Severe stenosis/complete occlusion of circle of Willis, moyamoya vessels narrow, extracranial collaterals begin to from
5	Prominence of extracranial collaterals
6	Complete carotid occlusion

Magnetic resonance imaging (MRI)/magnetic resonance angiography (MRA) typically ensues, at times demonstrating acute infarcts (best seen with diffusion-weighted imaging [DWI]). The "ivy sign"—sulcal linear hyperintensity—seen on T2 fluid-attenuated inversion recovery (FLAIR) is representative of slow flow. Diminished flow voids in the internal carotid artery (ICA), middle cerebral artery (MCA), and anterior cerebral artery (ACA) territories and prominent collateral flow voids in the basal ganglia and thalamus are characteristic of moyamoya.

Angiograms have been the imaging modality of choice to assess the severity of disease. In their classic 1969 study, Suzuki and Takaku[2] stratify the angiographic appearance of moyamoya disease into six stages (**Table 15.4**). Appropriate visualization of basal collaterals, small vessel occlusions, and associated vascular pathology often requires conventional digital subtraction angiography (DSA).

Identification of preexisting spontaneous collaterals from the external carotid circulation is critical for surgical planning, and external carotid artery (ECA) injections should be administered and internal carotid and vertebral artery imaging should be performed. The risk of angiography in moyamoya patients is not significantly different from the risk in patients with other cerebrovascular disease, with overall complication rates of less than 1%.

Other diagnostic evaluations that may be useful in patients with moyamoya include electroencephalography (EEG) and cerebral blood flow studies. Specific alterations of EEG recordings are usually observed only in pediatric patients and include posterior or centrotemporal slowing, a hyperventilation-induced diffuse pattern of monophasic slow waves (called "build-up"), and a characteristic "rebuild-up" phenomenon. Rebuild-up looks identical to the build-up slow waves seen in non-moyamoya patients, but differs in the timing of its presentation. Build-up occurs during hyperventilation, whereas rebuild-up occurs after its completion, indicating a diminished cerebral perfusion reserve.

Cerebral blood flow studies, including xenon-CT, positron emission tomography (PET), and single photon emission computed tomography (SPECT) with acetazolamide challenge, may be employed in the initial diagnostic evaluation and to assess subsequent response to surgery. Xenon-CT has been used to measure cerebral blood flow both prior to and following treatment; its shortcomings include a long acquisition time, limited availability, and susceptibility to motion artifact. PET imaging typically demonstrates reduced regional cerebral blood flow, an elevation of regional oxygen extraction fraction, and an elevation of regional cerebral blood volume. SPECT imaging in moyamoya helps to determine regional cerebral blood flow, particularly in vessels that are not seen angiographically. These studies may help to quantify blood flow, serve as a baseline prior to the institution of treatment, and occasionally aid in treatment decisions.

◆ Surgical Treatment and Results

There is no known treatment that reverses the primary disease process, and current treatments are designed to prevent strokes by improving blood flow to the affected cerebral hemisphere. Improvement in cerebral blood flow may protect against future strokes (both ischemic and hemorrhagic), effect a concurrent reduction in moyamoya collaterals, and reduce symptom frequency. Early diagnosis and surgical treatment are paramount to halt the relentless progression of moyamoya. Medical management with aspirin may help prevent embolic phenomena from microthrombus formation at stenotic sites. It is used at many institutions and as a continued treatment following surgery. Limited experience with calcium channel blockers suggests that they may alleviate headaches. However, care must be taken to avoid hypotension. Although there is a role for medication in the management of moyamoya, medical therapy should not be substituted for definitive surgical treatment.

There is ample evidence supporting the premise that revascularization surgery provides significant and durable reductions in stroke frequency to patients with moyamoya. Hallemeier et al[25] demonstrated a reduction from 65% to 17% in the 5-year risk of stroke among symptomatic moyamoya patients undergoing surgery.

The arteriopathy of moyamoya primarily affects the ICA while sparing the ECA. Surgical treatment of moyamoya typically uses the ECA as a source of new blood flow to the ischemic hemisphere. Two general methods of revascularization are employed: direct and indirect. In direct revascularization, a branch of the ECA (usually the superficial temporal artery [STA]) is directly anastomosed to a superficial cortical artery (usually the MCA). Indirect techniques involve the placement of vascularized tissue supplied by the ECA such as dura, temporalis muscle, or the STA itself in direct contact with the brain, leading to an in-growth of new blood vessels to the underlying cerebral cortex.

Regardless of the technique selected, all patients with moyamoya disease and moyamoya syndrome should be considered for operative treatment. Early definitive treatment with surgical revascularization—before irreversible neurologic deficits occur—is the single best option for preserving good neurologic function. Other than the rare patient with complex medical conditions precluding an operation or the individual with an unclear diagnosis, the presence of moyamoya should prompt a discussion about timely surgical therapy, particularly in pediatric patients.

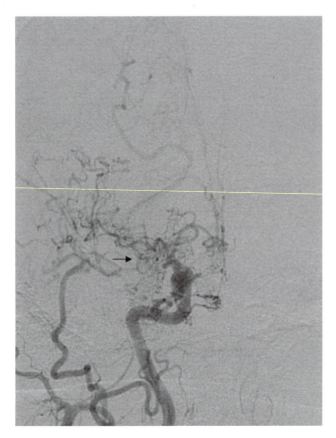

Fig. 15.1 This 52-year-old man with severe stenosis of the right supraclinoid internal carotid artery (ICA) and occlusion of the main stem of the right middle cerebral artery (MCA) and A1 presented with transient episodes of left-sided numbness. Moyamoya collateralization is seen *(arrow)*.

Direct Revascularization

Direct revascularization, most commonly via an STA-MCA bypass, is more ideally suited for adult patients with moyamoya, as the caliber of their vessels not only makes the procedure more feasible, but also facilitates an early, hemodynamically, significant amount of revascularization through the graft (**Figs. 15.1 and 15.2**). This approach allows for an immediate increase in blood flow to ischemic brain and a theoretical decrease in the hemodynamic load on moyamoya vessels as supported by increased perfusion seen on perfusion imaging, potentially decreasing the risk of subsequent hemorrhage.

Following a skin incision over the course of the parietal branch of the STA, the artery is dissected from surrounding connective tissue, and a craniotomy is turned, centered over the sylvian fissure. The dura is opened and a suitable M4 recipient branch is identified originating from or near the sylvian fissure, often overlying the temporal lobe. A temporary clip is carefully placed across the proximal STA, and the distal vessel is then cut obliquely. Temporary clips are then placed to trap a segment of the recipient MCA branch (**Fig. 15.3**) and, following a linear arteriotomy in the MCA (**Fig. 15.4**), an

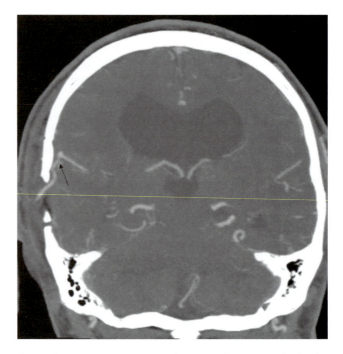

Fig. 15.2 Postoperative computed tomography angiography (CTA) demonstrating patency of his superficial temporal artery (STA)-MCA anastomosis *(arrow)*.

end-to-side anastomosis is performed with interrupted 10-0 nylon (**Fig. 15.5**). The temporary clips are then removed from the recipient MCA branch (taking care to flush out any air or thrombus), and, in turn, the STA. Craniotomy closure minimizes compression on the STA by ensuring a wide entry site through the bone.

Patients are maintained on aspirin postoperatively and hydrated, often at 1.25 to 1.5 times the maintenance level, assuming there are no preexisting medical conditions that predispose the patient to fluid overload. Blood pressure control to maintain normotension (usually in an intensive care

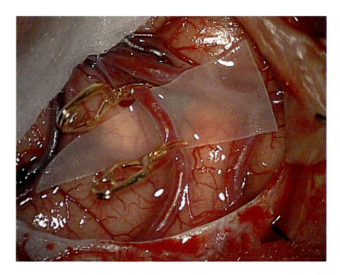

Fig. 15.3 Temporary clips are placed to trap a segment of M4.

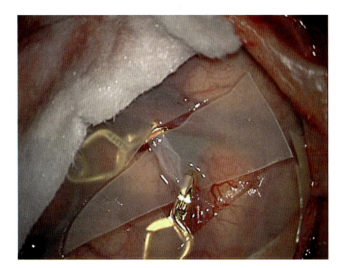

Fig. 15.4 A linear arteriotomy is made in the trapped MCA segment.

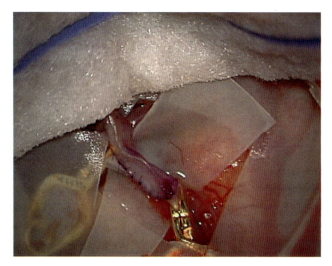

Fig. 15.5 Completed end-to-side anastomosis.

unit with use of an arterial line) should be maintained to preserve bypass flow and to prevent hyperperfusion. Up to 36% of patients may exhibit transient postoperative deficits owing to hyperperfusion.[27] Fujimura et al[27] reported adult onset and hemorrhagic presentation as significant risk factors for postoperative hyperperfusion.

Multiple surgical series have reinforced the efficacy of an STA-MCA bypass in the treatment of ischemic moyamoya in adults. In the original STA-MCA bypass study of Karasawa et al,[28] after a mean follow-up of 7.7 years, 53% of patients were asymptomatic and 29% of patients were significantly improved. Up to 80% of patients who presented with ischemic symptoms in the study of Okada et al[29] were asymptomatic after a mean follow-up period of 5.6 years.

Surgical results for patients presenting with the hemorrhagic form of the disease are mixed with 28% (39/138) of nonoperated patients in the study of Fujii et al[30] suffering rehemorrhage as compared with 19% (29/152) of patients treated with bypass. Although 67% of patients had a good long-term recovery over a mean follow-up of 7.8 years, 21% of patients in the study of Okada et al[29] died from rehemorrhage despite a bypass. In contrast Kawaguchi et al[31] reported no rehemorrhage or strokes over a mean period of 7.7 years after an STA-MCA bypass **(Table 15.5).**

The use of a direct bypass has also been reported in the pediatric population. Golby et al[32] reported a small series of 12 pediatric patients treated with direct bypass in which 83% had resolution of their symptoms, with the remaining 17% demonstrating some symptomatic improvement. Although this approach may be appropriate in selected patients, there are potential limitations to the widespread application of this technique to the entire pediatric population. Efficacy of direct bypass may be reduced by proximal stenosis that limits the distribution of blood supply from the single revascularized MCA branch. Temporary occlusion of an MCA branch during the procedure may interfere with already existent leptomeningeal collaterals, increasing the risk of perioperative stroke. The execution of the anastomosis may be tech-

nically impossible in small children with minuscule STA branches. Importantly, even if the bypass can be completed, the blood supply may be limited by the small caliber of the vessel, making long-term patency and adequacy of supply to the cortex questionable.

Indirect Revascularization

Although adults are usually good candidates for direct anastomosis, we routinely employ a version of indirect revascularization—pial synangiosis—in our pediatric moyamoya cases.[3] Of note, we have also had success with the application of this indirect technique to selected adult patients as well.

A wide variety of indirect approaches to revascularization have been described **(Table 15.6).** Methods include omental transposition, bur holes, encephalomyosynangiosis (EMS), encephalogaleo(periosteal)synangiosis (EGPS), encephaloduroarteriomyosynangiosis (EDAMS), and encephaloduroarteriosynangiosis (EDAS), including a variant utilized at Children's Hospital Boston: pial synangiosis. In all cases, the general principle centers on the concept of placing vascularized tissue supplied by the external carotid in contact with the brain, allowing for the ingrowth of new blood vessels into the cortex. A large meta-analysis of revascularization surgery for pediatric moyamoya reported the use of indirect procedures in 73% of cases (plus 23% combined with direct anastomosis).[33] Of 669 hemispheres treated, 98% were stable or improved whereas only 2% were worse at follow-up. Evidence of graft-derived revascularization was demonstrated radiographically in 83% of cases. These indirect approaches are generally less invasive, require shorter operative times, can be used for any vascular distribution, and do not require temporary vessel clamping—all of which likely contribute to reduced complications with this approach.

Since the serendipitous finding of neovascularization through a bur hole made for a ventriculostomy in a moyamoya patient, several studies have demonstrated their potential efficacy in treatment of moyamoya disease.[34,35] Kawaguchi et al[34]

Table 15.5 Surgical Series of Moyamoya Disease Treated by STA-MCA Anastomosis

Study	Pts	Mean Age (Years)	Presenting Sx	Follow-Up (Years)	Outcome
Golby et al, 1999[32]	12	Ped	42% stroke 25% TIA 25% TIA + stroke 8% seizure	2.9	83% Sx resolved 17% improved Sx
Hanggi et al, 2008[45]	9	36	89% TIA 11% Hem		67% improved 22% same 11% worse
Karasawa et al, 1978[28]	17	10 Ped 7 adult	88% ischemic 12% ischemic + SAH	1.3–4.1	53% ASx 29% significantly improved 6% slightly improved 12% same
Kawaguchi et al, 2000[31]	6	43	100% Hem	7.7	100% same/improved 0% repeat stroke/bleed
Mesiwala et al, 2008[46]	39	34	85% ischemic 13% Hem 3% ASx	3.6	95% same/improved 20% rebleed if Hem presentation 19% repeat TIA 5% mortality (1 MI, 2 remote bleeds)
Okada et al, 1998[29]	15	39	67% TIA 20% RIND 13% stroke	5.6	80% ASx 7% IPH—recovered 7% Mod disabled from initial insult 7% mortality (IPH)
Okada et al, 1998[29]	15	42	100% Hem	7.8	67% good recovery 14% moderately disabled 21% mortality (IPH)

Abbreviations: ASx, asymptomatic; Hem, hemorrhage; IPH, intraparenchymal hemorrhage; Pts, patients; RIND, reversible ischemic neurologic deficit; Sx, symptoms; TIA, transient ischemic attack.

Table 15.6 Modern Indirect Revascularization Methods

Method	Description	Advantages	Shortcomings
EDAS	STA with galeal cuff laid on cortical surface	Relative ease compared with direct bypass Known long-term efficacy	Unclear efficacy for ACA territory Suboptimal use of all potential collateralization sources
Pial synangiosis	EDAS + wide opening of arachnoid and suturing of STA to cortical surface	Opening of arachnoid and pial suturing allowing for improved revascularization	Unclear efficacy for ACA territory
EMS	Temporalis muscle laid over exposed cortex following arachnoid opening	Expedient No arterial dissection required Patients lacking a good donor vessel	Large craniotomy Seizures Mass effect
EDAMS	Combination of EDAS and EMS	Theoretical combined effects	Data has not clearly shown synergistic results
EGPS	Galea and periosteum inserted inter-hemispherically and sutured to dura	Potential ACA territory revascularization	Technically challenge with unclear efficacy for MCA territory revascularization
Bur holes	Multiple bur holes made	Simplicity Safety Potential ACA/PCA territory revascularization	Variable efficacy Pseudomeningoceles

Abbreviations: ACA, anterior cerebral artery; EDAMS, encephaloduroarteriomyosynangiosis; EDAS, encephaloduroarteriosynangiosis; EPGS, encephalogaleo(periosteal)synangiosis; EMS, encephalomyosynangiosis; MCA, middle cerebral artery; PCA, posterior cerebral artery; STA, superficial temporal artery.

reported the use of multiple (one to four) bur holes employed in 10 adults. All 10 patients demonstrated symptomatic improvement over a mean follow-up of 2.9 years without recurrent ischemic or hemorrhagic events.[34] Sainte-Rose et al[35] reported the use of multiple bur holes (10 to 24 per hemisphere) in 14 patients with ischemic symptoms; no patients had recurrent ischemic attacks over a mean follow-up of 4.2 years. Five of 18 procedures were complicated by pseudomeningocele formation, though only one required lumbar drainage.

Encephalomyosynangiosis (EMS) entails the placement of the temporalis muscle directly over exposed cortex following opening of the arachnoid. The dura is then sewn over the temporalis muscle. Limitations to this approach include a requisite large craniotomy, potential postoperative seizures, and mass effect. Takeuchi et al[36] reported the use of EMS in 10 pediatric patients. Four of seven patients with preoperative TIAs had no recurrence symptoms, whereas the remaining three had a significant reduction in the frequency of their TIAs. Irikura et al[37] performed EMS on 24 hemispheres in 13 pediatric cases. At least one third of the MCA distribution demonstrated vascularization in 75% of cases.

Encephalogaleo(periosteal)synangiosis (EGPS) is an analogous approach to EMS to facilitate ACA territory revascularization.[38] An S-shaped scalp incision is made 2 cm anterior to the coronal suture, and the galea and periosteum are dissected and incised in a zigzag pattern. A craniotomy is turned crossing the superior sagittal sinus, and the dura is incised separately over both hemispheres. The apex of the galea is then inserted as deeply as possible (with care taken not to injure bridging veins) and sutured to the dura. Kim et al[39] compared EDAS alone to the combination of EDAS and EGPS in 159 pediatric moyamoya cases. Patients undergoing EGPS demonstrated superior ACA territory vascularization (79% versus 16% of patients with at least one-third filling of the ACA territory) and favorable ACA territory outcome (62% versus 36%). However, overall clinical outcomes were not statistically significantly different between the two groups (85% with good outcomes for EDAS and EGPS compared with 74% for EDAS alone).

Encephaloduroarteriosynangiosis (EDAS) entails dissection of a branch of the STA with a galeal cuff, followed by craniotomy and dural opening to lay the vessel on the cortical surface. The galeal cuff is then sutured to the dural edges. Multiple surgical series have demonstrated the safety and durable reduction in symptoms in patients treated with this technique (**Table 15.7**). Radiographically, up to 65% of patients had over two thirds of their MCA territory revascularized via EDAS.[3]

Encephaloduroarteriomyosynangiosis (EDAMS) is a combination of EDAS and EMS. Some authors make additional cuts in the dura and fold the flaps inward to contact the cortex, promoting middle meningeal artery involvement in the neovascularization.[40] Kinugasa et al[40] employed EDAMS in 17 patients (28 hemispheres), reporting asymptomatic clinical outcomes in 47%, symptomatic improvement in 29%, unchanged clinical status in 18%, and worsened clinical status in 6% over a mean 3-year follow-up.

Our modification to EDAS, pial synangiosis, was recently reported for a large series of 143 pediatric patients with moyamoya.[3] We begin by marking out the course of the posterior parietal branch of the STA that is selected because most of the MCA distribution lies beneath it. We use the microscope immediately in the arterial dissection. The incision is made down to subcutaneous tissue directly over the vessel at its distal point. After the artery is identified, it is dissected with a pediatric hemostat and fine bipolar cautery to divide the side branches. A cuff of periadventitial tissue is maintained along the course of the artery, which is useful in suturing the vessel to the cortex and appears to facilitate additional ingrowth of collaterals. The temporalis muscle is opened in a cruciate fashion, a large craniotomy is turned, and the dura is opened into six separate flaps and then retracted with care taken to preserve middle meningeal collaterals. The arachnoid is opened widely over as much of the exposure as possible under high power. This aspect of the operation is crucial and serves the dual purpose of removing a mechanical barrier to the ingrowth of new vessels while also increasing exposure of the graft to growth factors known to be in the cerebrospinal fluid. The STA is then fixed to the cortical surface by four to six interrupted 10-0 nylon sutures (**Fig. 15.6**). This series of sutures minimizes graft movement, further encouraging collateral development. The dura is then laid on the brain surface without suturing and covered with saline-soaked Gelfoam. This allows collateralization via cut edges of the dura. The bone flap is replaced (leaving wide openings for the entry and exit of the STA), and the temporalis muscle is approximated in the axial plane only to avoid STA compression (**Fig. 15.7**). Meticulous hemostasis is critical.

Postoperatively, patients are kept well hydrated, and pain is carefully controlled to minimize potential hyperventilation from crying. Aspirin is restarted on the first postoperative day. Notably, the one patient in our pial synangiosis series that did not receive postoperative aspirin had an ischemic event.[3] Similarly, in the direct revascularization series of Golby et al,[32] a group of patients whose TIAs resumed after aspirin cessation had resolution of their symptoms once the medication was restarted.

In our 2004 report of 143 pediatric patients undergoing pial synangiosis, 63% of patients were independent without significant disability whereas only 2% of patients died over a mean follow-up of 5.1 years.[3] Notably, functional status at the time of surgery was a key determinant of long-term functional status, as all patients with presenting Glasgow Outcome Scale (GOS) scores of zero remain at zero at follow-up. Overall, only 3% of patients exhibited a decline in their neurologic status after surgery, whereas the prevalence of patients having strokes decreased from 67% preoperatively to 7.7% postoperatively. The long-term rate of stroke was 5% among patients with at least 5 years of follow-up. Stratified results for patients with moyamoya syndrome and Down syndrome and sickle cell disease[12] demonstrate similar benefits of pial synangiosis.

Combined Direct and Indirect Revascularization Methods

Multiple surgical series in the literature have reported on the efficacy of combining direct and indirect revascularization

Table 15.7 Encephaloduroarteriosynangiosis in the Treatment of Pediatric Moyamoya Disease

Study	Pts	Presenting Sx	Mean Follow-Up (Years)	Outcome	Revascularization*
Han et al, 1997[18]**	17	46% CVA 46% Hem 8% TIA	1	20% ASx 47% minor Sx 13% persistent Sx 13% same 7% worse	
Imaizumi et al, 1998[50]	10	70% TIA 30% non-TIA	18.8	40% ASx 10% Occ TIA/HA 10% mild disabled 10% Mod disabled 2% severely disabled 10% dead	90% effective
Isono et al, 2002[47]	11		8.3+	73% ASx 27% mild-mod deficits 0% postop CVA	92% "good"
Kim et al, 2007[17]	12	67% TIA + CVA 17% TIA 17% CVA	0.3–5	59% ASx 8% minimal Sx 25% improved but with Sx 8% same/unchanged	38% grade A 50% grade B 13% grade C
Kim et al, 2002[39]	67	58% TIA + CVA 28% TIA 8% CVA 6% Hem	3.8	40% ASx 34% Sx gone, preop deficit 19% Sx less frequent 7% same/worse 10% ischemic event	83% grade A+B 17% grade C
Matsushima et al, 1992[41]	10	85% TIA 15% CVA		23% ASx 46% improved 31% same	15% grade A 46% grade B 38% grade C
Nakashima et al, 1997[48]	41		11	62% ASx 23% improved 15% same	45% excellent 40% moderate 15% localized
Olds et al, 1987[14]	10		3.5	40% ASx 50% same/improved 10% worse—TIAs	
Scott et al, 2004[3]***	143	68% CVA 43% TIA Seizure 6% HA 6% Chorea 4% ASx 4% Hem 3%	5.1	63% without Sig disability 9% mild deficits 10% Mod deficits 4% Mod-severe deficits 1% died 3% Worse GOS than preop	65% grade A 25% grade B 10% grade C
Tripathi et al, 2007[49]	8	50% 2+ CVA 25% 1 CVA 13% TIAs 13% seizures	2	100% excellent recovery 0% CVA/TIA	

Abbreviations: Asx, asymptomatic; CVA, cerebrovascular accident (stroke); GOS, Glasgow Outcome Scale score; HA, headache; Hem, hemorrhage; Mod, moderate; Pts, patients; Sig, significant; TIA, transient ischemia attack.

*Grade A, more than two-thirds middle cerebral artery (MCA) territory filling; grade B, one- to two-thirds MCA territory filling; grade C, less than one-third MCA territory filling.

**Adult cases were also incorporated.

***The pial synangiosis method was employed.

methods for the treatment of moyamoya (**Table 15.8**). In the study of Karasawa et al,[16] 104 patients were followed over a mean period of 9.6 years after direct bypass and EMS, with 83% having good outcomes. Multiple small series have reported no ischemic events after the perioperative period following an STA-MCA bypass combined with EMS.[41–43]

Closer scrutiny of bypass flow results, however, demonstrates that many pediatric patients derive most of their

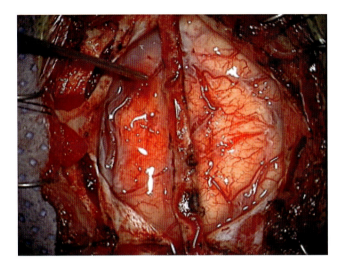

Fig. 15.6 Pial synangiosis. The STA is fixed to the cortical surface by interrupted 10-0 nylon sutures.

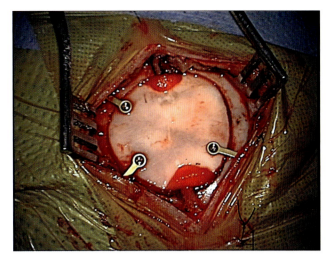

Fig. 15.7 Pial synangiosis. The bone flap is replaced, leaving wide openings for the entry and exit of the STA, and the temporalis muscle will be approximated in the axial plane only to avoid STA compression.

Table 15.8 Surgical Series Employing Combined Direct and Indirect Revascularization Techniques

Study	Pts	Age	Presenting Sx	Modalities	Mean Follow-Up (Years)	Periop Events	Outcome
Czabanka et al, 2008[44]	20	10 Ped 10 Adult	TIAs	STA-MCA EMS	2		67% improved 33% same
Fujimura et al, 2008[51]	9	Ped	56% TIA 44% CVA, TIA	STA-MCA EMS	2	6% Periop TIA 6% silent CVA	By hemisphere: 82% ASx 18% Reduction in Sx
Fujimura et al, 2009[27]	58	Adult		STA-MCA EMS	2	29% TIA* 7% HA*	All improved
Houkin et al, 1996[19]	35	Adult	69% Hem 31% ischemic	STA-MCA EDAMS	6.4		13% Hem rebled 18% ischemic bled No recurrent ischemia
Karasawa et al, 1992[16]	104	Ped	55% TIA 42% CVA 3% other	STA-MCA EMS	9.6	2% CVA	45% complete recovery 38% marked improvement 12% slight improvement 3% no change 2% worse
Kim et al, 2006[38]	8	Mixed	38% TIA 25% VF deficit 25% seizures 12% HA	STA-MCA EDAMS	2	12% TIA	75% excellent 25% fair due to preop Sx
Matsushima et al, 1992[41]	6	Ped	100% TIA	STA-MCA EMS		17% TIAs	All ASx
Mizoi et al, 1996[42]	23	Mixed		STA-MCA EMS	3.4	9% TIAs	No events in follow-up
Sakamoto et al, 1997[43]	10	Ped	100% TIA	Bilat double STA-MCA EMS	4	40% TIA	No events in follow-up
Suzuki et al, 1997[15]	38	Ped	82% TIA/seize 11% Chorea 3% HA 4% Other	STA-MCA EDAMS EMS Bur holes		3% CVA	81% TIA gone in 1 yr 19% TIA less frequent 75% choreoathetosis gone

Abbreviations: ASx, asymptomatic; CVA, cerebrovascular accident (stroke); Hem, hemorrhage; Pts, patients; Sx, symptoms; TIA, transient ischemic attack; VF, visual field.

*From symptomatic cerebral hyperperfusion.

revascularization from the indirect bypass, whereas adult patients tend to derive their supply from the direct bypass. The study of Czabanka et al[44] reported poor direct bypass flow in 60% of pediatric patients but good or moderate indirect bypass (EMS) revascularization in 100% of patients. In contrast, 53% of adults had poor revascularization via their EMS. Houkin et al[19] reported effective flow via direct bypass in 90% of adult patients; effective revascularization via EDAMS was only seen in 38% of adult patients. In contrast, 100% of pediatric EDAMS afforded effective revascularization, in contrast to 68% of direct bypasses performed in this population. Mizoi et al[42] demonstrated that the effectiveness of indirect procedures declined with advancing age; no patients older than 40 in this study had good collateral formation via indirect methods, in contrast to 64% of pediatric patients. On the other hand, all patients 30 years of age or older had medium or high flow through their direct bypasses, in contrast to only 54% of pediatric patients having medium flow (the remainder had poor flow).

◆ Conclusion

Moyamoya is an increasingly recognized cause of stroke in both children and adults. Characteristic radiographic findings confirm the diagnosis, and recognition of the disease early in its course with prompt institution of therapy is critical to providing the best outcome for patients. Revascularization surgery appears to be effective in preventing stroke in most patients with moyamoya. We have found pial synangiosis to be an effective approach for revascularization in pediatric moyamoya disease, whereas we employ both direct STA-MCA bypass and pial synangiosis for adults.

References

1. Takeuchi K, Shimizu K. Hypoplasia of the bilateral internal carotid arteries. Brain Nerve. 1957;9:37–43
2. Suzuki J, Takaku A. Cerebrovascular "moyamoya" disease. Disease showing abnormal net-like vessels in base of brain. Arch Neurol 1969;20:288–299
3. Scott RM, Smith JL, Robertson RL, Madsen JR, Soriano SG, Rockoff MA. Long-term outcome in children with moyamoya syndrome after cranial revascularization by pial synangiosis. J Neurosurg 2004;100(2, Suppl Pediatrics)142–149
4. Baba T, Houkin K, Kuroda S. Novel epidemiological features of moyamoya disease. J Neurol Neurosurg Psychiatry 2008;79:900–904
5. Kuriyama S, Kusaka Y, Fujimura M, et al. Prevalence and clinicoepidemiological features of moyamoya disease in Japan: findings from a nationwide epidemiological survey. Stroke 2008;39:42–47
6. Han DH, Kwon OK, Byun BJ, et al; Korean Society for Cerebrovascular Disease. A co-operative study: clinical characteristics of 334 Korean patients with moyamoya disease treated at neurosurgical institutes (1976–1994). Acta Neurochir (Wien) 2000;142:1263–1273, discussion 1273–1274
7. Hung CC, Tu YK, Su CF, Lin LS, Shih CJ. Epidemiological study of moyamoya disease in Taiwan. Clin Neurol Neurosurg 1997;99(Suppl 2):S23–S25
8. Wetjen NM, Garell PC, Stence NV, Loftus CM. Moyamoya disease in the midwestern United States. Neurosurg Focus 1998;5:e1
9. Uchino K, Johnston SC, Becker KJ, Tirschwell DL. Moyamoya disease in Washington State and California. Neurology 2005;65:956–958
10. Yonekawa Y, Ogata N, Kaku Y, Taub E, Imhof HG. Moyamoya disease in Europe, past and present status. Clin Neurol Neurosurg 1997;99(Suppl 2):S58–S60
11. Wakai K, Tamakoshi A, Ikezaki K, et al. Epidemiological features of moyamoya disease in Japan: findings from a nationwide survey. Clin Neurol Neurosurg 1997;99(Suppl 2):S1–S5
12. Smith ER, McClain CD, Heeney M, Scott RM. Pial synangiosis in patients with moyamoya syndrome and sickle cell anemia: perioperative management and surgical outcome. Neurosurg Focus 2009;26:E10
13. Kurokawa T, Tomita S, Ueda K, et al. Prognosis of occlusive disease of the circle of Willis (moyamoya disease) in children. Pediatr Neurol 1985;1:274–277
14. Olds MV, Griebel RW, Hoffman HJ, Craven M, Chuang S, Schutz H. The surgical treatment of childhood moyamoya disease. J Neurosurg 1987;66:675–680
15. Suzuki Y, Negoro M, Shibuya M, Yoshida J, Negoro T, Watanabe K. Surgical treatment for pediatric moyamoya disease: use of the superficial temporal artery for both areas supplied by the anterior and middle cerebral arteries. Neurosurgery 1997;40:324–329, discussion 329–330
16. Karasawa J, Touho H, Ohnishi H, Miyamoto S, Kikuchi H. Long-term follow-up study after extracranial-intracranial bypass surgery for anterior circulation ischemia in childhood moyamoya disease. J Neurosurg 1992;77:84–89
17. Kim DS, Kang SG, Yoo DS, Huh PW, Cho KS, Park CK. Surgical results in pediatric moyamoya disease: angiographic revascularization and the clinical results. Clin Neurol Neurosurg 2007;109:125–131
18. Han DH, Nam DH, Oh CW. Moyamoya disease in adults: characteristics of clinical presentation and outcome after encephalo-duro-arterio-synangiosis. Clin Neurol Neurosurg 1997;99(Suppl 2):S151–S155
19. Houkin K, Kamiyama H, Abe H, Takahashi A, Kuroda S. Surgical therapy for adult moyamoya disease. Can surgical revascularization prevent the recurrence of intracerebral hemorrhage? Stroke 1996;27:1342–1346
20. Ikezaki K, Fukui M, Inamura T, Kinukawa N, Wakai K, Ono Y. The current status of the treatment for hemorrhagic type moyamoya disease based on a 1995 nationwide survey in Japan. Clin Neurol Neurosurg 1997;99(Suppl 2):S183–S186
21. Kobayashi E, Saeki N, Oishi H, Hirai S, Yamaura A. Long-term natural history of hemorrhagic moyamoya disease in 42 patients. J Neurosurg 2000;93:976–980
22. Yoshida Y, Yoshimoto T, Shirane R, Sakurai Y. Clinical course, surgical management, and long-term outcome of moyamoya patients with rebleeding after an episode of intracerebral hemorrhage: An extensive follow-Up study. Stroke 1999;30:2272–2276
23. Saeki N, Nakazaki S, Kubota M, et al. Hemorrhagic type moyamoya disease. Clin Neurol Neurosurg 1997;99(Suppl 2):S196–S201
24. Kuroda S, Ishikawa T, Houkin K, Nanba R, Hokari M, Iwasaki Y. Incidence and clinical features of disease progression in adult moyamoya disease. Stroke 2005;36:2148–2153
25. Hallemeier CL, Rich KM, Grubb RL Jr, et al. Clinical features and outcome in North American adults with moyamoya phenomenon. Stroke 2006;37:1490–1496
26. Kuroda S, Hashimoto N, Yoshimoto T, Iwasaki Y; Research Committee on Moyamoya Disease in Japan. Radiological findings, clinical course, and outcome in asymptomatic moyamoya disease: results of multicenter survey in Japan. Stroke 2007;38:1430–1435
27. Fujimura M, Mugikura S, Kaneta T, Shimizu H, Tominaga T. Incidence and risk factors for symptomatic cerebral hyperperfusion after superficial temporal artery-middle cerebral artery anastomosis in patients with moyamoya disease. Surg Neurol 2009;71:442–447
28. Karasawa J, Kikuchi H, Furuse S, Kawamura J, Sakaki T. Treatment of moyamoya disease with STA-MCA anastomosis. J Neurosurg 1978;49:679–688
29. Okada Y, Shima T, Nishida M, Yamane K, Yamada T, Yamanaka C. Effectiveness of superficial temporal artery-middle cerebral artery anastomosis in adult moyamoya disease: cerebral hemodynamics and clinical course in ischemic and hemorrhagic varieties. Stroke 1998;29:625–630
30. Fujii K, Ikezaki K, Irikura K, Miyasaka Y, Fukui M. The efficacy of bypass surgery for the patients with hemorrhagic moyamoya disease. Clin Neurol Neurosurg 1997;99(2, Suppl 2)S194–S195
31. Kawaguchi S, Okuno S, Sakaki T. Effect of direct arterial bypass on the prevention of future stroke in patients with the hemorrhagic variety of moyamoya disease. J Neurosurg 2000;93:397–401
32. Golby AJ, Marks MP, Thompson RC, Steinberg GK. Direct and combined revascularization in pediatric moyamoya disease. Neurosurgery 1999;45:50–58, discussion 58–60
33. Fung LW, Thompson D, Ganesan V. Revascularisation surgery for paediatric moyamoya: a review of the literature. Childs Nerv Syst 2005;21:358–364
34. Kawaguchi T, Fujita S, Hosoda K, et al. Multiple burr-hole operation for adult moyamoya disease. J Neurosurg 1996;84:468–476
35. Sainte-Rose C, Oliveira R, Puget S, et al. Multiple bur hole surgery for the treatment of moyamoya disease in children. J Neurosurg 2006;105(6, Suppl)437–443

36. Takeuchi S, Tsuchida T, Kobayashi K, et al. Treatment of moyamoya disease by temporal muscle graft 'encephalo-myo-synangiosis'. Childs Brain 1983;10:1–15
37. Irikura K, Miyasaka Y, Kurata A, et al. The effect of encephalo-myo-synangiosis on abnormal collateral vessels in childhood moyamoya disease. Neurol Res 2000;22:341–346
38. Kim DS, Yoo DS, Huh PW, Kang SG, Cho KS, Kim MC. Combined direct anastomosis and encephaloduroarteriogaleosynangiosis using inverted superficial temporal artery-galeal flap and superficial temporal artery-galeal pedicle in adult moyamoya disease. Surg Neurol 2006;66:389–394, discussion 395
39. Kim SK, Wang KC, Kim IO, Lee DS, Cho BK. Combined encephaloduroarteriosynangiosis and bifrontal encephalogaleo(periosteal)synangiosis in pediatric moyamoya disease. Neurosurgery 2002;50:88–96
40. Kinugasa K, Mandai S, Kamata I, Sugiu K, Ohmoto T. Surgical treatment of moyamoya disease: operative technique for encephalo-duro-arterio-myo-synangiosis, its follow-up, clinical results, and angiograms. Neurosurgery 1993;32:527–531
41. Matsushima T, Inoue T, Suzuki SO, Fujii K, Fukui M, Hasuo K. Surgical treatment of moyamoya disease in pediatric patients—comparison between the results of indirect and direct revascularization procedures. Neurosurgery 1992;31:401–405
42. Mizoi K, Kayama T, Yoshimoto T, Nagamine Y. Indirect revascularization for moyamoya disease: is there a beneficial effect for adult patients? Surg Neurol 1996;45:541–548, discussion 548–549
43. Sakamoto H, Kitano S, Yasui T, et al. Direct extracranial-intracranial bypass for children with moyamoya disease. Clin Neurol Neurosurg 1997; 99(2, Suppl 2)S128–S133
44. Czabanka M, Vajkoczy P, Schmiedek P, Horn P. Age-dependent revascularization patterns in the treatment of moyamoya disease in a European patient population. Neurosurg Focus 2009;26:E9
45. Hanggi D, Mehrkens JH, Schmid-Elsaesser R, Steiger HJ. Results of direct and indirect revascularization for adult European patients with Moyamoya angiopathy. Acta Neurochir Suppl (Wien) 2008;103:119–122
46. Mesiwala AH, Sviri G, Fatemi N, Britz GW, Newell DW. Long-term outcome of superficial temporal artery-middle cerebral artery bypass for patients with moyamoya disease in the US. Neurosurg Focus 2008;24:E15
47. Isono M, Ishii K, Kamida T, Inoue R, Fujiki M, Kobayashi H. Long-term outcomes of pediatric moyamoya disease treated by encephalo-duro-arterio-synangiosis. Pediatr Neurosurg 2002;36:14–21
48. Nakashima H, Meguro T, Kawada S, Hirotsune N, Ohmoto T. Long-term results of surgically treated moyamoya disease. Clin Neurol Neurosurg 1997;99(2, Suppl 2)S156–S161
49. Tripathi P, Tripathi V, Naik RJ, Patel JM. Moya Moya cases treated with encephaloduroarteriosynangiosis. Indian Pediatr 2007;44:123–127
50. Imaizumi T, Hayashi K, Saito K, Osawa M, Fukuyama Y. Long-term outcomes of pediatric moyamoya disease monitored to adulthood. Pediatr Neurol 1998;18:321–325
51. Fujimura M, Kaneta T, Tominaga T. Efficacy of superficial temporal artery-middle cerebral artery anastomosis with routine postoperative cerebral blood flow measurement during the acute stage in childhood moyamoya disease. Childs Nerv Syst 2008;24:827–832

16

Craniectomy Rationale: Outcomes Data and Surgical Techniques

Sameer A. Sheth, Sunil A. Sheth, and Christopher S. Ogilvy

Pearls

- Space-occupying edema leading to transtentorial herniation is the leading cause of death immediately following massive cerebral infarction.
- Although maximal cerebral edema is thought to occur around day 2 to day 4, fatal cerebral herniation can occur as early as within 24 hours of ischemia.
- According to the best class I data currently available, decompressive craniectomy reduces the risk of mortality by 50%, and the risk of severe disability or death by 42%, compared with the best medical therapy, for patients <60 years old undergoing surgery <48 hours after stroke ictus.
- The data do not support exclusion of patients from surgical consideration based on laterality of infarct or presence/absence of aphasia
- Decompressive craniectomy should include a large craniectomy (≥12 cm anterior-posterior) and duraplasty, with the possible additional inclusion of an anterior temporal lobectomy

◆ Epidemiology and Natural History

Massive strokes producing life-threatening space-occupying edema represent one of the most challenging and fatal neurologic diseases, and comprise 1 to 10% of all ischemic strokes.[1] These infarcts typically involve the majority of the middle cerebral artery (MCA) distribution, with the occasional addition of the anterior (ACA) or posterior (PCA) cerebral artery territories. The malignant edema associated with these events usually reaches a peak 2 to 4 days following the ictus, but can manifest as early as within the first 24 hours[2] (**Fig. 16.1**). Despite optimal medical management in intensive care settings, the mortality rate from strokes of this size is approximately 80%.[3] The distribution of mortality rates is bimodal, with an early peak within the first 3 to 6 days, followed by a second

peak during the 2nd and 3rd weeks after stroke.[4] Mortality during the first peak is primarily due to transtentorial herniation from edema-related increased intracranial pressure (ICP) within a fixed-volume skull. Delayed mortality is often a result of complications related to both hospitalization, such as pneumonia, as well as medical comorbidities, such as myocardial infarction and heart failure.

Given the severity of this disease and the benefit of early intervention, several predictors of progression to malignant edema have been identified, the most important of which is the size of the stroke. An infarct volume greater than 145 cc measured by diffusion-weighted magnetic resonance imaging (MRI) within 14 hours of stroke onset has high sensitivity (100%) and specificity (94%) for predicting progression to life-threatening edema. Combining diffusion-weighted imaging (DWI) with apparent diffusion coefficient (ADC) imaging can increase specificity to almost 100%.[5] Other radiographic and clinical predictors include computed tomography (CT) showing stroke volume >50% of the MCA territory, National Institutes of Health Stroke Scale (NIHSS) >20 on admission, development of nausea/vomiting within 24 hours of onset of infarction, systolic blood pressure ≥180 mm Hg 12 hours after the onset, and a history of hypertension or heart failure.[6,7]

◆ Medical Management of Massive Cerebral Infarction

Massive cerebral infarction is a devastating disease, and patients with this condition require intensive monitoring on an inpatient unit. The guidelines that apply to the care of all patients with ischemic stroke with respect to blood pressure and glucose control, nutrition, and pulmonary embolus prophylaxis are still relevant in these patients. Although medical management is rarely therapeutic for massive cerebral infarc-

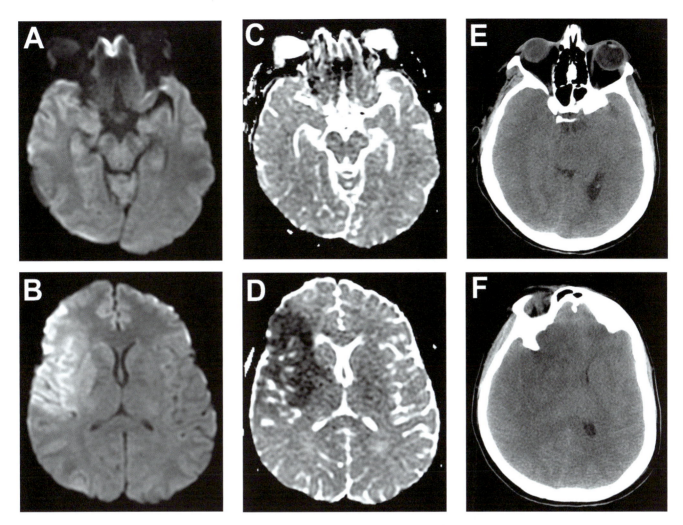

Fig. 16.1 Malignant cerebral edema. A magnetic resonance imaging (MRI) scan is shown of a 31-year-old woman obtained within 1 hour of the development of left face/arm/leg weakness. Diffusion-weighted imaging (DWI) sequence images **(A,B)** and the corresponding apparent diffusion coefficient (ADC) images **(C,D)** demonstrate a right middle cerebral artery (MCA) distribution infarct with a volume of greater than 50% of the MCA territory. There is no midline shift or uncal herniation. Despite aggressive medical management, malignant edema developed, with a consequent rapid decline in neurologic exam. A computed tomography (CT) scan obtained 19 hours after stroke onset shows evidence of malignant edema and consequent midline shift and uncal herniation **(E,F).**

tion, several measures can be taken to treat increased ICP through minimally invasive means (**Table 16.1**).

The mainstays of medical therapy include control of agitation and pain, and osmotic therapy with mannitol and hypertonic saline.[8] Although mannitol is widely used, class I data on its efficacy in reducing morbidity and mortality after stroke is not available.[9] Hypertonic saline, however, has been shown to reduce ICP, and carries the additional benefit of counteracting mannitol-induced hyponatremia, as often results from multiple administrations of the osmotic diuretic. Glycerol has also been used as an osmotic agent in the treatment of elevated ICP. Barbiturates reduce cerebral metabolism, and the resultant decrease in cerebral blood flow may theoretically decrease edema. The decrease in ICP is usually short-lived, however, and often carries with it a deleterious decrease in cerebral perfusion pressure (CPP). Thus, barbiturates should be used with caution in stroke patients.

Table 16.1 Medical Management for Malignant Cerebral Edema

Therapies with some evidence of benefit
Mannitol
Hypertonic saline
Barbiturates
Hypothermia

Therapies with little evidence of benefit
Steroids
Hyperventilation

Additional complementary measures have been tested to aid in the treatment of raised ICP, although data on these techniques are varied. Hyperventilation is a commonly used procedure aimed at decreasing ICP by inducing cerebral vasoconstriction to reduce cerebral blood flow. This method has been successful in reducing ICP acutely, but its effects are not typically long-lasting and have not resulted in improvements in neurologic outcome or mortality for stroke patients, possibly due to the attendant decrease in CPP. Other medical interventions include alkalinizing cerebrospinal fluid with tromethamine and reducing vasogenic edema with corticosteroids. Although these therapies have shown some benefit in select patient populations, they lack strong clinical evidence and so cannot be advocated for all stroke patients. Mild to moderate hypothermia has shown some early positive results, and although further characterization of the technique and its protocol are required, this maneuver may represent a viable therapy in the near future.[9]

◆ Evidence for the Role of Decompressive Craniectomy

Effect on Mortality and Functional Outcome

The employment of trephinations or craniectomies to relieve brain swelling is among the oldest practices in the history of neurosurgery. Following its increasingly common use in the management of severe head trauma, decompressive craniectomy (DC) was first used to treat ischemic stroke-related malignant edema in the 1970s and early 1980s.[10–12] For the following two decades, several retrospective uncontrolled series were published addressing the question of whether DC provided benefit. Compared with the 80% mortality described for best medical therapy, these studies uniformly showed lower mortality rates, ranging from 11 to 34% with series including more than four patients. The fraction of patients with a good functional outcome, however, varied widely from 8 to 57% for series including more than four patients.

Gupta et al[13] reviewed studies in the literature from 1970 to 2003 in which data for individual patients were available; they found 13 series with 138 patients. The pooled results demonstrated an overall mortality rate of 24%. They further separated the results into "good" (Barthel Index [BI] ≥60; modified Rankin Scale [mRS] ≤3; or Glasgow Outcome Scale [GOS] ≥4) and "poor" (BI <60; mRS >3; GOS <4) functional outcomes (see **Table 16.2** for an explanation of the outcome scales). With this dichotomization, 42% of all patients experienced a good functional outcome, and 58% experienced a poor outcome, including those who died. Subgroup analyses showed that patient age >50 predicted poor outcome, with 80% poor outcomes in the older group compared with 32% poor outcomes in the age group ≤50. Time between stroke ictus and surgery, presence of uncal herniation signs preoperatively, and laterality did not affect functional prognosis, but the available data for the latter two comparisons were sparse.

One of the larger early series not included in the above review was that of Schwab et al,[14] which included 63 DC

Table 16.2 Measures of Functional Outcome

Modified Rankin Scale (mRS)

0	No symptoms	
1	No significant disability	Able to perform all usual duties and activities
2	Slight disability	Difficulty with some usual activities, but independent with personal affairs
3	Moderate disability	Requiring assistance for walking
4	Moderately severe disability	Requiring assistance for bodily needs
5	Severe disability	Bedridden, incontinent, requiring constant nursing care
6	Death	

Glasgow Outcome Scale (GOS)

1	Death	
2	Persistent vegetative state	Unresponsive, no interaction with environment
3	Severe disability	Follows commands, unable to live independently
4	Moderate disability	Lives independently, unable to return to work or school
5	Good recovery	Able to return to work or school

Barthel Index (BI)*

0–10	Feeding	Unable (0), requires assistance (5), independent (10)
0–5	Bathing	Dependent (0), independent (5)
0–5	Grooming	Requires assistance with face/hair/teeth care (0), independent (5)
0–10	Dressing	Dependent (0), requires assistance (5), independent (10)
0–10	Bowels	Incontinent (0), occasional accident (5), continent (10)
0–10	Bladder	Incontinent/catheterized (0), occasional accident (5), continent (10)
0–10	Toilet use	Dependent (0), requires assistance (5), independent (10)
0–15	Transfers (bed to chair)	Unable (0), major help (5), minor help (10), independent (15)
0–15	Mobility (on level surfaces)	Immobile or <50 yards (0), wheelchair independent (5), walks with one person's help (10), independent (15)
0–10	Stairs	Unable (0), requires assistance (5), independent (10)

* Total score is the sum of the subcategories.

patients. The authors reported an overall mortality of 27%, and relatively good functional outcomes, with a mean BI score of 65. They additionally found that surgery within the first 24 hours after stroke led to a reduced mortality of 16%, compared with 34% if surgery was performed after 24 hours. Within the early surgery group, only 13% had signs of uncal herniation, compared with 75% in the late surgery group.

To answer persistent questions about the role of DC and the prognostic factors affecting patient selection, three randomized controlled trials were initiated in Europe in the mid-2000s. The DECIMAL (Decompressive Craniectomy in Malignant Middle Cerebral Artery Infarcts) trial was initiated in France,[15] the DESTINY (Decompressive Surgery for the Treatment of Malignant Infarction of the Middle Cerebral Artery) trial in Germany,[16] and the HAMLET (Hemicraniectomy After Middle Cerebral Artery Infarction With Life-Threatening Edema Trial) in the Netherlands.[17] These trials enrolled patients 18 to 55 or 60 years of age with a unilateral stroke occupying at least two thirds or 145 cc of the MCA distribution. Patients were randomized to receive either DC or best medical therapy, including all of the management options discussed in the previous section.

Both DECIMAL and DESTINY were aborted prematurely in early 2006 when a preliminary analysis demonstrated significant reduction in mortality in the surgical arm. Rather than subject further patients to the unnecessary risk of randomization, data from these two studies, along with the patients enrolled to that point in HAMLET, were pooled for analysis, a decision facilitated by the trials' largely similar design. By that time, DECIMAL had enrolled 38 patients, DESTINY 32 patients, and HAMLET 23 patients. In the pooled data ($N = 93$), a total of 42 patients were treated medically and 51 surgically. Mortality was 71% in the medical arm compared with 22% in the surgical arm, a significant absolute risk reduction of 50%.[18]

In terms of the functional outcome of survivors, surgery resulted in a larger fraction of patients with only slight disability (mRS 2) than did medical management (14% versus 2%), but also produced a larger number of survivors with moderately severe disability (mRS 4; 31% versus 2%). Therefore surgery resulted in a significant absolute risk reduction of death or severe disability (mRS >4) of 51%, from 76% to 25%. But because of the large number of DC survivors with mRS 4, the trials did not individually show a significant reduction in the risk of moderately severe disability or worse (mRS >3). In the pooled data, however, there was a small but significant absolute risk reduction of mRS >3 related to surgery of 23%, from 79% to 57%.[18]

The HAMLET trial continued to enroll patients well into 2007, and results were published in early 2009.[19] Of the 64 patients enrolled, 32 underwent DC, and 32 were treated medically. Again, a significant absolute risk reduction of 38% for mortality was afforded by DC, from 59% for patients treated medically to 22% for patients treated surgically. The functional outcome of survivors in this study was poorer compared with the other two randomized trials. The fraction of patients with moderately severe disability (mRS 4) was higher in the surgical arm (34% versus 16%), as was the fraction of patients with severe disability (mRS 5; 19% versus 0%).

The HAMLET publication also pooled its completed data with that of DESTINY and DECIMAL for a revised aggregate result ($N = 134$). This meta-analysis represents the best class I evidence to date available on this topic. The results confirmed the significant reduction in mortality risk of 50% in patients undergoing DC, from 71% to 21%. Risk for avoiding severe disability or death (mRS >4) was also reduced by 42%, from 75% to 33%. Risk for avoiding an outcome worse than moderately severe disability (mRS >3) was reduced just short of significance, by 16%, from 76% to 60%. All these results are summarized in **Table 16.3**.

Table 16.3 Randomized Controlled Trials of Decompressive Craniectomy for Malignant Edema from Massive Ischemic Stroke

RCT*	Publication	N	Decrease in Mortality (ARR†)	Decrease in Poor Functional Outcome (ARR†)
DECIMAL	Vahedi et al, 2007[15]	38	53%	28% for mRS >3 (NS); 53% for mRS >4
DESTINY	Juttler et al, 2007[16]	32	36%	20% for mRS >3 (NS); 43% for mRS >4
Combined analysis of DECIMAL, DESTINY, and early HAMLET results	Vahedi et al, 2007[18]	92	50%	23% for mRS >3; 51% for mRS >4
HAMLET	Hofmeijer et al, 2009[19]	64	38%	0% for mRS >3 (NS); 19% for mRS >4 (NS)
Combined analysis of DECIMAL, DESTINY, and HAMLET results	Hofmeijer et al, 2009[19]	134	50%	16% for mRS >3 (NS); 42% for mRS >4

Abbreviations: ARR, absolute risk reduction; DECIMAL, Decompressive Craniectomy in Malignant Middle Cerebral Artery Infarcts trial; DESTINY, Decompressive Surgery for the Treatment of Malignant Infarction of the Middle Cerebral Artery trial; HAMLET, Hemicraniectomy After Middle Cerebral Artery Infarction With Life-Threatening Edema Trial; mRS, modified Rankin Scale score; N, number of patients; RCT, randomized controlled trial.

*Two additional trials, HeaDDfirst (Hemicraniectomy and Durotomy Upon Deterioration From Infarction-Related Swelling Trial) and HeMMI (Hemicraniectomy for Malignant MCA Infarcts) were also initiated and are mentioned here for the sake of completeness. The first was aborted after 26 patients enrolled, with results pending, and the second has no available recent update.[30]

†Values are significant ($p < .05$), unless denoted by NS (nonsignificant). All results are 1-year outcomes.

Prognostic Factors Affecting Outcome Following Decompressive Craniectomy

Several prognostic factors have been consistently observed to affect outcome following DC. The early uncontrolled trials were divided on the question of whether earlier surgery leads to improved morbidity and mortality, with some finding a benefit for early surgery[14] and others not.[13] The three randomized trials mentioned above observed a definite benefit for early surgery. In a subgroup analysis of the data mentioned above, they found that the reduced risk of severe disability or death attributable to DC only pertained to patients who underwent surgery within the first 48 hours following stroke ictus. Patients receiving surgery after that time point had outcomes similar to their medically treated counterparts.[19] Explicitly, the absolute risk reduction for mortality was 59% (78% for the medical arm, 19% for the surgical arm) in the early group, compared with an insignificant 8% (36% in the medical arm, 27% in the surgical arm) in the late group.

It may be the case that prognosis is actually related to whether transtentorial herniation has occurred, rather than to an arbitrary number of hours from stroke onset. The randomized trials did not perform a subgroup analysis based on the presence or absence of clinical signs of herniation prior to surgery. One retrospective study of 71 patients compared outcomes in DC patients who received surgery before versus after neurologic deterioration related to herniation.[20] Compared with the late surgery group, the early surgery group had significantly higher Glasgow Coma Scale (GCS) score (11.2 versus 6.6, $p <.05$) and lower rate of anisocoria (0% versus 90%, $p <.01$) preoperatively. Their 6-month follow-up data showed a nonsignificant trend toward reduction in mortality in the early group (19% versus 28%), and a significant improvement in GOS and BI scores. Notably, the difference in time from ictus to surgery between the two groups was insignificant (2.48 days in the early group, 2.76 days in the late group), further suggesting that the important prognostic factor was presence or absence of herniation, rather than absolute time from stroke onset. In another uncontrolled series, patients who underwent "ultra-early" DC within 6 hours of ictus had fewer preoperative signs of herniation compared with patients who underwent surgery after 6 hours, and benefited from significantly lower rates of mortality and higher 6-month BI scores.[21] It is difficult to separate the factors of presence of herniation and absolute timing in the available literature, and the ethical grounds for a new randomized controlled trial poised to evaluate the question seem tenuous, given the well-described benefit of early surgery.

Another prognostic factor for DC survivors that has been well established is the benefit of younger age. Several uncontrolled series demonstrated improved outcomes in patients under the age of 50[13] or 60.[20,22] The randomized trials DECIMAL, DESTINY, and HAMLET excluded patients older than 60, but found that the morbidity and mortality benefit of DC did apply to patients who were 51 to 60 years old.[19]

Several studies have investigated the effect of stroke laterality on functional outcome. Despite the notion that a large dominant hemisphere stroke would produce unsalvageable functional deficit, a difference in prognosis attributable to laterality has not been found. Several series[13,14,20] and the randomized trials[15-19] found no difference in risk based on whether the stroke affected the dominant or nondominant hemisphere.

Summary and Recommendations

There is clear class I evidence for the benefit of early decompressive craniectomy in reducing mortality in patients under 60 years of age with malignant edema secondary to unilateral ischemic stroke, regardless of laterality. Given these data, the United Kingdom nationalized health service has adopted the recommendation that patients <60 years old with MCA infarct volume >145 cc and NIHSS score >15 be referred for DC within 24 hours, and for surgery to be performed within 48 hours.[23] For patients not fulfilling these criteria, the decision should be individualized, bearing in mind that the data suggest poorer outcomes. An algorithm outlining the suggested management for patients with stroke-related malignant cerebral edema is depicted in **Fig. 16.2**. Because of the demonstrated benefit of early surgery, this possibility should be discussed early in the treatment course with families of patients likely to develop life-threatening edema.

The data do not support exclusion of patients from surgical consideration based on laterality of the stroke or the presence or absence of aphasia. Surgery should be performed within approximately 48 hours of stroke onset to maximize the likelihood of benefit. The benefit of early surgery may be related to prevention of neurologic deterioration from transtentorial herniation, but that causality is not clear. The reduction in mortality associated with DC comes at the price of an increased fraction of survivors with moderately severe or severe disability. Whether this trade-off produces an overall improvement in functional outcome depends to a large degree on somewhat subjective divisions of what in reality is a continuum of patient outcomes. This question is further clouded by the lack of consensus regarding the metric with which to assess functional outcome, and how to incorporate the psychological effects of residual functional deficits, which are difficult to characterize.[24] Given the partial trade-off between mortality and functional outcome, a candid discussion incorporating the patient's and family's wishes is essential for guiding the decision of whether to perform decompressive craniectomy.

◆ Surgical Technique

Once the decision has been made for surgical intervention, a thorough preoperative evaluation should commence. Blood loss is often low enough to not require keeping crossmatched blood in the operating room. Thus, unless other relevant comorbidities are present, a type-and-screen logged in the blood bank is usually sufficient. Coagulopathies and metabolic derangements should be identified and corrected if present. In this patient population, special attention should be paid to the potential prior administration of fibrinolytic therapy, such as tissue-type plasminogen activator (tPA), or antiplatelet medications, such as aspirin or clopidogrel. Invasive pro-

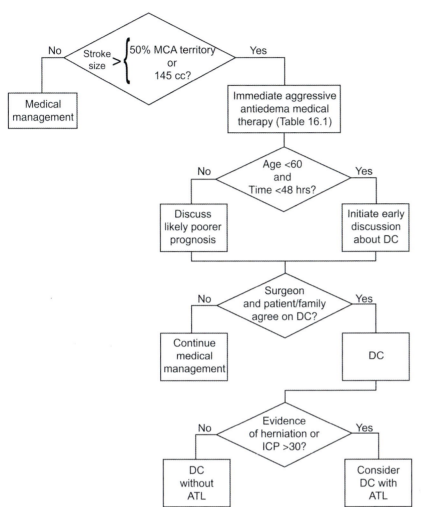

Fig. 16.2 Decision-making algorithm for management of massive MCA infarct. A suggested algorithm for the management of space-occupying edema secondary to a large MCA stroke is depicted. The decision points are based on the best available class I data (see text). ATL, anterior temporal lobectomy; DC, decompressive craniectomy; ICP, intracranial pressure.

cedures following intravenous tPA administration should be delayed for 24 hours if possible, and a platelet transfusion to reverse a functional platelet disorder should be considered in the latter case. To the degree permitted, cardiac risk should be stratified and optimized.

In the operating room, the patient is positioned supine after the induction of general anesthesia. The head is turned laterally, with the aid of a shoulder roll if necessary, and affixed with a three-pin head frame (**Fig. 16.3A**). Care should be taken to avoid excessive kinking of the neck and consequent pressure on the contralateral jugular vein, which would impede cerebral venous drainage.

A hemicraniectomy involving the area of the frontal, parietal, and temporal lobes is the procedure of choice for unilateral decompression. This is most often performed with a curvilinear question mark–shaped incision (**Fig. 16.3A**). The incision should extend sufficiently inferiorly to permit later identification of the zygoma. Using the midline as the medial extent of the incision ensures that the sagittal suture will be visible when placing bur holes. The anterior limit should be just behind the hairline for cosmesis. The incision should curve posteriorly enough to allow for a minimum 12-cm

anterior-posterior dimension of the craniectomy. Making the skin flap slightly larger than the planned bone flap facilitates future cranioplasty surgery.

After anterior reflection of the skin flap and temporalis muscle (**Fig. 16.3B**), burr holes are placed inferiorly in the temporal squamous bone just superior to the zygomatic process to access the floor of the middle fossa, anteriorly in the keyhole to access the floor of the anterior fossa, and posteriorly along the superior temporal line at the edge of the skin flap. Additional burr holes are placed medially, approximately 1 cm lateral to the sagittal sinus. The dura is stripped from the inner table, and the burr holes connected with a foot-plated bit. The bone flap is then removed, and can be stored in a –80°C freezer or via a separate incision in the abdomen. A craniectomy smaller than approximately 12 cm risks herniation of the brain through the cranial defect with consequent venous infarct and exacerbation of edema (**Fig. 16.3C**). Hemostasis is achieved with bipolar cautery, paying particular attention to the middle meningeal artery, and the optional placement of dural tenting sutures around the bone edge. Remaining portions of the sphenoid wing are removed with rongeurs to provide access to the temporal lobe. If

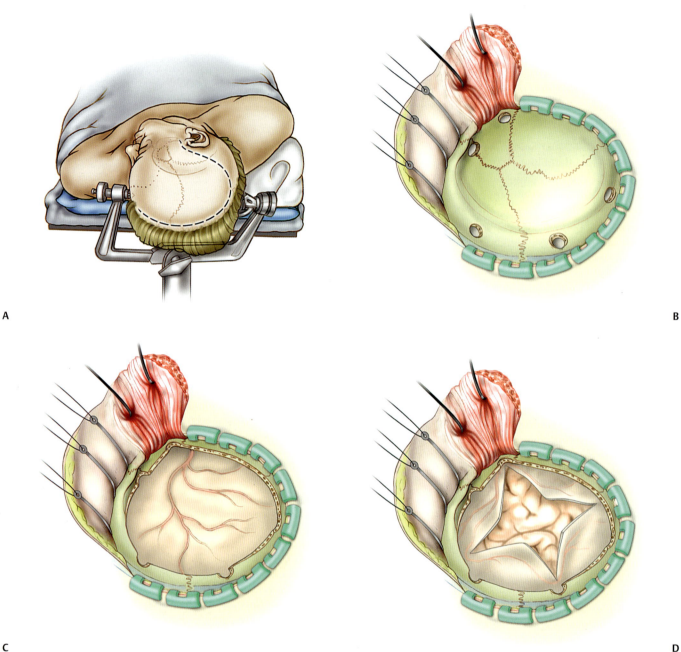

A

B

C

D

Fig. 16.3 Surgical technique. **(A)** The patient is positioned supine with the head turned, and a large question mark–shaped incision is typically used. **(B)** Retraction of the skin and temporalis muscle provides access to the cranium overlying the frontal, temporal, and anterior parietal lobes. **(C)** Burr holes are placed just superior to the zygoma to access the floor of the middle fossa, in the keyhole to access the floor of the anterior fossa, at the posterior margin of the incision near the level of the superior temporal line, and just lateral to the sagittal suture, accommodating a craniectomy at least 12 cm in the anterior-posterior dimension. **(D)** A stellate dural opening should be performed to maximize volume expansion. If an anterior temporal lobectomy is planned for further decompression, a corticectomy is performed in the middle temporal gyrus, approximately 4 to 5 cm posterior to the temporal tip. The neocortex and subjacent white matter are removed anteriorly toward the temporal tip and inferiorly toward the floor of the middle fossa. The amygdala, uncus, and mesial temporal structures are gently aspirated or peeled off the arachnoid.

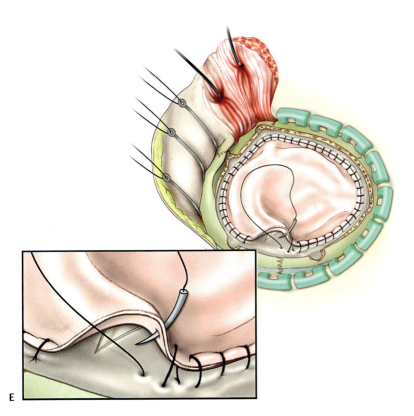

E

mastoid air cells are visible, they should be waxed. The dura is then opened in a stellate fashion, taking care to avoid damaging underlying brain and vessels (**Fig. 16.3D**). At this point the minimal decompression has been achieved.

In many cases, further decompression of the brainstem is performed with an anterior temporal lobectomy (ATL). Suggested indications for this procedure are ICP >30 if a pressure monitor is present,[21] or radiographic or clinical evidence of transtentorial uncal herniation. In decompressive surgery, the goal of an ATL is removal of the uncus and mesial temporal lobe. A corticectomy is performed in the middle temporal gyrus beginning 4 to 5 cm posterior to the temporal tip, and extended anteriorly to the tip. The corticectomy is then carried inferiorly to the floor of the middle fossa. The neocortex and underlying white matter are aspirated, followed by the subcortical anterior temporal structures, including the amygdala. Further neocortical removal, such as meticulous dissection of the superior temporal gyrus and skeletonization of the insula, is not required.

Mesially, it is critical to identify the arachnoid plane marking the medial extent of the temporal lobe. Care should be taken to preserve the integrity of this arachnoid barrier, to avoid damaging the brainstem and structures in the ambient cistern. The uncus can be gently aspirated or peeled off the arachnoid, completing the decompression. The third cranial nerve, PCA and/or posterior communicating artery, and midbrain may be visible beyond the arachnoid plane. The fourth cranial nerve is often visible along the tentorial edge. If uncal herniation has already occurred, complete removal of the uncus requires reaching beyond the tentorial edge, which is required for an adequate decompression.

For closure, a duraplasty rather than primary closure should be performed, either with autologous pericranium or synthetic material,[25] to allow expansion of the edematous brain.[26] For similar reasons, the temporalis muscle and fascia may be left unapproximated.[27] An ICP monitor or ventricular drain may be left in place if desired. The galea and skin are closed in layers.

The most common complications following DC include subdural hygroma, with an incidence of up to 50%, and infection or osteomyelitis of the bone flap, with an incidence of 1 to 6%.[23] Latent hydrocephalus may also occur, requiring cerebrospinal fluid (CSF) diversion at the time of cranioplasty.

◆ Cranioplasty

Reconstruction of the cranial defect produced by craniectomy usually takes place weeks to months after the craniectomy. This procedure is not only cosmetically appealing, but also protects the brain and obviates the constant need for a helmet. The first choice for material is the patient's autologous bone flap. If the bone flap is not available or infected, a prefabricated custom-made synthetic flap may be used. In this case, planning should begin well in advance of the surgical date to allow enough time for the patient to have the appropriate imaging study, and for the synthetic flap to be constructed. There does not seem to be a difference in operative time or infectious risk between these two options.[28]

In the operating room, the original incision is reopened, and the skin flap is separated from the duraplasty material. This separation may be aided by the use of synthetic rather

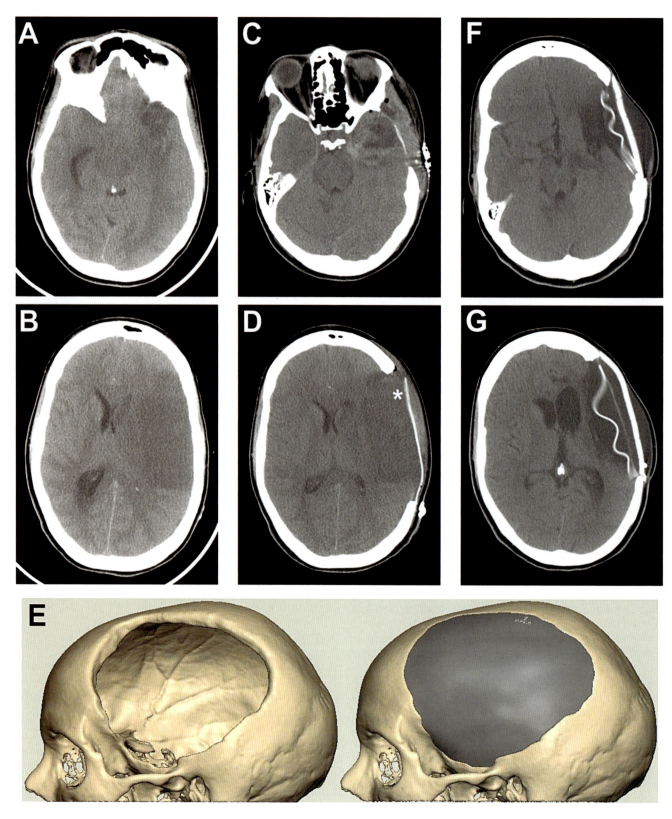

Fig. 16.4 Case illustration. These images pertain to the case of a 34-year-old woman described in the text. **(A,B)** Noncontrast head CT showing large left MCA stroke with edema and resultant midline shift and uncal herniation. **(C,D)** Head CT immediately following left decompressive craniectomy and anterior temporal lobectomy showing resolution of midline shift and brainstem compression. The bright curvilinear structure denoted with an asterisk is a Gore-Tex dural substitute. **(E)** Three-dimensional reconstruction of a thin-cut CT obtained to fashion a custom-made cranioplasty (shown in gray). **(F,G)** Head CT following cranioplasty.

than autologous duraplasty during the craniectomy.[25] The bony edge of the cranial defect is identified circumferentially. As mentioned above, this step is facilitated by planning a skin flap larger than the bone flap. The replacement flap is then affixed to the skull in at least three places with titanium or resorbable plates and screws, and the galea and skin are closed.

The development of communicating hydrocephalus is not uncommon following DC for stroke. If persistent, it usually requires CSF shunting. There is emerging evidence that performing cranioplasty earlier (a few weeks) rather than later (a few months) may reduce the need for CSF diversion.[29]

◆ Case Illustration

A 34-year-old woman with a history of infertility on Lupron (depot formulation of leuprolide, a gonadotropin-releasing hormone agonist) suffered the acute onset of decreased responsiveness, drowsiness, right hemiparesis, and urinary incontinence. She was quickly taken to a local hospital, where a noncontrast head CT was unremarkable. The diagnosis of seizure and consequent postictal state was entertained, but an electroencephalogram (EEG) showed only left-sided slowing without epileptiform discharges. The patient had a brief episode of complete heart block for which she received temporary pacing wires. As her exam did not improve over the next day, a repeat head CT was obtained, which showed an extensive left MCA stroke with 3 mm of midline shift. By that time she was not following commands, had slight pupillary asymmetry, and was plegic on the right. She received 65 g mannitol, was intubated, and urgently transferred to our facility for further care.

She arrived at the Massachusetts General Hospital Neuroscience Intensive Care Unit approximately 42 hours after the onset of stroke symptoms. Upon examination, her vitals were stable with sinus rhythm on pressure control ventilation. Off propofol, she had a GCS score of E1VTM5 and an NIHSS score of 24. She did not consistently follow commands. The left pupil was 2 mm larger than the right, but still reactive. Oculocephalic reflexes were not present, but she had corneal, cough, and gag reflexes. Her left side moved spontaneously, but her right arm extensor postured and the right leg triple flexed to painful stimuli. She was immediately taken for a head CT, which showed a large left MCA stroke (**Fig. 16.4A,B**).

Given the patient's young age, stroke burden, and developing evidence of herniation, the option of decompressive craniectomy was discussed with her family. They elected to proceed, and she was taken emergently for left hemicraniectomy, approximately 44 hours after stroke ictus. She underwent left hemicraniectomy, a 4-cm anterior temporal lobectomy, and placement of a bolt-type right frontal parenchymal ICP monitor. Postoperative CT scan is shown in **Fig. 16.4C,D**.

Immediately postoperatively, her GCS improved to E2VTM5, with equal and reactive pupils. Within 2 days she was opening her eyes to name and occasionally spontaneously, regarding the examiner, and intermittently following simple commands on the left. The ICP monitor was removed on post-operative day 4. She was transferred to an inpatient rehabilitation center on postoperative day 17, at which point she was reliably following two- or three-step commands. She had some spontaneous speech production, but with significant difficulty naming objects. Her right facial droop was mild, but her right arm and leg remained plegic. By the time she was discharged from rehab 29 days later, she could articulate short phrases, and walk 120 to 150 feet with a quad cane. The etiology of her stroke remained in question, with possibilities including cryptogenic embolus, or hypercoagulable state secondary to hormonal manipulation.

She presented for cranioplasty 3 months later, by which time her expressive aphasia improved enough to allow her to answer questions and respond in short sentences, but still with word-finding difficulty. Her right arm remained plegic, but she had antigravity strength in the right leg. Because an intraoperative culture from the bone flap grew *Propionibacterium acnes,* it had been discarded, and a thin-cut head CT had been obtained for custom synthetic cranioplasty construction (**Fig. 16.4E**). Surgery was uneventful, and the postoperative head CT was stable other than left ventriculomegaly (**Fig. 16.4F,G**). She was discharged home the next day, with planned follow-up for the detection of latent hydrocephalus.

References

1. Moulin DE, Lo R, Chiang J, Barnett HJ. Prognosis in middle cerebral artery occlusion. Stroke 1985;16:282–284
2. Qureshi AI, Suarez JI, Yahia AM, et al. Timing of neurologic deterioration in massive middle cerebral artery infarction: a multicenter review. Crit Care Med 2003;31:272–277
3. Hacke W, Schwab S, Horn M, Spranger M, De Georgia M, von Kummer R. 'Malignant' middle cerebral artery territory infarction: clinical course and prognostic signs. Arch Neurol 1996;53:309–315
4. Silver FL, Norris JW, Lewis AJ, Hachinski VC. Early mortality following stroke: a prospective review. Stroke 1984;15:492–496
5. Oppenheim C, Samson Y, Manaï R, et al. Prediction of malignant middle cerebral artery infarction by diffusion-weighted imaging. Stroke 2000; 31:2175–2181
6. Kasner SE, Demchuk AM, Berrouschot J, et al. Predictors of fatal brain edema in massive hemispheric ischemic stroke. Stroke 2001;32:2117–2123
7. Krieger DW, Demchuk AM, Kasner SE, Jauss M, Hantson L. Early clinical and radiological predictors of fatal brain swelling in ischemic stroke. Stroke 1999;30:287–292
8. Carter BS, Rabinov JD, Pfannl R, Schwamm LH. Case records of the Massachusetts General Hospital. Weekly clinicopathological exercises. Case 5-2004 - a 57-year-old man with slurred speech and left hemiparesis. N Engl J Med 2004;350:707–716
9. Bardutzky J, Schwab S. Antiedema therapy in ischemic stroke. Stroke 2007;38:3084–3094
10. Kjellberg RN, Prieto A Jr. Bifrontal decompressive craniotomy for massive cerebral edema. J Neurosurg 1971;34:488–493
11. Ivamoto HS, Numoto M, Donaghy RM. Surgical decompression for cerebral and cerebellar infarcts. Stroke 1974;5:365–370
12. Rengachary SS, Batnitzky S, Morantz RA, Arjunan K, Jeffries B. Hemicraniectomy for acute massive cerebral infarction. Neurosurgery 1981; 8:321–328
13. Gupta R, Connolly ES, Mayer S, Elkind MS. Hemicraniectomy for massive middle cerebral artery territory infarction: a systematic review. Stroke 2004;35:539–543
14. Schwab S, Steiner T, Aschoff A, et al. Early hemicraniectomy in patients with complete middle cerebral artery infarction. Stroke 1998;29:1888–1893
15. Vahedi K, Vicaut E, Mateo J, et al; DECIMAL Investigators. Sequential-design, multicenter, randomized, controlled trial of early decompressive craniectomy in malignant middle cerebral artery infarction (DECIMAL Trial). Stroke 2007;38:2506–2517
16. Jüttler E, Schwab S, Schmiedek P, et al; DESTINY Study Group. Decompressive Surgery for the Treatment of Malignant Infarction of the

Middle Cerebral Artery (DESTINY): a randomized, controlled trial. Stroke 2007;38:2518–2525

17. Hofmeijer J, Amelink GJ, Algra A, et al; HAMLET investigators. Hemicraniectomy after middle cerebral artery infarction with life-threatening Edema trial (HAMLET). Protocol for a randomised controlled trial of decompressive surgery in space-occupying hemispheric infarction. Trials 2006;7:29

18. Vahedi K, Hofmeijer J, Juettler E, et al; DECIMAL, DESTINY, and HAMLET investigators. Early decompressive surgery in malignant infarction of the middle cerebral artery: a pooled analysis of three randomised controlled trials. Lancet Neurol 2007;6:215–222

19. Hofmeijer J, Kappelle LJ, Algra A, Amelink GJ, van Gijn J, van der Worp HB; HAMLET investigators. Surgical decompression for space-occupying cerebral infarction (the Hemicraniectomy After Middle Cerebral Artery infarction with Life-threatening Edema Trial [HAMLET]): a multicentre, open, randomised trial. Lancet Neurol 2009;8:326–333

20. Mori K, Nakao Y, Yamamoto T, Maeda M. Early external decompressive craniectomy with duroplasty improves functional recovery in patients with massive hemispheric embolic infarction: timing and indication of decompressive surgery for malignant cerebral infarction. Surg Neurol 2004;62:420–429, discussion 429–430

21. Cho DY, Chen TC, Lee HC. Ultra-early decompressive craniectomy for malignant middle cerebral artery infarction. Surg Neurol 2003;60:227–232, discussion 232–233

22. Chen CC, Cho DY, Tsai SC. Outcome of and prognostic factors for decompressive hemicraniectomy in malignant middle cerebral artery infarction. J Clin Neurosci 2007;14:317–321

23. Kakar V, Nagaria J, John Kirkpatrick P. The current status of decompressive craniectomy. Br J Neurosurg 2009;23:147–157

24. Curry WT Jr, Sethi MK, Ogilvy CS, Carter BS. Factors associated with outcome after hemicraniectomy for large middle cerebral artery territory infarction. Neurosurgery 2005;56:681–692, discussion 681–692

25. Horaczek JA, Zierski J, Graewe A. Collagen matrix in decompressive hemicraniectomy. Neurosurgery 2008;63(1, Suppl 1)ONS176–ONS181, discussion ONS181

26. Yoo DS, Kim DS, Cho KS, Huh PW, Park CK, Kang JK. Ventricular pressure monitoring during bilateral decompression with dural expansion. J Neurosurg 1999;91:953–959

27. Park J, Kim E, Kim GJ, Hur YK, Guthikonda M. External decompressive craniectomy including resection of temporal muscle and fascia in malignant hemispheric infarction. J Neurosurg 2009;110:101–105

28. Lee SC, Wu CT, Lee ST, Chen PJ. Cranioplasty using polymethyl methacrylate prostheses. J Clin Neurosci 2009;16:56–63

29. Waziri A, Fusco D, Mayer SA, McKhann GM II, Connolly ES Jr. Postoperative hydrocephalus in patients undergoing decompressive hemicraniectomy for ischemic or hemorrhagic stroke. Neurosurgery 2007;61:489–493, discussion 493–494

30. Hutchinson P, Timofeev I, Kirkpatrick P. Surgery for brain edema. Neurosurg Focus 2007;22:E14

17

Carotid Endarterectomy: Decision Analysis and Surgical Technique

Jay U. Howington

Pearls

- A surgeon's technique for carotid endarterectomy should be tailored to his or her comfort as there is no "right" technique other than the one that minimizes morbidity and mortality.
- The initial dissection of the carotid bifurcation should be done only after the distal internal carotid has been secured to prevent thromboembolic complications as well as to assess the need for shunting.
- Never rely on only one noninvasive imaging modality for the evaluation of the degree of the carotid stenosis.
- Understand the individual patient's natural history compared with the potential risks of endarterectomy, bearing in mind that a good surgeon is a reluctant surgeon.

Extracranial carotid revascularization aims at preventing ischemic events caused by atherosclerotic thromboembolic events or hemodynamic compromise. The evidence for carotid endarterectomy (CEA) as a safe and effective procedure for the primary and secondary prevention of stroke has its foundation in several studies published in the 1990s. These include the North American Symptomatic Carotid Endarterectomy Trial (NASCET), the European Carotid Stroke Trial (ECST), and the Asymptomatic Carotid Artery Study (ACAS)[1-3] These studies represent level I data demonstrating that patients with symptomatic high-grade (70 to 99%) carotid stenosis and those with asymptomatic stenosis ranging from 60 to 99% benefit from carotid endarterectomy when compared with medical therapy. The details of these studies as well as the subsequent subgroup analyses are covered extensively in Chapter 5. The take-home message of these studies is that CEA is a safe and effective operation for the treatment of high-grade carotid stenosis when performed by experienced surgeons with low complication rates. However, the decision to operate on a patient's carotid artery should be based on more than just a simple measurement of the degree of stenosis. This chapter reviews the indications for CEA as a revascularization procedure and describes the general operative technique and perioperative management of these patients. Carotid artery stenting (CAS) and effective management are reviewed in Chapter 32 and elsewhere in this volume.

◆ Initial Evaluation

Carotid stenosis, like all atherosclerotic disease, is the result of a combination of genetics and lifestyle choices. Similarly, the natural history of extracranial carotid atherosclerosis depends on the same factors. Patients who are at a higher risk for developing carotid stenosis are also at an increased risk for stroke from that stenosis. The initial evaluation of patients with carotid disease must be done bearing in mind the risk factors for both carotid stenosis as well as for stroke from carotid stenosis. For the most part, patients are referred to a carotid surgeon after the diagnostic workup has begun. For those patients who are asymptomatic, a bruit is usually heard by a primary care physician, prompting a carotid ultrasound, which in turn leads to either a referral or further imaging. Symptomatic patients either present with a transient ischemic attack (TIA) that is retinal or hemispheric or have had a stroke, and then the imaging protocol varies. Suffice it to say, carotid duplex ultrasonography remains the current standard for the initial, noninvasive, assessment of the extracranial circulation. The place of ultrasound in the imaging workup of ischemic stroke is covered extensively in Chapter 11, but a brief review is necessary to define its role when deciding to operate.

The sensitivity and specificity for spectral analysis of carotid duplex–derived waveforms for detecting carotid stenosis ranging from ≥50% to 99% varies from 90% to 95% when compared with conventional angiography.[4] The spectral criteria

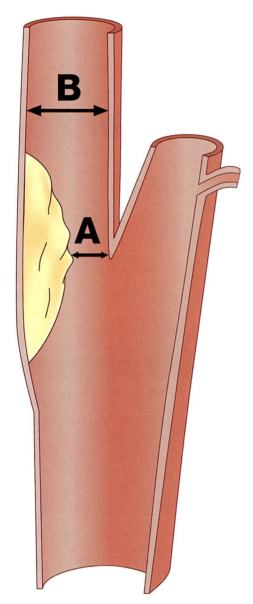

Fig. 17.1 The method used to measure the degree of carotid stenosis in the North American Symptomatic Carotid Endarterectomy Trial (NASCET). The diameter of the stenotic segment **(A)** is divided by the diameter of the internal carotid artery distal to the stenosis where the walls are parallel **(B)** and subtracted from 1.

published by Strandness[5] at the University of Washington is probably the most commonly used by ultrasound laboratories throughout the United States to grade carotid stenosis and classifies the stenosis as normal; 1 to 15%, 16 to 49%, 50 to 79%, 80 to 99% stenosis; or complete occlusion. The University of Washington criteria focus on the peak systolic velocity (PSV) of the internal carotid artery (ICA), the amount of spectral broadening during the deceleration phase of systole, and the amount of plaque present, and these criteria are usually found at the bottom of a carotid duplex report. When using these criteria, duplex ultrasonography is extremely sensitive in detecting occlusive disease, but several short-

comings make the University of Washington criteria less than ideal in the evaluation of carotid disease.

The technique for degree of stenosis measurement as used in NASCET has become the standard method for determining carotid stenosis **(Fig. 17.1)**.[1] The University of Washington criteria used the carotid bulb instead of the distal internal carotid as the reference diameter; therefore, these criteria tend to overestimate the degree of stenosis. The range of stenosis provided by these criteria are too broad and do not fit with indications published by NASCET and ACAS. Symptomatic ICA stenosis ranging from ≥70 to 99% is best treated with endarterectomy and medical management, whereas ACAS demonstrated benefit from endarterectomy in patients with asymptomatic ICA stenosis ranging from ≥60 to 99%.[1,2] Because of this shortcoming, Moneta's group[6–8] sought to establish other criteria for detecting ICA stenosis with a greater degree of accuracy. These criteria include the end diastolic velocity (EDV) and the ICA/common carotid artery (CCA) PSV ratio **(Table 17.1)**.

These criteria do increase the diagnostic accuracy of carotid ultrasound, but ultrasound leaves much to be desired when it comes to evaluating the level/location of the stenosis, proximal and distal anatomy, as well as the status of any collateral flow. Because of these shortcomings, it is the author's view that performing a CEA based on carotid ultrasound as the sole imaging modality is, at best, a poor decision. Patients with an ultrasound that suggests a high-grade stenosis should have at least one other confirmatory study before the decision to intervene is made. Adjuvant imaging modalities include computed tomography angiography (CTA), magnetic resonance angiography (MRA), and digital subtraction angiography (DSA).

Digital subtraction angiography has long been considered the gold standard in the evaluation of the cerebrovasculature, but it does have two significant drawbacks: it is invasive and therefore carries the risk of arterial injury, and the contrast dye is nephrotoxic. Conventional catheter-based angiography

Table 17.1 Consensus Panel Gray Scale and Doppler Ultrasound Criteria for ICA Stenosis[6]

Degree of Stenosis (%)	Primary Parameters			Additional Parameters	
	ICA PSV (cm/sec)	Plaque Estimate (%)		ICA/CCA PSV Ratio	ICA EDV (cm/sec)
Normal	<125	None		<2.0	<40
<50	<125	<50		<2.0	<40
50–69	125–230	≥50		2.0–4.0	40–100
≥70–99	>230	≥50		>4.0	>100
Occlusion	Undetectable	Visible, no lumen		N/A	N/A

Abbreviations: CCA, common carotid artery; EDV, end diastolic velocity ICA, internal carotid artery; N/A, not applicable; PSV, peak systolic velocity.

exposes the patient to the risk of a disabling stroke, and the incidence of transient or permanent neurologic deficits ranges from 0.17 to 2.63%.[9–11] A recent study of 2243 patients undergoing cerebrovascular DSA for surveillance after intracranial aneurysm treatment found a very low (0.43%) complication rate.[11] Although DSA does carry some risk, the benefits include the ability to measure the degree of stenosis exactly, evaluate proximal and distal anatomy, as well as evaluate the status of collateral flow **(Fig. 17.2).** Both CTA and MRA can provide similar information regarding proximal and distal anatomy, but collateral flow can only be inferred as both tests are not truly dynamic evaluations. CTA does carry the risks of radiation exposure and nephrotoxicity, and some patients

may not be able to have an MRA due to metallic implants or foreign bodies. That being said, both modalities have been compared with DSA extensively, and the pooled sensitivity and specificity for the diagnosis of a carotid stenosis that is ≥70% using CTA were found to be 85% and 93%, respectively.[12] For the diagnosis of the same degree of carotid stenosis, MRA had a pooled sensitivity of 95% and a pooled specificity of 90%.[13] The accuracy of either of these modalities is good enough to be used as a confirmatory test following a carotid ultrasound that suggests a high-grade carotid stenosis. Catheter-based angiography should be used when there is a discrepancy between the carotid ultrasound findings and those of the confirmatory test.

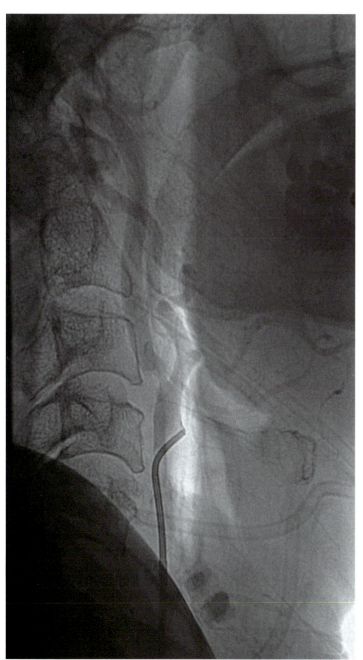

A

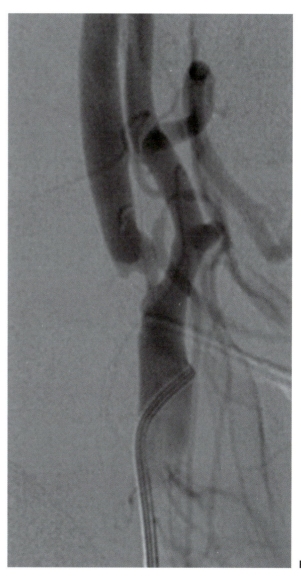

B

Fig. 17.2 **(A,B)** Lateral angiograms of a right common carotid artery injection. The unsubtracted image **(A)** shows the anatomic location of the stenosis at C3–4 and slightly inferior to the angle of the mandible. The subtracted image **(B)** clearly demonstrates the 72% stenosis at the origin of the internal carotid artery (ICA). (*continued on next page*)

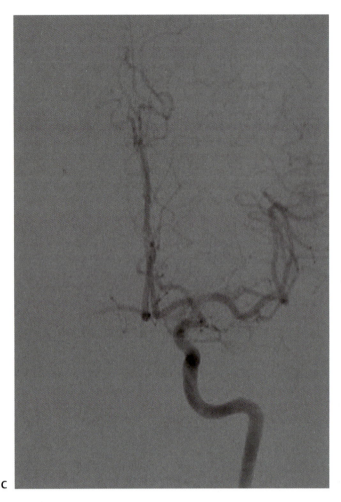

C

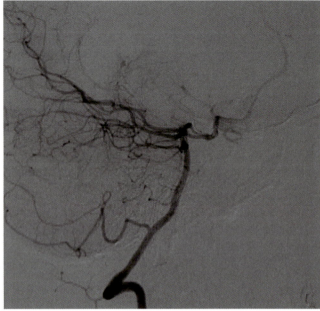

D

Fig. 17.2 (*continued*)   **(C)** This anteroposterior (AP) intracranial view of the left ICA in the same patient demonstrates the collateral flow through the anterior communicating artery to the right anterior cerebral artery including the A1 segment. **(D)** The lateral intracranial angiogram of a right vertebral artery injection in the same patient shows further collateral flow through the right posterior communicating artery to both the right anterior and middle cerebral arteries. An endarterectomy was performed on this patient and a video of that operation accompanies this chapter.

◆ Initial Decisions: Symptomatic Carotid Stenosis

Many patients are referred to carotid surgeons with the diagnosis of "symptomatic carotid stenosis," when in reality they are asymptomatic. The confusion exists because patients experience a "symptom" that is not referable to the carotid. Examples include dizziness, generalized weakness, syncope or near-syncope, and positive visual changes (floaters or scotoma). These do not qualify as symptomatic carotid ischemic events. The symptom has to be a transient or permanent focal neurologic deficit involving the ipsilateral hemisphere or retina in order for the carotid stenosis to be labeled symptomatic. The distinct separation between symptomatic and asymptomatic carotid stenosis is crucial to assessing a patient's risk because any extrapolation on the natural history with medical management or on the benefits of revascularization is based on clear-cut definitions of the terms *symptomatic* and *asymptomatic.*

The degree of stenosis along with the presence or absence of symptoms, referable to the carotid stenosis, are the main factors to consider when deciding to intervene on a patient with ICA stenosis. A brief review of just how they shape that decision is also in order. The results of NASCET and ECST demonstrated that those patients with symptomatic carotid stenosis in the range of 70 to 99% benefited from CEA when compared with medical therapy.[1,3] Those patients with a 50 to 69% stenosis also benefited, but there was only a 4.6% absolute risk reduction in ipsilateral ischemic stroke at 5 years compared with the 16% absolute risk reduction for stroke in the 70 to 99% subgroup. Those patients with near occlusions had no substantial benefit at 5 years. Rothwell et al[14] performed a meta-analysis using patient-level data from NASCET and ECST and found that the greatest benefit from endarterectomy was in this high-grade stenosis group, with a 16% absolute risk reduction for stroke at 5 years (p <.001). Observations from NASCET also suggested that the benefit from CEA was greater in those patients who had a stroke as opposed to a TIA and if the ischemic event was hemispheric versus retinal.[1] The findings of the NASCET and ECST studies led to the conclusion that the immediate risk of surgery is outweighed by the long-term reduction in stroke as a result of the revascularization of high-grade stenotic lesions. This conclusion, of course, is predicated on the achievement of an acceptably low surgical morbidity and mortality rate by the operating surgeon.

The American Heart Association Stroke Council ad hoc committees have published guidelines on the acceptable risk of

CEA.[15-17] They recommend that the combined risk of perioperative stroke and death should not exceed 3% for asymptomatic patients, 5% for patients with TIA, 7% for patients with stroke, and 10% for patients with recurrent stenosis if the benefits of CEA are to outweigh its inherent risks. In certain patient subgroups the risk of CEA is higher than 6%, and risk/benefit analysis becomes much more complicated than simply assuming that symptomatic high-grade ICA stenosis equals a CEA.

Factors such as surgeon experience, presenting symptoms, patient age and sex, medical comorbidities, anatomy, and plaque morphology all play a role in making the decision to perform a CEA. It is difficult to sort out whether the operative risk for CEA differs much among surgeons because of variables such as case mix and chance effects caused by the relatively small numbers in each surgeon's experience. It is known, however, that surgeons who perform a large number of endarterectomies tend to have better outcomes than do those surgeons who perform CEA infrequently.[18,19] There is no hard-and-fast rule as to how many CEAs one needs to perform in a given year to achieve satisfactory outcomes, and these criteria are usually left to the credentialing committee at each individual institution. Competency with regard to CEA for symptomatic ICA stenosis is usually based on the benchmark of a complication rate of ≤6%.[17] Any complication rate higher than this should prompt a thorough review of the surgeon's experience. The risks of CEA depend on the patients' clinical presentation, their overall medical condition, and the surgeon's personal experience and outcome data.

The multiple analyses by Rothwell et al[14,20-23] regarding CEA for symptomatic carotid stenosis found that the nature of the presenting event had a statistically significant effect on the operative risk associated with CEA (**Table 17.2**). Urgent CEA for crescendo TIAs or stroke in evolution is associated with a much higher risk than elective CEA, and it is felt that this discrepancy is due to several factors: the plaque in the carotid is considered acutely unstable with overlying thrombus; the risk of acute cardiac complications is increased from either systemic inflammation or atherosclerotic plaque instability; the patients lack the normal preoperative evaluation with correction of medical comorbidities; and there already might be irreversible ischemic damage.[22,24-26] The combined risk of neurologic and cardiovascular complications following urgent CEA is high but not prohibitively so given the natural history of patients with unstable symptoms. When deciding to perform a CEA in an urgent/emergent fashion, the surgeon should be cognizant of the heightened risk associated with this scenario and take whatever steps possible to optimize the patient prior to the operation. Surgery for stroke is associated with a higher risk than surgery for TIA, and surgery for TIA is associated with a higher risk than that for ocular events only. The benefit of CEA, however, is directly related to the risk of the operation in these patients.

Both NASCET and ECST included very small numbers of patients in their 80s or older because of the perceived risks of CEA, risks of general anesthesia, and the presumed shorter life expectancy.[1,3] The general thinking is that these patients are more at risk for stroke and have an increased morbidity and mortality secondary to stroke than does the younger

Table 17.2 Results of a Systematic Review of the Studies Reporting the Operative Risks of Stroke or Death Due to Carotid Endarterectomy Based on Presenting Symptom[14,20-23]

Presenting Event	Number of Studies	Number of Operations	Absolute Risk (%)	p Value
Symptomatic	95	36,482	5.1	<.001
Urgent	12	208	19.2	<.001
Stroke	50	7634	7.1	<.001
Cerebral TIA	24	8138	5.5	<.001
Ocular event	18	1784	2.8	<.001
Nonspecific	24	1751	4.2	<.001
Asymptomatic	60	14,399	2.8	<.001
Redo surgery	12	914	4.4	<.001

Abbreviation: TIA, transient ischemic attack.

population. Subgroup analysis of these studies have subsequently shown that the risk seen in these patients is not so much related to chronologic age as it is "physiologic" age.[27,28] The elderly population tends to have more medical comorbidities, and this increases their risk of perioperative mortality but not the risk of perioperative stroke. When evaluating an elderly patient for a CEA, life expectancy and the yearly risk of stroke must be compared with the risk of CEA. Currently, there is no real justification for withholding CEA from elderly patients who are otherwise physiologically fit to undergo the operation.

The subgroup analyses of both NASCET and ECST demonstrated a decreased benefit of CEA in women due in part to the higher operative risk.[1,3,23,29] In a meta-analysis, the overall odds of stroke and death were actually increased twofold in women, and one of the main reasons offered for this dramatic difference is that female carotid arteries are smaller than those in their male counterparts.[23,29] The smaller size of the artery may create a more technically demanding operation for the surgeon, and one may theorize that a smaller artery is more prone to hemodynamic changes. Also, population studies have shown that women at any age have a lower risk for stroke compared with men of the same age.[30] The results of NASCET and ECST support the principle that patients with lower risk profiles for stroke benefited less from CEA than those with higher risk profiles. The only problem with that notion is that although the perioperative risks for women undergoing CEA were higher than those for men, they experienced a similar long-term benefit from CEA.[29] So it goes without saying that the surgeon should factor in these gender differences during the risk assessment for female patients.

The benefit of cervicocerebral angiography over carotid ultrasound is that it yields a full evaluation of the vessels above and below the lesion as well as the level of the stenosis. Lesions that are at or above the C2 level are often difficult to expose, as are lower-lying lesions. Extremely proximal or distal lesions are usually better suited for carotid angioplasty

Table 17.3 Indications for Carotid Endarterectomy in Patients with Asymptomatic Disease[15]

For patients with a surgical risk <3% and life expectancy of at least 5 years:

1. Proven indications: ipsilateral carotid endarterectomy is acceptable for stenotic lesions (≥60% diameter reduction of distal outflow tract with or without ulceration and with or without antiplatelet therapy, irrespective of contralateral artery status, ranging from no disease to occlusion [grade A recommendation])

2. Acceptable indications: unilateral carotid endarterectomy simultaneous with coronary artery bypass graft for stenotic lesions (≥60% with or without ulcerations with or without antiplatelet therapy irrespective of contralateral artery status [grade C recommendation])

3. Uncertain indications: unilateral carotid endarterectomy for stenosis ≥50% with B or C ulcer irrespective or contralateral internal carotid artery status (grade C recommendation)

For patients with a surgical risk of 3 to 5%, or as high as 5 to 10%, no proven indications are acknowledged

and stenting, as the risk for cranial nerve injury is high with CEA and virtually nonexistent for CAS. Patients with isolated hemispheres by angiography need intraoperative shunting, which can increase the risk of CEA in the form of vessel dissection. Patients with contralateral ICA occlusions are also at risk of ischemia during CEA if they do not have a patent contralateral posterior communicating artery. Finally, patients with intracranial aneurysms found incidentally during the workup for the carotid stenosis are theoretically at increased risk of rupture once the pressure gradient across the proximal stenosis is removed.[31,32] Other factors, though not strictly "anatomic," affect a patient's anatomy in ways that definitely increase the risk of neurovascular injury during CEA. The scar tissue associated with previous neck surgery or irradiation increases the technical demands of CEA. These factors and others are listed in **Table 17.3**. Although none of the above anatomic findings are absolute contraindications for CEA, their associated risks must be considered, especially in light of advances in CAS.

Prabhakaran et al[33] found that plaque surface irregularity portended a threefold increase in ischemic stroke. They found that plaque surface irregularity, even after adjusting for degree of stenosis and plaque thickness, is an independent predictor of ischemic stroke. Patients with irregular or ulcerative symptomatic high-grade stenosis are at an increased risk of ischemic stroke when compared with those with nonulcerative lesions, but plaque irregularity is not clearly associated with an increased risk of stroke perioperatively with CEA.[23] This subgroup of patients benefits greatly from CEA.

◆ Risk Assessment: Asymptomatic Carotid Stenosis

The above-mentioned factors—degree of stenosis, surgeon experience, patient age and sex, medical comorbidities, anat-

omy, and plaque morphology—also play a key role in the risk/benefit analysis of a patient with asymptomatic high-grade ICA stenosis, but one must realize that the benefit of CEA over medical therapy is not nearly as demonstrable as it is in the symptomatic group.[2,15,21,34,35] Probably more than in any other scenario in medicine, CEA for asymptomatic ICA stenosis falls under the rubric of "first do no harm." The benefit of CEA in these patients varies with the degree of stenosis, as it does in the symptomatic group, except that neither the ACAS nor the Medical Research Council's Asymptomatic Carotid Surgery Trial (ACST) showed increasing benefit from surgery with increasing degree of stenosis within the 60 to 99% range. These studies did not specifically address the effect of degree of stenosis on perioperative risk, but the ECST study did demonstrate that the risk of stroke increases with the degree of stenosis, with the implication being that patients with severe stenosis may comprise a subgroup in whom CEA provides greater benefit.[3]

The overall complication rate in the ACAS trial was extremely low, at 2.3%, and half of this was due to complications of preoperative angiography.[2] The actual perioperative complication rate was 1.5%, and it should be noted that the surgeons in the study were carefully selected. The current recommendation is that the operating surgeon should have a ≤3% complication rate with CEA for asymptomatic patients.[15] To put this another way, the number of patients needed to undergo CEA to prevent one disabling or fatal stroke within 5 years is approximately 40. The ability to discern which asymptomatic patients are at risk for perioperative complications is crucial and depends heavily on surgeon experience.

The current guidelines put forth by the American Heart Association's Stroke Council involving CEA for asymptomatic carotid stenosis state that there is a proven indication for CEA in patients with ICA stenosis ≥60% in whom the surgical risk is <3% and who have a life expectancy of at least 5 years.[15] The complete recommendations are listed in **Table 17.3**. The reason that the 5-year life expectancy is part of the proven indications is that both ACAS and ACST had end points at the 5-year mark. Also, data from both studies suggest no benefit from CEA in the elderly (>75 years) population, as roughly half of these patients died within the subsequent 5 years from causes unrelated to the ICA stenosis. Subsequent publications have refuted this notion somewhat, stating that in elderly patients with limited comorbidities CEA remains the gold standard for the treatment of high-grade asymptomatic stenosis.[27,36,37] The risk of perioperative stroke is no different from that in the younger population, and there is only a slight increase in perioperative mortality, resulting in only a minimal increase in risk of stroke and death combined. Elderly patients with a life expectancy of at least 5 years will benefit from CEA as a means of preventing stroke. Nonelderly women patients, unlike the older population in general, have an increased risk of perioperative stroke but no increased risk of perioperative mortality when compared with men of the same age.[27] Once beyond the immediate perioperative period, women experience the same benefit of stroke prevention as do men. As with CEA in symptomatic females, the mechanism for the increased perioperative stroke rate remains largely unexplained.

Table 17.4 Anatomic Risk Factors for Carotid Endarterectomy

Carotid bifurcation above C2

Carotid bifurcation below C5

Tandem stenosis either proximal or distal

Previous neck surgery

Previous neck irradiation

Cervical immobility

Contralateral occlusion/isolated hemisphere

Contralateral vocal cord paralysis

Presence of tracheostomy stoma

Table 17.5 Complications of CEA

Stoke	Hypotension
Myocardial infarction	Hyperperfusion syndrome
Death	Intracerebral hemorrhage
Cranial nerve injury	Seizures
Wound hematoma	Recurrent stenosis
Hypertension	Infection

As mentioned above, anatomic risk factors exist for CEA and must be considered in the decision-making process. An asymptomatic patient with high-grade ICA stenosis and concomitant anatomic risk factors (**Table 17.4**) represents a unique challenge in risk/benefit analysis. The benefit of revascularization exists, but the risks of CEA could outweigh those benefits. In these cases either CAS or aggressive medical management (total cholesterol level ≤200 mg/dL, low-density lipoprotein ≤100 mg/dL, antiplatelet therapy, appropriate management of hypertension and diabetes, lifestyle adjustments) might be a more reasonable alternative. The effects of plaque morphology on stroke risk published by Prabhakaran et al[33] also must be factored in when evaluating the asymptomatic carotid stenosis patient. A smooth concentric stenosis has a lower risk than does an eccentric ulcerated stenosis. The medical management of peripheral vascular disease has changed with the incorporation of newer medications from that which constituted the medical arms of the major CEA trials, and there is speculation that these newer medications could change the management of asymptomatic carotid stenosis in high anatomic risk patients. In fact, a recent literature review demonstrated that in some patients current vascular disease medical intervention is at least as effective in preventing TIA and stroke associated with ICA stenosis as the combination of medical management and CEA used in the surgical trials.[38]

◆ Complications of Carotid Endarterectomy

The various complications of CEA have been studied and published extensively, as it is the most frequently performed noncardiac vascular procedure, and, as stated above, the complication rate must be kept low to keep the beneficial effects of CEA higher than those of medical therapy.[15] The complications can be divided into those directly incurred during the operation and those that occur in a delayed fashion secondary to the hemodynamic changes after CEA. These are listed in **Table 17.5** as a quick reference to be used when discussing the operation with patients. The risks of stroke and death have been covered already, and it should be noted that after stroke, myocardial infarction is the second most common cause of perioperative morbidity and mortality. It is thought that most patients with atherosclerotic disease in the ICA have concomitant disease in the coronary arteries. The hemodynamic changes that take place with general anesthesia and the manipulation of the carotid bulb during the operation can aggravate an already tenuous situation. Vasoactive drugs used during the operation can also stress the myocardium. These cardiovascular fluctuations are usually transient, but they can be significant enough to increase myocardial oxygen demand to the point where it exceeds oxygen delivery, thus resulting in ischemia or infarction. Patients with a history of cardiac disease are at much greater risk for myocardial infarction in the CEA perioperative period than those patients with either asymptomatic disease or no cardiac disease whatsoever.[39]

Cranial nerve injuries are the most common complication of CEA, occurring in up to 50% of patients.[40] Fortunately, the vast majority of these injuries are transient or minor, but they can be devastating. The resultant deficits need to be appreciated if the surgeon is to present an honest complication rate. The transverse cervical nerves that innervate the anterior cervical triangle are almost universally transected during CEA to provide adequate exposure, but the resulting anesthesia usually resolves within 6 months. Transection of these nerves is a necessary part of the operation and should not be considered a complication. Injury to the greater auricular nerve with ensuing anesthesia/dysesthesia over the ear lobe and in the angle of the jaw, however, is largely avoidable. In cases of high carotid bifurcations, the posterior aspect of the incision should be extended toward the mastoid to better expose and safely mobilize the nerve. Another nerve that is vulnerable during high exposures is the marginal mandibular branch of the facial nerve. This branch is responsible for the depressor function of the angle of the mouth, and as with the greater auricular nerve, curving the incision toward the mastoid reduces the incidence of injury. The spinal accessory nerve runs along the underside of the sternocleidomastoid muscle and is usually not seen during routine exposure of the carotid sheath; nevertheless, one should not place excessive pressure on this muscle with retraction. Injury to the hypoglossal nerve results in ipsilateral deviation of the tongue upon protrusion. The nerve usually crosses the ICA approximately 4 cm beyond the bifurcation, but this varies. Careful exposure of the nerve as well as a keen awareness of its usual course provides the surgeon with the best chance to protect it. Neurapraxic injuries resolve within 6 to 12 months, and with instances of transection the nerve should be repaired primarily. Finally, the vagus nerve is intimately associated with the carotid artery and jugular vein within the carotid sheath, and injury to it or its branches may result in difficulties with phonation. Specific maneuvers intended to protect these nerves are discussed below.

Hemodynamic instability is particularly common with CEA and can lead to further complications including both hypo- and hyperperfusion. The carotid atheroma itself impairs the baroreceptor activity of the carotid sinus, and surgical manipulation of it or the artery can alter the body's capacity to adjust accordingly to the hemodynamic demands following revascularization.[41] Also, presurgical hypertension is the single most important determinant for the development of postoperative hypertension.[15,41] Another factor that puts patients at risk for hemodynamic instability following CEA is the impairment of cerebral autoregulation that often accompanies the long-standing hypoperfusion associated with high-grade stenosis. The capillary bed in these patients may not be able to provide the vasoconstriction needed in response to the normal or elevated blood pressure that follows correction of the stenosis. The increase in blood flow coupled with normal or elevated perfusion pressure results in edema and hemorrhage. The syndrome of cerebral hyperperfusion occurs in roughly 1% of patients and classically presents 2 to 7 days after CEA as headache, neurologic deficits, or seizures.[15,41] If left untreated, intracerebral hemorrhage can occur. Patients with preoperative hypertension are the most at risk, and their pressure should be managed aggressively until they become hemodynamically stable.

Postoperative infections are relatively rare with CEA, as it is considered a clean procedure. In most institutions, antibiotics are administered as a single dose preoperatively and then for the next 24 hours depending on the length of stay. If an infection does occur, it is usually superficial and can be managed with oral antibiotics. Management of deeper infections in the setting of a patch grafts is not well documented in the literature because they are so rare. Wound hematomas, on the other hand, were documented in 5.5% of the patients in the NASCET study.[1] Most were superficial and caused only minor discomfort. Larger hematomas or those that expand quickly should be handled emergently. If the airway is maintained, the patient should be taken back to the operating room and the wound immediately explored. If there is airway compromise, the surgeon should not hesitate to explore the wound at the bedside. Patients with larger necks might be more difficult to assess, and in these cases, an anteroposterior (AP) cervical film should easily reveal whether the trachea is deviated or not. Meticulous attention to hemostasis is usually all that is needed once the suture line is finished, and the effects of heparin should not need to be reversed with protamine to achieve this end. Any obvious defect in the suture line on the artery should be treated with a suture; otherwise, Gelfoam, Surgicel, or a topical thrombin used separately or in combination with gentle pressure should suffice. Achieving hemostasis in patients on aggressive antiplatelet therapy can often be difficult, and a small drain placed away from the suture line will further decrease the risk of subsequent hematoma. Platelets should be transfused only in the most extenuating circumstances. Gentle pressure applied to the wound site during extubation will also serve to minimize the risk of hematoma.

In cases of a new hemispheric neurologic deficit in the immediate postoperative period, a prompt evaluation is mandatory to identify a reversible cause. If the operation itself was uneventful or not technically demanding, the incidence of a problem at the operative is extremely low. After a neurologic assessment, the patient should be taken immediately for a computed tomography (CT) scan to rule out an intracerebral hemorrhage. If no hemorrhage is seen, intravenous anticoagulation should be reinstituted and the patient taken for cerebral angiography. Should the angiogram demonstrate cervical carotid irregularities or thrombosis, these should be treated with surgical exploration. If there is an intracranial occlusion, then appropriate steps are taken by the neuro-interventionalist to restore flow. In those cases in which there is a strong suspicion that the problem is at the arteriotomy site, one may choose to forgo the above algorithm in favor of surgical exploration. It is the author's practice to allow patients to awaken from anesthesia in the operating room so that they can demonstrate satisfactory neurologic function.

◆ Timing of Surgery

In the past, there was a general rule that one should wait for 4 to 6 weeks before performing a CEA on someone who presented with a stroke.[1] The idea behind this was that the newly infarcted brain would be more vulnerable to further ischemic insult associated with CEA or that it would not be able to adequately respond to restored flow, and an intracerebral hemorrhage would ensue. Rerkasem and Rothwell[42] recently reviewed the available literature on this topic published between 1980 and 2008 and found that there was no evidence of any increased risk attributable to surgery in the subacute phase in patients with TIA or stroke. This was particularly true in patients in whom CEA was performed within 1 week of a nondisabling stroke that was stable. Patients with crescendo TIA or stroke in evolution, on the other hand, are at a much increased risk of stroke with CEA, but the risk of stroke with medical management is also very high. Unfortunately, no definitive data on how this particular subset of patients should be handled exists. Patients with truly disabling strokes that are stable will likely benefit from a rehabilitation period prior to CEA. This time allows the brain to heal, and after 4 to 6 weeks the risk of further neurologic deficit with CEA approximates that seen in patients with minor deficits or TIAs.[42] Patients with stable, minor strokes can be safely treated with CEA within a week of their event as long as other potential comorbidities are optimized prior to, during, and after the operation.

◆ Controversies

There are several controversies surrounding the technique of CEA that should be mentioned. These include patch angioplasty versus primary closure, whether or not to place an arterial shunt during the endarterectomy, and how best to monitor the patient's neurologic status during the operation. Other debates exist with regard to CEA, but they are beyond the scope of this chapter. Before reviewing the viewpoints involved in each of these controversies, it is important to recall the old adage that it is a poor surgeon who blames his tools. There is no absolute "right" way to perform a CEA, and each surgeon's particular technique should be the result of the multiple factors that shape his or her surgical training. Bond et al[43] published a meta-analysis of small randomized trials of primary closure, vein patch, or synthetic patch, and found that patch angioplasty reduced the risk of perioperative stroke or death with no difference between the vein and synthetic groups. Proponents of patch angioplasty argue that this technique increases the luminal diameter of the reconstructed artery and thereby decreases the chance of postoperative thrombotic occlusion and recurrent stenosis secondary to intimal hyperplasia. Those against the routine use of patch angioplasty point to the increased operative time needed to sew two suture lines, the cost of the synthetic patch, the morbidity associated with the harvest of autologous vein, and the fact that with meticulous microsurgical technique the arteriotomy can be reapproximated with minimal loss of the original luminal diameter.[44] Aneurysmal degeneration **(Fig. 17.3)**, patch rupture and potential foreign-body reaction are also potential drawbacks of patch angioplasty. Some reserve the use of patch angioplasty for specific instances: a small (<4 mm) ICA, an extended arteriotomy, irregular arteriotomy, recurrent stenosis, or concomitant repair of a distal kink or loop.

Carotid surgeons fall into three basic groups with regard to the topic of intraoperative arterial shunting: those who shunt in every case, those that never shunt, and those who shunt selectively. Intraoperative arterial shunting theoretically prevents low cerebral blood flow during CEA by maintaining antegrade flow in the ICA. Aside from maintaining flow, proponents of universal shunting argue that it eliminates the dependence on intraoperative monitoring and creates a more relaxed environment in the operating room in which extra time can be taken for things such as surgical education and thorough inspection of the intima and arteriotomy closure. There is little doubt that the above factors are positive, but placing a shunt is not without risk. Those who decry the use of shunting during CEA cite the risks of distal dissection, thromboembolic complications, and unrecognized shunt malfunction, and they also claim that shunts are probably not required in the majority of CEAs.[45] Many use shunting only when there is a change in the neurophysiologic monitoring that does not respond to appropriate hemodynamic alterations or cerebral protective agents. A shunt can be a valuable adjunct during CEA, but it should be used with caution and an awareness of its risks.

The best assessment of neurologic function remains the neurologic examination, and this is true when monitoring for possible ischemia during CEA. The information gained from serial neurologic assessment of patients operated upon with regional anesthesia and sedation is more accurate and readily available than information on any other monitoring technique, but it requires patients to be sedated, but not so much that they cannot cooperate with the exam or main-

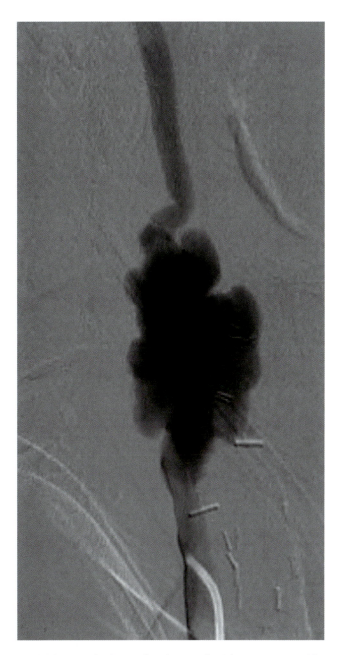

Fig. 17.3 Lateral subtracted angiogram of a right common carotid artery in a patient recently treated with a carotid endarterectomy (CEA) and vein patch angioplasty who presented 2 weeks postoperatively with an expanding pulsatile neck mass. The pseudoaneurysm was treated urgently with a covered stent.

tain their airways. With adequate preparation and patient education, awake CEA can be performed safely, but many surgeons choose not to because of the added complexity involved. The use of continuous electroencephalography (EEG) in conjunction with somatosensory evoked potentials (SSEPs) is another way to evaluated cerebral perfusion during CEA. Both EEG and SSEPs demonstrate loss of amplitude and frequency when cerebral blood flow decreases to a certain level.

The drawback for both of these modalities is that they assess relatively large vascular territories for ischemia and may not detect microemboli. Also, in patients with sizable preoperative infarcts, these neurophysiologic monitoring techniques have trouble detecting further neuronal dysfunction in the area immediately surrounding the infarct. The benefit of this type of monitoring is that cerebral perfusion can be evaluated prior to the arteriotomy by clamping the ICA distal to the lesion and then proceeding with the more proximal dissection. Any change in the EEG or SSEPs can then be addressed with hemodynamic alterations. A continued decrease despite increasing systemic blood pressure can be readily reversed by releasing the clamp, and the necessary steps for the placement of a shunt can be taken in an unhurried fashion. Preoperative evaluation of collateral flow with a cerebral angiogram also helps the surgeon in the planning of what steps to take to reduce cerebral ischemia (**Fig. 17.2C,D**). Again, there is no "right" way to perform a CEA. If the particular technique employed by an individual surgeon accomplishes the goal of revascularization with a low morbidity and mortality rate, then that technique is "right" for that surgeon.

◆ Operative Technique

The author has personally tried many different surgical techniques for CEA including both loupe magnification and the operating microscope, patch angioplasty and primary repair, and both general and regional anesthesia, and has at present adopted the standard use of 3.5× loupe-magnification, general anesthesia with EEG and SSEPs, and the selective use of shunting and patch angioplasty. This technique has been used in over 200 CEA procedures with a 30-day stroke rate of 2% in the combined asymptomatic and symptomatic populations. As previously mentioned, there is no absolute correct technique for CEA, and the style described below reflects a combination of different techniques that the author believes works best for him and his patients.

As with any surgical procedure, a complete understanding of the pertinent anatomy remains the foundation of any carotid endarterectomy. This means not only the anatomic knowledge of the neck but also the vascular anatomy proximal and distal to the lesion. The location of the stenosis, the proximal and distal extent of the plaque, the location and orientation of the superior thyroid artery as well as aberrant branches, and the presence or absence of intracranial collateral flow should be established prior to the operation. Knowledge of the level of the bifurcation helps to tailor the size and orientation of the incision, and a complete preoperative understanding of the patient's vascular anatomy is necessary for the surgeon to achieve complete vascular control throughout the procedure. Meticulous anatomic dissection is vital to identify and protect all vulnerable structures, and every effort must be made to ensure that the field remains bloodless. This can be easily accomplished with the routine use of both monopolar and bipolar electrocautery. There is rarely an indication for vascular clips. These add unnecessarily to the

cost of the operation, and any sizable vessels requiring more than electrocautery can be ligated with silk ties.

Once the patient is under general anesthesia and the EEG/SSEP monitoring is established, the patient is positioned with the head extended and rotated away from the side of the operation. Three safety straps are place across the patient's chest, abdomen, and thighs so that the table can be tilted approximately 10 degrees further away from the side of the lesion. The surgeon stands on the side of the stenosis, with the assistant on the opposite side. The added tilt allows for a flat operative field and better visibility for assistant. After the skin is prepped in the standard fashion, 1% lidocaine with epinephrine is injected subcutaneously under the planned incision. If at all possible, the author tries to make the incision tangentially within one of the creases of the neck. This heals more cosmetically than a more vertical incision made along the anterior border of the sternocleidomastoid muscle, and when placed appropriately provides generous exposure.

The initial incision is made through the dermis, and hemostasis is maintained with monopolar electrocautery. The dissection is then carried down to, and through, the platysma using electrocautery. This muscle is then undermined on both sides to provide enough edge for its reapproximation at the conclusion of the operation. A self-retaining retractor with dull points is then placed under the edges of the platysma. The dull points minimize the potential for vascular injury. Depending on the size of the patient, there is a variable amount of fat underneath the platysma, and this can be easily dissected through down to the anterior border of the sternocleidomastoid using scissors and electrocautery. The dissection then proceeds down the sternocleidomastoid to the level of the jugular vein, taking care to realize that the spinal accessory nerve can be encountered here. The retractor may be repositioned so that the lateral blade rests under the sternocleidomastoid, but the medial blade should not be moved to a deeper level where the laryngeal nerves may be injured. The surgeon's attention should now move to the medial edge of the jugular vein, as mobilizing the vein away from the carotid within the carotid sheath is the next step. The common facial vein and possibly other small veins are usually encountered at this point, and they need to be ligated with silk ties and divided so that the jugular can be retracted laterally to expose the bifurcation of the carotid. Once an adequate plane is developed between the jugular and the carotid, the lateral blades of the retractor can be used to retract the vein. A second retractor is placed orthogonally to the initial retractor but at a more superficial level.

The anesthesiologist then administers 5000 U of intravenous heparin before any further dissection is performed. Attention is then focused toward the dissection of the distal ICA. As the plane between the jugular laterally and the ICA medially is developed, the superior root of the ansa cervicalis, or descendens hypoglossi, is encountered. This nerve will lead the surgeon superiorly to the hypoglossal nerve, which is usually found just deep to the inferior belly of the digastric muscle. The hypoglossal crosses the ICA and the branches of the external carotid artery (ECA) and can be mobilized by releasing the nerve from its adventitial attachments. The nerve can be mobilized further by sectioning the descendens hypoglossi, tying a silk tie to the proximal end, and then pulling that superiorly. Ligation and division of the small artery and vein of the sternocleidomastoid will also allow for further mobilization of the hypoglossal. Identification and mobilization of the nerve is crucial to avoid any trauma to it and the resultant palsy. Circumferential dissection of the distal ICA should be done only beyond the visible or palpable plaque. Doing so will avoid manipulation of the plaque, which could cause thromboembolic complications. The distal ICA is dissected using a small right-angle clamp, and a vessel loop is passed around the vessel twice and then tagged off with a hemostat. A small aneurysm clip is then placed proximal to the vessel loop, and both the EEG technician and the anesthesiologist are notified. Clamping the ICA this early in the operation accomplishes two goals: it prevents thromboembolic complications during the subsequent dissection of the bifurcation and underlying plaque, and it enables the EEG technician to recognize any loss in power ipsilateral to the lesion. If there is a change detected on EEG, the anesthesiologist is asked to take steps necessary to elevate the mean arterial pressure and augment collateral flow. If this does not cause a correction in the EEG, the aneurysm clip is removed and arrangements are made for the placement of a shunt.

With the ICA clamped, the surgeon's attention can then be focused on the dissection of the external and common carotid arteries. Dissection of the ECA is usually done at the level of the take-off of the superior thyroid artery, and this small branch is tied off separately. The ECA is then turned laterally and the aneurysm clip applied. This maneuver allows the clip to rest in a flush position away from the arteriotomy line, minimizing the chance that it will be an obstacle during the arteriotomy closure. The common carotid is then dissected in a circumferential manner proximal to the palpable plaque, and a vessel loop is passed around it twice. A DeBakey clamp is then placed distal to the vessel loop with special attention not to include the vagus in the cross clamp. The retractors and clamp are covered with surgical towels to prevent inadvertent entanglement with suture, suction tubing, etc. There is rarely a need to dissect circumferentially around the bifurcation, as the vagus nerve can be injured here, and excessive mobilization of the artery can lead to a postoperative kink. If manipulation of the carotid sinus causes any change in the patient's vital signs, the sinus is injected with 2 cc of 1% plain lidocaine. Usually, any change in the vital signs is transient and will not require lidocaine at the sinus.

A small arteriotomy is made with a No. 11 blade in the distal common carotid, and at this point the suction is placed in the opening. This results in the collapse of the artery distal to the plaque, which serves as a guide to the distal extent of the arteriotomy. Pott's scissors are then used to extend the arteriotomy in both directions. At this stage, the aneurysm clip on the ICA is release to verify back flow and then reapplied. This is not a necessary step, but it does serve to bolster confidence in sufficient collateral flow.

The surgeon then grabs the lateral wall of the artery with Gerald forceps and develops a plane between the intima and the plaque with a small dissector. The assistant then holds the plaques as the plane is developed toward the posterior wall. The same is done with the medial side of the artery. The plaque is then cut with Pott's scissors and reflected superiorly while the dissector is used to separate the plaque from the arterial wall. A small right-angle clamp is used to develop this plane in the proximal ECA and is then used to perform a modified eversion endarterectomy of the ECA. The remainder of the plaque is then dissected free from the intima until it feathers out distally. One should not chase the plaque distal to the arteriotomy, as visibility is poor. Any flap seen distally after the plaque is removed should be treated with a tack-down suture of double-armed 6-0 Prolene placed from the inside of the vessel out. Ring-tipped forceps are then used to remove any remaining atheroma, and the endarterectomy bed is then inspected while irrigating with heparinized saline. During this maneuver, any wisps of atheroma remaining can be easily identified and removed.

Should a shunt be required, the author prefers the Argyle shunt (Covidien, Mansfield, MA). There are other shunts on the market, and they all work just as well. No matter the type of shunt used, the surgeon should be comfortable using it. A Rummel-type tourniquet is used on the vessel loops on both the ICA and the common carotid. A silk tie is secured around the shunt at its midpoint, and this provides an identifiable reference point should the shunt move once it is placed. The shunt is first passed proximally, and once blood flow is established and all of the air is out of the shunt, it is passed distally. The tourniquets are secured, and the tag ends of the vessel loops are secured out of the way. The EEG technician will invariably see a correction in the EEG.

The arteriotomy is then reapproximated primarily from distal to proximal. The initial anchor stitch is placed using both arms of the suture and passing from the inside to the out. The author prefers to tie this knot using instruments, as this will provide a longer working length of suture for the closure. Each pass of the needle is made as close as possible to the edge of the arteriotomy and advanced almost a millimeter with each new pass. This closure technique is very similar to the one employed in the microsurgical technique, and if done well will render a suture line that is almost invisible once completed. Such small bites obviate the need for a patch angioplasty in all but the smallest of ICAs. After passing the final stitch, the suture is held loosely and the ICA clamp is released to flush out any debris distal to the clamp as well as any air in the endarterectomy. The final knot is tied with the clamp still released, and the suture line is inspected for any possible leaks. The aneurysm clip is then reapplied, and the common carotid clamp is released followed by the ECA clamp. Sufficient time (10 seconds) is allowed to pass for any debris to be flushed into the ECA tree before releasing the ICA clamp. The tie on the superior thyroid artery is then removed. The suture line is once more inspected, with any major bleeding point treated with a 6-0 Prolene and a figure-8 stitch. Otherwise, any oozing is treated with antibiotic irrigation followed by Surgicel and gentle pressure for 5 minutes. The heparin is never reversed; the Surgicel is left on the suture line. Patients on dual antiplatelet therapy will have more oozing in general than patients on aspirin only and will benefit from placing a TLS® drain (Stryker, Kalamazoo, MI) in the operative bed.

The retractors are removed, and meticulous attention is then paid toward hemostasis. Any bleeding points at this stage of the operation can usually be stopped with bipolar electrocautery. The platysma is then reapproximated primarily with 2-0 Vicryl in a running fashion, and the skin with 4-0 Monocryl in a running subcuticular fashion. The skin is then reapproximated with Dermabond in women and with Mastisol followed by Steri-Strips in men. The reason for the distinction between the sexes is that the beard on a man can elevate and detach the Dermabond. The patient is then allowed to awaken from anesthesia to the point at which an adequate neurologic assessment can be performed prior to going to the recovery room.

◆ Conclusion

In the treatment of extracranial carotid disease, the most difficult aspect is deciding who will benefit from a CEA. A proper understanding of cervicocerebral vascular anatomy and cerebral physiology is mandatory for any surgeon performing CEA. Carotid surgeons must also assess their results to ensure that their complication rate does not exceed 3%. It is only when the morbidity and mortality of the operation are this low that the benefits of CEA outweigh the risks. The decision to operate on an asymptomatic patient should always be tempered with the potential benefits of modern medical therapy and endovascular techniques as well as the Hippocratic notion of "first do no harm." The techniques described in this chapter have been successful in achieving acceptable outcomes, but they are in no way meant to be thought of as a "standard." There are as many technical variations in CEA as there are surgeons, and the only standard is that of a good outcome.

References

1. Beneficial effect of carotid endarterectomy in symptomatic patients with high-grade carotid stenosis. North American Symptomatic Carotid Endarterectomy Trial Collaborators. N Engl J Med 1991;325:445–453
2. Endarterectomy for asymptomatic carotid artery stenosis. Executive Committee for the Asymptomatic Carotid Atherosclerosis Study. JAMA 1995;273:1421–1428
3. Randomised trial of endarterectomy for recently symptomatic carotid stenosis: final results of the MRC European Carotid Surgery Trial (ECST). Lancet 1998;351:1379–1387
4. Ratliff DA, Hames TK, Humphries KN, Birch S, Chant AD. The reliability of Doppler ultrasound techniques in the assessment of carotid disease. Angiology 1985;36:333–340
5. Strandness D Jr. Duplex Scanning in Vascular Disorders. New York: Raven Press, 1990
6. Grant EG, Benson CB, Moneta GL, et al. Carotid artery stenosis: grayscale and Doppler US diagnosis–Society of Radiologists in Ultrasound Consensus Conference. Radiology 2003;229:340–346
7. Moneta GL, Edwards JM, Chitwood RW, et al. Correlation of North American Symptomatic Carotid Endarterectomy Trial (NASCET) angiographic definition of 70% to 99% internal carotid artery stenosis with duplex scanning. J Vasc Surg 1993;17:152–157, discussion 157–159
8. Moneta GL, Edwards JM, Papanicolaou G, et al. Screening for asymptomatic internal carotid artery stenosis: duplex criteria for discriminating 60% to 99% stenosis. J Vasc Surg 1995;21:989–994
9. Earnest FT IV, Forbes G, Sandok BA, et al. Complications of cerebral angiography: prospective assessment of risk. AJR Am J Roentgenol 1984;142:247–253
10. Pryor JC, Setton A, Nelson PK, Berenstein A. Complications of diagnostic cerebral angiography and tips on avoidance. Neuroimaging Clin N Am 1996;6:751–758
11. Ringer AJ, Lanzino G, Veznedaroglu E, et al. Does angiographic surveillance pose a risk in the management of coiled intracranial aneurysms? A multicenter study of 2243 patients. Neurosurgery 2008;63:845–849, discussion 849
12. Koelemay MJ, Nederkoorn PJ, Reitsma JB, Majoie CB. Systematic review of computed tomographic angiography for assessment of carotid artery disease. Stroke 2004;35:2306–2312
13. Nederkoorn PJ, van der Graaf Y, Hunink MG. Duplex ultrasound and magnetic resonance angiography compared with digital subtraction angiography in carotid artery stenosis: a systematic review. Stroke 2003;34:1324–1332
14. Rothwell PM, Eliasziw M, Gutnikov SA, et al; Carotid Endarterectomy Trialists' Collaboration. Analysis of pooled data from the randomised controlled trials of endarterectomy for symptomatic carotid stenosis. Lancet 2003;361:107–116
15. Biller J, Feinberg WM, Castaldo JE, et al. Guidelines for carotid endarterectomy: a statement for healthcare professionals from a special writing group of the Stroke Council, American Heart Association. Stroke 1998;29:554–562
16. Goldstein LB, Adams R, Becker K, et al. Primary prevention of ischemic stroke: A statement for healthcare professionals from the Stroke Council of the American Heart Association. Stroke 2001;32:280–299
17. Sacco RL, Adams R, Albers G, et al; American Heart Association; American Stroke Association Council on Stroke; Council on Cardiovascular Radiology and Intervention; American Academy of Neurology. Guidelines for prevention of stroke in patients with ischemic stroke or transient ischemic attack: a statement for healthcare professionals from the American Heart Association/American Stroke Association Council on Stroke: co-sponsored by the Council on Cardiovascular Radiology and Intervention: the American Academy of Neurology affirms the value of this guideline. Stroke 2006;37:577–617
18. Killeen SD, Andrews EJ, Redmond HP, Fulton GJ. Provider volume and outcomes for abdominal aortic aneurysm repair, carotid endarterectomy, and lower extremity revascularization procedures. J Vasc Surg 2007;45:615–626
19. Rothwell PM, Warlow CP. Interpretation of operative risks of individual surgeons. European Carotid Surgery Trialists' Collaborative Group. Lancet 1999;353:1325
20. Bond R, Rerkasem K, Naylor AR, Abu Rahma AF, Rothwell PM. Systematic review of randomized controlled trials of patch angioplasty versus primary closure and different types of patch materials during carotid endarterectomy. J Vasc Surg 2004;40:1126–1135
21. Rothwell PM. Endarterectomy for symptomatic and asymptomatic carotid stenosis. Neurol Clin 2008;26:1079–1097, x
22. Rothwell PM, Giles MF, Chandratheva A, et al; Early use of Existing Preventive Strategies for Stroke (EXPRESS) study. Effect of urgent treatment of transient ischaemic attack and minor stroke on early recurrent stroke (EXPRESS study): a prospective population-based sequential comparison. Lancet 2007;370:1432–1442
23. Rothwell PM, Slattery J, Warlow CP. Clinical and angiographic predictors of stroke and death from carotid endarterectomy: systematic review. BMJ 1997;315:1571–1577
24. Karkos CD, Hernandez-Lahoz I, Naylor AR. Urgent carotid surgery in patients with crescendo transient ischaemic attacks and stroke-in-evolution: a systematic review. Eur J Vasc Endovasc Surg 2009;37:279–288
25. Karkos CD, McMahon G, McCarthy MJ, et al. The value of urgent carotid surgery for crescendo transient ischemic attacks. J Vasc Surg 2007;45:1148–1154
26. Wilson SE, Mayberg MR, Yatsu F, Weiss DG. Crescendo transient ischemic attacks: a surgical imperative. Veterans Affairs trialists. J Vasc Surg 1993;17:249–255, discussion 255–256
27. Bond R, Rerkasem K, Cuffe R, Rothwell PM. A systematic review of the associations between age and sex and the operative risks of carotid endarterectomy. Cerebrovasc Dis 2005;20:69–77
28. Perler BA. The impact of advanced age on the results of carotid endarterectomy: an outcome analysis. J Am Coll Surg 1996;183:559–564
29. Alamowitch S, Eliasziw M, Barnett HJ; North American Symptomatic Carotid Endarterectomy Trial (NASCET); ASA Trial Group; Carotid Endarterectomy (ACE) Trial Group. The risk and benefit of endarterectomy in women with symptomatic internal carotid artery disease. Stroke 2005;36:27–31
30. Wolf PA, D'Agostino RB, Belanger AJ, Kannel WB. Probability of stroke: a risk profile from the Framingham Study. Stroke 1991;22:312–318

31. Julien TH. CJ: Simultaneous carotid occlusive disease and intracranial aneurysm. In: Loftus CM, Kresowik TF, eds. Carotid Artery Surgery. New York: Thieme, 2000

32. Stern J, Whelan M, Brisman R, Correll JW. Management of extracranial carotid stenosis and intracranial aneurysms. J Neurosurg 1979;51:147–150

33. Prabhakaran S, Rundek T, Ramas R, et al. Carotid plaque surface irregularity predicts ischemic stroke: the northern Manhattan study. Stroke 2006;37:2696–2701

34. Halliday A, Mansfield A, Marro J, et al; MRC Asymptomatic Carotid Surgery Trial (ACST) Collaborative Group. Prevention of disabling and fatal strokes by successful carotid endarterectomy in patients without recent neurological symptoms: randomised controlled trial. Lancet 2004;363:1491–1502

35. Helton TJ, Bavry AA, Rajagopal V, Anderson RD, Yadav JS, Bhatt DL. The optimal treatment of carotid atherosclerosis: a 2008 update and literature review. Postgrad Med 2008;120:103–112

36. Schneider JR, Droste JS, Schindler N, Golan JF. Carotid endarterectomy in octogenarians: comparison with patient characteristics and outcomes in younger patients. J Vasc Surg 2000;31:927–935

37. Usman AA, Tang GL, Eskandari MK. Metaanalysis of procedural stroke and death among octogenarians: carotid stenting versus carotid endarterectomy. J Am Coll Surg 2009;208:1124–1131

38. Abbott AL. Medical (nonsurgical) intervention alone is now best for prevention of stroke associated with asymptomatic severe carotid stenosis: results of a systematic review and analysis. Stroke 2009;40:e573–e583

39. Riles TS, Kopelman I, Imparato AM. Myocardial infarction following carotid endarterectomy: a review of 683 operations. Surgery 1979;85:249–252

40. Forssell C, Kitzing P, Bergqvist D. Cranial nerve injuries after carotid artery surgery. A prospective study of 663 operations. Eur J Vasc Endovasc Surg 1995;10:445–449

41. Stoneham MD, Thompson JP. Arterial pressure management and carotid endarterectomy. Br J Anaesth 2009;102:442–452

42. Rerkasem K, Rothwell PM. Systematic review of the operative risks of carotid endarterectomy for recently symptomatic stenosis in relation to the timing of surgery. Stroke 2009;40:e564–e572

43. Bond R, Rerkasem K, AbuRahma AF, Naylor AR, Rothwell PM. Patch angioplasty versus primary closure for carotid endarterectomy. Cochrane Database Syst Rev 2004;2:CD000160

44. Myers SI, Valentine RJ, Chervu A, Bowers BL, Clagett GP. Saphenous vein patch versus primary closure for carotid endarterectomy: long-term assessment of a randomized prospective study. J Vasc Surg 1994;19:15–22

45. Ojemann RG, Heros RC. Carotid endarterectomy. To shunt or not to shunt? Arch Neurol 1986;43:617–618

18

Microsurgical Revascularization of Extracranial Vertebral Artery

Ricardo A. Hanel, Leonardo B.C. Brasiliense, Felipe C. Albuquerque, and Robert F. Spetzler

Pearls

- Occlusive disease of the extracranial vertebral artery (VA) is a common finding.
- Both thromboembolic and hemodynamic symptoms can occur. Very often symptoms are associated with contralateral VA disease or anatomic variation (e.g., hypoplasia, absent V4 segment).
- V1 segment stenosis treatment options include angioplasty/stenting (higher incidence of restenosis), vertebral artery to carotid artery transposition, and vertebral artery endarterectomy.
- V2 segment lesions are often related to extrinsic compression and require direct exposure/decompression.
- V3 segment lesions (bow hunter's syndrome) are often related to soft tissue compression and can be treated by either decompression, C1-C2 fusion, or both.

The natural history and role of surgical revascularization in the treatment of cervical atherosclerotic carotid disease to prevent stroke are well established.[1,2] The same, however, cannot be said about lesions involving the extracranial vertebral artery (VA). The different segments of the extracranial VA (V1, V2, and V3) can be affected by various conditions, individualized or combined, including atherosclerotic disease, extrinsic compression, and excessive mobility.

Atherosclerotic occlusive disease of the extracranial VA is a common finding on diagnostic imaging, but its actual incidence in the general population is unknown, although it has been estimated to vary from 25 to 40% of studied subjects.[3,4] Symptoms of posterior circulation ischemia are seldom as readily recognized as symptoms related to anterior circulation ischemia. This difficulty in diagnosis is related to the wide variety of complaints reported by patients and to the association of these complaints with those attributable to other body systems. Although the course of disease of the VA can often be asymptomatic, two thirds of patients have stroke as their presenting symptom.[4] For patients who present with transient ischemic attacks of the posterior circulation, the presence of VA disease represents a 25 to 35% risk of stroke over 5 years[4] with a high risk of mortality.[5] Although atherosclerotic disease can involve any segment of the VA, it is most frequently found at its origin.

There is no consensus regarding the best treatment for atherosclerotic disease or extrinsic compression of the VA. The efficacy of medical management with antiplatelet and anticoagulation agents has varied.[3–7] Indirect evidence from the anterior and intracranial circulation indicates that revascularization might be a better alternative for these patients.[1,2,8] In the late 1950s, surgical revascularization for the proximal VA via primary endarterectomy of the vertebral and subclavian arteries,[9] transposition of the VA to the common carotid artery (CCA),[10] and graft interposition[10] were introduced. The lack of supporting evidence from randomized trials, the negative results of the extracranial-to-intracranial bypass trial,[11] difficulties in diagnosis, and the advent of endovascular techniques probably prevented the widespread use of surgical revascularization for proximal vertebral artery conditions. Angioplasty and stenting for stenosis of the origin of the VA were introduced as safe alternatives to surgical revascularization.[12] However, the alarming rate of restenosis in as many as 43% of the cases receiving bare-metal stents for lesions at the origin of the VA[13] led investigators to question the long-term efficacy of such intervention. Drug-eluting stents have been used to overcome this problem.[14] Recently, many concerns have been raised about long-term outcomes and the possibility of a higher incidence of delayed thrombosis associated with drug-eluting stents.[15] The mid- and long-term outcomes of patients with drug-eluting stents placed to treat stenosis of the origin of the VA remain to be seen.

Surgical alternatives for the V2 segment, such as the anterior and anterolateral approach, have been described.[16] For the V3 segment, direct decompression has been described both associated and not associated with fusion.[17] The bony and ligamentous encasement and mobility of the V2 and V3 make endoluminal revascularization of these segments problematic.

This chapter analyzes the indications, technique, and results associated with microsurgical revascularization of the extracranial VA, with emphasis on the proximal vessel, given the high incidence of disease involving this segment.

◆ Anatomy

The proximal extracranial VA typically originates from the superior-posterior wall of its respective subclavian artery. The VA also can have an anomalous origin from multiple sites, including the aortic arch and the CCA.

In the classic arch configuration, the first segment of the VA begins at its origin along the posterior-superior border of the subclavian artery and extends to its entrance into the transverse foramen of the sixth cervical vertebra. The second segment extends from the sixth to the second cervical vertebra, traveling through the transverse foramen of each vertebral level. This segment can be extremely tortuous, which can make it difficult to place a stent in the middle or distal portions of the extracranial VA. The third segment of the VA is rostral to the second cervical vertebra, terminating at the point at which the artery pierces the dura mater. The fourth and final segment, the intradural segment, extends from the entrance of the VA into the cranial compartment to its junction with the contralateral VA to form the basilar artery. The posterior inferior cerebellar artery (PICA) usually originates from this intradural segment.

In an estimated 7% of patients, the VA ends anomalously at the PICA.[18] The rami of the anterior spinal artery also originate from this final segment and join to form the anterior spinal artery. In some patients, the PICA is absent and its territory will be fed by the ipsilateral anterior inferior cerebellar artery or the contralateral PICA.

Muscular branches usually originate from the second and third segments of the VA. These branches typically supply the dorsal cervical musculature and often communicate with branches of the thyrocervical trunk or external carotid artery, especially in the presence of an occlusion of the CCA or VA. It is important to recognize the location of these branches to avoid their perforation during manipulation of a catheter or wire. The presence of cervical muscular collateral vessels has been associated with improved clinical outcomes in symptomatic patients.[4]

◆ Clinical Manifestations

Cerebral ischemia is classified into two main categories on the basis of the duration of neurologic symptoms. A typical transient ischemic attack begins abruptly and lasts 5 to 20 minutes but can continue as long as 24 hours. A stroke is defined as any ischemic event with symptoms lasting longer than 24 hours.

Vertebrobasilar ischemia can result from embolic, thrombotic, and hemodynamic mechanisms. It is essential to classify the patient's neurologic symptoms into one of these categories based on the clinical time course of symptoms to determine the target of initial investigational studies and treatment. Embolism is the most frequent cause of vertebrobasilar ischemia and manifests with sudden maximal onset of neurologic symptoms. Embolism most commonly affects distal high-flow vasculature, which in the vertebrobasilar system usually involves the posterior cerebral arteries, primarily those associated with vision. Symptoms of embolic ischemia can resolve quickly, especially if rapid spontaneous lysis of the embolus occurs. Embolic stroke is most often associated with postinfarction intracerebral hemorrhage. Embolic ischemia is most often associated with a lesion at the origin of the VA.[4] For the V2 and V3 segments, symptoms are often associated with specific head movements. A history of vertebrobasilar symptoms referable to a particular head position must be considered highly suspicious for the diagnosis of bow hunter's syndrome. Tissington Tatlow and Bammer[19] described a series of maneuvers to isolate symptoms caused by head positioning relative to the torso from those caused by head positioning alone. The maneuvers were intended to distinguish traditional vestibular system–associated vertigo and nausea from symptoms related to vascular compromise.

Thrombotic cerebral ischemia usually has a relatively slow, fluctuating course until the patient's symptoms become maximally severe. This progressive course can occur over hours to days as the size of the thrombus increases or decreases. Thrombotic occlusive lesions are often associated with focal stenosis or ulceration of atherosclerotic plaque because these lesions are predisposed to platelet aggregation and thrombus formation.

Low-flow hemodynamic symptoms develop as a result of a critical stenosis or of tandem stenoses that reduce distal perfusion pressure. The reduction is such that a moderate decrease in mean arterial blood pressure or a sudden increase in resistance causes a precipitous drop in distal perfusion pressure beyond the level of the stenosis. When that decreased blood flow is insufficient to support normal neuronal function, neurologic symptoms occur. Vertebrobasilar insufficiency, which is the term used for transient, low-flow vertebrobasilar ischemic symptoms, is often positional and may be associated with a stereotypical movement such as extension or rotation of the head in a particular direction. These transient episodes can be caused by isolated atherosclerosis or severe cervical spondylosis that narrows the transverse foramina.[20] If ischemia is prolonged, it can lead to frank infarction. Vertebrobasilar insufficiency also can be caused by subclavian-steal syndrome, in which there is high-grade stenosis or occlusion of the subclavian artery proximal to the origin of the VA. When using the affected arm, the patient develops stereotypical, low-flow hemodynamic vertebrobasilar symptoms as a result of retrograde flow in the ipsilateral VA. Thus, the subclavian artery "steals" blood from the posterior fossa to feed the arm musculature.

A constellation of symptoms is referable to vertebrobasilar ischemia because of the potential involvement of neural tissue representing fine motor control, balance, cranial nerve function, vision, strength, and level of consciousness. Vertebrobasilar symptoms are often confused with dysfunction of other body systems. The true hallmark of vertebrobasilar ischemia is the simultaneous manifestation of multiple symptoms, the most common of which are vertigo and visual dysfunction.[7] Episodic perioral numbness or paresthesias are also specific signs of vertebrobasilar ischemia. Other potential symptoms include ataxia, dysarthria, syncope, headache, nausea, vomiting, tinnitus, bilateral motor or sensory complaints, and cranial nerve dysfunction. Cranial nerve dysfunction can result in facial palsy, dysphagia, aspiration, dysarthria, diplopia, nystagmus, facial numbness, or torticollis. Specific syndromes associated with occlusion of a particular vessel, such as lateral medullary syndrome (Wallenberg), are well described.[21]

◆ Indications for Treatment

No randomized data are available regarding the benefit of revascularization of the extracranial VA in preventing stroke. However, data extrapolated from case series[10,22,23] and cervical carotid trials[1] support such interventions by microsurgical or endoluminal means.

As with any treatment, the risks associated with surgical intervention must be outweighed by its potential benefits. The severe consequences of vertebrobasilar infarction necessitate a lower threshold for intervention when compared with anterior circulation disease of a similar angiographic severity. However, the need to intervene is tempered by the anatomic consideration of the posterior circulation as a confluence of two vessels and the large number of patients who remain asymptomatic despite occlusion of one extracranial VA. In an attempt to clarify the indications and benefits of treatment in this population, the Vertebral Artery Stenting Trial will randomize patients with symptomatic stenosis involving the origin of the VA to receive best medical treatment or endovascular revascularization (i.e., stenting).[24] The general guidelines below are followed at our institution.

Symptomatic Patients

The cause of symptoms attributed to vertebrobasilar ischemia must be determined to be embolic, thrombotic, or hemodynamic. Routine cerebrovascular imaging begins with diffusion and perfusion-weighted magnetic resonance imaging (MRI) of the head to determine the presence of a possible vertebrobasilar flow deficit or infarct. Vascular imaging is usually performed with computed tomography angiography (CTA) or MRI. The first is preferred, given the well-known false-positive results for VA origin stenosis on MRI. CTA is very valuable during investigation for extrinsic compression at V2 because of the strong correlation between bony and vascular anatomy. When V2 and V3 segment compression is suspected to be associated with certain head positions, cerebral angiography with head motion can be used to elucidate the level of compression.

At our institution, symptomatic patients with a single, causative atherosclerotic lesion involving the V1 segment that measures more than 50% stenosis on digital subtraction angiography undergo angioplasty and stenting. Both are performed during a single session. In patients with tandem lesions, the decision to treat one or both lesions depends on whether the symptoms are thought to be embolic or hemodynamic. For tandem lesions associated with embolic symptomatology, the bias for treatment is toward origin, higher grade, or ulcerated lesions. Cerebral blood flow analysis (positron emission tomography, single photon emission computed tomography, or computed tomography [CT] perfusion), with and without acetazolamide, can help assess whether compromise of the reserve indicates a hemodynamically significant lesion. V2 and V3 segment lesions are analyzed case by case, with extrinsic compression being treated by microsurgical decompression preferentially.

Asymptomatic Patients

Advances in imaging technology have increased the diagnosis of asymptomatic VA occlusive disease. Most asymptomatic patients do not require treatment. Several groups of asymptomatic patients, however, have indications for endovascular treatment because of their elevated risk for stroke. As mentioned, treatment should be considered because patients with extracranial VA occlusive disease typically first present with a stroke and not with a warning transient ischemic attack. Furthermore, high rates of morbidity and mortality are associated with vertebrobasilar strokes.[25] Patients with high-grade (>70% stenosis) lesions or a progressive increase in the severity of their stenosis have a high risk of stroke. Thus, patients with either feature would benefit from treatment, especially those with disease involving the dominant or a single VA.

◆ Microsurgical Revascularization of Extracranial Vertebral Artery

The surgical technique for revascularization and/or decompression of the extracranial VA is detailed elsewhere.[23,26,27] In recent years, therapeutic options such angioplasty and stenting have also been discussed with surgical candidates.

Some general principles for cerebrovascular revascularization developed by the senior author (R.F.S.) apply to revascularization of the extracranial VA. All patients are placed on aspirin (81 to 325 mg) before the procedure. Surgery is performed with the patient under general anesthesia, with normal physiologic parameters maintained during the case. Somatosensory evoked potentials and electroencephalography are used routinely. Intravenous heparin (50 to 70 U /kg) is given at least 5 minutes before occlusion of a major vessel. Barbiturate-induced burst suppression is induced before vascular clamping and maintained during the period of occlusion. The operative microscope is used during the final stages of vascular dissection and throughout vascular clamping, endarterectomy, and anastomosis. Microsuction (MicroVac, PMT Corp., Chanhassen, MN) is routinely applied to the anastomosis bed to improve overall visualization.

◆ Surgical Technique for Proximal Vertebral Artery Revascularization

Our preferred route is the supraclavicular approach for revascularization of the proximal VA (**Figs. 18.1, 18.2, 18.3, 18.4, and 18.5**). A linear incision, 6 to 8 cm long and centered at the clavicular head of the sternocleidomastoid (SCM) muscle, is placed approximately 2.5 cm above and parallel to the clavicle. The clavicular head of the SCM is isolated, ligated, and divided (**Fig. 18.6**). Lateral dissection usually stops before the phrenic nerve is exposed. The recurrent laryngeal nerve and sympathetic trunk are often exposed and must be handled carefully. Occasionally, brachial plexus structures are visualized and must be handled appropriately. First, the CCA is identified. Once the carotid sheath is opened, the CCA can be exposed and individualized. The internal jugular vein (IJV) is also identified and retracted laterally. When the procedure involves the left side, the thoracic duct requires special attention. This vessel-like structure, which is located on the fat pad deep to the IJV, should be ligated and divided to prevent the development of a lymphatic fistula. A smaller endolymphatic duct on the right side also may require ligation.

The VA can be identified using anatomic landmarks. Often the thyrocervical trunk, which originates from the subclavian artery, is first visualized during dissection. Its identification and proximal dissection leads to the subclavian artery and, just medial to the trunk, to the VA. The VA can be differentiated from the thyrocervical and costocervical trunk by the lack of branches on its proximal segment. In as many as 90% of the cases, the VA enters the foramen transversarium at the

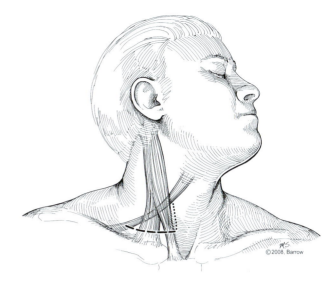

Fig. 18.1 Position of skin incision for the supraclavicular approach for proximal revascularization of the vertebral artery. Additional distal exposure can be obtained by extending the incision on the anterior border of the sternocleidomastoid muscle (*dotted line*). (Courtesy of the Barrow Neurological Institute.)

level of C6. Palpation of the transverse process of C6 helps guide localization and identification of the vessels. Given the presence of disease at the origin of the VA, the lack of pulsation of the vessel can sometimes be misleading. At this point, the VA and CCA are identified and isolated. The entire VA,

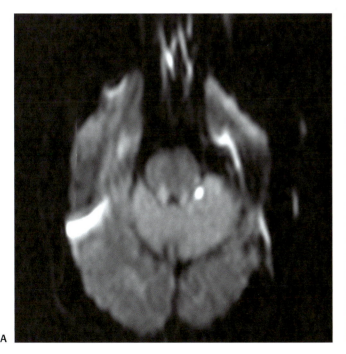

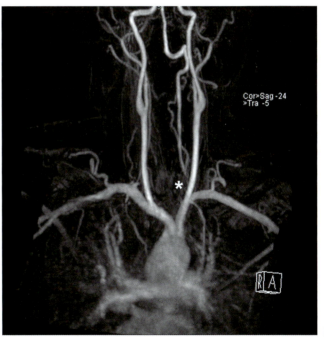

Fig. 18.2 A 41-year-old man presented with recurrent transient ischemic attacks of the vertebrobasilar artery despite maximal medical therapy. **(A)** Axial magnetic resonance imaging (MRI) showed a diffusion restrictive lesion in the distribution of the left posterior inferior cerebellar artery (PICA). **(B)** Magnetic resonance angiography (MRA) showed the absence of the right vertebral artery (VA) and a severely stenotic, possibly occluded, proximal left VA (*asterisk*). (*continued on next page*)

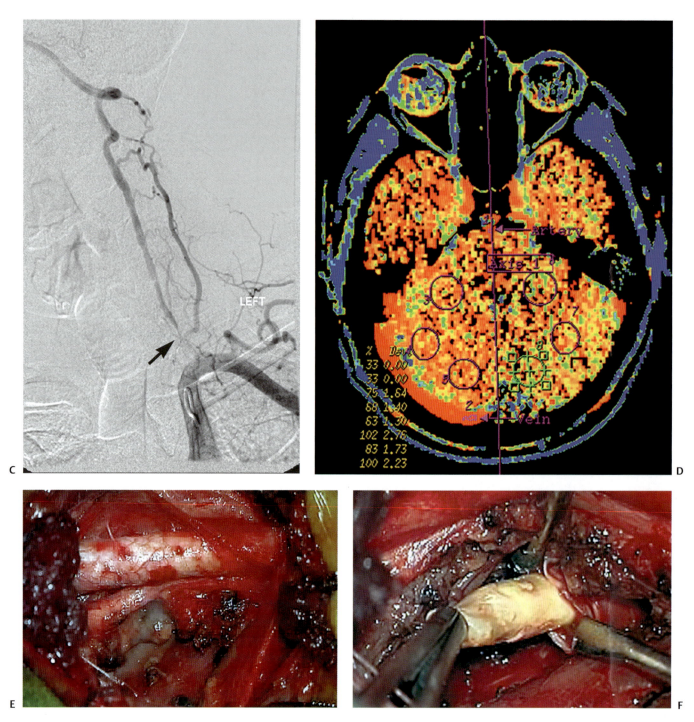

Fig. 18.2 (*continued*)   (**C**) Digital subtraction angiography showed complete occlusion of the left VA with recanalization via the thyrocervical branches (*arrow*). (**D**) Perfusion computed tomography showed hypoperfusion of the distribution of the left PICA. (**E**) The patient underwent a supraclavicular approach for (**F**) a left VA endarterectomy.

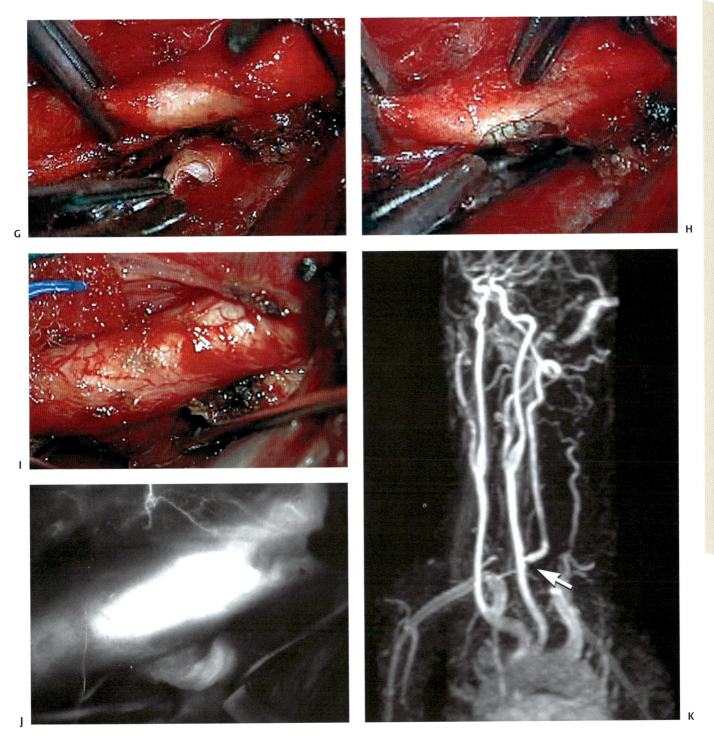

G

H

I

J

K

Fig. 18.2 (*continued*) (**G**) The resected end of the VA was positioned in preparation for the anastomosis. (**H**) The end of the VA was sutured to the side of the common carotid artery (CCA) to achieve (**I**) a left VA-to-CCA transposition. (**J**) Intraoperative indocyanine green videoangiogram and (**K**) postoperative MRA showed a patent anastomosis (*arrow*) and good revascularization of the left VA. (Courtesy of the Barrow Neurological Institute.)

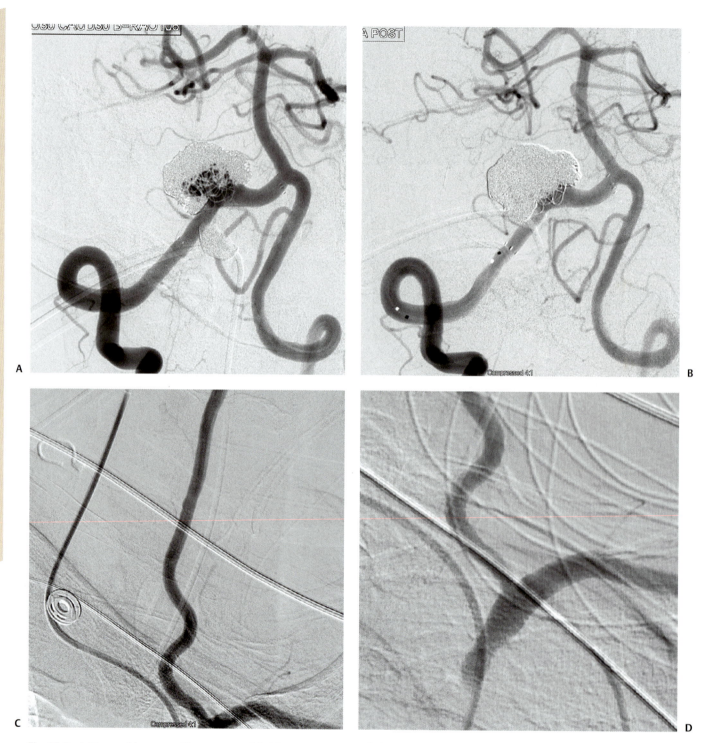

Fig. 18.3 A 58-year-old woman with a recurrent right VA aneurysm after **(A)** stent-assisted coiling underwent retreatment with **(B)** coiling. During angiography she was noted to have a subclavian steal **(C)** through the left VA related to **(D)** proximal occlusion of the left subclavian artery. Left VA-to-CCA transposition was indicated to reduce the demand for blood flow in the right VA, which harbored the aneurysm.

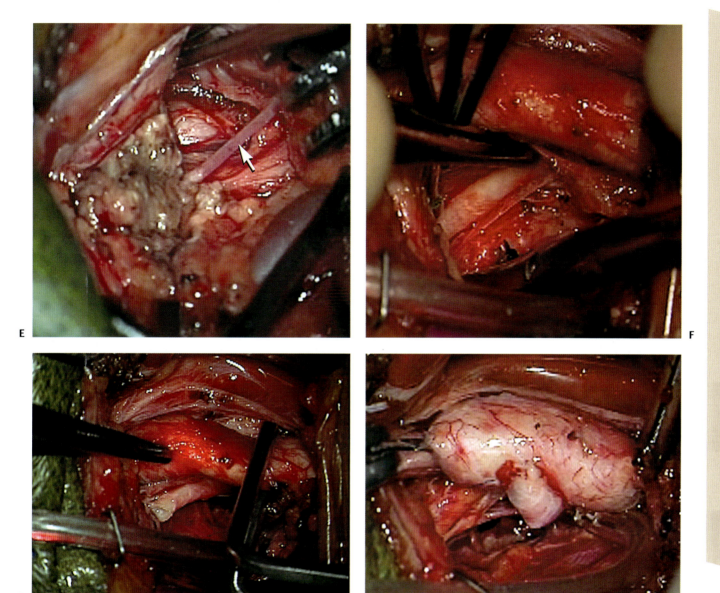

Fig. 18.3 (*continued*) (**E**) A left supraclavicular approach was performed, exposing the thoracic duct (*arrow*). (**F**) The left VA was sectioned, and (**G**) the CCA was prepared for (**H**) the left VA-to–left CCA transposition. (*continued on next page*)

from its origin to its entrance into the transverse foramen, is dissected and liberated from adhesions to facilitate manipulation during anastomosis.

When an isolated endarterectomy is planned, more extensive dissection of the subclavian artery is necessary. Its other branches at this level, namely the thyrocervical trunk and internal mammary artery, are carefully isolated. The ostial atherosclerotic plaque involving the origin of the VA is usually associated with subclavian plaque, which may require a concomitant subclavian endarterectomy (**Fig. 18.7**).

For a VA transposition, the CCA is, by far, the site most often used for the implant (**Fig. 18.8**). Another option in patients with a low carotid bifurcation is the thyrocervical trunk or the external carotid artery.

The initial step for a VA-to-CCA transposition is ligation of the VA at its origin with a hemoclip. Once the vessel is ligated, it is divided and the lumen is inspected. At this point, one of two scenarios is found: complete vessel occlusion or significant stenosis by thromboatheroma. In this situation, conventional thromboendarterectomy is conducted. If no backflow is obtained thereafter, the surgeon may consider a Fogarty maneuver or vessel ligation. If, however, backflow is present and no major plaque is initially identified, the VA is clamped (temporary aneurysm clip) at the level of the transverse foramen, and the lumen is irrigated with heparinized saline.

Next, the CCA is clamped proximally and distally to the planned level of the arteriotomy. The vascular clamps are

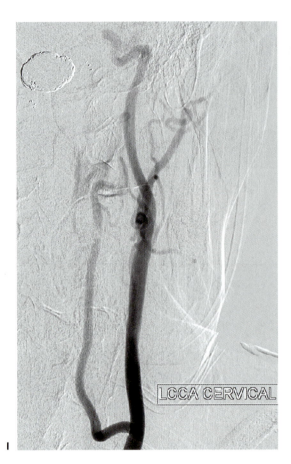

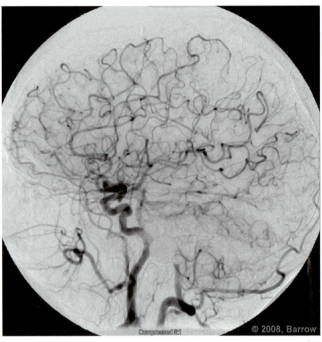

Fig. 18.3 (*continued*) (**I**) Postoperative angiogram confirmed patency of the anastomosis and showed good intracranial flow (**J**). (Courtesy of the Barrow Neurological Institute.)

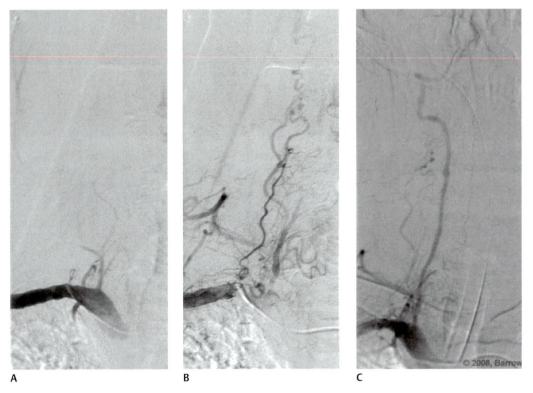

Fig. 18.4 Early (**A**) and late (**B**) cerebral angiograms showed symptomatic occlusion of the right VA in a 68-year-old man. Revascularization was successful via (**C**) an endarterectomy of the VA. (Courtesy of the Barrow Neurological Institute.)

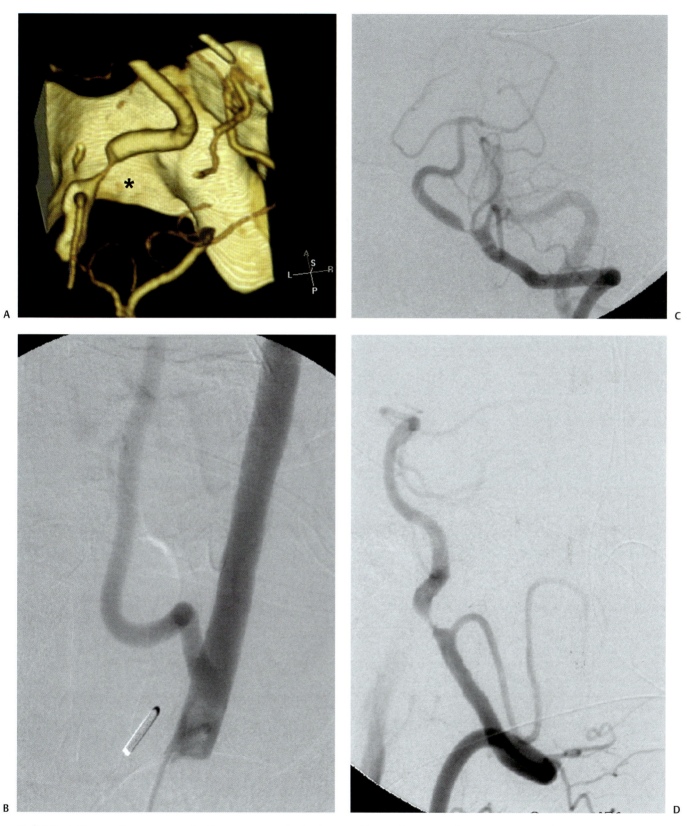

Fig. 18.5 A 78-year-old man presented with recurrent vertebrobasilar insufficiency 15 years after a left VA-to-CCA transposition. **(A)** Computed tomography angiography showed the presence of de novo intracranial stenosis *(asterisk).* **(B)** Cerebral angiography showed no evidence of stenosis at the transposition site, but anteroposterior **(C)** and lateral **(D)** angiographic views revealed severe stenosis of the left intracranial VA distal to the posterior inferior cerebellar artery. *(continued on next page)*

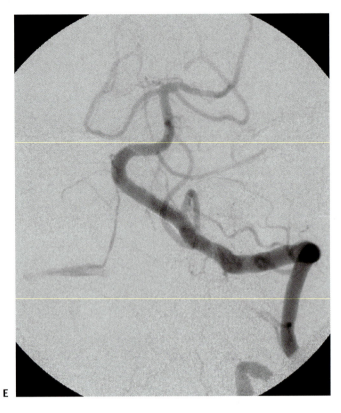

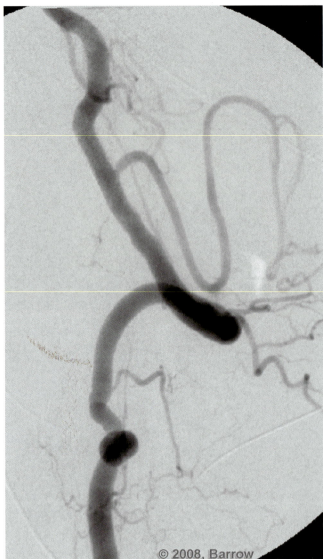

© 2008, Barrow

E

F

Fig. 18.5 (*continued*)   Anteroposterior (**E**) and lateral (**F**) angiographic images showed successful revascularization after angioplasty and stenting. (Courtesy of the Barrow Neurological Institute.)

usually placed in position to rotate the CCA slightly laterally. This maneuver enables a more posteriorly seated anastomosis. Arteriotomy is initiated with a No. 11 blade and completed with an arteriotomy punch 4 to 4.5 mm in diameter. The diameter of the VA is compared with the carotid opening and adjusted by fish-mouthing as needed. In the initial cases of this series, the senior author (R.F.S.) used polar tacking sutures at the superior and inferior ends of the circular anastomosis. More recently, however, a continuous looping suture with 7-0 monofilament Prolene has been applied successfully. This strategy increases the surgeon's ability to manipulate the vessel being implanted.

Once one side of the anastomosis is performed, the suture line and lumen are inspected. The second side is performed in a similar fashion. Before the suture line is closed, the distal VA is temporarily unclamped and allowed to back bleed. The arterial lumen is filled with pure heparin. All arterial clamps are released. Small bleeding points at the suture line are usually self-limiting and can be controlled with the use of Sur-

gifoam (Johnson & Johnson, New Brunswick, NJ) in locum. Indocyanine green videoangiography is performed when available. Careful hemostasis is obtained, and the wound is closed in layers. The clavicular head of the SCM is reapproximated, and the overlying wound is closed.

◆ Microsurgical Revascularization Versus Angioplasty and Stenting of the Proximal Vertebral Artery

To compare the modalities [microsurgery and endoluminal (stenting)] available for revascularization of atherosclerosis of the proximal VA, the immediate periprocedural and long-term results must be addressed.

For both modalities the immediate goals include a technically successful angiographic result (<50% residual stenosis) without neurologic or procedure-related complications and a successful clinical outcome associated with resolution of

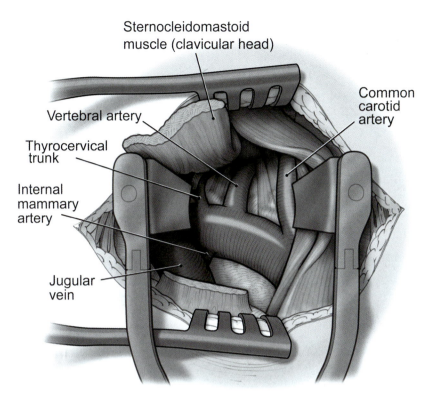

Sternocleidomastoid
muscle (clavicular head)

Vertebral artery

Thyrocervical
trunk

Internal
mammary
artery

Jugular
vein

Common
carotid
artery

Fig. 18.6 Illustration showing the subclavian exposure, with identification of the main vessel and branches (VA and thyrocervical trunk). In this demonstration, both heads of the sternocleidomastoid muscle were divided completely. (Courtesy of the Barrow Neurological Institute.)

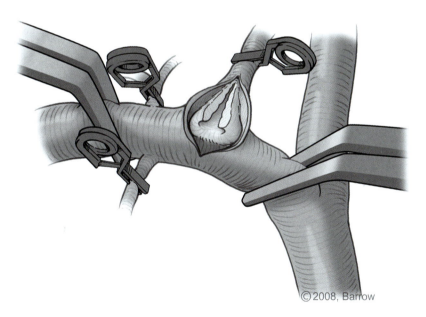

© 2008, Barrow

Fig. 18.7 Illustration showing an endarterectomy of the right VA. Plaque extends into the subclavian artery. (Courtesy of the Barrow Neurological Institute.)

the patient's symptoms. In these terms, microsurgical revascularization of the VA has an inherently higher risk of complications related to tissue manipulation such as Horner's syndrome, lymphatic injury, VA thrombosis, laryngeal nerve injury, wound hematoma, or wound infection. For obvious reasons, patients undergoing VA stenting are not exposed to such risks.

Both modalities are similar in terms of successful revascularization of the target vessel and resolution of symptoms. Success rates range from 93 to 98% for both.[10,13,23,28,29] Diaz et al[10] described 55 patients undergoing microsurgical revascularization for disease of the proximal VA with revascularization of the target vessel in all cases. Symptoms resolved in all but two patients. Using angioplasty and stenting, Albuquerque et al[28] achieved a technical success rate of 97% in 33 treated patients.

The essential issues regarding method of choice for proximal revascularization of the VA is the durability of the endo-

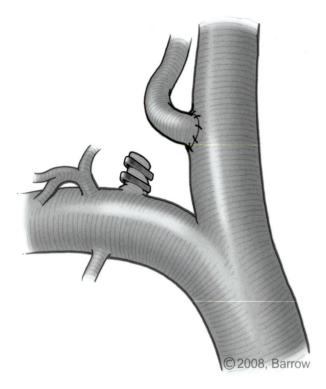

© 2008, Barrow

Fig. 18.8 Illustration showing a right VA-to–right CCA transposition. (Courtesy of the Barrow Neurological Institute.)

III Open Surgical Approaches

luminal method, namely, stenting and the possible occurrence of new symptoms.

Given the presence of intravascular stent, the assessment for restenosis at this location typically requires catheter-based angiography, although CTA can provide good-quality noninvasive imaging. In microsurgical cases, CTA or magnetic resonance angiography (MRA) with contrast usually provides an excellent assessment.

Although Chastain et al[30] reported a 10% incidence of restenosis in their 49 treated cases with a mean follow-up of 25 months, many other studies have consistently reported higher rates.[13,28] Albuquerque et al[27] reported restenosis (>50% diameter stenosis) in 13 (43%) of their patients at a mean follow-up of 16.2 months. In the Stenting of Symptomatic Atherosclerotic Lesions in the Vertebral or Intracranial Arteries (SSYLVIA) trial, 14 (78%) of 18 patients receiving treatment for extracranial VA stenosis underwent 6-month postprocedural angiographic follow-up.[13] Of those 14 patients, 6 (43%) showed evidence of in-stent stenosis. Half of these recurrent lesions completely occluded the vessel. Of the 18 patients, two (11%) developed stroke in the vascular distribution of the treated extracranial VA. Both of these patients had shown angiographic evidence of restenosis.

The advent of drug-eluting stents has revolutionized the endovascular treatment of coronary artery disease.[25] Its value has been advocated for treating lesions of the VA.[14,31] Although the introduction of such stents brought promising results in the treatment of coronary artery disease, concerns about delayed stent endothelialization and thrombosis have been raised.[15] Larger series of patients with disease at the origin of the VA need to be evaluated before recommendations can be made regarding the use of drug-eluting stents for such applications.

The long-term durability of microsurgical revascularization is well described,[23,32] but the description of the imaging follow-up available from those series is sparse. Hanel et al[32] treated 29 patients with revascularization of the proximal VA, most via VA-to-CCA transposition, endarterectomy, or both. There were no periprocedural strokes or deaths in this series. At a mean follow-up of 29 months, only 7% of the patients had new or recurrent vertebrobasilar symptom. Based on follow-up imaging of almost 50% of the cases, recurrent stenosis was present in only one of the 14 cases.[33]

◆ **Surgical Technique for Microsurgical Decompression of V2 Segment**

Although the anterolateral approach for the V2 segment has been described,[26] the simple anterior approach is our method of choice for decompression of V2 **(Fig. 18.9).** Instead of working lateral to the carotid sheath as described by George et al[27] in their anterolateral approach, we prefer to work medially to these structures, similar to a routine anterior cervical decompression and fusion (ACDF).

A standard anterior cervical discectomy and transverse cervical incision are planned at the level of compression. If more than two levels are involved, the skin is incised parallel to the anterior border of the SCM muscle. The approach proceeds similarly to an ACDF, with blunt dissection of the pretracheal fascia. The longus colli muscle is dissected further laterally to expose the anterior aspect of the transverse process. Careful dissection is needed to avoid iatrogenic injury of the VA between two adjacent transverse processes. Once these landmarks are identified, the bony structures forming the canal are drilled with a high-speed drill with diamond burs in a standard egg-shell technique. Wide exposure of the vessel (180 degrees) is the goal. Special attention is needed to prevent residual medial compression. Once the bony decompression is completed, the sheath containing the VA should be open, given occasional compression of the vessel by these fibrous structures.

◆ **Microsurgical Treatment of V3 Compression**

When symptoms are caused by rotation at C1-C2 **(Fig. 18.10),** a logical surgical approach is to perform fusion and fixation at that level **(Fig. 18.11).**[34] Fusion at C1-C2 has been associated with resolution of symptoms.[17,34] The disadvantage of this approach, however, is that neck rotation can be limited by as much as 50 to 70%.[17] In one series, patients whose rotational movements were extremely reduced experienced significant discomfort. Overall, however, the patients were satisfied with the surgery because the symptoms of bow hunter's stroke did not return.[17]

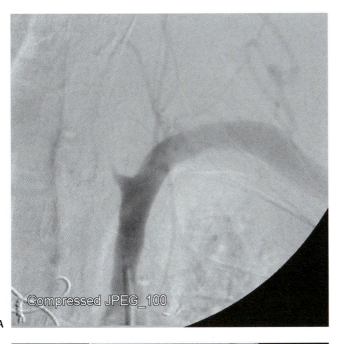

A

Fig. 18.9 A 69-year-old man presented with a 2-month history of new onset of daily intermittent vertigo/dizziness and episodes of syncope when he turned his head to the right. Noninvasive imaging suggested stenosis of the left VA. Cerebral angiograms showed complete occlusion at the origin of the VA **(A)** and significant stenosis of the rightV2 segment when he rotated his head to the right (**B**, right VA, neutral; **C**, rotation). The patient underwent decompression of the right VA via an anterior approach, and his symptoms resolved completely.

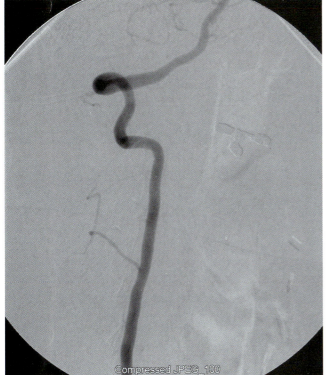

B

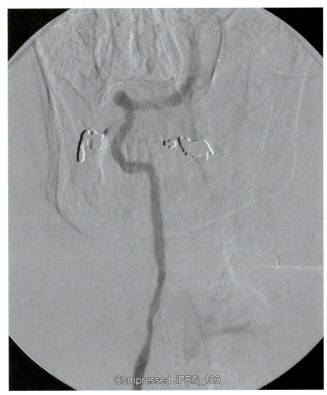

C

An alternate treatment is surgical decompression of the VA. Shimizu et al[35] used a posterior approach to the arch of C1 (**Fig. 18.12**) to release the VA from its points of fixation in the transverse foramen and sulcus arteriosus by performing a hemilaminectomy. Patients exhibited no further symptoms after surgery, and no rotary obstruction was apparent at that level on postoperative angiography. Surgical intervention to decompress fibrous bands[36] or osteophytic spurs[37] appears to offer long-term relief from symptoms, but no large series are available. Other approaches, including the anterolateral approach for decompression of the atlantoaxial VA, have also been described.[38]

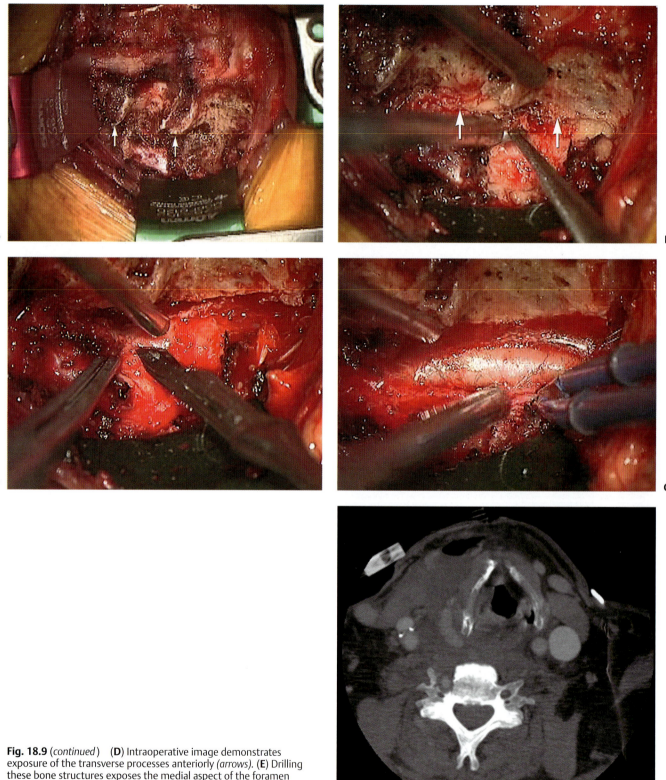

Fig. 18.9 (*continued*)   (**D**) Intraoperative image demonstrates exposure of the transverse processes anteriorly *(arrows)*. (**E**) Drilling these bone structures exposes the medial aspect of the foramen *(arrows)*. When the VA sheath is opened (**F**)**,** the vessel is exposed (**G**)**.** Postoperative CT angiography (**H**) confirmed good decompression of the vessel. (Courtesy of the Barrow Neurological Institute.)

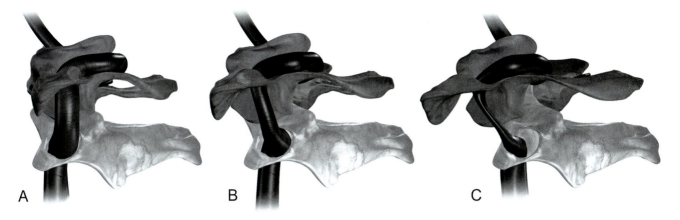

Fig. 18.10 Lateral views of motion at the atlantoaxial joint in neutral posterior **(A)** and with 10 degrees **(B)** and 20 degrees **(C)** of rotation show progressive narrowing of the VA with increased rotation. (Courtesy of the Barrow Neurological Institute.)

Fig. 18.11 C1-C2 posterior cervical fusion with transarticular screw and Sonntag-Dickman wiring used to immobilize the C1-C2 articulations. (Courtesy of the Barrow Neurological Institute.)

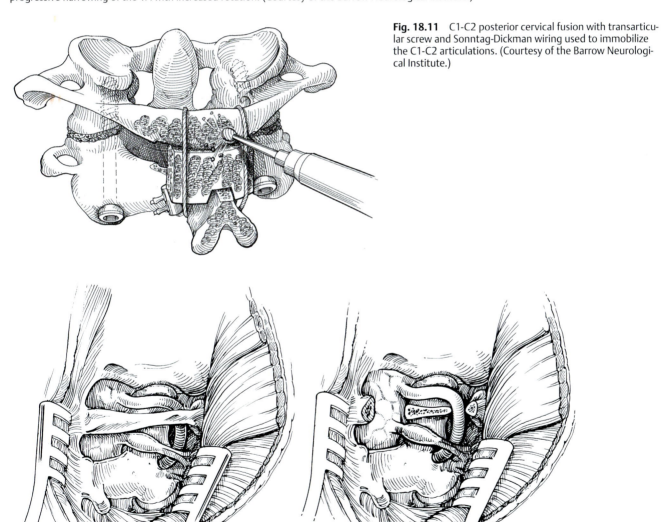

Fig. 18.12 Schematic exposure of the vertebral artery at C1-C2 **(A)** with decompression of the vessel after C1 hemilaminectomy and liberation of fibrous ligaments **(B).** (Courtesy of the Barrow Neurological Institute.)

Matsuyama et al[17] compared the efficacy of C1-C2 posterior fusion in eight patients to decompression of the VA alone in nine patients. Range of motion was reduced in those who underwent surgical fusion, but their symptoms did not recur. Conversely, of the nine patients who underwent VA decompression alone, three (33%) patients experienced recurrent symptoms and subsequently underwent surgical fusion. In these patients, dynamic angiography showed that the VA on the operated side was still occluded with head rotation. One patient developed a right cerebellar infarction between operations.

The senior author (R.F.S.) uses posterior decompression of the VA as a first-line surgical therapy to avoid compromising cervical range of motion. Postoperative dynamic angiography readily tests surgical efficacy. If patients subsequently fail clinically or on diagnostic evaluation, a stabilization and fusion procedure is considered. In all cases, patients undergoing surgical treatment must be informed of the advantages and disadvantages of both surgical options.

◆ Conclusion

Microsurgical treatment is a viable option for atherosclerotic and extrinsic stenotic disease of the extracranial VA. Careful case selection with all available modalities should lead to improved overall outcomes.

References

1. Beneficial effect of carotid endarterectomy in symptomatic patients with high-grade carotid stenosis. North American Symptomatic Carotid Endarterectomy Trial Collaborators. N Engl J Med 1991;325:445–453
2. Randomised trial of endarterectomy for recently symptomatic carotid stenosis: final results of the MRC European Carotid Surgery Trial (ECST). Lancet 1998;351:1379–1387
3. Hass WK, Fields WS, North RR, Kircheff II, Chase NE, Bauer RB. Joint study of extracranial arterial occlusion. II. Arteriography, techniques, sites, and complications. JAMA 1968;203:961–968
4. Wityk RJ, Chang HM, Rosengart A, et al. Proximal extracranial vertebral artery disease in the New England Medical Center Posterior Circulation Registry. Arch Neurol 1998;55:470–478
5. Moufarrij NA, Little JR, Furlan AJ, Williams G, Marzewski DJ. Vertebral artery stenosis: long-term follow-up. Stroke 1984;15:260–263
6. McDowell FH, Potes J, Groch S. The natural history of internal carotid and vertebral-basilar artery occlusion. Neurology 1961;11:153–157
7. Whisnant JP, Cartlidge NE, Elveback LR. Carotid and vertebral-basilar transient ischemic attacks: effect of anticoagulants, hypertension, and cardiac disorders on survival and stroke occurrence—a population study. Ann Neurol 1978;3:107–115
8. The Warfarin-Aspirin Symptomatic Intracranial Disease (WASID) Study Group. Prognosis of patients with symptomatic vertebral or basilar artery stenosis. Stroke 1998;29:1389–1392
9. Cate WR Jr, Scott HW Jr. Cerebral ischemia of central origin: relief by subclavian-vertebral artery thromboendarterectomy. Surgery 1959;45:19–31
10. Diaz FG, Ausman JI, de los Reyes RA, et al. Surgical reconstruction of the proximal vertebral artery. J Neurosurg 1984;61:874–881
11. The EC/IC Bypass Study Group. Failure of extracranial-intracranial arterial bypass to reduce the risk of ischemic stroke. Results of an international randomized trial. N Engl J Med 1985;313:1191–1200
12. Fessler RD, Wakhloo AK, Lanzino G, Qureshi AI, Guterman LR, Hopkins LN. Stent placement for vertebral artery occlusive disease: preliminary clinical experience. Neurosurg Focus 1998;5:e15
13. SSYLVIA Study Investigators. Stenting of Symptomatic Atherosclerotic Lesions in the Vertebral or Intracranial Arteries (SSYLVIA): study results. Stroke 2004;35:1388–1392
14. Boulos AS, Agner C, Deshaies EM. Preliminary evidence supporting the safety of drug-eluting stents in neurovascular disease. Neurol Res 2005;27(Suppl 1):S95–S102
15. Maisel WH. Unanswered questions—drug-eluting stents and the risk of late thrombosis. N Engl J Med 2007;356:981–984
16. Bruneau M, Cornelius JF, George B. Anterolateral approach to the V2 segment of the vertebral artery. Neurosurgery 2005;57(4, Suppl)262–267, discussion 262–267
17. Matsuyama T, Morimoto T, Sakaki T. Comparison of C1-2 posterior fusion and decompression of the vertebral artery in the treatment of bow hunter's stroke. J Neurosurg 1997;86:619–623
18. Amarenco P, Hauw JJ. Anatomy of the cerebellar arteries. Rev Neurol (Paris) 1989;145:267–276
19. Tissington Tatlow WF, Bammer HG. Syndrome of vertebral artery compression. Neurology 1957;7:331–340
20. Hardin CA. Vertebral artery insufficiency produced by cervical osteoarthritic spurs. Arch Surg 1965;90:629–633
21. Adams R, Victor M, Ropper A. Principles of Neurology. New York: McGraw-Hill, Health Professions Division, 1997:793–806
22. Berguer R, Flynn LM, Kline RA, Caplan L. Surgical reconstruction of the extracranial vertebral artery: management and outcome. J Vasc Surg 2000;31(1 Pt 1):9–18
23. Spetzler RF, Hadley MN, Martin NA, Hopkins LN, Carter LP, Budny J. Vertebrobasilar insufficiency. Part 1: Microsurgical treatment of extracranial vertebrobasilar disease. J Neurosurg 1987;66:648–661
24. Compter A, van der Worp HB, Schonewille WJ, et al. VAST: Vertebral Artery Stenting Trial. Protocol for a randomised safety and feasibility trial. Trials 2008;9:65
25. Abizaid A, Costa MA, Blanchard D, et al; Ravel Investigators. Sirolimus-eluting stents inhibit neointimal hyperplasia in diabetic patients. Insights from the RAVEL Trial. Eur Heart J 2004;25:107–112
26. Albuquerque FC, Spetzler RF. Vertebral artery revascularization. Operative Techniques in Neurosurgery. 2001;4:195–201
27. George B, Blanquet A, Alves O. Surgical exposure of the vertebral artery. Operative Techniques in Neurosurgery. 2001;4:182–194
28. Albuquerque FC, Fiorella D, Han P, Spetzler RF, McDougall CG. A reappraisal of angioplasty and stenting for the treatment of vertebral origin stenosis. Neurosurgery 2003;53:607–614, discussion 614–616
29. Wehman JC, Hanel RA, Guidot CA, Guterman LR, Hopkins LN. Atherosclerotic occlusive extracranial vertebral artery disease: indications for intervention, endovascular techniques, short-term and long-term results. J Interv Cardiol 2004;17:219–232
30. Chastain HD II, Campbell MS, Iyer S, et al. Extracranial vertebral artery stent placement: in-hospital and follow-up results. J Neurosurg 1999;91(4):547–552
31. Qureshi AI, Kirmani JF, Hussein HM, et al. Early and intermediate-term outcomes with drug-eluting stents in high-risk patients with symptomatic intracranial stenosis. Neurosurgery 2006;59:1044–1051, discussion 1051
32. Diaz F, Ausman JI. Surgical therapy in vascular brain stem diseases. In: Hofferberth B, Brune G, Sitzer G, eds. Vascular Brain Stem Diseases. Basel, Switzerland: Bertelsmann Foundation, 1990:270–281
33. Hanel RA, Brasiliense LB, Spetzler RF. Microsurgical revascularization of proximal vertebral artery: a single-center, single-operator analysis. Neurosurgery 2009;64:1043–1050, discussion 1051
34. Ford FR. Syncope, vertigo and disturbances of vision resulting from intermittent obstruction of the vertebral arteries due to defect in the odontoid process and excessive mobility of the second cervical vertebra. Bull Johns Hopkins Hosp 1952;91:168–173
35. Shimizu T, Waga S, Kojima T, Niwa S. Decompression of the vertebral artery for bow-hunter's stroke. Case report. J Neurosurg 1988;69(1):127–131
36. Mapstone T, Spetzler RF. Vertebrobasilar insufficiency secondary to vertebral artery occlusion from a fibrous band. Case report. J Neurosurg 1982;56:581–583
37. Sheehan S, Bauer R, Meyer J. Vertebral artery compression in cervical spondylosis. Arteriographic demonstration during life of vertebral artery insufficiency due to rotation and extension of the neck. Neurology 1960;10:968–986
38. Fox MW, Piepgras DG, Bartleson JD. Anterolateral decompression of the atlantoaxial vertebral artery for symptomatic positional occlusion of the vertebral artery. Case report. J Neurosurg 1995;83:737–740

19

Aortic Arch Surgery: Indications, Decision Analysis, and Surgical Technique

Mark D. Morasch and Joseph G. Adel

Pearls

◆ An aberrant right subclavian artery can be associated with a nonrecurrent recurrent vagus nerve and Ortner's syndrome, a right-sided thoracic duct, and an anomalous right vertebral origin.
◆ The treatment of Takayasu's arteritis, in the acute, inflammatory phase, is nonoperative. These patients should be managed initially, and for as long as clinically possible, with steroids.
◆ Patients with single trunk disease with a suitable ipsilateral donor vessel are well managed with cervical reconstruction of the diseased vessel via transposition or bypass, regardless of comorbid risk. Otherwise healthy patients with multi-trunk disease or no suitable ipsilateral donor vessel should be considered for aortic arch–based reconstruction via sternotomy. Poor-risk patients with significant comorbid conditions or with a history of sternotomy may best be treated endoluminally or with cross-neck bypasses.

Atherosclerotic occlusive disease involving the branches of the aortic arch is common in patients over the age of 65. The Joint Study of Arterial Occlusions reported that one third of patients undergoing arteriography are found to have significant lesions involving one or more of the vessels supplying blood to the head and arms.[1] Occlusive diseases affecting the brachiocephalic trunk vessels make up a relatively small fraction of them however. Furthermore, repair of occlusive lesions of the proximal brachycephalic vessels accounts for less than 10% of the operations performed on the extracranial cerebrovasculature. Despite this, and despite the fact that these vessels are relatively difficult to image using noninvasive technology, substantive data has accumulated regarding the natural history of the disease, and significant experience with surgical reconstruction has accrued over the past four decades. After two decades of experience with endoluminal therapy for treatment of arch branch disease, some useful data regarding angioplasty and stenting has now become available as well.

◆ Anatomy

The arch branches normally develop as three separate trunks taking origin from the proximal aorta within the superior mediastinum. The conventional definition includes the innominate artery, the subclavian arteries up to the origins of the vertebral arteries, and the common carotid arteries proximal to their bifurcations. The innominate artery and the left common carotid originate in close proximity to one another and ascend in the neck on either side of the trachea. The left subclavian artery is the third of three trunks and it originates posterior and to the left of the left common carotid. The vagus and right recurrent laryngeal nerves cross the anterior aspect of the right subclavian artery adjacent to the innominate bifurcation. On the left, the vagus and phrenic nerves cross one another between the left common carotid and the left subclavian under the cover of the pleura.

Anatomic variations are common, seen in over 20% of patients. The most common variation is the bovine-type aortic arch, where the first and second branches (innominate and left carotid) arise from a common ostium (16%) or as a single trunk (8%). The left vertebral artery originates as a separate branch arising from the aortic arch between the left common carotid and the left subclavian in 6% of the population. Developmental anomalies of the trunk vessels are less common. The arch configuration with an aberrant right subclavian artery that arises as the fourth of four vessels occurs in approximately 0.5% of individuals. A so-called truncus bi-carotidus, where the two carotids take origin together and the two subclavian vessels arise as one in a two-trunk configuration, occurs even less frequently. Retroesophageal subclavian arteries (RSAs), which are always found in association with these two configurations, occur with the same incidence of approximately 0.5%. In rare cases, certain symptom complexes including dysphagia (dysphagia lusoria) and chronic cough (from tracheal compression) can develop in patients with developmental errors and aberrant anatomy. Adjacent to the origin of an aberrant right subclavian artery there may be congenital dilatation of the wall called a diverticulum of Kommerell. This aortic wall outpouching is a remnant of the developmental right fourth aortic arch. The right inferior laryngeal nerve is not "recurrent" in patients with an aberrant right subclavian; instead, the nerve exits the vagus higher in the neck and takes a more direct route to the larynx resting on the wall of the right common carotid artery. A thoracic duct that empties into the right jugulosubclavian confluence should also be expected.

Developmental anomalies can also be found in conjunction with a right-sided or a double aortic arch. A mirror image of the left arch configuration occurs in most individuals with a right-sided arch. Right-sided arch anomalies are often associated with congenital cardiac abnormalities but they can occur in isolation as well.

◆ Epidemiology and Natural History

Atherosclerosis is, by far, the most common disease affecting the brachiocephalic vessels. Occlusive lesions less commonly result from inflammatory diseases such as Takayasu's arteritis or can be the result of exposure to therapeutic radiation. The vessels also can dissect or become aneurysmal. More distally, the subclavian arteries can be damaged from the long-term effects of thoracic outlet syndrome. Symptoms from nonatherosclerotic diseases such as Takayasu's or radiation-induced arteritis, dissections, aneurysms, and congenital lesions account for less than 20% of the disease that requires intervention.[2–6] Atherosclerotic lesions tend to cause occlusive and embolic symptoms equally, whereas vessel obliteration from arteritis tends only to cause symptoms related to hemodynamic insufficiency.

Occlusive lesions involving the brachiocephalic trunks tend to develop in a younger age group than atherosclerotic occlusive lesions elsewhere in the extracranial cerebrovascular circulation. Mean and median ages are commonly reported to range from 50 to 61 years. Single-vessel atherosclerotic occlusive disease involving the brachiocephalic trunks is often seen in younger adults (fifth decade), whereas patients with extensive or multiple trunk involvement tend to be older. The usual male preponderance noted with other atherosclerotic vascular conditions may not be found with disease of the brachiocephalic trunks. Females were treated in 53% of cases in one large series.[2,3] Cigarette smoking is certainly a significant risk factor for the development of atherosclerotic occlusive disease involving these vessels. Smoking is identified as a risk factor in 82% of all patients who require intervention.[2] Concomitant coronary artery disease (CAD) is present in one quarter to two thirds of patients who present for supraaortic trunk reconstruction. In one report, 63% of patients had significant CAD and 15% had undergone a previous myocardial revascularization.[2] In the same report, 47% of pa-

tients undergoing transthoracic reconstruction were hypertensive, and a smaller percentage (15%) were diabetic.

Atherosclerotic occlusive disease involving the brachiocephalic trunks can be either uni- or multifocal involving just one or more than one trunk vessel. In addition, the distribution of atherosclerosis within a single vessel can often be segmental in nature. Severe disease is defined as a >75% diameter stenosis. In addition, in symptomatic patients, a deep ulcerated plaque or a thrombus within the arterial lumen is also considered a severe lesion even though the defect may be <75% diameter. Severe lesions can be seen developing within and isolated to a single vessel. Alternatively, when the disease is seen in multiple trunks, the occlusive process is likely an extension of disease originating within the aortic arch that has "spilled over" into the vessel ostia. In one series of 283 transthoracic and cervical revascularizations of the brachiocephalic vessels, significant disease was present in more than a single vessel in 40% of cases.[3] All three of the trunks were critically diseased in 13%. Revascularization of unifocal disease was necessary in 60% of cases. When disease was limited to one trunk, the left subclavian artery was the vessel most commonly found to be involved with disease.

When multiple trunks are involved, patients usually develop symptoms of vertebrobasilar ischemia from low flow. Single-trunk disease manifests more commonly as hemispheric or upper extremity emboli. Isolated proximal disease within the subclavian artery can lead to symptomatic subclavian–vertebral steal, whereas innominate occlusion can result in steal from the anterior cerebral circulation (carotid-subclavian steal). Obliteration of the common carotid lumen can occur in a retrograde fashion following occlusion of the carotid bifurcation and internal carotid artery. Alternatively, an occlusion originating in a lesion in the proximal common carotid may eventually propagate distally into the bifurcation. The internal carotid not uncommonly remains patent in this situation. Duplex or delayed arteriographic images may show that the internal carotid is perfused anterograde via retrograde external carotid flow.

The traditional description of aneurysms of the brachiocephalic trunks refers to those of syphilitic etiology. Nowadays aneurysms of syphilitic origin have virtually disappeared. Most of the aneurysms of the innominate artery (IA) encountered today are associated with concomitant dilatation of the proximal ascending aorta or of the thoracoabdominal aorta. Posttraumatic false aneurysms of the brachiocephalic vessels are uncommon, and they are usually the result of rupture of the intima-media complex during deceleration in motor vehicle accidents. These pseudoaneurysms usually involve the origin of the IA. An occasional aneurysm is seen in association with Takayasu's disease. The most serious problems in patients with congenitally anomalous anatomy such as RSA are related to development of aneurysmal disease. These lesions usually involve the diverticulum at the origin of this artery (Kommerell).

Takayasu's arteritis frequently involves all three vessels proximally. The true etiology of this inflammatory disease has not been elucidated but it is known predominantly to affect females in their second and third decades of life. The hypertrophic occlusive lesions of Takayasu's disease have a smooth surface with a low embolic potential, and most symptoms relate to low flow as the disease progresses to multivessel occlusion. The histologic appearance of the lesions depends on the phase of the disease. They appear intensely inflammatory during the acute phase and more sclerotic when the disease is "burned out." The inflammatory process is usually most noticeable in the adventitial and medial layers of the involved vessels.

Giant cell arteritis rarely affects the proximal brachiocephalic trunks. Occasionally it does involve the more distal subclavian arteries and can be differentiated from Takayasu's by its location and by the fact that it affects a much older patient population.

Irradiated arteries develop an accelerated form of atherosclerosis as a result of radiation injury to the vessels. The rate at which the process develops depends on the radiation dose range. The brachiocephalic trunks may be involved after radiotherapy for, among other diseases, breast cancer, intrathoracic tumors, and Hodgkin's lymphoma.

Isolated brachiocephalic trunks dissection is rare, but type A aortic arch dissections may disrupt or extend into the trunk vessels impinging on cerebrovascular or upper extremity flow or prompting local thrombus, which can embolize. Like dissections elsewhere, chronic aneurysmal changes can develop over time, but this is rare.

◆ Indications for Reconstruction

Indications for revascularization of the brachiocephalic trunks are multiple. Symptomatic atherosclerotic occlusive disease may manifest as ocular, hemispheric, or vertebrobasilar transient ischemic attack (TIA) or stroke. Commonly patients present with a combination of both anterior and posterior cerebrovascular ischemic symptoms. In addition, some patients present with symptoms of upper extremity ischemia. Patients may develop varying degrees of arm ischemia, ranging from the claudication observed in patients with subclavian steal to limb-threatening ischemia resulting from extensive arterial occlusion or emboli. A third, less common problem is that of myocardial ischemia from the phenomena of coronary steal, which can develop in patients with innominate or subclavian disease proximal to an internal mammary revascularization of the coronary arteries. Rarely, patients with developmental anomalies involving the arch vessels require surgery to treat symptoms arising from esophageal or tracheal compression or for the treatment of symptomatic aneurysmal changes in or near the trunk vessels. True, asymptomatic, degenerative aneurysms involving the normally configured trunks are very rare, but when found they should be repaired in good-risk patients to prevent emboli to the brain or, less likely, vessel rupture.

Asymptomatic severe (>75%) atherosclerotic lesions of the innominate or common carotid arteries should be repaired in patients who present a reasonable risk (including patients with common carotid occlusion and a patent bifurcation), for the same reasons we repair asymptomatic severe carotid bifurcation stenoses. Asymptomatic lesions in the proximal subclavian artery should also be repaired in patients contemplating myocardial revascularization via an internal mammary artery and in patients with bilateral subclavian artery disease to permit and facilitate blood pressure management.

In general, no operation should be undertaken on patients with Takayasu's arteritis while in an active phase. An active state is usually signaled by the presence of the constitutional symptoms associated with acute inflammation and an elevated erythrocyte sedimentation rate. Steroid therapy usually treats the acute inflammatory process and makes attempts at surgical reconstruction much safer.

Of particular note, in our institution over the last 5 years, the most common indication for surgical manipulation of the brachiocephalic trunks has been to prepare patients with thoracic and thoracoabdominal aortic aneurysms, dissections, or traumatic tears for an endovascular stent-graft repair. Subclavian artery and even left common carotid artery transpositions as well as complete arch debranching procedures are not infrequently performed in order to preserve vertebral and left upper extremity flow while extending the proximal neck "landing zone" prior to endograft deployment.

◆ Disease Treatment

Four broad-based approaches have been developed for the treatment of brachiocephalic trunk lesions, each with distinct advantages and disadvantages: medical management, direct transthoracic reconstruction, remote cervical reconstruction, and endovascular recanalization (**Table 19.1**). Medical management includes the use of antiplatelet medications as with carotid bifurcation disease. The addition of statin medications along with smoking cessation may even lead to some plaque regression. The treatment for acute exacerbations of inflammatory diseases like Takayasu's includes the use of high-dose steroids tapered over time.

Surgical transthoracic revascularization may be chosen in good-risk patients with isolated innominate artery stenosis or occlusion and in patients with disease that involves multiple trunks. Remote cervical and endovascular techniques are alternatives to direct reconstruction and should be considered in patients with single-vessel disease that involves the carotid or subclavian arteries and in patients who have previously undergone a median sternotomy or who have a prohibitive medical comorbidity. Endoluminal therapies have become more commonplace over the last decade and clearly represent a less invasive alternative.

Direct Reconstruction

Direct reconstruction of the brachiocephalic trunks is approached through a complete or partial median sternotomy (**Fig. 19.1**). The cervical target vessels are easily exposed through this same full or partial sternotomy via an extension of the incision onto the neck as necessary.

Endarterectomy remains an option for reconstruction, particularly for isolated middle or distal innominate stenoses. Lesions that involve the more proximal vessel are more difficult to manage with endarterectomy. The majority of atherosclerotic lesions of the innominate do involve the proximal

Table 19.1 Surgical Treatment Options

Procedure	Procedure Choice Based on Symptomatic Patient Indication	Considerations
Direct Reconstruction		
Aorto-innominate/carotid bypass	• Good surgical risk	• Mainly cardiopulmonary
	• No suitable ipsilateral donor vessel	• Technically challenging
		• Excellent durability
Cervical Reconstructions		
Carotid to subclavian (ipsilateral) bypass	• Poor surgical risk	• Moderate to good durability
Subclavian to carotid (ipsilateral) bypass	• Prior sternotomy	• Cervical nerve injury risk
Subclavian to carotid transposition	• Good ipsilateral donor vessel	• Thoracic duct injury
Carotid to carotid bypass		
Endoluminal Reconstructions		
Innominate stent	• Poor surgical risk	• Poor to moderate durability
Common carotid stent	• Poor ipsilateral donor vessel	• Stent fracture
Subclavian angioplasty/stent		

portion of the vessel; these lesions are contiguous with the atherosclerotic plaque that extends over the dome of the aortic arch and insinuates, as well, into the origin of the left common carotid and subclavian arteries. In this common situation, endarterectomy of the IA requires division, under direct view, of the plaque as it blends with the aortic arch atheroma. This divided intima media can easily separate and become the origin of a dissection if it is not properly tacked. Another disadvantage of innominate endarterectomy follows from the fact that in 24% of patients, the origin of the IA and left common carotid artery are shared in a bovine configuration. In this circumstance, clamping the origin of the IA will also impinge upon left common carotid artery flow and result in unacceptable brain ischemia. Furthermore, to perform an adequate endarterectomy of these often-calcified innominate lesions, the plane from which the plaque must be removed mandates leaving an extremely thin wall through which sutures often tear or cause leaks. There are very few indications for IA endarterectomy today except in the rare circumstance of a lesion involving just the middle or distal innominate artery where the surgeon does not wish to dissect the ascending aorta or open the pericardium.

Bypasses that take origin from the ascending aorta tend to be safer and less demanding technically than endarterectomy (**Fig. 19.2**). With few exceptions, the aorta 4 to 6 cm above the aortic valve is usually spared disease, even if the rest of the aortic arch is involved. After the pericardium is open and a sufficient length of the ascending aortic arch is exposed, a partial occlusion Lemole-Strong clamp can be placed on the anterior wall of the ascending aorta, and a bypass conduit (usually a 9- or 10-mm prosthesis) is anastomosed to it. The proximal anastomosis is easier and less likely to leak if the systolic blood pressure can be maintained below 110 mm Hg. Also, heparin should be held until after

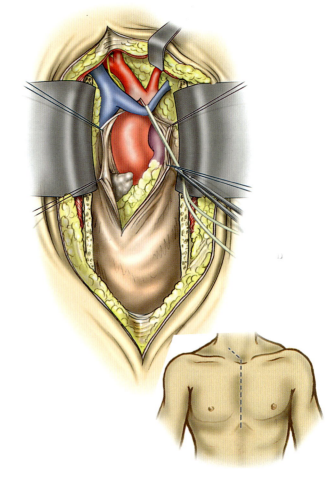

Fig. 19.1 Exposure for an aortocarotid bypass.

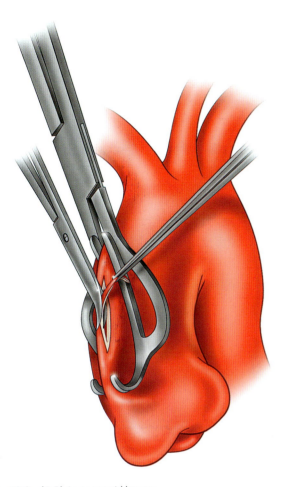

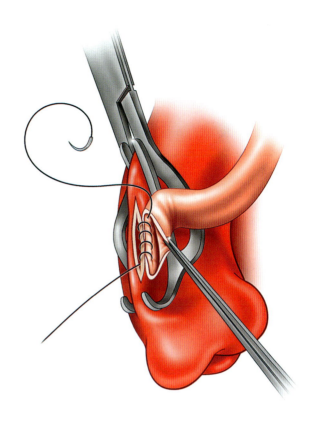

Fig. 19.2 (A,B) Aortocarotid bypass.

the graft is sewn in place and the clamp has been removed. Much of the morbidity of the transthoracic approach is related to embolization from the clamp site in the ascending aorta. It is important that the proximal anastomotic site be well flushed to prevent particle embolization and that the patient be placed in the Trendelenburg position when the clamp is removed to prevent air embolization. Heparin is administered when the suture line is hemostatic.

The bypass conduit is then passed behind the brachiocephalic vein to reach the target vessel. When bypasses to more than one trunk vessel are planned, it is better to use sequential bypass grafting with hand-sewn limbs rather than utilize commonly manufactured bifurcated grafts. We use this approach because this type of limb arrangement (**Fig. 19.3**) has a smaller diameter than does a commercially available bifurcated graft. The side arms of sequential bypasses can be oriented in such a fashion so as not to crowd the thoracic inlet. These side branches can then be routed to any of the proximal trunks or up to a carotid bifurcation.

The anterior approach to the proximal left subclavian artery, a posterior mediastinal structure, can be difficult. To dissect the proximal left subclavian artery through a median sternotomy usually requires ligation and division of the innominate vein to separate the sternal edges enough to permit dissection of the posterior mediastinum. Dividing the innominate vein should be avoided whenever possible, as significant arm swelling has been noted in some patients following this maneuver. Once the reconstruction is completed, the thymus, which has been divided through the midline or flipped laterally, is interposed between the sternum and the prosthetic graft. An alternative is to approach the proximal subclavian through a high posterolateral thoracotomy, although a cervical approach usually has as much utility. Our preference is to transpose the left subclavian into the bypassed left common carotid artery as a separate reconstruction as described below.

Cervical Reconstruction

Cervical reconstruction is the surgical technique of choice for single lesions involving the common carotid or subclavian arteries. Multiple remote cervical bypasses should also be considered for patients with multiple trunk involvement if there are contraindications to a transthoracic or an endovascular approach. When there is a usable ipsilateral "source vessel," an arterial transposition is the first choice (**Fig. 19.4**).

The subclavian artery may be transposed to the adjacent carotid or vice versa. Not only is preservation of the vertebral

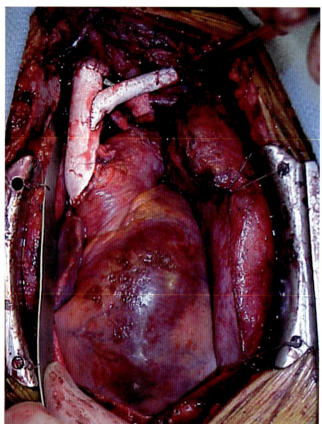

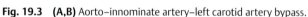

Fig. 19.3 **(A,B)** Aorto–innominate artery–left carotid artery bypass.

artery critical, but it is equally important to mobilize and preserve the valuable internal mammary artery (IMA) when performing a subclavian transposition. In the reverse, a common carotid to subclavian artery transposition, an adequate length of proximally narrowed common carotid artery can easily be mobilized to transpose it to the adjacent subclavian artery.

Arterial transpositions are completed through a short, transverse cervical incision above the clavicle. The dissection is performed between the two heads of the sternocleidomastoid muscle. After dividing the omohyoid muscle, the jugular vein and vagus nerve are reflected laterally, and the common carotid mobilized circumferentially and reflected medially. On the left, the thoracic duct is identified, ligated, and divided. On the right, multiple cervical lymphatic channels must also be tied. After dividing the vertebral vein, the subclavian artery and its proximal branches can be controlled. Once heparin has been administered, the subclavian or common carotid can be transected, depending on which vessel is to be reimplanted **(Fig. 19.5).** Care must be taken when ligating the proximal end of the divided trunk vessel. If control is lost in the chest or mediastinum, the consequences clearly can be devastating. A punch arteriotomy is created in the side of the donor vessel, and the end-to-side anastomosis is completed.

Occasionally it is not feasible to do a straightforward arterial transposition, often because the vertebral artery takes off early from the left subclavian. Another indication for carotid-subclavian bypass is proximal subclavian disease in a patient with symptomatic coronary steal and a patent internal mammary artery graft. The arterial clamps are placed clearly beyond the IMA to avoid myocardial ischemia. In this case, a short bypass to or from the common carotid to or from the retroscalene segment of the subclavian artery should be performed. Bypasses are performed, most expediently, just lateral to the clavicular head of the sternocleidomastoid muscle. The jugular vein is reflected medially to expose the common carotid. The subclavian artery is identified more distally than during transposition by dividing the anterior scalene muscle. The bypass is completed, usually using a prosthetic conduit, by performing sequential clamping and anastomoses **(Fig. 19.6).** Prosthetic conduits clearly outperform autogenous vein with regard to long-term patency of these bypasses.[7]

If an extra-anatomic approach is considered and the only source vessel is on the opposite side of the neck, the midline should be crossed using a retropharyngeal **(Fig. 19.7)** rather than a pre-sternal or pre-tracheal path.[8] The retropharyngeal route is shorter and more direct. Pre-tracheal or pre-sternal

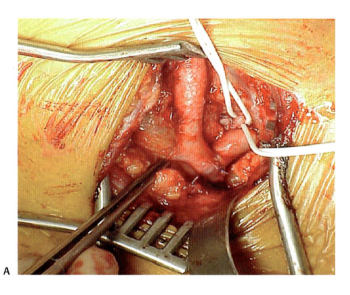

Fig. 19.4 **(A,B)** Subclavian artery–common carotid artery transposition.

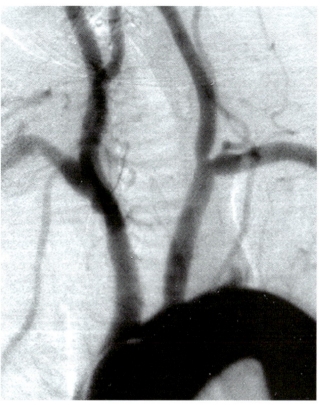

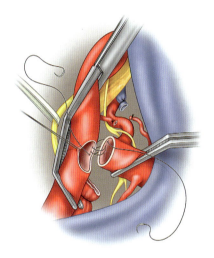

Fig. 19.5 Subclavian to common carotid transposition.

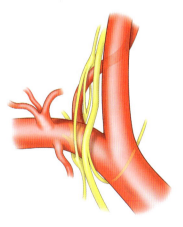

Fig. 19.6 Carotid-subclavian bypass.

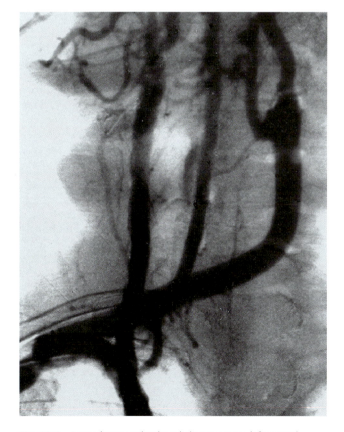

Fig. 19.7 Retropharyngeal right subclavian artery–left carotid bifurcation bypass.

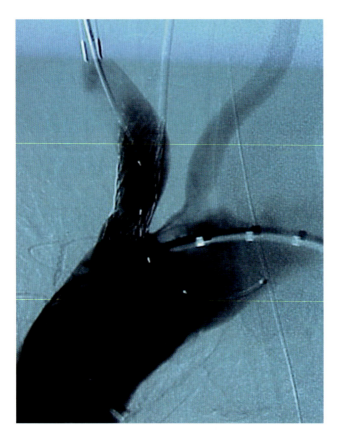

Fig. 19.8 Retrograde innominate artery angioplasty and stent in a patient with a prior sternotomy.

routing of a bypass graft can result in erosion of overlying skin and will become obtrusive if the patient ever requires a sternotomy or a tracheotomy. Long subclavian-subclavian, axillary-axillary, and femoro-axillary bypasses should also be avoided unless there is no other alternative because their patency rates are significantly poorer.

Endovascular Repair

Endoluminal therapies can be undertaken in antegrade fashion from the femoral artery or, in the case of innominate (**Fig. 19.8**) or subclavian lesions, percutaneously and in a retrograde fashion, from the brachial artery. Perhaps equally common would be retrograde treatment of common carotid or innominate lesions via surgical exposure as a lone procedure or during carotid bifurcation exposure for carotid endarterectomy.

Endovascular recanalization, introduced during the early 1980s, is performed under fluoroscopic control via remote arterial access with wires, catheters, and angioplasty balloons that are directed to the target trunk lesion. As an alternative, to prevent embolization Queral and Criado[9] advocate an open retrograde approach where the common carotid arteries are exposed in the neck and surgically controlled. Significantly more experience has been accumulated in the treatment of subclavian lesions than in the treatment of ca-

rotid or innominate disease, but this is likely due to the higher incidence of left subclavian lesions. Despite conflicting evidence for the routine use of metallic intravascular stents, deployment has become a routine adjuvant to balloon angioplasty in the proximal segments of these vessels, and covered stent grafts may soon have a role as well. Stents should not be placed in the postvertebral subclavian artery because of the significant risk of stent compression. Uniformly, luminal stenoses are treated with more success than are complete vessel occlusions (the incidence of rethrombosis of an occluded subclavian that has been recanalized by angioplasty and stent is as high as 50% in 8 months). Calcified lesions and long stenoses may also be problematic. It should also be noted that once a subclavian artery that has undergone endovascular treatment develops restenosis, a second and earlier restenosis is likely.

◆ Complications and Outcomes

The combined stroke and death rate for direct reconstruction of the arch branches should be less than 10% and in Berguer's[2] report, the 10-year patency rate was excellent at 88%. These patients can expect a median stroke-free life expectancy greater than 10 years.

There are two distinct subgroups of patients regarding short-term outcome following cervical reconstruction. First, there are patients with complex or extensive extracranial disease in whom reconstruction is performed preferentially through the neck because of a variety of relative contraindications to a transthoracic approach. Second, there are patients with a single lesion of the subclavian or common carotid artery who are choice candidates for a straightforward, limited cervical operation. In one review, the authors were surprised to find that the two groups fared equally well with regard to long-term patency and survival.[3] The more complex group, however, did experience a significantly greater perioperative stroke/death rate. In this series, virtually all patients were rendered asymptomatic. The primary 10-year patency rates compared favorably with other published series at 82%.[3,10,11] Stroke-free survival was 84% at 10 years.[3] It is important to note that there were no late failures in the group that underwent arterial transposition. The long-term patency rates for arterial transposition, when performed by surgeons with experience, is virtually 100%

Despite over 20 years of endoluminal experience, until recently the reports have been sporadic, and patient series have reported only small numbers of cases. The largest series published in the literature often combine immediate and short-term results of innominate, subclavian, and common carotid interventions together, making it difficult to interpret the results.[9,10,12] Some authors enthusiastically suggest that patient morbidity is markedly reduced when compared with open surgical reconstruction. Close scrutiny suggests, however, that overall complication rates are actually very similar to those for open reconstruction, and long-term durability of endoluminal therapy is probably inferior. This conclusion is hard to come by because reporting standards do not yet exist, nearly all of the endoluminal papers were not published with

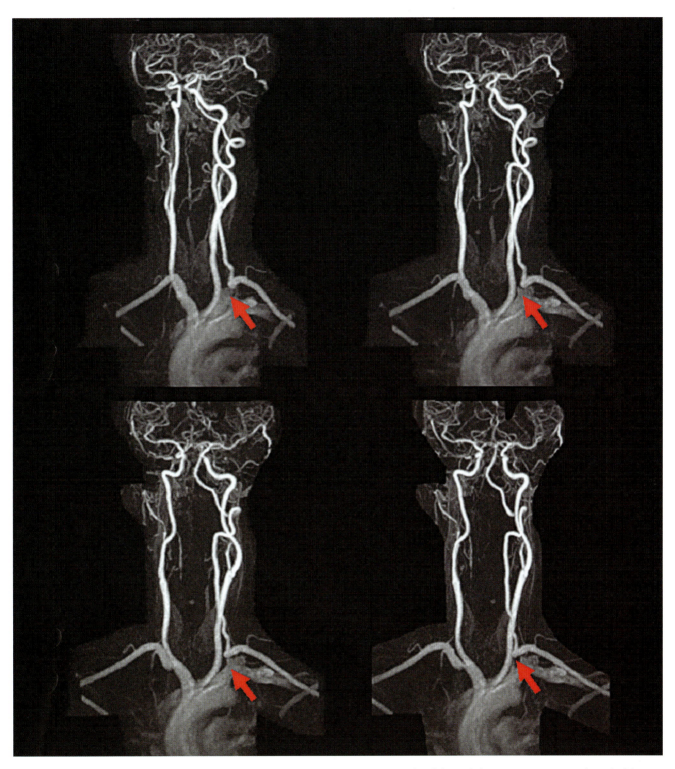

Fig. 19.9 Preoperative three-dimensional reconstruction magnetic resonance angiography of the neck demonstrating stenosis *(arrow)* of the proximal left subclavian artery with distal reconstruction.

intent-to-treat reporting, and long-term patient follow-up and well-documented patency data for angioplasty and stent placement is lacking. Primary success rates range from 73 to 100%, and complication rates range from 0 to 10%.[12–21] Mortality following endovascular treatment is rare. Henry et al[12] reported percutaneous endoluminal treatment of 113 subclavian lesions from a percutaneous femoral or brachial approach. Initial technical success was 91% for stenotic lesions and 47% in occluded vessels. As with most interventional techniques, success was defined as a residual narrowing of 30% or less. The complication rate was 5.3%. The clinically significant recurrence rate was 16% after a mean of 4.3 years. Tyagi et al[22] dilated 61 pre- and postvertebral subclavian lesions, with a 90% initial success rate and a 5.4% complication rate. Schillinger[23] retrospectively identified 115 patients who were treated for atherosclerotic subclavian disease (patients

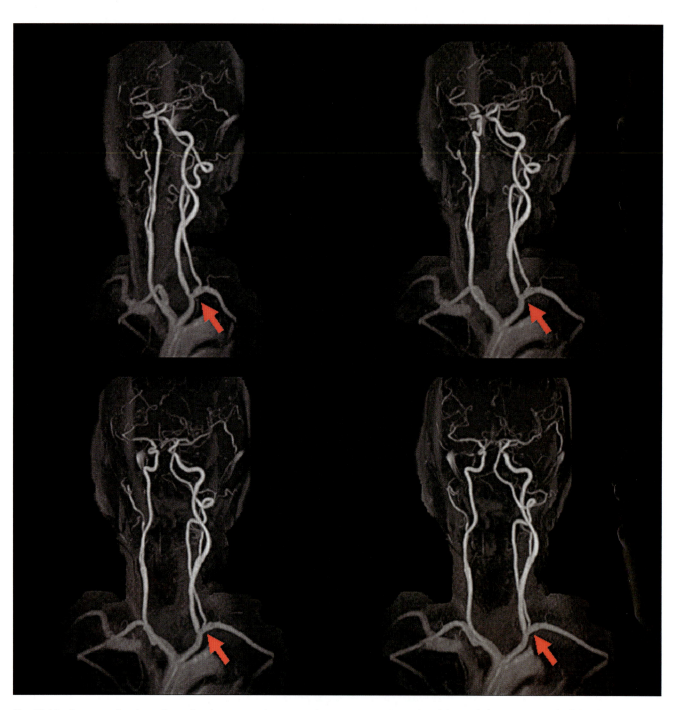

Fig. 19.10 Postoperative three-dimensional reconstruction magnetic resonance angiography of the neck demonstrating the left subclavian artery emanating (arrow) from the left common carotid artery.

with arteritis were excluded) over a 15-year period. Initial success was achieved in 85%. Complete occlusion and long lesions correlated with low success rate. Four-year patency rates were 59% in arteries with stents and 68% in arteries without stents. Sullivan et al[24] achieved initial success in 94% of patients with subclavian ($n = 66$), carotid ($n = 14$), or innominate ($n = 7$) lesions, and a broad range of complications occurred in 21% of the patients. This group concluded that the short- and long-term results of treatment favor surgical therapy, especially when the lesions were complete occlusions.

It should be noted that stent fracture following the endoluminal treatment of innominate lesions now appears to be a significant problem. If patients are followed long enough, the incidence of stent fracture is likely greater than 50%. The constant motion that occurs between the relatively fixed innominate and the mobile arch leads to metal fatigue over time. Fractures are seen less frequently in the left common carotid and left subclavian. Endoluminal treatment of arteritis, despite marginal success in some small case series,[22] should be condemned due to poor short- and mid-term patency results.

◆ Conclusion

Similar to the outcome data for the group of patients who undergo carotid bifurcation endarterectomy, long-term outcome data suggest that about one half of patients who undergo surgical reconstruction of the brachiocephalic vessels are still alive after 10 years.[2,3] Based on these data, good-risk surgical candidates with appropriate indications for intervention should undergo standard revascularization by competent surgeons utilizing techniques with proven long-term patency. Endovascular repair and remote bypass should be considered in patients with higher cardiopulmonary risk or limited life expectancy. Additionally, it is important to design one's approach based on the particular patient's anatomy.

◆ Case Illustration

A 62-year-old woman presented with occasional left upper extremity coldness and numbness, dizziness, and light-headedness. Her past medical history was significant for hypertension, hyperlipidemia, and right V3-V4 vertebral artery dissection and occlusion with secondary right medullary infarct and mild right-sided weakness. The patient was on aspirin and Plavix for the above diagnosis when she presented. Her physical examination was significant for a large left–right systolic blood pressure discrepancy in the upper extremities, left-sided carotid bruit, delayed left radial pulse, and chronic mild right hemiparesis. Imaging revealed left subclavian artery stenosis in addition to the chronic right vertebral artery occlusion (**Fig. 19.9**). Doppler ultrasonography was consistent with early subclavian steal syndrome on the left. Given the significant symptoms and findings, the patient was taken to the operating room where a left subclavian to common carotid artery transposition was performed. Postoperatively, she had a rapid recovery and was discharged on Plavix. The patient was noted at the 9-month postoperative follow-up (**Fig. 19.10**) to be doing well and to be symptom free.

References

1. Blaisdell WF, Clauss RH, Galbraith JG, Imparato AM, Wylie EJ. Joint study of extracranial arterial occlusion. IV. A review of surgical considerations. JAMA 1969;209:1889–1895
2. Berguer R, Morasch MD, Kline RA. Transthoracic repair of innominate and common carotid artery disease: immediate and long-term outcome for 100 consecutive surgical reconstructions. J Vasc Surg 1998; 27:34–41, discussion 42
3. Berguer R, Morasch MD, Kline RA, Kazmers A, Friedland MS. Cervical reconstruction of the supra-aortic trunks: a 16-year experience. J Vasc Surg 1999;29:239–246, discussion 246–248
4. Kieffer E, Sabater J, Koskas F. Brachiocephalic arterial reconstruction. In: Yao JST, Pearce WH, eds. Arterial Surgery. Stamford, CT: Appleton and Lange, 1996:141–162
5. Kieffer E, Sabatier J, Koskas F, Bahnini A. Atherosclerotic innominate artery occlusive disease: early and long-term results of surgical reconstruction. J Vasc Surg 1995;21:326–336, discussion 336–337
6. Rhodes JM, Cherry KJ Jr, Clark RC, et al. Aortic-origin reconstruction of the great vessels: risk factors of early and late complications. J Vasc Surg 2000;31:260–269
7. Ziomek S, Quiñones-Baldrich WJ, Busuttil RW, Baker JD, Machleder HI, Moore WS. The superiority of synthetic arterial grafts over autologous veins in carotid-subclavian bypass. J Vasc Surg 1986;3:140–145
8. Berguer R. Revascularization across the neck using the retropharyngeal rout. In: Veith FJ, ed. Current Critical Problems in Vascular Surgery, Vol. 7. St. Louis: Quality Medical Publishing, 1996
9. Queral LA, Criado FJ. The treatment of focal aortic arch branch lesions with Palmaz stents. J Vasc Surg 1996;23:368–375
10. Moore WS, Malone JM, Goldstone J. Extrathoracic repair of branch occlusions of the aortic arch. Am J Surg 1976;132:249–257
11. Vogt DP, Hertzer NR, O'Hara PJ, Beven EG. Brachiocephalic arterial reconstruction. Ann Surg 1982;196:541–552
12. Henry M, Amor M, Henry I, Ethevenot G, Tzvetanov K, Chati Z. Percutaneous transluminal angioplasty of the subclavian arteries. J Endovasc Surg 1999;6:33–41
13. Becker GJ, Katzen BT, Dake MD. Noncoronary angioplasty. Radiology 1989;170(3 Pt 2):921–940
14. Bogey WM, Demasi RJ, Tripp MD, Vithalani R, Johnsrude IS, Powell SC. Percutaneous transluminal angioplasty for subclavian artery stenosis. Am Surg 1994;60:103–106
15. Crowe KE, Iannone LA. Percutaneous transluminal angioplasty for subclavian artery stenosis in patients with subclavian steal syndrome and coronary subclavian steal syndrome. Am Heart J 1993;126:229–233
16. Erbstein RA, Wholey MH, Smoot S. Subclavian artery steal syndrome: treatment by percutaneous transluminal angioplasty. AJR Am J Roentgenol 1988;151:291–294
17. Hadjipetrou P, Cox S, Piemonte T, Eisenhauer A. Percutaneous revascularization of atherosclerotic obstruction of aortic arch vessels. J Am Coll Cardiol 1999;33:1238–1245
18. Mathias KD, Lüth I, Haarmann P. Percutaneous transluminal angioplasty of proximal subclavian artery occlusions. Cardiovasc Intervent Radiol 1993;16:214–218
19. Millaire A, Trinca M, Marache P, de Groote P, Jabinet JL, Ducloux G. Subclavian angioplasty: immediate and late results in 50 patients. Cathet Cardiovasc Diagn 1993;29:8–17
20. Motarjeme A, Keifer JW, Zuska AJ, Nabawi P. Percutaneous transluminal angioplasty for treatment of subclavian steal. Radiology 1985;155: 611–613
21. Rodriguez-Lopez JA, Werner A, Martinez R, Torruella LJ, Ray LI, Diethrich EB. Stenting for atherosclerotic occlusive disease of the subclavian artery. Ann Vasc Surg 1999;13:254–260
22. Tyagi S, Verma PK, Gambhir DS, Kaul UA, Saha R, Arora R. Early and long-term results of subclavian angioplasty in aortoarteritis (Takayasu disease): comparison with atherosclerosis. Cardiovasc Intervent Radiol 1998;21:219–224
23. Schillinger M, Haumer M, Schillinger S, Ahmadi R, Minar E. Risk stratification for subclavian artery angioplasty: is there an increased rate of restenosis after stent implantation? J Endovasc Ther 2001;8(6):550–557
24. Sullivan TM, Gray BH, Bacharach JM, et al. Angioplasty and primary stenting of the subclavian, innominate, and common carotid arteries in 83 patients. J Vasc Surg 1998;28:1059–1065

20

Microsurgery for Unruptured Intracranial Aneurysms

Andrew F. Ducruet, Philip M. Meyers, and Robert A. Solomon

Pearls

- With rare exceptions, all symptomatic unruptured aneurysms should be treated.
- Small, incidental aneurysms <5 mm should be managed conservatively in most cases.
- Patients <60 years of age with aneurysms ≥5 mm should be offered treatment unless there is a significant contraindication.
- Large, incidental aneurysms >10 mm should treated in all healthy patients <70 years of age.
- Microsurgical clipping rather than endovascular coiling should be the first choice in low-risk cases (young patients with small, anterior circulation aneurysms).

The management of unruptured intracranial aneurysms (UIAs) remains one of the most controversial topics in neurosurgery. Multiple efforts have been undertaken both to determine the natural history of this condition and to define the risks of UIA surgery as related to patient age, aneurysm size, and location.[1–3] Based on our interpretation of the literature and our experience treating patients with cerebral aneurysms, in this chapter we present a management algorithm for patients presenting with UIA. These recommendations are based on careful patient selection and the integration of the latest microsurgical and endovascular techniques. We employ a working collaboration of an experienced team of microvascular and endovascular neurosurgeons at a tertiary medical center with high case volume, as well as a decision-making paradigm committed to offering only low-risk treatments. In certain cases where both treatment and natural history carry a high risk, such as with complex giant aneurysms in an older patient, conservative management is elected.

◆ Epidemiology and Natural History

Intracranial aneurysms (IAs) are common lesions, occurring in 1 to 6% of the population and affecting equal numbers of women and men younger than 40 years, whereas women are affected more frequently in older age groups.[4] IAs are believed to result from intrinsic aberrations of the cerebral vasculature in which the integrity of the internal elastic lamina is compromised, engendering muscular defects in the adjacent layers of the tunica media and adventitia that augment the pathologic effects of chronic hemodynamic stress on the arterial wall. The tendency toward development of IAs is likely partly genetic, as multiple inherited conditions are associated with a diagnosis of IAs, including autosomal-dominant polycystic kidney disease, fibromuscular dysplasia, Marfan syndrome, and Ehlers-Danlos syndrome type IV.[5] A familial inheritance pattern, however, has been noted in only approximately 2% of IA.[5] Therefore, it is likely that a multifactorial etiology exists, reflecting the interaction of environmental factors, such as cigarette smoking, atherosclerosis, or hypertension, overlying a congenital predisposition.

Unruptured intracranial aneurysms are typically discovered incidentally, as the majority of these lesions are asymptomatic prior to rupture. However, neurologic symptoms, either acute or chronic, may spur diagnosis, particularly in the case of larger aneurysms and those undergoing acute expansion. Acute neurologic symptoms referable to UIA include ischemia, headache, seizures, and cranial neuropathies. Chronic neurologic symptoms such as headache, visual deficits, weakness, and facial pain may also occur. Regardless of symptomatology, the vast majority of UIAs are identified through noninvasive computed tomography (CT), magnetic resonance imaging (MRI), CT angiography, and MR angiography. However, as digital subtraction angiography (DSA) affords better visualization of aneurysm and parent vessel geometry, as well as the subtle anatomic relationships of the perforators, DSA remains the gold standard for definitive diagnosis and is often preferred in planning an elective operation for an UIA.

The annual risk of rupture of a UIA has been estimated to range from 0.1 to 8% or higher and is the subject of significant controversy. The publication of retrospective results from the International Study of Unruptured Intracranial Aneurysms

Authors (Year)	Number of Patients	Number of Aneurysms	Mean Follow-Up (years)	Rate of Rupture
ISUIA Investigators (1998)	1449	1937	8.3	Group 1: *<10 mm: 0.05%/yr* *≥10 mm: 1%/yr* Group 2: *<10 mm: 0.5%/yr* *≥10 mm: 1%/yr*
Rinkel et al (1998)	3907	N/A	N/A	Overall: 1.9%/yr *<10 mm: 0.7%/yr* *>10 mm: 4%/yr*
Juvela et al (2001)	142	181	18.1	10.5% at 10 yrs 23% at 20 yrs 30.3% at 30 yrs
Wiebers et al (2003)	1692	2686	4.1	Group 1: *<7 mm: 0%/yr* *7–12 mm: 2.6%/yr* *13–24 mm: 14.5%/yr* *≥25 mm: 40%/yr* Group 2: *<7 mm: 2.5%/yr* *7–12 mm: 14.5%/yr* *13–24 mm: 18.4%/yr* *≥25 mm: 50%/yr*

Abbreviations: N/A, not available.

(ISUIA), purporting a dramatically low risk of acute subarachnoid hemorrhage (aSAH) from aneurysms <10 mm, engendered a debate favoring observation for the vast majority of small UIAs.[6] However, several key investigations, including the subsequent prospective ISUIA,[6] the study by Juvela et al[7] with 18-year follow-up, and the comprehensive meta-analysis by Rinkel and colleagues,[2] suggest a higher rate of hemorrhage. These studies warrant careful review to help establish the natural history of UIA **(Table 20.1).**

The ISUIA is an ongoing collaboration of major neurosurgical centers attempting to delineate the natural history and interventional outcomes for UIA. The first of the two landmark papers arising from this study assessed the natural history of UIA in a retrospective fashion.[6] These patients were divided into two groups: 727 who had no history of aSAH (group 1), and 722 who had a history of aSAH from a different lesion (group 2). The rupture rates for UIA in these cohorts were drastically lower than in the previous estimates **(Table 20.1).** The authors found that increasing size and location (posterior circulation and posterior communicating artery [PCoA]) were significantly associated with rupture for group 1, whereas location (basilar tip) and increasing age were predictive of rupture for group 2. Although this study evaluated a large number of aneurysms across several centers, it has several serious design flaws and has since been discredited by the authors themselves.[8] The cohort of patients comprising this retrospective evaluation was subjected to a very significant selection bias, as all patients had already been evalu-

ated for surgery and selected for observation. As a result, it is likely that the majority of the patients harbored extremely low-risk aneurysms due to location (cavernous carotid aneurysms were identified in groups 1 and 2 at rates of 16.9% and 9.5%, respectively) or size (in groups 1 and 2, aneurysms of 2 to 5 mm were identified in 32.7% and 61.2% of patients, respectively). In addition, it is likely that the patients were medically ill, with increased deaths due to causes other than aSAH. Moreover, patients whose lesions were originally selected for conservative management may have crossed over to surgical treatment due to new symptoms. This crossover would remove patients who were imminently at risk for aSAH, lowering the observed rupture rate.

The second ISUIA study[8] was a prospective evaluation of the natural history of UIA. In this analysis, there were 1077 patients in group 1 and 615 patients in group 2 as previously defined. The total risk of rupture for patients in both groups 1 and 2 was calculated excluding those with aneurysms in the cavernous internal carotid artery (ICA) **(Table 20.1).** This prospective ISUIA also contained selection bias; for example, of the 1692 patients, 534 crossed to a therapeutic intervention and were removed from follow-up. In a significant portion of these crossover patients, the management strategy was likely changed because of either an increase in aneurysm size or the development of new symptoms. As well, 193 patients (11%) died of causes other than aSAH; these patients were excluded. It is also troubling that 52 of these patients died of intracranial hemorrhage, and it is not clear whether there was adequate evaluation to ensure that these hemorrhages were not due to aneurysms. In short, some caution is indicated when extrapolating these data to the population at large.

Rinkel et al[2] published an invaluable analysis of the natural history of UIA through a thorough review of the literature published between 1955 and 1996. To estimate the prevalence of UIA, data were summed from 23 studies that evaluated 56,304 patients. The overall prevalence of these lesions in adults with no known risk factors was 2.3%. For analysis of the bleeding rate of UIA, the authors identified nine studies including 3907 patients (**Table 20.1**). The large number of patients analyzed makes this study an important investigation into the natural history of UIA. Additionally, these results are strengthened by the fact that their estimates of the prevalence of and incidence of bleeding in UIA corroborate very closely with the known incidence of aSAH.

Juvela and colleagues[7] provide a comprehensive observational study that lacks the inherent bias of surgical selection found in ISUIA, as they examined all patients with UIA seen at their institution over a given time period. This study was possible because it was department policy to manage all UIA conservatively prior to 1979. In addition, Finland's socio-medical structure facilitated 100% follow-up to record the outcome over a longer period of time than in any other study. The cumulative rupture of aSAH is depicted in **Table 20.1**. Aneurysm size and patient age (inversely) were significant predictors of aSAH, as was active cigarette smoking. Major flaws in this study were the small total number and ethnic homogeneity of the patients and the overwhelming proportion (92%) of patients with prior aSAH. Despite these major flaws, the lack of a surgical selection bias and the outstanding long-term follow-up make this a valuable contribution to our understanding of the bleeding rates for UIA.

When interpreting the literature reporting the natural history of UIA, there are several factors to consider. For example, studies tend to break down aneurysms into size categories. It is unlikely that such a cutoff will result in substantially different rupture rates. In actuality, the risk of bleeding most likely reflects a nonlinear continuum of increasing risk with greater aneurysm size. Additionally, it is important to realize that aneurysms are likely not static in size. For instance, Juvela et al[1,7,9] found that in 31 of 87 (36%) patients, the size of conservatively managed aneurysms increased by >3 mm over a mean follow-up of 18.9 years. The relative effect of aneurysm growth on our ability to estimate hemorrhage risk is unknown, but it would be reasonable to assume that a growing aneurysm has an increased risk of rupture. Also, any estimation of rupture risk must take into account the aneurysm location. For instance, the results of the ISUIA demonstrate that aneurysms of the posterior communicating artery (PCoA) and posterior circulation display a much higher risk of rupture than those of the middle cerebral artery (MCA) and ICA. The literature indicates that posterior circulation, PCoA, and anterior communicating artery (ACoA) aneurysms carry the highest risk of subarachnoid hemorrhage (SAH), whereas aneurysms of the cavernous ICA carry an extremely low risk.[6,8]

Despite conflicting data in the literature, we recommend that the natural history of a given UIA should be assessed in each individual case. For instance, family history, smoking, excessive alcohol consumption, female sex, previous aSAH, presence of symptoms attributable to the lesion, aneurysm location, and lesion size have all predicted a worse natural history.[9,10] Any risk/benefit analysis of intervention must take into account the patient's life expectancy and medical co-morbidities. Despite these concerns, it is helpful to have a general algorithm for predicting rupture risk that may then be adjusted depending on risk factors. Our general estimate for the yearly risk of SAH for an UIA is approximately 1% for lesions 7 to 10 mm in diameter. The risk of rupture grows logarithmically as aneurysm size increases.

◆ Indications for Treatment

When determining a management paradigm for an UIA, one must weigh the natural history of the condition against the risks of intervention. Although there are no strict guidelines, certain factors may represent indications for treatment of UIA. Although 7 mm is the average size of ruptured aneurysms, and smaller aneurysms may exhibit a lower risk of rupture, we generally advocate treatment for aneurysms ≥5 mm in diameter. This criterion ensures that 99% of patients with aneurysms that should be treated will be offered treatment. In addition to size, any neurologic symptoms attributable to an aneurysm are generally considered a strong indication for surgery. Depending on the exact symptoms, many surgeons would favor urgent rather than elective treatment.

Additionally, it is our experience that there is a phenomenon of excessive psychological stress in patients with UIA. Even when patients fall into a subgroup of minimal treatment benefit and are appropriately counseled, they often insist on treatment. Although rigorous studies of this issue have yet to be performed, it appears that the psychological stress associated with having a UIA is enough to compel a patient to forgo the recommended conservative management for the peace of mind of treatment. These patients may be borderline candidates, and such strong feelings on the patients' part indicating quality-of-life issues may tilt the risk/benefit analysis toward intervention.

◆ Techniques of Treatment

Microsurgical Clipping

Microsurgical clipping remains the gold standard for exclusion of UIA from the circulation. It is our opinion that patients younger than 60 years of age with non-giant, anterior circulation aneurysms should be offered microsurgical clipping as the first-line treatment (**Fig. 20.1**). This contention is supported by several large published series that report high rates of total aneurysm obliteration and low rates of recurrence.[11,12] Furthermore, it is well accepted that successful surgical clipping translates into long-standing aneurysm obliteration and low subsequent rates of aSAH from a treated lesion.

The success of microsurgery is also measured in terms of the surgical outcome, which has been independently associ-

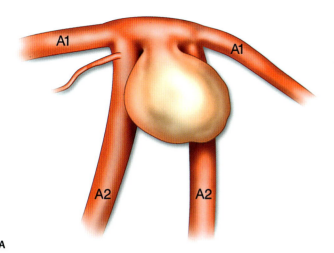

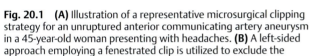

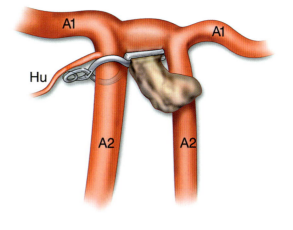

A
B

Fig. 20.1 **(A)** Illustration of a representative microsurgical clipping strategy for an unruptured anterior communicating artery aneurysm in a 45-year-old woman presenting with headaches. **(B)** A left-sided approach employing a fenestrated clip is utilized to exclude the aneurysm from the circulation, while sparing the recurrent artery of Heubner and preserving flow through the ipsilateral A2 segment. HU, recurrent artery of Huebner.

ated with patient age, aneurysm size, and location. Surgical outcomes are favorable for small, anterior circulation aneurysms in young patients. For example, in our prior series of 202 consecutive cases, we observed a 50% morbidity and mortality after surgery in unruptured giant basilar aneurysms compared with a 13% rate in giant anterior circulation aneurysms.[3] Our morbidity and mortality was 0% for aneurysms less than 10 mm, 6% for aneurysms between 10 and 25 mm, and 20% for aneurysms >25 mm. By comparison, Drake[13] reported a 15% morbidity and mortality rate in nongiant posterior circulation aneurysms compared with 39% for giant posterior circulation lesions. He also reported a 14.3% rate of morbidity and mortality after surgical treatment of asymptomatic UIA in the posterior circulation, relative to 0% morbidity in the anterior circulation. By comparison, the more recent ISUIA reports a relative risk of 2.6 for poor outcome for aneurysms larger than 12 mm in diameter, and an increase of 2.4 in relative risk was observed in patients older than 50 years of age.[8] Surgical risk factors have thus been identified, which might suggest alternative methods of aneurysm treatment in specific populations.

Endovascular Treatment

Endovascular treatment is a favored therapeutic option for patients >60 years of age with extensive medical comorbidities, or for patients with an aneurysm geometry that is not suitable for microsurgical treatment. Evaluating the relative success of endovascular treatment for UIA is complicated by the inherent selection bias in nearly all of the reports of endovascular management, and varying philosophies and techniques across institutions. The efficacy of endovascular therapy is measured in the same way as for surgery, by examining the rate of complete aneurysm occlusion as well as the rate of posttreatment rupture. Most studies evaluating endovascular occlusion rates report complete aneurysmal obliteration in

approximately 50 to 70% of aneurysms and near-complete occlusion (>90%) in approximately 90% of aneurysms immediately postembolization.[14] In the follow-up ISUIA, aneurysm obliteration was complete in 51%, partial in 21%, not achieved in 23%, and unknown in 5% of patients.[8] Importantly, aneurysm occlusion evolves over time because of progressive thrombosis, coil compaction, and vessel remodeling. This variability in occlusion over time demands follow-up surveillance through repeat angiography or noninvasive imaging.

Although endovascular obliteration of small aneurysms with small necks has been convincingly demonstrated, it is considerably more difficult to achieve angiographic obliteration of aneurysms with a fundus/neck ratio of <2. Recently, techniques have been developed to assist with coil embolization of these aneurysms, including balloon- and stent-assisted coiling. Balloon-assisted coiling involves inflating a temporary nondetachable balloon to occlude both the parent artery and the aneurysm prior to coil embolization, to achieve denser coil packing. Many centers have adopted these techniques successfully for wide-necked aneurysm; however, the technique is thought to be associated with an increase in thromboembolic events.[15] As a result, stent-assisted techniques have been developed. Stent-assisted coiling is similar to balloon remodeling except that it provides a more permanent means of preventing coil prolapse. However, the deployment of a stent in tortuous vessels is technically challenging. In response to this, self-expanding flexible stents designed to navigate the tortuous intracranial vasculature have been developed. But the risk of thromboembolic events is not trivial, and the potential of in-stent stenosis demands the institution of antiplatelet agents that can lead to hemorrhagic complications.

Another recent advance in endovascular treatment of UIA involves stent placement to achieve circumferential parent artery reconstruction, with the goal of diverting flow to promote aneurysm thrombosis. This technique has been recently exploited using the Pipeline Embolization device (EV3, Inc.,

Plymouth, MN), a self-expanding, microcatheter-delivered mesh device that has 30 to 35% metal surface area coverage when fully deployed. A recent series of 53 patients harboring large, wide-necked aneurysms treated with the Pipeline device was presented demonstrating near 100% occlusion at 12-month follow-up with impressively low complication rates.[16] We anticipate that as this strategy and other endovascular technology continue to improve, the indications for endovascular treatment of UIA will continually expand.

Bypass Procedures

Although most aneurysms can be isolated from the circulation using microsurgical clipping or coil embolization alone, some otherwise untreatable lesions require revascularization to facilitate safe and effective treatment. These techniques are applied in cases of a complex aneurysm in which balloon test occlusion demonstrates inadequate collateral cerebral blood flow and in which there is a need for hunterian ligation, trapping, and/or prolonged temporary occlusion.

Several different surgical approaches have been employed to bypass aneurysms that are not ideal for direct clip ligation or endovascular coiling. The most common techniques include extracranial-intracranial (EC-IC) bypass procedures such as a superficial temporal artery to middle cerebral artery graft. These include pedicled arterial grafts such as the superficial temporal artery or occipital artery, providing low-flow, or free grafts including the saphenous vein or radial artery, which allow for high-flow bypass. For some carefully selected giant aneurysms, application of an EC-IC bypass may also lead to flow redirection, which can result in spontaneous thrombosis of the aneurysm. Other grafting options include creative applications of side-to-side revascularization of vessels including the MCA or anterior cerebral artery (ACA) branches. Combined endovascular and microsurgical treatment has also been employed in the treatment of large and complex aneurysms. In this case, surgical bypass is followed by staged aneurysm occlusion. We anticipate that the above revascularization techniques will remain in use at the high-volume centers to which the most complex aneurysms are referred.

Deep Hypothermic Circulatory Arrest

For the treatment of complicated UIA not amenable to conventional clipping, total circulatory arrest with hypothermic cerebral protection may be employed. This high-risk procedure must be performed at centers equipped with the sophisticated intra- and postoperative neurosurgical and cardiothoracic care required. Although the advent of endovascular techniques and innovative bypass procedures has limited the application of this technique, anatomic and morphologic factors remain that dictate the need for open intervention with direct surgical clipping. These factors include aneurysms with large neck-to-dome ratios, thrombosed aneurysms, and those with critical perforators arising from the dome or neck. In these rare cases, deep hypothermic circulatory arrest provides cerebral neuroprotection coupled with a blood-free operative field and a collapsed aneurysm dome. As both the cardiac bypass and the hypothermia lead to an increased risk of complications, patient selection is critical to achieving acceptable patient outcome.

Our experience suggests that the ideal patient for aneurysm clipping under circulatory arrest is <60 years old and harbors few medical comorbidities. Individuals with large aneurysms in the ACoA, ICA bifurcation, or PICA, midbasilar, or vertebral arteries with an absence of thrombus or calcium are most likely to experience favorable outcomes.[17] Optimally, circulatory arrest should be limited to 30 minutes. Additionally, the avoidance of extreme hypothermia (<17°C) coupled with rapid postoperative awakening and neurologic assessment decreases the likelihood of life-threatening hematomas. Given the poor natural history of giant aneurysms, the procedure is indicated for patients with high-risk lesions not amenable to endovascular treatment, normothermic clipping, or cerebral bypass procedures.

Conservative Therapy

Conservative therapy for UIA encompasses two different paradigms. Despite improvements in microsurgical clipping and rapidly developing advances in endovascular therapies, certain aneurysms are better managed conservatively. The size (usually giant), character (calcified), and anatomic configuration (encompassing critical perforators arising from the dome of the aneurysm, and patients who would not be able to tolerate a bypass, or in whom bypass is not technically feasible) cause even the safest treatment risk to outweigh the natural history risk of these few lesions. A second class of lesion is the asymptomatic, small aneurysm, <5 mm, discovered incidentally. These aneurysms are best followed serially for expansion prior to definitive treatment. Despite these recommendations, it must be noted that in practice many ruptured aneurysms are found to be <5 mm in size, and thus further study is necessary to better define which aneurysms are at high risk for rupture.

◆ Outcome Following Aneurysm Treatment

An appreciation of the complication rates of microsurgical and endovascular repair of UIA, the resulting clinical outcome, as well as the risk for recanalization posttreatment is critical in weighing the risk of a given procedure against the natural history of the disease. Although the morbidity and mortality of aneurysm surgery depends on the particular neurosurgeon and medical center, several studies have attempted to formulate currently acceptable values. As Bederson et al[18] pointed out in their 2000 review, these values range from 0 to % for death and from 4 to 15% for complications. A comprehensive meta-analysis of outcomes following UIA surgery was published by Raaymakers et al[19] in 1998. The authors of this paper reported 2.6% mortality and 10.9% morbidity rates in 2460 patients, substantially higher than those quoted in a prior meta-analysis by King et al.[20] In general, complications tended to be serious, with half of affected individuals becoming dependent on others for their activities of daily living. Mortality rates varied substantially, with 62% of studies reporting no deaths, whereas other studies demonstrated death rates as high as 29%. As a general trend, mortality rates were lower in more recent studies and in those with a greater proportion of anterior circulation lesions. Giant aneurysm surgery carried a poor prognosis. Specifically, the authors found the following mortality and morbidity rates: giant posterior circulation aneurysms (9.6% and 37.9%); giant anterior circulation aneurysms (7.4% and 26.9%); non-giant posterior circulation aneurysms (3.0% and 12.9%); and non-giant anterior circulation aneurysms (0.8% and 1.9%). When comparing the findings of these studies it is important to note that the earlier report by King et al excluded symptomatic lesions, which tend to carry a worse prognosis. Moreover, the cohort of lesions reviewed by King et al contained a higher proportion of small aneurysms located in the anterior circulation, which are technically less demanding to treat.

The morbidity and mortality of surgery for UIA was one of the main outcomes assessed in the ISUIA studies.[6,8] The initial cohort studied consisted of 1172 patients, of whom 211 had a prior history of SAH.[6] The authors found age-dependent outcomes, as the morbidity and mortality at 1-year follow-up for patients younger than 45 was 6.5%; for those ages 45 to 64, it was 14.4%, and for those older than 64, it was 32%. Surprisingly, 3.1% of the treated patients without prior aSAH died from operative-related complications compared with only 0.9% of those with a history of aSAH. Close inspection, however, reveals that the latter group was on average younger (47 versus 53 years old) and harbored smaller aneurysms (27% versus 51% of lesions >10 mm) located more often in the anterior circulation (83.4% versus 73.6%). It is unclear whether these cohort differences are enough to account for this discrepancy in postsurgical outcomes, particularly because the presence of medical comorbidities, a known risk factor, was not recorded in ISUIA.

The follow-up ISUIA study assessed outcomes of both surgical and endovascular treatment of UIA. The surgical arm evaluated 1591 patients at 7 days, discharge, 30 days, and yearly.[8] Findings included 1.8% and 12.0% mortality and morbidity at 30 days, and 2.7% and 10.1% mortality and morbidity at 1 year. In this cohort, asymptomatic patients younger than 50 years of age with UIA <24 mm in diameter located in the anterior circulation had the lowest rates of surgical risk (5 to % at 1 year). For comparison, the follow-up ISUIA study also presented outcome data following endovascular treatment. This study assessed 409 patients without a history of aSAH who underwent coiling of a UIA. Findings included 2.0% and 7.4% mortality and morbidity, respectively, at 30 days, and 3.4% and 6.4% mortality and morbidity, respectively, at 1 year. Once again, rates of poor outcomes were higher in older (>50 years) patients with posterior circulation aneurysms >25 mm. When comparing these results to those of other studies, it is important to recognize that both ISUIA studies incorporated major cognitive impairment in their analysis, which was not considered in prior papers.

Discussion has also centered on the rates of recurrence of treated UIA, and the relevance of the angiographic recurrence to the risk of rebleeding, as well as the need for repeated procedures for surveillance of recurrent lesions. In the case of surgery, microsurgical clipping has been demonstrated to provide definitive long-term treatment of cerebral aneurysms. David et al[21] reviewed 160 surgically managed aneurysms that underwent late angiographic follow-up (mean 4.4 years postoperatively), and found only 1.5% of initially obliterated lesions exhibited recurrence. In aneurysms with known residual, 25% enlarged on follow-up imaging. Eight new lesions developed in six patients. This translates into a 0.52% annual rupture rate for completely clipped aneurysms and a 1.8% annual rate of de novo aneurysm formation. Tsutsumi et al[22] have also investigated this topic. In 1999 they published their data after following 115 patients with surgically treated unruptured aneurysm for an average of 8.8 years. Although four patients suffered aSAH, only one patient bled from a successfully clipped aneurysm, leading to a 0.10% annual regrowth rate for completely clipped aneurysms and a 0.20% annual rate of de novo aneurysm formation. In 2001 the same authors published their data after following 140 patients with surgically treated aneurysms (88 ruptured, 52 unruptured) for an average of 9.3 years and found a 0.26% annual regrowth rate for completely clipped aneurysms and a 0.89% annual rate of de novo aneurysm formation.[23] In 2004 Akyuz et al[12] reviewed 166 open surgical clipping cases with late angiography (mean 47 months postoperative). The authors demonstrated a 99.4% aneurysm cure rate; of the 159 aneurysms confirmed to be occluded on immediate postoperative angiogram, 158 remained obliterated on follow-up imaging.

In contrast, the recurrence rate of coiled aneurysms has been reported to be much higher. In 2002, Ng et al[24] quoted a 23% recanalization rate in 30 coiled aneurysms with 1-year angiographic follow-up. That same year, Thornton et al[25] obtained angiographic 1-year follow-up on 143 coiled aneurysms and documented a 1.8% recanalization rate for completely occluded aneurysms and a 28% recanalization rate for incompletely occluded ones. In 2003, Raymond et al[26] cited a 33.6% recanalization rate in 383 coiled aneurysms with 12.3-month mean angiographic follow-up. More recently, Murayama et al[27] reported their 11-year experience with embolization of cerebral aneurysms using the Guglielmi detachable coil (GDC) technology. After analyzing 6- and 12-month angiographic follow-up images for 916 coiled aneurysms, the authors demonstrated a 20.9% overall recanalization rate. The patients were divided into two groups: group A included the authors' initial 5-year experience with 230 patients harboring 251 aneurysms, and group B included the subsequent 6-year experience with 588 patients harboring 665 aneurysms. Complete occlusion was obtained in only 55% of aneurysms, with neck remnants present in 35.4% of lesions. Complications occurred in 9.4% of cases. The results reveal both a higher complete embolization rate and lower recanalization rate in group B patients as compared with those in group A (56.8% and 17.2% versus 50.2% and 26.1%, respectively), likely a reflection of improved technique, greater experience, and advanced GDC technology. Of note, recanalization was related to the size of the dome and neck of the aneurysm. In small aneurysms (4 to 10 mm) with small necks (<4 mm), the overall recanalization rate was only 5.1%.

In contrast, for small aneurysms with wide necks (≤4 mm) the overall recanalization rate was 20%. Moreover, among large aneurysms (11–25 mm) and giant aneurysms (>25 mm) the overall recanalization rate was 35% and 59.1%, respectively. These data strongly suggest that although clinical and postembolization outcomes in patients treated with the GDC system have improved over time, larger lesions with wider necks continue to carry a high risk for recanalization.

◆ Controversy (Clip Versus Coil)

No prospective, randomized multicenter trial has compared surgical and endovascular treatment of UIA. As a result, the appropriate treatment choice for a given UIA remains controversial. The choice of a particular treatment modality for each individual case should take into account size, location, anatomic characteristics, medical comorbidities, and the skill of the operator (**Table 20.2**). Additionally, as discussed previously, the risks of microsurgery and endovascular treatment must be weighed against the natural history of the disease. Furthermore, when considering the treatment of a UIA, we view the risk of incomplete treatment and recurrence, coupled with the need for careful surveillance for recurrent lesions, as a critically important distinguishing feature between clipping and coiling. Although some prospective data exist on the relative safety and immediate angiographic efficacy of these two techniques, significant selection bias and heterogeneous patient populations complicates meaningful direct comparison.

Several small, nonrandomized studies have undertaken to compare outcomes of UIA treated by endovascular and surgical means, and have demonstrated varying results. Johnston et al[28] performed a single-center blinded comparison of patients with UIA who received surgical (n = 68) or endovascular (n = 62) treatment. All aneurysms in this study were deemed by a panel of surgeons and interventionalists to be amenable to either surgical or endovascular treatment. A higher frequency of postprocedural disability was reported in patients who underwent surgery compared with those treated endovascularly (25% versus 8%). Additionally, length of stay and hospital costs were greater for the surgical patients. The same group then reviewed 2069 patients with UIA in a statewide database of California hospital discharges. Adverse outcomes were more frequent in the 1669 patients treated with surgery (25%) than in the 400 who underwent endovascular therapy (10%). In-hospital death was also more frequent after surgery than endovascular treatment (3.5% versus 0.5%), and length of stay and hospital costs were greater after surgery. Furthermore, adverse outcomes significantly declined over time for endovascular therapy (26% in 1991 to 4% in 1998) but not for surgery (26% in 1991 versus 21% in 1998), likely due to developments in technology and increasing interventionalist experience.

These data contrast with those from more recent work by Hoh et al.[29] In this study, the investigators compared aneurysm coiling and clipping from 565 patients treated at a single institution over a 2.5-year period. The investigators demonstrated a shorter length of hospital stay in coiled patients; however, coiling was associated with higher hospital costs in both ruptured and UIA, reflecting the increasing costs of endovascular technology over time. In a prospective, multicenter observational study, Brilstra et al[30] measured the effect of surgical or endovascular treatment of UIA on functional health, quality of life, anxiety, and depression. In the surgical group of 32 patients, 97% of aneurysms were successfully treated and 12% had a permanent complication. At 3 months postoperative, quality of life had improved but had not returned to baseline. In the endovascular group of 19 patients, 16 of 19 aneurysms (84%) were occluded by 90% or more, and none of the surviving patients had complications with permanent deficits. However, one patient died from rupture of an aneurysm previously treated endovascularly. Quality of life in the other 18 patients after 3 months and 1 year was similar to that before treatment. In the short term, surgical treatment seems to have a negative effect on functional health and quality of life, compared with a potentially increased rate of posttreatment hemorrhage in coiled patients.

◆ Management Recommendations

In 2000, the Stroke Council of the American Heart Association issued a scientific statement with the following recommendations for the management of UIA[18]: "In consideration of the apparent low risk of hemorrhage from incidental small (<10 mm) aneurysms in patients without previous SAH, treatment rather than observation cannot be generally advocated." This statement is now clearly antiquated, and it is time for a new consensus committee to issue updated rec-

Table 20.2 Summary of Treatment Modalities for Unruptured Intracranial Aneurysm

Treatment Modality	Characteristics Favoring	Characteristics Disfavoring
Microsurgical Clipping	Young age	Posterior circulation location
	Lack of medical comorbidity	
	Anterior circulation location	
Endovascular Coiling	Advanced age	Large neck-to-dome ratio
	Extensive medical comorbidity	Critical branch emerging from dome
	Posterior circulation location	

ommendations. The most conclusive data regarding the natural history of UIA is from ISUIA[6,8] and Juvela et al's[7] Helsinki experience. Murayama et al's experience with aneurysm regrowth after coil embolization provides important insight for comparison to the relative permanence of surgical clipping. Raaymaker et al's[19] meta-analysis of the literature on surgical morbidity for clipping of UIA aligns almost exactly with our own published data[3] and ongoing experience. These data sets and our own experience provide an invaluable, although imperfect, framework for the following structured guidelines (**Fig. 20.2**):

1. With rare exceptions, all symptomatic unruptured aneurysms should be treated. Extensive medical comorbidity, advanced age, and anatomic configuration of the aneurysm may contraindicate intervention when treatment risks approach 25%.
2. Small, incidental aneurysms <5 mm should be managed conservatively in most cases. An important exception to this rule involves those young patients with severe psy-

chological disturbances secondary to harboring an UIA. In such patients, particularly those psychologically crippled by their condition, definitive treatment can be justified and is often pursued.

3. Patients <60 years of age with aneurysms >5 mm should be offered treatment unless there is a significant contraindication. Although 7 mm was the cut-off in the ISUIA data, there are limitations to using such an exact measurement. Certainly, aneurysms less than 7 mm in diameter are known to infrequently rupture. The accuracy of measurement, even with angiographic data, is at least ±2 mm. Therefore, if 7 mm is used as a cutoff, some aneurysms will not be treated that should be treated. Rather, we suggest using a standard error of measurement below this cutoff, so that the 99% of patients at risk for rupture are offered treatment. When managing older patients (≥60 years of age), the decision to treat becomes less clear. In these situations, lesion location plays a critical role, as ACoA, PCoA, and basilar apex aneurysms carry higher rupture risk than aneurysms in other locations. Thus, we strongly advocate

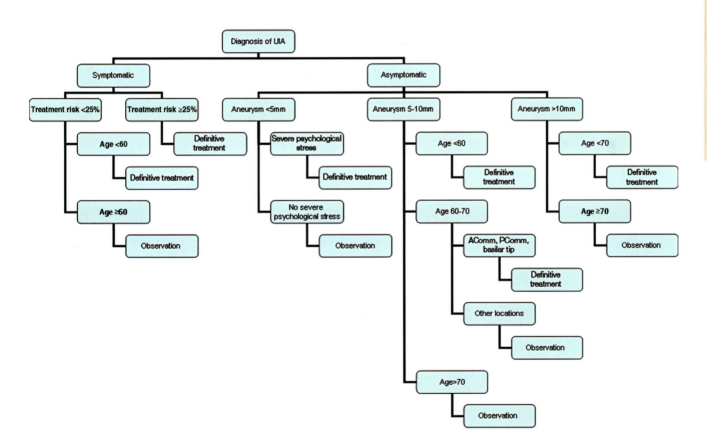

Fig. 20.2 Flowchart depicting our treatment paradigm for an unruptured intracranial aneurysm (UIA). Although this serves as a general management strategy, specific characteristics of both the patient and the aneurysm in question may occasionally lead to deviation from this paradigm.

treatment of such lesions, even in older healthy individuals, as there is low associated treatment morbidity.

4. Large, incidental aneurysms >10 mm should be treated in all healthy patients <70 years of age. The indications are less compelling in older individuals.

5. Microsurgical clipping rather than endovascular coiling should be the first choice in low-risk cases (young patients with small, anterior circulation aneurysms). In these cases, the risk of open microsurgery and endovascular surgery is about the same in terms of stroke and death, although endovascular coiling is less invasive. On the other hand, surgical clipping provides a repair that is at least an order of magnitude more durable than coiling. In cases where the invasion of clipping and the 6 weeks of recuperation do not pose an undue risk or hardship, clipping is the preferred option.

6. Very large and giant aneurysms, and aneurysms with high neck-to-dome ratios, generally benefit more from surgical approaches than from endovascular treatment. In the most complex aneurysms, combined approaches such as arterial bypass techniques followed by proximal endovascular occlusion, have proven invaluable.

7. Endovascular coiling represents a reasonable alternative that should be instituted whenever surgical intervention carries high risk such as with elderly or medically ill patients and in anatomically unfavorable situations. The improvement in stent/coil technology offers an excellent alternative in this group of poor surgical candidates, even in those aneurysms with wide necks and unfavorable neck/dome ratios.

◆ Case Illustrations

The following case illustrations demonstrate the treatment paradigms and follow-up strategies employed for the management of two representative UIAs at our institution.

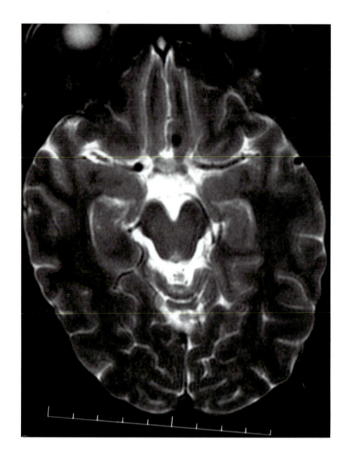

Fig. 20.3 Magnetic resonance imaging reveals a flow void representing the aneurysm in the region of the anterior communicating artery.

Microsurgical Treatment

A 42-year-old woman with an incidental diagnosis of an aneurysm discovered on MRI obtained after her sister suffered a subarachnoid hemorrhage **(Fig. 20.3)**. Diagnostic angiog-

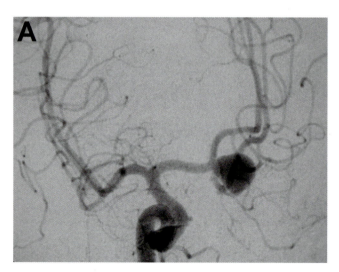
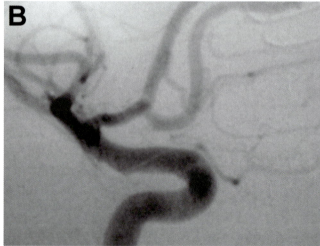

Fig. 20.4 **(A)** Digital subtraction angiography (DSA) reveals the presence of the anterior communicating aneurysm, approximately 1 cm in largest dimension, with a relatively narrow neck. **(B)** Intraoperative angiogram demonstrates complete obliteration of the aneurysm.

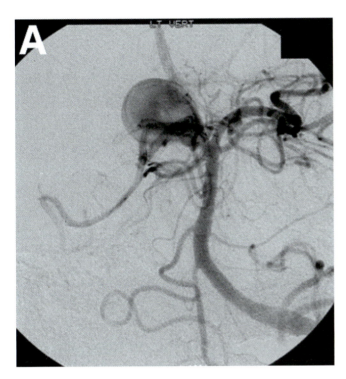
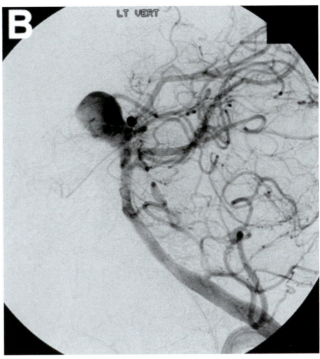

Fig. 20.5 Frontal **(A)** and lateral **(B)** DSA projections reveal the large, fusiform aneurysm incorporating the parent P1 vessel in the origin of the aneurysm.

raphy revealed an approximately 1-cm-diameter true ACoA aneurysm filling from the right **(Fig. 20.4A)**. Given the size and geometry of the aneurysm, and its relatively narrow neck, either endovascular or microsurgical treatment was deemed appropriate. Microsurgical clipping was elected. The aneurysm was completely obliterated by the placement of a clip over the neck of the aneurysm, with postoperative angiography revealing no significant residual filling **(Fig. 20.4B)**. She awoke from the procedure without neurologic deficits and has remained clinically stable without further imaging.

Endovascular Treatment

A 46-year-old woman presents complaining of a progressive right-sided hemicranial headache, without evidence of subarachnoid hemorrhage on admission head CT. Diagnostic angiogram revealed a 20- × 16- × 14-mm fusiform aneurysm of the right posterior cerebral artery (PCA) **(Fig. 20.5)**. Given the location and anatomic configuration of the aneurysm, endovascular treatment was undertaken **(Fig. 20.6)**. A Neuroform stent (Boston Scientific, Natick, MA) was deployed across the base of the aneurysm, and a total of 25 coils were placed in the aneurysm sac. Postembolization angiogram revealed only a small neck remnant, and the patient awoke without neurologic deficit **(Fig. 20.7)**. Follow-up angiogram at 6 months

revealed recanalization of the aneurysm **(Fig. 20.8)**, and an additional nine coils and an additional Neuroform stent were placed in a single procedure. Over the subsequent 4 years, an additional three stents and 21 coils have been placed to counter multiple episodes of recanalization, but at last follow-up the aneurysm remains stable and occluded.

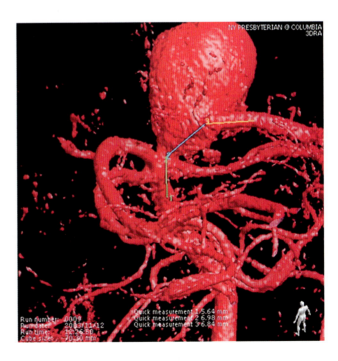

Fig. 20.6 Three-dimensional angiographic reconstruction more clearly delineates the aneurysm geometry as well as the relationship of the aneurysm to the parent artery.

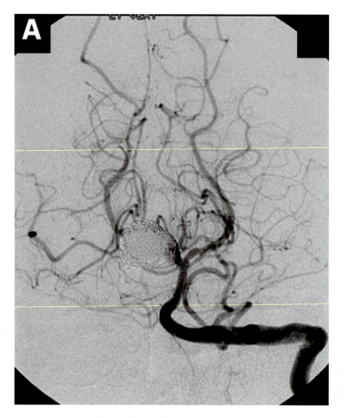
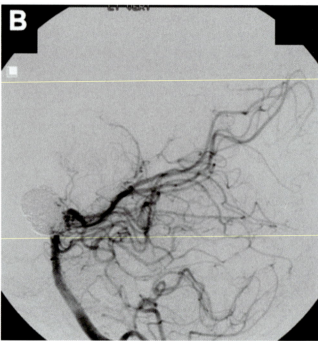

Fig. 20.7 Frontal **(A)** and lateral **(B)** DSA projections following stent-assisted coil embolization reveal only a small neck remnant.

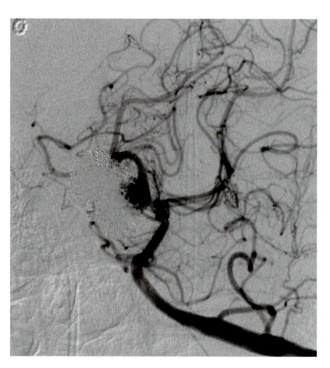

Fig. 20.8 Follow-up angiogram reveals progressive coil compaction and aneurysm recanalization that was treated with placement of multiple additional stents and coils.

References

1. Juvela S, Porras M, Poussa K. Natural history of unruptured intracranial aneurysms: probability of and risk factors for aneurysm rupture. J Neurosurg 2000;93:379–387
2. Rinkel GJ, Djibuti M, Algra A, van Gijn J. Prevalence and risk of rupture of intracranial aneurysms: a systematic review. Stroke 1998;29:251–256
3. Solomon RA, Fink ME, Pile-Spellman J. Surgical management of unruptured intracranial aneurysms. J Neurosurg 1994;80:440–446
4. Weir B. Unruptured intracranial aneurysms: a review. J Neurosurg 2002;96:3–42
5. Krischek B, Inoue I. The genetics of intracranial aneurysms. J Hum Genet 2006;51:587–594
6. International Study of Unruptured Intracranial Aneurysms Investigators. Unruptured intracranial aneurysms—risk of rupture and risks of surgical intervention. N Engl J Med 1998;339:1725–1733
7. Juvela S, Porras M, Heiskanen O. Natural history of unruptured intracranial aneurysms: a long-term follow-up study. J Neurosurg 1993;79: 174–182
8. Wiebers DO, Whisnant JP, Huston J III, et al; International Study of Unruptured Intracranial Aneurysms Investigators. Unruptured intracranial aneurysms: natural history, clinical outcome, and risks of surgical and endovascular treatment. Lancet 2003;362:103–110
9. Juvela S, Poussa K, Porras M. Factors affecting formation and growth of intracranial aneurysms: a long-term follow-up study. Stroke 2001;32: 485–491
10. Broderick JP, Sauerbeck LR, Foroud T, et al. The Familial Intracranial Aneurysm (FIA) study protocol. BMC Med Genet 2005;6:17
11. Thornton J, Bashir Q, Aletich VA, Debrun GM, Ausman JI, Charbel FT. What percentage of surgically clipped intracranial aneurysms have residual necks? Neurosurgery 2000;46:1294–1298, discussion 1298–1300
12. Akyüz M, Tuncer R, Yilmaz S, Sindel T. Angiographic follow-up after surgical treatment of intracranial aneurysms. Acta Neurochir (Wien) 2004; 146:245–250, discussion 250
13. Drake CG. Progress in cerebrovascular disease. Management of cerebral aneurysm. Stroke 1981;12:273–283

14. Pouratian N, Oskouian RJ Jr, Jensen ME, Kassell NF, Dumont AS. Endovascular management of unruptured intracranial aneurysms. J Neurol Neurosurg Psychiatry 2006;77:572–578
15. Nelson PK, Levy DI. Balloon-assisted coil embolization of wide-necked aneurysms of the internal carotid artery: medium-term angiographic and clinical follow-up in 22 patients. AJNR Am J Neuroradiol 2001;22:19–26
16. Lylyk P, Miranda C, Ceratto R, et al. Curative endovascular reconstruction of cerebral aneurysms with the pipeline embolization device: the Buenos Aires experience. Neurosurgery 2009;64:632–642, discussion 642–643, quiz N6
17. Mack WJ, Ducruet AF, Angevine PD, et al. Deep hypothermic circulatory arrest for complex cerebral aneurysms: lessons learned. Neurosurgery 2007;60:815–827, discussion 815–827
18. Bederson JB, Awad IA, Wiebers DO, et al. Recommendations for the management of patients with unruptured intracranial aneurysms: a statement for healthcare professionals from the Stroke Council of the American Heart Association. Stroke 2000;31:2742–2750
19. Raaymakers TW, Rinkel GJ, Limburg M, Algra A. Mortality and morbidity of surgery for unruptured intracranial aneurysms: a meta-analysis. Stroke 1998;29:1531–1538
20. King JT Jr, Berlin JA, Flamm ES. Morbidity and mortality from elective surgery for asymptomatic, unruptured, intracranial aneurysms: a meta-analysis. J Neurosurg 1994;81:837–842
21. David CA, Vishteh AG, Spetzler RF, Lemole M, Lawton MT, Partovi S. Late angiographic follow-up review of surgically treated aneurysms. J Neurosurg 1999;91:396–401
22. Tsutsumi K, Ueki K, Usui M, Kwak S, Kirino T. Risk of subarachnoid hemorrhage after surgical treatment of unruptured cerebral aneurysms. Stroke 1999;30:1181–1184
23. Tsutsumi K, Ueki K, Morita A, Usui M, Kirino T. Risk of aneurysm recurrence in patients with clipped cerebral aneurysms: results of long-term follow-up angiography. Stroke 2001;32:1191–1194
24. Ng P, Khangure MS, Phatouros CC, Bynevelt M, ApSimon H, McAuliffe W. Endovascular treatment of intracranial aneurysms with Guglielmi detachable coils: analysis of midterm angiographic and clinical outcomes. Stroke 2002;33:210–217
25. Thornton J, Debrun GM, Aletich VA, Bashir Q, Charbel FT, Ausman J. Follow-up angiography of intracranial aneurysms treated with endovascular placement of Guglielmi detachable coils. Neurosurgery 2002;50:239–249, discussion 249–250
26. Raymond J, Guilbert F, Weill A, et al. Long-term angiographic recurrences after selective endovascular treatment of aneurysms with detachable coils. Stroke 2003;34:1398–1403
27. Murayama Y, Nien YL, Duckwiler G, et al. Guglielmi detachable coil embolization of cerebral aneurysms: 11 years' experience. J Neurosurg 2003;98:959–966
28. Johnston SC, Wilson CB, Halbach VV, et al. Endovascular and surgical treatment of unruptured cerebral aneurysms: comparison of risks. Ann Neurol 2000;48:11–19
29. Hoh BL, Chi YY, Dermott MA, Lipori PJ, Lewis SB. The effect of coiling versus clipping of ruptured and unruptured cerebral aneurysms on length of stay, hospital cost, hospital reimbursement, and surgeon reimbursement at the university of Florida. Neurosurgery 2009;64:614–619, discussion 619–621
30. Brilstra EH, Rinkel GJ, van der Graaf Y, et al. Quality of life after treatment of unruptured intracranial aneurysms by neurosurgical clipping or by embolisation with coils. A prospective, observational study. Cerebrovasc Dis 2004;17:44–52

21

Microsurgery for Ruptured Aneurysms

Rossana Romani, Martin Lehecka, Mika Niemelä, Jaakko Rinne,
Tomi Niemi, Reza Dashti, and Juha Hernesniemi

Pearls

- The patient's head should be elevated above heart level, with systolic blood pressure around 100 mm Hg. The head position, incision, and bone flap should be tailored according to the location and orientation of the aneurysm.
- A slack brain is achieved by high-quality modern neuroanesthesia and the release of cerebrospinal fluid (CSF) from the basal cisterns, the lamina terminalis, and ventricular drainage.
- Continuous hemostasis is maintained throughout the procedure under a mouth-piece–controlled operating microscope with high magnification.
- Sufficient proximal control for safety, frequent use of temporary clips to soften the aneurysm, meticulous dissection of the aneurysm, use of the shortest possible clip (usually 1.5 times the neck width) to prevent branch occlusions and kinking of the parent artery, intraoperative confirmation of aneurysm occlusion, and branch patency with indocyanine green (ICG) angiography and micro-Doppler are hallmarks of a successful surgery.
- Immediate postoperative computed tomography (CT), computed tomography angiography (CTA), or digital subtraction angiography (DSA) are performed for quality control. Young patients, especially those with multiple aneurysms or with a family history of intracranial aneurysms, should be followed to exclude possible de novo aneurysms in the long run.

tured aneurysms are estimated to have an approximately 1% rupture rate per year.[5] Risk factors for aneurysm rupture include female gender; smoking; older age; high blood pressure; large aneurysm size; aneurysm location, especially posterior circulation location; country of origin; and history of subarachnoid hemorrhage.[4]

After the International Subarachnoid Aneurysm Trial (ISAT)[6,7] study, there has been a strong increase in the use of the endovascular techniques that have been overshadowing the most recent developments of microvascular neurosurgery. As endovascular techniques remain expensive, and not all of the aneurysms can be treated using them, there is still a place for high-quality microsurgery. Our philosophy when treating both anterior and posterior circulation aneurysms using microneurosurgery is to apply microsurgical techniques that are "simple, fast, and preserve normal anatomy."[8,9]

We review here the microneurosurgical experience of the senior author (J.H.) at two of the five Finnish neurosurgical units, the Kuopio and Helsinki University Hospitals, which have treated more than 10,000 intracranial aneurysms since the beginning of the microneurosurgical era in Finland in the mid-1970s. At present, in our institutions approximately 350 ruptured aneurysms are treated each year, most of them using state-of-the-art microneurosurgery.[10]

◆ Epidemiology and Natural History

The worldwide overall incidence of aneurysmal subarachnoid hemorrhage (SAH) is approximately 6 to 10 per 100,000 person-years, but in some countries, such as Finland and Japan, is as high as 16 to 20 per 100,000 person-years.[1] SAH caused by intracranial aneurysm rupture has a 50% overall mortality, and one third of the survivors suffer from significant neurologic deficits.[2]

Risk factors for aneurysmal SAH are smoking, hypertension, excessive use of alcohol, and family history.[3,4] Unrup-

◆ Indications

All patients of southern and eastern Finland come to Helsinki and Kuopio, which are two of the five neurosurgical units of Finland with a catchment area of nearly 3 million people. These two units cannot select their patients, in contrast to many metropolitan hospitals, which show a strong patient selection in their reports. Admitting all patients, including those with a poor grade and elderly patients with aneurysmal SAH for treatment from a defined catchment area, means that we face a management mortality of 20 to 35%, even when

Table 21.1 Frequency of Aneurysm Sites in the Finnish Population

Location of the aneurysms	%
Middle cerebral artery	38
Anterior communicating artery	26
Internal carotid artery	23
Pericallosal artery	6
Vertebrobasilar arteries	7

our surgeons have extensive experience and use the most sophisticated treatment methods. Depending on the selection of patients, treatment mortality can be between 1% and 25%, or even higher. These figures are highly influenced by the preoperative patient condition, the practitioners' treatment skills, and the length of the follow-up.

◆ Selection of Patients for Active Treatment

Our policy is to treat all SAH patients in the acute phase as soon as possible, usually during the first 24 hours after the aneurysm rupture. Nearly half (45%) of all patients are operated on within 24 hours. Distribution of intracranial aneurysms in the Finnish population according to their site of origin is represented in **Table 21.1**.

Patients with expansive hematomas, in our population most often due to ruptured middle cerebral artery (MCA) aneurysm,[11] are operated on immediately. We operate even on patients with fixed, dilated pupils if the patient is young and the pupil dilatation has been present for only a very short time. Microsurgical clipping is preferred in these patients, as it allows also the removal of the hematoma and application

of the extraventricular drain (EVD). The EVD can be placed either through the lamina terminalis during the surgery or through an additional cortical puncture. We prefer the former method.[12] Especially patients with poor grade should have no treatment delays, and are treated during the first day. Multivariate analysis shows that among patients with ruptured aneurysms, the major determinants of outcome are preoperative grade, intracerebral hematoma (ICH) or intraventricular hematoma (IVH) on initial computed tomography (CT) scan, and preoperative hydrocephalus[13] **(Table 21.2)**. In addition, perioperative aneurysmal rupture, occlusion of major vessels, postoperative hematoma, and perforator injury are also related to unfavorable outcome.

◆ Preoperative Treatment

Before the ruptured aneurysm has been secured, systolic arterial blood pressure must be controlled, and blood pressures above 160 mm Hg should be treated with labetalol. At the same time, a systolic pressure that is too low will not provide sufficient perfusion pressure and should be prevented as well. In patients with an intracranial space-occupying hematoma, a higher blood pressure can be allowed to secure adequate cerebral perfusion pressure. The transmural pressure of the aneurysm sac is one of the determinants of the risk of rebleeding, and as it cannot be measured individually, the accepted blood pressure remains to be determined individually. In all SAH patients arterial blood pressure is measured invasively. In conscious patients, spontaneous breathing is usually adequate, but in patients with a Glasgow Coma Scale (GCS) score of 8 or less, an artificial airway and controlled ventilation are indicated. Adequate anesthesia is required before intubation to prevent rebleeding, because laryngoscopy and intubation induce a stress response with an increase in blood pressure. Sedation using propofol should be considered in patients under controlled ventilation.

Tranexamic acid (1 g IV every 6 hours up to 3 days) is administered to prevent rebleeding until clipping. Nimodipine (PO or IV) is given to all patients with ruptured aneurysms to

Table 21.2 Glasgow Outcome Scale (GOS) score at 3 Months After Microsurgical Treatment of Ruptured Aneurysm Correlated with Preoperative WFNS Grade in Patients Treated in Helsinki 2001–2003

WFNS	GR	%	MD	%	SD	%	GOS PVS	%	Death	%	Total	%
1	154	73	36	17	12	6	2	1	4	2	208	42
2	43	48	19	21	20	22	2	2	5	6	89	18
3	7	26	7	26	8	30	0	0	5	19	27	5
4	19	21	26	30	26	31	1	1	12	14	84	17
5	6	7	12	14	28	33	15	18	24	28	85	17
	229	46	100	20	94	19	20	4	50	10	493	

Abbreviations: GOS, Glasgow Outcome Scale; GR, good recovery; MD, moderate disability, SD, severe disability; PVS, persistent vegetative state; WFNS, World Federation of Neurosurgical Societies grading.

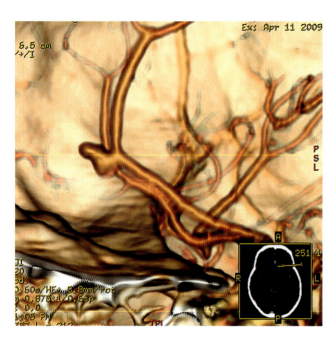

Fig. 21.1 Preoperative sagittal view of a three-dimensional (3D) computed tomography angiography (CTA) showing a ruptured, left pericallosal aneurysm.

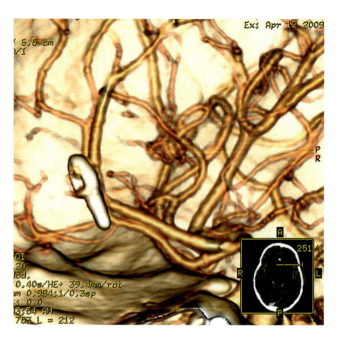

Fig. 21.2 Postoperative sagittal view of a 3D CTA showing a perfect clipping of the ruptured pericallosal aneurysm.

prevent vasospasm. A more detailed description of our anesthesiologic principles in treatment of SAH patients are described elsewhere.[14]

◆ Neuroradiologic Investigations

Since the late 1970s, CT has been the primary diagnostic tool for detecting SAH and for determining the presence of an ICH or hydrocephalus. Digital subtraction angiography (DSA) has been replaced by CT angiography (CTA) at our department

since the year 2000 as the primary imaging method for detecting intracranial aneurysms.[14] CTA is fast and noninvasive, and it gives information about bony landmarks and provides accurate diagnosis of aneurysms larger than 2 mm. Furthermore, three-dimensional (3D) CTA images provide a surgical view of the aneurysms[15] **(Fig. 21.1).** Postoperatively, all patients undergo CT and CTA[16] **(Fig. 21.2).** CTA is used during the follow-up to determine the presence of aneurysm remnants or regrowth **(Fig. 21.3).** DSA is reserved for complex, giant, or previously coiled aneurysms, and it can be used also intraoperatively during the surgery.

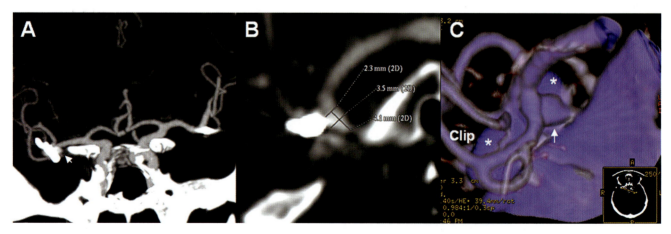

Fig. 21.3 Coronal two-dimensional (2D) CTA **(A),** oblique view of a 2D CTA **(B),** and oblique view of 3D CTA **(C)** showing a right middle cerebral artery (MCA) bifurcation aneurysm that was ruptured and clipped (*) in 1988. The aneurysm recurred (arrow) during the follow-up and it was diagnosed by CTA.

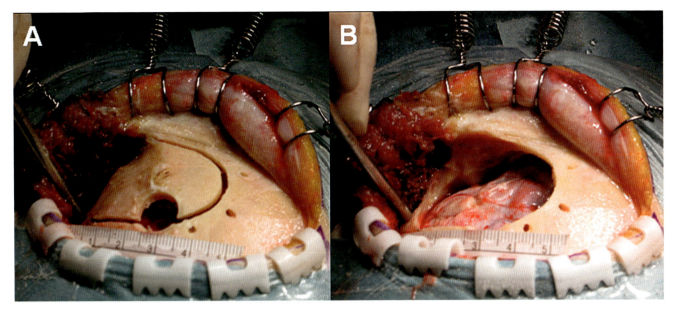

Fig. 21.4 Intraoperative view of a left lateral supraorbital approach **(A)** and the dura exposed **(B)**.

◆ Surgical Techniques

Anterior Circulation Aneurysms

Surgical Approaches

We operate on nearly all aneurysms of the anterior circulation, except those of the pericallosal artery, using the lateral supraorbital (LSO) approach. The LSO approach has been used by the senior author (J.H.) for more than 25 years in treatment of both vascular[18–24] and neoplastic lesions of the anterior cranial fossa.[17,18] This approach is a less invasive modification of the pterional approach. It is located more frontally, with the bone flap of approximately 3 × 4 cm in diameter **(Figs. 21.4 and 21.5)**. We do not use the orbitozygomatic approach or any of its different modifications mainly because in our experience the removal of the orbital roof causes swelling of the orbital contents and thereby takes much (or all) of the extra space achieved.

The LSO approach has been described in detail elsewhere.[19] Briefly, the head is fixed to the Sugita frame and (1) elevated clearly above the cardiac level; (2) rotated 15 to 30 degrees toward the opposite side according to the position of the aneurysm; (3) extended or slight flexed depending on the height of the aneurysm from the skull base; and (4) tilted laterally to make the proximal part of the sylvian fissure nearly vertical. We adjust the position of the fixed head and body during the operation as needed. After minimal shaving and injection of a local anesthetic combined with Adrenaline for vasoconstriction, a 7- to 9-cm-long, curved skin incision is placed just behind the hairline. A one-layer skin-muscle flap is retracted frontally with spring hooks, and the superior orbital rim and the anterior zygomatic arch are exposed. The extent of the craniotomy de-

pends on the surgeon's experience and preference. It may be tailored according to the location and the size of the aneurysm. Usually, a small LSO craniotomy is all that is necessary, but for giant aneurysms a slightly larger bone flap is planned. A single bur hole is placed just under the temporal line in the bone, that is, the superior insertion of the temporal muscle. A bone flap of 3 × 4 cm is detached mostly by a side-cutting drill, and the basal part is partially drilled to remove most of the sphenoid wing **(Fig. 21.5)**. The dura is incised curvilinearly with the base in the frontobasal direction, and dural edges are elevated using multiple stitches, extended over cra-

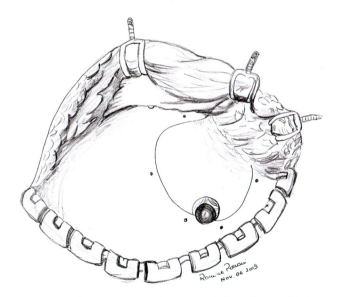

Fig. 21.5 Schematic drawing showing a right lateral supraorbital (LSO) approach.

niotomy dressings. From this point on, all surgery is performed under the operating microscope, including the skin closure. The LSO approach is simple and fast with little removal of the skull base; the whole approach takes only 10 to 15 minutes. Our record in performing this LSO craniotomy from skin to skin in an unruptured MCA aneurysm is 25 minutes, with uneventful recovery of the patient. A fast operation is naturally not the major goal in itself, but it allows more operations to be performed in a single operating room during a single day, thereby being more cost-effective, and potentially the risk of the infection is lower. Our experience is that clean surgery is fast, and it results in a good outcome for the patient.

The LSO approach, like any other approach for ruptured aneurysms, requires a slack and relaxed brain, achieved by modern neuroanesthesia[20] to minimize brain retraction.[18] For paraclinoid aneurysms or those of the posterior communicating artery (PCoA) close to the anterior clinoid, an intradural clinoidectomy with ultrasonic bone curette (Sonopet Omni, Model UST-2001 Ultrasonic Surgical System, Synergetics, Inc., Miwatec Co., Kawasaki, Japan) is performed to have the proximal control of the aneurysm. The anterior clinoid is not removed routinely, but the decision is made only after the initial inspection of the anatomic relation between the aneurysm and the parent artery.

Distal anterior cerebral artery (DACA) aneurysms or pericallosal aneurysms differ from other anterior circulation aneurysms in the sense that they require a different approach, namely the interhemispheric approach.[21–25] This can be done with the patient either lying supine with the head in neutral position and elevated approximately 20 degrees above the heart level, or placed in the lateral park bench position with the head elevated and tilted upward. We prefer the supine position. For most DACA aneurysms the skin incision is curvilinear over the midline behind the coronal suture. A single bur hole is placed on the midline, and a paramedian bone flap is placed slightly over the midline to facilitate retraction of the falx medially. The size of the bone flap, usually 3 to 4 cm in diameter, depends both on the surgeon's experience and on the presence of an ICH. A flap too small may not provide sufficient room for working between the bridging veins. The dura is opened under the microscope as a C-shaped flap with its base at the midline. Nowadays, we recommend the use of a neuronavigator to help intraoperative localization of the aneurysm inside the interhemispheric fissure, which does not have a good anatomic landmark.

Intracerebral Hematoma

In cases of a large hematoma and lack of space after the LSO or interhemispheric approaches, a small cortical incision is made, avoiding the eloquent areas, and the hematoma is partially removed to gain space.[21–24,26–30] Caution is needed as this may cause rerupture of the aneurysm, which would be very difficult to control through the hematoma cavity without proper proximal control. It is important to apply only minor force in removing the ICH, and in the immediate vicinity of the aneurysm the hematoma should be left in place until proximal and distal control have been achieved.

Treatment of Acute Hydrocephalus

In the presence of acute hydrocephalus, an EVD is placed to reduce intracranial pressure (ICP). This can be done before surgery or, in cases of severe brain swelling and lack of space after craniotomy, through a separate puncture.[21–24,26–30]

In the presence of a red, angry, swollen brain, as is often the case in acute SAH, the first step is to relax the brain by removing cerebrospinal fluid (CSF) from the basal cisterns. If only a limited amount of CSF can be removed from the basal cisterns, opening of the lamina terminalis can be used to achieve slack brain intraoperatively. After opening the carotid and optic cisterns, dissection is continued following the ipsilateral optic nerve with a gentle retraction of the frontal lobe. The lamina terminalis with its gray-bluish appearance is behind the optic chiasm and can be fenestrated by using sharp bipolar or microscissor.[12] The opening of the lamina terminalis usually can be performed in all ruptured anterior circulation aneurysms except in downward projecting anterior communicating artery (ACoA) aneurysms, which could rupture due to dissection near the optic chiasm. In these cases, the Liliequist membrane is opened to remove additional CSF. This technique can be used also for internal carotid artery (ICA) aneurysms if necessary. The other exception is pericallosal artery aneurysms, which are approached using the interhemispheric route. In pericallosal aneurysms with severe brain edema, a conventional ventricular puncture at the border of the craniotomy is preferred, but in less severe cases a small callosotomy and opening of the lateral ventricle can be used to release additional CSF.

After the aneurysm has been clipped, in cases where it is necessary to monitor the ICP or to remove CSF, a thin ventricular catheter (small, radiopaque barium-impregnated ventricular catheter, Medtronic reference number 41207; Medtronic, Inc., Minneapolis, MN) is inserted through the fenestration of the lamina terminalis into the third ventricle.[12]

Aneurysm Dissection and Temporary Clipping

Internal carotid artery aneurysms, except those of the ICA bifurcation, rarely require opening of the sylvian fissure. In ICA bifurcation and a proximal MCA aneurysm of the M1 type, the proximal part of the sylvian fissure is opened.[26,30] Dissection of the sylvian fissure is more difficult in the presence of a swollen brain in acute SAH. Opening of the sylvian fissure starts with a small arachnoid incision of 2 mm using a sharp needle acting as an arachnoid knife at the frontal lobe side of the sylvian veins, and physiologic saline is injected using a handheld syringe to expand the plane for further dissection—the water dissection technique.[31] Sharp bipolar, suction, microscissor, and small cottonoids are used to open the fissure from inside out, carefully mobilizing the vascular structures and pushing them to either side. For MCA bifurcation aneurysms, the sylvian fissure is opened directly over the aneurysm, and the aneurysm is approached from the distal direction.[27] ACoA aneurysms are usually approached from the side of the dominant A1.[29] Both ipsilateral and contralateral A1s are visualized by careful mobilization and retraction of the frontal lobe. Small resection of the gyrus rectus is usually necessary to see the whole aneurysm and, more importantly, origins of both pericallosal arteries. The gyrus rectus is identified on the medial side of the ipsilateral olfactory tract. Pia is opened with microscissors or sharp bipolar forceps, and gyrus tissue is carefully removed by suction, usually less than 1 cm in length and a few millimeters in depth. Pia and arachnoid planes have to be preserved in the interhemispheric fissure to protect the aneurysm, the recurrent artery of Heubner (RAH), and the A2 branches.[29]

The aneurysm base is dissected using microscissors and a microdissector so that the pilot clip can be inserted safely. Especially in ruptured aneurysms it is wise to use temporary clips (proximal and distal) during the dissection to avoid intraoperative rupture and profuse bleeding. The duration of each temporary occlusion should be kept as short as possible; usually a duration of 5 minutes is well tolerated. For ICA aneurysms, the temporary clips are placed at the ICA just below the base of the aneurysm and distally on either the ICA directly or possibly the MCA and the anterior cerebral artery (ACA), while trying to preserve the flow into the PCoA or the anterior choroid artery. For MCA aneurysms, the proximal temporary clip is placed on the M1 segment and the distal one(s) on one or several of the M2 branches depending on the location of the aneurysm.[26,27,32] ACoA aneurysms usually require temporary clipping of both A1s.[29] The temporary clips should always be placed on arterial segments free of perforators, irrespective of the aneurysm in question. With the temporary clips in place, a first permanent clip is inserted, the so-called pilot clip. With this clip in place, the aneurysm can be reshaped using bipolar coagulation and exchanged for a final clip.

Final clipping may require repetitive use of temporary clips until the optimal final clip configuration has been reached. If reshaping is not considered, the length of the final clip should be 1.5 times the width of the aneurysm base as measured from the preoperative angiograms. The direction, shape, and length of the final clip(s) should be assessed carefully so as not to sever any branches or perforators. If the first clip slides exposing some of the neck, another clip can be placed proximally to the first one for complete aneurysm exclusion (double clipping).

After final clipping, the aneurysm sac is opened by a needle or scissors to ensure complete occlusion. At the same time a small piece of aneurysm wall can be removed for scientific purposes.[33]

Sometimes in distal aneurysms such as the distal MCA[32] or pericallosal artery aneurysms,[22–25] it may be difficult to find the aneurysm, as there are no good anatomic landmarks near the aneurysm to be used for orientation. In these cases, neuronavigation can be useful in planning the craniotomy and finding the aneurysm.

Posterior Circulation Aneurysms

Surgical Approaches

Basilar tip aneurysms, with superior and anterior projection, located at or above the posterior clinoid process, can be treated by using the LSO or pterional approach.

All basilar tip aneurysms located below the posterior clinoid process and those with posterior projection are treated in our institution using the subtemporal approach. This approach has been adopted by the senior author (J.H.) since the 1980s and was refined during his training period with Drake and Peerless,[34,35] who used the subtemporal approach in 80% of 1234 patients with basilar bifurcations aneurysm treated between 1959 and 1992.

For the subtemporal approach, the patient is placed in the park-bench position. The head is fixed in a Sugita frame and (1) elevated above the cardiac level; (2) the upper shoulder is retracted; and (3) the head is tilted downward toward the floor. We usually prefer the right (nondominant) side, unless the projection, the complexity of the aneurysm, scarring from earlier operations, a left occulomotor palsy, a left-sided blindness, or right hemiparesis requires an approach from the dominant side.[35] Spinal drainage (or ventriculostomy) is mandatory; usually drainage of 50 to 100 mL of CSF is enough to achieve a slack brain before the dura is opened. The skin incision starts above the zygomatic arch approximately 1 cm anterior to the tragus and is either linear, going cranially 7 to 8 cm, or curvilinear above the ear. A small craniotomy (usually 3 × 3 cm) is performed, and the dura is opened. The temporal lobe is mobilized starting from the temporal pole moving posterior. The retraction of the temporal lobe should be slowly increased. The trick of the proper use of the subtemporal approach lies in gaining access quickly to the tentorial edge without significant compression of the temporal lobe. At the tentorial edge, more CSF can be removed and the brain relaxed further. The elevation of the uncus with the retractor exposes the opening to the interpeduncular cistern and the third nerve, which can be mobilized by disconnecting the arachnoid bands surrounding it. Postoperative occulomotor palsy is difficult to predict, as sometimes it occurs after only minimal dissection, and other times it does not occur despite significant manipulation.

With only the uncal retraction of the third nerve, the opening into the interpeduncular cistern remains narrow. More room can be obtained by lifting the tentorium in the lateral direction by placing a suture in the edge of the tentorium in front of the insertion and the intradural course of the fourth nerve. Instead of tying a suture, often a very difficult task, a small aneurysm clip can be used to obtain the same result[36] **(Fig. 21.6).** If necessary, the tentorium can be divided posterior to the insertion of the IV nerve, elevated and fixed also with a small aneurysm clip(s) to gain better access for temporary clipping of the basilar artery (BA). In situations with a low-lying basilar bifurcation, dividing of the tentorium remains absolutely necessary, and a more posterior approach with a larger bone flap is planned from the beginning of the operation. After arachnoid bands are cut and further CSF is removed, the peduncle can be gently retracted with dissecting instruments and cottonoids to see the basilar artery and the base of the aneurysm. The posterior clinoid process does not need to be removed when the subtemporal approach is used.

Midbasilar aneurysms are the most difficult ones to reach, requiring extensive skull base approaches. A transpetrosal presigmoid approach can be used, but it has the disadvantages

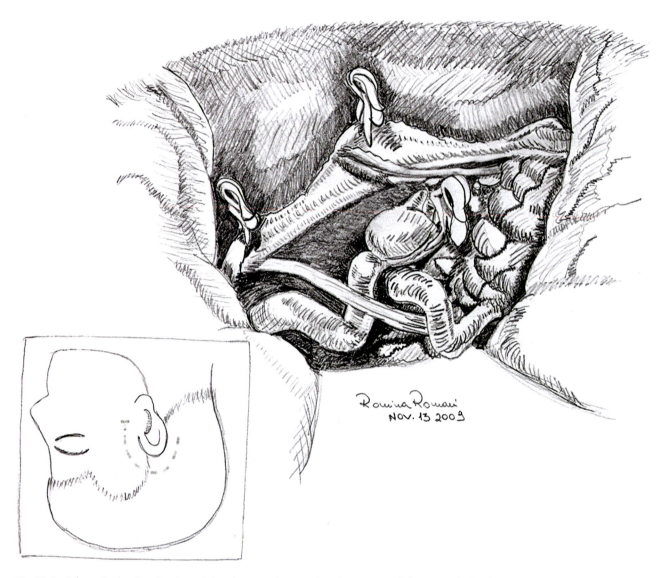

Fig. 21.6 Schematic drawing showing a right subtemporal approach with retraction of the tentorial edge by Yaşargil clips which are sharp and penetrate the dura well.

of possible damage of the cranial nerves, CSF leakage problems, and prolonged operative time.

Most of the vertebral artery (VA) posterior inferior cerebellar artery (PICA) aneurysms (usually 10 mm or more above the foramen magnum) can be treated by a simple lateral sub-occipital craniotomy, and there is usually no need for a far lateral extension.[18,37]

Aneurysm Dissection and Temporary Clipping

The spinal drainage is closed when the basal cisterns are opened and CSF can be drained from there. Temporary clipping is safe and useful to reduce the tension of the aneurysm sac for dissection, coagulation, and aneurysm clipping. For basilar bifurcation aneurysms, the temporary clip is applied on the basilar artery, and, depending on the size and com-

plexity of the aneurysm, on one or both PCoAs. If there is not enough space for a temporary clip, we now use adenosine (0.4 mg/Kg IV) to gain a few seconds of marked hypotension with possible cardiac arrest, enabling the surgeon to clip the aneurysm once it becomes softer and smaller.[18] In complex BA aneurysms both the temporary clipping and the adenosine may be used.

Basilar Aneurysm Dissection

The major difficulties with a basilar bifurcation aneurysm lie behind the sac. Rarely does the aneurysm stand free in the interpeduncular space; usually it is half-buried in the interpeduncular fossa. The main difficulty in basilar aneurysms is their involvement with perforators, which are usually attached to the posterior wall of cranial-projecting basilar tip aneurysms, the most common orientation, or backward-projecting basilar tip aneurysms. In addition, the forward-projecting basilar tip aneurysms may sometimes be attached to the clivus.[35]

Clearing the base of P1 prepares the way for the all-important task of finding and separating the perforators. Most of the perforators arise from P1 near its origin and course obliquely upward and backward on the side and back of the neck and waist of the sac. They are often free or only lightly adherent to small sacs, but are usually adherent sometimes densely to large aneurysms. Not infrequently, one or more perforators arising from the upper basilar artery course upward on the back of the neck. Getting behind the neck usually requires gentle retraction forward of the waist of the aneurysm dome with the sucker tip, while using the small curved dissector to clear and separate any perforators clinging to the back of the neck. Usually, the perforators can be teased off, but occasionally one or more can be quite adherent to a thin-walled neck. More forceful dissection to free them is made less dangerous by temporary basilar artery occlusion. Ordinarily, the neck can be displaced forward enough to see across the interpeduncular fossa to the opposite peduncle, the origin of the opposite P1, and the root of the opposite third nerve. Adherent perforators must be separated upward far enough so that the posterior clip blade can slip inside them without kinking or tearing their origin.[34,35]

The neck of an aneurysm is completely obliterated when the clip blades fall across the neck in parallel with the parent bifurcation and there is less risk of kinking P1, particularly with large necks. This ideal placement is more likely to occur with the subtemporal exposure (and is identical to the principles used to treat the much more common middle cerebral artery bifurcation aneurysms). Clips placed more perpendicular to this crotch often leave tags of the neck in front and behind ("dog ears"), as the sides of the neck are approximated and the bifurcation crimped. "Dog ears" of residual necks have grown, in our and others' experience, into new aneurysms.

The upward curve of P1 only stands free beside small aneurysms, but is usually densely adherent to larger sacs. With the design of the fenestrated clip in 1969 by Drake, P1 can be left adherent to the sac but open in the aperture while the blades fall across the neck of the aneurysm. Some perforators or the third nerve may be included safely in the aperture. Blades longer than necessary may occlude the opposite P1 or its perforators. As the posterior blade is passed behind the neck, while using temporary basilar occlusion to soften a dangerously thin neck, one must be certain that there are no perforators inside the clip. As the blades are allowed to close and narrow the neck, the opposite P1 will come into view so that final alignment can be made before final closure. Not infrequently with the first placement, the blades will be too high or too low on the opposite side, and it is sobering to realize how often one or more perforators are found caught under the blade even when the surgeon is sure that all the perforators have been seen and separated.

If single fenestrated clip blades cannot be positioned perfectly without concern for the P1 origins or perforators, then a shorter fenestrated one should be placed so as to occlude

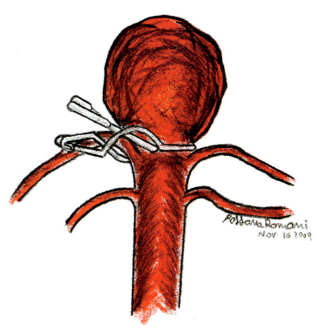

Fig. 21.7 Schematic drawing showing the tandem clipping with a straight clip and a ring clip techniques (by C.G. Drake) used especially in broad-base basilar bifurcation aneurysms and large and giant aneurysms and other sites.

accurately the far two thirds of the neck, leaving the near neck, P1, and perforators open in the fenestration. After that it usually is simple to separate this open but narrowed portion of the neck from P1 and the perforators, and occlude it by adding a tandem straight clip (i.e., Drake's tandem clip)[34] (**Fig. 21.7**).

When approaching subtemporally, bipolar coagulation is occasionally useful to shrink and firm up bulbous or otherwise awkward necks of aneurysms, but the fear of occlusion of nearby or hidden perforators always remains. In clipping superior cerebellar artery (SCA) and proximal posterior cerebral artery (PCA) aneurysms, the perforators are usually of less concern, but the height and direction of the aneurysm, in addition to its size, warrant careful preoperative planning. Local papaverine is applied after clipping of the aneurysm to prevent local vasospasm due to manipulation.

◆ Intraoperative Monitoring

Since 2006 we have been using intraoperative fluorescent videoangiography with indocyanine green (ICG) in all aneurysm surgeries. It has proved to be very useful in verifying the flow in the parent artery and perforating branches, and in detecting incomplete occlusions of the aneurysm[38] (**Fig. 21.8**). However, the technique has its limitations in aneurysms with calcified or atherosclerotic wall and in hidden corners. Everything should be exposed for visualization. In addition to ICG, microvascular Doppler is also always used. Intraoperative DSA is useful in complex, giant, or partially thrombosed aneurysms with thick walls.

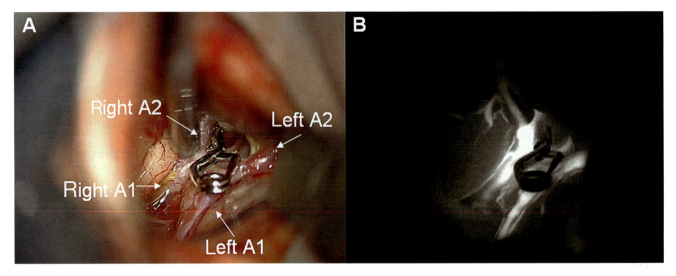

Fig. 21.8 Intraoperative view of a small ruptured anterior communicating artery (ACoA) aneurysm after clipping **(A)** and during the indocyanine green (ICG) angiography showing the flow inside both A2s **(B).**

◆ Bypass Techniques

Certain aneurysms cannot be occluded directly, and different flow diversion techniques using bypass surgery with subsequent exclusion of the aneurysm from circulation are necessary. Bypass techniques are gaining more importance in aneurysm surgery, but because these surgeries are infrequent and at the same time very complex, centralization of such difficult cases into dedicated, high-volume cerebrovascular centers is necessary. The bypass methods need still much refinement. The goal should be to develop a technique as simple as possible, which could be performed under local anesthesia with very short operative times.

◆ Large and Giant Aneurysms

Large or giant saccular and all nonsaccular, calcified, or thrombosed aneurysms still present a considerable challenge in their treatment. These aneurysms need a variety of different treatment methods including direct clipping, trapping, bypass, endovascular, and conservative treatments. With endovascular treatment using coils or stent-assisted coils, the base of the large or giant aneurysm often remains open, and the aneurysms regularly regrow during the follow-up period. Microneurosurgical clipping often provides a more permanent treatment of the aneurysm neck as well as reduction of the mass effect caused by the aneurysm itself. In the same way as with bypass surgery, treatment of complex and giant aneurysms should be centralized because they often require very specialized techniques such as crushing the base with a vascular clamp,[39] or excision of the aneurysm and reconstruction of the vessels using interposition grafts.

◆ Considerations for Skull Base Approaches

If needed, anterior or posterior clinoid processes can be removed simply with the help of an ultrasonic aspirator (Sonopet Omni, Model UST-2001 Ultrasonic Surgical System, Synergetics™, Inc., Miwatec Co., Kawasaki, Japan). The Sonopet safely results in more space available to improve proximal control or to free the base of the aneurysm than would be achieved with drilling. These maneuvers are very useful in treating parasellar carotid aneurysms or those of the basilar tip. We have tried the orbitozygomatic approach and its different modifications but have not regularly used them. In our experience, the removal of the orbital roof causes swelling of the orbital contents that fill most (or all) of the extra space achieved.[18]

Most of the VA-PICA aneurysms, located ≥10 mm above the foramen magnum, can be treated by a simple "tic" (lateral suboccipital) craniotomy, and there is no need for a far lateral extension, which should be reserved only for the aneurysms at the level of foramen magnum.[37] The midbasilar region is the most difficult to approach by open surgery, and it generally requires an extensive skull base approach.[40–42] If necessary, transpetrosal and presigmoid approaches can be used, but their use should be limited due to the high risk of cranial nerve deficits or postoperative CSF leakage problems, not to mention the prolonged operative time.[18]

◆ Considerations for Coiling

Helsinki has become an international microsurgical training center for cerebrovascular surgery. More than 200 neurosurgeons from around the world come each year to observe and to learn from our large experience. Nearly all ruptured aneurysms and three fourths of posterior circulation aneurysms are treated by open microneurosurgery. We recently reviewed our experience of 82 previously coiled aneurysms that were re-treated with clipping; 15 of these aneurysms were operated on during the first month after coiling.[43] Coiling is performed in Helsinki mainly when the experienced vascular neurosurgeon is away attending conferences. In the ISAT study, the risk of recurrent bleeding during long-term follow-up has been higher with coiling than with clipping,[44] even if we certainly see in our large Finnish experience recurrences also after clipping. With our large experience of more than 12,000 cerebral aneurysm patients treated, perfect clipping of the aneurysm(s) is a safe and fast procedure enabling us to treat also patients with expanding hematomas and severe hydrocephalus. We recommend coiling for those centers where microsurgical expertise is limited or lacking.

◆ Postoperative Care

All SAH patients are treated at the neurointensive care unit (NICU) postoperatively. Blood pressure is monitored invasively. ICP is measured via ventriculostomy, as indicated, and cerebral perfusion pressure (CPP) is optimized. Electrocardiogram (ECG), oxygen saturation, and, in intubated patients, end-tidal CO_2 tension are monitored continuously. A central venous line is necessary postoperatively. In poor-grade patients or in those suffering from vasospasm, a more detailed hemodynamic monitoring (e.g., cardiac output, systemic vascular resistance) is required to guide the administration of vasoactive drugs and intravenous fluids. Phenylephrine is the most commonly administered drug to maintain CPP. However, SAH may lead to myocardial insufficiency, and the addition of dopamine or the combination of noradrenaline and dobutamine may be necessary to achieve hemodynamic stability. Urine output is measured hourly. In patients with high ICP, or SAH from the ACoA, there is increased risk of developing diabetes insipidus. Therefore, arterial blood gas analysis, plasma sodium, and potassium concentration are assessed four times a day during the stay in the NICU.

In addition to general care, special attention is paid to the prevention and treatment of arterial vasospasm, with the greatest risk occurring up to 14 days after the initial aneurysm rupture. The risk of vasospasm is evaluated individually. In most cases, the duration of stay in the NICU depends on the above-mentioned risk for delayed cerebral ischemia. Transcranial Doppler may be a good tool for evaluating vasospasm in some cases. The classical triple H principles (hypertension, hemodilution, hypervolemia) are achieved by keeping patients normo- or mildly hypervolemic by infusion of Ringer's acetate (with or without tetrastarch) 3000 to 4000 mL per day with additional sodium 20 to 40 mmol/L. In patients with a low risk for vasospasm, systolic arterial pressure (SAP) is kept at or above 120 mm Hg, in medium-risk patients above 130 to 140 mm Hg, and in high-risk patients above 160 mm Hg[20] **(Table 21.3)**.

Table 21.3 Postoperative Care of Aneurysmal Subarachnoid Hemorrhage (SAH) in Helsinki Neurosurgical Intensive Care Unit (ICU)[20]

Prevention/treatment of vasospasm

Nimodipine oral/IV.

Hypertension: phenylephrine, norepinephrine or dopamine/dobutamine

Hemodilution: Hct 0.3. Ringer's acetate (+NaCl)/tetrastarch

Prevention of vasospasm:

HH: 1–2; Fischer: 1–2; SAP >110–120 mm Hg, normovolemia

HH: 1–2; Fischer: 3–4; SAP >140 mm Hg, normovolemia

HH: 3–5; Fischer: 3–4; SAP >140–160 mm Hg, slight hypervolemia

Treatment of vasospasm:

"Triple H" (hypertension; hypervolemia; hemodilution): RR >160–180 mm Hg

Pulmonary/airway management

Oxygen/ventilatory support as needed: normoventilation, SaO_2 >95%, PaO_2 >13 kPa

Pneumonia, aspiration: antibiotics

Pulmonary edema: noncardiogenic/cardiogenic, PEEP, furosemide, dobutamine

Seizures

Previous antiepileptic drugs (lorazepam or levetiracetam)

No routine prophylaxis

Electrolytes and glucose

Correct abnormalities

Hyponatremia: SIADH, CSW syndrome

B-glucose 5–8 mmol/L

Sedation, postoperative pain and fever

Propofol and/or dexmedetomidine patients under mechanical ventilation

Benzodiazepines

Opioids: oxycodone

Paracetamol

Active cooling as needed

NSAIDs: 5–7 days post-SAH

Thromboembolism

Antiembolic or pneumatic compression stockings

Individually LMWH 5–7 days postcraniotomy

Source: From Randell T, Niemelä M, Kyttä J, et al. Principles of neuroanesthesia in aneurysmal subarachnoid hemorrhage: the Helsinki experience. Surg Neurol 2006;66:382–388.
Abbreviations: CSW, cerebral salt-wasting; Hct, hematocrit; HH, Hunt-Hess; LMWH, low molecular weight heparin; NSAID, nonsteroidal antiinflammatory drug; PEEP, positive end-expiratory pressure; SAP, systolis arterial pressure; SIADH, syndrome of inappropriate antidiuretic hormone hypersecretion.

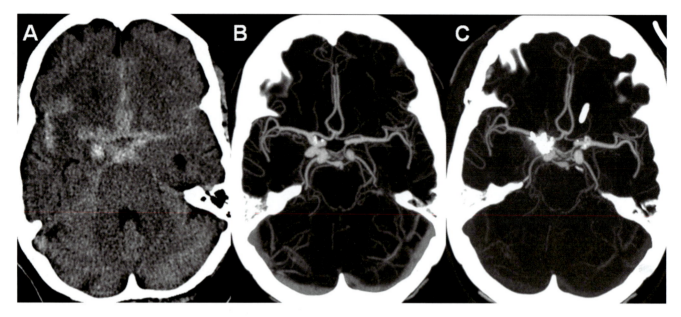

Fig. 21.9 **(A)** Subarachnoid hemorrhage (SAH) after rupture of the right internal carotid artery (ICA)–posterior communicating artery (PCoA) aneurysm. Axial 2D CTA reconstruction showing the aneurysm before **(B)** and after **(C)** clipping.

◆ Illustrative Cases

Case 1: Ruptured ICA-PCoA Aneurysm

A 73-year-old woman presented with sudden headache, nausea, and vomiting. A CT scan showed SAH (Fischer 3). The patient was intubated because of aspiration pneumonia. A CTA scan showed a right-sided, medium-sized PCoA aneurysm which was clipped on the same day. After the operation, the patient developed hydrocephalus, which was treated initially with frontal ventriculostomy, and later the patient received a ventriculoperitoneal shunt. The patient was discharged in good condition 13 days after the operation **(Fig. 21.9)**.

Case 2: Ruptured M1 Aneurysm

A 47-year-old woman became suddenly confused and nauseous, and was admitted to a local hospital, where CT/CTA scans showed SAH with left temporal hematoma (Fischer 4) caused by a small, ruptured M1 left-sided aneurysm. After transfer to our department, an EVD was placed and a left LSO craniotomy performed with clipping of the aneurysm and removal of the ICH. Postoperative CTA confirmed the exclusion of the aneurysm **(Fig. 21.10)**. The patient gradually improved during hospitalization and was transferred after 3 weeks to another hospital for rehabilitation.

Case 3: Ruptured ACoA and Unruptured Right M1 Aneurysm

A 54-year-old man presented with a sudden headache recurring after 6 days and vomiting. He went to a local hospital where a CT scan revealed an SAH (Fischer 3). CTA showed two aneurysms: ruptured ACoA and unruptured M1 on the right. One day after admission, a right LSO approach was undertaken with clipping of both aneurysms. Postoperative neuroradiologic examinations confirmed the exclusion of both aneurysms **(Fig. 21.11)**. The patient was discharged 9 days after the operation in good condition.

Case 4: Ruptured Pericallosal Aneurysm

A 32-year-old man had a severe headache followed by a transitory hemiparesis. A CT scan revealed SAH (Fischer 3), and a CTA the presence of a ruptured aneurysm of the left pericallosal artery **(Fig. 21.1)**, which was clipped via a right frontal paramedial craniotomy after placing an EVD. Postoperative examinations confirmed exclusion of the aneurysm without complications **(Fig. 21.2)**, and the patient was discharged after 11 days.

Case 5: Ruptured Basilar Tip Aneurysm

A 37-year-old man had a severe headache, and a CT scan showed SAH (Fischer 3). The intact patient was referred to our department 3 weeks later from another country for the treatment of a medium-sized basilar tip aneurysm, which was clipped via a subtemporal approach. Postoperative CTA confirmed complete occlusion of the aneurysm **(Fig. 21.12)**. The outcome was uneventful, and the patient was discharged after 1 week.

Case 6: Ruptured Basilar–Superior Cerebellar Artery Aneurysm

A 44-year-old man presented with progressive headache followed by a sudden fall. A CT scan revealed SAH (Fischer 3).

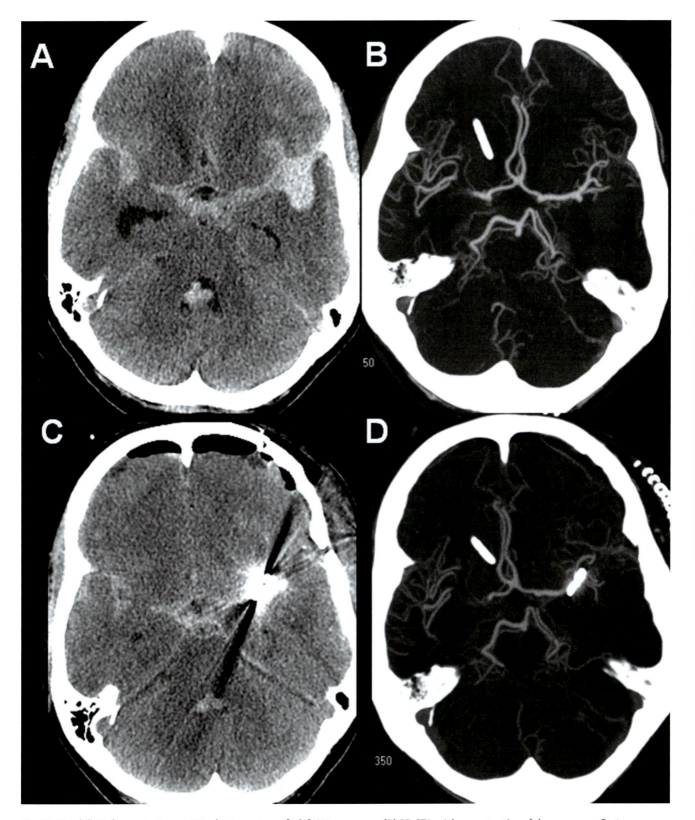

Fig. 21.10 **(A)** CT demonstrating an SAH due to rupture of a left M1 aneurysm. **(B)** 2D CTA axial reconstruction of the aneurysm. Post-operative CT **(C)** and axial 2D CTA **(D)** showing perfect closure of the aneurysm.

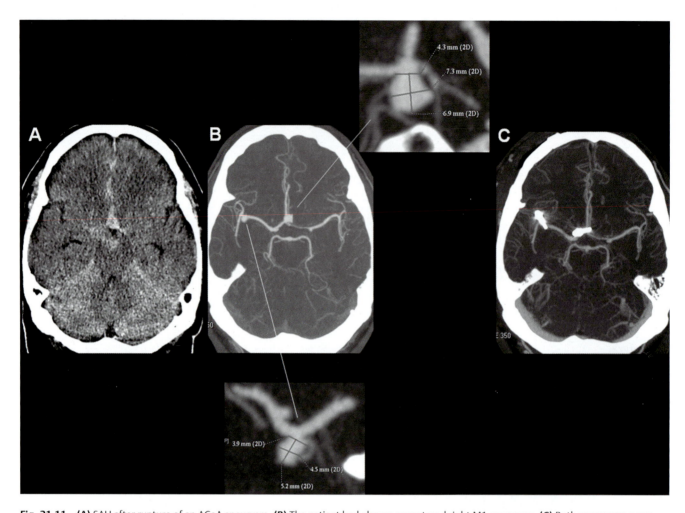

Fig. 21.11 **(A)** SAH after rupture of an ACoA aneurysm. **(B)** The patient had also an unruptured right M1 aneurysm. **(C)** Both aneurysms were successfully clipped during the same operation.

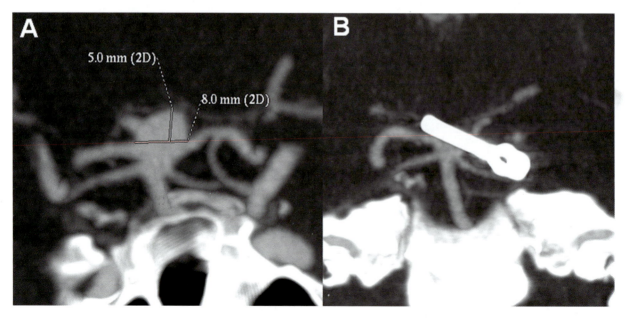

Fig. 21.12 Coronal 2D CTA showing a basilar tip aneurysm that ruptured 3 weeks earlier before **(A)** and after **(B)** successful clipping.

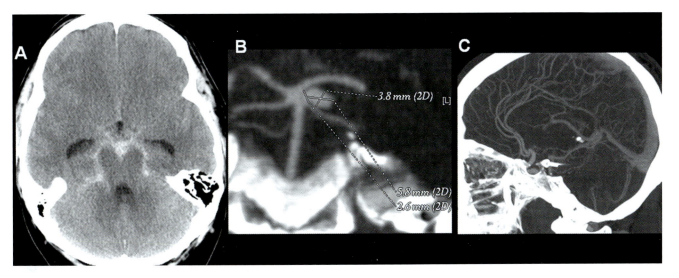

Fig. 21.13 **(A)** SAH due to a ruptured left superior cerebellar artery (SCA)–basilar artery (BA) aneurysm. **(B)** It is completely clipped, as shown on a 2D sagittal CTA **(C)**.

The patient was transferred to our department, presenting with a strong headache without neurologic deficits. A CTA showed a ruptured BA-SCA aneurysm on the left side. The patient underwent a left subtemporal approach and clipping of the aneurysm on the day of admission. Postoperative CT and CTA showed complete occlusion of the aneurysm without complications **(Fig. 21.13)**. The patient was discharged 16 days after the operation with a slight left third nerve palsy.

Case 7: Ruptured Vertebrobasilar Junction Aneurysm

A 63-year-old man complained of a severe headache followed by vomiting and brief loss of consciousness. CT and CTA revealed the presence of a ruptured right-sided vertebrobasilar junction aneurysm. On admission, the patient was in good general condition. The day after, he underwent a right-sided suboccipital craniotomy with clipping of the aneurysm. Postoperative radiologic examination showed complete occlusion of the aneurysm **(Fig. 21.14)**. He was discharged 10 days after the operation in good condition.

◆ Future Directions

Patients should be referred to dedicated neurovascular centers to minimize technical and medical complications. In spite of the increased use of endovascular methods in the treatment of (especially) posterior circulation aneurysms, a perfect clip closing the base of the aneurysm still remains the most long-lasting cure for the aneurysm.[44] In the future we need to develop very simple bypass techniques, both low flow and high flow, for the combined treatment of many complex aneurysms. Then we will be able to stop using some

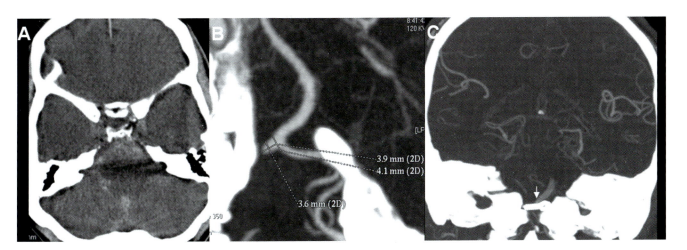

Fig. 21.14 **(A)** SAH due to a vertebrobasilar junction aneurysm **(B)**. It is successfully clipped (arrow) **(C)**.

of the most extensive skull base approaches in favor of minimally invasive approaches. "Simple, clean, and preserving normal anatomy" should be our universal goal.[8,9]

The best time to treat an aneurysm is before its rupture. Now we work in an era of minimally invasive techniques, but the future will be an era of biologic solutions and of identifying aneurysms before their rupture. We are studying how to identify the gene defect carriers,[45] and thereafter follow those patients who can develop these often deadly sacks. We also need to identify rupture-prone aneurysms with, for example, molecular imaging to identify inflammatory changes in the aneurysm wall. This goal can be achieved by understanding the pathobiology of the aneurysm wall itself, for example, the role of inflammation in the growth and rupture, to be able to image molecular changes.[33] The research on the aneurysm wall has just begun, and eventually after some decades may make both microsurgical and endovascular approaches completely obsolete. In fact, we believe that in the future, many, if not most, aneurysms will be treated by local delivery of a specific agent to strengthen the aneurysm wall, and eventually with pharmaceutical therapy. Ultimately, obtaining a simple and inexpensive method to identify unruptured aneurysms in the population will improve the management outcome for aneurysm patients more than any technical innovation or improvements in surgical skills.

References

1. van Gijn J, Rinkel GJ. Subarachnoid haemorrhage: diagnosis, causes and management. Brain 2001;124(Pt 2):249–278
2. Schievink WI. Intracranial aneurysms. N Engl J Med 1997;336:28–40
3. Juvela S, Porras M, Poussa K. Natural history of unruptured intracranial aneurysms: probability of and risk factors for aneurysm rupture. J Neurosurg 2000;93:379–387
4. Juvela S. Prehemorrhage risk factors for fatal intracranial aneurysm rupture. Stroke 2003;34:1852–1857
5. Juvela S, Poussa K, Porras M. Factors affecting formation and growth of intracranial aneurysms: a long-term follow-up study. Stroke 2001;32:485–491
6. Molyneux AJ, Kerr RS, Yu LM, et al; International Subarachnoid Aneurysm Trial (ISAT) Collaborative Group. International Subarachnoid Aneurysm Trial (ISAT) of neurosurgical clipping versus endovascular coiling in 2143 patients with ruptured intracranial aneurysms: a randomised comparison of effects on survival, dependency, seizures, rebleeding, subgroups, and aneurysm occlusion. Lancet 2005;366:809–817
7. Campi A, Ramzi N, Molyneux AJ, et al. Retreatment of ruptured cerebral aneurysms in patients randomized by coiling or clipping in the International Subarachnoid Aneurysm Trial (ISAT). Stroke 2007;38:1538–1544
8. Hernesniemi J, Niemelä M, Dashti R, et al. Principles of microneurosurgery for safe and fast surgery. Surg Technol Int 2006;15:305–310
9. Hernesniemi J, Niemelä M, Karatas A, et al. Some collected principles of microneurosurgery: simple and fast, while preserving normal anatomy: a review. Surg Neurol 2005;64:195–200
10. Yaşargil MG. Microneurosurgery, Vol. 2: Clinical Considerations, Surgery of the Intracranial Aneurysms, and Results. New York: Thieme, 1984
11. Rinne J, Hernesniemi J, Niskanen M, Vapalahti M. Analysis of 561 patients with ruptured 690 middle cerebral artery aneurysms: anatomic and clinical features as correlated to management outcome. Neurosurgery 1996;38:2–11
12. Lehto H, Dashti R, Karataş A, Niemelä M, Hernesniemi JA. Third ventriculostomy through the fenestrated lamina terminalis during microneurosurgical clipping of intracranial aneurysms: an alternative to conventional ventriculostomy. Neurosurgery 2009;64:430–434, discussion 434–435
13. Lehecka M, Niemelä M, Seppänen J, et al. No long-term excess mortality in 280 patients with ruptured distal anterior cerebral artery aneurysms. Neurosurgery 2007;60:235–240, discussion 240–241
14. Kangasniemi M, Mäkelä T, Koskinen S, Porras M, Poussa K, Hernesniemi J. Detection of intracranial aneurysms with two-dimensional and three-dimensional multislice helical computed tomographic angiography. Neurosurgery 2004;54:336–340, discussion 340–341
15. Lehecka M, Porras M, Dashti R, Niemelä M, Hernesniemi JA. Anatomic features of distal anterior cerebral artery aneurysms: a detailed angiographic analysis of 101 patients. Neurosurgery 2008;63:219–228, discussion 228–229
16. Kivisaari RP, Porras M, Ohman J, Siironen J, Ishii K, Hernesniemi J. Routine cerebral angiography after surgery for saccular aneurysms: is it worth it? Neurosurgery 2004;55:1015–1024
17. Romani R, Lehecka M, Gaal E, et al. Lateral supraorbital approach applied to olfactory groove meningiomas: experience with 66 consecutive patients. Neurosurgery 2009;65:39–52, discussion 52–53
18. Hernesniemi J, Romani R, Niemelä M. Skull base and aneurysm surgery. Surg Neurol 2009;71:30–31
19. Hernesniemi J, Ishii K, Niemelä M, et al. Lateral supraorbital approach as an alternative to the classical pterional approach. Acta Neurochir Suppl (Wien) 2005;94:17–21
20. Randell T, Niemelä M, Kyttä J, et al. Principles of neuroanesthesia in aneurysmal subarachnoid hemorrhage: The Helsinki experience. Surg Neurol 2006;66:382–388, discussion 388
21. Lehecka M, Dashti R, Hernesniemi J, et al. Microneurosurgical management of aneurysms at the A2 segment of anterior cerebral artery (proximal pericallosal artery) and its frontobasal branches. Surg Neurol 2008;70:232–246, discussion 246
22. Lehecka M, Dashti R, Hernesniemi J, et al. Microneurosurgical management of aneurysms at A3 segment of anterior cerebral artery. Surg Neurol 2008;70:135–151, discussion 152
23. Lehecka M, Dashti R, Hernesniemi J, et al. Microneurosurgical management of aneurysms at A4 and A5 segments and distal cortical branches of anterior cerebral artery. Surg Neurol 2008;70:352–367, discussion 367
24. Lehecka M, Lehto H, Niemelä M, et al. Distal anterior cerebral artery aneurysms: treatment and outcome analysis of 501 patients. Neurosurgery 2008;62:590–601, discussion 590–601
25. Hernesniemi J, Tapaninaho A, Vapalahti M, Niskanen M, Kari A, Luukkonen M. Saccular aneurysms of the distal anterior cerebral artery and its branches. Neurosurgery 1992;31:994–998, discussion 998–999
26. Dashti R, Rinne J, Hernesniemi J, et al. Microneurosurgical management of proximal middle cerebral artery aneurysms. Surg Neurol 2007;67:6–14
27. Dashti R, Hernesniemi J, Niemelä M, et al. Microneurosurgical management of middle cerebral artery bifurcation aneurysms. Surg Neurol 2007;67:441–456
28. Dashti R, Hernesniemi J, Lehto H, et al. Microneurosurgical management of proximal anterior cerebral artery aneurysms. Surg Neurol 2007;68:366–377
29. Hernesniemi J, Dashti R, Lehecka M, et al. Microneurosurgical management of anterior communicating artery aneurysms. Surg Neurol 2008;70:8–28, discussion 29
30. Lehecka M, Dashti R, Romani R, et al. Microneurosurgical management of internal carotid artery bifurcation aneurysms. Surg Neurol 2009;71:649–667
31. Nagy L, Ishii K, Karatas A, et al. Water dissection technique of Toth for opening neurosurgical cleavage planes. Surg Neurol 2006;65:38–41, discussion 41
32. Dashti R, Hernesniemi J, Niemelä M, et al. Microneurosurgical management of distal middle cerebral artery aneurysms. Surg Neurol 2007;67:553–563
33. Tulamo R, Frösen J, Junnikkala S, et al. Complement activation associates with saccular cerebral artery aneurysm wall degeneration and rupture. Neurosurgery 2006;59:1069–1076, discussion 1076–1077
34. Drake CG, Peerless SJ, Hernesniemi J. Surgery of Vertebrobasilar Aneurysms: London, Ontario Experience on 1767 Patients. New York: Springer, 1996
35. Hernesniemi J, Ishii K, Niemelä M, Kivipelto L, Fujiki M, Shen H. Subtemporal approach to basilar bifurcation aneurysms: advanced technique and clinical experience. Acta Neurochir Suppl (Wien) 2005;94:31–38
36. Hernesniemi J, Ishii K, Karatas A, et al. Surgical technique to retract the tentorial edge during subtemporal approach: technical note. Neurosurgery 2005;57(4, Suppl)E408, discussion E408
37. Hernesniemi J. Distal PICA aneurysms. J Neurosurg 2003;98:1144, author reply 1144
38. Dashti R, Laakso A, Niemelä M, Porras M, Hernesniemi JA. Microscope-integrated near-infrared indocyanine green videoangiography during surgery of intracranial aneurysms: the Helsinki experience. Surg Neurol 2009;71:543–550, discussion 550
39. Navratil O, Lehecka M, Lehto H, et al. Vascular clamp-assisted clipping of thick-walled giant aneurysms. Neurosurgery 2009;64(3, Suppl)113–120, discussion 120–121

40. Hernesniemi J, Karatas A, Niemelä M, et al. Aneurysms of the vertebral artery (VA). Zentralbl Neurochir 2005;66:223–229, author reply 230
41. Hernesniemi J, Karatas A, Ishii K, Niemelä M. Anteroinferior cerebellar artery aneurysms: surgical approaches and outcomes—a review of 34 cases. Neurosurgery 2005;57:E601, author reply E601
42. Hernesniemi J, Vapalahti M, Niskanen M, Kari A. Management outcome for vertebrobasilar artery aneurysms by early surgery. Neurosurgery 1992;31:857–861, discussion 861–862
43. Romani R, Lehto H, Laakso A, et al. Microsurgery for previously coiled aneurysms: experience with 81 patients. Neurosurgery 2011;68(1): 140–153, discussion 153–154
44. Molyneux AJ, Kerr RS, Birks J, et al; ISAT Collaborators. Risk of recurrent subarachnoid haemorrhage, death, or dependence and standardised mortality ratios after clipping or coiling of an intracranial aneurysm in the International Subarachnoid Aneurysm Trial (ISAT): long-term follow-up. Lancet Neurol 2009;8:427–433
45. Bilguvar K, Yasuno K, Niemelä M, et al. Susceptibility loci for intracranial aneurysm in European and Japanese populations. Nat Genet 2008;40:1472–1477

22

Clipping of Complex and Giant Aneurysms

Christopher S. Eddleman, Rudy J. Rahme, Salah G. Aoun, Andrew J. Fishman, H. Hunt Batjer, and Bernard R. Bendok

Pearls

◆ Giant intracranial aneurysms (GIAs) are defined as aneurysms with a fundal width of 2.5 cm or more. Complex intracranial aneurysms are defined as intracranial aneurysms that cannot be managed with standard surgical or interventional techniques due to their configuration or anatomic characteristics.

◆ Revascularization strategies can simplify the treatment of complex and giant aneurysms.

◆ The successful management of patients with complex and giant intracranial aneurysms (CGIAs) requires meticulous planning during every phase of the treatment. The team should include surgeons with expertise in microsurgery, interventional techniques, cranial base surgery, and neurotology. Additionally, consultants should be available in the fields of primary care, neurology, neuroradiology, and critical care. Intraoperatively, the expertise of neuroanesthesiology, neurophysiologists, and specialized nursing is paramount. Occasionally, expertise from plastic and reconstructive surgery is beneficial as well.

◆ Treatment of CGIAs is broadly classified as either constructive or deconstructive. Constructive strategies focus on preserving the blood flow through the parent artery and preserving distal flow while excluding the aneurysm from the cerebral circulation. Deconstructive strategies usually involve a hunterian ligation of the proximal inflow artery, with or without cerebral revascularization.

◆ Computed tomography angiography (CTA) can be utilized postprocedurally to assess patency of a bypass graft.

The treatment of complex and giant intracranial aneurysms (CGIAs) has long been considered one of the most challenging areas in cerebrovascular neurosurgery. Early surgical experience, even in the most experienced hands, was often ineffective, with high morbidity and mortality rates. Preoperative imaging studies were poor and lacked sufficient detail. Not surprisingly, many of these lesions were discovered incidentally during exploratory surgery for symptomatic mass effect and were not readily treatable. Those lesions for which treatment was attempted mostly resulted in poor outcomes.

In recent decades, pioneering advancements and innovations in microsurgical and endovascular techniques as well as in diagnostic imaging have transformed the management of these formidable lesions, resulting in acceptable and durable clinical and radiographic outcomes. Although endovascular techniques continue to mature, a substantial population of intracranial aneurysms remains intractable to a simple endovascular option or is prone to substantial recurrence rates. Therefore, mastery of microsurgical techniques and carefully planned, often multidisciplinary, surgical strategies for CGIAs continue to be necessary.

◆ Aneurysm Characteristics

Giant intracranial aneurysms (GIAs) are defined as aneurysms with a fundal width of 2.5 cm or more. The incidence of GIAs has been reported to be approximately 5% of all intracranial aneurysms.[1] Most GIAs present in the fifth and sixth decades of life, with a slight female predominance. According to data from the International Study of Unruptured Intracranial Aneurysms (ISUIA), the 5-year cumulative rupture risk is 6.4% for cavernous giant aneurysms, 40% for anterior circulation aneurysms, and 50% for posterior circulation giant aneurysms.[2] It should be noted that these data are for asymptomatic aneurysms. Symptomatic aneurysms carry a much higher risk.

Complex intracranial aneurysms are defined as intracranial aneurysms that cannot be managed with standard surgical or interventional techniques due to their anatomic characteristics or relationship to surrounding anatomy (**Table 22.1 and Fig. 22.1**). CGIAs can require prolonged temporary occlusion time or sacrifice of a significant parent artery for definitive therapy. They may also exert significant mass effect on the surrounding brain or nervous structures, and often

Table 22.1 Definition of Complex Intracranial Aneurysm

Lesion Description

Giant (>25 mm)

Presence of extensive thrombus or calcifications

Vital arterial branches emanating from either fundus or neck

Deep location

Aberrant shape or configuration (fusiform, dissecting, or serpentine)

Procedure Requirements

Extended temporary occlusion time

Performance of cerebral revascularization or reimplantation

Suction decompression

Cranial nerve involvement

Previous treatment (microsurgery or endovascular)

Sacrifice of parent artery

require complex surgical exposures to gain safe access and vascular control. Hybrid endovascular and open techniques can be used to treat some of these lesions. Previous treatment can render what was once a simple aneurysm a complex aneurysm. The incidence and characterization of CGIAs are difficult to estimate due to the subjective nature of the term as well as to the variability of their morphologic and anatomic presentations. Outcome measures are confounded by the technical skill required for successful treatment and the complexity of the required surgical or endovascular repair.

◆ Patient and Aneurysm Selection

The successful management of patients with CGIAs requires meticulous planning during every phase of treatment. Preoperatively, the patient should be evaluated and optimized with regard to medical comorbidities to avoid unanticipated complications. In addition to experienced cerebrovascular skull base neurosurgeons, the team should include medical and neurology consultants, neuroradiologists and interventionalists, neuroanesthesiologists, intraoperative neurophysiologists, and a variety of surgical partners including surgeons with cranial base/neurotology experience, and occasionally a plastic and reconstructive surgeon to help plan and execute the often complex approach and help handle reconstruction issues.

Although the ISUIA has provided some basic grounds for treatment recommendations, CGIAs can have characteristics that defy categorization based on size alone. Irregular aneurysm contour, for example, may render a lesion more prone to rupture than predicted by ISUIA data alone. Moreover, medical comorbidities and the patient's wishes based on family history and psychological burden should be taken into account when making treatment decisions.

Surgical treatment of CGIAs can be required for lesions that have limited or no endovascular options, have failed endo-

vascular therapy, require hunterian ligation or trapping, are at high risk for recurrence with endovascular therapy, are associated with significant intrasaccular thrombus, are associated with branch vessels which require revascularization, or are associated with significant mass effect. Some CGIAs may require a hybrid approach involving both surgical and endovascular techniques for a successful treatment. An example of this is suction-decompression of paraclinoidal or cavernous aneurysms using an endovascular balloon catheter. Alternatively, some CGIAs are best treated via endovascular means because significant surgical morbidity exists, there are confounding medical comorbidities, or because of the patient's or family's wishes. Finally, some CGIAs have neither surgical nor endovascular solutions, such as some fusiform or serpentine lesions, and thus are not treated.

◆ Cerebral Revascularization and Blood Flow Alteration

Challenging CGIA cases that require prolonged temporary occlusion times or involve parent artery sacrifice may require prophylactic augmentation of collateral blood flow through bypass grafting or other forms of revascularization.[3–15] Options include extracranial-to-intracranial and intracranial-to-intracranial bypasses. In-situ or harvested grafts can be utilized, such as the superficial temporal artery, occipital artery, radial artery, and saphenous vein. Careful patient selection has proven to be the most prominent predictor of successful revascularization strategies. Factors to be considered for revascularization include the amount of blood flow required (low- versus high-flow grafts) and the site of delivery. For CGIAs of the proximal internal carotid, bypass candidates undergo a balloon test occlusion (BTO) to assess blood flow dynamics, collateralization, and vascular reserve (**Table 22.2**). Occasionally, BTO can be considered for more distal intracranial aneurysms (intracranial BTO).

After completion of a diagnostic angiogram, a balloon is placed just proximal to the aneurysm in question and inflated. Temporary flow occlusion is confirmed, and the reserve supply from leptomeningeal and circle of Willis vessels is qualitatively analyzed as are flow dynamics including venous washout. Although an angiographic study of the collateral circulation is helpful, it does not assess the impact on the patient's clinical examination. As such, clinical changes are assessed by monitoring the patient's clinical examination during a hypotensive challenge as well as by electroencephalogram (EEG) and single-pass single photon emission computed tomography (SPECT) imaging. Typically, clinical exams are performed at baseline and every 5 minutes after balloon inflation. If the patient tolerates all forms of provocative testing, then the parent artery in question can be sacrificed with minimal risk of postoperative complications. However, in some cases the need for a prophylactic bypass procedure may be necessary regardless of the results of a BTO, especially when prolonged temporary occlusion times are anticipated. Furthermore, in younger patients, a bypass may be considered to prevent a possible de novo aneurysm formation that may result from altered hemodynamics (e.g., anterior com-

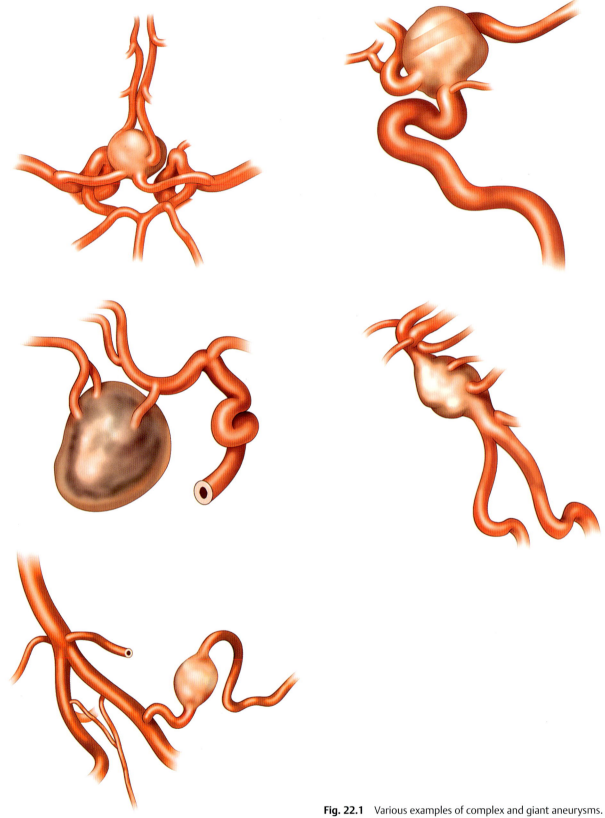

Fig. 22.1 Various examples of complex and giant aneurysms.

Table 22.2 Bypass Indication by Balloon Test Occlusion

Bypass procedure indicated	BTO and SPECT results
PAO without bypass	No clinical failure to balloon occlusion; no SPECT abnormalities
Low-flow bypass	Failure to tolerate balloon occlusion during hypotensive state with/without EEG changes; no SPECT abnormalities; poor angiographic collateralization
High-flow bypass	Failure of all clinical exams; SPECT abnormalities

Abbreviations: BTO, balloon trial occlusion; EEG, electroencephalogram; PAO, parent artery sacrifice; SPECT, single photon emission computed tomography.

municating artery [ACoA] aneurysm formation years after carotid artery occlusion). The BTO is also useful in determining the most adequate type of graft (high flow versus low flow). If the patient tolerates the clinical exams but not the hypotensive challenge, or demonstrates asymmetric cerebral blood flow on SPECT, then the patient would benefit from a low-flow revascularization procedure. However, if the patient develops significant deficits at normotension during the BTO, then a high-flow bypass, usually using a harvested radial artery or saphenous vein graft, may be a better option. Patients who cannot tolerate any temporary occlusion or in cases requiring the need for a jump revascularization graft to avoid interruption in distal blood flow, the excimer laser-assisted nonocclusive anastomosis (ELANA) procedure has been shown to be safe and effective in experienced hands.[16,17] Finally, maintenance of in-situ vessels can be accomplished in innovative ways. Efferent vessels emanating from the aneurysmal fundus or neck may be reimplanted (end-to-side) or attached through a side-to-side anastomosis to either the proximal parent artery or to another surrounding vessel. This strategy ensures adequate size matching and flow requirements.

Intraoperative graft patency monitoring can be assessed with indocyanine green (ICG) videoangiography, micro-Doppler ultrasound, or intraoperative angiography.[3] ICG is a noninvasive means to assess flow patency whereby a fluorescent dye is injected intravenously and visualized during the surgical procedure using a filter attached to the operating microscope. Patients undergoing accompanying revascularization procedures are placed on aspirin therapy for at least a week before the revascularization procedure. However, if the procedure is planned within a week, the patient can be loaded with aspirin at the time of the procedure. In cases of hypercholesterolemia, a statin can be administered pre- and postoperatively as it has been proven to affect long-term graft patency.[18]

One of the primary concerns during complex vascular lesions surgery is the acute and delayed ischemic complications that might result from temporary occlusion. Temporary flow arrest or permanent parent artery sacrifice may be necessary for the treatment of complex and giant aneurysms.

For patients who can tolerate little if any disruption in cerebral perfusion as determined by a BTO, cerebral revascularization can be helpful. In certain cases, bypass may be required solely to provide necessary cerebral blood flow during extended temporary occlusion times during aneurysmorrhaphy. Alternatively, when a parent artery sacrifice is necessary and sufficient collateral supply does not exist, permanent revascularization is necessary. Furthermore, some efferent vessels distal to the lesion may not be salvageable without bypass techniques. In cases in which efferent branches emanate from the fundus or very close to the neck and sacrifice of these branches would have a significant effect on the patient's neurologic status, reimplantation or regional reanastomosis of these efferent branches into other parent arteries can sometimes substitute for a bypass procedure. However, if several efferent branches exist, a bypass to one branch may be necessary while reimplanting the remaining branches to other local arteries.

Alteration of cerebral blood flow can also facilitate the manipulation and treatment of GIAs. Minimizing or completely stopping inflow to these lesions can convert them into soft, pliable sacs that can be more easily manipulated. Several techniques have been developed over the last several years to render these giant lesions safer and easier to treat. One option is deep hypothermic circulatory arrest. This technique has seen a recent resurgence due to the wider availability of advanced intraoperative critical care. Disadvantages include the additional personnel required, as well as the potential added complications of cerebral edema, thromboembolism, and coagulopathy.[19,20] Alternatively, a hypothermic low-flow cardiopulmonary bypass technique has been used to sustain a reduced cardiac output of approximately 500 mL/min.[21] This technique renders the aneurysmal sac more pliable without the added risk of complete circulatory arrest. In recent years, a simpler pharmacologic blood flow reducing technique has been utilized. Adenosine, a fast-acting nucleoside, has been used to induce bradycardia and asystole for several seconds, thereby shutting down cardiac output temporarily. This simple technique can allow the prepared surgeon enough time to manipulate the aneurysm without the need for more invasive measures. This is especially beneficial in those patients who cannot tolerate temporary occlusion or those with severe atheromatous disease. Finally, endoluminal balloons can be used for temporary occlusion of the afferent vessel to the aneurysm. This endovascular approach provides access to segments of the parent artery, obviating the need of a complex open approach to the petrous carotid or proximal vertebral artery.

◆ Surgical Techniques and Treatment Strategies

Overview of Surgical Approaches

One of the most important aspects in the surgical treatment of CGIAs is the preoperative planning, which should anticipate potential pitfalls and complications. Developing thoughtful plans for optimal exposure of the surrounding parenchyma

Table 22.3 Selection of Surgical Approach for Aneurysm Location

Surgical Approaches	Types of Aneurysms Treated
Pterional	ACA, ACoA, ICA, PCoA, MCA, BA
OZ/FTOZ	ACA, ACoA, ICA, PCoA, MCA, BA
Interhemispheric	Distal ACA
Subtemporal/transtemporal/extended	BA, PCA, SCA
Translabyrinthine/transpetrosal	BA, PCA, SCA
Supralabyrinthine	BA, PCA, SCA
Retrosigmoid/extended	BA, PCA, SCA, VA, AICA
Far lateral/extended	VA, AICA, PICA

Abbreviations: ACA, anterior cerebral artery; ACoA, anterior communicating artery; AICA, anterior inferior cerebellar artery; BA, basilar artery; FTOZ, frontotemporo-orbitozygomatic; ICA, internal carotid artery; MCA, middle cerebral artery; OZ, orbitozygomatic; PCA, posterior cerebral artery; PCoA, posterior communicating artery; PICA, posterior inferior cerebellar artery; SCA, superior cerebellar artery; VA, vertebral artery.

and vasculature and for possible revascularization is necessary for success. Minimizing brain retraction through a combination of physiologic and pharmaceutical brain relaxation techniques as well as precise selection of the surgical approach reduces intraoperative risks in these complex procedures.

Although minimally invasive surgical approaches have been popularized over the last several years, these approaches potentially limit the exposure of CGIAs in a way that may present significant challenges if complications occur. Tailored cranial-base exposures have seen a resurgence due to their potential for greater visualization of relevant anatomy and minimization of brain manipulation. Advances in neuronavigation enable more precise tailoring of cranial drilling. Complete exposure facilitates wide visualization of both the afferent and efferent vessels so that application of temporary clips does not restrict the surgical view during clip reconstruction and revascularization. **Table 22.3** provides a general outline of approach selection determined by the location of the aneurysm. Although several different surgical approaches can be utilized exclusively or in combination, the best choice will be influenced by the specific nature of the lesion and the anticipated challenges in vascular reconstruction. Factors to be considered include bypass requirements, overall size, the degree of mass effect, and the location of the planned proximal and distal control.

Pterional Approaches, Modifications, and Extensions

For decades, the workhorse surgical approach to the circle of Willis has been the standard pterional craniotomy. With this surgical approach and its modifications, together with variations in head rotation, most proximal anterior circulation lesions can be exposed and treated with adequate visualiza-

tion and workspace. In addition, some posterior circulation aneurysms, such as those in the basilar apex, posterior cerebral artery (PCA), and superior cerebellar artery (SCA), can be treated using this standard surgical approach; however, in many instances, this corridor may be limiting. Frequently, complex lesions of the posterior circulation may require more room for lesion manipulation or clip placement, and therefore may require a more tailored surgical approach. Modifications of the pterional approach include orbitozygomatic, orbitobasal, and fronto-orbital (**Fig. 22.2**). These modifications usually increase the working space, sometimes only by several millimeters, but that may make the difference between ease and struggle when handling a complex lesion.

Interhemispheric Approaches, Modifications, and Extensions

For lesions of the distal anterior cerebral artery circulation, interhemispheric approaches are usually used. They can range from just anterior to the coronal suture to transbasal approaches through the frontal sinuses, depending on the specific location of the lesion.

Subtemporal/Transtentorial Approaches, Modifications, and Extensions

A useful alternative for upper basilar artery aneurysms is the subtemporal approach (**Fig. 22.3**). Lesions of the PCA and SCA can also be well visualized with this approach. This approach typically involves placing the patient in the lateral position with the cranial vertex tilted approximately 20 to 30 degrees to the floor. Typically, a lumbar drain is placed preoperatively to allow adequate brain relaxation in conjunction with hyperosmolar (mannitol and/or 3% sodium) solution administration. Brain relaxation is necessary to minimize the need for brain retraction while maximizing working space in this confined anatomic area.

Retrosigmoid Approach/Far Lateral Approach, Modifications, and Extensions

Lesions of the midbasilar artery, posterior inferior communicating artery (PICA), anterior inferior communicating artery (AICA), and vertebrobasilar (VB) junction are usually best approached through a retrosigmoid posterior fossa craniotomy and its extensions (**Fig. 22.4**). These approaches are grouped together as extensions of the far lateral approaches and are tailored specifically to the needs of the individual lesion.

◆ Aneurysm Treatment Strategies

Treatment of complex and giant intracranial aneurysms can be broadly classified as either constructive or deconstructive (**Fig. 22.5**). Constructive strategies preserve blood flow through the parent artery and preserve distal flow while excluding the aneurysm from the cerebral circulation using clip

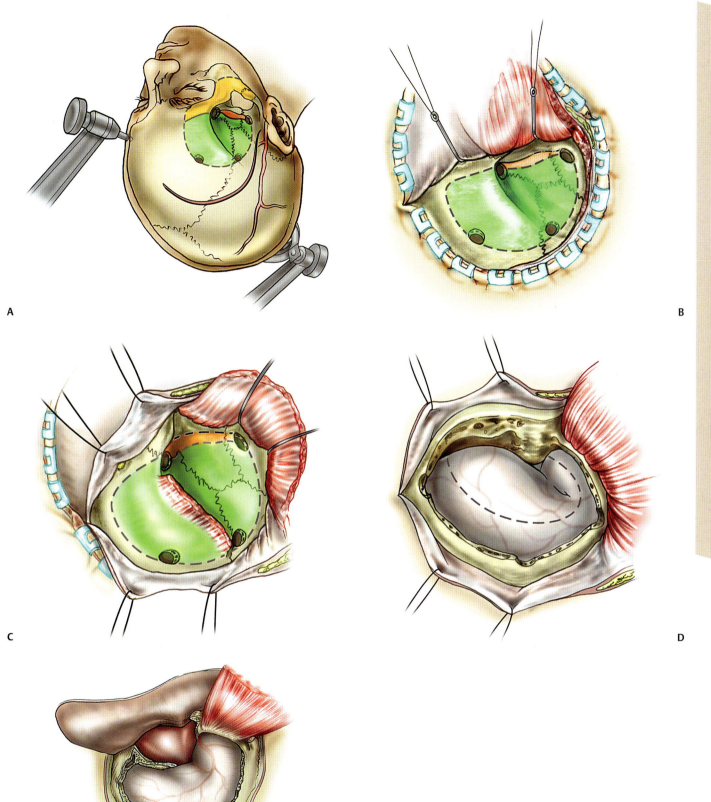

A

B

C

D

E

Fig. 22.2 **(A)** Standard pterional approach (green) with orbito-zygomatic extension (yellow). **(B)** Standard pterional approach with muscle retraction and burr holes. **(C)** Standard pterional approach with a more anterior and inferior reflexion of the muscle. **(D)** Dural incision. **(E)** Exposure of the orbito-zygomatic approach.

22 Clipping of Complex and Giant Aneurysms

295

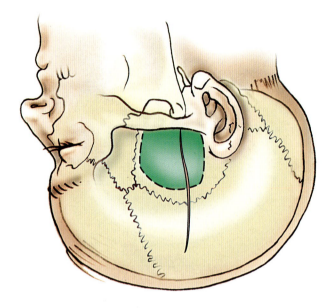

Fig. 22.3 Standard subtemporal approach.

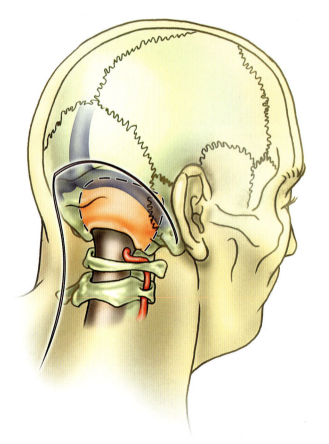

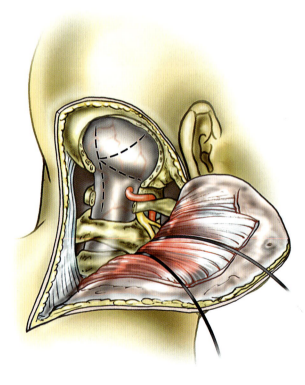

A

B

Fig. 22.4 **(A,B)** The retrosigmoid approach. **(A)** Skin incision. **(B)** Dural incision.

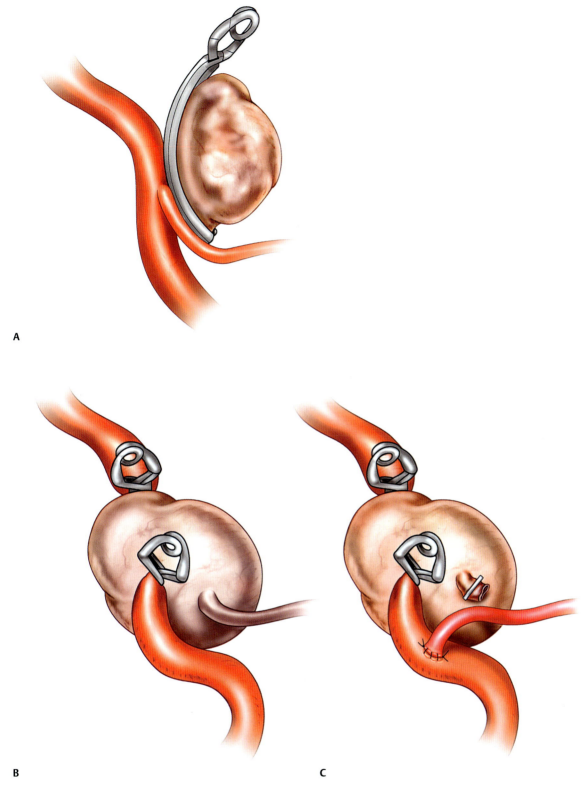

A

B

C

Fig. 22.5 **(A–C)** Aneurysm clipping. Constructive **(A)** and deconstructive **(B)** strategies. **(C)** With reimplantion.

reconstruction strategies through various clip reconstruction configurations. Deconstructive strategies involve proximal occlusion of the parent artery (hunterian ligation) or trapping with or without cerebral revascularization.

Constructive strategies require surgical exposure of the neck of the aneurysm, afferent and efferent vessels, and adequate proximal and distal control. A cranial base resection might be needed to achieve this exposure. For example, the anterior clinoid process can be removed with a microdrill in the case of large or complex supraclinoid ophthalmic artery aneurysms. It is imperative that clip placement does not threaten the surrounding vessels or nervous structures due to the lack of total visualization. Therefore, the surgeon must be able to see the blades of the clips well enough to establish that they are free and clear of any vital structures and that the aneurysm is completely secured.

Large and giant aneurysms often require some form of decompression to allow aneurysm clips to be placed effectively. This can be achieved by trapping the aneurysm with temporary clips with the patient in burst suppression. The aneurysm can then be decompressed with either a needle on a syringe, or incised with a scalpel and decompressed with either a suction or ultrasonic aspirator (if intraluminal clot is present). Aneurysms of the paraclinoid region present a unique challenge with regard to decompression in that proximal control requires cervical carotid artery access with either open exposure or an endovascular catheter. These maneuvers temporarily soften the fundus and enable the surgeon to manipulate the aneurysm and gather up the tissue. In this state, the anatomy can be more easily examined so that proper placement of clips is ensured to safely reconstruct the parent artery conduit.

A wide variety of clip sizes, shapes, and configurations are available (**Fig. 22.6**). Most CGIAs require several clips for adequate neck coverage as well as clip support to prevent slippage. Fenestrated aneurysm clips are available to clip around vital structures while still maintaining adequate closing force. Fenestrated clips are also incorporated in multi-clip reconstructions to compress deeper elements without being impeded by more proximal redundant or thickened tissue (**Fig. 22.7**). Modern aneurysm clips are highly adaptable to variable aneurysm wall thicknesses. The amount of aneurysmal tissue present also determines the kind of clip reconstruction that can be accomplished. Large or giant thrombotic aneurysms often require an aneurysmorrhaphy so that redundant tissue can be removed, leaving enough neck tissue that can be gathered and clipped without narrowing of the parent artery lumen. However, large and giant aneurysmal sacs can limit the closure of the neck due to wall adherence to adjacent structures. As closure of the clip blades is attempted, the clip can slide down onto the parent artery. This could significantly narrow or occlude the parent artery lumen. It is very important to avoid removing too much of the aneurysm sac, as too little aneurysm tissue available to provide a firm grasp by the clip blades can also lead to narrowing of the parent artery, predisposing it to thromboembolic complications. Calcifications in the aneurysmal neck are also problematic, in that the clip blades do not fully close, often leaving a small passageway for leakage. Further, calcifications can also pro-

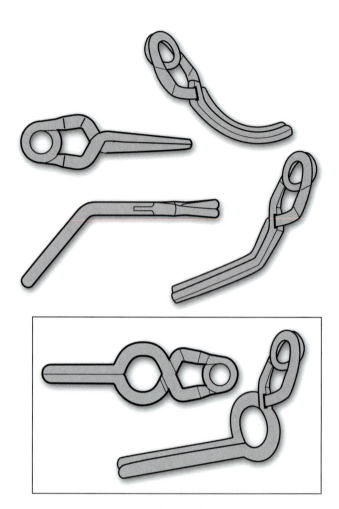

Fig. 22.6 Aneurysm clips and their configurations.

mote clip slippage toward either the fundus or parent artery. These calcifications can be softened by several repeated closings of a clip near the neck. To further reduce clip slippage, bolster clips can be added (**Fig. 22.8**). In occasional situations, crushing the neck with dissection instruments can be highly effective in creating a "seat" for facilitation of clip closure. This procedure must be done carefully and judiciously, as it risks arterial dissection in the parent vessel.

Some CGIAs require the sacrifice of a major parent artery. Hunterian ligation and trapping strategies have been used effectively for decades and have been shown to be highly effective for the treatment of intracranial aneurysms. Cerebral revascularization procedures may accompany deconstructive strategies for CGIAs depending on the tolerance of a preoperative BTO or anatomic assessment. If a high-flow bypass graft is used, it is important to occlude the parent artery immediately after completing the anastomosis, as competitive blood flow may cause the graft to thrombose.

Complex aneurysms that cause mass effect may be decompressed prior to trapping, to allow for adequate visualization of all afferent and efferent vessels. If the primary goal is to relieve mass effect, then opening and decompression can be

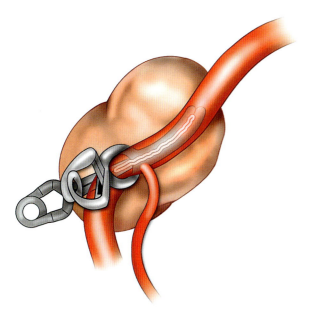

A

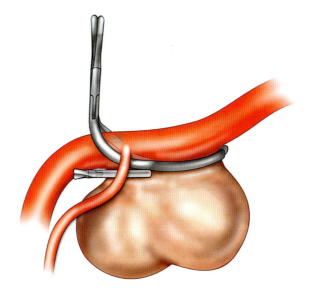

B

Fig. 22.7 **(A,B)** Fenestrated clip application.

performed after trapping. Important branches can then be reimplanted or anastomosed into the surrounding efferent trunks (**Fig. 22.9**).

◆ Previously Treated Aneurysms

With the increase in endovascular management of intracranial aneurysms, the number of lesions that require retreat-

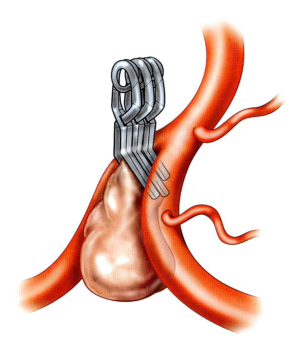

Fig. 22.8 Tandem clips configuration.

ment has also increased. Reasons include either the misappropriation of endovascular therapy or simply the failure of endovascular treatment, which includes incomplete occlusion or regrowth of the aneurysm through recanalization or continued aneurysmal tissue remodeling.[22–27] Coil-induced inflammation may also play a role. Surgically treated lesions can also present as either recurrences or remnants, although this is rare.[22–27] Scarring from previous treatment can complicate dissection of the aneurysmal neck, subarachnoid space, associated vessels, and perforators. When removal of a previously placed clip is required, it is uncomplicated, especially if several months or years have passed since the primary procedure. The degree of scarring and tissue reorganization should be factored into the timing of retreatment. A previously coiled lesion can be stiff, metallic, nonpliable, and surrounded by friable tissue. Part of the coil mass may be protruding into the subarachnoid space or resting in the aneurysmal neck, complicating the placement of aneurysm clips. Removal of the coil mass is still almost always unnecessary (**Fig. 22.10**). Revascularization strategies may be needed in select cases.

◆ Postoperative Considerations

As with all aneurysm patients, close postoperative monitoring is essential in the first 24 hours after the procedure. Monitoring usually occurs in the intensive care unit. A computed tomography angiography (CTA) scan can be performed the following morning to ensure patency of any bypass graft that might have been utilized. All aspects of patient care are tightly monitored. If a bypass procedure was performed, patients are usually maintained on aspirin therapy indefinitely and, depending on mobility, on prophylactic doses of subcutaneously administered heparin beginning 24 to 48 hours

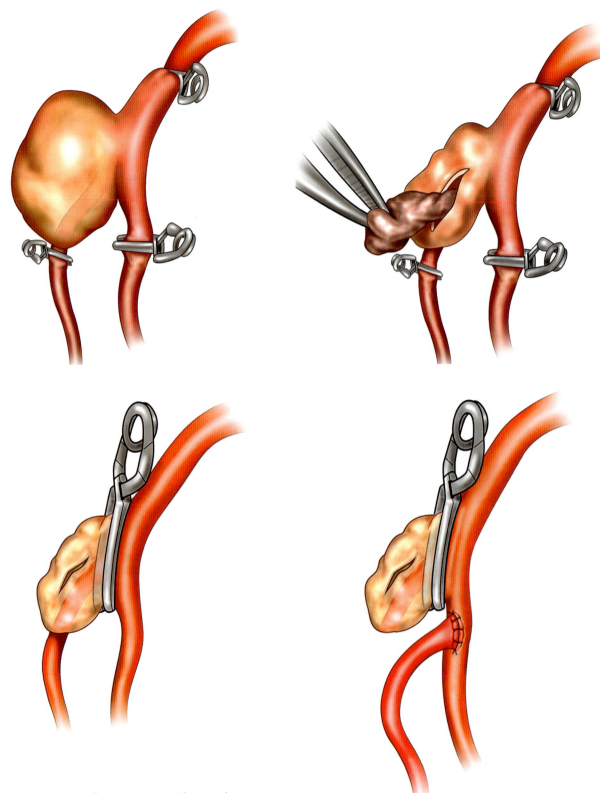

A

B

C

D

Fig. 22.9 **(A–D)** Trapping of giant aneurysm with revascularization and reimplantation.

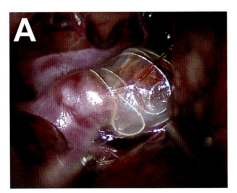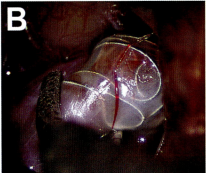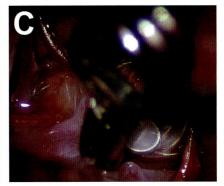

Fig. 22.10 **(A–C)** Previously coiled aneurysm with adequate neck for clipping.

postoperatively. Blood pressure should usually be maintained at normopressure. If there is concern for the patency of the graft at any point during the immediate postoperative period, a cerebral angiogram can be performed with endovascular interventions performed if necessary (infusion of vasodilators and/ or angioplasty).

◆ **Future Directions**

Endoscopic-assisted microsurgery has played an increasing role in the treatment of intracranial tumors over the last several years and is slowly being explored to the treatment of intracranial vascular disease. Although unlikely to ever replace microsurgery, endoscopic assistance may enable improved visualization around vascular tissues.[28] A resurgence in bypass procedures is currently underway as alternative bypass approaches are being refined such as the ELANA and the sutureless ELANA (SELANA) techniques.[16,29] These techniques allow either prophylactic or permanent bypass procedures to be completed without interruption of distal cerebral blood flow, which may reduce complications related to ischemic events in patients who have little reserve collateral blood flow.

Computed tomography (CT) and magnetic resonance imaging (MRI) continue to improve in spatial and temporal resolutions, as does the software that allows manipulation of these images. Imaging layering will continue to improve such that multimodal imaging sources can be combined to offer the best imaging information without the need for other imaging personnel. These imaging modalities and techniques will also be incorporated into the modern operating room setups. The modernized operating room will allow a multifaceted array of equipment available to the operating surgeon including improved ability to examine films, advanced microscope imaging with picture-in-picture displays, availability of integrated endovascular and endoscopic technologies, and advanced neuroanesthesia equipment and techniques. In particular, advances in neuroanesthesia will be focused on improving patient outcome and decreasing complications and morbidity and mortality rates through optimal hemodynamic control during complex surgeries. Adenosine-induced flow arrest to facilitate complex aneurysm clipping is one such ex-

ample.[30] In select cases, this technique allows for aneurysm clipping under safe conditions, shielding the patient from the risk of uncontrolled intraoperative aneurysm rupture and hemorrhage.

The most significant potential breakthrough will take place outside the operating room, in the establishment of preemptive screening strategies. Genomewide association studies are well underway, and specific high-risk loci and single nucleotide polymorphisms have already been identified.[31-34] Environmental risk factors, most notably cigarette smoking, have come into better focus. As our understanding of intracranial aneurysm behavior evolves, our approach to this disease will invariably become more sophisticated, individualized, and focused on each person's and each aneurysm's specific characteristics. Nonetheless, we are still far from being able to develop rational screening protocols for the population. It is conceivable, however, that in the future a person's risk of aneurysm formation, growth, or rupture will be assessed using an individualized computational method that will account for environmental, morphologic, and genetic factors.

◆ **Conclusion**

In spite of dramatic technologic development and progressing endovascular capabilities, there will continue to be a need for open cerebrovascular solutions. Major challenges will be confronted to ensure that a highly technically trained multidisciplinary team is in place at key institutions. How do we ensure that such individuals will be well trained and practiced if volumes of less complex cases are diluted by regional decentralization? How can we ensure that neurosurgeons will be highly trained in this subspecialty with further encroachment on duty hours during training? How will "health care reform" focused on zero tolerance for surgical complications impact our ability to serve as a "court of last appeal" for those affected with severe cerebrovascular pathologies? Will our partner hospitals allow us to take on these complicated patients? Will we be forced to ration available resources only to those young healthy patients with simpler problems? These are indeed the challenges of the next decade in cerebrovascular neurosurgery. In the meantime, we must continue to advocate for our patients' best interests. These efforts coupled with surgical creativity in the development of new and innovative strategies will serve our specialty and our public well.

References

1. Fox JL. Intracranial Aneurysms. New York: Springer-Verlag, 1983
2. Wiebers DO, Whisnant JP, Huston J III, et al; International Study of Unruptured Intracranial Aneurysms Investigators. Unruptured intracranial aneurysms: natural history, clinical outcome, and risks of surgical and endovascular treatment. Lancet 2003;362:103–110
3. Surdell DL, Hage ZA, Eddleman CS, Gupta DK, Bendok BR, Batjer HH. Revascularization for complex intracranial aneurysms. Neurosurg Focus 2008;24:E21
4. Quiñones-Hinojosa A, Lawton MT. In situ bypass in the management of complex intracranial aneurysms: technique application in 13 patients. Neurosurgery 2008;62(6, Suppl 3)1442–1449
5. Mohit AA, Sekhar LN, Natarajan SK, Britz GW, Ghodke B. High-flow bypass grafts in the management of complex intracranial aneurysms. Neurosurgery 2007;60(2, Suppl 1)ONS105–ONS122, discussion ONS122–ONS123
6. Russell SM, Post N, Jafar JJ. Revascularizing the upper basilar circulation with saphenous vein grafts: operative technique and lessons learned. Surg Neurol 2006;66:285–297
7. Lawton MT, Quiñones-Hinojosa A. Double reimplantation technique to reconstruct arterial bifurcations with giant aneurysms. Neurosurgery 2006;58(4, Suppl 2)ONS-347–ONS-353, discussion ONS-353–ONS-354
8. Quiñones-Hinojosa A, Du R, Lawton MT. Revascularization with saphenous vein bypasses for complex intracranial aneurysms. Skull Base 2005;15:119–132
9. Quiñones-Hinojosa A, Lawton MT. In situ bypass in the management of complex intracranial aneurysms: technique application in 13 patients. Neurosurgery 2005;57(1, Suppl)140–145, discussion 140–145
10. Sekhar LN, Stimac D, Bakir A, Rak R. Reconstruction options for complex middle cerebral artery aneurysms. Neurosurgery 2005;56(1, Suppl)66–74, discussion 66–74
11. Kawashima M, Rhoton AL Jr, Tanriover N, Ulm AJ, Yasuda A, Fujii K. Microsurgical anatomy of cerebral revascularization. Part I: anterior circulation. J Neurosurg 2005;102:116–131
12. Kawashima M, Rhoton AL Jr, Tanriover N, Ulm AJ, Yasuda A, Fujii K. Microsurgical anatomy of cerebral revascularization. Part II: posterior circulation. J Neurosurg 2005;102:132–147
13. Ponce FA, Albuquerque FC, McDougall CG, Han PP, Zabramski JM, Spetzler RF. Combined endovascular and microsurgical management of giant and complex unruptured aneurysms. Neurosurg Focus 2004;17:E11
14. Evans JJ, Sekhar LN, Rak R, Stimac D. Bypass grafting and revascularization in the management of posterior circulation aneurysms. Neurosurgery 2004;55:1036–1049
15. Wanebo JE, Zabramski JM, Spetzler RF. Superficial temporal artery-to-middle cerebral artery bypass grafting for cerebral revascularization. Neurosurgery 2004;55:395–398, discussion 398–399
16. Streefkerk HJ, Bremmer JP, Tulleken CA. The ELANA technique: high flow revascularization of the brain. Acta Neurochir Suppl (Wien) 2005; 94:143–148
17. Langer DJ, Vajkoczy P. ELANA: Excimer Laser-Assisted Nonocclusive Anastomosis for extracranial-to-intracranial and intracranial-to-intracranial bypass: a review. Skull Base 2005;15:191–205
18. Dagher NN, Modrall JG. Pharmacotherapy before and after revascularization: anticoagulation, antiplatelet agents, and statins. Semin Vasc Surg 2007;20:10–14
19. Dorotta I, Kimball-Jones P, Applegate R II. Deep hypothermia and circulatory arrest in adults. Semin Cardiothorac Vasc Anesth 2007;11: 66–76
20. Levati A, Tommasino C, Moretti MP, et al. Giant intracranial aneurysms treated with deep hypothermia and circulatory arrest. J Neurosurg Anesthesiol 2007;19:25–30
21. Bendok BR, Getch CC, Frederiksen J, Batjer HH. Resection of a large arteriovenous fistula of the brain using low-flow deep hypothermic cardiopulmonary bypass: technical case report. Neurosurgery 1999;44: 888–890, discussion 890–891
22. Waldron JS, Halbach VV, Lawton MT. Microsurgical management of incompletely coiled and recurrent aneurysms: trends, techniques, and observations on coil extrusion. Neurosurgery 2009;64(5, Suppl 2)301–315, discussion 315–317
23. Tirakotai W, Sure U, Yin Y, et al. Surgery of intracranial aneurysms previously treated endovascularly. Clin Neurol Neurosurg 2007;109:744–752
24. König RW, Kretschmer T, Antoniadis G, et al. Neurosurgical management of previously coiled recurrent intracranial aneurysms. Zentralbl Neurochir 2007;68:8–13
25. Veznedaroglu E, Benitez RP, Rosenwasser RH. Surgically treated aneurysms previously coiled: lessons learned. Neurosurgery 2004;54:300–303, discussion 303–305
26. Zhang YJ, Barrow DL, Cawley CM, Dion JE. Neurosurgical management of intracranial aneurysms previously treated with endovascular therapy. Neurosurgery 2003;52:283–293, discussion 293–295
27. Thornton J, Dovey Z, Alazzaz A, et al. Surgery following endovascular coiling of intracranial aneurysms. Surg Neurol 2000;54:352–360
28. Profeta G, De Falco R, Ambrosio G, Profeta L. Endoscope-assisted microneurosurgery for anterior circulation aneurysms using the angle-type rigid endoscope over a 3-year period. Childs Nerv Syst 2004;20:811–815
29. Bremmer JP, Verweij BH, Van der Zwan A, Reinert MM, Beck HJ, Tulleken CA. Sutureless nonocclusive bypass surgery in combination with an expanded polytetrafluoroethylene graft. Laboratory investigation. J Neurosurg 2007;107:1190–1197
30. Bebawy JF, Gupta DK, Bendok BR, et al. Adenosine-induced flow arrest to facilitate intracranial aneurysm clip ligation: dose-response data and safety profile. Anesth Analg 2010;110:1406–1411
31. Yasuno K, Bilguvar K, Bijlenga P, et al. Genome-wide association study of intracranial aneurysm identifies three new risk loci. Nat Genet 2010; 42:420–425
32. Deka R, Koller DL, Lai D, et al; FIA Study Investigators. The relationship between smoking and replicated sequence variants on chromosomes 8 and 9 with familial intracranial aneurysm. Stroke 2010;41:1132–1137
33. Bilguvar K, Yasuno K, Niemelä M, et al. Susceptibility loci for intracranial aneurysm in European and Japanese populations. Nat Genet 2008; 40:1472–1477
34. Helgadottir A, Thorleifsson G, Magnusson KP, et al. The same sequence variant on 9p21 associates with myocardial infarction, abdominal aortic aneurysm and intracranial aneurysm. Nat Genet 2008;40:217–224

23

Surgical Management of Intracranial Arteriovenous Malformations

Christopher S. Eddleman, Rudy J. Rahme, Bernard R. Bendok, and H. Hunt Batjer

Pearls

- Selection of intracranial arteriovenous malformation (iAVM) patients for treatment must consider lesional and patient-specific features including size, morphology, associated aneurysms or venous stenosis, location, age, and patient expectations.
- Endovascular embolization strategies may include progressive blood flow reduction with liquid embolics, aneurysm treatment, and deep feeder embolization, when feasible.
- Acute, life-threatening hematomas should be managed with the intent to decompress the brain and leave the iAVM intact, if possible.
- Intraoperative bleeding is best managed by a thorough three-dimensional knowledge of the lesion and arterial feeding system, microclips, and a return to an accurate dissection plan.

Intracranial arteriovenous malformations (iAVMs) are uncommon congenital vascular malformations, consisting of a tangled network of dilated arteries and abnormal veins; however rare, they still are responsible for the majority of spontaneous intracranial hemorrhages in young adults.[1-3] Management of iAVMs was once limited to observation and/or surgical therapy. Over the last couple decades, the number of treatment modalities has substantially increased to the point where nowadays most iAVMs are managed with multimodality and combinational therapies. Currently, lesions once thought untreatable, such as deep parenchymal, brainstem, and giant (Spetzler-Martin grade IV, V, or VI) lesions, are now amenable to treatment in various ways.[4-6] Combinations of endovascular, radiosurgical, and microsurgical approaches have been well documented in the literature. Although the modalities of treatment have multiplied and advanced, the natural history of iAVMs has remained somewhat controversial, making the distinction of which lesions should be treated sometimes difficult at best. Furthermore, the use of noninva-sive imaging has increased in volume and sophistication over the last several years, increasing the number of iAVMs detected, therefore placing more importance on the ability to distinguish which iAVMs warrant treatment. Despite the multitude of approaches for iAVM therapy, microsurgical resection remains the gold standard in terms of durability and minimization of recurrence and rehemorrhage risks. The most important aspect of treating these lesions is the development of a comprehensive and individualized strategy for each patient and lesion.

◆ Epidemiology

Intracranial AVMs are thought to be congenital lesions with one-tenth the incidence rate of intracranial aneurysms. The true incidence is difficult to assess because the coding system of the International Classification of Diseases (ninth revision) does not classify iAVMs separately, often grouping these lesions with several other kinds of intracranial vascular malformations, including but not limited to cavernous malformations and unruptured aneurysms. Furthermore, initial admissions for intracerebral hemorrhage or seizure can often go unrecognized as being caused by the presence of an iAVM. Several autopsy series have reported prevalence data ranging from 5 to 613 AVM cases per 100,000.[3,7,8] Retrospective studies have shown the iAVM incidence to be 0.51 to 5 per 100,000.[9-11] Prospective studies, such as the New York Islands Arteriovenous Malformation Hemorrhage Study and the Manhattan Stroke Study, reported that the average annual iAVM detection rate was 1.34 per 100,000 person-years (95% confidence interval [CI], 1.18–1.49) and 0.55 per 100,000 person-years (95% CI, 0.11–1.61), respectively.[12,13] Despite relative agreement between retrospective and prospective studies on the incidence and prevalence of iAVMs in the general population, the actual patient burden of iAVMs may never be known due to the underreported incidence of asymptomatic iAVMs or hidden iAVMs in the setting of fatal or very large hemorrhages without angiographic evaluation. Although relatively rare, these lesions are an important and preventable cause of hemorrhagic stroke, death, and disability in a relatively young patient cohort.

◆ Natural History

The natural history of iAVMs remains a controversial topic. Intracranial AVMs are a heterogeneous group of vascular malformations that elicit highly variable characteristic behavior and that depend on the angioarchitectural features of the lesions themselves, such as large parent artery feeders, associated venous stenosis, nidal or pre-nidal associated aneurysms, and so on. Furthermore, iAVMs present clinically in a variety of ways, most commonly hemorrhage, seizure, headache, or focal neurologic deficits, or can be found incidentally. Hemorrhage rates for iAVMs range from 2 to 4%[1,14]; however, it can increase in certain specific circumstances, such as pregnancy, previous hemorrhage, progressive venopathy, or intranidal aneurysms that are arterial or venous.

In the New York Island study, Stapf and colleagues[13,15] reported that hemorrhagic presentation, older age, deep location, and exclusive deep drainage were independent predictors of hemorrhage. The highest risk population had a hemorrhage rate up to 34% within a mean follow-up of only a few months. Young patients with superficial iAVMs and superficial venous drainage were noted to have lower hemorrhagic risk. These observations suggested that the hemorrhagic risk is a dynamic characteristic of iAVMs and likely depends on both local and systemic hemodynamic changes. In contrast, Hernesniemi et al[1] recently reported that the highest risk of hemorrhage was found in young patients during the first 2 years after initial diagnosis. The annual hemorrhage risk is 4.6%, during those 2 years and decreases to 1.6% in subsequent years. Both studies, however, did agree that previous hemorrhage, deep location, and exclusively deep venous drainage were independently associated with a higher rupture risk. Timely management was advised for lesions that fit this description. However, the treatment of the more benign iAVMs (e.g., located in non-eloquent or superficial regions, exclusively superficial venous drainage, and no prior history of hemorrhage) is particularly controversial due to the lack of knowledge on the natural history of these lesions. For a more complete understanding of the natural progression of iAVMs, future studies will require long-term follow-up (>15 years) because the incidence and annual hemorrhage risk is low. Studies involving follow-up periods of <5 years are unlikely to provide the information necessary to correctly elucidate the true natural history of iAVMs. In addition, radiographic subtleties such as nidal aneurysms, venous stenosis, and angiomatous versus embryonal morphology should be carefully studied. At this time, the discussion of the natural history of iAVMs versus the surgical risks involved can be difficult to compare and contrast based solely on the litera-

ture and often becomes reliant on the experience and intuition of the treating physicians.

◆ Patient and Lesion Selection

The decision to treat an intracranial AVM must involve balanced considerations of both lesional and patient characteristics (**Table 23.1**). When to treat an intracranial AVM is often a more difficult question than how to treat, except when patients present with hemorrhage, unrelenting seizure, or progressive neurologic deficits. Patient-specific factors such as age, comorbidities, weight, occupation, psychological burden, and risk aversion must be completely evaluated. Lesion-specific factors such as size, functional eloquence of location, venous stenosis, associated aneurysms, corridors of access, angiomatous changes, and dysplastic arterial supply must be carefully assessed (**Fig. 23.1**). Asymptomatic iAVMs that present with angioarchitectural features associated with higher hemorrhagic risks, such as venous stenosis, associated aneurysms, and deep drainage, are recommended for evaluation and possible intervention. Subsequently, a risk-benefit paradigm can be assembled predicated on a best-guess analysis of natural history risk if left untreated. Intracranial AVMs that are cortically based, that involve only superficial drainage, and that do not involve eloquent cortex have a low surgical morbidity. However, the superficial drainage may be draped over the nidus and pose increased surgical risks. In the same fashion, a deep AVM may pose a higher surgical risk, but if associated with a previous hemorrhage, the hematoma may provide a surgical corridor that decreases associated surgical morbidity. Deep venous drainage, which has traditionally been associated with increased surgical morbidity, may in fact be advantageous such that these veins do not im-

Table 23.1 Patient/Lesion Selection
Patient-specific factors
Age
Comorbidities
Weight
Occupation
Psychological burden
Risk aversion
Lesion-specific factors
Size
Functional eloquence of location
Venous stenosis
Associated aneurysms
Corridors of access
Angiomatous changes
Dysplastic arterial supply

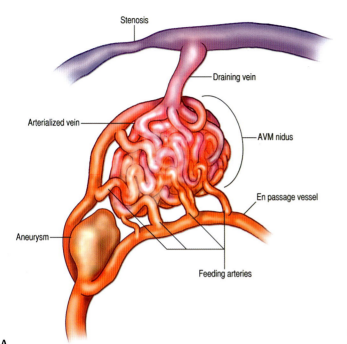

A

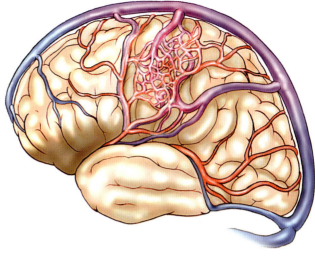

B

Fig. 23.1 Arteriovenous malformation (AVM): arterial feeders, proximal aneurysm, nidus, draining veins, and venous stenosis.

pede surgical resection of the nidus. AVMs that are anatomically within an eloquent area, as shown by functional imaging, will likely pose significant surgical risk and are often relegated to alternative treatments. In an earlier report, Pollock et al classified AVM patients into four groups, based on rupture risk:

1. Low-risk AVMs: no history of a prior bleed, >1 draining vein, and a compact nidus
2. Intermediate-low–risk AVMs: no history of a prior bleed, 1 draining vein, and/or a diffuse nidus
3. Intermediate-high–risk AVMs: history of a prior bleed, >1 draining vein, and a compact nidus
4. High-risk AVMs: history of a prior bleed, 1 draining vein, and/or a diffuse nidus

The low-risk group had an annual rupture risk of approximately 1.3% and a 40-year risk of 33%, whereas the high-risk group had an approximately 9% annual risk and a 40-year risk of 98%. The authors used a predictive formula that assumed that each hemorrhage is an independent event and that there are no deaths from AVM hemorrhage:

$$\text{Cumulative hemorrhage rate} = 1 - (\text{Annual risk of no bleed})^{\text{No. of years}}$$

However, surgical morbidity and mortality weighed against the natural history of the disease are not the only factors to be taken into account when making treatment decisions. The patient's wishes and expectations must also be considered. Despite the fact that the annual hemorrhage risk of most iAVMs is small, it is the lifetime accumulation of risk that should be discussed and compared with an upfront proce-

dure risk. Patients often have difficulty comprehending lifetime risk potentials regarding death and disability, but the concepts must be communicated.

◆ Surgically Important Angioarchitectural Characteristics

Detailed assessment of the iAVM angioarchitecture is critical to the success of surgical management. Preoperative imaging provides the angioarchitectural features, such as arterial feeder localization, nidal morphology, and draining venous patterns, which the surgeon will be required to know and anticipate at every point during the surgical resection (**Fig. 23.1**). The iAVM nidus can be classified into compact, diffuse, or a combination, usually characterized by separated pedicles, occurring naturally, from previous treatment (endovascular or radiosurgery), or from previous hemorrhage. A compact nidus is desirable from a surgical perspective and usually allows a more manageable resection because there is little to no brain parenchyma involved within the nidus, and a perinidal subarachnoid dissection plane can be more easily established. Arteriovenous malformations with a diffuse nidus are inherently more difficult to manage surgically, particularly if near eloquent tissue because of the indistinct nature of the nidus and the intervening brain parenchyma between tufts of the nidus. The characterization of the arterial supply to an iAVM nidus is also extremely important, as it will dictate not only the nidus location, but also what to anticipate during surgical resection. An attempt must be made to preoperatively identify the presence of *en passage* vessels because inadvertent ligation of these vessels can put distal tissue at risk. Parasylvian iAVMs, in particular, routinely have middle cerebral artery (MCA) trunks that feed the malformation but continue on to supply other vital parts of the brain. Further, deep-feeding vessels can be anticipated and better controlled when the iAVM nidus itself or the apex is located near an ependymal surface. These feeders must be anticipated to avoid significant bleeding, which can be difficult to control and can quickly fill the ventricular system. Lastly, extracranial arterial feeders should be identified because these feeding vessels can usually be preoperatively embolized. Extracranial feeding arteries with transosseous components can complicate the craniotomy and, if not anticipated, can lead to serious epidural bleeding during dissection and elevation of the bone flap.

Identification and characterization of the venous angioarchitecture of the iAVM is as important as or even more important than the identification and characterization of the arterial system. Although superficial draining veins usually portend a lower hemorrhage risk profile, they can often make surgical resection more difficult, especially if they are draped across the surgical field. Retraction of these superficial veins and repetitive coagulation near them can increase the turgor of the iAVM, in spite of progressive deafferentation, thereby increasing the risk of intraoperative hemorrhage. Deep draining veins, although thought to increase the hemorrhage risk, actually provide a surgical advantage, as they will not be in the surgical field when dissecting the iAVM nidus. If superficial in origin, the main draining vein should be identified and protected throughout the surgical resection of the nidus, as it will be the last vessel ligated. However, depending on the pedicle construction of the iAVM nidus, there may be more than one main draining vein. These draining veins should also be maintained until all of the feeding arteries to that particular pedicle are ligated and cut. Premature ligation of important draining veins puts the pedicle at higher risk of congestion, leading to potential intraoperative rupture. As the procedure progresses, it is sometimes necessary to ligate a vein even while arterial supply persists. Placing a temporary clip on the vein and observing the iAVM and palpating it for turgor assessment can give vital information as to the safety of dividing a particular draining vein.

◆ Preoperative Embolization

Endovascular therapy of iAVMs offers great assistance to the surgical treatment.[16–26] Strategies for endovascular therapy include the embolization of flow-related and peri-nidal aneurysms, progressive flow reduction to reduce the hemodynamic impact of "sudden" iAVM obliteration, and selective obliteration of deep feeding. Rarely, iAVMs may be cured by endovascular therapy alone, but partially treated iAVMs are thought to maintain similar hemorrhagic risks as untreated lesions.

Intracranial aneurysms are associated with iAVMs in approximately 30% of cases, half of which are on arterial feeders and half are located in the nidus itself.[5,27–31] The timing of treatment of these aneurysms has been often debated. At our institution, we follow a few basic rules to determine the treatment of aneurysms associated with AVMs. If the aneu-

rysm is associated with a pedicle of the AVM or located on the proximal circle of Willis and thought to be the cause of hemorrhage, then that aneurysm is treated acutely. If the aneurysm is located within the AVM nidus and is thought to have ruptured, then the aneurysm is treated early, if feasible. If the aneurysm is located on the proximal feeding arteries to the nidus and treatment of the AVM may put the aneurysm at risk of rupture by increasing outflow resistance and transmural gradient, then the aneurysm is treated via endovascular or microsurgical means, if feasible prior to AVM treatment. Finally, if inaccessible aneurysms exist that are thought to be flow-related and small, usually on the order of <3 mm, they are usually left alone and typically resolve on their own once the AVM is treated.

Careful study of the lesional morphology and the specific surgical problems that will be encountered help set the stage for developing an endovascular strategy for each unique patient. The progressive development of endovascular techniques and embolic agents has transformed the surgical management of these lesions. Each trip to the endovascular suite, however, may carry a 5 to 8% risk of ischemic or hemorrhagic complications (likely lower in careful hands). Large, high-flow iAVMs may be selected for slow, repetitive embolization procedures with 1 to 3 weeks between each treatment to allow for incremental flow redistribution to the surrounding brain tissue. For smaller lesions, embolization may target medial and lateral posterior choroidal feeders, for example, as these are the deepest areas to access during resection. We prefer aggressive embolization in parasylvian iAVMs as it allows for intraoperative road mapping and preservation of *en passage* vessels. The value of embolization of eloquent iAVM margins is that the surgical planes can be developed with more precision. External feeders are embolized to simplify the craniotomy, as mentioned above. In many small cortical iAVMs with superficial arterial supply, the risk of embolization may not be justified unless endovascular cure is the goal. The bottom line is that the treating surgeon should serve as the "captain of the ship" and define the strategic goals and end points of the endovascular component.

◆ Surgical Management of Arteriovenous Malformations

The most common clinical presentation of iAVMs is hemorrhage. However, in most cases, it is advised to wait until the hematoma begins to resolve, often several weeks after hemorrhage, before definitive surgical resection of an iAVM is initiated. This is a safe strategy, as the risk of early rebleeding is extremely low. Hematomas can often obscure the iAVM nidus, result in fragmentation of the nidus, or promote edema of the surrounding brain parenchyma, which can also further complicate a precise resection. However, the resultant hematoma can occasionally present with life-threatening mass effect and require emergent evacuation **(Fig. 23.2)**. The craniotomy in this situation should be constructed to facilitate either acute or delayed iAVM resection. Normally the initial surgical goal is to relieve mass effect while leaving the iAVM undisturbed, due to the low risk of early rehemorrhage. Re-

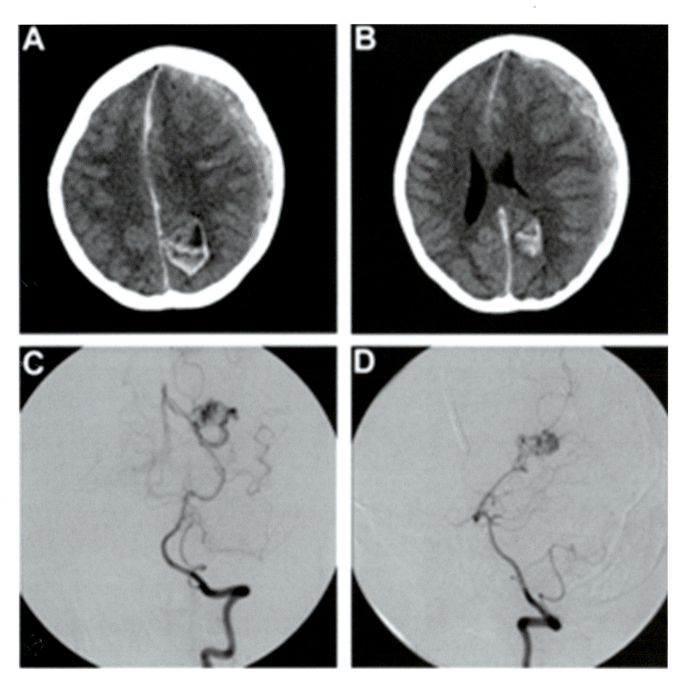

Fig. 23.2 **(A–D)** Ruptured AVM.

evaluation of the iAVM should be delayed after evacuation to allow reduction in postoperative edema, resolution of residual hematoma, decompression of the iAVM nidus, and recanalization of previously thrombosed or spastic arterial supply to the iAVM, enabling a more complete determination of the angioarchitecture. A definitive plan can be implemented within 4 to 6 weeks from the initial hemorrhage.

One of the most important aspects in the surgical treatment of iAVMs is the planning of the procedure, which is often multifaceted, entailing a surgical approach, anatomic definition, localization of feeding arteries and draining veins, extirpation,

and anticipation of potential pitfalls and complications (**Fig. 23.3**). The selection of the appropriate surgical corridor should allow the surgeon adequate exposure of the iAVM while maximizing the working space for visualization and lesional manipulation. Brain relaxation and minimization of brain retraction can be facilitated by the neuroanesthesia team (see Chapter 13) with proper head position and cerebrospinal fluid (CSF) drainage. Several different surgical approaches can be utilized depending on the location of the iAVM.

The location of the iAVM nidus can be divided into superficial, lobar, subcortical-deep, and posterior fossa regions. The

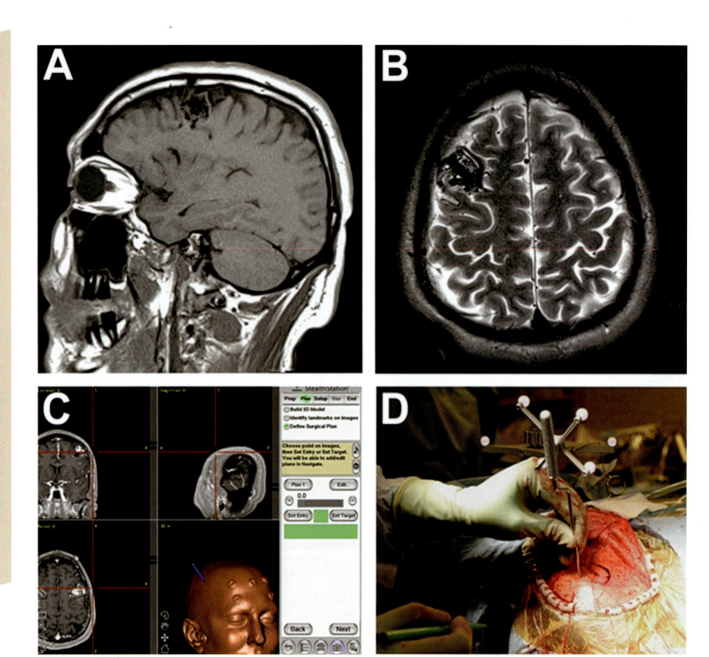

Fig. 23.3 (A–D) Operative plan: position, incision, bone flap, and dural opening.

subcortical-deep locations include the basal ganglia, thalamus, and intraventricular regions. The posterior fossa includes the vermis, cerebellar hemispheres, tonsils, and brainstem. Each location presents specific challenges when approaching, defining, and resecting the iAVM nidus; however, several surgical principles can be applied to all iAVMs irrespective of their primary location.

Surgical Procedures and Considerations

After securing the head in a three-point clamp device, whether radiolucent or opaque, depending on the potential use of intraoperative angiography, strategic positioning of the head

can provide several upfront advantages to the operating surgeon. Positioning the head above the heart provides maximum venous outflow as long as the neck has some extension to ensure unobstructed flow through the jugular veins. Further, positioning the head such that the working area sits in a plane that is comfortable for the surgeon to work in during the procedure is paramount (we prefer and recommend that the surgeon be seated during the microsurgical phases of the operation). Localization of the iAVM nidus can be done with a neuronavigation system so that the skin flap can accommodate an adequate bone flap. In the era of minimally invasive approaches, we caution against using too small a craniotomy. Adequate exposure beyond the margins of an AVM is needed to allow safe control of the AVMs vascular supply and venous drainage throughout all phases of the procedure, especially in the unfortunate situation where deep bleeding occurs, resulting in brain expansion and loss of exposure.

Before the skin incision is made, all required surgical instruments, including retractors, aneurysm clips and mini-clips, various nonstick bipolar coagulators, the micro-Doppler, and microdissection tools should be available and their functionality checked. In the case of deep iAVMs, long instruments should also be available. After the skin incision is made and the skin flap reflected and protected from potential ischemia, the location of the iAVM should again be localized with the neuronavigation system to ensure proper sizing of the bone flap, which again should be made to encompass the entire area around the iAVM. An adequately sized craniotomy will ensure proper visualization of all surrounding feeding arteries, draining veins, as well as normal brain parenchyma and vasculature. Making the dural opening can be dangerous and should be undertaken with caution, especially in cases of superficial iAVMs where arachnoidal adhesions often bind the iAVM vasculature to the dura. In addition, there are often small dural feeding vessels that should be coagulated and divided. The dural opening should be circumferential and reflected toward a major sinus for protection or in a manner to maximize visualization of the working area. It

should also be made some distance away from the cortical aspect of the iAVM if possible, so that important feeding vessels can be preserved and not transected during the opening or the reflection of the dura. Once the dura is reflected, all of the superficial arterial feeders and draining veins should be identified. If the iAVM is located subcortically or deep, neuronavigation should once again be used to ensure that the most direct subarachnoid and trans-sulcal trajectory to the lesion is planned.

The initial phase of dissection is the arachnoid plane (**Fig. 23.4**) around the cortical arterial feeders, draining veins and surrounding vasculature. Identification of the vasculature is very important as it will define the initial phases of the dissection. For all superficial vessels, each one should be identified as a feeding artery, draining vein, or normal vasculature. Frequently, arterialized draining veins can appear similar to their arterial counterparts. Sometimes neuronavigation can distinguish between these vessels. If there is a question as to whether a particular vessel is an arterial feeder or an arterialized draining vein, further dissection toward the nidus will usually clarify the anatomy. Indocyanine green (ICG) video-angiography (**Fig. 23.5**) can also assist in this distinction.[32] Small vascular clips can also be used to temporarily occlude feeding arteries until their involvement or path to the iAVM

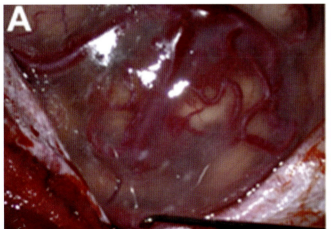
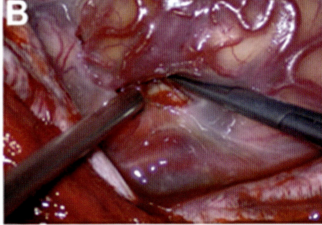
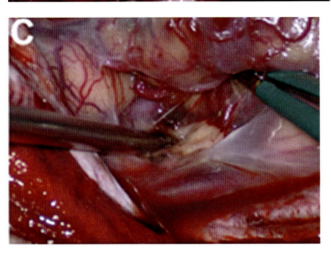

Fig. 23.4 (A–C) Arachnoid dissection.

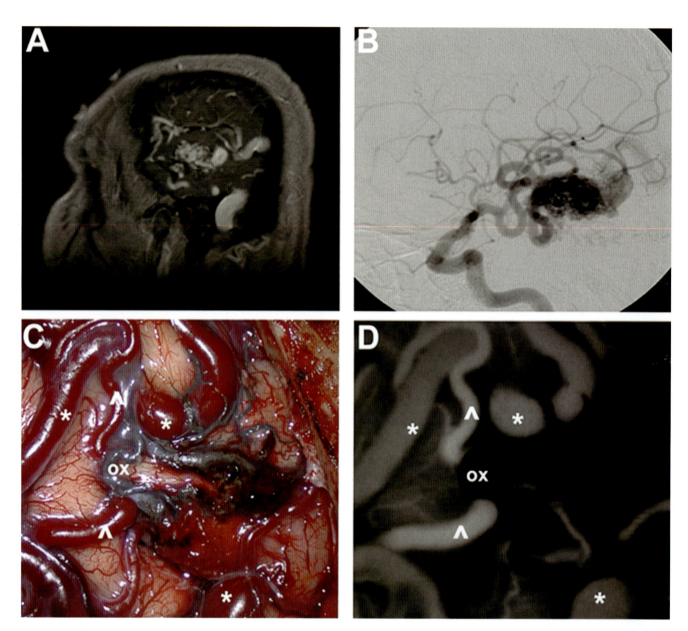

Fig. 23.5 **(A–D)** Indocyanine green (ICG) videoangiography. The "OX," arrowheads, and asterisks were added to facilitate comparison of the two images.

nidus can be clarified. Normally, these vessels are highly tolerant of temporary occlusion with minimal effects on the surrounding brain parenchyma; however, the clips should be reopened intermittently to avoid possible ischemic complications in situations where the relationship of the vessel to the nidus is difficult to discern quickly. If the iAVM is located subcortically, superficial vessels can be followed into a surrounding sulcus or fissure toward the iAVM nidus. Once the superficial vasculature is identified and dissected and the margins of the nidus are clarified, the next phase of the dissection can begin.

Once the supplying and draining vessels of the iAVM have been identified and the superficial arterial feeders ligated, a pial-arachnoid plane around the nidus should be carefully established, working in a stepwise circumferential manner,

maintaining the patency of the draining veins and carefully coagulating, ligating, dividing, and/or clipping the arterial feeders along the way only at their entry point into the nidus (with care to preserve *en passage* vessels). Frequently, except in pediatric patients, a plane or rim of gliotic brain tissue will define the boundaries of the iAVM nidus. In this parenchymal phase of dissection, it is very important to dissect the nidus in a spiral fashion, paying careful attention so as not to develop a deeper plane at any point, as bleeding, if encountered, is much more difficult to control and visualize with limited exposure. In other words, "Don't dig a hole!" **(Fig. 23.6).**

Once an adequate parenchymal plane is developed, retraction against the iAVM, and not the surrounding brain, can begin. If the drainage system of the nidus has been main-

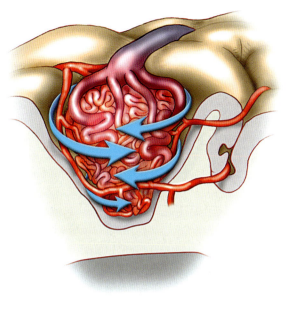
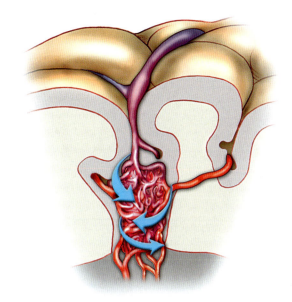

A

B

Fig. 23.6 **(A,B)** Parenchymal dissection.

tained, the nidus should be a pliable mass. However, the nidus should not be forcibly retracted, as deep arterial feeders are small and friable and can be easily torn resulting in unantici- pated hemorrhage. Further, the use of certain liquid embol- ics can make retraction of the nidus more difficult and less compressible. Polyvinyl alcohol is very compliant, isobutyl 2-cyanoacrylate is rock-like, and n-butyl 2-cyanoacrylate and Onyx (eV3, Inc, Plymouth, MN) are intermediate. Dissection planes can be maintained using either Kendall Telfa (Covi- dien, Mansfield, MA) or cotton pledgets as the parenchymal dissection proceeds. The dissection plane is continued along the iAVM nidus toward the apex of the lesion. As the nidus is manipulated in an effort to define dissection planes, although always tempting, bipolar coagulation on the nidus itself should be used cautiously as the nidal complex of vessels contains both feeding arteries and draining veins, so that premature coagulation of the main draining may lead to rupture of the nidus. Disruption or coagulation of a significant number of venous loops can increase nidal congestion and lead to pre- mature rupture. Further, translocating feeding arteries from the apex may be torn open leading to difficult-to-control hemorrhaging. If significant hemorrhage does occur during this phase of the resection, the most common cause is that the nidus has been entered (**Fig. 23.7**). The surgeon should place cotton in the area of hemorrhage and back up to re- define the dissection plane. Compression or retraction of the nidus can sometimes decrease the bleeding enough to local- ize the source. However, small feeding arteries toward the apex of the nidus are difficult to control due to their retrac- tion into the parenchyma and high pressure of blood supply. Bipolar electrocautery is often ineffective in these locations due to the inability to heat blood in these high-flow situa- tions. Small AVM clips should be used, as they are the most effective tools for hemostasis, as this stops flow, facilitating coagulation and division of the vessel.

If the apex of the nidus abuts an ependymal surface, it is often helpful to open up the ventricle around the lesion so that the deep arterioles can be coagulated against the ven- tricular wall. The ventricle should be protected with cotton pledgets so that any blood will not track into the ventricular system. As with the superficial dissection, the draining veins, if located deeply, should be maintained until complete dis- connection of the arterial supply. As the disconnection nears completion, the turgor in the drainage system should begin to lessen and the appearance of the color should reflect mixed arterialization. Small AVM clips can be systematically applied to the apex of the nidus, and the dissection plane is carried around the deepest aspects of the iAVM. Hemorrhage en- countered at this point most commonly represents retained iAVM nidus. If the bleeding cannot be controlled, it is impera- tive that the iAVM be removed so that the resection cavity can be explored and the source of hemorrhage identified. Before complete nidal extirpation, the turgor of the nidus should be examined after temporary clipping of the final draining vein. If, after several minutes of temporary occlusion, the nidal turgor does not increase, the draining vein should be ligated and divided followed by removal of the iAVM nidus (**Fig. 23.8**). ICG angiography is also useful to confirm deafferentation.

The resection cavity should be meticulously inspected for complete hemostasis. A Valsalva maneuver can be performed to test for hemorrhage of previously ligated feeding vessels. Although several limitations exist with respect to visualizing residual iAVM nidus within brain tissue, ICG videoangiog- raphy can be used to inspect the resection cavity for early venous drainage or retained tufts of arterial feeders. Some institutions utilize intraoperative angiography at this point, which is still the gold standard for imaging residual iAVM nidus. If our index of suspicion is low, we typically maintain careful blood pressure control and perform definitive angi- ography the following morning.

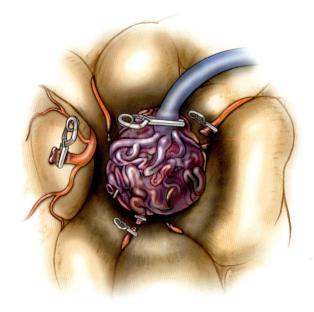

Fig. 23.7 Hemostasis.

◆ Surgical Complications

As with most complex vascular lesions, a prepared surgeon can often avoid or minimize most complications that can occur during the surgical resection of an intracranial arteriovenous malformation (**Table 23.2**). However, if complications do occur, they should be approached in a systematic fashion so that all potential causes can be dealt with in an effective and efficient manner.

In the setting of an acutely ruptured iAVM, surgical evacuation of the hematoma is often recommended when extensive mass effect is produced, resulting in neurologic compromise. In most situations, it is recommended that only the hematoma be evacuated and that the iAVM nidus be left undisturbed until there is sufficient time for proper radiographic evaluation and recovery from the likely resultant brain edema from the rupture itself. Resection of iAVMs in the acute setting brings with it increased risk of residual

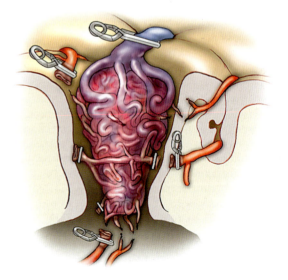

A

B

Fig. 23.8 **(A,B)** Clipping of the final draining vein and delivery of the AVM.

Table 23.2 Complications of Arteriovenous Malformation Surgery

Intraoperative hemorrhage

Nidal violation

Small friable/fragile arterial feeders

Nidal rupture/venous congestion

Residual nidus

Aneurysm rupture

Brain edema

Intraventricular hemorrhage

Hydrocephalus

Occlusive hyperemia

Postoerative hemorrhage

Normal pressure perfusion breakthrough

Residual nidus

Aneurysm rupture

Neurologic deficits

nidus, as parts of the nidus can be compressed by the hematoma and not initially recognized, and the risk of damage to the surrounding normal brain parenchyma, as edematous brain is more vulnerable to injury in these situations. Surgical planning in the acute phase should also include preparation for the subsequent procedure of iAVM resection. As such, the skin incision and bone flap planning should incorporate what will be planned for future resection, even though it may be considered large with respect to that needed for the hematoma evacuation. On the other hand, iAVM resection can be considered in the acute setting if the location of the nidus is within or immediately adjacent to the hematoma, is small and compact, and has straightforward morphology accessible to the operating surgeon. Once the hematoma is removed, time can be taken to stabilize the patient; the edematous brain, intracranial hemodynamics, and intracranial pressure can be allowed to normalize, and the patient can receive a multidisciplinary workup for more appropriate surgical and possibly adjunctive endovascular or radiosurgical planning.

Intraoperative complications of iAVM resection demand the most from the surgeon because these complications require not only recognition but also fast, efficient, and effective management. Given the high-flow nature of these vascular lesions, intraoperative bleeding, minor or major, is a necessary expectation. Minimization of intraoperative bleeding can be accomplished to some degree through adjunctive measures such as endovascular embolization. Before the iAVM resection begins, careful measures are taken to minimize bleeding complications. Maximizing venous drainage from the brain can aid in decreasing possible congestion that may occur during resection as well as carefully mapping out and identifying cortical draining veins, often through wall thickness, color, and pulsatility. Inadvertent sacrifice of draining veins

can occur through transection, retraction, and thrombosis, which can lead to nidal congestion, thus increasing the chances for intraoperative rupture.

Intraoperative bleeding can result for many reasons, and iAVM surgeons must systematically eliminate all causes so that significant complications do not occur. It cannot be overemphasized that the most important characteristics that a surgeon must have are patience and persistence, as these traits are paramount when dealing with intraoperative hemorrhagic complications during iAVM resection. The most common cause of persistent bleeding during resection of an iAVM is thought to be due to violation of the nidus. The operating surgeons must constantly reassure themselves that the plane of dissection does not violate the nidus. At any point where violation of the nidus is thought to occur, the surgeon must first stop dissection and reidentify the nidal margins. It may be necessary to increase the width of the dissection plane to fully appreciate the nidal margins or provide enough working space to contend with continued hemorrhaging. If the nidus has been entered, tamponading the nidus with either a suction tip or a brain retractor can often quell the persistent bleeding, at least enough to identify the source of hemorrhage. Further, it is important to identify the proximal supply to a bleeding site because it may be located at some distance from the bleeding point in the nidus, and wasteful time may be spent trying to coagulate or ceasing a bleeding point that may be in reality impossible to complete.

As dissection of the iAVM nidus continues, the deeper arterial feeders are often the most difficult to control, due to deep location, limited visualization, and friable and fragile nature of these arterial feeders. Tamponade and bipolar electrocautery are often ineffective with regard to obtaining hemostasis in this area due to the high-flow nature of these vessels as well as retraction of arterial feeders into the surrounding white matter, making bleeding control difficult at best. Small clips or miniclips may be more effective in controlling deep feeder hemorrhage. Also, exposure of some length of the arterial feeders may lend these vessels to bipolar electrocautery such that the blades of the bipolar can be applied to a visualized length of vessel rather than just across the diameter. If the operating surgeon cannot control hemorrhage, several other techniques can be used to facilitate hemostasis. It is often helpful in these situations if there are two surgeons, both armed with large-bore suctions, who understand the basic principles of hemorrhage control. A cell saver should be considered in extreme situations so that the blood can be returned to the patient. Further, it is important to obtain wide margins so that the bleeding site can be adequately visualized.

Although not frequently required, aggressive measures may be necessary to control bleeding during the resection of an iAVM, which may include early delivery of the nidus, partial or complete lobectomy, or ventriculostomy. All of these measures are intended to widen the working area such that bleeding can be sufficiently controlled. Temporary clips on major trunks can be beneficial as delivery of the nidus is anticipated. Lastly, control of excessive hemorrhaging can sometimes be aided by the neuroanesthesiologists. Adenosine can be used to pause the heart for several seconds, which may be enough time to get control of the bleeding. Furthermore, the amount of blood flow required by the brain can be reduced by either placing the patient into burst suppression or temporarily reducing the blood flow through pharmacologic means, such as with adenosine. Significant persistent bleeding after removal of the iAVM nidus usually indicates residual nidus. Whether due to the angiomatous nature of the nidus or from disconnection during the resection, a residual nidus may be hidden in the depths of the resection bed or in a surrounding sulcus. Although intraoperative catheter angiography is the gold standard for detecting a residual nidus, ICG videoangiography may be used in select cases to observe early venous drainage, although this modality of intraoperative imaging cannot be used to look through tissue and thus has significant limitations. Intraoperative ultrasound is another imaging modality that can be used to detect residual iAVM nidus. A residual nidus will often be an irregular, edematous zone in the resection cavity. Meticulous inspection of the resection bed is paramount so that suspicious areas can be inspected through exploration, minor blood pressure elevation, and intraoperative imaging modalities. During significant and prolonged bleeding, the neuroanesthesiologist must maintain vigilance to ensure that coagulopathy does not develop.

Although intraoperative rupture or persistent bleeding from either arterial feeders or the nidus itself is the most common complications in iAVM surgery, significant brain edema and subsequent swelling can also occur during resection and should be anticipated. Several nonsurgical complications, for example, compromised venous outflow leading to hypercapnia, can lead to brain edema and thus should be ruled out if the brain begins to appear edematous. Once the nonsurgical causes of edema are eliminated, surgical complications must be considered, including intraparenchymal hemorrhage, obstructive hydrocephalus, and occlusive hyperemia. Intraparenchymal hemorrhage can result from an isolated part of the nidus without venous drainage or retracted arterial feeders cut during the nidus dissection. Although large intraparenchymal hematomas are unlikely to develop without the notice of the operating surgeon, some can expand through sulcal or falcine planes, allowing adequate space for significant expansion. If the hemorrhage expands into the ventricular system, obstructive hydrocephalus may occur and develop quickly, thus requiring the emergent placement of a ventricular drain intraoperatively. It is therefore reasonable to know what ventricular access is available during iAVM resection, thus minimizing the time interval between need and placement of a ventricular catheter. However, hemorrhage into the ventricular system may be occult and may be manifested only through changes in the vital signs or brain distention. Therefore, it is imperative that the operating surgeon be aware of the clinical signs of intraventricular hemorrhage so that such a complication can be anticipated. Intraoperative ultrasound can be used quickly and is highly effective at identifying intraparenchymal and intraventricular hemorrhage in these situations. Once intraparenchymal, intraventricular hemorrhage, and hydrocephalus have been factored out as a cause of increasing brain edema, occlusive hyperemia must be considered. Although controversial, dys-

function of autoregulation in the surrounding brain and its blood supply is thought to contribute to reactive edema once an iAVM nidus has been removed. Normal perfusion pressure breakthrough (NPPB), proposed by Spetzler et al,[33] is characterized by persistently edematous and bleeding brain around the margins of resection. The blood supply to these areas is thought to have exhausted the compensatory regulation of blood flow due to ischemic steal effects by the iAVM, resulting in hyperemia after iAVM resection and subsequent edema and hemorrhage. Management of this condition consists of minimizing the metabolic demands of the brain and inciting cerebral protection through pharmacologic means, including electroencephalogram (EEG) burst suppression, cerebral perfusion pressure (CPP)/intracranial pressure (ICP) control, and rigorous systolic blood pressure (SBP) management.

◆ Surgical Outcomes

Ultimately, the most important aspect of the surgical treatment of iAVMs is the clinical outcome. Spetzler and Martin[2] originally based their ubiquitous grading scale on the morbidity and mortality associated with surgical treatment alone (**Table 23.3**). However, the modern management of iAVMs involves multimodal therapy, rendering the morbidity statistics reported by Spetzler and Martin less applicable. Furthermore, this grading scheme only took into account those patients who were treated, thereby likely biasing the results. Finally, the Spetzler-Martin grading scheme did not take into account the variability of lesions within each classification that can have a profound effect on surgical difficulty as well as outcome. As a result, surgical outcomes have been difficult to assign to iAVMs of a particular grade. Careful analysis of angioarchitectural features that have been related to surgical morbidity, such as nidal diffuseness and deep perforator

Table 23.3 Surgical Outcomes of Arteriovenous Malformation Resection

Grade	No. of Patients	No Deficit (%)	Minor Deficit* (%)	Major Deficit# (%)
I	23	100	0	0
II	21	95	5	0
III	25	84	12	4
IV	15	73	20	7
V	16	69	19	12
Total	100	86	10	4

*Minor deficits include temporary increase in visual field deficit, aphasia, weakness, dysphagia, or increased brainstem deficit, aphasia, ataxia or trigeminal deficit.

#Major deficits include hemiparesis, homonymous hemianopsia, severe neurological deficit, or major aphasia.

Source: Adapted from Spetzler RF, Martin NA. A proposed grading system for arteriovenous malformations. J Neurosurg 1986;65:476–483.

arterial supply, should be more rigorously analyzed before finalizing the discussion of surgical risks. Moreover, the use of multimodal therapy and its variable applications has also complicated outcomes reporting. Despite this, multiple case series involving multimodal therapy of iAVMs have been reported in the literature over the last decade. In most case series, low-grade (I or II) iAVMs have low morbidity rates, ranging between 1% and 3%,[34–36] unless located in the brainstem, thalamus, or basal ganglia, which present with higher operative risks of permanent morbidity, 6 to 13%.[5,6,37,38] Grade III AVMs represent a highly variable group of AVMs and should be considered on an individual basis.[8,39] Multimodal therapy including surgical management of high-grade AVMs (IV and V) have improved over the last several years due to the reduction of intraoperative hemorrhage, enhanced embolization techniques, catheters and agents, improved angioarchitectural mapping, microsurgical techniques, and the use of improved intraoperative imaging.[8,40–42] As a result, the ability to treat high-grade AVMs has improved but with persisting risks associated with surgical resection, 5 to 23%.

◆ Postoperative Considerations

In the postoperative period, close postoperative monitoring is essential in the first 24 to 48 hours after resection of an iAVM. Monitoring occurs in the intensive care unit under the supervision of a neurosurgical and neurocritical care team. If an intraoperative angiogram is not performed, a follow-up angiogram should be performed the following morning to ensure radiographic success of the procedure and to rule out any residual iAVM nidus that may remain. Blood pressure monitoring is strict. Serial neurologic examinations are done to ensure that delayed neurologic deficits can be detected. Postoperative complications such as retrograde thrombosis, hemorrhagic venous infarction, and clinical seizures can occur and must be anticipated. Acute changes in the neurologic exam can be due to any of the above complications. Most postoperative seizures can be controlled with antiepileptic medications. Although rare, recurrence of iAVMs in pediatric and adolescent patients does occur, and follow-up imaging is recommended to rule out such an occurrence. Follow-up imaging is usually performed at 12 months and 60 months and then again at 20 years of age in the pediatric population. In patients who are neurologically devastated from the initial rupture, prolonged immobility must be expected, and the complications that occur in the postoperative period, such as respiratory infections and deep venous thromboses (DVT), must be accounted for. Aggressive pulmonary care and prophylactic DVT therapy should be highly considered after the acute postoperative period.

◆ Future Directions

Intracranial arteriovenous malformations are complex vascular lesions that require a multimodal approach for complete anatomic and physiologic understanding. The future of iAVM surgery will involve integrating both sets of informa-

tion for use in the operating room. Computed tomography (CT) and magnetic resonance imaging (MRI) continue to improve in both spatial and temporal resolution, as does the software that allows manipulation of these images. Image layering and integration with the surgical microscope will continue to evolve and become incorporated into the modern operating room. As endovascular techniques and equipment continue to progress as well as the agents used, adjunctive therapy for preoperative embolization will continue to provide more complete embolization of the iAVM nidus as well as aid in the identification of the nidal margins through specialized imaging available on modern microscopes. The combination of the innovations mentioned above will certainly lead to reduced complications in surgical resections of iAVMs as well as more complete resections.

◆ Conclusion

The surgical management of intracranial arteriovenous malformations continues to progress as fast as technology will allow. Continued education regarding the technical demands of the operating surgeon will be more necessary in the future as endovascular and radiosurgical techniques are used more frequently to treat such lesions. Anticipating the potential complications as well as knowledge of the successful surgical techniques for iAVM surgery allow the neurosurgeon the most complete and effective approach to surgical management of iAVMs.

References

1. Hernesniemi JA, Dashti R, Juvela S, Väärt K, Niemelä M, Laakso A. Natural history of brain arteriovenous malformations: a long-term follow-up study of risk of hemorrhage in 238 patients. Neurosurgery 2008; 63:823–829, discussion 829–831
2. Spetzler RF, Martin NA. A proposed grading system for arteriovenous malformations. J Neurosurg 1986;65:476–483
3. Stapf C, Mohr JP, Pile-Spellman J, Solomon RA, Sacco RL, Connolly ES Jr. Epidemiology and natural history of arteriovenous malformations. Neurosurg Focus 2001;11:e1
4. Duckworth EA, Gross B, Batjer HH. Thalamic and basal ganglia arteriovenous malformations: redefining "inoperable." Neurosurgery 2008; 63(1, Suppl 1)ONS63–ONS67, discussion ONS67–ONS68
5. Gross BA, Bendok BR, Hage ZA, Awad IA, Batjer HH. Advances in open neurovascular surgery 2007. Stroke 2009;40:324–326
6. Gross BA, Duckworth EA, Getch CC, Bendok BR, Batjer HH. Challenging traditional beliefs: microsurgery for arteriovenous malformations of the basal ganglia and thalamus. Neurosurgery 2008;63:393–410, discussion 410–411
7. Laakso A, Dashti R, Seppänen J, et al. Long-term excess mortality in 623 patients with brain arteriovenous malformations. Neurosurgery 2008; 63:244–253, discussion 253–255
8. van Beijnum J, Bhattacharya JJ, Counsell CE, et al; Scottish Intracranial Vascular Malformation Study Collaborators. Patterns of brain arteriovenous malformation treatment: prospective, population-based study. Stroke 2008;39:3216–3221
9. ApSimon HT, Reef H, Phadke RV, Popovic EA. A population-based study of brain arteriovenous malformation: long-term treatment outcomes. Stroke 2002;33:2794–2800
10. Berman MF, Hartmann A, Mast H, et al. Determinants of resource utilization in the treatment of brain arteriovenous malformations. AJNR Am J Neuroradiol 1999;20:2004–2008
11. Jessurun GA, Kamphuis DJ, van der Zande FH, Nossent JC. Cerebral arteriovenous malformations in the Netherlands Antilles. High prevalence of hereditary hemorrhagic telangiectasia-related single and multiple cerebral arteriovenous malformations. Clin Neurol Neurosurg 1993;95: 193–198

12. Stapf C, Labovitz DL, Sciacca RR, Mast H, Mohr JP, Sacco RL. Incidence of adult brain arteriovenous malformation hemorrhage in a prospective population-based stroke survey. Cerebrovasc Dis 2002;13:43–46

13. Stapf C, Mast H, Sciacca RR, et al; New York Islands AVM Study Collaborators. The New York Islands AVM Study: design, study progress, and initial results. Stroke 2003;34:e29–e33

14. Ondra SL, Troupp H, George ED, Schwab K. The natural history of symptomatic arteriovenous malformations of the brain: a 24-year follow-up assessment. J Neurosurg 1990;73:387–391

15. Stapf C, Mast H, Sciacca RR, et al. Predictors of hemorrhage in patients with untreated brain arteriovenous malformation. Neurology 2006;66: 1350–1355

16. Andrews BT, Wilson CB. Staged treatment of arteriovenous malformations of the brain. Neurosurgery 1987;21:314–323

17. Cronqvist M, Wirestam R, Ramgren B, et al. Endovascular treatment of intracerebral arteriovenous malformations: procedural safety, complications, and results evaluated by MR imaging, including diffusion and perfusion imaging. AJNR Am J Neuroradiol 2006;27:162–176

18. Deveikis JP. Endovascular therapy of intracranial arteriovenous malformations. Materials and techniques. Neuroimaging Clin N Am 1998;8: 401–424

19. Gailloud P. Endovascular treatment of cerebral arteriovenous malformations. Tech Vasc Interv Radiol 2005;8:118–128

20. Hartmann A, Mast H, Choi JH, Stapf C, Mohr JP. Treatment of arteriovenous malformations of the brain. Curr Neurol Neurosci Rep 2007;7: 28–34

21. Hartmann A, Mast H, Mohr JP, et al. Determinants of staged endovascular and surgical treatment outcome of brain arteriovenous malformations. Stroke 2005;36:2431–2435

22. Jahan R, Murayama Y, Gobin YP, Duckwiler GR, Vinters HV, Viñuela F. Embolization of arteriovenous malformations with Onyx: clinicopathological experience in 23 patients. Neurosurgery 2001;48:984–995, discussion 995–997

23. Katsaridis V, Papagiannaki C, Aimar E. Curative embolization of cerebral arteriovenous malformations (AVMs) with Onyx in 101 patients. Neuroradiology 2008;50:589–597

24. Lawton MT, Hamilton MG, Spetzler RF. Multimodality treatment of deep arteriovenous malformations: thalamus, basal ganglia, and brain stem. Neurosurgery 1995;37:29–35, discussion 35–36

25. van Rooij WJ, Sluzewski M, Beute GN. Brain AVM embolization with Onyx. AJNR Am J Neuroradiol 2007;28:172–177, discussion 178

26. Weber W, Kis B, Siekmann R, Kuehne D. Endovascular treatment of intracranial arteriovenous malformations with onyx: technical aspects. AJNR Am J Neuroradiol 2007;28:371–377

27. Cockroft KM, Thompson RC, Steinberg GK. Aneurysms and arteriovenous malformations. Neurosurg Clin N Am 1998;9:565–576

28. Liu Y, Zhu S, Jiao L, Wang H, Li X, Li G. Cerebral arteriovenous malformations associated with aneurysms—a report of 10 cases and literature review. J Clin Neurosci 2000;7:254–256

29. Nakahara I, Taki W, Kikuchi H, et al. Endovascular treatment of aneurysms on the feeding arteries of intracranial arteriovenous malformations. Neuroradiology 1999;41:60–66

30. Redekop G, TerBrugge K, Montanera W, Willinsky R. Arterial aneurysms associated with cerebral arteriovenous malformations: classification, incidence, and risk of hemorrhage. J Neurosurg 1998;89:539–546

31. Westphal M, Grzyska U. Clinical significance of pedicle aneurysms on feeding vessels, especially those located in infratentorial arteriovenous malformations. J Neurosurg 2000;92:995–1001

32. Killory BD, Nakaji P, Gonzales LF, Ponce FA, Wait SD, Spetzler RF. Prospective evaluation of surgical microscope-integrated intraoperative near-infrared indocyanine green angiography during cerebral arteriovenous malformation surgery. Neurosurgery 2009;65:456–462, discussion 462

33. Spetzler RF, Wilson CB, Weinstein P, Mehdorn M, Townsend J, Telles D. Normal perfusion pressure breakthrough theory. Clin Neurosurg 1978; 25:651–672

34. Kiriş T, Sencer A, Sahinbaş M, Sencer S, Imer M, Izgi N. Surgical results in pediatric Spetzler-Martin grades I-III intracranial arteriovenous malformations. Childs Nerv Syst 2005;21:69–74, discussion 75–76

35. Morgan MK, Rochford AM, Tsahtsarlis A, Little N, Faulder KC. Surgical risks associated with the management of Grade I and II brain arteriovenous malformations. Neurosurgery 2007;61(1, Suppl)417–422, discussion 422–424

36. Pavesi G, Rustemi O, Berlucchi S, Frigo AC, Gerunda V, Scienza R. Acute surgical removal of low-grade (Spetzler-Martin I-II) bleeding arteriovenous malformations. Surg Neurol 2009;72:662–667

37. Sasaki T, Kurita H, Kawamoto S, Nemoto S, Kirino T, Saito I. Clinical outcome of radiosurgery, embolization and microsurgery for AVMs in the thalamus and basal ganglia. J Clin Neurosci 1998;5(Suppl):95–97

38. Yamada K, Mase M, Matsumoto T. Surgery for deeply seated arteriovenous malformation: with special reference to thalamic and striatal arteriovenous malformation. Neurol Med Chir (Tokyo) 1998;38(Suppl): 227–230

39. Lawton MT; UCSF Brain Arteriovenous Malformation Study Project. Spetzler-Martin grade III arteriovenous malformations: surgical results and a modification of the grading scale. Neurosurgery 2003;52:740–748, discussion 748–749

40. Chang SD, Marcellus ML, Marks MP, Levy RP, Do HM, Steinberg GK. Multimodality treatment of giant intracranial arteriovenous malformations. Neurosurgery 2003;53:1–11, discussion 11–13

41. Chang SD, Marcellus ML, Marks MP, Levy RP, Do HM, Steinberg GK. Multimodality treatment of giant intracranial arteriovenous malformations. Neurosurgery 2007;61(1, Suppl)432–442, discussion 442–444

42. Natarajan SK, Ghodke B, Britz GW, Born DE, Sekhar LN. Multimodality treatment of brain arteriovenous malformations with microsurgery after embolization with onyx: single-center experience and technical nuances. Neurosurgery 2008;62:1213–1225, discussion 1225–1226

24

Cavernoma

Murat Gunel

Pearls

- Cerebral cavernous malformations (CCMs) are relatively common vascular defects consisting of dilated loops of capillary-like channels lacking intervening neural parenchyma. They are seen in approximately 1 in 200 individuals and account for 8 to 15% of all vascular malformations of the central nervous system (CNS).
- Cerebral cavernous malformations are a result of a genetic disorder that can be either sporadic or familial; 96% of all mutations in the familial form of the disease are secondary to mutations in one of the three genes in the CCM family: *CCM1*, or *KRIT1*; *CCM2*, or malcavernin; or *CCM3*, also known as the Programmed Cell Death-10 gene.
- Only 20 to 30% of all patients with cavernomas are symptomatic; they typically present headaches, seizures, or focal neurologic deficits, most commonly in the third to fifth decades of life. Asymptomatic patient commonly present after incidental detection of lesions on imaging studies conducted for unrelated reasons.
- Treatment options for CCMs are limited to expectant management; medical management, which is confined to the use of antiepileptic drugs for seizure control; and complete surgical resection. Of these, surgery is the only option that can be completely curative.
- For brainstem cavernomas, thin-cut T1 images through the brainstem often reveal where the lesion comes to the surface, which is helpful in operative planning. Intraoperatively, there is a discoloration of the pial surface of the brainstem from hemosiderin, which guides the surgeon to the point of entry. It is advisable to leave the gliotic plane intact (unlike with supratentorial lesions) to reduce the risk of neurologic deficit.

◆ Description

Cerebral cavernous malformations (CCMs) are vascular malformations composed of intertwined clusters of abnormally dilated capillary-like channels. These vascular channels consist of a single layer of endothelial cells and lack structural elements of mature vessels, including elastin and smooth muscle. Typically, no normal parenchyma is found in between the sinusoidal vascular spaces **(Fig. 24.1)**. Unlike normal cerebral vessels, the endothelial cells are often devoid of tight junctions. Additionally, other elements of the blood–brain barrier, including astrocytic foot processes and pericytes, are also either diminished or completely missing.[1–3] Consequently, cavernous malformations are "leaky," and frequently there are microhemorrhages at and surrounding the lesion site.[1] Whereas many of these bleeds remain clinically silent, they nonetheless impact the surrounding brain parenchyma over time, causing reactive gliosis as well as hemosiderin deposits that accumulate as blood is metabolized.

Macroscopically, CCMs are reddish-purple in color and variable in size, ranging from 1 mm to several centimeters in diameter. They are often multilobular and encapsulated by a variable layer of fibrous adventitia, giving them their characteristic mulberry-like appearance. Due to the recurrence of microhemorrhages and associated blood metabolism, CCM lesions are dynamic, both increasing and decreasing in size over time.

Although most common intracranially, CCMs can be found in any component of the central nervous system (CNS), including the spinal cord, cranial nerves, ventricles, and retina, and rarely in other organs, including the skin.

◆ Epidemiology

Before the advent of magnetic resonance imaging (MRI), CCMs were definitively diagnosed only at autopsy or during surgery, and were thus thought to be rare. An MRI-based study showed a 0.4% prevalence of CCMs,[4] in agreement with an earlier autopsy study.[5] With the improvement of diagnostic acumen, CCMs are now recognized as common lesions, affecting one in every 200 people and accounting for 8 to 15% of all vascular malformations of the CNS.[6,7]

Cerebral cavernous malformations occur in both sporadic and familial forms. Sporadic cases almost never involve more

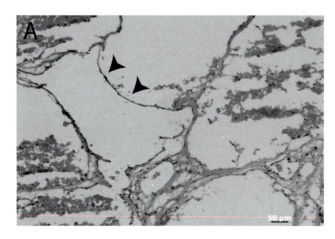

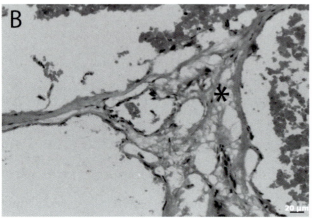

Fig. 24.1 Hematoxylin and eosin (H&E) stains showing histology of cavernous malformations. **(A)** A single layer of endothelium *(arrowheads)* surrounds sinusoidal spaces containing thrombosed blood. **(B)** There is no normal brain parenchyma between layers of endothelium *(asterisk)*.

than two lesions, and family history is absent. On the other hand, the familial form usually manifests as multiple lesions in the setting of a strong family history of neurologic disease. Regardless of disease type, the vast majority of CCMs occur in the brain, primarily in the supratentorial compartment (63–90% of lesions)[6] and the posterior fossa (7.8–35.8%), with the brainstem being the most common site infratentorially (9–35%).[8] Spinal CCMs are rare, but their exact frequency is unknown, and can be extra- or intramedullary as well as extradural or intradural.

Cerebral cavernous malformations are associated with developmental venous malformations (DVMs) in up to 100% of cases,[8] making CCM plus DVM the most common mixed cerebrovascular lesion (**Fig. 24.2**).[9] This co-occurrence has implications for surgical treatment (see below).

◆ Natural History

The clinical presentation and progression of CCMs vary widely among individuals, and depend on the location of the lesion and the presence and extent of hemorrhage. Although previously believed to be congenital, CCMs have been shown to develop de novo.[10] Once present, lesions are dynamic,[10] growing and shrinking in size as microhemorrhages occur and are resorbed, and as vessels thrombose and recanalize.[11] Lesion development and sequelae therefore remain unpredictable, as host, environmental, and genetic factors combine to produce the resulting clinical manifestation.

Although CCMs are common, only 20 to 30% of individuals with lesions will ever become symptomatic.[4] Those who do typically remain asymptomatic until the third to fifth decades of life, presenting with seizures, headaches, progressive neurologic defects, or cerebral hemorrhages.[4] Seizures are the most common symptom, especially in patients with lesions in the frontal and temporal lobes. Simple, complex partial, and generalized seizures have been reported in patients with supratentorial CCMs.[12] The median age of an individual's first seizure is 42 ± 4 years.[13] The estimated risk of suffering a seizure is 1 to 2% per year.[13] Infratentorial CCMs, particularly those arising in the brainstem, tend to become symptomatic at smaller sizes, and usually manifest as progressive neurologic deficit.[14]

Although a sudden gross hemorrhage is the most feared CCM complication, this event is infrequent, with an estimated annual risk between 0.25% and 6%[13] that varies with an individual's presenting symptom and with several features inherent to the lesion. Patients diagnosed either incidentally on routine imaging or after presenting with seizures have the lowest bleeding risk (0.4–2%). This risk increases to 5% over the following year when an individual presents with a symptomatic hemorrhage.[15] Hemorrhage risk also varies with the size and location of the lesion, as well as with patient age. Larger and deeper lesions are more likely to bleed than smaller, superficial ones, and younger patients tend to have a higher bleeding risk than older patients. Furthermore, higher rates of hemorrhage have been reported during pregnancy.[4]

Gross hemorrhages from CCMs usually present with focal neurologic deficits. These deficits are typically maximal at the onset of the bleed and tend to resolve gradually as the hemorrhage undergoes organization and absorption. Recurrent episodes of hemorrhage are associated with progressive worsening of neurologic deficits and an increased risk of permanent neurologic impairment.[16]

◆ Radiographic Findings

Magnetic resonance imaging remains the radiographic tool of choice for detecting CCMs. Lesions typically appear as a mixture of high and low T1 and T2 signals surrounded by hemoglobin degradation products such as methemoglobin, hemosiderin, and ferritin, depending on the age of the surrounding blood, and these different components give lesions their typical mulberry or popcorn appearance with a surrounding dark halo composed mostly of hemosiderin from chronic bleeds (**Fig. 24.3**).

Based on imaging characteristics, CCMs have been categorized into four types, each associated with a pathologic correlate that explains the lesion's radiographic findings. Type I

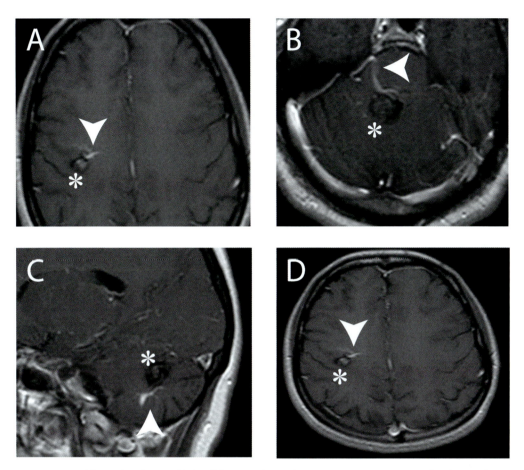

Fig. 24.2 Axial **(A,B,D)** and sagittal **(C)** gadolinium-enhanced magnetic resonance imaging (MRI) scans show cavernous malformations *(asterisk)* with associated developmental venous malformations *(arrowhead)*. This is the most common mixed cerebrovascular lesion.

lesions are characterized by isolated subacute hemorrhage that causes a rim of hemosiderin-stained macrophages and gliotic brain to form a capsule around the lesion, visualized as a hypointense rim on T2-weighted imaging. Type II cavernomas, which are characterized by multiple recurrent hemorrhages, typically have loculated areas of hemorrhage and thrombosis, giving them a reticulated mixed signal core on both T1- and T2-weighted imaging. In type III CCMs, a hypointensity surrounded by a hypointense rim is seen on imaging due to hemosiderin staining within and around the lesion after chronic resolved hemorrhages. These lesions are also seen as markedly hypointense on gradient echo MRI. Type IV lesions are either poorly or not at all visualized on T1- or T2-weighted MRI. They are visible on gradient echo MRI, however, where they appear as a small, punctuate hypointense foci. This grouping system provides prognostic value, as 93% of type I and II lesions become symptomatic, whereas only 33% of type III and IV lesions have associated symptoms.[17]

Computed tomography (CT) is less useful as a diagnostic tool for CCMs, as the majority of findings are nonspecific. CCMs typically appear as nonenhancing heterogeneous lesions, corresponding to either hemorrhage or calcification, but can also be seen as isodense or hypodense cystic lesions, with or without a nodule. Hypodense areas can further ap-

pear surrounding the cavernoma, representing edema, hemosiderin, or even atrophy.[18] Lack of specific findings on CT emphasizes the need to adapt imaging modalities to the study of CCMs.[18] Nonetheless, CT remains an ideal tool when ruling out acute hemorrhages.

Angiography is also of little diagnostic help, as CCMs are usually angiographically occult. Some lesions may show a subtle blush, and larger lesions may appear as an avascular mass on angiography.[12] In the context of hemorrhage, however, the presence of DVMs, which can be easily recognized on angiography, should alert the clinician to the possibility of a coexistent CCM.

◆ Genetics

Although the heritable nature of CCMs has been well recognized since its original description, the extent of the familial nature of cavernomas was greatly underappreciated until the advent of MRI. By allowing detection of asymptomatic lesions, the use of MRI helped to elucidate the prevalence of the disease within families, and thus provided insight into the genetics underlying the disorder. It is now established that the genetic mode of inheritance of familial CCM is auto-

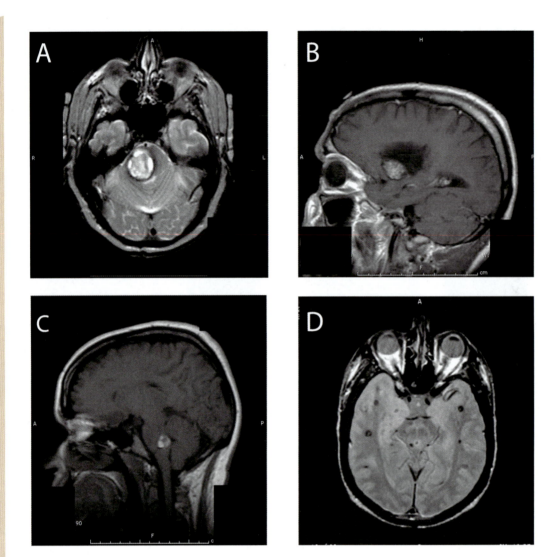

Fig. 24.3 MRI characteristics of cerebral cavernous malformations (CCMs). **(A)** Axial T2-weighted MRI reveals a large pontine CCM with a surrounding hemosiderin ring. **(B,C)** Sagittal T1-weighted images shows hyperintense supratentorial **(B)** and infratentorial **(C)** lesions likely indicative of subacute blood. **(D)** Gradient echo images show multiple small cavernous malformations in this Hispanic patient with a mutation in the *CCM1* gene.

somal dominant with variable expressivity and a high degree of penetrance.

The difference in the number of lesions seen in sporadic and familial cases suggests that the underlying molecular pathophysiology follows Knudson's two-hit hypothesis. In this model, the first hit (mutation) is inherited, whereas the second hit is acquired, thus leading to earlier onset of more severe disease in familial forms.

Genetic linkage analyses identified three loci at which mutations have been found to cause CCM development: chromosomes 7q *(CCM1)*, 7p *(CCM2)*, and 3q *(CCM3)*.[19] Subsequent positional cloning experiments led to the identification of Krev1 interaction trapped protein-1 (KRIT1), as the *CCM1* gene, *MGC4607* (or malcavernin) as the *CCM2* gene, and Programmed Cell Death-10 *(PDCD10)* as the *CCM3* gene. It should be kept in mind, however, that mutations in these three genes account for 96% of all familial forms of the dis-

ease, leaving the possibility of a fourth disease-causing gene yet to be discovered.[20]

KRIT1 was the first of the CCM genes to be discovered on chromosome 7q21 and contains 16 exons that encode the 736 amino acid protein KRIT1. KRIT1 has several domains implicated in protein–protein interactions, including three ankyrin, one FERM, and three NPXY domains that are thought to participate in binding to microtubules, integrins, and other cell signaling molecules.[12] Over 90 distinct frameshift or nonsense mutations have been detected to date, causing premature insertion of a termination codon, and suggesting loss of KRIT1 protein function as the underlying genetic mechanism. KRIT1 is expressed in neurons and astrocytes in the brain as well as in the endothelium of arteries and capillaries of various organs,[21] and in vivo studies suggest that CCM1 plays an essential role in vascular development. Ccm1$^{-/-}$ mice have vascular abnormalities that are incompatible with life and result in embryonic lethality associated with defects of arterial morphogenesis.[22] Although Ccm1[+/−] mice appear normal, in a background lacking p53 function, approximately half of the heterozygotes develop vascular lesions of the brain resembling cavernous malformations or capillary telangiectasias.[23]

The *CCM2* gene is *MGC4607*, or malcavernin. *MGC4607* is a 10-exon gene located on chromosome 7p13 and encoding the CCM2 protein. Like *CCM1*, most *CCM2* mutations result in premature termination of protein translation, again suggesting loss of function as the underlying genetic mechanism. The expression pattern of *CCM2* is similar to that of *CCM1*, localizing to neurons, astrocytes, and the arterial endothelium. Although its function is not completely known, CCM2 has significant homology to OSM, a protein in rodents that is responsible for osmo- and mechanosensing of the extracellular matrix. In humans, at least in certain settings, CCM2 appears to play a role as a scaffolding protein, using p38 signaling to convey information about environmental stress.[24] In addition, in vivo studies predict that CCM2 has a major angiogenic role because *Ccm2* knockout mice, similar to the *Ccm1* mutants, die during embryogenesis. In addition, approximately 10% of *Ccm2* heterozygotes develop vascular lesions.[25] In conditional *Ccm2* mutants, cardiovascular pathology results when *Ccm2* is inactivated in the endothelium but not when it is inactivated in either neural or smooth muscles cells,[26] further supporting the hypothesis that CCM is primarily a disease of the endothelium. These studies suggest that CCM2 acts autonomously in the endothelium, potentially affecting cell junctions with subsequent effects on vessel formation and integrity.[26]

Finally, *PDCD10* was identified as being the causative gene in CCM3 families. This seven-exon gene is located on 3q26 and encodes a 212 amino acid protein. Similar to *CCM1* and *CCM2*, all variants in *CCM3* identified to date are nonsense mutations. Interestingly, the expression pattern of CCM3 parallels that of CCM1 and CCM2, being present in the arterial endothelium as well as in neurons and astrocytes.[27] In vitro studies of CCM3 suggest that it is pro-apoptotic.[28] Recent in vivo studies using zebrafish show that CCM3 plays a role in vascular development, as *CCM3* knockout animals developed the same cardiovascular dilations seen in *CCM1* and *CCM2* knockout animals.[29]

The identification of the three CCM genes and the elucidation of the function of their encoded proteins have provided unprecedented insight into CCM pathophysiology and has begun to define the molecular pathways underlying these lesions. Further mechanistic insight into CCM signaling will have significant implications for CCM patients, potentially leading to new medical treatment algorithms in the future.

◆ Treatment Options

Treatment options for CCM include expectant management, medical management, and surgical resection. These options are summarized below; however, it should be kept in mind that these are general guidelines, and that each patient must be considered individually.

Expectant Management

Expectant management of CCMs consists of follow-up MRI at regular intervals, usually once every 1 to 2 years. New images are compared with older ones to detect lesion changes such as expansion or hemorrhage, and the need for intervention is discussed if such findings are present. When deciding on this form of management, several features of both the patient and lesion must be considered. Patients who are poor surgical candidates, including older patients and those with multiple comorbidities, are usually best treated with expectant management. For younger, healthier individuals, however, the location of the lesion and its presenting symptoms play a bigger role. Lesions that are surgically higher risk are usually handled expectantly, as are lesions in eloquent brain regions, because surgical manipulation can be neurologically damaging. In general, asymptomatic patients, especially those who are older at the time of diagnosis and therefore have a lower lifetime benefit from surgery, should be offered expectant management, whereas younger, symptomatic patients should undergo a surgical resection. Finally, patients with the familial form of the disease who have multiple cavernomas are usually managed expectantly, and surgery is considered only if lesions are causing significant symptoms.

Medical Management

Medical management of CCMs is similar to that of expectant management in the sense that it also involves routine imaging, but it also includes the use of medication to alleviate symptoms secondary to cavernomas. At this time, however, medications for symptomatic relief are limited to antiepileptics to control seizure activity related to a lesion. This treatment is appropriate for patients who have acquired a seizure disorder secondary to their cavernoma, but the lesion is either low risk for hemorrhage and thus not requiring surgical intervention, or is in a location not amenable to surgical resection. Patients with multiple cavernomas in which the seizure focus cannot be determined, as well as patients with multiple seizure foci that are not surgically accessible, are also well suited for this treatment option. Not all patients' seizures can be controlled by antiepileptics, however, and surgical intervention should be considered for these patients should their seizures become intractable.

Surgical Management

Surgical management of CCMs is accomplished ideally through a complete lesionectomy. As the only curative option for cavernomas, surgery offers patients several advantages. Not only is a patient's hemorrhage risk immediately eliminated if the entire lesion is removed, but seizures usually cease and most neurologic deficits completely resolve within weeks to months after lesion removal. These benefits need to be weighed against the morbidity and mortality inherent to the surgery itself. Therefore, before deciding on surgical management, the risks of the procedure, which vary for each individual based on underlying health conditions and lesion characteristics mainly determined by location, should be determined, as should the expected lifetime benefit of CCM removal. Surgical management is reserved for those patients in whom the benefits of surgery outweigh the risks of the procedure.

Although most surgical cases need to be determined on an individual basis, certain lesion characteristics are associated with low operative risk and are thus more amenable to surgical intervention. Lesion location is one such feature. Solitary, superficial lesions can be removed with very few complications other than those of general anesthesia, and thus these patients often elect surgical management. Infratentorial lesions, as well as those in close proximity to eloquent structures, are higher risk for surgical morbidity with respect to neurologic functioning. These lesions themselves are also associated with a greater risk, though, because a large bleed in such areas could be neurologically devastating. To lessen the surgical risk associated with these lesions, general practice for deep infratentorial lesions is to postpone surgery until the lesion reaches the pial surface through repeat bleeds. The tracking of blood to the pial surface provides a plane of access to the lesion, and facilitates lesion removal with less operative morbidity.

A patient's presenting symptoms are also important to consider when deciding whether to surgically remove a lesion. Seizures, for example, are a common presentation of CCMs, especially for those located in the supratentorial compartment. Such lesions are often considered for surgical resection when they are identified as the cause of seizures in patients whose seizures are refractory to medical treatment.

Overt hemorrhage, another common CCM presentation, can occur in both supratentorial and infratentorial lesions. In supratentorial lesions, acute hemorrhages are usually taken to surgery based on the rate of the patient's neurologic decline and the foreseeable consequences of mass effect from the hemorrhage. If blood interferes with the ability to detect a possible CCM on imaging, surgery can be deferred, provided surgical decompression is not immediately required. In these patients, two options can be considered: the patient can undergo elective exploration soon after the event, or expectant management can be continued until a definitive diagnosis is made. Expectant management is most appropriate for patients in whom craniotomies are high risk, and begins with a follow-up MRI 2 to 6 weeks after the event. Surgical resection is also recommended for infratentorial lesions with this presentation, but aside from lesions requiring immediate intervention, this option should be considered only after the patient has suffered from two or more hemorrhages.

Although these treatment recommendations are not necessarily applicable to every patient, they provide a set of guidelines to consider when contemplating the management of a specific patient. As further research is performed on CCMs and new treatment options explored, these suggestions will likely change. Regardless of how patients are treated, however, they should all receive counseling on the disease. This includes warning them of the symptoms suggestive of a hemorrhage, instructing them to appropriately seek medical attention, as well as avoiding use of anticoagulants, because they increase the potential for serious sequelae

should a hemorrhage occur. Women of reproductive age should be advised of the possible increase in hemorrhage risk during pregnancy.[4]

◆ Radiosurgery Versus Microsurgical Treatment

The use of radiosurgery in treating CCMs remains controversial.[14] Because it is the only intervention for CCMs aside from surgery, it has been considered for treating CCMs in surgically difficult areas or in patients who are not operative candidates. Without an imaging modality able to detect total lesion occlusion,[30] however, it is impossible to determine whether this treatment is curative. Instead, efficacy of the procedure must be judged on clinical observation of postprocedural hemorrhage rates. Although some studies report decreased hemorrhage rates following radiosurgery,[31,32] others, including some of these same studies, show an increased complication rate following this treatment, including permanent neurologic deficits.[33] Patients in one study had to undergo surgical resection of their lesions after radiosurgery failed to completely eliminate their cavernomas.[33] Furthermore, histologic evaluation of surgically resected CCMs from patients treated with radiosurgery anywhere from 1 to 10 years prior, failed to demonstrate complete obliteration. Indeed, the main histologic finding observed in previously radiated CCM specimens is only the presence of fibrinoid necrosis.[34] Based on these clinical and pathologic results, there is no current evidence that radiosurgery is an effective treatment for CCMs.

◆ Surgical Technique

The surgical goal of CCM removal is to completely excise the lesion while minimizing contact with normal brain tissue and preserving the branches of the associated venous anomaly that does not appear to be draining the CCM. Preoperative and potentially intraoperative MRIs are essential in realizing this goal. The preoperative MRI assists in planning the surgical approach that allows for the best visualization of the lesion. For lesions that are not immediately visible upon exposure of the brain, an intraoperative MRI with stereotactic images may assist in localizing the lesion. Preoperative functional MRI (fMRI) data can also be co-registered with stereotactic images and can provide useful intraoperative information regarding borders of eloquent cortex for supratentorial lesions.

Once the CCM is visualized, bipolar cauterization is used to enter and shrink the lesion. Acute, subacute, and chronic blood is frequently seen within the cavernoma and should be suctioned from the lesion. A gliotic pseudocapsule typically provides a surgical plane along which the lesion can be resected, and by working circumferentially around the lesion in this plane, the CCM will eventually be freed from surrounding tissue. If a pseudocapsule is absent from the lesion, the malformed capillaries must be gently dissected from the surrounding parenchyma with microdissectors, taking care to avoid any damage to neighboring venous anomalies. Finally, before closing, the surgical site should be carefully inspected for evidence of satellite lesions and cavernoma remnants. If present, they should be coagulated or resected regardless of location, but with appropriate caution in infratentorial lesions. If there is any doubt as to whether these findings are related to the cavernoma in infratentorial lesions, it is best to err on the side of caution and remove only tissue that is known to stem from the CCM. The same concept applies to removing hemosiderin-stained parenchyma, which can be freely resected in supratentorial lesions as long as it is far from areas of critical function. In infratentorial lesions, these must be considered on a case-by-case basis, partially depending on whether the patient has a history of seizures. Once all CCM remnants are removed, closure can proceed in the typical fashion, followed by transfer of the patient to the appropriate intensive care unit. All patients should have a postoperative MRI shortly after surgery. The MRI should be scrutinized for evidence of lesion remnants, and, if residual cavernoma is present in a region that is surgically accessible, the patient should return to the operating room for removal of the remainder of the lesion. If evidence of residual lesion is completely absent, the patient should be cured, and no further neurosurgical follow-up is necessary unless the patient becomes symptomatic, suggesting incomplete removal or development of a new lesion.

◆ Outcomes

Patients undergoing surgical removal of CCMs generally have good outcomes, with low neurologic morbidity and minimal mortality. The risks involved with operative management vary greatly depending on location, with supratentorial lesions having the lowest associated risks. Because seizures are a common symptom among patients with supratentorial cavernomas, several studies have investigated the outcome of seizures after resection of these lesions. In one of the largest studies, lesions were removed completely from the 168 study participants. In the first 3 years after surgery, 65% of subjects were cured of disabling seizures, with half of them remaining completely seizure-free during this time. No mortality occurred, and mild postoperative neurologic deficits were seen in only 12 patients.[35] These results suggest that removal of supratentorial CCMs is not only a relatively safe option, but that this procedure is also an effective treatment for the majority of patients experiencing seizures due to a lesion in this area.

Although infratentorial cavernomas are usually associated with higher surgical morbidity and mortality than supratentorial lesions, the benefits of surgical management of these lesions, in experienced hands, may still outweigh the risks. In one retrospective study of 100 patients with brainstem cavernomas, only 12% of cases had significant complications that extended beyond the postoperative period. In addition, at follow-up 36 months later, only 9% of these patients had postoperative outcomes that were worse than their preoperative state. In contrast, neurologic functioning of 42% of patients who were managed conservatively declined over a

36-month interval.[8] These results suggest that even though surgery for infratentorial lesions may have a greater associated risk, the long-term benefit of surgery may outweigh that of conservative management. Although these findings are important to consider when deciding on the optimal treatment plan for a patient, each case must be dealt with on an individual basis.

References

1. Clatterbuck RE, Eberhart CG, Crain BJ, Rigamonti D. Ultrastructural and immunocytochemical evidence that an incompetent blood-brain barrier is related to the pathophysiology of cavernous malformations. J Neurol Neurosurg Psychiatry 2001;71:188–192
2. Tu J, Stoodley MA, Morgan MK, Storer KP. Ultrastructural characteristics of hemorrhagic, nonhemorrhagic, and recurrent cavernous malformations. J Neurosurg 2005;103:903–909
3. Wong JH, Awad IA, Kim JH. Ultrastructural pathological features of cerebrovascular malformations: a preliminary report. Neurosurgery 2000; 46:1454–1459
4. Robinson JR, Awad IA, Little JR. Natural history of the cavernous angioma. J Neurosurg 1991;75:709–714
5. Otten P, Pizzolato GP, Rilliet B, Berney J. 131 cases of cavernous angioma (cavernomas) of the CNS, discovered by retrospective analysis of 24,535 autopsies. Neurochirurgie 1989;35:82–83, 128–131
6. Giombini S, Morello G. Cavernous angiomas of the brain. Account of fourteen personal cases and review of the literature. Acta Neurochir (Wien) 1978;40:61–82
7. Lonjon M, Roche JL, George B, et al. Intracranial cavernoma. 30 cases. Presse Med 1993;22:990–994
8. Porter RW, Detwiler PW, Spetzler RF, et al. Cavernous malformations of the brainstem: experience with 100 patients. J Neurosurg 1999;90: 50–58
9. Abe T, Singer RJ, Marks MP, Norbash AM, Crowley RS, Steinberg GK. Coexistence of occult vascular malformations and developmental venous anomalies in the central nervous system: MR evaluation. AJNR Am J Neuroradiol 1998;19:51–57
10. Clatterbuck RE, Moriarity JL, Elmaci I, Lee RR, Breiter SN, Rigamonti D. Dynamic nature of cavernous malformations: a prospective magnetic resonance imaging study with volumetric analysis. J Neurosurg 2000; 93:981–986
11. Scott RM, Barnes P, Kupsky W, Adelman LS. Cavernous angiomas of the central nervous system in children. J Neurosurg 1992;76:38–46
12. Simard JM, Garcia-Bengochea F, Ballinger WE Jr, Mickle JP, Quisling RG. Cavernous angioma: a review of 126 collected and 12 new clinical cases. Neurosurgery 1986;18:162–172
13. Del Curling O Jr, Kelly DL Jr, Elster AD, Craven TE. An analysis of the natural history of cavernous angiomas. J Neurosurg 1991;75:702–708
14. Bertalanffy H, Benes L, Miyazawa T, Alberti O, Siegel AM, Sure U. Cerebral cavernomas in the adult. Review of the literature and analysis of 72 surgically treated patients. Neurosurg Rev 2002;25:1–53, discussion 54–55
15. Brown RD Jr, Flemming KD, Meyer FB, Cloft HJ, Pollock BE, Link ML. Natural history, evaluation, and management of intracranial vascular malformations. Mayo Clin Proc 2005;80:269–281
16. Samii M, Eghbal R, Carvalho GA, Matthies C. Surgical management of brainstem cavernomas. J Neurosurg 2001;95:825–832
17. Zabramski JM, Wascher TM, Spetzler RF, et al. The natural history of familial cavernous malformations: results of an ongoing study. J Neurosurg 1994;80:422–432
18. Houtteville JP. The surgery of cavernomas both supra-tentorial and infra-tentorial. Adv Tech Stand Neurosurg 1995;22:185–259
19. Dubovsky J, Zabramski JM, Kurth J, et al. A gene responsible for cavernous malformations of the brain maps to chromosome 7q. Hum Mol Genet 1995;4:453–458
20. Labauge P, Laberge S, Brunereau L, Levy C, Tournier-Lasserve E. Hereditary cerebral cavernous angiomas: clinical and genetic features in 57 French families. Société Française de Neurochirurgie. Lancet 1998;352: 1892–1897
21. Guzeloglu-Kayisli O, Amankulor NM, Voorhees J, Luleci G, Lifton RP, Gunel M. KRIT1/cerebral cavernous malformation 1 protein localizes to vascular endothelium, astrocytes, and pyramidal cells of the adult human cerebral cortex. Neurosurgery 2004;54:943–949, discussion 949
22. Whitehead KJ, Plummer NW, Adams JA, Marchuk DA, Li DY. Ccm1 is required for arterial morphogenesis: implications for the etiology of human cavernous malformations. Development 2004;131:1437–1448

23. Plummer NW, Gallione CJ, Srinivasan S, Zawistowski JS, Louis DN, Marchuk DA. Loss of p53 sensitizes mice with a mutation in Ccm1 (KRIT1) to development of cerebral vascular malformations. Am J Pathol 2004;165:1509–1518

24. Uhlik MT, Abell AN, Johnson NL, et al. Rac-MEKK3-MKK3 scaffolding for p38 MAPK activation during hyperosmotic shock. Nat Cell Biol 2003; 5:1104–1110

25. Plummer NW, Squire TL, Srinivasan S, et al. Neuronal expression of the Ccm2 gene in a new mouse model of cerebral cavernous malformations. Mamm Genome 2006;17:119–128

26. Whitehead KJ, Chan AC, Navankasattusas S, et al. The cerebral cavernous malformation signaling pathway promotes vascular integrity via Rho GTPases. Nat Med 2009;15:177–184

27. Tanriover G, Boylan AJ, Diluna ML, Pricola KL, Louvi A, Gunel M. PDCD10, the gene mutated in cerebral cavernous malformation 3, is expressed in the neurovascular unit. Neurosurgery 2008;62:930–938, discussion 938

28. Chen L, Tanriover G, Yano H, Friedlander R, Louvi A, Gunel M. Apoptotic functions of PDCD10/CCM3, the gene mutated in cerebral cavernous malformation 3. Stroke 2009;40:1474–1481

29. Voss K, Stahl S, Hogan BM, et al. Functional analyses of human and zebrafish 18-amino acid in-frame deletion pave the way for domain mapping of the cerebral cavernous malformation 3 protein. Hum Mutat 2009;30:1003–1011

30. Kim DG, Choe WJ, Paek SH, Chung HT, Kim IH, Han DH. Radiosurgery of intracranial cavernous malformations. Acta Neurochir (Wien) 2002; 144:869–878, discussion 878

31. Hasegawa T, McInerney J, Kondziolka D, Lee JY, Flickinger JC, Lunsford LD. Long-term results after stereotactic radiosurgery for patients with cavernous malformations. Neurosurgery 2002;50:1190–1197, discussion 1197–1198

32. Kondziolka D, Lunsford LD, Flickinger JC, Kestle JR. Reduction of hemorrhage risk after stereotactic radiosurgery for cavernous malformations. J Neurosurg 1995;83:825–831

33. Karlsson B, Kihlström L, Lindquist C, Ericson K, Steiner L. Radiosurgery for cavernous malformations. J Neurosurg 1998;88:293–297

34. Gewirtz RJ, Steinberg GK, Crowley R, Levy RP. Pathological changes in surgically resected angiographically occult vascular malformations after radiation. Neurosurgery 1998;42:738–742, discussion 742–743

35. Baumann CR, Acciarri N, Bertalanffy H, et al. Seizure outcome after resection of supratentorial cavernous malformations: a study of 168 patients. Epilepsia 2007;48:559–563

25

Intracranial Dural Arteriovenous Fistulas

Brian J. Jian, Vineeta Singh, and Michael T. Lawton

Pearls

◆ A dural arteriovenous fistula (DAVF) is an abnormal connection between an artery or arteries that supply the dura mater and a vein or venous sinus contained within the leaflets of dura, not in the brain parenchyma, with similar hemodynamics to a brain arteriovenous malformation (AVM): low resistance, high flow arteriovenous shunting, and a susceptibility to hemorrhage that is three to five times greater than brain AVMs.

◆ Dural arteriovenous fistulas are acquired lesions that develop in response to venous pathology: venous hypertension, caused by any venous outflow occlusion, impairs cerebral perfusion and produces venous ischemia; angiogenesis factors such as hypoxia-inducible factor-1 (HIF-1) and vascular endothelial growth factor (VEGF) are released as a compensatory response; and aberrant angiogenesis leads to DAVF formation, arteriovenous shunting, and exacerbation of underlying venous hypertension (angiogenesis hypothesis).

◆ Borden type I DAVFs drain anterograde into the associated dural venous sinus or meningeal veins; type II DAVFs drain into dural venous sinuses or meningeal veins, but also have retrograde drainage into cortical veins; and type III DAVFs drain exclusively into cortical veins, without venous sinus or meningeal venous drainage. Borden types II and III are associated with increased hemorrhage risk, and treatment is indicated for these patients.

◆ Dural arteriovenous fistulas are categorized as supratentorial, tentorial, and infratentorial. Supratentorial lesions include superior sagittal sinus and sphenoparietal sinus DAVFs, ethmoidal DAVFs, and carotid-cavernous fistulas; tentorial lesions include galenic, straight sinus, torcular, tentorial sinus, superior petrosal sinus, and incisural DAVFs; and infratentorial DAVFs include transverse-sigmoid sinus, marginal sinus, and inferior petrosal sinus DAVFs.

◆ Surgical treatment of DAVFs consists of following the arterialized cortical draining vein retrograde to the DAVF, and then interrupting the fistulous connection between the arteries in the dura and the draining vein or veins, typically with a clip or cautery on the venous side of the fistula.

Dural arteriovenous fistulas (DAVF) are fascinating lesions. Very simply, a DAVF is an abnormal connection between an artery or arteries that supply the dura mater and a vein or venous sinus contained within the leaflets of dura. DAVFs have similar hemodynamics to brain arteriovenous malformations (AVMs), with low-resistance, high-flow arteriovenous shunting. These dangerous hemodynamics make DAVFs susceptible to hemorrhage similar to brain AVMs, often with an annual rupture risk that is three to five times greater than that of brain AVMs. The fistula resides in the dura and not in the brain parenchyma, distinguishing it from a brain AVM. Intracranial DAVFs are not nearly as common as brain AVMs, with an incidence that is one-tenth that of AVMs. DAVFs have been observed repeatedly to form in patients and can be induced experimentally with venous hypertension in animals, lending themselves to laboratory investigation. Similarities between DAVFs and brain AVMs have led to misnomers for this lesion, such as dural AVM, but it is now clear that this lesion is not a congenital malformation resulting from an embryologic mishap but an acquired lesion with a pathogenesis that is increasingly understood. Similarities between the clinical presentation of and angiographic findings in patients with DAVFs and brain AVMs can also lead to misdiagnosis of DAVFs and mistakes in management. This chapter reviews the pathogenesis, natural history, management options, and surgical techniques associated with DAVFs. These lesions can be treated safely and effectively with endovascular, microsurgical, and combined techniques, but they require a sharp diagnostic eye to plan interventions appropriately.

◆ Pathogenesis

Several hypotheses for DAVF pathogenesis have been proposed, the most common one being that of intrinsic arteriovenous channels in dura mater opening up in response to an inciting event such as venous sinus thrombosis. Pathologic and radiologic studies have identified arteriovenous communications normally present in dura mater.[1] Meningeal arteries give rise to a rich anastomotic network of vessels on the outer or periosteal surface of the dura, with arterial branches to the skull, arterioles to the dura, secondary anastomotic arteries, and arteriovenous (AV) shunts. These intrinsic AV shunts are susceptible to changes in venous pressure, and increases in pressure in the venous sinuses can open these shunts to initiate arteriovenous flow. Growth of dural arteries, for example during organization of the thrombus causing a venous sinus occlusion, enlarges these arteriovenous shunts and stimulates DAVF formation.

Another hypothesis suggests that DAVFs develop from dysautoregulation of the dural arterioles.[2] In the setting of chronic venous hypertension, dural arterioles vasodilate in response to elevated back pressures on the venous side. Over time, maximally dilated sphincters in arterioles lose autoregulatory control, turning normal capillary connections into AV shunts and a DAVF. This hypothesis also implicates intrinsic dural channels that become dysfunctional in response to venous hypertension. The initiation of AV shunt flow generates positive feedback for DAVF enlargement.

Inflammation caused by venous sinus thrombosis was one of the earliest explanations of DAVF pathogenesis. Angiographically, patients presenting with an acute sinus thrombosis and no angiographic evidence of DAVF were observed on follow-up studies to have recanalized their sinus and developed a new DAVF. Pathologic studies of resected DAVF specimens demonstrated inflammatory activity, organization of thrombus, and recanalization of venous sinus, to varying degrees. Although it is easy to assume that inflammation triggered DAVF formation in these cases, venous sinus thrombosis is not an infrequent problem and the incidence of DAVF formation is low in these patients. In addition, animal models have demonstrated that sinus thrombosis alone is not sufficient for DAVF formation; venous hypertension is also required with sinus thrombosis.[3]

Angiogenesis was implicated in the pathogenesis of DAVFs when surgical specimens were observed to have neovascular activity in the overall inflammatory reaction to venous sinus thrombosis.[4] An angiogenesis hypothesis proposes that DAVF formation results from newly formed connections between dural arteries and venous sinuses, rather than from preexisting connections opening or becoming dysfunctional. Originally, angiogenesis was considered a by-product of inflammation, but inflammatory angiogenesis at the site of sinus thrombosis fails to explain the not infrequent formation of a DAVF remote from the site of venous sinus thrombosis.

An alternative angiogenesis hypothesis proposes that DAVF formation is a response to abnormal cerebral circulation. Angiogenesis activity in dural specimens was shown to be related to elevated venous sinus pressure and angiographic DAVF formation in a rat model, establishing for the first time a causal link between noninflammatory angiogenesis and venous hypertension.[5] This study by Lawton et al also demonstrated regression of DAVFs with elimination of venous hypertension. This angiogenesis hypothesis suggests that venous hypertension, which might be caused by any venous outflow occlusion, impairs cerebral perfusion and produces venous ischemia. Angiogenesis is triggered as a compensatory response, but aberrant angiogenesis may lead to DAVF formation. In this hypothesis, AV shunting exacerbates underlying venous hypertension and initiates a vicious cycle.

Subsequent investigation found increased expression of known angiogenesis factors such as vascular endothelial growth factor (VEGF) in astrocytes using similar animal models[6–8] and in surgically resected DAVFs.[9] Recently, expression of the upstream regulator of angiogenesis, hypoxia-inducible factor-1 (HIF-1), demonstrated a rapid increase in response to venous hypertension, located in endothelial cells in parasagittal venules adjacent to the hypertensive sinus.[8] These studies confirm the link between venous hypertension and angiogenesis, but suggest a hemodynamic mechanism rather than an ischemic mechanism (**Fig. 25.1**). DAVF pathogenesis is far from solved, but existing evidence clarifies that this is an acquired lesion with a dynamic clinical course.

◆ Risk Factors for Dural Arteriovenous Fistula Formation

Based on this understanding of DAVF pathogenesis, cerebral venous thrombosis and conditions contributing to it are risk factors for DAVF formation. Inherited predispositions to thrombosis include factor V Leiden mutation,[10,11] MTHFR C677T mutation,[12] and prothrombin gene *20210* mutation.[13] Patients who have both factor V Leiden and prothrombin gene *20210* mutations are at a higher risk of developing venous thrombosis than those with either one alone.[14–16] These mutations have been reported in patients with DAVFs,[17–20] and a study found a higher frequency of prothrombin gene *20210A* mutation in patients with DAVF compared with controls.[20] In our experience, approximately one third of patients with DAVF test positively for thrombophilia (factor V Leiden, MTHFR, and/or prothrombin gene mutations).[21] In addition, these patients are more likely to present with venous sinus thrombosis or occlusion and with focal neurologic deficits. Based on these findings, we routinely test for factor V Leiden and prothrombin gene mutation in DAVF patients to help manage possible thrombotic complications. Some authors have suggested following blood levels of D-dimer as an indication of acute venous thrombosis in DAVF patients.[22] Although we are particularly interested in cerebral venous thrombosis and its role in the pathogenesis of DAVFs, it should be noted that angiographic venous occlusion is present in only approximately 20% of all DAVF patients.

Head trauma is the most obvious cause of DAVF formation, with development of symptoms such as a loud cranial bruit[23] at the time of injury and confirmed angiographically. The most common traumatic fistula is a direct communication between the internal carotid artery (ICA) and the cavernous sinus (carotid-cavernous fistula [CCF]), resulting from basilar skull fractures, dissections that ruptures into the cavernous sinus, direct penetrating trauma, or iatrogenic causes (e.g., transsphenoidal surgery, percutaneous trigeminal rhizotomy, or catheter angioplasty). Trauma may also involve the cranial convexity and injure superior sagittal and transverse sinuses.

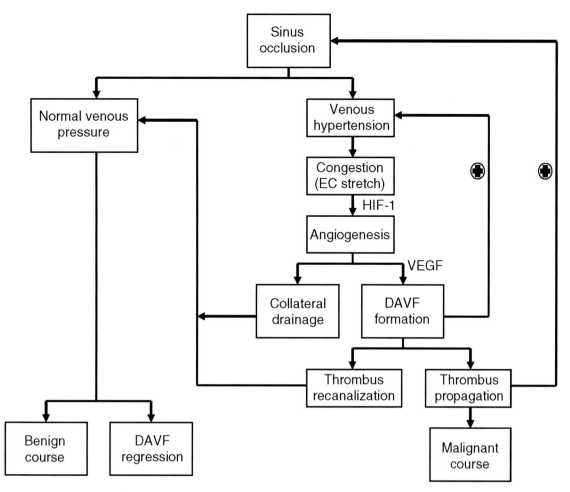

Fig. 25.1 Summary of the angiogenesis hypothesis for the pathogenesis of dural arteriovenous fistulas (DAVFs). An obstruction to venous outflow, like a sinus thrombosis, would produce venous hypertension in some patients. Venous hypertension congests the cerebral circulation and stretches venous endothelial cells, which increases expression of hypoxia inducible factor-1 (HIF-1). This signal triggers angiogenesis activity and vascular endothelial growth factor (VEGF) expression, DAVF formation, and arteriovenous shunting into the dural sinuses. Arterialization of the venous sinuses exacerbates venous hypertension and may also exacerbate outflow occlusion by promoting thrombus propagation. A vicious cycle is initiated that enlarges the DAVF, and causes retrograde cortical venous drainage and a malignant clinical course. In contrast to this pathophysiology, physiologic angiogenesis attempts to increase relieve venous congestion and establish collateral venous drainage around an obstructed sinus. DAVFs not exposed to venous hypertension would have a benign clinical course or may even regress. EC, endothelial cell.

Posttraumatic DAVFs may present with clinical symptoms weeks to years after the head trauma.

Cranial surgery has been associated with DAVF formation, especially meningioma resection.[24–26] We have observed small DAVFs after ventriculostomy and after craniotomy for routine vascular cases, when postoperative angiography is performed to assess complete aneurysm clipping or AVM resection. These DAVFs are probably due to local trauma, but DAVFs have been reported remote from the surgical site.

Dural arteriovenous fistulas are more common in women than men. In our experience with 400 patients, 57% were women and 43% were men. CCFs were even more likely in women (7:1 female predominance), suggesting a hormonal risk. However, this predominance is modest (2:1) in other locations such as the transverse-sigmoid sinus,[27,28] and eth-moidal DAVFs have a male predominance. An increased frequency of DAVF diagnosis has been noted during pregnancy,[29] suggesting pregnancy may predispose women to DAVF development. Most women with DAVFs develop their first symptoms later in pregnancy or in the peripartum period. Estrogen may play a role in DAVF formation, based on reports of worsened symptoms in premenstrual women with DAVFs,[30] a higher prevalence of DAVF in postmenopausal women,[31] and regression of DAVF with oral estrogen.[32] The risk of estrogen in DAVF formation remains unproven.

Other rare causes of DAVF formation are chronic otitis media, hypertension, and arterial dysplasias such as Ehlers-Danlos syndrome (type IV), neurofibromatosis, and Rendu-Osler-Weber disease. Some DAVFs have no identifiable cause, and these lesions are considered spontaneous in origin.

◆ Dural Arteriovenous Fistula Classification and Natural History

Numerous classifications have been reported to help understand the varied anatomy and behavior of these diverse lesions. Djindjian and Merland were the first to propose a classification system for intracranial DAVFs, analyzing the number of fistulas, the direction of blood flow, and the venous drainage pattern. Cognard later proposed a system of five types based on drainage or reflux: anterograde venous sinus drainage (type I), reflux into cortical veins (type II), retrograde cortical venous drainage (type III), retrograde cortical venous drainage with venous ectasia (type IV), and spinal venous drainage (type V). The University of California at San Francisco (UCSF) grading system divides DAVFs into four grades: DAVFs with normal anterograde venous sinus drainage without venous restriction or cortical venous drainage (grade 1); DAVFs with both anterograde and retrograde venous sinus drainage with or without cortical venous drainage (grade 2); DAVFs with retrograde venous sinus drainage and cortical venous drainage (grade 3); and DAVFs with only retrograde cortical venous drainage (grade 4).

The number and subtleties of these classifications tends to confuse rather than simplify the angiographic interpretation of these lesions. The Borden classification unifies and simplifies these other classification and has become the more accepted system.[33] Type I DAVFs drain anterograde into the associated dural venous sinus or meningeal veins. Type II DAVFs drain into dural venous sinuses or meningeal veins, but also have retrograde drainage into cortical veins. Type III DAVFs drain exclusively into cortical veins, without venous sinus or meningeal venous drainage.

The purpose of this classification is to identify DAVFs with increased risk of hemorrhage, thereby identifying those patients in need of treatment. Borden types II and III are associated with increased hemorrhage risk, and treatment is indicated in these patients. In addition to helping select patients for treatment, the Borden classification provides general guidelines for treatment. Type 1 DAVFs are treated with transarterial embolization or surgical skeletonization of the venous sinuses if venous drainage needs to be preserved. Type II DAVFs are treated by interruption of the arterialized draining cortical vein and occlusion or excision of the venous sinus. Type III DAVFs are treated by interruption of the arterialized draining cortical vein. Unlike with brain AVMs, DAVFs do not require resection, and the draining vein can be safely occluded without excising the dura containing the lesion.

◆ Clinical Presentation

Pathologic consequences of DAVF include arterialization of the venous system at the site of fistula, which can lead to venous hypertension and congestion, and can induce cerebral ischemia and hemorrhage. Some DAVFs can be benign, presenting as an incidental angiographic finding or minor symptoms like headache or pulsatile tinnitus from turbulent blood flow through the shunt. Some DAVFs can be malignant, presenting with progressive neurologic deterioration from venous ischemia or acute deterioration from intracranial hemorrhage.

The variety of symptoms is wide and also includes double vision, visual obscuration, focal neurologic deficits, seizures, and progressive dementia.[34–39] Pulsatile tinnitus, headache, and visual disturbances were the three most common presenting symptoms in our cohort of DAVF patients.[21]

Type of presentation and severity of symptoms are determined by the location of the fistula, the anatomy of venous drainage, and resultant alterations in cerebral hemodynamics. Alterations in hemodynamics depend on the volume of shunt flow and the degree of compromise of venous outflow. The exact mechanism has not been fully investigated and the relation to patient's symptoms is not always clear.[40–42] The annual risk of hemorrhage from a DAVF with cortical venous drainage is as high as 19% annually. Mortality and neurologic morbidity associated with hemorrhagic presentation has been estimated to be 20 to 30%. Cortical venous drainage and posterior fossa location of the DAVF were independent predictors of a hemorrhagic presentation.[21]

Dural arteriovenous fistula patients present at a mean age of 50 to 60 years. No sex predilection has been established, although men appear more likely than women to present with hemorrhage. An underlying DAVF should be suspected in patients with nontraumatic intracerebral hemorrhage (ICH) with a subarachnoid component.[21] Women with DAVF more commonly present with pulsatile tinnitus than do men, whereas men usually present with nontraumatic intraparenchymal and subarachnoid hemorrhage.[21]

◆ Types of Dural Arteriovenous Fistulas

Our surgical experience with DAVFs consists of 81 patients, and half of these patients had DAVFs located in the tentorium (Table 25.1). We categorized the tentorial DAVFs into six types: galenic, straight sinus, torcular, tentorial sinus, superior petrosal sinus, and incisural DAVFs. Therefore, DAVFs do not differentiate neatly into the usual supra- and infratentorial categories like many other intracranial lesions, and instead we consider DAVFs as supratentorial, tentorial, and infratentorial.

Supratentorial DAVFs include superior sagittal sinus and sphenoparietal sinus DAVFs, ethmoidal DAVFs, and carotid-cavernous fistulas. Infratentorial DAVFs include transverse-sigmoid sinus, marginal sinus, and inferior petrosal sinus DAVFs.

In decreasing order of frequency, the common types of DAVFs are carotid-cavernous fistula, transverse-sigmoid sinus, and superior sagittal DAVFs. However, these lesions are amenable to endovascular therapy, and the common types of DAVFs in our surgical experience are different. In decreasing order of frequency, the common types of DAVFs treated surgically are straight sinus, transverse-sigmoid sinus, and ethmoidal DAVFs.

Supratentorial Dural Arteriovenous Fistulas

Carotid-Cavernous Fistulas

A CCF is any abnormal communication between the ICA, external carotid artery (ECA), or any of their branches and the

Table 25.1 Patient Distribution of Dural Arteriovenous Fistulas (DAVFs) Categorized by Location During a 12-Year Period

DAVF	Patients	%
Supratentorial		
Superior sagittal sinus	7	8.6
Carotid-cavernous sinus	1	1.2
Ethmoidal	11	13.6
Sphenoparietal sinus	5	6.2
Tentorial		
Galenic	7	8.6
Straight sinus	14	17.3
Torcular	8	9.9
Tentorial sinus	2	2.5
Superior petrosal sinus	8	9.9
Incisural	2	2.5
Infratentorial		
Transverse-sigmoid sinus	13	16.0
Marginal sinus	3	3.7
Inferior petrosal sinus	0	0.0
Total	81	100.0

cavernous sinus. CCFs can be classified hemodynamically into high-flow and low-flow fistulas, or anatomically into direct and indirect fistulas. The Barrow classification recognizes four types of CCF: type A is a direct fistula between the intracavernous ICA and cavernous sinus; type B is a dural AV shunt between intracavernous branches of the ICA (such as the branches from the meningohypophyseal trunk or inferolateral trunk) and the cavernous sinus; type C is a dural AV shunt between meningeal branches of the ECA (such as the accessory middle meningeal artery or ascending pharyngeal artery) and the cavernous sinus; and type D is a dural AV shunt between intracavernous branches of both the ICA and ECA and the cavernous sinus. Type A CCFs usually occur in the setting of head trauma or as a result of a ruptured cavernous ICA aneurysm. These fistulas have high-flow and produce symptoms related to venous engorgement of the orbit, including pulsatile exophthalmos, chemosis, cranial nerve III, IV and VI paresis, and rarely glaucoma and visual loss. Types B, C, and D CCFs usually occur spontaneously or following minor trauma with symptoms that are less severe and more insidious in their onset. These indirect CCFs may occur at any age, but are more commonly present in women older than 40 years and may be associated with conditions such as vascular Ehlers-Danlos syndrome, hypertension, hypercoagulability, or pregnancy, among others.[43,44] Their pathogenesis has been hypothesized in some cases to be related to prior, clinically silent, thrombosis of the cavernous sinus with subsequent formation of aberrant vascular connections during recanalization.[43]

Type A CCFs require treatment to prevent progressive visual loss, reverse unsightly exophthalmos, or eliminate intolerable bruits or pain. The treatment is endovascular, occluding the fistula with a detachable balloon deployed from a microcatheter in the ICA and inflated in the fistula. These CCFs can also be occluded transvenously with coils in the cavernous sinus, deployed using microcatheters that reach the fistula via the internal jugular vein and inferior petrosal sinus.

Cavernous sinus DAVFs (types B, C, and D) have a benign natural history and often resolve spontaneously. Carotid self-compression (20 seconds, three to four times per hour when awake, using the contralateral hand) may promote thrombosis of the DAVF, but is contraindicated in patients with high-grade carotid stenosis or ulcerative plaques. Endovascular intervention is indicated in patients with visual deterioration, progressive intraocular hypertension, obtrusive diplopia, proptosis with corneal exposure, or intolerable bruit. ECA feeding arteries can be embolized safely in patients with types C and D CCFs, usually resulting in cures. Persistent lesions can be treated additionally with transvenous embolization. Selective catheterization of ICA feeding arteries is more difficult, and embolization is associated with an increased risk of cerebral emboli, but type B lesions are rare. Refractory CCFs that fail endovascular therapy and remain with retrograde cortical venous drainage may require surgical intervention to occlude the vein and interrupt the fistula (**Fig. 25.2**).

Superior Sagittal Sinus Dural Arteriovenous Fistula

Superior sagittal sinus (SSS) DAVFs are uncommon, but the difficulty in curing these lesions endovascularly makes them more prevalent in surgical series. In our experience, seven of 81 patients (9%) had SSS DAVFs with high-risk features. These lesions can present with pulsatile tinnitus, signs of raised intracranial pressure, or signs of raised cavernous sinus pressure from diversion of venous outflow. Local symptoms, such as focal seizures or focal neurologic deficits, can result in venous engorgement or varix formation and mass effect.

Superior sagittal sinus DAVFs are supplied by middle meningeal arteries or their branches. Scalp arteries (superficial temporal and occipital arteries) can also supply these DAVFs, as can cortical arteries. Venous drainage is primarily to the SSS, but these can be Borden type II or III lesions with cortical venous drainage through convexity veins. SSS DAVFs can be embolized transarterially with ease, but numerous meningeal feeding arteries make them difficult to cure. Fistulas with cortical venous drainage can also be difficult to cure endovascularly because there is typically poor access from the venous side.

Superior sagittal sinus DAVFs requiring surgery are exposed with a midline craniotomy over the sinus and the fistula. Cutting the craniotomy flap over the sinus requires careful preservation of the dura, particularly in older patients with adherent dura. Two separate flaps may be needed to first expose the ipsilateral dura and to allow the sinus to be dissected from the inner table of skull before crossing the midline with the second flap. Surgical management of the fistula depends on its Borden type. Type I SSS DAVFs are treated by skeletonizing the SSS extensively, eliminating the arterial

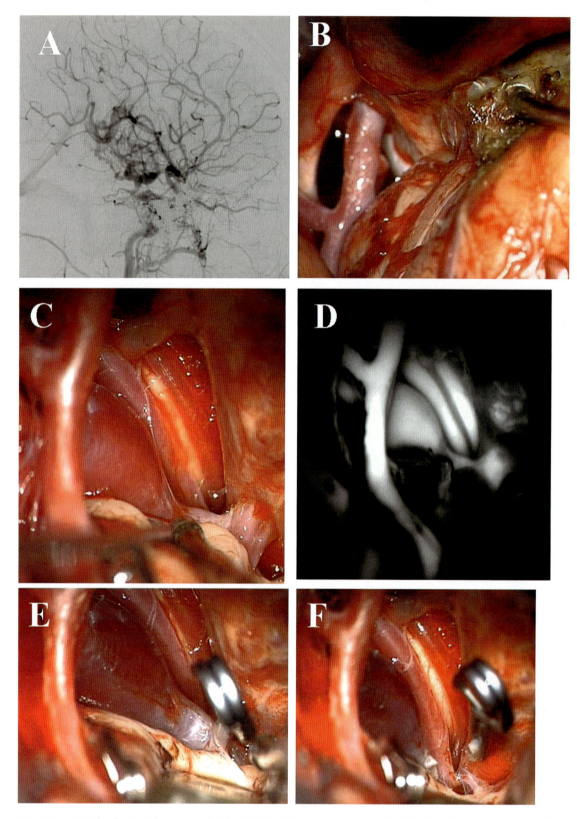

Fig. 25.2 Example of a carotid-cavernous fistula (CCF) that failed endovascular therapy. **(A)** This 8-year-old girl had multiple endovascular coiling treatments of her CCF, and persistent deep venous drainage to the basal vein of Rosenthal remained (right internal carotid artery angiogram, lateral view). **(B)** A right orbitozygomatic craniotomy exposed the lateral wall of cavernous sinus, where coils were seen. **(C)** The arterialized vein was identified at the tentorial edge and **(D)** indocyanine green videoangiography confirmed shunt flow. **(E)** The DAVF was interrupted with an aneurysm clip on the vein as it exited the tentorial dura, and **(F)** the vein was cut.

supply while preserving normal flow in the sinus. Type III SSS DAVFs are treated by interrupting the fistula on its venous side as it exits the sinus, usually by clipping the vein, cauterizing it, and dividing it. Type II SSS DAVFs are treated with a combination of skeletonization of the sinus and interruption of arterialized veins.

Sphenoparietal Sinus Dural Arteriovenous Fistulas

Sphenoparietal sinus DAVFs are also uncommon in the overall cohort of DAVF patients, with an incidence around half that of SSS DAVFs. We encountered five patients in our surgical cohort. Like SSS DAVFs, sphenoparietal sinus DAVFs are supplied by middle meningeal arteries or their branches, and by scalp arteries. Venous drainage is primarily into sylvian veins that can course posteriorly toward the vein of Labbé, inferiorly under the temporal lobe, or superiorly toward the SSS.

These lesions are exposed with a standard pterional craniotomy. In our experience, these DAVFs are typically Borden type III lesions that can be treated with simple interruption of the arterialized draining vein as it exits the dura over the sylvian fissure (**Fig. 25.3**).

Ethmoidal Dural Arteriovenous Fistulas

Ethmoidal DAVFs are located on the floor of the anterior cranial fossa, adjacent to the cribriform plate. The fistula is supplied by anterior ethmoidal arteries, and it drains directly into cortical veins at the frontal pole. Unlike all the other DAVFs, ethmoidal DAVFs are not associated with a venous sinus. This unusual anatomy accounts for their propensity to hemorrhage.

We previously reported an experience with 16 patients with ethmoidal DAVFs, the largest in the literature.[45] Half of our patients presented with hemorrhage. Nonhemorrhagic presentations included headaches, decreasing visual acuity, and diminished sense of smell and taste. Male predominance is also striking, with 11 men in our series (69%). The mean age was 62 years.

The anterior ethmoidal artery that feeds these DAVFs is a branch from the ophthalmic artery, which is in turn a branch from the ICA. Feeding arteries can arise unilaterally (50% of our patients) or bilaterally (50% of our patients). Branches from the ECA, namely the superficial temporal artery and internal maxillary artery, can also supply these lesions.

Endovascular treatment of ethmoidal DAVFs has not been widely performed for several reasons. First, selective catheterization of the ophthalmic and ethmoidal arteries is difficult due to the small caliber and tortuous course of these arteries. Second and most importantly, embolization of the central retinal artery, also a distal branch of the ophthalmic artery, can complicate the procedure and devastate a patient's vision. Third, unlike embolization of other DAVFs whose blood supply originates from the ECA, embolization of ethmoidal DAVFs through an ICA branch carries the risk of embolic agents refluxing into the cerebral circulation. These obstacles have deterred most endovascular surgeons from treating ethmoidal DAVFs. The endovascular results that have been published suggest that endovascular management of ethmoidal DAVFs has a small but clinically significant risk to vision, is rarely effective in curing the fistula, and does not eliminate the need for surgery.

These DAVFs are exposed through a bifrontal craniotomy and a subfrontal approach (**Fig. 25.4**). The patient is placed in the supine position with the head extended slightly. A bicoronal skin incision is needed to mobilize the scalp flap inferiorly enough for a low craniotomy. Pericranium is harvested during the approach to make it available for covering the frontal sinus, if it has been entered. Ethmoidal DAVFs are exposed optimally with a craniotomy flap whose medial border is either right on the superior sagittal sinus or crosses over to the contralateral side. Midline exposure enables the dura to be opened to the edge of the superior sagittal sinus and gives easy access to the interhemispheric fissure. The craniotomy flap is extended inferiorly as close to the anterior cranial fossa floor as possible. Crossing the midline with this cut sometimes requires drilling down the ridge of bone on the inner table in the midline.

Freeing the bone flap from the underlying dura can be difficult, given the age of many of these patients and the adherence of their dura. In these cases, the bone flap is divided adjacent to the superior sagittal sinus to visualize directly and dissect the sinus from the bone flap. The inner table of frontal bone in the inferior midline is drilled until flat, which increases visualization along the anterior cranial fossa floor and eliminates the need for frontal lobe retraction.

The critical maneuver is the interruption of the fistulous connection between the arteries perforating the dura around the cribriform plate and the draining vein or veins. The cortical draining vein is identified early during the dissection as it enters the superior sagittal sinus and followed retrograde to the DAVF. When present, the venous varix is encountered during the dissection and is typically the site of hemorrhage in patients who bled. Excessive manipulation or evacuation of the hematoma is avoided to prevent bleeding from the varix before the fistula is controlled.

Numerous arteries in the dura of the anterior cranial fossa floor and falx typically merge into a dilated draining vein. The vein is coagulated and divided. Occasionally there are posterior ethmoidal feeding arteries that are obscured from view by the frontal lobe or the varix, but nonetheless contribute fistulous flow. If persistent arteriovenous shunting is observed in the draining vein, the vein just distal to the fistula should be dissected further to identify these posterior feeding arteries. Dissecting the varix is useful for this reason, but it does not need to be resected. Excision of dura involved with the fistula and adjacent bone is not necessary.

After the DAVF is occluded, any associated hematoma can be evacuated completely without risk of rupturing the varix. Manipulation of the olfactory bulbs and tracts is minimized to preserve olfaction. If the frontal sinus was entered during the exposure, sinus mucosa is exenterated and the sinus is packed with Gelfoam. A vascularized pericranial flap is then laid down over the defect and sutured to the inferior frontal dura to block any communication with the intracranial compartment. The plated bone flap secures the pericranial flap's coverage of the defect.

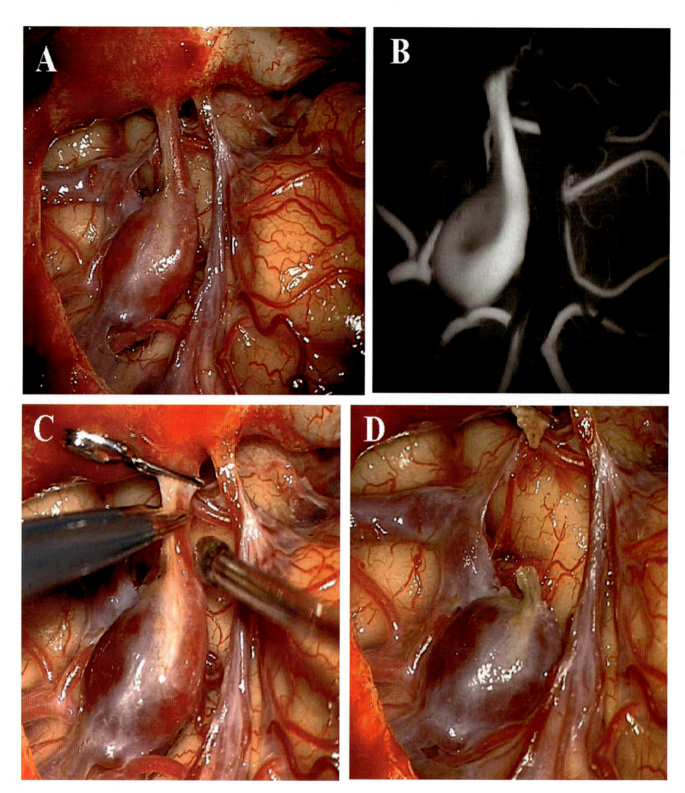

Fig. 25.3 Example of a sphenoparietal sinus DAVF. **(A)** A standard left pterional craniotomy exposed the sylvian fissure; the arterialized vein draining the fistula was identified. **(B)** Indocyanine green videoangiography confirmed shunt flow. **(C)** The DAVF was interrupted with an aneurysm clip on the vein as it exited the pterional dura, and **(D)** the vein was cut. Note the immediate color change of blood in the venous varix, confirming complete obliteration.

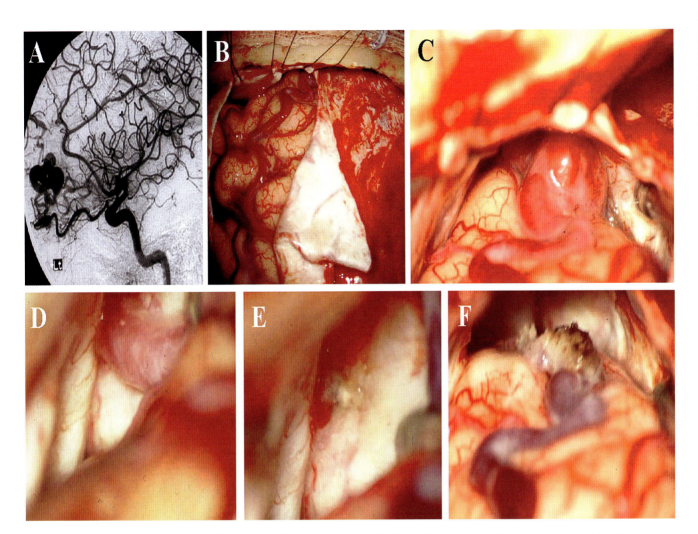

Fig. 25.4 Example of an ethmoidal DAVF. **(A)** Angiography demonstrates an ethmoidal DAVF feed by ethmoidal branches from the ophthalmic artery (left internal carotid artery injection, lateral view). **(B)** A low bifrontal craniotomy and removal of the inner table of inferior frontal bone widely exposes the anterior cranial fossa floor and the interhemispheric fissure without frontal lobe retraction. **(C)** Access to the fistula can be obscured by the venous varix, requiring the neurosurgeon to work carefully around it. **(D)** The arterialized vein is followed down to the fistulous site at the dura around the cribriform plate. **(E)** The draining vein is coagulated and interrupted, and **(F)** the varix and draining vein darken to confirm obliteration.

In our experience, surgical management has low associated risk, entails no risk to vision, affects a cure in all cases, and can contribute to good clinical outcomes in most patients. For these reasons, surgical management of ethmoidal DAVFs remains the treatment of choice.

Tentorial Dural Arteriovenous Fistulas

Tentorial DAVFs are rare and dangerous lesions.[46–52] In a meta-analysis of 377 patients with DAVF reported before 1989, tentorial DAVFs were less common than transverse-sigmoid sinus and cavernous sinus DAVFs (8% versus 63% and 12%, respectively), but tentorial DAVFs had the most aggressive neurologic behavior, with 97% causing hemorrhage or progressive focal neurologic deficits.[47] Tentorial DAVFs frequently have angiographic features associated with hemorrhage: retrograde drainage through cortical or subarachnoid veins, deep drainage through the vein of Galen, and venous varices. Consequently, tentorial DAVFs are treated aggressively when diagnosed, even in the absence of presenting hemorrhage.[50]

Tentorial DAVFs are difficult to cure with endovascular therapy. Their arterial supply is extensive, involving meningeal arteries from the ICA and the vertebral artery that are difficult to cannulate and riskier to embolize than ECA feeders. Transvenous navigation to deeper locations around the tentorium is difficult. More importantly, tentorial DAVFs often drain exclusively to subarachnoid veins rather than to their associated sinus (Borden type III), which prevents transvenous access.[46] Therefore, the management of tentorial DAVFs may require microsurgical interruption, unlike most other DAVFs.[48,53–60]

We categorize tentorial DAVFs into six types, based on anatomic location, dural base, associated venous sinus, and

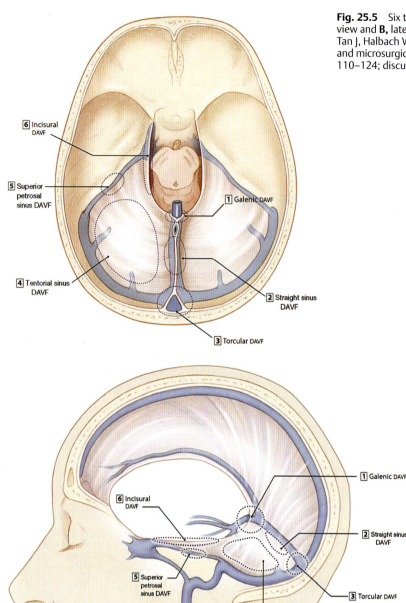

Fig. 25.5 Six types of tentorial dural arteriovenous fistulas (**A,** axial view and **B,** lateral view). (From Lawton M, Sanchez-Mejia RO, Pham D, Tan J, Halbach W. Tentorial arteriovenous fistulae: operative strategies and microsurgical results for six types. Neurosurgery 2008;62(3 Suppl 1): 110–124; discussion 124–125. Reprinted by permission.)

direction of venous drainage **(Fig. 25.5).** Galenic DAVFs (type 1) are located in the midline at the posterior margin of the tentorial incisura, associated with the vein of Galen as it enters the anterior falcotentorial junction, with venous drainage that can be supratentorial, infratentorial, or both **(Fig. 25.6).** Straight sinus DAVFs (type 2) are located in the midline along the falcotentorial junction, associated with the straight sinus, with drainage to veins on the undersurface of the tentorium. Torcular DAVFs (type 3) are located in the midline at the posterior margin of the falcotentorial junction, associated with the torcular, with supratentorial venous drainage. Tentorial sinus DAVFs (type 4) are located in the body of the tentorium, associated with the tentorial sinus,

with supratentorial drainage to occipital veins. Superior petrosal sinus DAVFs (type 5) are located laterally where the tentorium joins the dura of the middle cranial fossa, associated with the superior petrosal sinus, with infratentorial drainage to the petrosal vein and its tributaries. Incisural DAVFs (type 6) are located along the free edge of tentorium, not clearly associated with a venous sinus, with drainage into supratentorial veins in and around the ambient cistern.

Galenic Dural Arteriovenous Fistulas

Galenic DAVFs are the most complex of the six types of tentorial fistulas. The galenic region is the deepest location; the

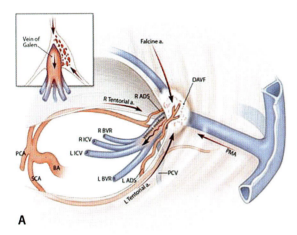

A

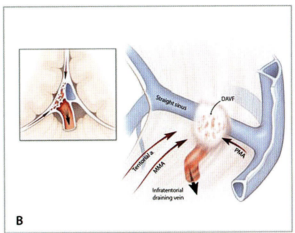

B

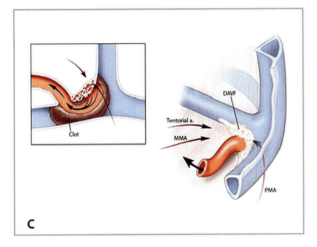

C

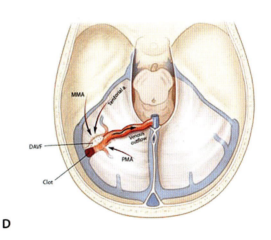

D

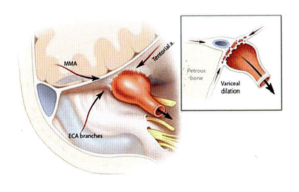

E

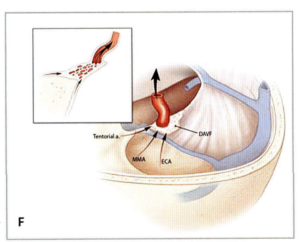

F

Fig. 25.6 Anatomy of tentorial dural arteriovenous fistulas by type. **(A)** Galenic DAVF (type 1). **(B)** Straight sinus DAVF (type 2). **(C)** Torcular DAVF (type 3). **(D)** Tentorial sinus DAVF (type 4). **(E)** Superior sagittal sinus DAVF (type 5). **(F)** Incisural DAVF (type 6). a., artery; ADS, artery of Davidoff and Schecter; BA, basilar artery; BVR, basal vein of Rosenthal; DAVF, dural arteriovenous fistula; ECA, external carotid artery; ICV, internal cerebral vein; L, left; MMA, middle meningeal artery; PCA, posterior cerebral artery; PCV, precentral cerebellar vein; PMA, posterior meningeal artery; R, right; SCA, superior cerebellar artery.

confluence of falx and tentorium creates awkward barriers and surgical blind spots; arterial inflow arrives from all directions; and venous outflow can be difficult to decipher, particularly when veins are tortuous or variceal. Consequently, a panoramic exposure is required that only the posterior interhemispheric approach **(Fig. 25.7)** can provide.[61] This approach is performed with the patient in the lateral position through a torcular craniotomy that exposes the superior sagittal sinus, both transverse sinuses, and the torcular. After opening the dura, the dependent occipital lobe is retracted by gravity, and the interhemispheric fissure opens widely without a retractor **(Fig. 25.8)**. Cuts in the falx above the straight sinus, and bilaterally in the tentorium parallel to the straight sinus, skeletonize the straight sinus and transform this unilateral, supratentorial exposure into a bilateral, supra- and infratentorial exposure. Anatomy in front of the fistula in the quadrigeminal and ambient cisterns can be visualized clearly.

Skeletonizing the straight sinus also de-arterializes galenic DAVFs. Transecting the tentorium obliterates supply from the tentorial arteries and ECA branches, whereas transecting the falx obliterates supply from the middle meningeal artery (MMA)/falcine arteries. Supply from the occipital artery is

already obliterated when the scalp flap is elevated, and posterior meningeal artery (PMA) can be interrupted along its course up the suboccipital dura to the torcular region. However, the goal of occluding the fistula is accomplished by interrupting the venous drainage, not by interrupting the arterial supply. Dural cuts are performed to widen the posterior interhemispheric corridor, visualize the galenic complex, and decipher the venous anatomy, not to de-arterialize the fistula.

Interruption of the fistula is completed by placing a clip on the vein draining the fistula, which requires meticulous microsurgical dissection of the venous anatomy. The vein of Galen and the internal cerebral veins are most prominent from the perspective of the posterior interhemispheric approach, but the internal cerebral vein is rarely the target for the occluding clip. The basal vein of Rosenthal and the precentral cerebellar vein are more commonly the target for the clip, but are also more difficult to visualize. The basal vein of Rosenthal is identified by dissecting lateral and inferior to the internal cerebral veins into the ambient cistern. The precentral cerebellar vein lies in a blind spot in the surgical corridor beneath the falcotentorial dura, but this untethered dura

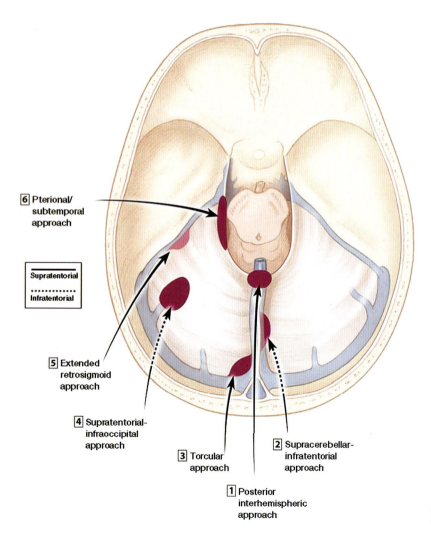

6 Pterional/ subtemporal approach

Supratentorial
Infratentorial

5 Extended retrosigmoid approach

4 Supratentorial-infraoccipital approach

3 Torcular approach

2 Supracerebellar-infratentorial approach

1 Posterior interhemispheric approach

Fig. 25.7 Summary of surgical approaches to tentorial dural arteriovenous fistulas.

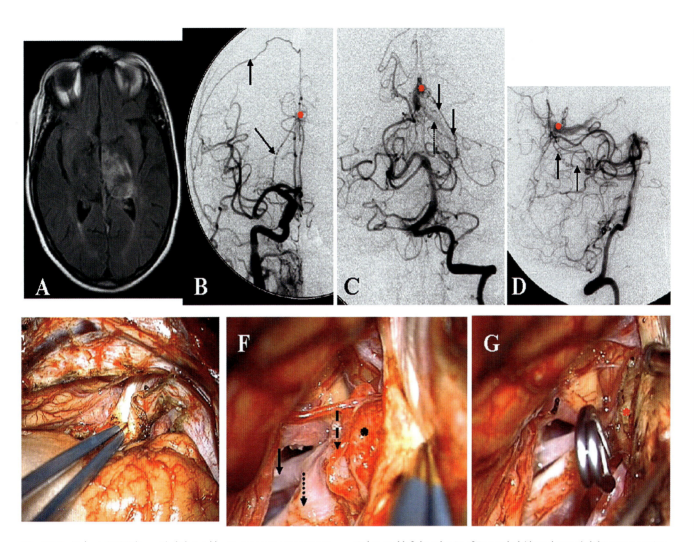

Fig. 25.8 Galenic DAVF (type 1). **(A)** Axial brain magnetic resonance imaging (MRI) (fluid-attenuated inversion recovery [FLAIR] sequence) showed increased signal in the left thalamus from retrograde venous drainage from the fistula to the vein of Galen, left basal vein of Rosenthal, and left internal cerebral vein. **(B)** Right internal carotid artery angiogram (anterior-posterior view) demonstrated arterial supply to the fistula *(red asterisk)* from the right tentorial artery *(dotted arrow)* and middle meningeal/falcine artery *(solid arrow)*. Left vertebral artery angiograms (**C,** anterior-posterior view, and **D,** lateral view) demonstrated arterial supply to the fistula *(red asterisk)* from the artery of Davidoff and Schecter *(solid arrows),* and drainage into the vein of Galen and left basal vein of Rosenthal *(dotted arrow)*. **(E)** Intraoperative photograph demonstrates the posterior interhemispheric approach, with the patient positioned laterally (left side down), gravity retraction of the left occipital lobe, and transection of the left tentorium and falx (at tips of bipolar forceps) to widen the exposure. **(F)** Reflection of the dura at the falcotentorial junction with the bipolar forceps visualized the fistula *(black asterisk)* and the vein of Galen complex (right basal vein of Rosenthal, *solid arrow;* right internal cerebral vein, *dotted arrow;* and artery of Davidoff and Schecter, *dashed arrow)*. **(G)** The straight sinus was already occluded, so the fistula *(red asterisk)* was interrupted with a clip placed on the vein of Galen as it exited the fistula.

can be mobilized aggressively to visualize the cerebellar veins. Veins that are red and dilated declare their participation in draining the fistula, whereas blue veins declare their participation in normal circulation. The connections between the fistulous dura and its arterialized draining veins are not always obvious from gross inspection of the extravascular anatomy.

Clip application is dictated by the straight sinus's patency, which must be determined preoperatively from the angiogram. All galenic DAVFs in our experience were Borden type III fistulas with retrograde drainage in the vein of Galen or its tributaries. However, not all straight sinuses were occluded in patients with galenic DAVFs; some straight sinuses had antegrade flow seen during the venous phase of the angiogram. A patent straight sinus requires vein of Galen preservation and clip application to occlude just the tributary vein draining the fistula, rather than the Galen trunk. Other tributary veins uninvolved with the fistulous outflow can continue to drain the deep cerebral circulation in an antegrade direction. In contrast, an occluded straight sinus allows clip application directly on the galenic trunk to occlude fistulous outflow, which usually requires less dissection and is easier to decipher.

The supracerebellar-infratentorial approach is an alternative approach to galenic DAVFs, which has the advantage of positioning the neurosurgeon on the same side of the tentorium as fistulas that drain inferiorly to cerebellar veins. However, the steep pitch of the tentorium at the vein of Galen creates a narrow attic with a very limited view, and a dilated, low-hanging vein of Galen can fill this small field.

Straight Sinus Dural Arteriovenous Fistulas

Compared with galenic DAVFs, straight sinus DAVFs are much simpler: they are not as deeply located; they usually drain out of a solitary vein; and they are exposed by opening the natural subarachnoid plane under the tentorium, without skeletonizing sinuses or dissecting venous complexes (**Fig. 25.6**). The supracerebellar-infratentorial approach with the patient in the sitting position is the ideal operative approach. With the sitting position, gravity retracts the cerebellum and opens this plane to facilitate visualizing the fistula, even in patients presenting with hemorrhage that have intraparenchymal clot, cerebellar swelling, and a tight surgical corridor (**Fig. 25.9**). The supracerebellar-infratentorial approach can be performed with the patient in the prone position, but retractors are needed, which risks avulsing the draining vein and causing brisk bleeding from a fistula not yet in view. Neurosurgeons often prefer placing the patient in the prone position because it allows them to sit while operating. However, the surgeon can still sit while operating on patients in the sitting position. The patient's back is positioned nearly vertical and the head is slouched forward to align the plane of the tentorium nearly horizontal. The surgeon sits on a rolling stool and supports his or her elbows on a free-standing arm brace raised to shoulder level, which relaxes the arms and stabilizes the hands. The dissection and fistula occlusion are usually brief, so this somewhat awkward position for the neurosurgeon is easily tolerated.

The suboccipital craniotomy extends from above the transverse sinuses and torcular superiorly to just above, but not to, the foramen magnum. Exposure of the torcular removes the bony ledge that would otherwise obscure the infratentorial plane. Dural tears and venous sinus injury can be dangerous, particularly with patients in the sitting position. Older patients with adherent dura may have sinuses that are not safe to cross with the craniotome, and instead may require a suboccipital craniotomy first, then dissection of the dura from the inner table of skull under direct visualization. Alternatively, bone overlying the sinuses can be drilled away with a diamond drill bit until the inferior margins of the venous sinuses are seen. We performed this approach in the sitting position in three patients in their 70s without complications from the venous sinuses or air embolism. Once the torcular is exposed, the dura is opened in a flap based on the transverse sinuses and tacking sutures that elevate the torcular. The arterialized vein draining the fistula is identified on the cerebellar surface by its red color and traced back to the fistula. Alternatively, the arterialized vein is seen in the subarachnoid space descending from the dura. The draining vein has a thickened wall and distinctive white color with red vasovasorum. A clip is applied to the draining vein as it exits the tentorial dura, and it is coagulated and cut.

Torcular Dural Arteriovenous Fistulas

We encountered eight patients with torcular DAVFs, but these few patients demonstrated the difference between treating a Borden type II and a type III fistula. Type III torcular fistulas that drain exclusively to adjacent veins are treated simply by clipping the arterialized veins as they exit the sinus. These superficial fistulas are exposed using a torcular craniotomy with the patient positioned prone and with minimal subarachnoid dissection. In contrast, type II fistulas that drain to torcular sinuses and to adjacent veins are considerably more difficult to treat. Arterialized draining veins are occluded the same way as with type III fistulas, but shunt flow into the torcular sinuses cannot be interrupted without sacrificing a major sinus. Therefore, skeletonization of the torcular is also required with type II fistulas to interrupt arterial inflow.[60]

There are a total of eight dural leaflets around the torcular that can harbor arterial supply: falx cerebri, bilateral tentorium (two), bilateral occipital dura (two), bilateral suboccipital dura (two), and falx cerebelli. Complete skeletonization of the torcular requires a total of 12 cuts in these eight dural leaflets, with four of the leaflets requiring two cuts: the occipital dura must be cut along the transverse sinus and the superior sagittal sinus, and the tentorium must be cut along the straight sinus and the transverse sinus. The torcular craniotomy exposes all of these leaflets, but some additional retraction is needed to make the tentorial incisions along the straight sinus.

Tentorial Sinus Dural Arteriovenous Fistulas

We differentiate tentorial sinus DAVFs as a distinct but poorly described type of tentorial fistulas. This lesion has not been described in the neurosurgical literature in part because the tentorial sinus is an obscure entity that is often detected but ignored on angiography and magnetic resonance imaging (MRI). Furthermore, the anatomy of the tentorial sinuses is highly variable, which might make it difficult to recognize different tentorial sinus DAVFs as being the same type. Rhoton's group[62] classified the tentorial sinus into four groups depending on whether venous tributaries originated from the cerebrum (group I), cerebellum (group II), the tentorium itself (group III), or incisura (group IV). In another anatomical study of 80 cadavers, Muthukumar and Palaniappan[63] found tentorial sinuses in 86% of specimens and classified them into three types depending on their location (medial or lateral) and size (small or large). Miabi et al[64] used contrast-enhanced MRI to identify 104 tentorial sinuses in 55 patients and define yet another classification scheme: venous candelabra (type 1), multiple independent veins (type II), and venous lakes within tentorium (type III). With so much confusion in the literature over a subtle and highly variable venous structure, it is no wonder that the association between the tentorial sinus and paramedian tentorial DAVFs has not been firmly established. Although we did not find any description of tentorial sinus DAVFs in the neurosurgical literature, it has been reported recently in the radiologic literature.[65]

Tentorial sinus DAVFs encountered in our experience had features implicating the tentorial sinus: none was associated

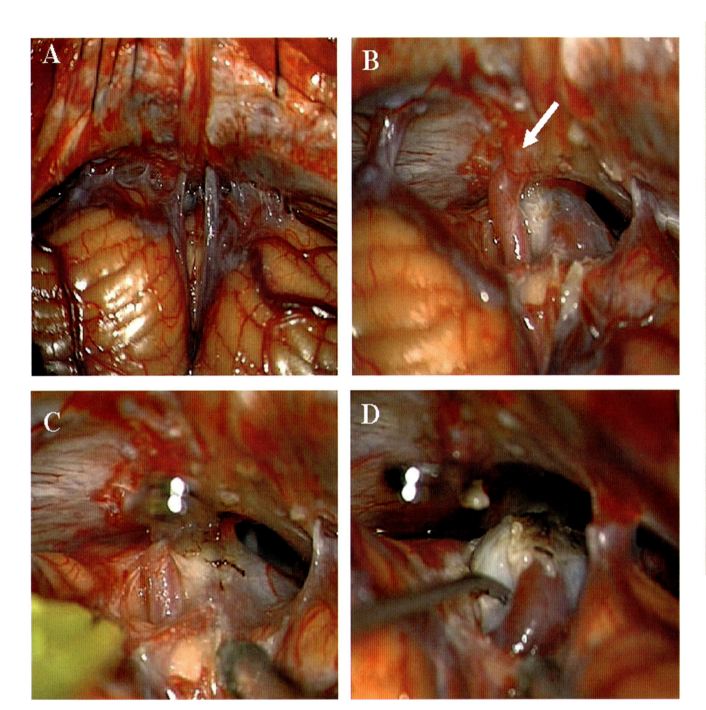

Fig. 25.9 Straight sinus DAVF (type 2). These DAVFs are supplied by the posterior meningeal artery and are drained by a vein coursing over the superior surface of the cerebellum, under the apex of the tentorium. **(A)** Intraoperative photograph demonstrates the supracerebellar-infratentorial approach, with the patient in the sitting position, torcular dura pulled superiorly with tacking sutures, and gravity retraction of the cerebellum to open the infratentorial plane. **(B)** The arterialized vein draining the fistula *(arrow)* is seen exiting the dura and coursing anteriorly to the galenic region. **(C)** The fistula was interrupted with a clip on this vein as it exited the tentorial dura, and **(D)** was then cut to obliterate the fistula.

with other dural sinuses (straight, superior petrosal, or transverse sinuses); some were laterally located, where the vein of Labbé might join the tentorial sinus under the temporal and occipital lobes; and others were medially located, where the medial variant of the tentorial sinus has been described.

The supratentorial-infraoccipital approach, as described by Smith and Spetzler[66] for posteromedial temporal lobe lesions, was used to expose tentorial sinus DAVFs. We prefer to position patients laterally rather than prone, with the head rotated downward to face the floor. A torcular craniotomy is important if the fistula is medially located, because a torcular craniotomy enables the dura to be opened widely and the occipital pole to be mobilized freely. More lateral DAVFs near the transverse-sigmoid junction may not need this midline exposure, and a unilateral temporal-occipital craniotomy taken down to or below the transverse sinus would suffice. Occlusion of the fistula is accomplished by interrupting the draining vein as it exits the tentorium.

Superior Petrosal Sinus Dural Arteriovenous Fistulas

Superior petrosal sinus DAVFs consistently drained infratentorially into the petrosal vein (Dandy's vein), making the extended retrosigmoid approach an ideal exposure.[67] More radical transpetrosal approaches are not necessary because only the draining vein needs to be exposed to interrupt the fistula. The patient is positioned laterally with the head slightly flexed and angled downward toward the floor, optimizing the view along the angle between tentorium and petrous face. We use a C-shaped scalp incision behind the ear, a limited posterior mastoidectomy, skeletonization of the sigmoid sinus with a diamond-bit drill, craniotomy rather than craniectomy, and anterior mobilization of the sigmoid sinus with the dural flap. These maneuvers enhance the exposure of a conventional retrosigmoid approach that does not drill the sigmoid sinus.[67] Feeding arteries from the ECA traverse the mastoid and petrous bones to make the drilling bloodier than with other lesions. These transosseous arteries are controlled easily with bone wax or drilling with a diamond bit.

If the fistula has ruptured and the cerebellum is swollen, cerebrospinal fluid should be released from the cisterna magna immediately after opening the dura to relax the cerebellum. Microsurgical dissection into the cerebellopontine angle leads to the arterialized petrosal vein, which is frequently variceal due to the high-flow nature of this fistula **(Fig. 25.10)**. The clip is applied as close to the petrous dura as possible, but not so close that closure of the blades avulses the vein. Draining veins distal to the clip should darken after the fistula is interrupted. The venous varix can sometimes hide an additional draining vein coursing medially toward the brainstem, so the varix should be mobilized and this medial territory inspected carefully. In our experience, half of these superior petrosal sinus DAVFs were Borden type II fistulas, with drainage medially into the superior petrosal sinus. Patency of this sinus can result in residual, but low-risk (Borden type I), shunting after occluding the draining petrosal vein, as in one patient in our experience.

Incisural Dural Arteriovenous Fistulas

Incisural DAVFs are the other type of tentorial fistulas not well characterized in the literature. Picard et al[68] described a "marginal tentorial sinus" that courses along the free edge of the tentorial incisura, is not present in most people, and receives venous tributaries from the basal vein of Rosenthal and lateral mesencephalic veins.[50] We hypothesize that incisural DAVFs are associated with this marginal tentorial sinus, and the lack of a clear association between this fistula and the venous sinus is due to the rarity of each entity. In our

large experience, this subtype was the least common, with just two patients.

Incisural DAVFs and tentorial sinus DAVFs are similar because both are associated with intrinsic tentorial sinuses, both have variable anatomy, and both drain supratentorially. However, we differentiated these two types because they require different surgical approaches. Tentorial sinus DAVFs are located infraoccipitally and are exposed through a torcular or occipital craniotomy. In contrast, exposure of incisural DAVFs calls for either a more anterior pterional-transsylvian approach or a lateral subtemporal approach. In our experience, the venous drainage from incisural DAVFs coursed posteriorly to the galenic system, but the fistulas were quite anterior, at the level of the uncus or supraclinoid ICA. Incisural DAVFs are also near the superior petrosal sinus and can be mistaken for the more common petrosal DAVF. However, the extended retrosigmoid approach used for petrosal DAVFs positions the neurosurgeon on the opposite side of the tentorium from an incisural DAVF, and even incising the tentorium was not sufficient to widen the exposure. Therefore, incisural DAVFs can be deceptive and require careful analysis of the venous drainage pattern on preoperative angiograms to be certain of their type and location along the incisura. We suspect that some of the difficulty in surgically obliterating superior petrosal sinus DAVFs relates to unrecognized differences between superior petrosal sinus and incisural DAVFs, and the erroneous selection of an infratentorial approach for incisural DAVFs.

Infratentorial Dural Arteriovenous Fistulas

Transverse-Sigmoid Sinus Dural Arteriovenous Fistulas

Transverse-sigmoid sinus DAVFs were the second most common DAVF in our overall experience, diagnosed in 142 of 402 patients (35%). Symptoms associated with these DAVFs include pulsatile tinnitus, headache, visual obscuration, seizures, and hemorrhage. In low-risk DAVFs with low-flow AV shunts and no cortical venous drainage, symptoms are limited to pulsatile tinnitus. In high-risk DAVFs with increased shunt flow and retrograde cortical venous drainage, symptoms related to venous hypertension ensue with increased intracranial pressure, venous ischemia, focal neurologic deficits, and seizures.

Transverse-sigmoid sinus DAVFs are amenable to endovascular therapy. Transvenous and transarterial approaches can be used alone or in combination to obliterate the fistulas. Obliteration rates with endovascular therapy alone are high, and in our experience only 13 patients have required surgical intervention. These patients typically have Borden type III lesions that persist after transarterial embolization and have poor transvenous access. Transverse-sigmoid sinus DAVFs are exposed with an extended retrosigmoid craniotomy that widely exposes the junction of these two sinuses by removing overlying bone with a diamond drill bit, as described above for superior petrosal sinus DAVFs. The dura is opened to identify the arterialized draining vein, which is clipped, cauterized, and divided. Skeletonization of the transverse, sigmoid, and superior petrosal sinuses is also required for Borden

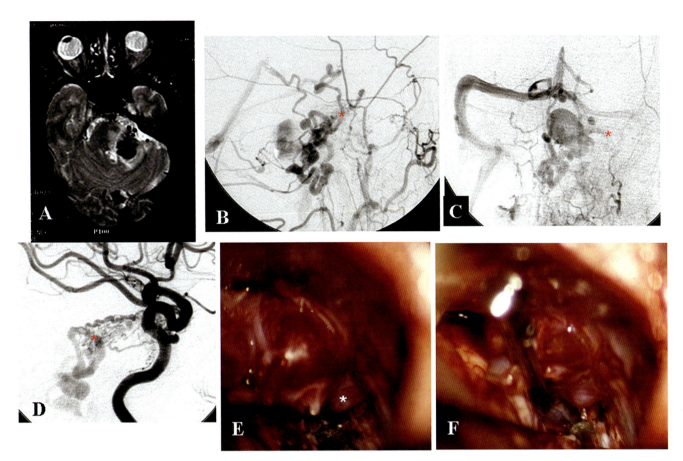

Fig. 25.10 Superior petrosal sinus DAVF (type 5). **(A)** Brain MRI (axial view, T2-weighted image) demonstrated a hematoma in the left cerebellar peduncle, surrounding edema, and dilated veins in the cerebellopontine angle. **(B)** Left external carotid artery angiogram (lateral view, showed arterial supply to the fistula *(red asterisk)* from the middle meningeal artery and transosseous perforators. **(C)** The venous phase of the angiogram (anterior-posterior view) showed the fistula's drainage through tortuous and variceal cerebellar veins. **(D)** Left internal carotid artery angiogram (lateral view) showed arterial supply to the fistula *(red asterisk)* from the tentorial artery. **(E)** Intraoperative photograph demonstrates the extended retrosigmoid approach, with the patient in the lateral position (right side down), the dura flapped against the transverse and sigmoid sinuses, and exposure of the angle between the petrous bone and the tentorial dura. The vein draining the fistula was visualized at this petrotentorial junction *(white asterisk).* **(F)** The fistula was interrupted with a clip on the draining vein.

type II lesions. Patients with Borden type I DAVFs are managed conservatively.

Marginal Sinus Dural Arteriovenous Fistulas

The marginal sinus resides at the foramen magnum, encircling the cervicomedullary junction and draining into the jugular veins or sigmoid sinuses. Marginal sinus DAVFs are supplied by branches from the vertebral artery, including the posterior meningeal artery and direct branches from the vertebral artery trunk. Ascending muscular branches from the vertebral artery and ECA branches can also contribute to these fistulas. These DAVFs are rare. Patients present with hemorrhage, signs of venous hypertension, or symptoms of medullary or spinal cord compression from dilated veins.

Marginal sinus DAVFs are amenable to endovascular therapy, using transvenous or transarterial approaches to obliterate the fistulas. Obliteration rates with endovascular therapy alone are high, and in our experience only three patients required surgical intervention. These DAVFs are exposed through a far-lateral craniotomy. The dural opening often occludes feeding arteries from the posterior meningeal artery. The approach provides access to the vertebral artery to identify additional feeders that arise from its subarachnoid segment. The arterialized vein is clipped, cauterized, and divided as it exits the dura overlying the occipital condyle.

Inferior Petrosal Sinus Dural Arteriovenous Fistulas

Inferior petrosal sinus DAVFs are rare lesions. They tend not to have leptomeningeal venous drainage, giving them a benign natural history. They have a low hemorrhage risk and can present with pain and cranial neuropathies. Management is often conservative. When treatment is necessary, endovascular therapy is highly successful. There have been no cases in our experience where surgical therapy has been needed for these lesions.

◆ Treatment Decision

The diverse clinical spectrum and variable natural history of these lesions demand an individualized approach to clinical decision making. Due to limited natural history data on these uncommon lesions, the decision to aggressively manage is usually solely based on the severity of neurologic symptoms and angiographic characteristics of DAVF. The recent literature suggests that DAVFs with cortical venous drainage and those located in the posterior fossa should be aggressively treated to prevent hemorrhage.[21] Besides hemorrhagic risk, the pathophysiology of chronic neurologic decline is thought to be due to venous hypertension based on computed tomography (CT), magnetic resonance imaging (MRI), and single photon emission computed tomography (SPECT) findings. Concern about hemorrhage drives clinical management decisions after the diagnosis of DAVF, but the injurious effects of venous hypertension are underappreciated and poorly understood.

Angiography has traditionally been used to diagnose DAVFs and stratify DAVFs into low- or high-risk groups based on patterns of venous drainage. Although angiography provides excellent anatomic resolution of the fistula site, supply, and drainage, it provides a crude assessment of cerebral perfusion. Positron emission tomography (PET) scanning has been used to evaluate hemodynamic and metabolic disturbances in patients with DAVF,[69] but this imaging modality is not readily available. Conventional MRI including magnetic resonance angiography (MRA) may show hypertrophied dural feeders, enlarged cortical veins, and even parenchymal signal changes suggestive of venous ischemia, but it does not directly measure alterations in cerebral perfusion. Dynamic susceptibility contrast-enhanced MRI has been useful in characterizing changes in cerebral perfusion in the setting of acute ischemic stroke and may be relevant to DAVFs. Preliminary evidence suggests that perfusion MRI may also be useful in the evaluation of DAVFs.[70] Perfusion CT scans may offer the best and easiest method for assessing the abnormal hemodynamics in these patients. It is readily available, quick, and often markedly abnormal in patients with venous hypertension or venous ischemia caused by DAVFs. Cerebral perfusion data may offer a method of assessing the extent of venous hypertension and venous ischemia, thereby offering a method of individualizing treatment decisions that goes beyond assessing hemorrhagic risk.

References

1. Kerber CW, Newton TH. The macro and microvasculature of the dura mater. Neuroradiology 1973;6:175–179
2. Terada T, Tsuura M, Komai N, et al. The role of angiogenic factor bFGF in the development of dural AVFs. Acta Neurochir (Wien) 1996;138:877–883
3. Herman JM, Spetzler RF, Bederson JB, Kurbat JM, Zabramski JM. Genesis of a dural arteriovenous malformation in a rat model. J Neurosurg 1995;83:539–545
4. Houser OW, Baker HL Jr, Rhoton AL Jr, Okazaki H. Intracranial dural arteriovenous malformations. Radiology 1972;105:55–64
5. Lawton MT, Stewart CL, Wulfstat AA, Derugin N, Hashimoto T, Young WL. The transgenic arteriovenous fistula in the rat: an experimental model of gene therapy for brain arteriovenous malformations. Neurosurgery 2004;54:1463–1471, discussion 1471
6. Shin Y, Nakase H, Nakamura M, Shimada K, Konishi N, Sakaki T. Expression of angiogenic growth factor in the rat DAVF model. Neurol Res 2007;29:727–733
7. Shen F, Fan Y, Su H, et al. Adeno-associated viral vector-mediated hypoxia-regulated VEGF gene transfer promotes angiogenesis following focal cerebral ischemia in mice. Gene Ther 2008;15:30–39
8. Zhu Y, Lawton MT, Du R, et al. Expression of hypoxia-inducible factor-1 and vascular endothelial growth factor in response to venous hypertension. Neurosurgery 2006;59:687–696, discussion 687–696
9. Uranishi R, Nakase H, Sakaki T. Expression of angiogenic growth factors in dural arteriovenous fistula. J Neurosurg 1999;91:781–786
10. Deschiens MA, Conard J, Horellou MH, et al. Coagulation studies, factor V Leiden, and anticardiolipin antibodies in 40 cases of cerebral venous thrombosis. Stroke 1996;27:1724–1730
11. Ridker PM, Miletich JP, Stampfer MJ, Goldhaber SZ, Lindpaintner K, Hennekens CH. Factor V Leiden and risks of recurrent idiopathic venous thromboembolism. Circulation 1995;92:2800–2802
12. Boncoraglio G, Carriero MR, Chiapparini L, et al. Hyperhomocysteinemia and other thrombophilic risk factors in 26 patients with cerebral venous thrombosis. Eur J Neurol 2004;11:405–409
13. Reuner KH, Ruf A, Grau A, et al. Prothrombin gene G20210–>A transition is a risk factor for cerebral venous thrombosis. Stroke 1998;29:1765–1769
14. Zöller B, García de Frutos P, Hillarp A, Dahlbäck B. Thrombophilia as a multigenic disease. Haematologica 1999;84:59–70
15. Martinelli I, Landi G, Merati G, Cella R, Tosetto A, Mannucci PM. Factor V gene mutation is a risk factor for cerebral venous thrombosis. Thromb Haemost 1996;75:393–394
16. De Stefano V, Martinelli I, Mannucci PM, et al. The risk of recurrent deep venous thrombosis among heterozygous carriers of both factor V Leiden and the G20210A prothrombin mutation. N Engl J Med 1999;341:801–806
17. Kraus JA, Stüper BK, Nahser HC, Klockgether T, Berlit P. Significantly increased prevalence of factor V Leiden in patients with dural arteriovenous fistulas. J Neurol 2000;247:521–523
18. Singh V, Meyers PM, Halbach VH, et al. Dural arteriovenous fistula associated with prothrombin gene mutation. J Neuroimaging 2001;11:319–321
19. Kraus JA, Stüper BK, Berlit P. Association of resistance to activated protein C and dural arteriovenous fistulas. J Neurol 1998;245:731–733
20. Gerlach R, Yahya H, Rohde S, et al. Increased incidence of thrombophilic abnormalities in patients with cranial dural arteriovenous fistulae. Neurol Res 2003;25:745–748
21. Singh V, Smith WS, Lawton MT, Halbach VV, Young WL. Risk factors for hemorrhagic presentation in patients with dural arteriovenous fistulae. Neurosurgery 2008;62:628–635, discussion 628–635
22. Izumi T, Miyachi S, Hattori K, Iizuka H, Nakane Y, Yoshida J. Thrombophilic abnormalities among patients with cranial dural arteriovenous fistulas. Neurosurgery 2007;61:262–268, discussion 268–269
23. Chaudhary MY, Sachdev VP, Cho SH, Weitzner I Jr, Puljic S, Huang YP. Dural arteriovenous malformation of the major venous sinuses: an acquired lesion. AJNR Am J Neuroradiol 1982;3:13–19
24. Feldman RA, Hieshima G, Giannotta SL, Gade GF. Traumatic dural arteriovenous fistula supplied by scalp, meningeal, and cortical arteries: case report. Neurosurgery 1980;6:670–674
25. Nabors MW, Azzam CJ, Albanna FJ, Gulya AJ, Davis DO, Kobrine AI. Delayed postoperative dural arteriovenous malformations. Report of two cases. J Neurosurg 1987;66:768–772
26. Watanabe A, Takahara Y, Ibuchi Y, Mizukami K. Two cases of dural arteriovenous malformation occurring after intracranial surgery. Neuroradiology 1984;26:375–380
27. Fermand M, Reizine D, Melki JP, Riche MC, Merland JJ. Long term follow-up of 43 pure dural arteriovenous fistulae (AVF) of the lateral sinus. Neuroradiology 1987;29:348–353
28. Houser OW, Campbell JK, Campbell RJ, Sundt TM Jr. Arteriovenous malformation affecting the transverse dural venous sinus—an acquired lesion. Mayo Clin Proc 1979;54:651–661
29. Toya S, Shiobara R, Izumi J, Shinomiya Y, Shiga H, Kimura C. Spontaneous carotid-cavernous fistula during pregnancy or in the postpartum stage. Report of two cases. J Neurosurg 1981;54:252–256
30. Lasjaunias P, Halimi P, Lopez-Ibor L, Sichez JP, Hurth M, De Tribolet N. Endovascular treatment of pure spontaneous dural vascular malformations. Review of 23 cases studied and treated between May 1980 and October 1983. Neurochirurgie 1984;30:207–223
31. Ohta T, Kajikawa H. Dural arteriovenous malformation (author's transl.). Neurol Med Chir (Tokyo) 1978;18:439–472
32. Lasjaunias P. Surgical neuroangiography: search for a speciality. AJNR Am J Neuroradiol 1987;8:581–582

33. Borden JA, Wu JK, Shucart WA. A proposed classification for spinal and cranial dural arteriovenous fistulous malformations and implications for treatment. J Neurosurg 1995;82:166–179
34. Lasjaunias P, Chiu M, ter Brugge K, Tolia A, Hurth M, Bernstein M. Neurological manifestations of intracranial dural arteriovenous malformations. J Neurosurg 1986;64:724–730
35. Datta NN, Rehman SU, Kwok JC, Chan KY, Poon CY. Reversible dementia due to dural arteriovenous fistula: a simple surgical option. Neurosurg Rev 1998;21:174–176
36. Matsuda S, Waragai M, Shinotoh H, Takahashi N, Takagi K, Hattori T. Intracranial dural arteriovenous fistula (DAVF) presenting progressive dementia and parkinsonism. J Neurol Sci 1999;165:43–47
37. Tanaka K, Morooka Y, Nakagawa Y, Shimizu S. Dural arteriovenous malformation manifesting as dementia due to ischemia in bilateral thalami. A case report. Surg Neurol 1999;51:489–493, discussion 493–494
38. Yamakami I, Kobayashi E, Yamaura A. Diffuse white matter changes caused by dural arteriovenous fistula. J Clin Neurosci 2001;8:471–475
39. Bernstein R, Dowd CF, Gress DR. Rapidly reversible dementia. Lancet 2003;361:392
40. Lalwani AK, Dowd CF, Halbach VV. Grading venous restrictive disease in patients with dural arteriovenous fistulas of the transverse/sigmoid sinus. J Neurosurg 1993;79:11–15
41. van Dijk JM, terBrugge KG, Willinsky RA, Wallace MC. Clinical course of cranial dural arteriovenous fistulas with long-term persistent cortical venous reflux. Stroke 2002;33:1233–1236
42. Cellerini M, Mascalchi M, Mangiafico S, et al. Phase-contrast MR angiography of intracranial dural arteriovenous fistulae. Neuroradiology 1999;41:487–492
43. Miller NR. Diagnosis and management of dural carotid-cavernous sinus fistulas. Neurosurg Focus 2007;23:E13
44. Desal HA, Toulgoat F, Raoul S, et al. Ehlers-Danlos syndrome type IV and recurrent carotid-cavernous fistula: review of the literature, endovascular approach, technique and difficulties. Neuroradiology 2005;47:300–304
45. Lawton MT, Chun J, Wilson CB, Halbach VV. Ethmoidal dural arteriovenous fistulae: an assessment of surgical and endovascular management. Neurosurgery 1999;45:805–810, discussion 810–811
46. Borden JA, Wu JK, Shucart WA. A proposed classification for spinal and cranial dural arteriovenous fistulous malformations and implications for treatment. J Neurosurg 1995;82:166–179
47. Awad IA, Little JR, Akarawi WP, Ahl J. Intracranial dural arteriovenous malformations: factors predisposing to an aggressive neurological course. J Neurosurg 1990;72:839–850
48. Lewis AI, Rosenblatt SS, Tew JM Jr. Surgical management of deep-seated dural arteriovenous malformations. J Neurosurg 1997;87:198–206
49. Lewis AI, Tomsick TA, Tew JM Jr. Management of tentorial dural arteriovenous malformations: transarterial embolization combined with stereotactic radiation or surgery. J Neurosurg 1994;81:851–859
50. Tomak PR, Cloft HJ, Kaga A, Cawley CM, Dion J, Barrow DL. Evolution of the management of tentorial dural arteriovenous malformations. Neurosurgery 2003;52:750–760, discussion 760–762
51. Zink WE, Meyers PM, Connolly ES, Lavine SD. Combined surgical and endovascular management of a complex posttraumatic dural arteriovenous fistula of the tentorium and straight sinus. J Neuroimaging 2004;14:273–276
52. Cognard C, Gobin YP, Pierot L, et al. Cerebral dural arteriovenous fistulas: clinical and angiographic correlation with a revised classification of venous drainage. Radiology 1995;194:671–680
53. Zhang JY, Cawley CM, Dion JE, Barrow DL. Surgical treatment of intracranial dural arteriovenous fistulas. In: Lawton M, Gress D, Higashida R, eds. Controversies in Neurological Surgery: Neurovascular Diseases. New York: Thieme, 2006
54. Hoh BL, Choudhri TF, Connolly ES Jr, Solomon RA. Surgical management of high-grade intracranial dural arteriovenous fistulas: leptomeningeal venous disruption without nidus excision. Neurosurgery 1998;42:796–804, discussion 804–805
55. Goto K, Sidipratomo P, Ogata N, Inoue T, Matsuno H. Combining endovascular and neurosurgical treatments of high-risk dural arteriovenous fistulas in the lateral sinus and the confluence of the sinuses. J Neurosurg 1999;90:289–299
56. Collice M, D'Aliberti G, Arena O, Solaini C, Fontana RA, Talamonti G. Surgical treatment of intracranial dural arteriovenous fistulae: role of venous drainage. Neurosurgery 2000;47:56–66, discussion 66–67
57. Ushikoshi S, Houkin K, Kuroda S, et al. Surgical treatment of intracranial dural arteriovenous fistulas. Surg Neurol 2002;57:253–261
58. Kattner KA, Roth TC, Giannotta SL. Cranial base approaches for the surgical treatment of aggressive posterior fossa dural arteriovenous fistulae with leptomeningeal drainage: report of four technical cases. Neurosurgery 2002;50:1156–1160, discussion 1160–1161
59. Kiyosue H, Hori Y, Okahara M, et al. Treatment of intracranial dural arteriovenous fistulas: current strategies based on location and hemodynamics, and alternative techniques of transcatheter embolization. Radiographics 2004;24:1637–1653
60. Sundt TM Jr, Piepgras DG. The surgical approach to arteriovenous malformations of the lateral and sigmoid dural sinuses. J Neurosurg 1983;59:32–39
61. Chi JH, Lawton MT. Posterior interhemispheric approach: surgical technique, application to vascular lesions, and benefits of gravity retraction. Neurosurgery 2006;59(1, Suppl 1)ONS41–ONS49, discussion ONS41–ONS49
62. Matsushima T, Suzuki SO, Fukui M, Rhoton AL Jr, de Oliveira E, Ono M. Microsurgical anatomy of the tentorial sinuses. J Neurosurg 1989;71:923–928
63. Muthukumar N, Palaniappan P. Tentorial venous sinuses: an anatomic study. Neurosurgery 1998;42:363–371
64. Miabi Z, Midia R, Rohrer SE, et al. Delineation of lateral tentorial sinus with contrast-enhanced MR imaging and its surgical implications. AJNR Am J Neuroradiol 2004;25:1181–1188
65. Horie N, Morikawa M, Kitigawa N, Tsutsumi K, Kaminogo M, Nagata I. 2D Thick-section MR digital subtraction angiography for the assessment of dural arteriovenous fistulas. AJNR Am J Neuroradiol 2006;27:264–269
66. Smith KA, Spetzler RF. Supratentorial-infraoccipital approach for posteromedial temporal lobe lesions. J Neurosurg 1995;82:940–944
67. Quiñones-Hinojosa A, Chang EF, Lawton MT. The extended retrosigmoid approach: an alternative to radical cranial base approaches for posterior fossa lesions. Neurosurgery 2006;58(4, Suppl 2)ONS-208–ONS-214, discussion ONS-214
68. Picard L, Bracard S, Islak C, et al. Dural fistulae of the tentorium cerebelli. Radioanatomical, clinical and therapeutic considerations. J Neuroradiol 1990;17:161–181
69. Iwama T, Hashimoto N, Takagi Y, et al. Hemodynamic and metabolic disturbances in patients with intracranial dural arteriovenous fistulas: positron emission tomography evaluation before and after treatment. J Neurosurg 1997;86:806–811
70. Fujita A, Nakamura M, Tamaki N, Kohmura E. Haemodynamic assessment in patients with dural arteriovenous fistulae: dynamic susceptibility contrast-enhanced MRI. Neuroradiology 2002;44:806–811

26

Spinal Dural Fistula

Albert J. Schuette, Charles M. Cawley, and Daniel L. Barrow

Pearls

- Delayed venous drainage from the artery of Adamkiewicz is present in the majority of patients presenting with spinal dural arteriovenous fistulas (DAVFs).
- In the 10 to 15% of cases where the spinal DAVF is supplied by a radiculomedullary artery that also supplies the anterior or posterior spinal arteries, open surgical obliteration is indicated.
- There has been no study demonstrating a difference in clinical symptoms in patients successfully treated by surgery or endovascular methods.
- In the past several years, intraoperative indocyanine green (ICG) near-infrared videoangiography has emerged as a rapid and safe alternative to spinal digital subtraction angiography (DSA) for confirmation of the obliteration of a fistula.
- There have been reports of late clinical deterioration following long periods of improvement or stabilization.

Spinal dural arteriovenous fistulas (DAVFs) are the most common heterogenous group of spinal vascular malformations, with varied natural histories, pathophysiologies, and treatment strategies.[1-3] Although these lesions represent a rare cause of myeloradiculopathy, they remain potentially curable if diagnosed in a timely fashion.[4,5] Due to the insidious nature of symptom onset, these patients rarely seek care from a neurosurgeon directly, but rather present to their primary care physician or neurologist. For that reason, knowledge of this disease must extend past the neurosurgical community. With advances in modern imaging through magnetic resonance imaging (MRI) and computed tomography (CT) angiography, there are now improved noninvasive means available for earlier diagnosis.[6] Along with advances in imaging, therapeutic options have been refined and include both endovascular and microsurgical options.[4,7,8] Both can be effective in obliterating the arteriovenous shunt.

◆ History (Table 26.1)

The earliest descriptions of spinal vascular malformations were made by Virchow in 1865, who described them as neo-plasms of the spine.[9] Gaupp characterized these lesions in 1888 as "hemorrhoids" of the pia mater.[2] These early descriptions led Fedor Krause to attempt the first exposure of one of these lesions in 1910. After the laminectomy, no attempt was made at treatment, and the patient had a poor outcome. Charles Elsberg in 1912 reported the first excision in a 13-year-old boy. Although this patient did not improve, a later attempt in 1916 in a densely paraplegic patient led to complete recovery in 3 months.[2] This surgery concentrated on removing a 2-cm section of abnormally dilated vein. This successful attempt, the first recorded in the literature, was performed on purely clinical grounds without any preoperative imaging. A later trend toward more aggressive surgery with extensive stripping of the dilated, arterialized veins failed to match the results of Elsberg's success and actually worsened the condition by exacerbating the underlying venous hypertension.

Sir Percy Sargent first correctly described the insidious neurologic decline through observations of his own patients and a review of the previous medical literature.[2] Diagnosis of this disorder relied on these clinical symptoms until the first preoperative diagnostic study for a spinal dural arteriovenous malformation was completed by Perthes in 1927 using Pantopaque myelography.[2,9] In 1926, Foix and Alajouanine described a rapidly progressing necrotic myelopathy that led to paraplegia and death. This syndrome, which bears their names, is believed to be due to an end-stage spinal DAVF.[9]

With a means of identifying these lesions, attempts were made to classify them based on anatomic structure. Cushing and Bailey in 1928 initially categorized these malformations as neoplasms and arteriovenous malformations.[9] Wyburn-Mason further refined this classification system in 1943 by differentiating the lesions into arteriovenous malformations (AVMs) and purely venous malformations.[2]

The development of spinal angiography and the field of interventional neuroradiology in the 1960s redefined spinal DAVFS and allowed for a detailed understanding of the angioarchitecture of these lesions. Centers in London, Paris, and the National Institutes of Health (NIH) in the United States collaborated in these advances, making way for improved

Table 26.1 Historic Milestones in the Treatment of Spinal Dural Fistulas

Author	Year	Contribution
Virchow	1865	Earliest description: "neoplasms of the spine"
Graupp	1888	Description as "hemorrhoids" of the pia mater
Krause	1910	First exposure of a spinal dural fistula
Elsberg	1913	Earliest attempt at treatment
Elsberg	1916	First successful surgical treatment
Perthes	1927	First diagnostic study with myelography
Cushing and Bailey	1928	First classification system
Various centers	1960s	Refinement of digital subtraction angiography
Kendall and Logue	1977	Localization of fistulous point to dural sleeve

preoperative planning and advanced treatment options.[9] Kendall and Logue[10] first localized the spinal DAVF to the dural sleeve in 1977. They described a simple means to treat this lesion with surgical interruption of the fistulous point.

Since that time, the most often utilized classification system categorizes vascular malformations in four basic groups. Spinal DAVFs are classified as a type I lesion and are the primary topic of this chapter.

◆ Classification

Purpose of Schemes

The drive to classify spinal vascular malformations began in earnest with the descriptions by Wyburn-Mason based on posthumous histopathology and has since been redefined by selective angiography.[9] Various classification schemes have been used since that time with varying nomenclature.[1,2,11] The most often used classification scheme differentiates spinal vascular malformations based on the location of the pathology, the arterial supply, and the venous drainage. This classification is valuable, not only for its simplicity, but also for its insight into the pathophysiology, natural history, and treatment options. Although this classification system works for most lesions, some spinal vascular malformations may incorporate multiple characteristics from various classes. We will mention the other classes of spinal AVMs briefly, as it is important to understand what distinguishes type I spinal DAVFs from other spinal vascular malformations.

Type I: Spinal Dural Arteriovenous Fistulas

Previously called angioma racemosum venosum by Wyburn-Mason, the type I spinal AVMs are DAVFs between a radicular artery and a medullary vein at the nerve root sleeve[2,9,12]

(**Fig. 26.1A**). These lesions are further classified into type Ia, where there is a single arterial feeder, and type Ib, where there are multiple fistulous points. The majority of spinal DAVFs are single arterial feeder types (Ia) and are low-flow lesions.[12] It has been reported that 3 to 12% of all spinal cord lesions are vascular in pathology. Of this group, approximately 70 to 80% are spinal DAVFs.[2,5] They occur most commonly in the lower thoracic and upper lumbar spine at the level of the conus medullaris. Type I spinal arteriovenous fistula (AVFs) are found predominantly in men over 40 years of age, with the median age being 57 years.

The lesion may have multiple arterial feeders but drain to a single draining vein. The fistulous point lies transdurally at the nerve sleeve, with the draining vein located intradurally.[3] Venous drainage from the fistula is directed rostrally in most cases. As a result of the fistula, the direction of flow reverses in the valveless medullary vein, and blood travels from the intradural medullary vein into the coronal venous plexus, which becomes engorged and dilated.[13] These dilated veins are present solely on the dorsal surface of the spinal cord in 85% of cases.[2] It is important to note that spinal DAVFs typically do not share blood supply with the neural parenchyma of the spinal cord.

Although most commonly located in the thoracic and upper lumbar spine, these lesions may be found throughout the spinal cord. In the cervical spine, the radicular feeding arteries may arise from the thyrocervical, costocervical, vertebral, or external carotid arteries. In the lower lumbar and sacral spine, arterial feeders can include branches from the iliac arteries. Spinal dural AVMs are believed to be acquired lesions, a belief supported by the age at presentation. Spinal DAVFs in young patients are very rare. There are also reports in the literature of patients undergoing diagnostic studies for disk disease with negative results, and later presenting with progressive myelopathy and a spinal DAVF.

Type II: Intramedullary Arteriovenous Malformations

Intramedullary AVMs are composed of a distinct, intramedullary nidus of vessels that is fed by the anterior or posterior spinal arteries (**Fig. 26.1B**). As with intracranial AVMs, there are direct connections between arteries and veins without intervening capillary beds. These congenital lesions are often referred to as glomus AVMs. Differing from spinal AVFs, intramedullary AVMs are high-flow and high-pressure systems.

Unlike type I lesions, intramedullary AVMs occur with equal incidence in both men and women and may be located throughout the spinal cord. They typically present in children and young adults with acute symptoms of hemorrhage from the AVM but ultimately may present at any age. Treatment often includes a combination of presurgical embolization and subsequent surgical resection.

Type III: Diffuse Spinal Arteriovenous Malformations

Diffuse, metameric, or juvenile AVMs are extensive congenital vascular malformations that tend to involve both intramedullary and extramedullary tissues[2] (**Fig. 26.1C**). These lesions may extend to the extraspinal tissues including the

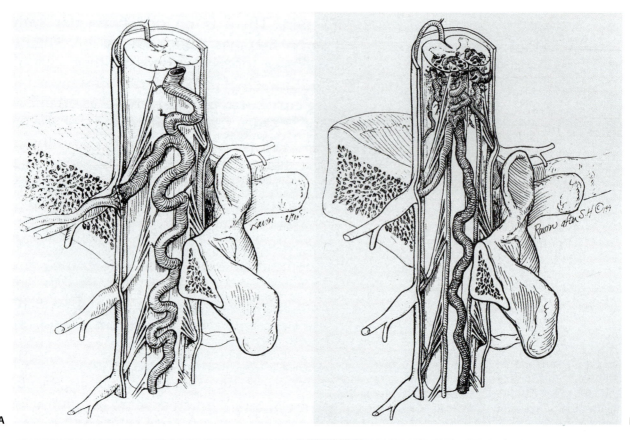

A

B

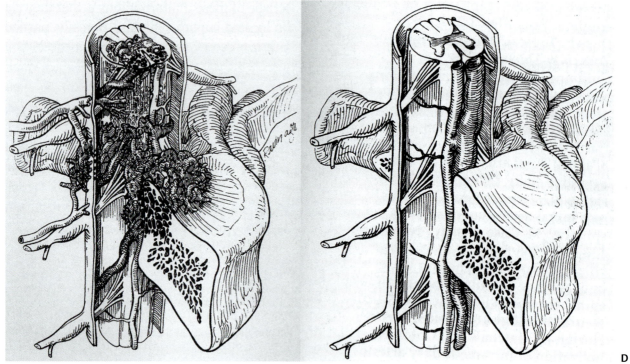

C

D

Fig. 26.1 **(A)** Drawing of a type Ia spinal dural arteriovenous fistula (DAVF). **(B)** Drawing of a type II spinal arteriovenous malformation (AVM) with an intramedullary nidus. **(C)** Drawing of a type III spinal AVM (juvenile type). **(D)** Drawing of a type IV intradural extramedullary AVF. (From Barrow DL, Awad IA, American Association of Neurological Surgeons. Spinal Vascular Malformations. Park Ridge, IL: American Association of Neurological Surgeons, 1999. Reprinted by permission from the American Association of Neurological Surgeons.)

Table 26.2 Treatment Options for Arteriovenous Malformations

Type	Anatomy	Presentation	Patient Characteristics	Location	Treatment
I	Fistulous point in nerve root sheath	Slowly progressive myelopathy: venous hypertension	Believed to be acquired; men over 40	Thoracic to upper lumbar	Surgery or endovascular treatment
II	Intramedullary compact nidus	Acute presentation with hemorrhage	Congenital: children and young adults typically	Throughout the spinal cord	Embolization with subsequent surgical resection
III	Intramedullary nidus with extra-spinal extension	Acute presentation	Adolescents and young adults	Cervical and thoracic spine	Similar to class II with worse outcomes
IV	Intradural extramedullary fistula Type A: single feeder with small venous enlargement Type B: multiple feeders with venous enlargement Type C: giant multipediculated feeders and large engorged veins	Progressive deficit from venous hypertension	All ages with no sex predilection	Type A: thoracic and lumbar spine Type C: cervical and thoracic spine	Type A: typically surgery Type B: endovascular or surgery Type C: typically endovascular with subsequent surgery for remnants

surrounding bone and skin. The least common of the spinal cord vascular malformations, they are also the most difficult to treat. These lesions normally present in adolescents and young adults and are characterized by their large size, high flow, and numerous feeding arteries. The nidus of the AVM is different from type II AVMs as it is large, loose, and interspersed within the spinal cord. There is functional spinal cord present inside the AVM, adding to the difficulty of treating these lesions. Cobb's syndrome refers to an extremely rare type III AVM that involves multiple embryologic layers.[2] Although the treatment for type III AVMs is similar to that for type II, outcomes are typically worse.

Type IV: Perimedullary Arteriovenous Fistulas

Type IV AVMs are intradural, extramedullary, direct arteriovenous fistulas from the anterior spinal, or, less commonly, the posterior spinal artery to the venous system on the pial surface of the cord.[11,14] Unlike type II and III AVMs, these lesions are completely outside the spinal cord (**Fig. 26.1D**). The resultant fistula leads to venous hypertension within the spinal cord. Perimedullary fistulas most commonly occur in the thoracolumbar region at the conus medullaris of the spinal cord. There is no sex predilection in type IV lesions. These congenital or acquired lesions may be subclassified as types IV-A, IV-B, or IV-C based on the size and flow characteristics. Treatment options are based on subclassification and are summarized in **Table 26.2**.

◆ Clinical Presentation and Natural History

Patients with spinal dural type I AVFs frequently experience pain as the initial symptom.[2,15] This pain is variable with ei-

ther back pain or radicular pain dominating. Along with pain, patients may present with any combination of weakness, sensory deficits, bladder or bowel symptoms, and sexual function loss. Aminoff and Logue[15] in 1974 found that one half of spinal AVF patients presented with back pain as the earliest symptom. One third of the patients in their study had lower extremity motor weakness or sensory deficits on initial presentation. Some estimates place the mean time from onset of symptoms to major motor dysfunction at 5 to 7 years.[2] The course of neurologic decline is generally progressive, but periods of remission may occur.[15] This illustrates the insidious nature of this disease course. Spinal DAVFs often differ from other vascular malformations of the spine in this time course of presentation.[2] Intramedullary AVMs present primarily in an acute manner, with sudden onset of neurologic deterioration due to hemorrhage from the AVM. Type III juvenile AVMs, due to their diffuse nature, may present with acute neurologic deterioration from the intramedullary component or more slowly due to the extramedullary component. Type IV spinal AVMs may present in a similar manner to type I spinal DAVFs, with progressive onset of myeloradiculopathy but with a higher incidence of acute worsening.

The neurologic symptoms from spinal DAVFs may mimic other more common disease processes, delaying accurate diagnosis[2,15] (**Table 26.3**). The presence of radicular or back pain commonly leads to a preliminary diagnosis of lumbar spondylosis, which is very common in the patient population harboring these lesions. Early onset of micturition difficulty and weakness should prompt a physician to look closely for other possible causes including a spinal dural AVM. With the relapsing and remitting time course of its symptoms, a patient initially may be diagnosed with demyelinating disease. It is important therefore to understand that spinal dural fistulas become symptomatic in an older age group than does demyelinating disease and are predominantly in men. These demographics are very different from those of the typical

Table 26.3 Symptoms Associated with Type I Dural Arteriovenous Fistula (DAVF)

Back pain

Radicular pain

Progressive weakness

Micturition difficulty

Saddle sensory loss

Hyperreflexia

Muscle spasms

Erectile dysfunction

Pulsatile tinnitus or cranial nerve palsies in cervical DAVF

demyelinating disease patient. Therefore, taking all this information together, the typical patient presenting with a spinal DAVF would be a middle-aged man with back pain progressing slowly to mixed upper and lower motor neuron deficits, saddle sensory loss, and some micturitional dysfunction. It is important to note that spinal DAVFs at the craniocervical junction may present with symptoms mimicking an intracranial fistula with pulsatile tinnitus and cranial nerve palsies.[2]

Without treatment, these lesions are progressively debilitating.[16] In 6 months after the onset of symptoms, nearly 20% of patients are severely disabled. This number swells to 50% in 3 years and 90% in 5 years.[18] In fact, at the 3-year mark, only 9% of patients had unrestricted activity. Death may follow from sepsis due to decubitus ulcers, urinary tract infections, and pneumonia.

◆ Pathophysiology

The proposed mechanisms for the progressive neurologic deterioration seen in spinal dural fistulas include venous thrombosis, vascular steal, compression by engorged and dilated veins, arachnoiditis, and pulsatile compression.[2,3,13] After early attempts to decompress the dilated veins failed, attention turned to venous outflow abnormalities. Currently, the pathophysiology of spinal DAVFs is believed to be venous hypertension and congestion. This venous hypertension stems from the reversal of flow in the radiculomedullary veins due to the fistulous connection. This increase in pressure is transmitted to the coronal venous plexus, ultimately causing poor venous drainage and stagnation of flow. Poor venous drainage can lead to poor tissue perfusion and cord hypoxia. Some have proposed that ischemia is the primary cause of the pain experienced by the patient. This accepted pathophysiologic process corresponds well with observations made by Foix and Alajouanine in 1926.[2,9,12]

Elegant studies in the past have demonstrated the increased pressure in the draining veins in the presence of a spinal DAVF. Hassler et al[13] showed that proximal draining venous pressures were 60 to 88% of the mean systolic arterial blood pressures, with a mean value of 74%. After treatment, venous

pressures dropped to 16 to 64% of the original value. This study also indicated that prior venous pressures were affected by systemic arterial pressures prior to treatment. Once the fistulous point was treated, pressures were independent of arterial pressure, demonstrating the return of normal spinal cord autoregulation. Interestingly, clinical symptoms and outcomes were not related to the measured pressures.

Spinal DAVFs occur most commonly in the lower thoracic and upper lumbar region of the spinal cord. This region, a watershed area of arterial blood flow, is also the most easily affected by increased venous pressures. This pathophysiologic mechanism is supported by the signs and symptoms seen in the clinical setting. Patients often describe a worsening of symptoms with exercise, likely due to increased demand. Pregnancy and posture may worsen symptoms as well, likely due to compression of draining veins or increased pressure on the venous system.

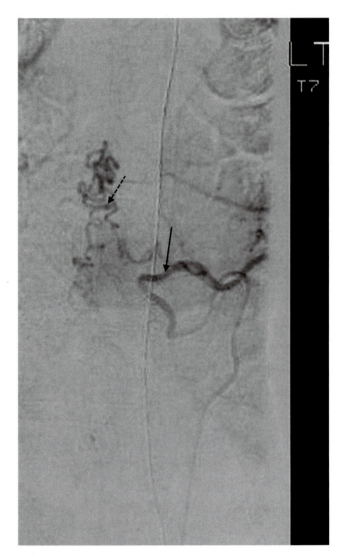

Fig. 26.2 Digital subtraction angiogram demonstrating a spinal DAVF at T7 on the left side. The solid arrow denotes the feeding artery and the dashed arrow denotes the draining vein.

◆ Diagnostic Imaging

Initially, the diagnosis of spinal DAVFs was made with exploratory laminectomy as demonstrated by Charles Elsberg.[2,12] Using spinal myelography, Perthes in 1927 first imaged a spinal DAVF. Since that time, MRI and selective diagnostic angiography have become the mainstay of diagnosis. Newer imaging techniques including improved MR angiography and intraoperative ICG videoangiography have further refined the diagnostic and routine follow-up process.[17,18]

Digital Subtraction Angiography

Biplane digital subtraction angiography (DSA) remains the gold standard for diagnosis of spinal DAVFs, providing superior anatomic and temporal resolution[1,2,5] **(Fig. 26.2)**. All patients suspected of having a spinal DAVF should undergo DSA to classify the lesion and establish the location and number of feeders to the fistula. The ability to examine arterial and venous phase images in high resolution is unique and valuable for evaluation of treatment options.[6] With improvements in endovascular treatment of these lesions, a diagnostic angiogram can easily lead to endovascular obliteration of the lesion. Because of the invasive nature of angiography, this test is typically the last diagnostic test ordered by a physician, usually after MRI and often as a confirmational test.

When obtaining a spinal DSA on a patient with a suspected DAVF, there are several important points to consider. A common femoral sheath is usually placed to easily allow catheter exchange. Multiple curved catheter tips are available to allow cannulation of arterial feeders in the cervical, thoracic, and lumbar regions. The angiogram must be continued into the late venous phase to identify late opacification of the fistula. Delayed venous drainage from the artery of Adamkiewicz is present in the majority of patients presenting with spinal DAVFs.[2] Given that a fistula may be fed from multiple levels (type I-B), levels adjacent to the fistula must be examined for additional feeding arteries. This can include the iliacs in the sacral spine as well as the costocervical, thyrocervical, and external carotid arteries in the cervical spine.

Computed Tomography Myelography and Angiography

Computed tomography myelography, initially the mainstay in the diagnosis of spinal DAVFs, has now yielded to MRI as the noninvasive imaging test of choice.[2,6,19] Although sensitive for detecting vessels in the subarachnoid space, myelography may identify normal arterial and venous structures[2] **(Fig. 26.3)**. CT myelography still plays a role in patients who are unable to undergo MRI. CT angiography plays an increasingly vital role in the diagnosis of spinal DAVFs.[6] Multidetector

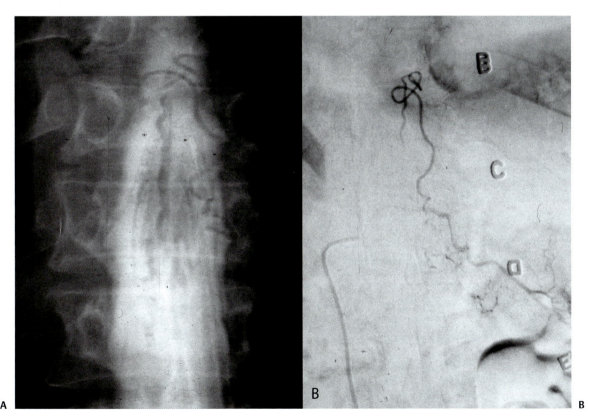

A   B   B

Fig. 26.3 **(A)** Computed tomography (CT) myelogram demonstrates enlarged vessels in the subarachnoid space. The arrow points to enlarged subarachnoid vessels. **(B)** Digital subtraction angiogram confirms the diagnosis of a spinal DAVF demonstrated on CT myelography.

spiral CT angiography has proven to be an excellent test for determining a fistulous point when compared with spinal angiography. At this time, the temporal and spatial resolution of CT angiography is still inferior to DSA, especially in examining arterial and venous phases of injections.

Magnetic Resonance Imaging and Magnetic Resonance Angiography

Magnetic resonance imaging is the initial imaging modality used to identify spinal DAVFs in the majority of patients.[2,6,19] The presence of enlarged subarachnoid vessels typically offers clues to the diagnosis of these lesions. These can be seen as serpiginous flow voids on T2-weighted imaging. Care should be taken to exclude the presence of pulsatile flow artifact from cerebrospinal fluid. Signal change in the cord parenchyma can be seen in both T1- and T2-weighted images (**Fig. 26.4**). In fact, the T2 signal change can be present over one to 11 vertebral segments and often down to the conus medullaris. Gilbertson et al[19] found that T2 signal change in the cord was present in all 30 patients with confirmed spinal DAVFs in their study. The administration of gadolinium leads to contrast enhancement in the same area as the T2 signal change. Studies have further shown that enhancement increases over time when MRIs are completed in a delayed fashion, further illustrating a delay in venous outflow. Unfortunately, MRI alone provides a static and nonspecific image.

Rapid time resolved magnetic resonance angiography (MRA) has been developed to improve temporal and maintain spatial resolution.[6,18] This technique allows visualization of large segments of fistulas while avoiding large doses of ionizing radiation. Unfortunately, the disadvantages include a poorer signal-to-noise ratio with the increase in temporal resolution, difficulty in detecting normal intramedullary vessels, a limitation in spatial resolution, and time-consuming and expensive postprocessing required for the images. Ali et al[18] demonstrated in a group of 11 patients that MRA correctly identified the fistulous site in the six patients with spinal DAVFs and correctly showed that the other five patients did not have spinal DAVFs. All results were confirmed with DSA. It should be noted that MRI can provide false localization, illustrating the importance of DSA as the gold standard.

There are reports of patients in the literature with angiographically occult spinal DAVF. Alleyne et al[20] reported three patients who presented with symptoms consistent with a spinal DAVF but no filling of the feeding artery during DSA. In these cases, CT and MRI demonstrated a possible fistula site, and surgical exploration was undertaken to treat the lesions.

Intraoperative Imaging

Intraoperative DSA has been used since the early 1990s to document complete obliteration of a spinal dural fistula[21] (**Fig. 26.5**). In the past several years, intraoperative ICG near-infrared videoangiography has emerged as a rapid and safe alternative to spinal DSA for confirmation of the obliteration of a fistula.[17] ICG angiography allows temporal resolution of the fistula with detailed spatial resolution. The primary

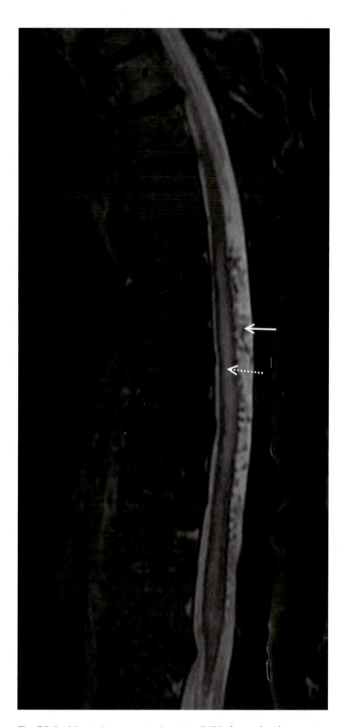

Fig. 26.4 Magnetic resonance imaging (MRI) shows the characteristic findings associated with a DAVF, including enlarged subarachnoid vessels *(solid arrow)* and T2 cord signal change *(dotted arrow)*.

advantages of this technique are its rapid use, taking several minutes to inject and view in the microscope, and low cost. It is important to note that the site of the fistula must be visible in the operative site as the ICG cannot be viewed through tissue or blood. ICG angiography also avoids further radiation to the patient and the operative team.

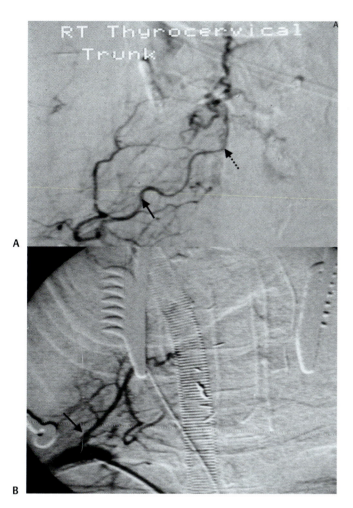

Fig. 26.5 **(A)** Angiogram illustrates a type IB spinal DAVF off the thyrocervical and costovertebral trunks. The solid arrow denotes the feeding artery and the dashed arrow denotes the draining vein. **(B)** Intraoperative angiogram demonstrates obliteration of the fistula.

Follow-Up Imaging

The follow-up imaging of choice varies in the literature. Most patients undergo a confirmatory angiogram either at the time of surgery or during the same admission. After confirmation of fistula occlusion, follow-up imaging is generally based on clinical improvement. In patients with a delay in recovery, a follow-up MRI or angiogram can be completed to determine treatment effectiveness. Reports in the literature show that MRA may contribute to postoperative assessment of fistula occlusion in the future.

◆ Treatment of Spinal Dural Arteriovenous Fistulas

Given the progressive course associated with spinal DAVFs, virtually all patients should be considered for treatment. As shown by Aminoff and Logue,[16] the neurologic prognosis of an untreated DAVF is poor, with 91% of patients severely disabled at 3 years after symptom onset. This indicates that a symptomatic DAVF should be treated as aggressively as possible.

The earliest recorded successful treatment of a spinal DAVF was performed by Charles Elsberg in 1916,[2] who removed a 2-cm segment of abnormally dilated vein. The patient made a dramatic recovery within 3 months of the surgery. Since that time, surgical results were inconsistent until an understanding of the pathology through angiography was completed. Surgical literature advanced with the work of Kendall and Logue[10] in 1977 and the subsequent work of Oldfield et al[22] in 1983.

These early works detailed the need for interruption of the arterialized draining vein. Since that time, both endovascular and surgical methods have been used to successfully obliterate the fistula with varying neurologic recoveries in afflicted patients. The choice between open surgical and endovascular therapy varies depending on the desire of the patient and the available expertise in a given institution.

Endovascular

With patients undergoing DSA routinely for evaluation and confirmation of the presence of a spinal DAVF, endovascular therapy provides a logical method for interruption of the fistula. Unfortunately, initial results for endovascular therapy were poor using polyvinyl alcohol, with recurrence rates up to 83%.[23,24] The development of liquid embolics has led to continued decreases in recurrence rates in the literature.[5,7]

The primary goal of endovascular therapy is to embolize the distal feeding artery, the complete nidus, and the proximal portion of the arterialized draining vein.[2,7,25] If occlusion occurs too proximally in the arterial feeder, there is a high rate of fistula persistence and recanalization. If excessive distal occlusion on the venous side occurs, the patient may have worsening of clinical symptoms due to an exacerbation of venous hypertension. The anatomy of the fistula must be taken into account prior to treatment. In the 10 to 15% of cases where the spinal DAVF is supplied by a radiculomedullary artery that also supplies the anterior or posterior spinal arteries, open surgical obliteration is indicated.[2] Endovascular therapy is of limited use in patients in whom the radicular artery is exceptionally tortuous, making canalization with a microcatheter extremely difficult or impossible.

As mentioned above, the use of liquid adhesive embolic agents such as N-butyl-2-cyanoacrylate (NBCA) and the Onyx liquid embolic system (eV3, Inc., Plymouth, MN) have shown higher success rates and lower recurrence rates from earlier studies (**Figs. 26.6 and 26.7**). Narvid et al[5] from the University of California at San Francisco reported a cure rate of 77% (27 of 35 patients) in patients undergoing initial endovascular exploration using primarily NBCA. Park et al[26] reported an initial endovascular success rate of 82.4% (14 of 17 patients). Two of these patients suffered recurrence from recanalization or collateral development (**Fig. 26.8**). Initial success rates in past studies have varied from 30 to 90%.[7,25] Nogueira et al[27] reported a small group of three patients treated with Onyx with no residual or recurrence.

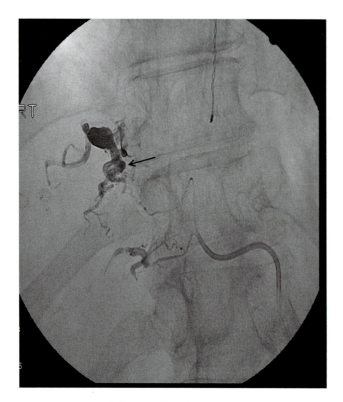

Fig. 26.6 Onyx embolization of a right T10 spinal DAVF. Arrow denotes the onyx cast.

difference in patient clinical symptoms in patients successfully treated by surgery or endovascular methods.

Surgical

The goal of surgical treatment of spinal DAVFs is disconnection of the fistula and the arterialized draining vein to relieve the venous hypertension.[22] Preoperative planning is essential to understand the location and anatomy surrounding the fistula. Care should be taken to note all the feeding arteries, as the laminectomy must include all involved levels. The surgeon should also recognize the direction of the draining vein; usually it is the rostral direction. Finally, great care must be taken to determine the correct level prior to incision. This can be completed with intraoperative fluoroscopy to count the spinal levels, neuronavigation, or preoperative marking by radiology.

After correct localization, the procedure involves a laminectomy or hemilaminectomy at the site of the fistula. The laminectomy must be taken laterally out to the facet to expose the nerve root, as the fistulous point typically lies dorsolaterally. Even if the facet capsule is violated, patients typically are not unstable after the procedure. The operating microscope is brought into the field at this time.

Prior to opening the dura, time should be taken to achieve meticulous hemostasis. The dura is opened and tacked back using a 4-0 Nurolon suture. The arachnoid can then be opened using an arachnoid blade. At this time, the dilated, engorged veins should be visible on the dorsal surface of the spinal cord. Using microdissectors the intradural contents can be carefully mobilized to expose the fistula **(Fig. 26.9)**.

Indocyanine green (ICG) videoangiography can be used to aid in identifying the fistula at this point.[17] The efferent arterialized vein is dissected, coagulated using bipolar cautery, and cut sharply. Attention is turned to the nidus, which is

After adequate treatment, patients who undergo endovascular therapy have improvement or stabilization of symptoms. Endovascular therapy has been associated with shorter hospital stays. The disadvantages of the procedure include higher documented recurrence rates as well as a need for radiation exposure. There has been no study demonstrating a

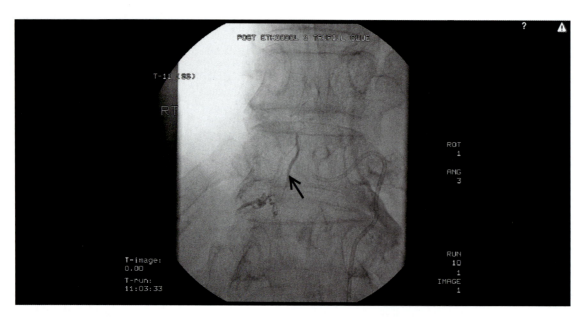

Fig. 26.7 *N*-butyl-2-cyanocrylate (NBCA) embolization *(arrow)* of a right T11 spinal DAVF.

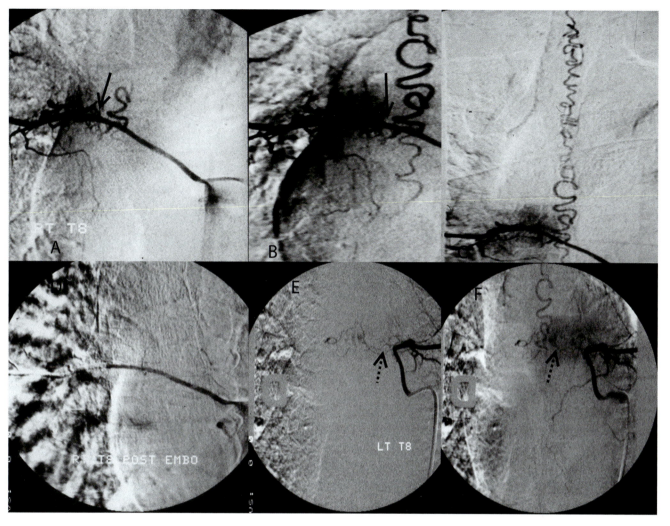

Fig. 26.8 Example of a recurrence of a spinal DAVF following embolization. **(A–C)** DSA demonstrates a spinal DAVF at T8 filling from the right *(solid arrow)*. **(D)** Postembolization angiogram demonstrates obliteration of the fistula. **(E,F)** Follow-up angiogram demonstrates a recurrence filling from the left T8 *(dotted arrow)*.

carefully coagulated and then inspected for other arterial feeders **(Fig. 26.10)**. Care must be taken to preserve both the radicular artery and the nerve root.

Several options are available to determine the completeness of the surgery. First, a surgeon can inspect the coronal venous plexus to ensure decreased engorgement and darkening, which occurs slowly over several minutes. Another option available to the surgeon is intraoperative Doppler ultrasonography, which can be easily brought onto the field for testing the venous plexus of the spinal cord.[28] A third option requires the previous placement of a wraparound sheath for intraoperative angiography. This method has been shown to be both effective and safe in the operating room setting.[21] Unfortunately, this method can be time-consuming due to the complicated nature of a spinal angiogram in the prone position. In the last several years, ICG videoangiography has emerged as a safe, reproducible, and rapid method to assess the adequacy of fistula disconnection.[17] As mentioned previously, ICG cannot be viewed through tissue or hematoma.

Therefore, all vessels in question must be visible in the operating microscope field.

The dura is closed in a watertight fashion. The lamina may be replaced using small titanium plates if it was preserved. The wound is closed in the usual fashion. In the recovery room, the patient should be assessed for signs of neurologic deficit. Further imaging can be obtained depending on the quality of intraoperative imaging and the clinical progression of the patient.

The results of surgical disconnection of spinal DAVFs have been studied in detail. The initial cure rates for surgery range from 84 to 98% in reports from 1999 and 2004.[2,4] A meta-analysis by Steinmetz et al[4] estimates surgical complication rates of 1.9%, slightly lower than those for endovascular treatment (3.7%). The primary disadvantage of surgery remains its invasive nature, with longer hospital stays documented in multiple reports.

Outcomes following surgical and endovascular therapy have been shown to be similar if the fistula is completely

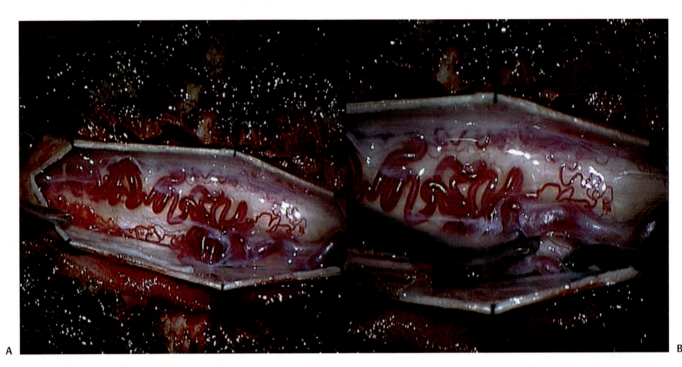

Fig. 26.9 **(A)** Microsurgical exposure of a type I spinal DAVF. Note the engorged coronal venous plexus present on the surface of the spinal cord *(solid arrow)*. **(B)** Identification of the fistulous site at the nerve root sleeve *(dotted arrow)*.

disconnected.[2,7] Multiple studies have shown improvement or stabilization of symptoms in the majority of cases. The degree of improvement is related to the preoperative functional status of the patient, reinforcing the need for early treatment.[2] Narvid et al[5] found significant improvement in neurologic outcomes in both endovascular and surgical groups.

They noted that bladder dysfunction, previously documented to be recalcitrant to treatment, and weakness both improved. Van Dijk et al[8] in 2002 showed that all patients included in the study had stable or improved neurologic examinations at an average of 33 months of follow-up. There have been reports of late clinical deterioration following long periods of

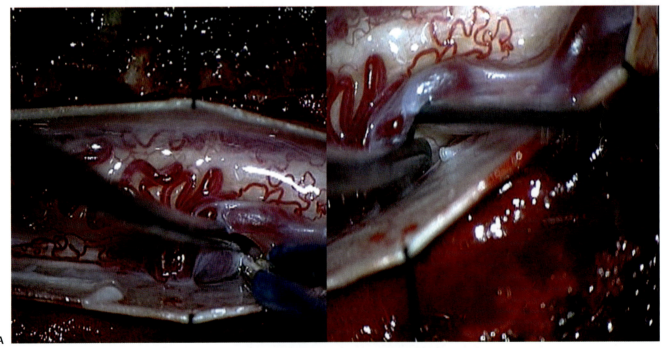

Fig. 26.10 **(A)** Coagulation of the fistulous point using bipolar cautery *(solid arrow)*. **(B)** Division of the fistula *(dotted arrow)*.

improvement or stabilization. Tacconi et al[29] in 1997 reviewed 25 patients and reported a long-term and delayed functional decline after successful treatment. The theory behind this deterioration is that a slow but progressive and irreversible decline is due to local vascular changes following the disconnection of the fistula.[29]

Radiosurgery

There have been reports of successful treatment of intramedullary spinal AVMs and intracranial DAVFs with radiosurgery.[30] At this time, there is insufficient data on the treatment of type I spinal DAVFs with stereotactic radiosurgery.

◆ Conclusion

Although there are numerous reports in the neurosurgical literature concerning spinal DAVFs, this pathologic entity continues to be misdiagnosed. Patients have symptoms for 1 to 2 years on average prior to diagnosis. Given that outcomes are directly related to pretreatment neurologic condition, it is imperative to make an early diagnosis. Modern imaging studies continue to make advances in detection, with noninvasive MRI, MRA, and CT angiography providing the diagnosis in many cases. Surgical intervention continues to be the most reliable method for permanent fistula disconnection, although improved liquid embolics and catheters have closed the gap significantly. Good outcomes after intervention can be achieved with both surgical and endovascular treatment.

References

1. Kim LJ, Spetzler RF. Classification and surgical management of spinal arteriovenous lesions: arteriovenous fistulae and arteriovenous malformations. Neurosurgery 2006;59(5, Suppl 3)S195–S201, discussion S3–S13
2. Barrow DL, Awad IA, American Association of Neurological Surgeons. Spinal Vascular Malformations. Park Ridge, IL: American Association of Neurological Surgeons, 1999
3. Aminoff MJ, Barnard RO, Logue V. The pathophysiology of spinal vascular malformations. J Neurol Sci 1974;23:255–263
4. Steinmetz MP, Chow MM, Krishnaney AA, et al. Outcome after the treatment of spinal dural arteriovenous fistulae: a contemporary single-institution series and meta-analysis. Neurosurgery 2004;55:77–87, discussion 87–88
5. Narvid J, Hetts SW, Larsen D, et al. Spinal dural arteriovenous fistulae: clinical features and long-term results. Neurosurgery 2008;62:159–166, discussion 166–167
6. Eddleman CS, Jeong H, Cashen TA, et al. Advanced noninvasive imaging of spinal vascular malformations. Neurosurg Focus 2009;26:E9
7. Dehdashti AR, Da Costa LB, terBrugge KG, Willinsky RA, Tymianski M, Wallace MC. Overview of the current role of endovascular and surgical treatment in spinal dural arteriovenous fistulas. Neurosurg Focus 2009;26:E8
8. Van Dijk JM, TerBrugge KG, Willinsky RA, Farb RI, Wallace MC. Multidisciplinary management of spinal dural arteriovenous fistulas: clinical presentation and long-term follow-up in 49 patients. Stroke 2002;33:1578–1583
9. Black P. Spinal vascular malformations: an historical perspective. Neurosurg Focus 2006;21:E11
10. Kendall BE, Logue V. Spinal epidural angiomatous malformations draining into intrathecal veins. Neuroradiology 1977;13:181–189
11. Spetzler RF, Detwiler PW, Riina HA, Porter RW. Modified classification of spinal cord vascular lesions. J Neurosurg 2002;96(2, Suppl)145–156
12. Klopper HB, Surdell DL, Thorell WE. Type I spinal dural arteriovenous fistulas: historical review and illustrative case. Neurosurg Focus 2009;26:E3
13. Hassler W, Thron A, Grote EH. Hemodynamics of spinal dural arteriovenous fistulas. An intraoperative study. J Neurosurg 1989;70:360–370
14. Barrow DL, Colohan AR, Dawson R. Intradural perimedullary arteriovenous fistulas (type IV spinal cord arteriovenous malformations). J Neurosurg 1994;81:221–229
15. Aminoff MJ, Logue V. Clinical features of spinal vascular malformations. Brain 1974;97:197–210
16. Aminoff MJ, Logue V. The prognosis of patients with spinal vascular malformations. Brain 1974;97:211–218
17. Raabe A, Beck J, Gerlach R, Zimmermann M, Seifert V. Near-infrared indocyanine green video angiography: a new method for intraoperative assessment of vascular flow. Neurosurgery 2003;52:132–139, discussion 139
18. Ali S, Cashen TA, Carroll TJ, et al. Time-resolved spinal MR angiography: initial clinical experience in the evaluation of spinal arteriovenous shunts. AJNR Am J Neuroradiol 2007;28:1806–1810
19. Gilbertson JR, Miller GM, Goldman MS, Marsh WR. Spinal dural arteriovenous fistulas: MR and myelographic findings. AJNR Am J Neuroradiol 1995;16:2049–2057
20. Alleyne CH Jr, Barrow DL, Joseph G. Surgical management of angiographically occult spinal dural arteriovenous fistulae (type I spinal arteriovenous malformations): three technical case reports. Neurosurgery 1999;44:891–894, discussion 894–895
21. Barrow DL, Boyer KL, Joseph GJ. Intraoperative angiography in the management of neurovascular disorders. Neurosurgery 1992;30:153–159
22. Oldfield EH, Di Chiro G, Quindlen EA, Rieth KG, Doppman JL. Successful treatment of a group of spinal cord arteriovenous malformations by interruption of dural fistula. J Neurosurg 1983;59:1019–1030
23. Hall WA, Oldfield EH, Doppman JL. Recanalization of spinal arteriovenous malformations following embolization. J Neurosurg 1989;70:714–720
24. Marsh WR. Vascular lesions of the spinal cord: history and classification. Neurosurg Clin N Am 1999;10:1–8
25. Medel R, Crowley RW, Dumont AS. Endovascular management of spinal vascular malformations: history and literature review. Neurosurg Focus 2009;26:E7
26. Park SB, Han MH, Jahng TA, Kwon BJ, Chung CK. Spinal dural arteriovenous fistulas: clinical experience with endovascular treatment as a primary therapeutic modality. J Korean Neurosurg Soc 2008;44:364–369
27. Nogueira RG, Dabus G, Rabinov JD, Ogilvy CS, Hirsch JA, Pryor JC. Onyx embolization for the treatment of spinal dural arteriovenous fistulae: initial experience with long-term follow-up. Technical case report. Neurosurgery 2009;64:E197–E198, discussion E198
28. Randel S, Gooding GA, Dillon WP. Sonography of intraoperative spinal arteriovenous malformations. J Ultrasound Med 1987;6:539–544
29. Tacconi L, Lopez Izquierdo BC, Symon L. Outcome and prognostic factors in the surgical treatment of spinal dural arteriovenous fistulas. A long-term study. Br J Neurosurg 1997;11:298–305
30. Sinclair J, Chang SD, Gibbs IC, Adler JR Jr. Multisession CyberKnife radiosurgery for intramedullary spinal cord arteriovenous malformations. Neurosurgery 2006;58:1081–1089, discussion 1081–1089

27

Surgical Approaches to Intracerebral Hemorrhage

Christopher S. Eddleman, Jennifer Jaffe, Rudy J. Rahme, H. Hunt Batjer, Bernard R. Bendok, and Issam A. Awad

Pearls

- Rapid correction of coagulopathies can reduce hematoma expansion with the use of appropriate reversal agents and in a timely fashion, which can reduce morbidity associated with volume expansion.
- The combination of both stereotactically placed catheters and open surgical evacuation can be done in a safe manner and lead to reduced morbidity in intracerebral hemorrhage (ICH) patients.
- Emergent hematoma evacuation remains a lifesaving intervention in younger patients with large ICH volume who are deteriorating clinically, and in patients with cerebellar ICH. These patients have generally been excluded from clinical trials.
- Volume reduction or enhanced clearance rate of hematoma may be the operative goals of interventions for ICH in most patients with stable ICH and slow neurologic decline, as opposed to immediate and complete hematoma evacuation.
- Intraventricular thrombolytics can be used safely and lead to increased clearing of intraventricular hemorrhage (IVH) and reduced rates of hydrocephalus without an increased risk of rehemorrhage. The effectiveness of this intervention is currently being tested in a phase III trial.

Spontaneous intracerebral hemorrhage (ICH), although accounting for only 10 to 30% of all stroke admissions to hospitals,[1–3] represents the most devastating and costly[1–3] type of stroke and harbors the poorest outcomes, with only approximately 20% of patients regaining any functional dependence at 6 months.[1,3] The great majority of hemorrhagic strokes consist of intracerebral hemorrhage with or without intraventricular hemorrhage (IVH) and have been associated with 30-day mortality rates ranging from 30 to 50%[2–9] and case disability rates above 80%.[10–13] As such, the societal and financial burden continues to pose a serious health care economic load. Unlike ischemic strokes for which noteworthy therapeutic progress has been made through acute thrombolysis and several effective medical and surgical approaches for secondary stroke prevention, the management of spontaneous ICH has remained controversial. As technology and surgical techniques have continued to evolve and improve, the question regarding surgical treatment for ICH continues to be reassessed. McKissock and colleagues[14] conducted the first prospective, randomized trial of surgical treatment of ICH in 1961 and raised the possibility that carefully selected patients may benefit from surgical therapy of ICH with and without accompanying IVH. This chapter discusses ICH and IVH, and the surgical management, outcomes, and future considerations and studies regarding this devastating type of stroke.

◆ Epidemiology

Intracerebral hemorrhage can be classified as primary or secondary. Primary ICH, accounting for over 70% of ICH cases, is typically the result of cerebral amyloid angiopathy (CAA) or chronic hypertension (hypertensive arteriopathy), most commonly in the elderly population.[1,4,15–18] There is a slight male dominance of the disease, and incidence rates are approximately twice as high in African-American, Hispanic, and Asian populations.[1,18–23] Primary ICH is often found in the deeper, subcortical areas of the brain. Secondary ICH often results from the use of anticoagulants or antithrombolytic agents, the presence of vascular anomalies, the use of illicit drugs, or from coagulation disorders, and is more often found in younger patients. Secondary ICHs are more commonly lobar in location[24] (**Fig. 27.1**).

The strongest risk factors for primary ICH are hypertension and advancing age. In addition, a wide variety of studies

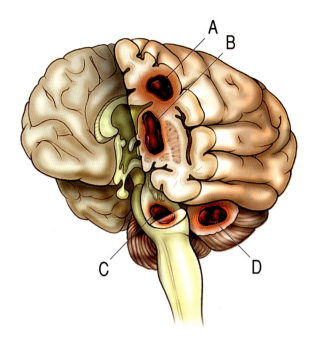

Fig. 27.1 Locations of intraparenchymal hemorrhage. A, lobar; B, basal ganglia; C, brainstem; D, cerebellum.

have demonstrated strong independent relationships of the Glasgow Coma Scale (GCS) score on presentation (inverse relationship), age, and ICH volume on outcome after ICH.[25–32] The independent and negative impact of associated IVH and its relationship to increased mortality have also been reported.[8,13,16,25–30,33–38] Clot location, smoking and drinking histories, cardiac disease, and diabetes are also related risk factors for ICH.[6,27,30]

Despite the suggested benefit of surgery in trauma-related ICH and the removal of subdural hematoma, the role of surgical intervention in nontraumatic, spontaneous ICH remains inconsistent in clinical practice. In spite of this discordant approach to patients with ICH, approximately 6000 to 7000 patients undergo operative removal of ICH annually.[39,40] Recent study suggested potential eligibility for ICH evacuation in up to 15% of prospectively screened ICH cases, with up to 30% of cases benefiting from drainage of associated IVH.[41] The goal of surgery in ICH and IVH is to decrease the size of the clot, reduce any mass effect, limit increases in intracranial pressure (ICP), and minimize the neurotoxic effects of blood-degradation products.

◆ Pathogenesis

Primary ICH is the result of chronic damage to the small blood vessels in the brain. The cerebral arterioles play an integral role in reducing blood pressure and pulse pressure in the microvasculature of the brain, but are susceptible to the effects of chronic hypertension. Chronic hypertension stimulates gradual, adaptive changes in an attempt to preserve the blood–brain barrier. Elevated blood pressure can lead to

smooth muscle hyperplasia, vascular remodeling, and eventually cellular death. When this occurs, the affected arterioles become largely fibrotic, lacking viable smooth muscle cells, which is characterized by fibrinoid necrosis and lipohyalinosis, leading to the formation of Charcot-Bouchard aneurysms, which make vessels more susceptible to rupture.[42] The small lenticulostriate vessels that originate as right-angle branches from the middle cerebral artery stem (a large diameter vessel with a vigorous, high pressure blood flow) are particularly susceptible to damage from hypertension.[43] These vessels penetrate into the basal ganglia, and thus when a rupture occurs, it more frequently involves the deeper regions of the brain including the basal ganglia, thalamus, subcortical white matter, and pons.

Hypertension is of particular importance not only because it can cause ICH, but also because it is a potentially modifiable risk factor, and is hence amenable to primary prevention strategies. Hypertension increases the risk of stroke by two to more than four times, independent of other risk factors. Elevation of either systolic or diastolic pressure is associated with greater risk.[44] Brott et al[17] suggested that population strategies to control hypertension could decrease the incidence of ICH by 39%.

Cerebral amyloid angiopathy is a very common finding in the brains of Alzheimer's disease (AD) patients and is recognized as a histopathologic attribute of the disease. CAA is the progressive process by which an amyloid protein deposits in the cerebral blood vessels, preferentially in the cortical and leptomeningeal arteries and arterioles, and results in degenerative vascular changes. The importance of CAA as a risk factor for ICH has become increasingly more significant in recent years as it was revealed that the same amyloid β (Aβ) peptide that was associated with AD was also responsible for a significant proportion of ICH (7–10%) occurring in nonhypertensive patients.[45] These degenerative changes have been associated with decreased vascular integrity and fragility, which increase the susceptibility to rupture.[46]

Until recently, the diagnosis of probable CAA was based on neuropathologic findings in a biopsy specimen or in tissue obtained during hematoma evacuation. Staining techniques with Congo red allows ready identification of amyloid in tissue samples. In the absence of neuropathologic confirmation, the diagnosis of probable CAA has been based on the finding of frequent hemorrhages, and sometimes microhemorrhages, in patients over 60 years of age, or in instances where there is a solitary hemorrhage with no other obvious cause. From a current radiologic standpoint, the most sensitive techniques for detecting microhemorrhages associated with CAA are by T2-weighted gradient echo (GRE) and susceptibility-weighted magnetic resonance imaging (MRI), as these can detect a loss of signal from the presence of hemosiderin in the foci of the microbleeds.

The *ApoE* gene on chromosome 21 has been associated with many cases of CAA and is polymorphic in humans, encoding one of three alleles designated ε2, ε3, or ε4.[47–50] Recent evidence suggests that although the ε3 allele is the normal genotype, the ε4 allele predisposes deposition of Aβ in the walls of the small blood vessels while the ε2 is associated with CAA-related hemorrhage.[51] It has also been shown that carriers of the ε2 or ε4 allele have an increased risk of recurrent ICH.[52,53] In addition, there may be an interaction between genetic and environmental factors that increases the risk of ICH in the presence of a genetic predisposition. It has been suggested that CAA patients exposed to clinical risk factors such as hypertension, antiplatelet/anticoagulant medication, and minor head trauma appear to be at most risk of lobar hemorrhage if those same patients were *ApoE* ε2 carriers than those who did not carry that allele.[50]

◆ Acute Resuscitation and Medical Management

The clinical presentation of ICH patients is highly variable but most often includes depressed mental status, focal neurologic deficits, and cardiovascular instability. After the primary survey of the patient, including the securing of an airway, assessment of breathing, and maintenance of adequate cerebral and systemic circulation and blood pressure, the patient can then be evaluated from a neurologic point of view.

Intracranial imaging with a noncontrast computed tomography (CT) scan of the head is the most common modality for evaluation of acute mental status and neurologic changes, and it is highly sensitive and specific for the diagnosis of ICH. Once the diagnosis of ICH has been made, then the management team can focus on the parameters that are important for minimizing hematoma expansion and secondary sequelae. At this point, it is important to consider potential etiologies of ICH. Once stabilization of the patient has occurred, other imaging modalities, such as computed tomography angiography (CTA) or MRI of the brain, can be used to delineate potential etiologic factors responsible for the ICH, such as aneurysm, arteriovenous malformation (AVM), tumor, and so on.

Intracranial Pressure Management

For patients who present with impaired level of consciousness (typically a GCS score <9) or for those whose neurologic exam is unreliable, intracranial pressure (ICP) monitoring should be considered. ICP can be monitored using a fiberoptic intraparenchymal monitor ("bolt") or an external ventricular drain (EVD). The bolt is more accurate and can be combined with an intraventricular monitor. The intraventricular component allows therapeutic drainage of cerebrospinal fluid (CSF) and accurate monitoring of ICP, especially in cases of ventricular obstruction. Optimizing the patient's position by elevation of the head while keeping the head midline and keeping the temperature <37°C, thus preventing hyperthermia and euvolemia, and draining CSF through the ventricular drain can be used to control ICP. Altering the carbon dioxide levels in the blood through mild hyperventilation can also alter the volume load and demand of the brain but should not be maintained for long periods of time. The effects of chronic hyperventilation can be compensated by metabolic acidosis over time, limiting its chronic effect on ICP, and increasing vulnerability to rebound hyperperfusion. Pharmacologic management of ICP may involve hyperosmotic solutions, for example, 3% sodium or mannitol. Diuretics can also lead to increased sodium levels and decreases in systemic volume. Finally, sedatives, paralytics, and barbiturates can be used to reduce the systemic and cerebral metabolic demands and thus reduce brain blood volume and facilitate ICP control

Blood Pressure Control

Patients with ICH often present with elevated systolic blood pressure (SBP) of >160 mm Hg. It has been shown that hematoma enlargement has been associated with elevated blood pressure and neurologic deterioration.[15,16] Further, elevated pressure has been associated with the expansion of the original hematoma, intraventricular extension, and worse overall outcome.[54–57] However, in the face of elevated ICP, the acute management of SBP can be a challenge; one must not decrease cerebral perfusion pressure (CPP) at the expense of BP management. The American Heart Association guidelines currently recommend blood pressure control if the SBP is >180 mm Hg or mean arterial pressure is >130 mm Hg. Several reports have suggested that reduced SBP within 6 hour was associated with improved mortality; however, these studies did not control for pretreatment GCS, ICH volume, and the presence of IVH—factors shown to be associated with increased morbidity and mortality. Acute and rapid reduction of SBP has also been shown to increase mortality primarily due to ischemic complications, both systemic and neurologic. Recent trials examining the effect of blood pressure control in patients with ICH have been completed. The Intensive Blood Pressure Reduction in Acute Cerebral Hemorrhage Trial (INTERACT) demonstrated no significant difference in neurologic deterioration at 72 hours between ICH groups who presented within 6 hour of onset and whose blood pressure was reduced to <180 mm Hg or <140 mm Hg; however, there was a trend toward reduction of ICH volume growth in patients whose blood pressure was more aggressively reduced.[58] Another trial, the Antihypertensive Treatment in Acute Cerebral Hemorrhage (ATACH) trial, did not preliminarily show a significant difference between three groups with targeted SBP targets.[59,60] Worster et al[61] recently reviewed the literature regarding whether early intensive lowering of blood pressure reduced hematoma volume and improved clinical outcomes, and found that although there are trends toward reduction in hematoma volume, there is no improvement in clinical outcomes. Therefore, it is currently reasonable to treat elevated blood pressures using the American Heart Association (AHA) guidelines. Ongoing clinical trials such as ATACH and INTERACT2 will continue to increase our understanding of the principles of blood pressure management in acute ICH.

Reversal of Coagulopathy

Hemostasis and correction of an underlying coagulopathy are important determinants of hematoma expansion. Patients who present with ICH often have been on some form of anticoagulant or antiplatelet therapy, thus presenting with an altered ability to maintain adequate hemostasis in the face of hemorrhage. It is estimated that approximately 15% of ICH cases are associated with warfarin use, which has been shown to increase the risk of ICH five to 10 times and doubles the risk of mortality and increases the risk of progressive bleeding and clinical deterioration. Furthermore, it has been shown that patients on warfarin therapy are associated with larger initial hematoma volumes and continue to expand for longer durations.[62] Some studies have also shown that antiplatelet agents increase the risk of ICH[63,64]; for example, aspirin therapy has been shown to increase the risk of ICH by approximately 40% and in combination with clopidogrel up to approximately 60%, but some studies have refuted this claim.[6,65,66] The cardiovascular benefits of these medications often outweigh their hemorrhage risks in most patients. However, when patients present with ICH and have been on anticoagulants, it is paramount to begin the correction of their coagulation parameters immediately so as to reduce the chance for hematoma expansion. In patients with mechanical heart valves or persistent atrial fibrillation requiring anticoagulant therapy, the patients' international normalized ratio (INR) can be lowered to 1.5 to 2 without a significant increase in stroke risk over a short period of time (<2 weeks).[67,68]

There have not been any prospective randomized studies addressing the efficacy of anticoagulant reversal protocols. The available reversal agents for reversal of anticoagulation are vitamin K_1, fresh frozen plasma (FFP), prothrombin complex conjugates (PCCs), and recombinant activated factor VII (rFVIIa). Vitamin K_1 administration, either intravenous or oral, has been shown to be effective but not in the early hours, making this agent ineffective for the hyperacute period.[69] Although the most common method of anticoagulant reversal has been the intravenous administration of FFP, the optimal dosing parameters have not been well established. Administration of FFP is normally delayed due to the requirement of compatibility testing and thawing of the blood products, which can significantly affect reversal; every 30-minute period that passes before administration has been shown to lead to a 20% reduction in the successful reversal of INR at 24 hours.[70] With ICH growth most commonly documented in the first hours after symptom onset, reversal of coagulopathy with FFP is often too slow for timely benefit. Furthermore, administration of FFP can be complicated with circulatory overload, allergic reactions, transfusion-related acute lung injury, citrate toxicity, and transmission of viral infections.[71] Although not available in the United States, but shown to be effective in several small European studies, PCC provides clotting factors that are deficient in anticoagulated patients and can reverse the INR in <30 minutes; however, improved clinical outcomes have also not been convincingly demonstrated.[71]

A promising agent in reduction of hematoma expansion has been rFVIIa, approved in the U.S. for bleeding complications of hemophilia. Several reports have documented rapid effective reversal of warfarin coagulopathy, allowing safe neurosurgical intervention in patients deteriorating from intracranial hemorrhage,[70-77] The impact of rFVIIa on ICH growth in coagulopathic patients has not been carefully evaluated, although it is increasingly used (compassionate off-label in-

dication) in deteriorating ICH patients and in cases requiring invasive interventions. Risks of thromboembolism with this agent have been reported,[78] but mostly in non-ICH patients, and there is particular concern about prothrombotic complications in patients with critical coronary disease, mechanical heart valves, cerebrovascular stenoses, or hypercoagulable states, so the potential benefits of rapid arrest of ICH growth must be carefully weighed against these risks on a case-by-case basis.[79]

There has been interest in the potential benefit of rFVIIa in preventing early ICH volume expansion in *noncoagulopathic* patients. Although administration of rFVIIa has been shown to significantly reduce the incidence of ICH volume expansion within 3 hours of symptom onset, the clinical benefit of reduced mortality and morbidity did not reach statistical significance in the phase III Factor Seven for Acute Hemorrhagic Stroke (FAST) study.[80-82] A very useful estimate of dose-related complications was provided in these studies. However, variant dosing of rFVIIa and lack of ICH risk stratification could have potentially masked benefits in some subgroups.[83] Further, this FAST approach did not control for additional measures of reducing mortality and morbidity such as blood pressure reduction and replacement of vitamin K–dependent factors, or adjuvant interventions for ICH or IVH volume reduction that could enhance clinical benefit. It is thought that the combination of strategies could potentially lead to decreased hematoma expansion and improved clinical outcomes.

Despite the optimal correction of the INR, the patient may remain coagulopathic due to insufficient levels of factor IX, not assessed or corrected by examining the INR or by inadequate platelet function, most often in patients on chronic aspirin or clopidogrel oral therapy. Reversal of platelet dysfunction is often initiated with one to two packs of single donor platelets. The evidence for adding desmopressin (de-amino-8-D-arginine vasopressin [DDAVP]) is lacking for efficacy. However, no published guidelines or general consensus exists regarding the reversal of antiplatelet agents in the face of ICH.[63,65,84,85] However, decreased platelet activity in patients with ICH has recently been associated with IVH extension and worse clinical outcomes.[86]

Surgical Management

Despite aggressive medical management, ICH continues to be associated with significant morbidity and mortality. Established factors associated with worse clinical outcomes include large initial hematoma volume with subsequent expansion, increased ICP, and intraventricular extension. Medical management has focused on the reduction of secondary injury by reducing hematoma expansion, which is thought to be reduced with aggressive blood pressure management, correction of coagulopathy, ICP control, and advancements in neurocritical care. However, some patients present with significant hematoma volumes, either initially or subsequently enlarged on follow-up imaging, such that surgical evacuation is warranted. Current clinical indications for surgical evacuation of spontaneous ICH include neurologic deterioration, expanding hematoma, uncontrollable ICP, or radiographic indications of impending brainstem herniation. However, many factors can confound the decision for surgical management such as age, medical comorbidities, neurologic status, patient's advanced directives, hematoma location, and cardiopulmonary stability at the time of presentation. As a result, patient selection for surgical management of ICH has been difficult and remains controversial. In spite of this, the surgical management of ICH with and without IVH has expanded over the last decade due to the improvement of surgical navigation systems, minimally invasive approaches, and improved control of blood pressure and coagulopathies, making surgical evacuation a viable option in a larger fraction of patients. Adjuvant critical care and medical interventions have also evolved, potentially altering outcome expectations.[41]

Open Surgical Evacuation of Intracerebral Hemorrhage

Given the higher incidence of mortality and severe morbidity as well as the monumental health care costs associated with the care of patients with spontaneous ICH, the significance of developing an alternative to medical management seemed paramount. The trauma surgery literature had demonstrated a clear benefit of evacuation intracranial hematomas.[87–90] The goals of surgical evacuating in patients with spontaneous ICHs, as with all patients with intracranial hematomas, are to remove the maximum amount of hematoma without injury to the surrounding normal brain, thus reducing mass effect, toxic burden of blood breakdown products, and ICP. Experimental models of ICH in animals demonstrated significant metabolic changes in the perihematomal brain tissue within 3 to 5 hours after blood infusion.[91] Further, other animal studies have shown that early reduction in mass effect of a lesion increases blood flow and reduces ischemic changes, resulting in improved neurologic outcomes.[92] Extending these findings into the clinical realm would be expected to result in similar outcomes. However, multiple previous randomized studies, including the largest multicenter randomized trial, the Surgical Trial in Intracerebral Hemorrhage (STICH), failed to demonstrate improved clinical outcomes in patients undergoing surgical evacuation versus best medical therapy.[93–96] The earliest surgical study of ICH evacuation came from McKissock and colleagues,[14] who reported worse clinical outcomes with surgical intervention. However, this study was confounded by the lack of appropriate imaging and the undetermined etiology of the hemorrhagic event. Subsequent studies by Juvela et al,[94] Batjer et al,[93] and Chen et al,[54] although showing a trend toward improved clinical outcomes, failed to demonstrate a statistically significant improvement in clinical and neurologic outcomes in patients with surgical evacuation of ICH versus medical therapy. The STICH trial[95] compared early surgery (within 24 hours of documentation of ICH acquired within 72 hours of ictus) with initial conservative management, although medically managed patients were available for surgical evacuation at the discretion of the treating physician, which occurred in 26% of patients due to neurologic deterioration. The primary outcome was death or disability at 6 months. Despite the insignificant benefit of early surgery as compared with initial conservative therapy, a subgroup analysis demonstrated a

possible benefit of surgical evacuation in patients who presented with superficial (<1 cm from cortical surface) hematomas. It was thought that earlier studies involving hematomas not located in or around the cortical surface necessitated the traversing of normal functioning parenchyma, leading to worse clinical and neurologic outcomes.

Advancements in technology have significantly improved the surgeon's ability to modify open surgical techniques of ICH evacuation. The introduction and progression of the surgical microscope facilitates better hemostasis and hematoma cavity exploration in cases where alternative etiologies are suspected. Neuronavigation has become ubiquitous in most academic and stroke centers and allows precise localization of the hematoma, and efficient design of the craniotomy bone flap and trajectory design such that minimal parenchyma is traversed. In the last several years, decompressive hemicraniectomy has also been used in conjunction with ICH evacuation to allow for subsequent brain swelling in cases of large hematomas. Despite these advancements in technology and the insignificant results of previous randomized trials for surgical evacuation of ICH, the secondary injuries that occur from hematomas spurred the development of minimally invasive surgical options.

Thrombolytic Evacuation of Intracerebral Hemorrhage

Historically, patients who present with smaller ICH volume (<20 cc) have a lower mortality and improved clinical outcome, thought to be due to reduced mass effect and destruction of vital brain parenchyma. Patients with large ICH volumes, as mentioned above, generally have poor outcomes with or without open surgical evacuation. Thus, the clinical question became could large ICH volumes be reduced through minimally invasive catheter techniques, as some of the high mortality and morbidity were thought to be secondary to the surgical procedure itself. Several small studies and case series exploited the possibility and feasibility of minimally invasive catheterization and evacuation of ICH, mostly using stereotactic image-guidance with CT or MRI. Despite the success of catheterization, the absolute results of these studies were mixed due to the heterogeneity of the patient population and surgical techniques utilized. To aid in the dissolution of the hematoma, some investigators injected thrombolytic agents into the catheters. Several investigators reported safe and successful reduction of clot burden with promising clinical outcomes. These results led to the proposal of a National Institutes of Health (NIH)-sponsored study to assess stereotactic guidance and minimally invasive approaches for the surgical evacuation of ICH. The Minimally Invasive Surgery Plus rtPA for Intracerebral Hemorrhage Evacuation (MISTIE) trial compares medical management alone to the placement of a stereotactically guided catheter through a burr hole into the hematoma, subsequently followed by a single aspiration and then by recombinant tissue-type plasminogen activator (rtPA) infusion into the catheter for 72 hours to medical management alone. The phase II trial is aimed at assessing safety and the preliminary treatment effect with varying doses of rTPA in comparison to endoscopic technique and best medical therapy alone (for more information, go to www

.mistietrial.com). Primary outcome measures include mortality rate and functional status at 1 year. Secondary outcome measures include quality-of-life measures and the incidence of infection, rebleeding, and procedure-related complications. Preliminary results from the first dose tier of this trial were recently presented and demonstrated that rtPA-treated cases achieved approximately a 50% reduction in ICH volume within 3 days, whereas there was no measurable ICH volume reduction in medically managed cases.[97] Hemorrhage was correlated to the placement of the catheter and rtPA administration, but well within prospectively acceptable rates. Although the techniques used for this study have been shown to be safe, early case analyses have demonstrated the importance of catheter placement for effectiveness of therapy and reduction of complications. This trial is ongoing with higher dose tiers and comparison with the endoscopic limb (discussed below).

With the advent of CT scans in the intensive care unit (ICU) and operating room, many teams are using real-time CT-guided placement of catheters in ICH or for trapped ventricles associated with IVH (see below). Advantages of this technique include immediate feedback on the extent of hematoma aspiration and the final placement of the catheter.

Endoscopic Approaches to Intracerebral Hemorrhage Evacuation

Alternative strategies to ICH evacuation were conceived in an attempt to improve the mortality experienced by both open surgical and medically managed ICH patients. Endoscopic evacuation with the assistance of stereotactic guidance or ultrasonic localization was developed in hopes of achieving improved neurologic outcomes. Auer and colleagues[98] reported the survival benefit of endoscopic evacuation with ultrasonic localization over medical management in patients with hematoma volumes greater than 50 mL, despite no additional improvement in mortality with smaller lesions. Further, patients treated with endoscopic evacuation had a more favorable recovery at 6 months. Nishihara et al[99] reported almost complete removal of hematomas in a cohort of patients presenting with volumes >40 mL without complications. Prasad et al[100] also reported significant reductions in mortality and morbidity in patients younger than 60 years who presented with initial hematoma volumes >50 mL. These positive results were thought to be due to reduced tissue damage compared to craniotomy, reduction of procedural blood loss, and reduction in procedure time. Further, better control of the hematoma cavity and more complete evacuation of the hematoma have been demonstrated, as compared with CT-guided stereotactic aspiration. To combine the advantages of endoscopic evacuation with stereotactic navigation, Miller et al[101] have recently demonstrated the safety and feasibility of combining the two modalities for patients with spontaneous ICH. Although the numbers of patients included in the endoscopic arm of this study were exceptionally small, the trend toward favorable hematoma evacuation and improvement in the mortality rate was superior to medical management and comparable to previous results by Auer et al[98] and Mendelow et al.[37]

The interest in and continued development of endoscopic techniques is clear. Continued development of endoscopic instruments for the specific use of hematoma evacuation is on the horizon, namely stereotactically guided endoscopes, more streamline endoscopic instruments, and stable pneumatic arms, which assist in the maintenance of the endoscope's position, thus allowing the surgeon to work with both hands and obviating the need for an assistant to hold the endoscopic camera. Furthermore, the inclusion of an endoscopic arm in the phase II MISTIE trial speaks to the importance of endoscopic assistance in ICH evacuation.

Intraventricular Hemorrhage

The devastating effects of hemorrhagic stroke are magnified when the blood extends into the ventricular system of the brain. This often occurs in association with deep, larger hematomas, and has been reported in 30 to 50% of ICH cases. Patients presenting to emergency departments with ventricular extension of blood often come with decreased levels of consciousness and poorer prognoses. Previous studies have reported that not only is the presence of IVH related to 30-day mortality rates,[102–107] but the volume of IVH is important to the overall outcome in ICH.[13] The presence of blood in the ventricular system disturbs a delicate balance of CSF circulation and ICP of the brain. The presence of blood can occlude the ventricles, which causes the system to obstruct CSF circulation and absorption, which in turn can compromise CPP. Furthermore, blood in the ventricular system may be related to direct mass effect on periventricular structures, causing surrounding edema and hydrocephalus.

To address the resultant issues of intraventricular blood, establishment of an external ventricular drainage system was introduced. The primary purpose of the insertion of an EVD by ventriculostomy (placing a catheter through the brain into the ventricle) is to measure and control ICP through CSF drainage. Because the insertion involves a surgical procedure, it poses a small risk of hemorrhage and increases the risk of infection, as the brain is being exposed to an open system in the process of placement of the catheter. Also, with clotted blood in the ventricles, the EVD catheter itself is likely to become occluded with blood. When this occurs, the EVD fails to perform its function to accurately measure ICP or drain CSF.

Early animal studies addressed the issue of catheter blockage and explored the use of intraventricular administration of thrombolytic agents through the EVD catheter. These studies hypothesized that the use of thrombolytics accelerated the resolution of the blood clot and prevented occlusion of the catheter, which decreased the prolonged EVD use and its associated risks/complications. An early study to address the effectiveness and safety of clot lysis was performed by Narayan et al.[108] Intracerebral-intraventricular hematomas were created by injecting 0.2 mL of clotted human blood into the frontal lobe and lateral ventricle of 57 rabbits. Investigational animals received 0.2 mL of urokinase (UK) solution immediately after injection, and control animals were given an equal volume of saline. Clot lysis was assessed after animal sacrifice at 3 hours postinjection and others at 24 hours. Those rabbits with UK injection experienced a greater clot lysis success rate (19 of 22) as compared with the control animals (3 of 13). There was no significant difference in results with these animals and with 22 other animals that were treated similarly 24 hours after clot injection. The group demonstrated that UK could be safely administered for clot lysis in the rabbit model, and a delay in therapy of up to 24 hours did not adversely influence the drug's effectiveness.

Pang and colleagues[109] conducted a series of canine studies to determine dosage of UK appropriate to lyse 10 mL of clotted intraventricular blood, and established a necessary dose of 10,000 IU. Subsequent studies addressed issues of safety by using a twofold excess dose (20,000 IU) in vivo every 12 hours for 4 days to evaluate systemic bleeding, hematology results, and localized bleeding at the site of catheter injection. This was performed on six adult dogs, resulting in no complications.[110] This led to an investigation comparing the rate of IVH resolution between 10 untreated control dogs and 10 case dogs treated with 20,000 IU every 4 hours; all the dogs had 10-mL intraventricular clots. Time to complete resolution for the treated dogs was significantly shorter than for the untreated dogs. Furthermore, eight of 10 control dogs developed hydrocephalus, whereas only two of 10 treated dogs developed the same complication. The authors concluded that intraventricular thrombolysis with UK significantly accelerated the resolution of blood, decreased the hydrocephalus, and improved the neurologic outcome.[111] A similar benefit of intraventricular thrombolysis was demonstrated in a porcine model using tissue-type plasminogen activator (tPA).[112]

Another group of researchers investigated the dose-effect relationship of tPA for the treatment of IVH in a rat model.[113] Autologous blood was injected into the left ventricles of 40 adults male rats to establish IVH, followed after 2 hours by injection of either saline or tPA in doses ranging from 0.25 to 2 µg directly into the IVH over the course of 3 hours. Twenty-four hours post–IVH induction, the brains were removed for study, revealing that dosages of 0.5 to 2 µg of tPA diminished the size of IVH in a dose-dependent manner, but only the smallest dose improved cerebral blood flow. None of the dosages improved ventricular dilation. Doses above 1 µg caused injuries, leading researchers to conclude that a safe, effective dosing ratio is 0.5 µg to treat every 5 µL of IVH.

With promising animal models of intraventricular thrombolysis supporting the hypothesis, thrombolysis was administered in humans. Case studies performed by different groups have had varying results in safety and efficacy in human subjects. The varying thrombolytic dose could partially explain the different results. Shen et al[114] used 12,000 to 96,000 IU daily in four subjects, all of whom developed an infection. Despite the complications, there were no deaths reported in this study, and the authors found the treatment to be safe and effective. Other authors using urokinase to treat IVH in conjunction with an EVD came to similar conclusions.[115–121] Several studies and case reports used tPA instead of UK, which was found to improve the outcomes.[102,112,123–131] An opposing view of the safety of tPA was presented by Schwarz et al.[132] In a small case series of two patients, there was re-

bleeding in both patients, and hydrocephalus, increased ICP, and coma occurred as well, causing the authors to caution against the use of tPA.

A shortcoming in all of these studies was the small sample sizes, and most of the studies lacked controls. A large-scale, randomized controlled study is needed to assess the safety and efficacy of thrombolysis in the setting of IVH, which has been realized in the Clot Lysis Evaluating Accelerated Resolution (CLEAR) IVH clinical trial. Although the complete analysis of the results of phase II of the CLEAR IVH trial has not yet been published, preliminary analysis indicates that placement of an EVD followed by intraventricular injection of low-dose rtPA (1 mg every 8 hours for a maximum of 4 days) resulted in dissolution of the clot an average of 24 hours before either 0.3 or 1 mg administered every 12 hours. The rate of symptomatic hemorrhage was not statistically different from that in the placebo group, although more hemorrhages were encountered when higher doses of rtPA were used.

Despite the positive directions that CLEAR-IVH seems to have established, other issues remain with regard to catheter placement. Placement of an EVD is not without its own set of potential complications.[133,134] Recent reports have demonstrated that although placement of a bedside EVD is a safe procedure, correct placement of the catheter can be difficult in cases where a midline shift is present, as is often the case with ICH patients, and there is a risk of hemorrhage related to catheter placement. Image-guided navigation can offer assistance in these cases, but the imaging increases the costs as well as the operating room time. Further, mass effect from the original hematoma can also lead to ventricular trapping, preventing communication between the catheter and some compartments within the ventricles. Thus, if rtPA is injected into one ventricle, it may or may not reach all aspects of the hematoma. In these cases, a second catheter may be warranted for complete IVH treatment. A second catheter is often best placed using image guidance with stereotaxy or in real time. These issues with IVH must be evaluated on a case-by-case basis and approached with the common goal of correct EVD placement so that rtPA is directed into the ventricular system in hopes of clot dissolution without added risks to the surrounding brain parenchyma.

Intraventricular thrombolysis will now be tested in a definitive phase III clinical trial, funded by the NIH, comparing EVD irrigation with rtPA and placebo, with primary end points of improving survival and reducing disability after obstructive IVH (for more information, go to www.CLEARIII.com). This trial will likely change neurosurgical practice, by either endorsing or discrediting the use of intraventricular thrombolysis. Meanwhile, many cases with obstructed ventricles and uncontrolled ICPs will continue to be treated on a case-by-case basis, considering the risks and potential benefit of intraventricular thrombolysis on a compassionate basis, when no other options are available.

◆ Conclusion

The surgical treatment of ICH has undergone many advancements in recent years. Despite the lack of clinical and surgical trials demonstrating a clear and significant benefit of aggressive evacuation, the trend with all modalities has resulted in improved clinical outcomes and reduced mortality.[41] As technology continues to advance at a rapid pace, and patient selection criteria become more refined, surgical evacuation of ICH continues to become a viable option in many patients. With the development of minimally invasive surgical techniques with neuronavigation, the use of thrombolytics, and improved control of hematoma volume, blood pressure, and coagulopathies, it is hoped that the treatment of spontaneous ICH will become a standard of care with acceptable improvement in both clinical and neurologic outcomes.

References

1. Broderick J, Connolly S, Feldmann E, et al; American Heart Association; American Stroke Association Stroke Council; High Blood Pressure Research Council; Quality of Care and Outcomes in Research Interdisciplinary Working Group. Guidelines for the management of spontaneous intracerebral hemorrhage in adults: 2007 update: a guideline from the American Heart Association/American Stroke Association Stroke Council, High Blood Pressure Research Council, and the Quality of Care and Outcomes in Research Interdisciplinary Working Group. Stroke 2007;38:2001–2023
2. Qureshi AI, Suri MF, Nasar A, et al. Thrombolysis for ischemic stroke in the United States: data from National Hospital Discharge Survey 1999–2001. Neurosurgery 2005;57:647–654, discussion 647–654
3. Mayer SA, Rincon F. Treatment of intracerebral haemorrhage. Lancet Neurol 2005;4:662–672
4. Broderick JP, Diringer MN, Hill MD, et al; Recombinant Activated Factor VII Intracerebral Hemorrhage Trial Investigators. Determinants of intracerebral hemorrhage growth: an exploratory analysis. Stroke 2007; 38:1072–1075
5. Fogelholm R, Avikainen S, Murros K. Prognostic value and determinants of first-day mean arterial pressure in spontaneous supratentorial intracerebral hemorrhage. Stroke 1997;28:1396–1400
6. Nilsson OG, Lindgren A, Brandt L, Säveland H. Prediction of death in patients with primary intracerebral hemorrhage: a prospective study of a defined population. J Neurosurg 2002;97:531–536
7. Park HS, Kang MJ, Huh JT. Recent epidemiological trends of stroke. J Korean Neurosurg Soc 2008;43:16–20
8. Razzaq AA, Hussain R. Determinants of 30-day mortality of spontaneous intracerebral hemorrhage in Pakistan. Surg Neurol 1998;50:336–342, discussion 342–343
9. Tuhrim S, Dambrosia JM, Price TR, et al. Prediction of intracerebral hemorrhage survival. Ann Neurol 1988;24:258–263
10. Adams HP Jr. Treating ischemic stroke as an emergency. Arch Neurol 1998;55:457–461
11. Bamford J, Dennis M, Sandercock P, Burn J, Warlow C. The frequency, causes and timing of death within 30 days of a first stroke: the Oxfordshire Community Stroke Project. J Neurol Neurosurg Psychiatry 1990; 53:824–829
12. Cooper D, Jauch E, Flaherty ML. Critical pathways for the management of stroke and intracerebral hemorrhage: a survey of US hospitals. Crit Pathw Cardiol 2007;6:18–23
13. Tuhrim S, Horowitz DR, Sacher M, Godbold JH. Volume of ventricular blood is an important determinant of outcome in supratentorial intracerebral hemorrhage. Crit Care Med 1999;27:617–621
14. McKissock W, Richardson A, Taylot J. Primary intracerebral haemorrhage: a controlled trial of surgical and conservative treatment in 180 unselected cases. Lancet 1961;2:221–226
15. Broderick JP, Brott TG, Tomsick T, Barsan W, Spilker J. Ultra-early evaluation of intracerebral hemorrhage. J Neurosurg 1990;72:195–199
16. Brott T, Broderick J, Kothari R, et al. Early hemorrhage growth in patients with intracerebral hemorrhage. Stroke 1997;28:1–5
17. Brott T, Thalinger K, Hertzberg V. Hypertension as a risk factor for spontaneous intracerebral hemorrhage. Stroke 1986;17:1078–1083
18. Bruno A, Carter S. Possible reason for the higher incidence of spontaneous intracerebral hemorrhage among Hispanics than non-Hispanic whites in New Mexico. Neuroepidemiology 2000;19:51–52
19. Ariesen MJ, Claus SP, Rinkel GJ, Algra A. Risk factors for intracerebral hemorrhage in the general population: a systematic review. Stroke 2003;34:2060–2065
20. Bruno A, Qualls C. Risk factors for intracerebral and subarachnoid hemorrhage among Hispanics and non-Hispanic whites in a New Mexico community. Neuroepidemiology 2000;19:227–232
21. Klatsky AL, Friedman GD, Sidney S, Kipp H, Kubo A, Armstrong MA. Risk of hemorrhagic stroke in Asian American ethnic groups. Neuroepidemiology 2005;25:26–31
22. Qureshi AI, Giles WH, Croft JB. Racial differences in the incidence of intracerebral hemorrhage: effects of blood pressure and education. Neurology 1999;52:1617–1621
23. Suzuki K, Kutsuzawa T, Takita K, et al. Clinico-epidemiologic study of stroke in Akita, Japan. Stroke 1987;18:402–406
24. Ruíz-Sandoval JL, Cantú C, Barinagarrementeria F. Intracerebral hemorrhage in young people: analysis of risk factors, location, causes, and prognosis. Stroke 1999;30:537–541
25. Cheung RT, Zou LY. Use of the original, modified, or new intracerebral hemorrhage score to predict mortality and morbidity after intracerebral hemorrhage. Stroke 2003;34:1717–1722
26. Godoy DA, Piñero G, Di Napoli M. Predicting mortality in spontaneous intracerebral hemorrhage: can modification to original score improve the prediction? Stroke 2006;37:1038–1044
27. Hemphill JC III, Bonovich DC, Besmertis L, Manley GT, Johnston SC. The ICH score: a simple, reliable grading scale for intracerebral hemorrhage. Stroke 2001;32:891–897
28. Masè G, Zorzon M, Biasutti E, Tasca G, Vitrani B, Cazzato G. Immediate prognosis of primary intracerebral hemorrhage using an easy model for the prediction of survival. Acta Neurol Scand 1995;91:306–309
29. Portenoy RK, Lipton RB, Berger AR, Lesser ML, Lantos G. Intracerebral haemorrhage: a model for the prediction of outcome. J Neurol Neurosurg Psychiatry 1987;50:976–979
30. Ruiz-Sandoval JL, Chiquete E, Romero-Vargas S, Padilla-Martínez JJ, González-Cornejo S. Grading scale for prediction of outcome in primary intracerebral hemorrhages. Stroke 2007;38:1641–1644
31. Weimar C, Benemann J, Diener HC; German Stroke Study Collaboration. Development and validation of the Essen Intracerebral Haemorrhage Score. J Neurol Neurosurg Psychiatry 2006;77:601–605
32. Weimar C, Roth M, Willig V, Kostopoulos P, Benemann J, Diener HC. Development and validation of a prognostic model to predict recovery following intracerebral hemorrhage. J Neurol 2006;253:788–793
33. Daverat P, Castel JP, Dartigues JF, Orgogozo JM. Death and functional outcome after spontaneous intracerebral hemorrhage. A prospective study of 166 cases using multivariate analysis. Stroke 1991;22:1–6
34. Hallevy C, Ifergane G, Kordysh E, Herishanu Y. Spontaneous supratentorial intracerebral hemorrhage. Criteria for short-term functional outcome prediction. J Neurol 2002;249:1704–1709
35. Lisk DR, Pasteur W, Rhoades H, Putnam RD, Grotta JC. Early presentation of hemispheric intracerebral hemorrhage: prediction of outcome and guidelines for treatment allocation. Neurology 1994;44:133–139
36. Qureshi AI, Suri MF, Nasar A, et al. Changes in cost and outcome among US patients with stroke hospitalized in 1990 to 1991 and those hospitalized in 2000 to 2001. Stroke 2007;38:2180–2184
37. Mendelow AD, Gregson BA, Fernandes HM, et al; STICH investigators. Early surgery versus initial conservative treatment in patients with spontaneous supratentorial intracerebral haematomas in the International Surgical Trial in Intracerebral Haemorrhage (STICH): a randomised trial. Lancet 2005;365:387–397
38. Wartenberg KE, Mayer SA. The STICH trial: the end of surgical intervention for supratentorial intracerebral hemorrhage? Curr Neurol Neurosci Rep 2005;5:473–475
39. Adeoye O, Woo D, Haverbusch M, et al. Surgical management and case-fatality rates of intracerebral hemorrhage in 1988 and 2005. Neurosurgery 2008;63:1113–1117, discussion 1117–1118
40. Fayad PB, Awad IA. Surgery for intracerebral hemorrhage. Neurology 1998;51(3, Suppl 3)S69–S73
41. Jaffe J, AlKhawam L, Du H, et al. Outcome predictors and spectrum of treatment eligibility with prospective protocolized management of intracerebral hemorrhage. Neurosurgery 2009;64:436–445, discussion 445–446
42. Jackson CA, Sudlow CL. Is hypertension a more frequent risk factor for deep than for lobar supratentorial intracerebral haemorrhage? J Neurol Neurosurg Psychiatry 2006;77:1244–1252
43. Takebayashi S. Ultrastructural morphometry of hypertensive medial damage in lenticulostriate and other arteries. Stroke 1985;16:449–453
44. Passero S, Ciacci G, Reale F. Potential triggering factors of intracerebral hemorrhage. Cerebrovasc Dis 2001;12:220–227
45. Petridis AK, Barth H, Buhl R, Hugo HH, Mehdorn HM. Outcome of cerebral amyloid angiopathic brain haemorrhage. Acta Neurochir (Wien) 2008;150:889–895
46. Vinters HV. Cerebral amyloid angiopathy. A critical review. Stroke 1987; 18:311–324

47. Garcia C, Pinho e Melo T, Rocha L, Lechner MC. Cerebral hemorrhage and apoE. J Neurol 1999;246:830–834

48. Greenberg SM. Cerebral amyloid angiopathy: prospects for clinical diagnosis and treatment. Neurology 1998;51:690–694

49. Maia LF, Vasconcelos C, Seixas S, Magalhães R, Correia M. Lobar brain hemorrhages and white matter changes: Clinical, radiological and laboratorial profiles. Cerebrovasc Dis 2006;22:155–161

50. McCarron MO, Nicoll JA, Stewart J, et al. The apolipoprotein E epsilon2 allele and the pathological features in cerebral amyloid angiopathy-related hemorrhage. J Neuropathol Exp Neurol 1999;58:711–718

51. McCarron MO, Nicoll JA. Apolipoprotein E genotype and cerebral amyloid angiopathy-related hemorrhage. Ann N Y Acad Sci 2000;903:176–179

52. O'Donnell HC, Rosand J, Knudsen KA, et al. Apolipoprotein E genotype and the risk of recurrent lobar intracerebral hemorrhage. N Engl J Med 2000;342:240–245

53. Tzourio C, Arima H, Harrap S, et al. APOE genotype, ethnicity, and the risk of cerebral hemorrhage. Neurology 2008;70:1322–1328

54. Chen ST, Chen SD, Hsu CY, Hogan EL. Progression of hypertensive intracerebral hemorrhage. Neurology 1989;39:1509–1514

55. Kazui S, Minematsu K, Yamamoto H, Sawada T, Yamaguchi T. Predisposing factors to enlargement of spontaneous intracerebral hematoma. Stroke 1997;28:2370–2375

56. Kazui S, Naritomi H, Yamamoto H, Sawada T, Yamaguchi T. Enlargement of spontaneous intracerebral hemorrhage. Incidence and time course. Stroke 1996;27:1783–1787

57. Ohwaki K, Yano E, Nagashima H, Hirata M, Nakagomi T, Tamura A. Blood pressure management in acute intracerebral hemorrhage: relationship between elevated blood pressure and hematoma enlargement. Stroke 2004;35:1364–1367

58. Anderson CS, Huang Y, Wang JG, et al; INTERACT Investigators. Intensive blood pressure reduction in acute cerebral haemorrhage trial (INTERACT): a randomised pilot trial. Lancet Neurol 2008;7:391–399

59. Lapchak PA, Araujo DM. Advances in hemorrhagic stroke therapy: conventional and novel approaches. Expert Opin Emerg Drugs 2007;12:389–406

60. Qureshi AI. Antihypertensive Treatment of Acute Cerebral Hemorrhage (ATACH): rationale and design. Neurocrit Care 2007;6:56–66

61. Worster A, Keim SM, Carpenter CR, Adeoye O; Best Evidence in Emergency Medicine (BEEM) Group. Does early intensive lowering of blood pressure reduce hematoma volume and improve clinical outcome after acute cerebral hemorrhage? J Emerg Med 2009;37:433–438

62. Flaherty ML, Tao H, Haverbusch M, et al. Warfarin use leads to larger intracerebral hematomas. Neurology 2008;71:1084–1089

63. Roquer J, Rodríguez Campello A, Gomis M, Ois A, Puente V, Munteis E. Previous antiplatelet therapy is an independent predictor of 30-day mortality after spontaneous supratentorial intracerebral hemorrhage. J Neurol 2005;252:412–416

64. Saloheimo P, Ahonen M, Juvela S, Pyhtinen J, Savolainen ER, Hillbom M. Regular aspirin-use preceding the onset of primary intracerebral hemorrhage is an independent predictor for death. Stroke 2006;37:129–133

65. Foerch C, Sitzer M, Steinmetz H, Neumann-Haefelin T. Pretreatment with antiplatelet agents is not independently associated with unfavorable outcome in intracerebral hemorrhage. Stroke 2006;37:2165–2167

66. Rosand J, Eckman MH, Knudsen KA, Singer DE, Greenberg SM. The effect of warfarin and intensity of anticoagulation on outcome of intracerebral hemorrhage. Arch Intern Med 2004;164:880–884

67. Andersen KK, Olsen TS, Dehlendorff C, Kammersgaard LP. Hemorrhagic and ischemic strokes compared: stroke severity, mortality, and risk factors. Stroke 2009;40:2068–2072

68. Sorensen SV, Dewilde S, Singer DE, Goldhaber SZ, Monz BU, Plumb JM. Cost-effectiveness of warfarin: trial versus "real-world" stroke prevention in atrial fibrillation. Am Heart J 2009;157:1064–1073

69. Huttner HB, Schellinger PD, Hartmann M, et al. Hematoma growth and outcome in treated neurocritical care patients with intracerebral hemorrhage related to oral anticoagulant therapy: comparison of acute treatment strategies using vitamin K, fresh frozen plasma, and prothrombin complex concentrates. Stroke 2006;37:1465–1470

70. Goldstein JN, Thomas SH, Frontiero V, et al. Timing of fresh frozen plasma administration and rapid correction of coagulopathy in warfarin-related intracerebral hemorrhage. Stroke 2006;37:151–155

71. Aiyagari V, Testai FD. Correction of coagulopathy in warfarin associated cerebral hemorrhage. Curr Opin Crit Care 2009;15:87–92

72. Aguilar MI, Hart RG, Kase CS, et al. Treatment of warfarin-associated intracerebral hemorrhage: literature review and expert opinion. Mayo Clin Proc 2007;82:82–92

73. Appelboam R, Thomas EO. Warfarin and intracranial haemorrhage. Blood Rev 2009;23:1–9

74. Freeman WD, Aguilar MI. Management of warfarin-related intracerebral hemorrhage. Expert Rev Neurother 2008;8:271–290

75. Goldstein JN, Rosand J, Schwamm LH. Warfarin reversal in anticoagulant-associated intracerebral hemorrhage. Neurocrit Care 2008;9:277–283

76. Ilyas C, Beyer GM, Dutton RP, Scalea TM, Hess JR. Recombinant factor VIIa for warfarin-associated intracranial bleeding. J Clin Anesth 2008;20:276–279

77. Kalina M, Tinkoff G, Gbadebo A, Veneri P, Fulda G. A protocol for the rapid normalization of INR in trauma patients with intracranial hemorrhage on prescribed warfarin therapy. Am Surg 2008;74:858–861

78. Dutton RP, Stein DM, Hess JR, Scalea TM. Recombinant factor VIIa and thromboembolic events. JAMA 2006;296:43–44, author reply 44

79. Awad IA, Cozzens J. Recombinant human Factor VIIa for intracerebral hemorrhage:Miracle drug or irrational exuberance? Neurosurgery 2006;58:N6

80. Mayer SA, Brun NC, Begtrup K, et al; FAST Trial Investigators. Efficacy and safety of recombinant activated factor VII for acute intracerebral hemorrhage. N Engl J Med 2008;358:2127–2137

81. Mayer SA, Brun NC, Begtrup K, et al; Recombinant Activated Factor VII Intracerebral Hemorrhage Trial Investigators. Recombinant activated factor VII for acute intracerebral hemorrhage. N Engl J Med 2005;352:777–785

82. Mayer SA, Brun NC, Broderick J, et al; Europe/AustralAsia NovoSeven ICH Trial Investigators. Safety and feasibility of recombinant factor VIIa for acute intracerebral hemorrhage. Stroke 2005;36:74–79

83. Mayer SA, Davis SM, Skolnick BE, et al; FAST trial investigators. Can a subset of intracerebral hemorrhage patients benefit from hemostatic therapy with recombinant activated factor VII? Stroke 2009;40:833–840

84. Leira R, Dávalos A, Silva Y, et al; Stroke Project, Cerebrovascular Diseases Group of the Spanish Neurological Society. Early neurologic deterioration in intracerebral hemorrhage: predictors and associated factors. Neurology 2004;63:461–467

85. Silva Y, Leira R, Tejada J, Lainez JM, Castillo J, Dávalos A; Stroke Project, Cerebrovascular Diseases Group of the Spanish Neurological Society. Molecular signatures of vascular injury are associated with early growth of intracerebral hemorrhage. Stroke 2005;36:86–91

86. Naidech AM, Bernstein RA, Levasseur K, et al. Platelet activity and outcome after intracerebral hemorrhage. Ann Neurol 2009;65:352–356

87. Bullock MR, Chesnut R, Ghajar J, et al; Surgical Management of Traumatic Brain Injury Author Group. Surgical management of acute epidural hematomas. Neurosurgery 2006;58(3, Suppl)S7–S15, discussion Si-iv

88. Bullock MR, Chesnut R, Ghajar J, et al; Surgical Management of Traumatic Brain Injury Author Group. Surgical management of acute subdural hematomas. Neurosurgery 2006;58(3, Suppl)S16–S24, discussion Si-iv

89. Firsching R, Frowein RA, Thun F. Intracerebellar haematoma: eleven traumatic and non-traumatic cases and a review of the literature. Neurochirurgia (Stuttg) 1987;30:182–185

90. Moulton RJ. Traumatic intracranial mass lesions: how soon for evacuation? Can J Surg 1992;35:35–37

91. Del Bigio MR, Yan HJ, Buist R, Peeling J. Experimental intracerebral hemorrhage in rats. Magnetic resonance imaging and histopathological correlates. Stroke 1996;27:2312–2319, discussion 2319–2320

92. Wagner KR, Xi G, Hua Y, et al. Ultra-early clot aspiration after lysis with tissue plasminogen activator in a porcine model of intracerebral hemorrhage: edema reduction and blood-brain barrier protection. J Neurosurg 1999;90:491–498

93. Batjer HH, Reisch JS, Allen BC, Plaizier LJ, Su CJ. Failure of surgery to improve outcome in hypertensive putaminal hemorrhage. A prospective randomized trial. Arch Neurol 1990;47:1103–1106

94. Juvela S, Heiskanen O, Poranen A, et al. The treatment of spontaneous intracerebral hemorrhage. A prospective randomized trial of surgical and conservative treatment. J Neurosurg 1989;70:755–758

95. Morgenstern LB, Frankowski RF, Shedden P, Pasteur W, Grotta JC. Surgical treatment for intracerebral hemorrhage (STICH): a single-center, randomized clinical trial. Neurology 1998;51:1359–1363

96. Zuccarello M, Brott TG, Derex L, et al. Early surgical treatment for supratentorial intracerebral hemorrhage: a randomized feasibility study. Stroke 1999;30:1833–1839

97. Morgan T, Zuccarello M, Narayan R, Keyl P, Lane K, Hanley D. Preliminary findings of the minimally-invasive surgery plus rt-PA for intracerebral hemorrhage evacuation (MISTIE) clinical trial. Acta Neurochir Suppl (Wien) 2008;105:147–151

98. Auer LM, Deinsberger W, Niederkorn K, et al. Endoscopic surgery versus medical treatment for spontaneous intracerebral hematoma: a randomized study. J Neurosurg 1989;70:530–535

99. Nishihara T, Morita A, Teraoka A, Kirino T. Endoscopy-guided removal of spontaneous intracerebral hemorrhage: comparison with computer tomography-guided stereotactic evacuation. Childs Nerv Syst 2007;23:677–683

100. Prasad K, Mendelow AD, Gregson B. Surgery for primary supratentorial intracerebral haemorrhage. Cochrane Database Syst Rev 2008; CD000200

101. Miller CM, Vespa P, Saver JL, et al. Image-guided endoscopic evacuation of spontaneous intracerebral hemorrhage. Surg Neurol 2008; 69:441–446, discussion 446

102. Bhattathiri PS, Gregson B, Prasad KS, Mendelow AD; STICH Investigators. Intraventricular hemorrhage and hydrocephalus after spontaneous intracerebral hemorrhage: results from the STICH trial. Acta Neurochir Suppl (Wien) 2006;96:65–68

103. Fountas KN, Kapsalaki EZ, Parish DC, et al. Intraventricular administration of rt-PA in patients with intraventricular hemorrhage. South Med J 2005;98:767–773

104. Hanley DF. Intraventricular hemorrhage: severity factor and treatment target in spontaneous intracerebral hemorrhage. Stroke 2009;40: 1533–1538

105. Ozdemir O, Calisaneller T, Hastürk A, Aydemir F, Caner H, Altinors N. Prognostic significance of third ventricle dilation in spontaneous intracerebral hemorrhage: a preliminary clinical study. Neurol Res 2008; 30:406–410

106. St Louis EK, Wijdicks EF, Li H, Atkinson JD. Predictors of poor outcome in patients with a spontaneous cerebellar hematoma. Can J Neurol Sci 2000;27:32–36

107. Steiner T, Diringer MN, Schneider D, et al. Dynamics of intraventricular hemorrhage in patients with spontaneous intracerebral hemorrhage: risk factors, clinical impact, and effect of hemostatic therapy with recombinant activated factor VII. Neurosurgery 2006;59:767–773, discussion 773–774

108. Narayan RK, Narayan TM, Katz DA, Kornblith PL, Murano G. Lysis of intracranial hematomas with urokinase in a rabbit model. J Neurosurg 1985;62:580–586

109. Pang D, Sclabassi RJ, Horton JA. Lysis of intraventricular blood clot with urokinase in a canine model: Part 1. Canine intraventricular blood cast model. Neurosurgery 1986;19:540–546

110. Pang D, Sclabassi RJ, Horton JA. Lysis of intraventricular blood clot with urokinase in a canine model: Part 2. In vivo safety study of intraventricular urokinase. Neurosurgery 1986;19:547–552

111. Pang D, Sclabassi RJ, Horton JA. Lysis of intraventricular blood clot with urokinase in a canine model: Part 3. Effects of intraventricular urokinase on clot lysis and posthemorrhagic hydrocephalus. Neurosurgery 1986;19:553–572

112. Mayfrank L, Lippitz B, Groth M, Bertalanffy H, Gilsbach JM. Effect of recombinant tissue plasminogen activator on clot lysis and ventricular dilatation in the treatment of severe intraventricular haemorrhage. Acta Neurochir (Wien) 1993;122:32–38

113. Wang YC, Lin CW, Shen CC, Lai SC, Kuo JS. Tissue plasminogen activator for the treatment of intraventricular hematoma: the dose-effect relationship. J Neurol Sci 2002;202:35–41

114. Shen PH, Matsuoka Y, Kawajiri K, et al. Treatment of intraventricular hemorrhage using urokinase. Neurol Med Chir (Tokyo) 1990;30:329–333

115. Akdemir H, Selçuklu A, Paşaoğlu A, Oktem IS, Kavuncu I. Treatment of severe intraventricular hemorrhage by intraventricular infusion of urokinase. Neurosurg Rev 1995;18:95–100

116. Coplin WM, Vinas FC, Agris JM, et al. A cohort study of the safety and feasibility of intraventricular urokinase for nonaneurysmal spontaneous intraventricular hemorrhage. Stroke 1998;29:1573–1579

117. Naff NJ, Hanley DF, Keyl PM, et al. Intraventricular thrombolysis speeds blood clot resolution: results of a pilot, prospective, randomized, double-blind, controlled trial. Neurosurgery 2004;54:577–583, discussion 583–584

118. Todo T, Usui M, Takakura K. Treatment of severe intraventricular hemorrhage by intraventricular infusion of urokinase. J Neurosurg 1991; 74:81–86

119. Torres A, Plans G, Martino J, et al. Fibrinolytic therapy in spontaneous intraventricular haemorrhage: efficacy and safety of the treatment. Br J Neurosurg 2008;22:269–274

120. Tung MY, Ong PL, Seow WT, Tan KK. A study on the efficacy of intraventricular urokinase in the treatment of intraventricular haemorrhage. Br J Neurosurg 1998;12:234–239

121. Ziai WC, Torbey MT, Naff NJ, et al. Frequency of sustained intracranial pressure elevation during treatment of severe intraventricular hemorrhage. Cerebrovasc Dis 2009;27:403–410

122. Deutsch H, Rodriguez JC, Titton RL. Lower dose intraventricular T-PA fibrinolysis: case report. Surg Neurol 2004;61:460–463, discussion 463

123. Findlay JM, Grace MG, Weir BK. Treatment of intraventricular hemorrhage with tissue plasminogen activator. Neurosurgery 1993;32:941–947, discussion 947

124. Findlay JM, Weir BK, Stollery DE. Lysis of intraventricular hematoma with tissue plasminogen activator. Case report. J Neurosurg 1991;74: 803–807

125. Goh KY, Poon WS. Recombinant tissue plasminogen activator for the treatment of spontaneous adult intraventricular hemorrhage. Surg Neurol 1998;50:526–531, discussion 531–532

126. Grabb PA. Traumatic intraventricular hemorrhage treated with intraventricular recombinant-tissue plasminogen activator: technical case report. Neurosurgery 1998;43:966–969

127. Hall B, Parker D Jr, Carhuapoma JR. Thrombolysis for intraventricular hemorrhage after endovascular aneurysmal coiling. Neurocrit Care 2005;3:153–156

128. Ionita CC, Ferrara J, McDonagh DL, Grossi P, Graffagnino C. Systemic hemostasis with recombinant-activated factor VII followed by local thrombolysis with recombinant tissue plasminogen activator in intraventricular hemorrhage. Neurocrit Care 2005;3:246–248

129. Kumar K, Demeria DD, Verma A. Recombinant tissue plasminogen activator in the treatment of intraventricular hemorrhage secondary to periventricular arteriovenous malformation before surgery: case report. Neurosurgery 2003;52:964–968, discussion 968–969

130. Rohde V, Schaller C, Hassler WE. Intraventricular recombinant tissue plasminogen activator for lysis of intraventricular haemorrhage. J Neurol Neurosurg Psychiatry 1995;58:447–451

131. Vereecken KK, Van Havenbergh T, De Beuckelaar W, Parizel PM, Jorens PG. Treatment of intraventricular hemorrhage with intraventricular administration of recombinant tissue plasminogen activator A clinical study of 18 cases. Clin Neurol Neurosurg 2006;108:451–455

132. Schwarz S, Schwab S, Steiner HH, Hacke W. Secondary hemorrhage after intraventricular fibrinolysis: a cautionary note: a report of two cases. Neurosurgery 1998;42:659–662, discussion 662–663

133. Gardner PA, Engh J, Atteberry D, Moossy JJ. Hemorrhage rates after external ventricular drain placement. J Neurosurg 2009;110:1021–1025

134. Kakarla UK, Kim LJ, Chang SW, Theodore N, Spetzler RF. Safety and accuracy of bedside external ventricular drain placement. Neurosurgery 2008;63(1, Suppl 1)ONS162–ONS166, discussion ONS166–ONS167

28

Radiosurgical Management of Arteriovenous Malformations

Douglas Kondziolka, Hideyuki Kano, Huai-che Yang, John C. Flickinger, and L. Dade Lunsford

---

Pearls

- Arteriovenous malformation (AVM) radiosurgery has its greatest role in the management of subcortical AVMs less than 3 cm in maximum diameter.
- Dose selection for AVM radiosurgery is mainly based on AVM volume and location, but the margin dose should rarely be below 16 Gy.
- The main limitation of AVM radiosurgery is hemorrhage during the latency interval before complete obliteration.
- If radiosurgery is performed for AVMs greater than 15 mL in volume, consideration should be given to volume or dose staging of the target.

Successful arteriovenous malformation (AVM) radiosurgery achieves complete AVM nidus obliteration, which leads to elimination of further hemorrhage risk.[1–3] While this goal is being achieved, there should be limited morbidity and no mortality from hemorrhage or radiation-induced brain injury. When these outcomes can be achieved with a high likelihood, a strong case can be made *for* radiosurgery. If clinical or angiographic factors argue *against* the achievement of these goals, then other strategies should be considered instead. Physicians who make an argument for radiosurgery cite one or more of the following factors: (1) radiosurgery is an effective therapy for the management of deep-brain AVMs; (2) radiosurgery is an effective therapy for residual AVMs after subtotal resection; (3) radiosurgery is worthwhile in attempting to lower management risks for AVMs in functional brain locations; (4) because embolization does not cure most AVMs, additional therapy such as radiosurgery may be required; (5) microsurgical resection may not be the best choice for some patients because of their general health; and (6) radiosurgery entails lower costs. Because radiosurgery is the first and only biologic AVM therapy, it represents the basis for future cellular approaches to vascular malformation diseases. For this reason, the future of radiosurgery may be impacted positively by the development of other biologic strategies such as brain protection or endothelial sensitization.

◆ Decision Making

Those who make an argument against the use of radiosurgery cite the following factors: (1) radiosurgery does not always work, especially when only partial AVM obliteration is achieved[4]; (2) brain hemorrhage may occur during the time it takes for radiosurgery to work; (3) radiation-related morbidity may cause functional neurologic deficits; (4) there may be long-term problems after brain irradiation[5]; and (5) resection may be a more cost-effective treatment over the long term.[6] Although all these factors can be debated, most neurosurgeons agree that the role of radiosurgery is greatest for patients with small-volume, deep-brain AVMs.[2] It has a lesser role for patients with larger and surgically accessible AVMs. In between these two extremes there exists much debate. The role of radiosurgery for patients with small but accessible AVMs is growing steadily.[7] For patients with large-volume yet deeply located AVMs, multimodality management often is required. Thus, whether radiosurgery should be considered in the management of an individual patient depends on the factors of AVM volume, brain location, prior hemorrhage history, patient age, and surgical resectability. These factors have been studied in detail by different groups as predictors of successful AVM outcomes or as reasons for radiosurgery failure.[3,8,9] The role of AVM obliteration and radiosurgical morbidity in decision making is addressed in further detail later in this chapter.

How Does Radiosurgery Work?

Radiosurgery is effective because single-fraction irradiation causes significant injury to the endothelial cells of blood vessels that compose the AVM.[10–12] Stereotactic definition of the AVM target ensures that these radiobiologic effects are limited to the malformation. Conformal radiosurgery allows irradiation of only a small volume of surrounding normal tissue in the region of radiation dose fall-off.[2] Dose-prescription formulas are used to help select an appropriate radiation dose depending on imaging and clinical factors.[13]

The immediate effect of radiosurgery is to damage the endothelial cells of the AVM vessels. Release of tissue-specific cytokines common to other forms of radiation-induced injury is likely to mediate such acute effects. Inflammatory cells mediate tissue repair in response to irradiation. Later, chronic inflammation consists of the ingrowth of granulation tissue that contains fibroblasts and new capillaries. These events may explain the delayed imaging changes sometimes observed after radiosurgery. Szeifert et al[14] identified the presence of actin-producing fibroblasts, so-called myofibroblasts, that are hypothesized to exert contractile properties and facilitate AVM obliteration. Contrast-enhanced magnetic resonance imaging (MRI) studies at this late stage after obliteration commonly show enhancement of the obliterated AVM. This finding does not indicate a "patent" AVM, but rather we believe it is a marker for the newly formed capillary network within the scarred AVM tissue remnant. Several reports have noted the rare, late finding of cyst formation at the AVM site, which probably represents expansion of the extracellular fluid space within the fibrosis.[5,15] Radiosurgery may impact on seizure control through irradiation of epileptogenic tissue or through correction of abnormal hemodynamic conditions.[16]

Results of Stereotactic Radiosurgery

Clinical Experience

At the University of Pittsburgh, 1129 AVM patients had gamma knife radiosurgery during a 20-year period. The mean patient age was 36 years (range 2–82). Prior intracranial hemorrhage was reported in 38% of patients (n = 424), headaches in 38%, and seizures in 28%. The wide variety of clinical presentations ensures discussion of the different treatment options in all patients. All referred vascular malformation cases are discussed at a weekly multidisciplinary conference. Intravascular embolization was performed in 206 patients (18%) before radiosurgery; 127 patients (11%) had already undergone one or more surgical procedures prior to radiosurgery. For some of these patients, the goal of surgery had been AVM resection, whereas for others the goal was hematoma removal. The median AVM volume was 3.4 mL (range 0.03–58 mL). The 50% isodose was used as the margin isodose in 81% of patients. Only 0.7% of patients were treated below the 50% isodose.

The Spetzler-Martin grading system was used to classify all AVMs according to size, critical location, and venous drainage. The most commonly referred patient was one with a small-volume, deeply located AVM (grade III, n = 380, 34%). The smallest category of patients had an AVM that was small, superficial, and noncritical in location (grade I, n = 27, 3.0%). In such patients we first recommend a resection unless the patient has a medical contraindication or refuses that recommendation. Eleven percent of patients (n = 121) had a grade VI AVM. The AVM was located totally within the parenchyma of the brainstem or thalamus. The mean dose delivered to the AVM margin was 18 Gy, and the mean maximum dose 34 Gy. Although there is no such thing as an "inoperable" AVM, we consider an AVM to be associated with an acceptably high risk for resection when it is located completely within the parenchyma of the brainstem, thalamus, or basal ganglia. In our series, 53 patients had brainstem AVMs, 97 had thalamic AVMs, and 68 had basal ganglia malformations.

When radiosurgery did not lead to complete AVM obliteration, we further discussion the merits of repeat radiosurgery or resection. At our center 118 patients underwent repeat radiosurgery for persistent AVM nidus after at least 3 years had elapsed since the first procedure. If, after 3 to 4 years, a residual AVM nidus with early venous drainage remains, then a second radiosurgical procedure should be performed.[17] We do not recommend additional management for patients who harbor only an early draining vein, as this feature resolves over an additional observation interval. In addition, we know of no patient who sustained a later hemorrhage when only an early draining vein was present. Some patients' angiograms show some abnormal-appearing vessels in the region of the irradiated AVM, without early venous drainage. This fine vascular blush may indicate the neocapillary network within the scarred malformation. Such findings also require no additional therapy.

Repeat radiosurgery is associated with a 70% probability of obliteration.[4,18] At the second procedure, only the small remnant needs to be irradiated, usually at a dose higher than the first dose delivered (especially if the initial AVM was large and the remnant is small, depending on location).

How Arteriovenous Malformation Obliteration Affects Decision Making

Whether an AVM can be successfully obliterated depends on whether proper stereotactic nidus definition can be performed followed by delivery of an adequate radiosurgery dose.[19] A complete analysis of 197 AVM patients with up to 3-year angiographic follow-up showed an overall complete obliteration rate of 72% after a single procedure. These results were stratified by volume. In 20 of 197 patients (10%) the targeted AVM nidus failed to obliterate totally. The most important reason for lack of complete obliteration was incomplete targeting.[18] An additional 35 patients (18%) had a residual AVM that was not included in the original treatment volume. Many of these patients then underwent a second radiosurgery procedure. Important obliteration factors were identified in this study: incomplete imaging-definition of the AVM, reappearance of AVM after initial compression by hematoma, and recanalization of a previously embolized nidus.

We and others advocate the use of multimodality imaging (MRI, magnetic resonance angiography [MRA], and conventional stereotactic angiography) to obtain the best results.[20] For the smallest AVM (less than 1.3 mL), 90% of patients had complete obliteration (45 of 50), and 98% had obliteration of the target (49 of 50). For AVMs between 1.4 and 3 mL, 41 of 49 patients had complete obliteration (84%) and 47 of 49 had obliteration of the included target (96%). These data indicate that the radiosurgical dose will achieve our goal with a high likelihood if we can accurately tailor it to the entire lesion margin (**Fig. 28.1**).

In a separate analysis of our data, we reported a multivariate analysis of AVM obliteration as related to dose and volume.[19] A clear dose response up to 25 Gy was identified. We concluded that large AVMs have low obliteration rates because of the combination of lower treatment doses used and the greater problems encountered with target definition. An analysis of 95 patients with thalamic or basal ganglia AVMs found similar obliteration rates when stratified by volume; overall, 80% of patients were cured after a single procedure. Thus, AVM volume not only means that more tissue exists to undergo obliteration, but that there may be additional challenges in stereotactic targeting.

Liscak et al[21] reported that AVM obliteration was achieved in 222 (67%) of 330 patients after the initial stereotactic radiosurgery (SRS) and in 47 (69%) of 68 patients who underwent repeat SRS. Final angiography verified complete obliteration by 12 to 96 months (median, 25 months). Smaller volume AVMs and the application of a higher margin dose resulted in a higher chance of obliteration. The risk of rebleeding after SRS was 2.1% annually until full obliteration. The risk of permanent morbidity after the initial and repeat SRS were 2.7% and 2.9%, respectively.[21] Subtotal obliteration of AVMs after SRS implies a complete angiographic disappearance of the AVM nidus but persistence of an early filling draining vein, indicating that residual shunting is still present; hence, per definition there is still a patent AVM, and the risk of bleeding is not eliminated. Yen et al[22] reported that there was no case of bleeding after the diagnosis of subtotally obliterated 159 AVMs (16 of 159 subtotally obliterated AVM patients underwent repeat SRS) at mean follow-up of 3.9 years after diagnosis of a subtotally obliterated AVM. The fact that none of the patients with subtotally obliterated AVMs suffered a rupture is not compatible with the assumption of an unchanged risk of hemorrhage for these lesions, and implies that the protection from rebleeding in patients with subtotal obliteration may be significant. Subtotal obliteration does not seem to be a stage of an ongoing obliteration. At least in some cases it represents an end point of this process, with no subsequent obliteration occurring. This observation requires further confirmation by open-ended follow-up imaging.

The optimal timing of gamma knife surgery (GKS) after AVM hemorrhage depends on identification of the target tissue. If a hematoma obscures identification of the nidus, then several months should elapse for blood to resorb. Maruyama et al[23] retrospectively studied 211 patients with AVMs who presented with hemorrhage and underwent GKS as the initial treatment. Patients were categorized into three groups according to the interval between the time of first hemorrhage and GKS, as follows: group 1, 0 to 3 months (70 patients); group 2, >3 to 6 months (62 patients); and group 3, >6 months (79 patients). After a median follow-up of 6.3 years, the rates of obliteration, hemorrhage after treatment, and complication were not significantly different between the three groups even though the patients with a longer interval before GKS (group 3) had more AVMs in eloquent areas and neurologic deficits. However, the numbers of patients with preoperative hemorrhage in the interval before GKS was significantly higher in group 3 (1, 3, and 20 patients in groups 1, 2, and 3, respectively). These results were similar in the analyses of 127 patients presenting with intracerebral hemorrhage (ICH). The authors concluded that no benefit was detected in waiting for hematoma absorption before performing GKS after a hemorrhage from an AVM. Because of higher hemorrhagic risk from performing GKS more than 6 months after hemorrhage, the authors recommend performing GKS within 6 months after hemorrhage (**Fig. 28.2**).[23]

Pikus et al[24] argued that the high rate of complete microsurgical resection in their 72-patient AVM series (99%) with an 8% rate of new permanent neurologic deficits, supported their belief that resection was better than radiosurgery for small AVMs. However, only three of their patients (4%) had AVMs in the basal ganglia, thalamus, or brainstem. Porter et al[6] constructed a decision analysis model based on obliteration estimates and morbidity rates for resection and radiosurgery. They concluded that resection conferred a clinical benefit because of early protection from hemorrhage. Radiosurgery became a superior treatment if the surgical morbidity rate exceeded 12%. They did not factor the use of second stage or repeat radiosurgery into their model, choosing to leave patients with subtotally obliterated AVMs unprotected for the rest of their expected life. This outcome is rare because most patients achieve complete obliteration but may require more than one procedure. Thus, how obliteration data are used and the brain locations from which they are obtained are important factors in deciding when to use the different techniques.

◆ How Radiosurgery Morbidity Affects Decision Making

Because immediate postradiosurgery complications are rare, many patients and physicians choose radiosurgery because of the rapid return to activities and employment. The risk of radiation necrosis with permanent neurologic deficit is 2 to 3% in most reports.[21,25] Postradiosurgery seizures are rare when we administer therapeutic levels of anticonvulsant medication to patients with supratentorial lobar AVMs. One must consider the chance for delayed morbidity after radiosurgery that corresponds with the time course for AVM obliteration. We found that the rate of developing any postradiosurgery imaging change at 2 to 7 years after radiosurgery is 30%.[9] We believe that the majority of these changes are hemodynamic or inflammatory. Most do not cause neurologic symptoms. Symptomatic imaging changes are found in 10%. These changes resolve in half the patients within 3 years of

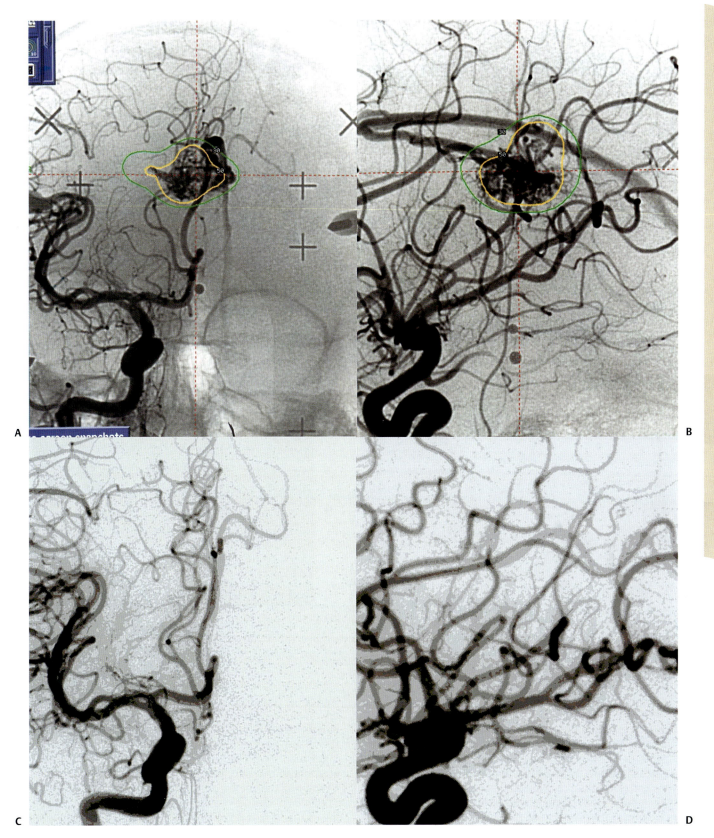

Fig. 28.1 **(A,B)** Right carotid angiograms at the time of radiosurgery (volume 2.3 cc, margin dose 23 Gy) in an 8-year-old boy who presented with hemorrhage from a corpus callosum arteriovenous malformation (AVM). **(C,D)** Twenty-six months later the carotid angiograms show complete obliteration.

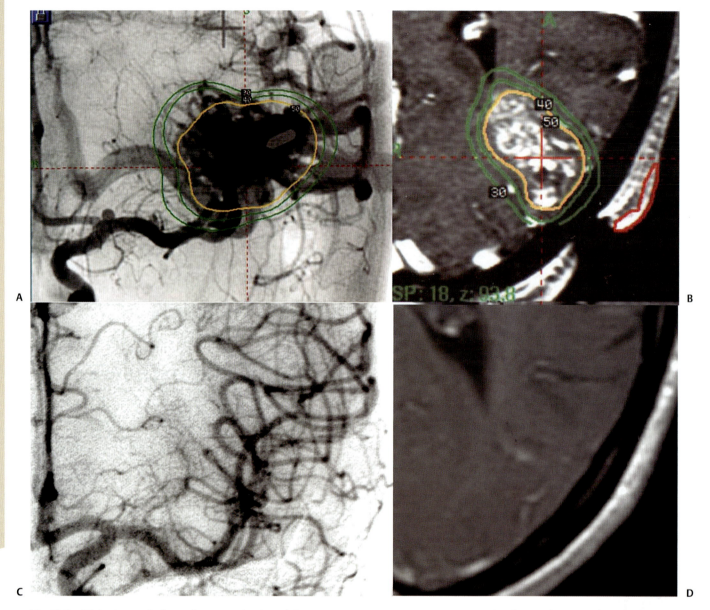

Fig. 28.2 **(A)** Angiogram before radiosurgery showing a left parieto-occipital AVM with a proximal aneurysm. **(B)** The radiosurgery dose plan (volume 5.6 cc, prescription dose 19 Gy) is shown on the magnetic resonance imaging (MRI) scan. Three years later the carotid angiogram **(C)** and MRI scan **(D)** show complete obliteration of AVM and disappearance of proximal aneurysm.

onset, as compared with a 95% resolution rate in patients with asymptomatic imaging findings **(Fig. 28.3)**.

There are several ways to predict the chance for adverse radiation effects. A multivariate analysis of imaging changes with various radiosurgical parameters found that the only significant independent correlation was the total volume of tissue that received ≥12 Gy.[8] Symptomatic imaging changes were correlated with the volume that received this dose and with location (brainstem versus nonbrainstem). Although radiosurgery may seem to be the only viable treatment option for intraparenchymal brainstem AVMs, a higher risk must be expected.

Finally, the persistent risk of hemorrhage during the obliteration latency interval remains one of the strongest argu-

ments against radiosurgery in some cases. Although Karlsson et al[17] reported protection from rehemorrhage in the interval prior to complete obliteration, neither the Pittsburgh nor the University of Florida series identified such a benefit.[26] Maruyama et al,[27] in a retrospective analysis involving 500 patients who had undergone radiosurgery for cerebral arteriovenous malformations, rehemorrhage decreased by 54% during the latency period and by 88% after obliteration. They did not cite the number of patients experiencing bleeding, and analyzed one hemorrhage event after SRS for each patient, because the Cox-proportional hazard method that they used in their series can allow only one event for each patient. This factor would have been affected by their outcomes.[27] In our experience the hemorrhage rate after radio-

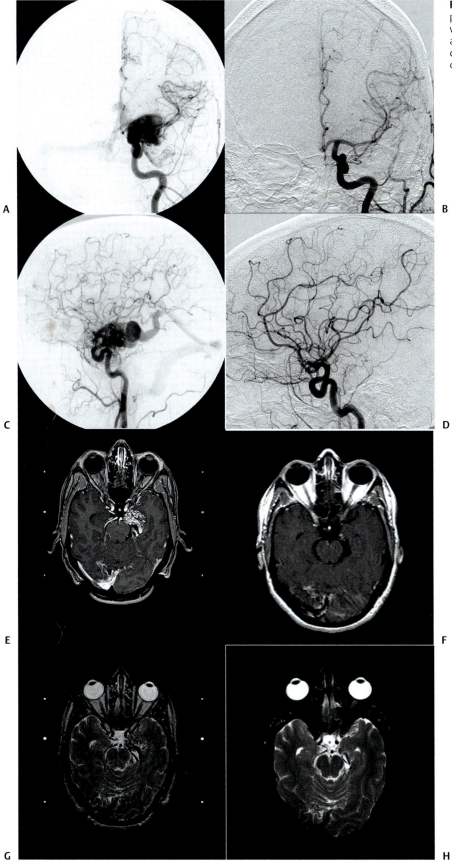

Fig. 28.3 **(A,C,E,G)** A 47-year-old woman presents with a left mesial temporal lobe AVM with varix. Eighteen months later the carotid angiograms **(B,D)** and MRI scans **(F,H)** show complete obliteration of AVM and disappearance of the varix.

surgery remains the same as the hemorrhage rate before radiosurgery until the AVM is obliterated. We have never observed a bleed after obliteration.

◆ Options for Large Arteriovenous Malformations: Staged Volume Radiosurgery and Embolization

We prospectively began to stage anatomic components to deliver higher single doses to symptomatic AVMs that were >15 mL in volume. Twenty-eight patients with large AVM underwent staged SRS at a median follow-up of 50 months after the last SRS. The median target volume was 12.3 mL at stage I and 11.5 mL at stage II. The median margin dose was 16 Gy at both stages. Four (14%) patients sustained a hemorrhage after SRS. Of 28 patients, 21 had follow-up of more than 3 years. Of these 21 patients, seven underwent repeat SRS and none had sufficient follow-up. Of 14 patients followed for more than 3 years, seven (50%) had total, four (29%) near total, and three (21%) had moderate AVM obliteration.[28]

We now recommend prospective staged radiosurgery for larger AVMs (volume staging), especially for patients who present with hemorrhage and who are not suitable for resection. With this approach, the AVM volume is divided into components to allow radiosurgery of smaller volumes at higher, more effective, and more tolerable doses. Forty-six patients have now undergone staged radiosurgery at our center. Irradiation of an entire large AVM at a low dose (below 15 Gy to the AVM margin) has such a low obliteration rate that it is probably not worthwhile. We separate the AVM radiosurgeries by 4 to 6 months to allow repair of sublethal deoxyribonucleic acid damage in normal brain.[29] There is evidence to suggest that even incompletely obliterated AVMs may become easier to resect after a period of several years. Perhaps prophylactic staged radiosurgery may facilitate eventual resection of AVMs previously considered untreatable.[30] This approach is a relatively new one, and the outcomes are being evaluated currently.

In the past, we used endovascular embolization to reduce the volume of the AVM nidus in preparation for eventual radiosurgery, usually 4 to 6 weeks later. In some patients, this strategy proved effective, and permanent occlusion of both the embolized portion and the irradiated portion was the result. We continue to perform embolization if there is a high likelihood of significant volume reduction following that procedure. Embolization must also be performed with a reasonable risk to benefit ratio. If our neurointerventional team does not believe that significant feeding artery and nidus occlusion is likely, we consider a staged radiosurgery approach.

◆ Conclusion

Arteriovenous malformation radiosurgery has been practiced for over 40 years and is now a common method to manage properly selected patients with brain AVMs. The techniques have been refined along with our understanding of the ex-

pected response. It is this understanding of expected outcomes that should facilitate a discussion of the pertinent issues for management of patients with AVMs. Some patients require multimodality approaches. All AVM patients should seek to understand whether stereotactic radiosurgery is an appropriate option for their problem.

References

1. Friedman WA, Bova FJ. Linear accelerator radiosurgery for arteriovenous malformations. J Neurosurg 1992;77:832–841
2. Lunsford LD, Kondziolka D, Flickinger JC, et al. Stereotactic radiosurgery for arteriovenous malformations of the brain. J Neurosurg 1991;75:512–524
3. Pollock BE, Flickinger JC, Lunsford LD, Maitz A, Kondziolka D. Factors associated with successful arteriovenous malformation radiosurgery. Neurosurgery 1998;42:1239–1244, discussion 1244–1247
4. Maesawa S, Flickinger JC, Kondziolka D, Lunsford LD. Repeated radiosurgery for incompletely obliterated arteriovenous malformations. J Neurosurg 2000;92:961–970
5. Yamamoto M, Jimbo M, Hara M, Saito I, Mori K. Gamma knife radiosurgery for arteriovenous malformations: long-term follow-up results focusing on complications occurring more than 5 years after irradiation. Neurosurgery 1996;38:906–914
6. Porter PJ, Shin AY, Detsky AS, Lefaive L, Wallace MC. Surgery versus stereotactic radiosurgery for small, operable cerebral arteriovenous malformations: a clinical and cost comparison. Neurosurgery 1997;41:757–764, discussion 764–766
7. Pollock BE, Lunsford LD, Kondziolka D, Maitz A, Flickinger JC. Patient outcomes after stereotactic radiosurgery for "operable" arteriovenous malformations. Neurosurgery 1994;35:1–7, discussion 7–8
8. Flickinger JC, Kondziolka D, Pollock BE, Maitz AH, Lunsford LD. Complications from arteriovenous malformation radiosurgery: multivariate analysis and risk modeling. Int J Radiat Oncol Biol Phys 1997;38:485–490
9. Flickinger JC, Kondziolka D, Maitz AH, Lunsford LD. Analysis of neurological sequelae from radiosurgery of arteriovenous malformations: how location affects outcome. Int J Radiat Oncol Biol Phys 1998;40:273–278
10. Flickinger JC, Kondziolka D, Lunsford LD, et al. A multi-institutional analysis of complication outcomes after arteriovenous malformation radiosurgery. Int J Radiat Oncol Biol Phys 1999;44:67–74
11. Schneider BF, Eberhard DA, Steiner LE. Histopathology of arteriovenous malformations after gamma knife radiosurgery. J Neurosurg 1997;87:352–357
12. Wu A, Lindner G, Maitz AH, et al. Physics of gamma knife approach on convergent beams in stereotactic radiosurgery. Int J Radiat Oncol Biol Phys 1990;18:941–949
13. Flickinger JC. An integrated logistic formula for prediction of complications from radiosurgery. Int J Radiat Oncol Biol Phys 1989;17:879–885
14. Szeifert GT, Kemeny AA, Timperley WR, Forster DM. The potential role of myofibroblasts in the obliteration of arteriovenous malformations after radiosurgery. Neurosurgery 1997;40:61–65, discussion 65–66
15. Hara M, Nakamura M, Shiokawa Y, et al. Delayed cyst formation after radiosurgery for cerebral arteriovenous malformation: two case reports. Minim Invasive Neurosurg 1998;41:40–45
16. Huang CF, Somaza S, Lunsford LD, et al. Radiosurgery in the management of epilepsy associated with arteriovenous malformations. Radiosurgery 1996;1:195–200
17. Karlsson B, Kihlström L, Lindquist C, Steiner L. Gamma knife surgery for previously irradiated arteriovenous malformations. Neurosurgery 1998;42:1–5, discussion 5–6
18. Pollock BE, Kondziolka D, Lunsford LD, Bissonette D, Flickinger JC. Repeat stereotactic radiosurgery of arteriovenous malformations: factors associated with incomplete obliteration. Neurosurgery 1996;38:318–324
19. Flickinger JC, Pollock BE, Kondziolka D, Lunsford LD. A dose-response analysis of arteriovenous malformation obliteration after radiosurgery. Int J Radiat Oncol Biol Phys 1996;36:873–879
20. Friedman WA, Bova FJ, Mendenhall WM. Linear accelerator radiosurgery for arteriovenous malformations: the relationship of size to outcome. J Neurosurg 1995;82:180–189
21. Liscák R, Vladyka V, Simonová G, et al. Arteriovenous malformations after Leksell gamma knife radiosurgery: rate of obliteration and complications. Neurosurgery 2007;60:1005–1014, discussion 1015–1016
22. Yen CP, Varady P, Sheehan J, Steiner M, Steiner L. Subtotal obliteration of cerebral arteriovenous malformations after gamma knife surgery. J Neurosurg 2007;106:361–369

23. Maruyama K, Koga T, Shin M, Igaki H, Tago M, Saito N. Optimal timing for gamma knife surgery after hemorrhage from brain arteriovenous malformations. J Neurosurg 2008;109(Suppl):73–76

24. Pikus HJ, Beach ML, Harbaugh RE. Microsurgical treatment of arteriovenous malformations: analysis and comparison with stereotactic radiosurgery. J Neurosurg 1998;88:641–646

25. Pollock BE, Meyer FB. Radiosurgery for arteriovenous malformations. J Neurosurg 2004;101:390–392, discussion 392

26. Pollock BE, Flickinger JC, Lunsford LD, Bissonette DJ, Kondziolka D. Hemorrhage risk after stereotactic radiosurgery of cerebral arteriovenous malformations. Neurosurgery 1996;38:652–659, discussion 659–661

27. Maruyama K, Kawahara N, Shin M, et al. The risk of hemorrhage after radiosurgery for cerebral arteriovenous malformations. N Engl J Med 2005;352:146–153

28. Sirin S, Kondziolka D, Niranjan A, Flickinger JC, Maitz AH, Lunsford LD. Prospective staged volume radiosurgery for large arteriovenous malformations: indications and outcomes in otherwise untreatable patients. Neurosurgery 2006;58:17–27, discussion 17–27

29. Firlik AD, Levy EI, Kondziolka D, Yonas H. Staged volume radiosurgery followed by microsurgical resection: a novel treatment for giant cerebral arteriovenous malformations: technical case report. Neurosurgery 1998;43:1223–1228

30. Steinberg GK, Chang SD, Levy RP, Marks MP, Frankel K, Marcellus M. Surgical resection of large incompletely treated intracranial arteriovenous malformations following stereotactic radiosurgery. J Neurosurg 1996;84:920–928

29

Revascularization of the Brain Using the ELANA Technique: History, Techniques, Indications, and Future Directions

T.P.C. van Doormaal, A. van der Zwan, and Cornelis A.F. Tulleken

Pearls

- The flow through a conventional, distal, low-flow bypass is often not sufficient. A conventional end-to-side attachment on a proximal cerebral artery to create a high-flow bypass carries a significant ischemic risk. This anastomosis can be safely performed with the excimer laser–assisted nonocclusive anastomosis (ELANA) technique.
- In the treatment of giant aneurysms of the anterior cerebral circulation, a high-flow ELANA bypass is a useful instrument. The outcomes for patients with giant aneurysms in the posterior circulation, however, are still grim because of the disease.
- In patients with hemodynamic cerebral ischemia and internal carotid artery occlusion, for whom there are no other treatment options left, a high-flow ELANA bypass has satisfying results. However, the benefit of a high-flow compared with a low-flow bypass in this subgroup has never been demonstrated in a prospective, randomized trial.
- The future of cerebral revascularization in general and ELANA in particular is firmly focused on creating a safe, minimally invasive, more easily performed anastomosis.

◆ History

The extra- to intracranial (EC-IC) bypass procedure was adopted by the international neurosurgical community after its introduction by Yasargil et al[1] in 1969. The technique involved attaching the superficial temporal artery (STA) to a distal middle cerebral arterial (MCA) branch vessel, and was primarily utilized as a cerebral blood flow augmentative procedure in the treatment of cerebral ischemia caused by an occlusion or inaccessible stenosis of the internal carotid artery (ICA).

In 1985, the EC-IC Bypass Study Group[2] found the procedure to be of no statistical benefit to patients when compared with aspirin treatment. Bypass was immediately discontinued as a treatment for cerebral ischemia. However, the procedure continued to be utilized for cerebral blood flow replacement as an adjunct to parent-vessel sacrifice in patients with aneurysms and tumors who had poor collateral circulation. The STA conduit and distal middle cerebral recipient were both relatively small arteries, and the volume of replacement flow was limited. Significant stroke complications have been noted in patients with apparently intact bypasses due to inadequate flow replacement. Strategies to improve flow replacement volume were subsequently developed.[3,4]

One important strategy to improve bypass flow is more proximal anastomosis placement on relatively large intracranial arteries. This concept of higher flow in more proximally located bypasses was mathematically confirmed by Hillen et al.[5] However, when placing a conventional anastomosis proximal to one of the main cerebral arteries, such as the ICA, the MCA, the posterior cerebral artery (PCA), or the basilar artery (BA), one of the main difficulties is the obligatory temporary occlusion of the recipient artery. This is accompanied by a significant risk of brain infarction.

In attempting to avoid ischemia during proximal anastomosis attachment, the senior author (C.A.F.T.) has been working with his team on a nonocclusive anastomosis procedure since 1979. In one of the first attempts to create a nonocclusive anastomosis, the donor artery was connected for approximately three quarters of its circumference to the recipient artery wall before opening the anastomosis[6] **(Fig. 29.1).** Scanning electromicroscopic examination of the anastomoses showed complete repair with almost perfect re-endothelialization after 3 weeks. This was a remarkable result, because

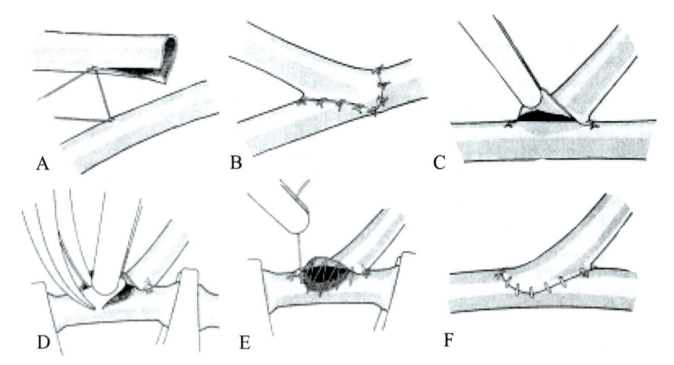

Fig. 29.1 One of the first attempts to create an anastomosis with minimal occlusion time. **(A)** A fish-mouth incision is made in the donor vessel and a suture is placed at the back of the longitudinal cut. **(B)** The graft is connected to the recipient vessel for three quarters of its circumference. **(C)** The remaining quarter is prepared for fast closing.

(D) The recipient vessel is temporarily occluded and opened at the anastomosis site. **(E)** The last quarter of the anastomosis is closed. **(F)** The temporary hemoclips are removed and the anastomosis is complete.

against all conventions in these anastomoses adventitial and medial layers of the recipient artery were exposed in the lumen of the anastomosis.

This procedure was further developed to a fully nonocclusive anastomosis, meaning that the recipient was never occluded during anastomosis creation, using a neodymium:

yttrium-aluminum-garnet (Nd:YAG) laser.[7] A sapphire tip coupled to the Nd:YAG laser catheter was introduced into a side branch of a bypass graft and created a hole in the recipient artery **(Fig. 29.2)**. After 65 rabbit experiments this technique was successfully used in one patient. However, to achieve an acceptable anastomosis, the adventitial layer and

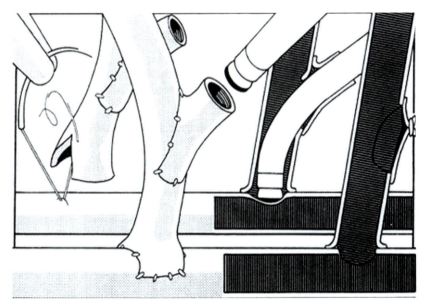

Fig. 29.2 The neodymium:yttrium-aluminum-garnet (Nd:YAG) laser facilitated the first totally nonocclusive anastomosis. First, the graft, with an artificial side branch, was sutured onto the wall of the recipient vessel. The Nd:YAG laser catheter was then inserted into the side branch and into the graft so that it could create an opening in the wall of the recipient vessel. (From Tulleken CA, Verdaasdonk RM, Berendsen W, Mali WP. Use of the excimer laser in high-flow bypass surgery of the brain. J Neurosurg 1993;78(3):477–480. Reprinted by permission.)

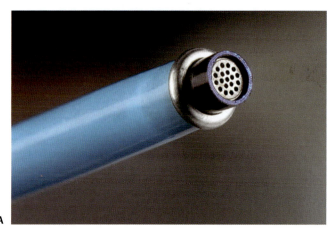
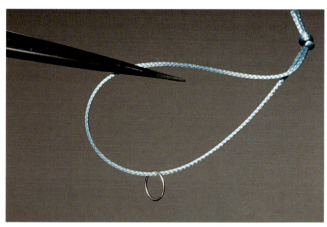

Fig. 29.3 **(A)** The ELANA catheter 2.0. The rim contains 200 laser fibers. The outside diameter is 2.0 mm. The metal surface inside (the "grid") contains holes, through which vacuum suction is applied when the catheter is in position to retrieve a round disk of arterial wall from the recipient artery wall. **(B)** The ELANA platinum ring. A 2.8-mm and a 2.6-mm version are currently available. ([**A**] from van Doormaal TP, van der Zwan A, Verweij BH, Langer DJ, and Tulleken CA. Treatment of giant and large internal carotid artery aneurysms with a high-flow replacement bypass using the excimer laser-assisted nonocclusive anastomosis technique. Neurosurgery 2008;62:1414. Reprinted by permission.)

a part of the medial layer of the recipient artery had to be removed at the site of anastomosis. This is a delicate microneurosurgical procedure, which is not without risk.

Therefore, we started to use an excimer laser (first the Tui-Laser, Coherent, Inc., Santa Clara, CA, and later the Spectranetics laser, Colorado Springs, CO), which became available at the University Medical Center of Utrecht, the Netherlands, in January 1991. With this technique, removal of the adventitial and medial layers of the recipient artery was no longer necessary. Our experiments on the common carotid artery (CCA) of the rabbit showed excellent results.[8] However, in the first 10 human patients, three bypasses occluded.[9] We went back to the laboratory, and started experimenting on the aorta of the rabbit, which is more comparable to the human distal ICA and MCA than the rabbit CCA. It was shown that a solid excimer laser catheter tip made holes in the wall of the aorta that were severely irregular. We therefore designed a laser catheter tip that consisted of two circular layers of fine laser fibers (diameter 60 mm), arranged around a thin-walled hollow catheter with a diameter of 2.2 mm.[10] This catheter has to be connected to a vacuum suction pump next to the excimer laser system **(Fig. 29.3)**. The idea was to punch out a full-thickness disk of arterial wall, which would then be removed when the laser catheter was withdrawn. The punched-out portion of the arterial wall remains attached to the tip, because of continuous suction through the laser catheter. This would create a perfectly round anastomosis. In the first experiments, however, we did not succeed in retrieving the disk that was cut out of the arterial wall by the laser. The disk always remained attached to the wall of the artery at the two lateral sides. We hypothesized that laser light might penetrate tissue more easily if it were applied perpendicularly, and that it might have difficulties in penetrating tissue to which it was applied more obliquely.

A simple and elegant solution to this problem was found. A platinum ring with a diameter of 2.8 mm was first sutured to the arterial wall, after which the donor vein was attached to the ring plus recipient artery **(Fig. 29.3)**. The ring created a flat surface for the laser catheter, which now could create a wide and perfectly round anastomosis. The technique was called the excimer laser–assisted nonocclusive anastomosis (ELANA) technique **(Fig. 29.4)**. Experimental results were excellent, after which more than 400 patients were operated on using the ELANA technique.[8,10–14]

◆ Techniques

Extracranial-Intracranial

The most frequently performed high-flow bypass in our institution is made between the external carotid artery (ECA) extracranially and the internal carotid artery (ICA) bifurcation intracranially. As donor graft we preferably use the saphenous vein. Harvesting should be performed with minimal manipulation of the vein.[15] We first make the ELANA anastomosis on the ICA using approximately 10 cm of vein graft. Since 1998, we suture the ELANA ring first to the vein graft before suturing it intracranially to the recipient artery. This reduces the number of technically difficult intracranial microsutures. After lasing the anastomosis and temporary clip placement, we make a conventional end-to-side anastomosis on the ECA using a second piece of vein graft. Subsequently, both ends of the bypass are sutured together end to end. This is performed at the spot where the bypass enters the intracranial space in a slight oblique fashion to prevent kinking of the bypass. An open conduit for the bypass is made in front of the ear, which is closed as the final step of the procedure after skin closure over the skull. We do not tunnel the bypass because we use this part of the bypass to control for twisting or vasospasms. Moreover, we measure flow through the bypass in front of the ear until the end of the procedure.

Other extracranial inflow anastomosis spots for an EC-IC high-flow bypass include the CCA, but only in cases of ICA

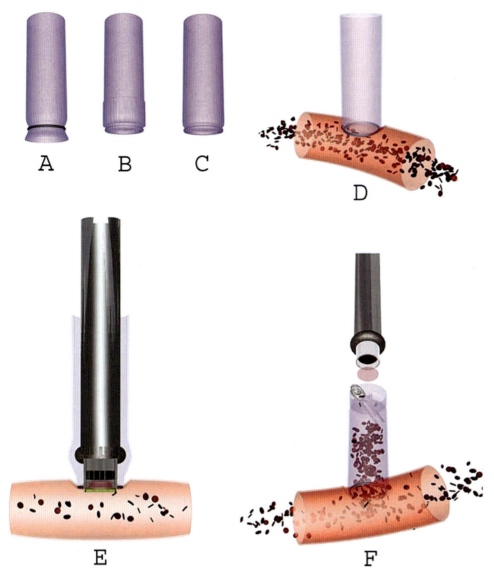

Fig. 29.4 The excimer laser–assisted nonocclusive anastomosis (ELANA) technique. First, a donor vessel (saphenous vein) is harvested from the leg. **(A–C)** A platinum ring with a diameter of 2.8 mm is attached to the outside of the donor vein with eight microsutures. **(D)** The ring and distal donor segment are attached to the recipient artery with eight microsutures followed by the passing of a laser suction catheter (the ELANA catheter 2.0) down the lumen of the open donor vessel. **(E)** The tip of the catheter is placed against the sidewall of the recipient vessel. After 2 minutes of active vacuum suction through the catheter, the laser portion of the catheter is activated during 5 seconds. **(F)** The laser broaches the recipient arterial wall and separates an arteriotomy flap from the recipient. The suction portion of the catheter maintains the small arteriotomy flap in contact with the catheter, thus preventing its migration into the lumen of the recipient. The catheter is removed from the donor lumen. When the newly created artificial side branch is occluded with a clip, the anastomosis is completed. Note that the recipient vessel was patent during the entire procedure. (From van Doormaal TP, van der Zwan A, Verweij BH, Langer DJ, Tulleken CA. Treatment of giant and large internal carotid artery aneurysms with a high-flow replacement bypass using the excimer laser-assisted nonocclusive anastomosis technique. Neurosurgery 2008;62:1414. Reprinted by permission.)

occlusion and hemodynamic cerebral ischemia, or the superior thyroid artery if the ECA wall is arteriosclerotic. In patients with hemodynamic cerebral ischemia who show extra- to intracranial collateral flow via the ophthalmic artery on preoperative angiographic studies, we construct a conventional end-to-side inflow anastomosis on the proximal STA.

Other outflow anastomosis spots for the ELANA technique include all cerebral arteries with a minimal diameter of 2.5 mm. If the recipient is smaller, an ELANA probably is not necessary because of collateral flow, and a conventional anastomosis can be made.

Intracranial-Intracranial

At the inflow side of an intra- to intracranial (IC-IC) bypass we perform per definition an ELANA anastomosis, because this anastomosis is constructed on a large proximal cerebral artery **(Fig. 29.4).** Therefore an important criterion for this bypass, next to a healthy looking recipient vessel wall surface, is enough surgical space at the bypass inflow site to suture the ELANA anastomosis. Moreover, there has to be enough intracranial space for a bypass conduit. At the distal side the character of the anastomosis depends on the size of the artery and the level of branching, with the same criteria as the outflow anastomosis of the high flow EC-IC bypass. If an IC-IC bypass is possible, we generally prefer it over an EC-IC bypass because a large surgical exposure using the ECA is avoided.

◆ Indications

ELANA bypass surgery is performed for various indications. Therefore, subtypes of patient groups should be specified to draw reliable conclusions about the clinical results.

Giant Aneurysms

The natural course of giant aneurysms is grim. A mortality and severe morbidity rate of 65 to 85% within 2 years due to mass effect of rupture is reported.[16] If an aneurysm is considered unclippable and uncoilable, we consider the aneurysm for cerebral revascularization. The main location for these aneurysms is the ICA before its bifurcation.[14] In patients harboring these aneurysms, first a balloon test occlusion of the ICA must be performed with a venous outflow study to observe if the patient tolerates definitive ICA occlusion. If the patient clinically does not tolerate the occlusion, or if asymmetry in venous outflow is more than 1 second, a revascularization procedure is indicated before definitive ICA occlusion. Generally, our first treatment plan in these patients is to create an EC-IC high-flow replacement bypass using the saphenous vein (**Fig. 29.5**).[14] We had a technical success rate of 97%

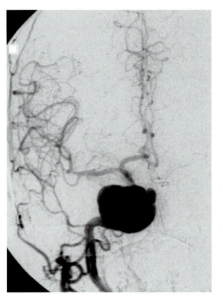 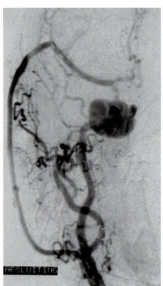

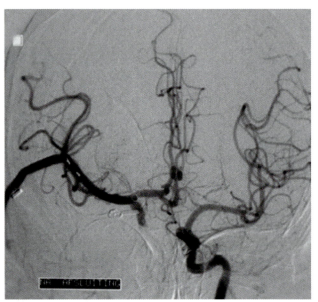

Fig. 29.5 Digital subtraction angiograms of a giant internal carotid artery (ICA) aneurysm treated with high-flow extracranial-intracranial (EC-IC) ELANA bypass and postoperative ICA occlusion. **(A)** Preoperative. **(B)** Postoperative. **(C)** After ICA balloon occlusion. (From van Doormaal TP, van der Zwan A, Verweij BH, Langer DJ, Tulleken CA. Treatment of giant and large internal carotid artery aneurysms with a high-flow replacement bypass using the excimer laser-assisted nonocclusive anastomosis technique. Neurosurgery 2008;62:1414. Reprinted by permission.)

A

B

C

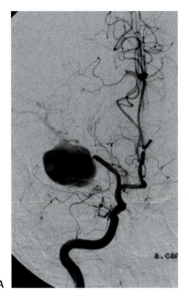
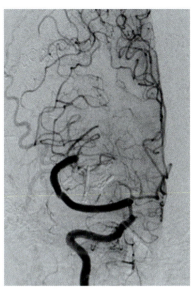

A

B

Fig. 29.6 **(A,B)** Digital subtraction angiograms of a giant middle cerebral artery (MCA) aneurysm treated with high-flow intracranial-intracranial (IC-IC) ELANA bypass (proximal ELANA anastomosis and a distal conventional anastomosis) and intraoperative aneurysm trapping. (From van Doormaal TP, van der Zwan A, Verweij BH, Han KS, Langer DJ, Tulleken CA. Treatment of giant middle cerebral artery aneurysms with a flow replacement bypass using the excimer laser-assisted nonocclusive anastomosis technique. Neurosurgery 2008;63(1):12-20. Reprinted by permission.)

in these patients and a functionally favorable outcome in 74% of these patients.

In patients harboring a giant aneurysm of the ICA bifurcation, the proximal MCA (M1-M2), the anterior communicating artery (ACoA), or the BA, a custom-made plan for a EC-IC or IC-IC bypass **(Fig. 29.6)** has to be formulated to rebuild the vascular architecture. The anatomy must be studied in detail to assess which vessels are approachable for bypass grafting. Nowadays not only conventional angiography, but also computed tomography (CT) perfusion and magnetic resonance angiography (MRA) are used to study this anatomy. Also, the flow that needs replacement has to be determined. This can be preoperatively assessed using MRA or the NOVA technique (VasSol Inc., River Forest, IL), or it can be intraoperatively assessed by measuring the flow through the inflow and outflow arteries using a Transonic Systems Inc. (Ithaca, NY) flow meter. In patients with a giant MCA aneurysm that was revascularized with a flow replacement ELANA bypass (EC-IC or IC-IC), a technical success rate of 91% and a functionally favorable outcome in 77% of the patients was achieved.[13]

In patients with a giant aneurysm in the posterior circulation, good results have not been achieved in terms of functional outcomes using any technique.[17] This is one of the future challenges in cerebral revascularization.

Symptomatic Carotid Artery Occlusion

Patients with transient ischemic attack (TIAs) or a minor disabling ischemic stroke associated with occlusion of the ICA and a compromised hemodynamic state of the brain have a risk of recurrent stroke as high as 9 to 18% per year.[18,19] In patients for whom there are no other treatment options, EC-IC bypass surgery may be considered. The STA-MCA bypass was shown not to be effective in preventing stroke in patients with symptomatic ICA occlusion in general in the EC-IC bypass trial.[2] On average, the STA-MCA bypass has been reported to result in a flow of 10 to 50 mL/min through the

bypass.[20] Assuming that a more proximal bypass would be more capable of preventing TIAs due to a high flow, we preferably operate on patients using a high-flow ELANA bypass.

We select patients with cerebral ischemia for revascularization based on several criteria. First, the symptoms of cerebral ischemia (not the retina only) have to be transient or at most moderately disabling (a modified Rankin scale [mRs] score of 3 or better). Second the symptoms have to be associated with carotid artery occlusion (CAO). We exclude patients with MCA stenosis based on unfavorable clinical results in the past. Third, the symptoms have to be present after documentation of the CAO despite antithrombotic medication or oral anticoagulants at most 6 months before surgery. Fourth, there has to be evidence of a possible hemodynamic origin of symptoms. This evidence could consist of symptoms classically associated with hemodynamic cause (limb shaking, symptoms subsequent to rising or exercise) or a border-zone infarct. Finally the patient should show a low transcranial Doppler (TCD) CO_2 reactivity.

If a patient meets our operative criteria, we preferably construct a high-flow EC-IC ELANA bypass. The inflow anastomosis is preferably made on the CCA. When collateral EC-IC ophthalmic artery flow is visible on the angiogram, we use the STA as the proximal artery. For the outflow anastomosis we use the ELANA technique on a large proximal intracranial artery like the ICA (bifurcation or just below) or the proximal MCA. We achieved a short-term technical success in 96% of these patients and a long-term favorable outcome (totally stroke free postoperatively) in 79%[21] (also based on partially unpublished data). However, the benefit of a high-flow compared with a low-flow bypass has never been shown in a prospective, randomized trial.

Two new prospective studies are currently being conducted to evaluate if the STA-MCA bypass combined with the best medical therapy better prevents subsequent ipsilateral stroke than the best medical therapy alone. Both studies use impaired regional cerebral blood flow following carotid artery occlusion (CAO) shown by a positron emission tomography (PET) oxygen extraction fraction (OEF) as an inclusion criterion. The first study, the Japanese EC-IC Bypass Trial (JET study) showed in its second interim analysis that bypass surgery seems superior to medical treatment in terms of stroke prevention.[22] However, definitive results of this study have not been published yet in the English-language literature. The second study, the Carotid Occlusion Surgery Study (COSS),[23] was terminated at the time of this publication. It is not expected that a significant advantage of surgery was found in this study. However, results have not been officially published yet. Both the JET and COSS study use a selection of the new techniques that currently facilitate identification of patients with a low or absent remaining capacity to compensate for impaired cerebral blood flow. These techniques include CO_2 reactivity measured with CT or TCD, CT and magnetic resonance imaging (MRI) before and after the administration of acetazolamide, xenon-enhanced CT, and single photon emission computed tomography (SPECT) and PET to assess the OEF.

◆ Future Directions

Research into the future direction of cerebral revascularization in general and ELANA in particular is firmly focused on creating a safe, minimally invasive, more easily performed anastomosis. Research is currently underway to develop a completely sutureless ELANA (SELANA) bypass that can be applied through minimal space. Other future strategies involve upscaling and downscaling the size of the ring, downsizing the size of the laser system, as well as varying the laser catheter design and energy to allow vessels of any caliber to be effectively anastomosed utilizing an ELANA system. This includes the adaptation of the ELANA or SELANA technique for application on the CCA, the extracranial ICA, the ECA, and the vertebral artery. This application is contemplated not so much because of the nonocclusive character of the technique, but more because of its technical simplicity and its favorable patency rate.

Additionally, artificial vessel technologies are being investigated to be combined with the ELANA or SELANA ring, to improve bypass quality, and to preclude the need for the vessel harvesting operation for the patient. Furthermore, tissue engineering technologies have begun to develop that may allow the creation of an actual, specifically engineered blood vessel from the patient's own tissues. These artificially produced autologous graft vessels could then be grown around an ELANA or SELANA ring, allowing them to be easily attached using the laser technique.

During the past 10 years there has been an explosion in devices and technologic advances in the field of neurointerventional/endovascular surgery. Although rapid advances in skull-base and minimally invasive approaches have occurred, fewer new devices have been developed for use in open surgery. The ELANA technique represents one of the few new surgical devices for use in vascular neurosurgery. However, the availability of this technique and the upcoming potential availability of a minimal invasive, simple, sutureless version should not lead to general adaptation of cerebral revascular-

ization in every neurosurgical clinic. Besides learning how to create an anastomosis, the neurosurgeon should be trained and regularly performing microanastomoses. To reach this goal, microsurgical training in a readily available vascular laboratory is increasingly needed for the dedicated surgeon. Specialized centers should be formed with close cooperation between highly trained neurosurgeons and neurointerventional specialists. The neurosurgeon in these centers should master different state-of-the-art cerebral revascularization techniques as much as the neuroradiologist should master all state-of-the-art endovascular techniques. Other nearby centers should refer patients and closely cooperate with the specialized center in terms of research and resident education. This will lead to the regular performance of technically difficult cerebral revascularization procedures by the same highly trained neurosurgeons and perioperative guidance by the same specialists, such as anesthesiologists, neurologists, intensivists, nurses, and medical technology staff. Moreover, it will stimulate new developments in the field of cerebral revascularization, and therefore lead to better functional outcomes for patients.

References

1. Yasargil MG. Microsurgery Applied to Neurosurgery. Stuttgart: Georg Thieme Verlag, 1969
2. The EC-IC bypass study. N Engl J Med 1987;317:1030–1032
3. Lawton MT, Hamilton MG, Morcos JJ, Spetzler RF. Revascularization and aneurysm surgery: current techniques, indications, and outcome. Neurosurgery 1996;38:83–92, discussion 92–94
4. Sekhar LN, Bucur SD, Bank WO, Wright DC. Venous and arterial bypass grafts for difficult tumors, aneurysms, and occlusive vascular lesions: evolution of surgical treatment and improved graft results. Neurosurgery 1999;44:1207–1223, discussion 1223–1224
5. Hillen B, Hoogstraten HW, Post L. A mathematical model of the flow in the circle of Willis. J Biomech 1986;19:187–194
6. Tulleken CA, Hoogland P, Slooff J. A new technique for end-to-side anastomosis between small arteries. Acta Neurochir Suppl (Wien) 1979;28: 236–240
7. Tulleken CA, van Dieren A, Verdaasdonk RM, Berendsen W. End-to-side anastomosis of small vessels using an Nd:YAG laser with a hemispherical contact probe. Technical note. J Neurosurg 1992;76:546–549
8. Tulleken CA, Verdaasdonk RM, Berendsen W, Mali WP. Use of the excimer laser in high-flow bypass surgery of the brain. J Neurosurg 1993;78:477–480
9. Tulleken CA, Verdaasdonk RM. First clinical experience with Excimer assisted high flow bypass surgery of the brain. Acta Neurochir (Wien) 1995;134:66–70
10. Tulleken CA, Verdaasdonk RM, Beck RJ, Mali WP. The modified excimer laser-assisted high-flow bypass operation. Surg Neurol 1996;46:424–429
11. Klijn CJ, Kappelle LJ, van der Zwan A, van Gijn J, Tulleken CA. Excimer laser-assisted high-flow extracranial/intracranial bypass in patients with symptomatic carotid artery occlusion at high risk of recurrent cerebral ischemia: safety and long-term outcome. Stroke 2002;33:2451–2458
12. Tulleken CA, Verdaasdonk RM, Mansvelt Beck HJ. Nonocclusive excimer laser-assisted end-to-side anastomosis. Ann Thorac Surg 1997;63(6, Suppl)S138–S142
13. van Doormaal TP, van der Zwan A, Verweij BH, Han KS, Langer DJ, Tulleken CA. Treatment of giant middle cerebral artery aneurysms with a flow replacement bypass using the excimer laser-assisted nonocclusive anastomosis technique. Neurosurgery 2008;63:12–20, discussion 20–22
14. van Doormaal TP, van der Zwan A, Verweij BH, Langer DJ, Tulleken CA. Treatment of giant and large internal carotid artery aneurysms with a high-flow replacement bypass using the excimer laser-assisted nonocclusive anastomosis technique. Neurosurgery 2008;62(6, Suppl 3) 1411–1418
15. Sundt TM III, Sundt TM Jr. Principles of preparation of vein bypass grafts to maximize patency. J Neurosurg 1987;66:172–180

16. Barrow DL, Alleyne C. Natural history of giant intracranial aneurysms and indications for intervention. Clin Neurosurg 1995;42:214–244
17. Streefkerk HJ, Wolfs JF, Sorteberg W, Sorteberg AG, Tulleken CA. The ELANA technique: constructing a high flow bypass using a non-occlusive anastomosis on the ICA and a conventional anastomosis on the SCA in the treatment of a fusiform giant basilar trunk aneurysm. Acta Neurochir (Wien) 2004;146:1009–1019, discussion 1019
18. Vernieri F, Pasqualetti P, Passarelli F, Rossini PM, Silvestrini M. Outcome of carotid artery occlusion is predicted by cerebrovascular reactivity. Stroke 1999;30:593–598
19. Grubb RL Jr, Powers WJ. Risks of stroke and current indications for cerebral revascularization in patients with carotid occlusion. Neurosurg Clin N Am 2001;12:473–487, vii
20. Nakayama N, Kuroda S, Houkin K, Takikawa S, Abe H. Intraoperative measurement of arterial blood flow using a transit time flowmeter: monitoring of hemodynamic changes during cerebrovascular surgery. Acta Neurochir (Wien) 2001;143:17–24
21. Klijn CJ, Kappelle LJ, van der Zwan A, van Gijn J, Tulleken CA. Excimer laser-assisted high-flow extracranial/intracranial bypass in patients with symptomatic carotid artery occlusion at high risk of recurrent cerebral ischemia: safety and long-term outcome. Stroke 2002;33:2451–2458
22. Ogasawara K, Ogawa A. JET study (Japanese EC-IC Bypass Trial). Nippon Rinsho 2006;64(Suppl 7):524–527
23. Grubb RL Jr, Powers WJ, Derdeyn CP, Adams HP Jr, Clarke WR. The Carotid Occlusion Surgery Study. Neurosurg Focus 2003;14:e9

IV

Neurointerventional Approaches

30

Endovascular Thrombolysis and Thrombectomy: Pharmacologic and Mechanical

Sabareesh K. Natarajan, Adnan H. Siddiqui, L. Nelson Hopkins, and Elad I. Levy

Pearls

- Neurologic outcome after stroke intervention depends on the volume of the ischemic brain, the time window to recanalization, the ability to have sustained flow restoration, and the morbidity of symptomatic intracranial hemorrhage (SICH) associated with the treatment.
- Current treatment options for acute ischemic stroke are aimed at an early and sustained restoration of flow to the penumbra, increasing the time window for treatment and decreasing the rates of SICH.
- Endovascular interventions, especially mechanical thrombolysis, are more efficient than intravenous (IV) or intraarterial (IA) pharmacologic thrombolysis in opening up the vessels without the increased risk of SICH associated with the use of pharmacologic thrombolysis.
- Although recanalization rates have increased with endovascular therapies, SICH rates also have increased, whereas outcomes have improved only marginally.
- Better standards and protocols for physiologic imaging with good reproducibility, improvements in mechanical revascularization strategies, and newer thrombolytics allow the selection of patients who may benefit from endovascular revascularization even up to 24 to 36 hours after stroke symptom onset.
- Better patient selection and addition of neuroprotective strategies may improve outcomes in the future.

◆ Epidemiology and Natural History of Acute Large Vessel Occlusions

Stroke remains the third most common cause of death in industrialized nations and the single most common reason for permanent adult disability.[1] Each year, approximately 795,000 Americans experience a new or recurrent stroke.[2] The direct and indirect costs of stroke for 2009 are estimated at $68.9 billion.[2] The incidence of new or recurrent strokes

per year is projected to rise to 1.2 million per year by 2025.[3] The only U.S. Food and Drug Administration (FDA)-approved medical therapy for acute stroke until recently was intravenous (IV) recombinant tissue-type plasminogen activator (rtPA) administered within 3 hours of symptom onset for patients eligible for thrombolysis.[4,5] However, <1% of acute ischemic stroke patients in the United States receive rtPA, primarily because of a delay in presentation for treatment.[6] Early reocclusion following thrombolysis has been demonstrated by transcranial Doppler imaging to occur in 34% of patients receiving IV rtPA and may result in neurologic worsening in many of these patients.[7-9]

Occlusion of the major intracranial arteries (carotid siphon, middle cerebral artery [MCA], vertebral artery, basilar artery) is an important cause of ischemic stroke.[10] The recanalization rates of IV rtPA for proximal, large-vessel arterial occlusions are poor and range from only 10% for internal carotid artery (ICA) occlusion to 30% for MCA occlusion.[11] Intravenous thrombolysis (IVT) is not as effective for thromboembolic obstruction of these large, proximal vessels as for more distal smaller vessels.[12] Outcomes after large intracranial vessel thromboembolic occlusion currently remain dismal and are associated with high morbidity and mortality.[13-16]

◆ Rationale for Intraarterial Pharmacologic and Mechanical Thrombolysis

The rationale for intraarterial (IA) thrombolytic therapy was based on the observation that most ischemic strokes were the consequence of thrombotic or thromboembolic arterial occlusions.[17] Angiographic studies demonstrated the presence of occlusive clots in up to 80% of ischemic strokes.[11] In the remaining 20% of stroke events, the putative underlying mechanism was a microthrombus not detected by angiogram or a thrombotic occlusion that spontaneously recanalized.

Recanalization Improves Outcomes and Is Better with Endovascular Therapy

In the Mechanical Embolus Removal in Cerebral Ischemia (MERCI) trial,[18] Multi MERCI trial,[19] and the combined analysis of Interventional Management of Stroke (IMS) I and II data,[20] the outcome, as measured by the modified Rankin Scale (mRS) score of at ≤2 at 3 months, was significantly better and the 3-month mortality was significantly lower in patients who had Thrombolysis in Myocardial Infarction (TIMI) score 2 or 3 recanalization (partial or complete recanalization, respectively) than in patients in whom vessels failed to recanalize after endovascular therapy. Rha and Saver[21] reviewed 53 studies encompassing 2066 patients and found good functional outcomes (mRS score ≤2) at 3 months were more frequent in patients with vessel recanalization than without vessel recanalization (odds ratio [OR], 4.43; 95% confidence interval [CI], 3.32–5.91). The 3-month mortality rate was reduced in patients whose vessels were recanalized (OR, 0.24; 95% CI, 0.16–0.35). Endovascular methods, particularly mechanical therapies, can achieve higher recanalization rates, and hence better outcomes.

Does the Time Window Between Symptom Onset and Treatment Affect Outcomes?

The European Cooperative Acute Stroke Study (ECASS) III trial[22] has demonstrated value for extending the time window for IV tissue-type plasminogen activator (tPA) to 4.5 hours. A recent meta-analysis by Lansberg et al[23] including data for patients treated in the 3- to 4.5-hour time window in ECASS I ($n = 234$), ECASS II ($n = 265$), ECASS III ($n = 821$), and the Alteplase Thrombolysis for Acute Noninterventional Therapy in Ischemic Stroke (ATLANTIS) ($n = 302$) showed that rtPA treatment was associated at 3 months with an increased chance of favorable outcome on a global outcome measure (a global OR test based on three individual outcome scales at day 90: mRS score 0 to 1, National Institutes of Health Stroke Scale [NIHSS] score 0 to 1, and Barthel Index >95; OR 1.31; 95% CI, 1.10–1.56; $p = .002$); and the mRS 0 to 1 (OR 1.31, $p = .008$) and mortality rates (OR 1.04; 95% CI, 0.75–1.43; $p = .83$) were not significantly different for intravenous thrombolysis (IVT) and placebo-treated patients. The new American Heart Association/American Stroke Association (AHA/ASA) guidelines[24] recommend evaluating patients for IV tPA 3 to 4.5 hours after stroke symptom onset using the same eligibility criteria as the 0- to 3-hour time window with application of additional exclusion criteria.

A meta-analysis conducted by Wardlaw et al[25] demonstrated higher benefit (compared with the risk of being dead or disabled) up to 6 hours after IVT, thus formally providing level-1 evidence, even in patients selected by "only" noncontrast computed tomographic (NCCT) imaging. The Prolyse in Acute Cerebral Thromboembolism (PROACT) trials[26,27] estab-

lished a benefit of IA thrombolysis up to 6 hours after stroke symptom onset, with an increase in recanalization rates. Mechanical revascularization strategies reestablish flow faster than thrombolytics and thus may increase the benefit of treatment even when there is a delay in presentation for treatment. The MERCI trial,[18,28] Multi MERCI trial,[19] and the Penumbra trial[29] show effectiveness of mechanical revascularization therapy up to 8 hours after stroke symptom onset. There is increasing evidence that identification of potentially salvageable brain tissue with advanced magnetic resonance imaging (MRI) and computed tomography (CT) may facilitate the selection of patients who can be effectively and safely treated beyond 8 hours post-ictus.[22,30–36] Although the evidence for a longer time window for treatment is increasing, the number needed to treat (NNT) increases with the time window, and the outcome is better if the treatment is initiated earlier.[37]

The most dreaded complication associated with revascularization therapy is symptomatic intracranial hemorrhage (SICH). The mortality rate after SICH in the National Institute of Neurological Disorders and Stroke (NINDS) trial was 47%.[4] The following IVT trials—NINDS, ATLANTIS, and ECASS II—show an increased hemorrhage rate of 6 to 8% with IV thrombolytics, compared with 1% with placebo.[38] Theoretically, mechanical revascularization strategies increase the benefit of therapy by increasing the recanalization rate and decrease the risk of SICH by avoiding the use of thrombolytics. This concept becomes increasingly relevant and important as the time window from stroke symptom onset increases.

On the basis of this concept and our experience, the first choice at our center is mechanical revascularization therapy for patients who present after 3 hours of stroke symptom onset and patients with wake-up strokes (in whom the time of stroke symptom onset is not known) after evaluating and confirming large vessel occlusion. IA pharmacologic thrombolysis is used only if the site of occlusion is distal and not reachable for mechanical therapy as an adjunct for distal embolization, if any, after mechanical therapy. Patients who do not meet the eligibility criteria for thrombolytic therapy, fail to improve neurologically after thrombolytic therapy, or who improve and then worsen (patients with reocclusion) are also candidates for mechanical revascularization therapies.

◆ Patient Selection and Complication Avoidance

The principles of patient selection and complication avoidance are the same. As described above, the most dreaded complication leading to poor prognosis is SICH. Better patient selection decreases complications including SICH. The three major criteria for selection of a patient for endovascular thrombolysis are (1) contraindication for IV tPA or neurologic condition did not improve or worsened after improvement with IV tPA (as discussed above); (2) a short time window from stroke symptom onset (as discussed above); and (3) the presence of an ischemic penumbra—the therapeutic target.

Table 30.1 Criteria for Defining the Ischemic Penumbra

Penumbral tissue is an area of hypoperfused, abnormal tissue with either physiologic or biochemical characteristics or both, consistent with cellular dysfunction but not cellular death.

The tissue is within the same ischemic territory as the infarct core.

The tissue can either survive or progress to necrosis.

Salvage of the tissue is associated with better clinical outcome.

The Penumbral Concept

Astrup et al[39] established the principle that potentially salvageable cerebral ischemic tissue is present around the ischemic core. The ischemic penumbra is defined as "ischemic tissue that is functionally impaired and is at risk of infarction and has the potential to be salvaged by reperfusion and/or other strategies. If it is not salvaged, this tissue is progressively recruited into the infarct core, which will expand with time into the maximal volume originally at risk." The criteria established for defining ischemic penumbra are shown in **Table 30.1**. Using MRI, up to 44% of stroke patients may have penumbral tissue after 18 hours.[40] Using positron emission tomography (PET), Markus et al[41] have shown salvageable penumbral tissue in stroke patients even 12 to 48 hours after stroke onset. Therefore, imaging of the penumbra may be relevant in selecting patients for thrombolytic therapy who present beyond the 3-hour time window.

Brain-tissue flow can be described by several parameters, including cerebral blood flow (CBF), cerebral blood volume (CBV), and mean transit time (MTT). CBV is defined as the total volume of flowing blood in a given volume in the brain, with units of milliliters of blood per 100 g of brain tissue. CBF is defined as the volume of blood moving through a given volume of brain per unit of time, with units of milliliters of blood per 100 g of brain tissue per minute. MTT is defined as the average transit time of blood through a given brain region, measured in seconds. "Core" is typically operationally defined as the CBV lesion volume, and "penumbra," as the MTT or CBF lesion volume.

Multimodal Computed Tomography Imaging to Assess the Penumbra

The obvious advantages of CT over other penumbral imaging techniques are its widespread availability, speed of imaging, cost-effectiveness, and accessibility in the emergency department. We use a combined multimodal CT stroke protocol consisting of NCCT, CT perfusion (CTP), and CT angiography (CTA) to select patients for endovascular thrombolysis. Other groups[42–44] have similarly noted benefits of combined CTA and CTP imaging in rapid assessment of acute stroke.

Noncontrast CT can occasionally identify the penumbra under some circumstances. Isolated focal swelling has been correlated with penumbral tissue and parenchymal hypoattenuation with the infarct core.[45] However, on NCCT, acutely hypoperfused regions often appear normal, and CTP is helpful in predicting the fate of ischemic tissue in these cases.[46] NCCT also helps in excluding the presence of hemorrhagic stroke or hemorrhage into an ischemic stroke, either of which is a contraindication to thrombolysis.

In patients who do not have an intracranial hemorrhage (ICH), an immediate CT angiogram from aortic arch to vertex, followed immediately by whole-brain CTP on a 320-slice CT scanner, is performed at our center. The newer 320-slice CTP scanner creates whole-brain perfusion maps and CTA within 5 to 10 minutes, has good resolution with fewer artifacts in the posterior fossa, and is comparable with MR perfusion imaging.[47] The newer 320-slice scanners provide a delay map that creates CBF and MTT maps without delay artifacts.[48,49]

In our experience, CTA has been found to be significantly better than MR angiography (MRA) with respect to resolution, detail, and avoidance of common MR artifacts secondary to low or turbulent flow phenomenon and vessel calcification. CTA helps in patient selection by evaluating the sites and nature of occlusion, the difficulty in access through the arch and extracranial vessel, and collateral circulation. CTA and CTP require the injection of less than 130 mL of iodinated contrast material, which is generally well tolerated, except for a low risk of nephropathy and in cases of a contrast allergy. Smith et al[50] have demonstrated the safety of this approach without previous determination of a serum creatinine level.

The passage of the contrast agent through the brain is recorded, and parametric maps of CBV, CBF, and contrast MTT are generated by CTP. Postprocessing software enables the calculation of absolute CBV and CBF values. Larger regions surrounding the core with decreased CBF and increased MTT (relative to the corresponding contralateral brain tissue >145%) are regarded as tissue at risk.[51,52] In our experience, patients with a penumbral volume of >50% of the occluded vessel territory benefit from endovascular thrombolysis if feasible. CTA assesses the collateral vessel status surrounding an irreversible infarct.[53]

Computed tomography perfusion imaging is also helpful in evaluating the ischemic core (very low CBF [>70% reduction], very low CBV [<2 mL/100 g])[51] and extremely prolonged transit time.[54–56] In our experience, patients with large ischemic cores and even small ischemic cores in the basal ganglia region have a high risk of SICH and poor outcome. We try to avoid endovascular thrombolysis in these patients, and if compelled to intervene due to the presence of a large penumbra, we avoid pharmacologic thrombolysis and glycoprotein (GP) IIb/IIIa antagonists. The disadvantages of CTP are its use of radiation, its incomplete validation, and the qualitative differences in postprocessing software.

Symptomatic Intracranial Hemorrhage

As discussed previously, SICH is the most dreaded complication after stroke revascularization. The mortality rate after SICH in the NINDS trial was 47%.[4] Pharmacologic thrombolytics have been shown to increase the risk of SICH.[38,57]

Hypertension during the first 24 hours after stroke revascularization and pretherapeutic hyperglycemia contribute to increased risk of SICH.[57] In PROACT II,[27] there was an increased risk of SICH in patients with a pretherapeutic glycemia value of >200 mg/dL. A glycemia value of >400 mg/dL represents a contraindication to pharmacologic thrombolysis. When dichotomized Alberta Stroke Program Early CT Scores (ASPECTSs) are assessed from NCCT, patients with low stroke burden (ASPECTS ≥7) on CT imaging incur less SICH after IVT and have a greater chance of gaining independence (mRS ≥2).[58] The use of CTP images, rather than NCCT, increases the prognostic accuracy of the ASPECT score, with final infarct mirroring CBV or CBF deficits when reperfusion is or is not achieved, respectively.[55] As discussed previously, we have found CTP to be very valuable in predicting SICH in our patients, and we try to avoid pharmacologic thrombolysis or any reperfusion therapy in patients at high risk for SICH based on these predictors on a case-by-case basis.

Although IV tPA between 3 and 4.5 hours after stroke symptom onset has been endorsed by the recent AHA/ASA guidelines,[24] we still believe that patients should be evaluated for IA therapies if they present with a large vessel occlusion or if they present for treatment after 3 hours of stroke symptom onset. At our center, patients presenting from 3 to 4.5 hours after stroke symptom onset who have no risks of SICH by clinical, radiologic, and physiologic data could be treated with IVT and endovascular thrombolysis. If patients are at higher risk of SICH, irrespective of the time window of presentation, mechanical thrombolysis would be the best therapy, and we defer from using pharmacologic thrombolysis in these patients after 3 hours. At our center, patients will NOT be evaluated for IA therapy if ALL of the following three criteria are present: (1) they present within 3 hours of stroke symptom onset, (2) they do not have a large vessel occlusion, and (3) their neurologic condition improves and does not worsen after IVT therapy.

◆ Revascularization Treatment Strategies

The current protocol for selection of treatment strategies for revascularization of acute ischemic stroke patients at our center is shown in **Table 30.2**.

Table 30.2 Patient Selection for Stroke Revascularization

Patients with a diagnosis of stroke will not be evaluated for intraarterial (IA) therapy if all of the following three criteria are present: they present within 3 hours of stroke symptom onset, they do not have a large vessel occlusion, and their neurologic condition improves and does not worsen after intravenous thrombolysis (IVT) therapy.

Patients who have contraindications for thrombolytic agents and have clinical or radiologic signs suggestive of high risk of symptomatic intracranial hemorrhage (SICH) are evaluated for mechanical revascularization strategies.

Patients who fail to improve by four National Institutes of Health Stroke Scale (NIHSS) points after 1 hour of IVT or worsen after improvement with IVT are evaluated for endovascular thrombolysis.

All patients who arrive between 3 and 24 hours of stroke onset, have wake-up strokes, or have a large vessel occlusion at presentation are evaluated for endovascular revascularization.

Patients without contraindications for intravenous (IV) tissue-type plasminogen activator (tPA) should be evaluated for IV tPA within 3 to 4.5 hours after stroke symptom onset with additional exclusion criteria, according to the new American Heart Association/American Stroke Association (AHA/ASA) guidelines,[24] and all these patients will be evaluated for endovascular thrombolysis.

The decision to perform a cerebral angiogram is made after assessing the following: premorbid status of the patient, computed tomography angiography (CTA) study from the heart to the head, computed tomography perfusion (CTP) study to evaluate the ischemic penumbra, and a cranial noncontrast computed tomography (NCCT) scan to exclude intracerebral hemorrhage (ICH).

A cerebral angiogram is performed and revascularization considered only if the patient had a premorbid modified Rankin Scale (mRS) ≤1, CTP studies show a penumbra of >50% of the volume of the territory of the occluded vessel, and CT does not show ICH.

Every patient considered for endovascular revascularization is given a bolus of IV heparin that is weight-adjusted to maintain the activated coagulation time at 250 seconds or greater. If the patient is not taking aspirin or clopidogrel (or ticlopidine), the patient will be treated with aspirin (enteric-coated, if necessary), 325 mg. Patients considered for stent placement will be given a loading dose of either clopidogrel (600 mg) or ticlopidine (1 g).

Endovascular revascularization options—intraarterial thrombolysis (IAT) with recombinant tissue-type plasminogen activator (rtPA), wire manipulation, Merci device (Concentric Medical, Inc.), Penumbra device (Penumbra Inc.)—are chosen depending on the site and length of occlusion, ability to use thrombolytics in the patient, presence of perfusion cores in the basal ganglia, and nature of the clot. We prefer to use mechanical revascularization strategies as the first choice in preference to IAT whenever possible.

IA glycoprotein (GP) IIb/IIIa is used for situations in which reocclusion due to thrombus formation is seen after recanalization.

Wingspan (Boston Scientific) or Enterprise (Cordis/Johnson & Johnson) stent placement is used as a bail-out in patients in whom vessels cannot be recanalized with current Food and Drug Administration (FDA)-approved modalities and who have an occlusion at a site that can be stented under Humanitarian Device Exemption and FDA-approved trials.

IAT and mechanical revascularization methods are combined when appropriate.

Patients are observed in the intensive care unit for 6 to 12 hours posttreatment, and a blood pressure of approximately 150/90 mm Hg is maintained to avoid reperfusion injury.

Table 30.3 Advantages and Disadvantages of Intraarterial Pharmacologic Thrombolysis

Advantages

1. Angiographic evaluation reveals the precise occlusion site and the extent of collaterals, and assesses the grade of recanalization during treatment.

2. An effective concentrated dose of thrombolytic agent is delivered directly to the thrombus, thus reducing the systemic side effects.

3. The approach facilitates combination with mechanical recanalization techniques.

Disadvantages

1. It is a time-consuming procedure that delays the initiation of treatment, compared with intravenous thrombolysis.

2. It entails manipulation of cervical and cranial vessels, with the risk of peri-interventional complications.

3. It demands highly specialized centers with high human and financial resources.

4. Direct endovascular access to the distal intracranial vasculature (e.g., distal M2 and M3 segments of the middle cerebral artery) is limited.

Intraarterial Pharmacologic Thrombolysis

To perform IA thrombolysis (IAT), a microcatheter is placed proximal to or directly into the thrombus. A long 6- or 7-French (F) sheath is placed into the femoral artery, and a 6F or 7F guiding catheter is advanced into the ICA or vertebral artery of the affected side. A microcatheter is then navigated to the occlusion site over a microwire. The theoretical advantages and disadvantages of IAT are presented in **Table 30.3**. Results for the important published interventional stroke trials are summarized in **Table 30.4** (NINDS[4] and ECASS III[22] data have been summarized for comparison in the same table).

Intraarterial Thrombolysis Trials

The safety and efficiency of IA administration in the treatment of acute ischemic stroke were evaluated in PROACT I.[26] The results of this trial suggested an enhanced recanalization with prourokinase and a positive trend toward better neurologic outcome and survival rate. The PROACT II trial[27] was a large-scale, multicenter, randomized (2:1), phase III trial that included 180 patients with angiographically confirmed M1 or M2 occlusion within the first 6 hours after symptom onset. Patients were randomized to receive 9 mg of IA prourkinase plus heparin (n = 121) or heparin only (n = 59). Excellent neurologic outcome (mRS ≤2) was achieved in 40% of the treated patients compared with 25% in the control group (absolute benefit, 15%; relative benefit, 58%; NNT, 7; p = .043). This study was able to demonstrate the beneficial effect of IAT on the recanalization and clinical outcome of patients with M1 and M2 occlusions.

Meta-Analysis of Intraarterial Thrombolysis Trials for Middle Cerebral Artery Occlusion

A meta-analysis of PROACT I and II data showed an OR of better outcome with treatment of 2.49 (p = .022), which was greater than the OR (2.13) in the original PROACT II analysis.[59] The Japanese Middle cerebral artery Embolism Local fibrinolytic intervention Trial (MELT)[60] studied safety and clinical efficacy of IA infusion of urokinase (UK) in patients with acute stroke treated within 6 hours of symptom onset. As in PROACT I and II, patients displaying angiographic occlusions of the M1 or M2 MCA segments were randomized. The trial was aborted prematurely by the steering committee after the approval of IV rtPA in Japan. A meta-analysis of PROACT I, PROACT II, and MELT, including 204 patients treated with IAT and 130 control patients, showed a lower rate of death or dependency at long-term follow-up within the IAT treatment group, compared with the control group (58.5% versus 69.2%; p = .03; OR, 0.58; 95% CI, 0.36–0.93).[61]

These studies established superiority of IAT within 6 hours over antithrombotic therapy for MCA M1 and M2 occlusions. There are no level-1 data of the efficacy of IAT for distal ICA or posterior circulation occlusion. The superiority of IAT over IVT has not been demonstrated by randomized clinical studies. The FDA did not approve prourokinase, and it is currently not available for clinical use. Current AHA/ASA guidelines[5,24] recommend the use of IAT with rtPA within 6 hours from symptom onset for selected patients who have a major stroke due to MCA occlusion and who are not eligible for IVT. Therefore, at present, this approach should not preclude IV administration of rtPA in all other eligible patients.

Special Situations

◆ Wake-Up Strokes

Approximately 16 to 28% of ischemic stroke patients awaken with their deficits.[62,63] In these wake-up strokes, the onset of symptoms is defined as the "time last seen well." Because this is the time the patient went to sleep, these patients, unfortunately, are usually placed outside the window for thrombolysis or ineligible for entry into reperfusion clinical trials. Barreto et al[64] reported that patients with wake-up stroke have better outcomes when they are treated. Adams et al,[65] in their post-hoc analysis of wake-up stroke in the Abciximab in Emergency Stroke Treatment Trial-II (AbESTT-II), reported poorer outcomes after treatment. In our series of 30 patients with stroke onset >8 hours and wake-up stroke (mean presentation NIHSS score 13) who were selected for treatment on the basis of CTP results, a combination of endovascular revascularization strategies resulted in a TIMI score 2 or 3 recanalization in 67% of patients, with a SICH rate of 10%.[66] At 3 months, 20% of patients improved to mRS <2, and the mortality was 33.3%.

◆ Posterior Circulation Stroke

Posterior circulation stroke differs in several aspects. The evolution of clinical symptoms is often gradual, making precise

Table 30.4 Summary of Important Published Interventional Stroke Trials; Data from IV Tissue-Type Plasminogen Activator Trials of the National Institute of Neurological Disorders and Stroke and the European Cooperative Acute Stroke Study (ECASS) III Are Included for Comparison

Study	No. of Patients	Type of Study	Treatment	Time Window from Symptom Onset (h)	Mean Presentation NIHSS	Recanalization Rate (%)	SICH Rate (%)	mRS ≤2 or ≤1* at 3 Months (%)	Mortality at 3 Months (%)	Main Results
NINDS[4]	333 (168 versus 165)	RCT	IV rtPA (0.9 mg/kg) versus placebo	0–3	14 versus 15	NR	6.4 versus 0.6	39 versus 26*	21 versus 24	1. No difference between groups at 24 hour (trend in favor of treatment) 2. Clinically significant improvement in functional status at 90 days in treated group (p = .30) 3. Significant difference in SICH rates (p < .001)
ECASS III[22]	821 (418 versus 403)	RCT	IV rtPA (0.9 mg/kg) versus placebo	3–4.5	10.7 versus 11.6	NR	2.4% versus 0.2%	52.4 versus 45.2*	7.7 versus 8.4	1. Significant improvement in functional status at 3 months (p = .04) 2. Significant difference in SICH rates (p = .008) 3. No difference in mortality (p = .68)
PROACT[26]	40 (26 versus 14)	RCT	IA r-prourokinase (6 mg) + IV heparin (high or low dose) versus IV heparin (high or low dose)	0–6	17 versus 19	57.7 versus 14.3	15.4 versus 7.1	30.8 versus 21.4*	26.9 versus 42.9	1. Significant higher recanalization efficacy with IAT (p = .17) 2. No significant difference in SICH (p = .64)
PROACT II[27]	180 (121 versus 59)	RCT	IA r-prourokinase (9 mg) + IV heparin (low dose) versus IV heparin (low dose)	0–6	17 versus 17	66 versus 18	10 versus 2	40 versus 25	25 versus 27	1. Significant better outcome at 3 months (p = .04) and significant higher recanalization rate (p < .001) in the treatment group 2. Difference in SICH not significant (p = .06)
IMS[103]	80 (IAT-62)	Prospec	IV rtPA (0.6 mg/kg) + IA rtPA (4 mg in clot + 9 mg/hr) (if clot identified by angiography after IVT) + low-dose IV heparin	0–3	18	56	6.30	43, 30*	16%	Results compared with NINDS rtPA and placebo arms 1. Significant better 3-month outcomes when compared with NINDS placebo OR >2 2. Difference in mortality or SICH not significant

Study	N	Type	Treatment	Hours		Recanalization (%)				Results
IMS II[81]	81 (IAT-55)	Prospec	IV rtPA (0.6 mg/kg) + IA rtPA (22 mg over 2 hour using EKOS or normal catheter) (if clot identified by angiography after IVT) + low-dose IV heparin	0–3	19	58	9.90	46	16	Results compared with NINDS rt-PA and placebo arms 1. Significant better 3-month outcomes when compared with NINDS placebo OR >2.7 2. Better outcomes in the recanalized cohort when compared with nonrecanalized (p = .046) 3. Difference in mortality or SICH not significant
MERCI[18,28]	141	Prospec	IA Merci (I generation) + IAT, no IVT	0–8	20	60.3 (48 device alone)	7.80	36	34	Better functional outcome at 3 months in recanalized patients when compared with nonrecanalized patients (p = .01)
Multi MERCI[19]	164	Prospec	IA Merci (I & II generation) + IAT + IVT allowed	0–8	19	68 (≤5 device alone)	9.80	36	26	Higher rates of recanalization with 2nd-generation devices
Penumbra[87]	125	Prospec	IA Penumbra + IAT	0–8	17	81.6 (device alone)	11.20	25	32.80	Higher rates of recanalization when compared with previous mechanical revascularization therapies

Abbreviations: ECASS, European Cooperative Acute Stroke Study; EKOS, MicroSonic Accelerated Thrombolytic System, EKOS Corp., Bothell, WA;[[AU: Table 4: is EKOS defined correctly?]] h, hours; IA, intraarterial; IAT, intraarterial thrombolysis; IMS, Interventional Management of Stroke; IV, intravenous; IVT, intravenous thrombolysis; MERCI, Mechanical Embolus Removal in Cerebral Ischemia; mRS, modified Rankin Scale; NINDS, National Institute of Neurological Disorders and Stroke; NR, not reported; PROACT, Prolyse in Acute Cerebral Thromboembolism; OR, odds ratio; Prospec, prospective; RCT, randomized controlled trial; rtPA, recombinant tissue-type plasminogen activator; SICH, symptomatic intracranial hemorrhage.

*mRS ≤1.

Note: Results are presented for treatment group versus control group for RCTs.

assessment of the onset of symptoms and of the time window for treatment difficult. Atherothrombosis (unstable plaque with thrombus) is more common. The risk of reocclusion after recanalization is therefore higher.[67-70] The natural history shows a poor outcome with a high mortality rate of 70 to 80% unless recanalization is achieved.[67,71] A meta-analysis of IAT in basilar artery occlusion[72] showed a recanalization rate of 64% and a mortality rate of 87% in nonrecanalized patients, with a significant ($p <.001$) reduction in mortality to 37% in recanalized patients. A meta-analysis of either IVT or IAT for basilar artery occlusion[73] showed that the likelihood of a good outcome was 2% without recanalization. Recanalization was achieved more frequently with IAT (65% versus 53%, $p = .05$), but the outcomes after IAT and IVT were similar. Levy et al[74] performed a meta-analysis for predictors of outcome after IAT for vertebrobasilar artery occlusion and found failure to recanalize was associated with a higher mortality rate (relative risk, 2.34; 95% CI, 1.48–3.71). Studies have suggested extending the time window for treatment beyond or up to 24 hours postictus.[69,75,76]

◆ Distal Internal Carotid Artery Occlusion

Small retrospective case series[13,14] show the safety and efficacy of IAT with acceptable recanalization rates and outcomes in patients with distal ICA occlusion. The ability to recanalize distal ICA occlusions is low because of a larger clot burden in these patients. They have a poor outcome because there is ischemia to the regions supplied by the perforators arising from the A1 and M1.

◆ Failure of Intravenous Thrombolysis

Intraarterial thrombolysis may be considered in cases of failure of IVT (e.g., lack of early improvement in neurologic status and NIHSS scores after the procedure).[77]

Glycoprotein IIb/IIIa Antagonists

The use of GP IIb/IIIa antagonists, such as abciximab, eptifibatide, or tirofiban, in ischemic stroke remains investigational. The Combined Approach to Lysis Utilizing Eptifibatide and rtPA in Acute Ischemic Stroke (CLEAR) trial[78] evaluated the combination of low-dose IV rtPA and eptifibatide in patients with NIHSS scores of >5 who presented within 3 hours of stroke onset. The study enrolled a total of 94 subjects, with 69 patients receiving the combination therapy and 25 patients receiving IV rtPA therapy. There was one (1.4%) SICH in the combination group and two (8.0%) in the standard treatment group ($p = .17$). There was a nonsignificant trend toward increased efficacy with the standard-dose rtPA treatment arm. The ReoPro Retavase Reperfusion of Stroke Safety Study Imaging Evaluation (ROSIE) is a National Institutes of Health (NIH)-sponsored phase II trial that is evaluating the use of IV reteplase in combination with abciximab for the treatment of MRI-selected patients with stroke within 3 to 24 hours from onset. Preliminary analysis of the first 21 patients enrolled has revealed no SICH or major hemorrhage.[79] Conversely, the AbESTT II trial, a phase III multicenter, randomized, double-blinded, and placebo-controlled study evaluating the safety and efficacy of abciximab in acute ischemic stroke treated within 6 hours after stroke onset or within 3 hours of awakening with stroke symptoms, was stopped early due to high rates of SICH or fatal ICH in the abciximab-treated patients (5.5% versus 0.5%, $p = .002$).[80] Data for the use of GP IIb/IIIa inhibitors in conjunction with IAT and mechanical revascularization are even more scant. We use these drugs at our center for reocclusion after reopening of the vessel to change the prothrombotic state to an antithrombotic state. When we do so, we try to maintain the activated coagulation time at less than 200 seconds to minimize bleeding.

Intravenous Thrombolysis and Intraarterial Thrombolysis Bridging Therapy

At many centers, accessible occlusions in the anterior circulation are treated with IAT, either in patients in whom reperfusion did not occur after IVT or even as a first line of treatment. In the IMS II trial,[81] combination IV and IA therapy resulted in a better outcome than did placebo treatment in the NINDS trial[4]; further, if secondary outcome measures (mRS score, NIHSS score, and Barthel Index) were considered, a statistically better outcome was seen with combination therapy in IMS II than with IV treatment in NINDS. Recanalization was achieved only after rescue IA therapy in most patients in the NINDS trial. A bridging strategy between IV and IA thrombolysis has the advantage of not delaying IV therapy, while identifying nonresponders with persisting large artery occlusion.

This approach is being tested in IMS III, with initial IV rtPA followed by artery reopening by thrombolysis or clot retrieval if vessel occlusion is demonstrated.[82] A summary of the trials using combination IVT and IAT (IMS I and IMS II) is included in **Table 30.4**.

Intraarterial Thrombolysis Versus Intravenous Thrombolysis

The outcome and morbidity of patients treated with IVT and IAT were compared at two different stroke treatment centers.[83] Patients were selected based on the presence of a hyperdense MCA sign on CT imaging, indicating an M1 occlusion. Fifty-five patients were treated with IAT using UK; 59 patients underwent IVT with rtPA. Although the time to treatment was significantly ($p = .0001$) longer in the IAT group (mean, 244 minutes) than in the IVT group (mean, 156 minutes), the study revealed a more frequent favorable outcome for patients treated with IA UK (53%) compared with patients treated with IVT (23%; $p = .001$). In addition, the mortality rate was reduced in the IAT group compared with the IVT group (4.7% versus 23%; $p = .001$).

Mechanical Thrombolysis or Embolectomy

The mechanical recanalization systems can be divided into two major groups, proximal or distal devices, according to where they apply force on the thrombus. Proximal devices

Table 30.5 Advantages and Disadvantages of Mechanical Thrombolysis

Advantages

1. Devices used for mechanical thrombolysis lessen and may even preclude the use of pharmacologic thrombolytics, thus reduce the incidence of symptomatic intracranial hemorrhage.

2. These devices may extend the treatment window beyond the limit of 6 to 8 hours.

3. Mechanical fragmentation of the clot increases the surface area of clot available for endogenous and exogenous fibrinolysis.

4. Recanalization time may be faster.

5. Devices used for mechanical thrombolysis may be effective for thrombi or other material resistant to thrombolytics that occlude the vessel.

6. Mechanical thrombolysis has emerged as the key option for patients who have contraindication for pharmacologic thrombolysis, such as recent surgery or abnormal hemostasis,[105] or have a late presentation.[18,19,28]

Disadvantages

1. It is technically difficult to navigate mechanical thrombolysis devices through the intracranial vasculature.

2. There is the risk of excessive trauma to the vasculature.

3. Distal embolization occurs from a fragmented thrombus.

apply force to the proximal base of the thrombus. This group includes various aspiration catheters. Distal devices approach the thrombus proximally but then are advanced by guidewire and microcatheter across the thrombus to be unsheathed distally, where force is applied to the distal base of the thrombus. This group includes snare-like, basket-like, or coil-like devices. In an animal model,[84] proximal devices were faster in application and associated with a low complication rate. The distal devices were more successful at removing thrombotic material, but their method of application and attendant thrombus compaction increased the risk of thromboembolic events and vasospasm.[85,86] Advantages and disadvantages of mechanical revascularization strategies overall are summarized in **Table 30.5**. The current FDA-approved embolectomy devices are the Penumbra device (proximal device) and the Merci retriever device (distal device).

Penumbra Device

From a procedural point of view, proximal devices like the Penumbra are comparable to IAT. Access is usually gained with a 6F to 8F sheath. After placement of the guiding catheter, the device is navigated to the proximal surface of the clot. This approach omits repetitive passing of the occlusion site. The Penumbra System (Penumbra Inc., Alameda, CA) consists of a microcatheter attached to continuous aspiration via a dedicated aspiration pump system. A microwire/separator with an olive-shaped tip is used to fragment the thrombus from proximal to distal. Direct thrombus extraction can also be attempted with a ring retriever while a balloon-guided catheter is used to temporarily arrest flow. Both microcatheter and separator are available in various sizes and diameters to adjust the device to different anatomic settings (**Fig. 30.1**). Angiographic images for a case in which this device was used to treat an occlusion of the MCA bifurcation are presented in **Fig. 30.2**.

McDougall et al[87] reported the results of a prospective multicenter single-arm trial of 125 patients with acute stroke who underwent revascularization with the Penumbra device. A TIMI score 2 or 3 recanalization was achieved in 81.6% patients with a SICH rate of 11.2%.

Merci Device

The Merci Retrieval System (Concentric Medical, Inc., Mountain View, CA) is a shaped wire constructed of nitinol. The flexible corkscrew-like tip can easily be delivered through a microcatheter into the vessel distal to the occlusion site. When deployed, it returns to its preformed coiled shape to ensnare the thrombus. The thrombus is bypassed and the retriever deployed from inside the catheter distal to the thrombus. The corkscrew-like tip is pulled back slowly to ensnare the clot as a corkscrew would ensnare a cork. The retriever is then retracted into the guide catheter under proximal flow

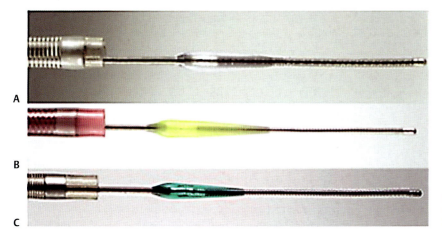

Fig. 30.1 Penumbra device. **(A)** Size 026. **(B)** Size 032. **(C)** Size 041. (Courtesy of Penumbra Inc., Alameda, CA.)

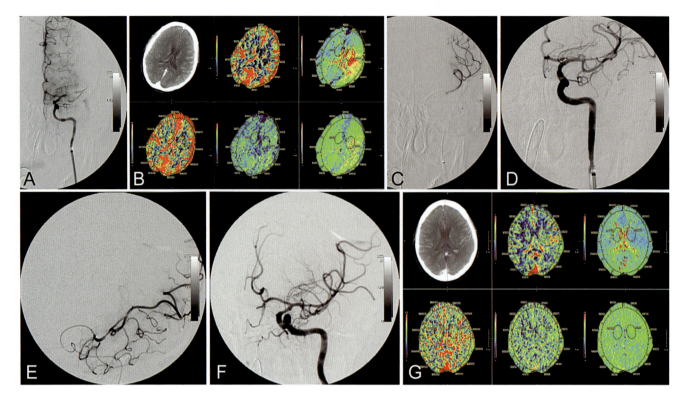

Fig. 30.2 **(A)** Selective angiogram of the left internal carotid artery (ICA) showing occlusion of the middle cerebral artery (MCA) bifurcation. **(B)** Computed tomography (CT) perfusion images showing minimal core (decreased cerebral blood volume [CBV]) and penumbra (increased cerebral blood flow [CBF], mean transit time [MTT], and time to peak [TTP]) in the left MCA territory. **(C)** Selective micro-run of the M2 vessel after the lesion has been crossed with a microcatheter. **(D)** Selective angiogram of the left ICA with the Penumbra device (Penumbra Inc., Alameda, CA) in the superior branch of the MCA showing good flow through the superior branch. **(E)** Selective angiogram of the inferior MCA branch with the Penumbra device in situ showing good flow. **(F)** Final angiogram showing Thrombolysis in Myocardial Infarction (TIMI) score 3 recanalization of the MCA bifurcation. **(G)** CT perfusion images after recanalization showing corrected CBF, MTT, and TTP maps.

arrest. Different versions of the device are available (**Fig. 30.3**). In the first-generation devices (X5 and X6), the nitinol wire was shaped in helical tapering coil loops. The second-generation devices (L4, L5, and L6) differ from the X devices by the inclusion of a system of arcading filaments attached to a nontapering helical nitinol coil, which has a 90-degree angle in relation to the proximal wire component. The third-generation devices (V series) have variable pitch loops under a linear configuration with attached filaments. The retriever device is deployed through a 2.4F microcatheter (14X or 18 L, Concentric Medical, Inc.). The recent addition of a 4.3F distal access catheter has provided additional coaxial support to the system, resulting in improved deliverability with the potential for simultaneous thromboaspiration as well. The devices are available in various diameters from 1.5 to 3 mm, depending on the caliber of the occluded vessel.

The use of Merci devices is technically more complex than the use of proximal types of devices. These devices are regularly used in combination with proximal balloon occlusion in the ICA, in addition to aspiration from the guiding catheter, to reduce the risk of distal thromboembolism. In general, an 8F to 9F sheath and a balloon catheter of similar size are used. After placement of the balloon catheter in the ICA, a microcatheter in combination with a microwire is navigated to the occlusion site. This catheter then has to be advanced beyond the thrombus. An injection of contrast material is recommended distal to the thrombus to estimate the length of the occlusion and to illustrate the anatomy of the distal vessel. The device is then introduced into the microcatheter and unsheathed behind the thrombus. The balloon at the tip of the guiding catheter is inflated. During slow retraction of the device and mobilization of the thrombus, aspiration is applied at the guiding catheter. The device and thrombus are retrieved into the guiding catheter, and the balloon is deflated. In clinical practice, the entire procedure often has to be repeated multiple times to recanalize the vessel. Furthermore, the application of the balloon catheter might be limited in cases of high-grade ICA stenosis. Angiographic images for a case in which this device was used to treat an acute M1 occlusion are presented in **Fig. 30.4**.

In 2004, the FDA approved the use of the Merci device for clot removal from intracranial vessels in patients with ischemic stroke. FDA approval was based on a review of the data obtained in the multicenter MERCI trial that involved 141 patients (mean age, 60 years; mean NIHSS score, 20) ineligible for standard thrombolytic therapy.[18,28] The time win-

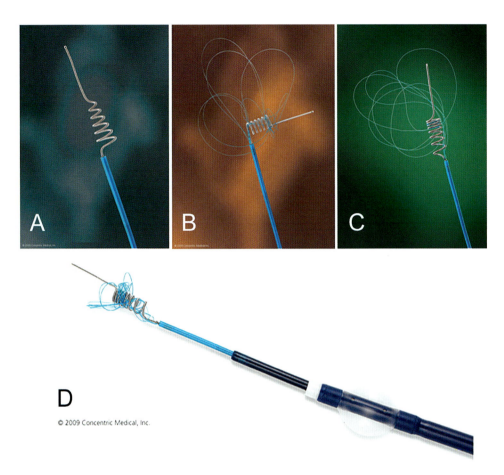

Fig. 30.3 Types of Merci devices. **(A)** Type X. **(B)** Type L. **(C)** Type V. **(D)** Catheter system. (Courtesy of Concentric Medical. Mountain View, CA.)

dow between onset of clinical symptoms and endovascular treatment was extended to 8 hours, compared with the 6-hour window usually applied for IAT. This trial reported a TIMI score 2 or 3 recanalization rate of 48% using the X-type

Merci retriever. SICH was found in 7.8% of the patients, mainly after treatment of ICA and MCA occlusions (in 90% of cases). In the study, the number of attempts to retrieve the clot was limited to six; a mean of 2.9 attempts was performed

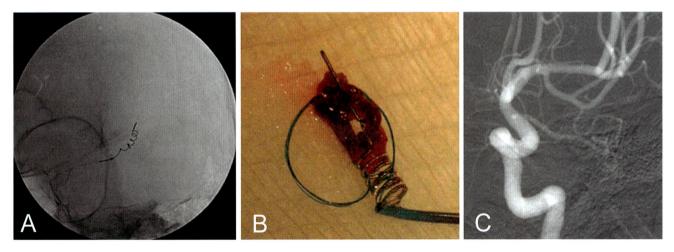

Fig. 30.4 Merci clot retriever device (Concentric Medical, Inc., Mountain View, CA) for a patient with an acute M1 occlusion. **(A)** Plain film during angiogram showing a Merci device in the M1. **(B)** Clot removed with the Merci retriever. **(C)** Post-Merci recanalization angiogram showing TIMI score 3 recanalization. (From Natarajan SK, Snyder KV, Siddiqui AH, Levy EI, Hopkins LN. Interventional management of acute ischemic stroke (Chapter 57). In: Haase J, Schafers H-J, Sievert H, Waksman R, eds. Cardiovascular Interventions in Clinical Practice. Oxford UK: Wiley Blackwell, 2010;609–628. Reprinted by permission.)

for recanalization. The mean procedure time was 2.1 hours. With respect to device-related complications, the study reported vessel perforations (4.2%), subarachnoid hemorrhage (SAH) (2.1%), and embolization of thrombotic material (2.1%).

The Multi MERCI trial[19] was a prospective, multicenter, single-arm registry that included 164 patients (mean age, 68 years; mean NIHSS score, 19) treated with different Merci retrieval systems (X5, X6, and L5). Again, the time window between onset of clinical symptoms and endovascular treatment was extended to 8 hours, and 92% of the patients were treated for an ICA or MCA occlusion. Patients with persistent large-vessel occlusion after IVT (with rtPA) were also included in the study, and adjunctive IAT (using rtPA) was allowed. In 55% of the interventions, mechanical thrombectomy led to recanalization (TIMI score 2 or 3). After adjunctive IAT, 68% of the target vessels were recanalized. Clinically significant device-related complications occurred in 5.5%, and the rate of SICH was 9.8%. At 90 days, 36% of the patients had a favorable outcome (mRS, 0–2) and the mortality rate was 34%. The Merci device has also increased recanalization rates with intracranial ICA occlusion.[88]

Stent-Assisted Thrombolysis

Self-expanding stents (SESs) designed specifically for the cerebrovasculature are available and can be delivered to target areas of intracranial stenosis with a success rate of >95% and an increased safety profile as they are deployed at significantly lower pressures than balloon-mounted coronary stents.[89] Advantages and disadvantages of stent-assisted revascularization are summarized in **Table 30.6**. Reocclusion after IVT (34%) and IA pharmacologic thrombolysis (17%) have been shown to be associated with poor outcome.[90]

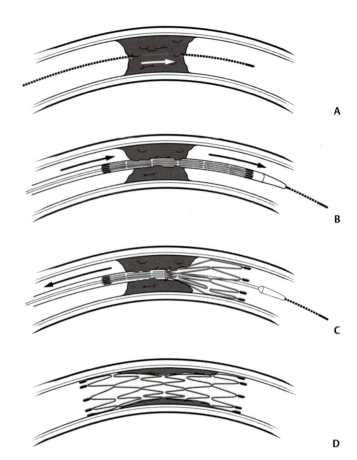

Fig. 30.5 Wingspan stent (Boston Scientific, Natick, MA) for recanalization. **(A)** Occlusive clot crossed with a microwire. **(B)** Placement of stent across the occlusion. **(C)** Deployment of stent, thus trapping the occlusion. **(D)** Recanalization. (From Levy EI, Mehta R, Gupta R, et al. Self-expanding stents for recanalization of acute cerebrovascular occlusions. AJNR Am J Neuroradiol 2007;28:816–822. Reprinted by permission.)

Table 30.6 Advantages and Disadvantages of Stent-Assisted Thrombolysis

Advantages

1. There is an immediate restoration of flow in the occluded vessel

2. There are high recanalization rates.

3. There are decreased chances of early reocclusion after treatment.

4. Stents with radial expansive force like the Wingspan (Boston Scientific) can be used in atherothrombotic lesions with proven safety.

Disadvantages

1. A great proportion of stroke is caused by emboli in a normal intracranial vessel, and hence may need only embolectomy and not a permanent scaffold.

2. Stent navigability and deployment is possible only in the proximal vessels around the circle of Willis and not in the distal intracranial vasculature.

3. Patients need to be on dual antiplatelet therapy for 3 months after stent placement; this may potentially increase the rate of intracranial hemorrhage.

A total of five intracranial SESs are currently available: (1) the Neuroform stent (Boston Scientific, Natick, MA), (2) the Enterprise stent (Cordis/Johnson & Johnson, Warren, NJ), (3) the Leo stent (Balt Extrusion, Montmorency, France), (4) the Solitaire/Solo stent (ev3, Irvine, CA), and (5) the Wingspan stent (Boston Scientific, Natick, MA) (**Figs. 30.5** and **30.6**). The first four devices are currently marketed for stent-assisted coil embolization of wide-necked aneurysms, whereas the Wingspan stent is approved for the treatment of symptomatic intracranial atherosclerotic disease. Both the Neuroform and the Wingspan stents have an open-cell design, whereas the Enterprise, Leo, and Solitaire/Solo stents have a closed-cell design. The closed-cell design allows resheathing of the stent after partial deployment (70% for Enterprise; 90% for Leo)[91,92] or even full deployment (Solitaire/Solo).[93]

Levy et al[94] described the use of the SES (Neuroform3 or Wingspan) to treat 18 patients with stroke (19 lesions) presenting with acute focal occlusions involving the MCA M1 and/or M2 segment (nine lesions), the ICA-T (seven lesions), or the vertebrobasilar system (three lesions). A TIMI score 2 or 3 revascularization was achieved in 15 of 19 lesions (79%).

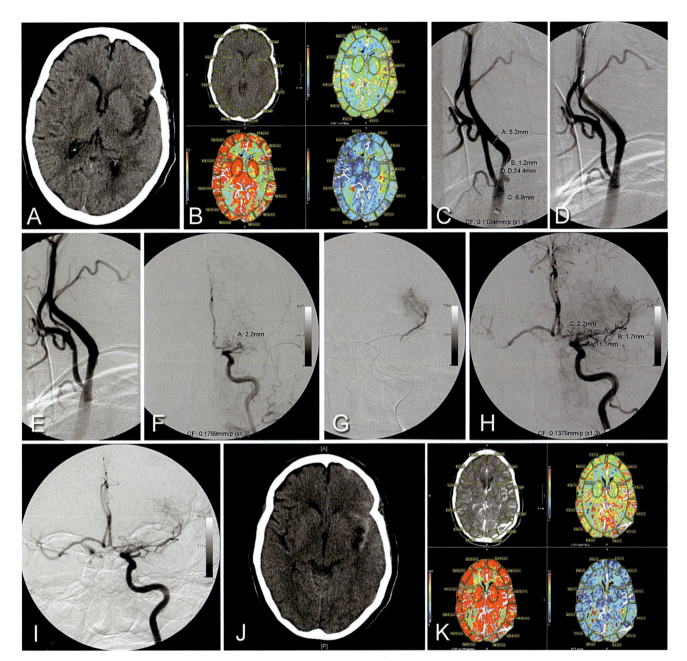

Fig. 30.6 **(A)** Noncontrast CT of the head showing hypodensity in the left basal ganglia region. **(B)** CT perfusion imaging showing minimal core in the left MCA territory with a surrounding penumbra. **(C)** Left common carotid artery injection showing 75% narrowing of the proximal portion of the left cervical ICA. **(D)** Placement of a 6- to 8- × 40-mm Xact stent (Abbott Laboratories, Abbott Park, IL) in the narrow segment with a distal protection device (EPI Embolic Protection Inc./ Boston Scientific, Natick MA). **(E)** Post-stent placement angiogram showing good flow through the left cervical ICA. **(F)** Selective injection of the left ICA showing left proximal M1 occlusion. **(G)** Selective micro-run of the left MCA branches after crossing the lesion with a microcatheter. **(H)** Angiogram showing narrowing of the left M1. **(I)** Angiogram after placement of a 4.5- × 22-mm self-expanding Enterprise stent (Cordis/Johnson & Johnson, Warren, NJ) across the M1 narrowing and TIMI score 3 flow in the distal MCA branches. **(J)** Noncontrast CT of the head postrevascularization showing minimal contrast staining/subarachnoid hemorrhage (SAH) in the left sylvian fissure (the patient improved and was not symptomatic for the SAH). **(K)** CT perfusion postrevascularization showing minimal core and disappearance of the penumbra.

The in-hospital mortality rate was 38.9% (7 of 18 patients). Four patients had mRS scores of ≤3 at the 3-month follow-up evaluation. Zaidat et al[95] evaluated the use of Neuroform (four patients) or Wingspan (five patients) stents in nine patients with acute stroke with occlusions involving the MCA (six lesions), ICA (two lesions), or the vertebrobasilar junction (one lesion). Complete (TIMI 3) and partial or complete (TIMI 2 or 3) recanalization occurred in 67% and 89% of the patients, respectively. There was one ICH (11%) and one acute in-stent thrombosis (successfully treated with abciximab and balloon angioplasty). The mortality rate was 33% (three of nine patients). All survivors achieved an mRS score of ≤2. Follow-up angiography was performed in four of the nine patients at a mean of 8 months (range, 2–14 months) and showed no stent restenosis.

A multicenter retrospective review of prospectively collected data of 20 acute ischemic stroke patients (mean presentation NIHSS score, 17) treated with the Enterprise stent as a bail-out procedure after current embolectomy options had been exploited showed 100% TIMI score 2 or 3 recanalization and improvement in NIHSS of ≥4 points at discharge in 75% of patients.[96] On the basis of this preliminary data, we received FDA approval for a pilot study, Stent-Assisted Recanalization in acute Ischemic Stroke (SARIS), to evaluate the Wingspan stent for revascularization in patients who did not improve after IVT or had a contraindication for IVT.[97] The average presenting NIHSS score was 14. Seventeen patients presented with a TIMI score of 0 and three patients with a TIMI score of 1. Self-expanding intracranial stents were placed in 19 of 20 enrolled patients. One patient experienced recanalization of the occluded vessel with positioning of the Wingspan stent delivery system prior to stent deployment. In two patients, the tortuous vessel did not allow tracking of the Wingspan stent. The more navigable Enterprise stent was used in both these cases. A TIMI score 2 or 3 recanalization was achieved in 100% of patients; 65% of patients improved >4 points in the NIHSS score after treatment. One patient (5%) had SICH and two had asymptomatic ICH. At 1-month follow-up, 12 of 20 (60%) patients had an mRS ≤2, and nine (45%) had an mRS ≤1. Mortality at 1 month was 25%. None of these patients died due to any cause related to stent placement; all deaths were due to the severity of the initial stroke and associated comorbidities.

Extracranial Carotid Revascularization

Acute strokes related to isolated proximal (extracranial) ICA occlusions typically have a better prognosis, given the compensatory collateral flow at the level of the external carotid artery (ECA)–ICA anastomosis (e.g., ophthalmic artery) and/or circle of Willis. However, patients with an incomplete circle of Willis or with tandem occlusions of the intracranial ICA–MCA often present with severe strokes and are potential candidates for emergent revascularization. Stent placement in the proximal cervical vessels may also be required to gain access to the intracranial thrombus with other mechanical devices or catheters. Furthermore, brisk antegrade flow is essential for the maintenance of distal vascular patency, as is particularly evident in patients with severe proximal steno-

ses who commonly develop rethrombosis after vessel recanalization. Recent case series have shown success and good outcome after endovascular treatment of acute ischemic stroke due to proximal extracranial ICA occlusions.[98–102] The distal intracranial lesions seen after stenting of extracranial lesions may be due to emboli caused by reopening of the occluded ICA. This could be prevented or at least minimized by using a balloon guide catheter, such as the Concentric guide (Concentric Medical, Inc.), or a sheath, such as the Gore flow-reversal device (WL Gore & Associates, Flagstaff, AZ), for temporary flow arrest or flow reversal with aspiration, especially when antegrade flow is restored. The operator needs to check to make sure that the inner diameter of the balloon guide catheter is large enough to accommodate the chosen stent system.

◆ Outcomes

The initial data from clinical studies of interventions for acute ischemic stroke appeared to suggest a proportional relationship between recanalization and good outcome. The recanalization rates following IVT are variously estimated at 26 to 40%. PROACT II[27] revealed 66% recanalization with 40% good outcome and 10% ICH in the IA-UK (thrombolytic) treatment group as compared with 18% recanalization with 25% good outcome and 3% ICH in the placebo group. IMS I[103] evaluated IA tPA alone and noted good outcomes in 43%, with a mortality rate of 16% and SICH rate of 6.1%. In this trial, revascularization was achieved in 51% of cases. IMS II[81] combined IA tPA with a ultrasonic delivery catheter with improvement in recanalization to 69%, good outcomes in 45%, and mortality of 16%, with SICH increasing to 11%. IMS III is ongoing. The MERCI trials[18,19,28] used single-arm prospective data (Multi MERCI) to reveal recanalization rates of 69.4% with good outcomes in 39%, mortality of 30%, and symptomatic ICH of 7.9%. Most recently, the Penumbra device was approved based on its recanalization rate of 81% (100% recanalization in those patients in whom the device could be successfully deployed into the occlusive lesion. However, counter to previous studies, the good outcome category (mRS ≤2) was only 25% with a mortality of 16.4% and symptomatic ICH in 11.2%.[29]

These data beg the question as to what is the relationship between recanalization and good outcomes. We hypothesize that it depends on what is being revascularized. Revascularizing ischemic core likely causes breakthrough hemorrhage, the risk of which will further increase in those situations in which thrombolytic therapies are utilized. This results in an increase in SICH rates concurrent with increasing revascularization rates, as noted above. Therefore, as the success of the revascularization strategy improves, more ICH occurs because of breakthrough bleeding in ischemic cores. Therefore, increasing recanalization does not simply improve outcomes.

Improved outcome rates, based on all the studies noted above, fluctuate from 25 to 45%. We hypothesize that part of the reason this number is relatively fixed is that all these studies had relied on a simple cranial NCCT. Therefore, as recanalization rates increase, good clinical outcomes rise and then fall because of the poor patient selection that is consistent in all these studies. We strongly believe that revascularization of large cores does not improve outcomes and leads to potentially worse outcomes secondary to ICH. It is also evident that the vast majority of patients who present with an acute ischemic stroke will have some area of established core infarct and a variable degree of penumbra. The precise risk-benefit ratio for intervention in the varied ratios of core versus penumbra is not known. On the basis of our experience, we believe that the relative benefit of revascularization recedes when the core exceeds 50% of at-risk territory, as has been discussed above.

Abundant preclinical studies have identified multiple mechanisms of ischemic brain injury and have provided evidence that strategies designed to counter these mechanisms can protect the ischemic brain. Rigorously conducted experimental studies in animal models of brain ischemia provide incontrovertible proof-of-principle that high-grade protection of the ischemic brain is an achievable goal. Nonetheless, many agents have been brought to clinical trial without a sufficiently compelling evidence-based preclinical foundation. Ginsberg[104] identified 160 clinical trials of neuroprotection for ischemic stroke conducted as of late 2007. Of these, only approximately 40 represent larger-phase completed trials, and fully one half of the latter utilized a window to treatment of >6 hours, despite strong preclinical evidence that this delay exceeds the likely therapeutic window of efficacy in acute stroke. Other shortcomings of these trials include the use of agents lacking robust, consistent preclinical efficacy; inability to achieve adequate dosing in humans; and suboptimal clinical and statistical design features. Rigorous preclinical testing and appropriate strategies for clinical trials may lead to evidence of benefit of neuroprotective strategies, either alone or in combination, that will improve outcomes after acute ischemic stroke intervention.

◆ Conclusion

Crucial determinants for neurologic outcome after acute ischemic stroke intervention are size and location of the ischemic brain area perfused by the occluded vessel, time window between onset of symptoms and revascularization, recanalization rate associated with a specific treatment, and occurrence of SICH. Although these determinants have been enlisted, the relationship between these variables is complex and the quantification of the most important determinant—size and location of the ischemic brain—and the identification of patients who would benefit from revascularization of potential salvageable brain and those who would be harmed by revascularization due to SICH are not standardized.

Even now, some expert stroke centers, including our center, routinely use mechanical thrombolysis in the setting of a highly organized system in partnership with an interventional team. Mechanical revascularization therapy in patients beyond standard clinical time windows and in wake-up strokes, if there is evidence of salvageable penumbral tissue on CT or MRI, is also being routinely practiced at these centers. However, this approach has not been established by level-1 evidence in the absence of a confirmatory trial, although there is increasing level-2 evidence supporting this concept. The future in the treatment of acute ischemic stroke is likely a combination of different mechanical and thrombolytic techniques, probably in a staged-escalation fashion.

References

1. Report of the WHO Task Force on Stroke and other Cerebrovascular Disorders. Stroke–1989. Recommendations on stroke prevention, diagnosis, and therapy. Stroke 1989;20:1407–1431
2. Lloyd-Jones D, Adams R, Carnethon M, et al; American Heart Association Statistics Committee and Stroke Statistics Subcommittee. Heart disease and stroke statistics—2009 update: a report from the American Heart Association Statistics Committee and Stroke Statistics Subcommittee. Circulation 2009;119:e21–e181
3. Broderick JP, William M. William M. Feinberg Lecture: stroke therapy in the year 2025: burden, breakthroughs, and barriers to progress. Stroke 2004;35:205–211
4. National Institute of Neurological Disorders and Stroke rt-PA Stroke Study Group. Tissue plasminogen activator for acute ischemic stroke. N Engl J Med 1995;333:1581–1587
5. Adams HP Jr, del Zoppo G, Alberts MJ, et al; American Heart Association; American Stroke Association Stroke Council; Clinical Cardiology Council; Cardiovascular Radiology and Intervention Council; Atherosclerotic Peripheral Vascular Disease and Quality of Care Outcomes in Research Interdisciplinary Working Groups. Guidelines for the early management of adults with ischemic stroke: a guideline from the American Heart Association/American Stroke Association Stroke Council, Clinical Cardiology Council, Cardiovascular Radiology and Intervention Council, and the Atherosclerotic Peripheral Vascular Disease and Quality of Care Outcomes in Research Interdisciplinary Working Groups: the American Academy of Neurology affirms the value of this guideline as an educational tool for neurologists. Stroke 2007;38:1655–1711
6. Barber PA, Zhang J, Demchuk AM, Hill MD, Buchan AM. Why are stroke patients excluded from TPA therapy? An analysis of patient eligibility. Neurology 2001;56:1015–1020
7. Alexandrov AV, Grotta JC. Arterial reocclusion in stroke patients treated with intravenous tissue plasminogen activator. Neurology 2002;59:862–867
8. Janjua N, Alkawi A, Suri MF, Qureshi AI. Impact of arterial reocclusion and distal fragmentation during thrombolysis among patients with acute ischemic stroke. AJNR Am J Neuroradiol 2008;29:253–258
9. Saqqur M, Molina CA, Salam A, et al; CLOTBUST Investigators. Clinical deterioration after intravenous recombinant tissue plasminogen activator treatment: a multicenter transcranial Doppler study. Stroke 2007;38:69–74
10. Benesch CG, Chimowitz MI; The WASID Investigators. Best treatment for intracranial arterial stenosis? 50 years of uncertainty. Neurology 2000;55:465–466
11. Wolpert SM, Bruckmann H, Greenlee R, Wechsler L, Pessin MS, del Zoppo GJ. Neuroradiologic evaluation of patients with acute stroke treated with recombinant tissue plasminogen activator. The rt-PA Acute Stroke Study Group. AJNR Am J Neuroradiol 1993;14:3–13
12. Saqqur M, Uchino K, Demchuk AM, et al; CLOTBUST Investigators. Site of arterial occlusion identified by transcranial Doppler predicts the response to intravenous thrombolysis for stroke. Stroke 2007;38:948–954
13. Arnold M, Nedeltchev K, Mattle HP, et al. Intra-arterial thrombolysis in 24 consecutive patients with internal carotid artery T occlusions. J Neurol Neurosurg Psychiatry 2003;74:739–742
14. Jansen O, von Kummer R, Forsting M, Hacke W, Sartor K. Thrombolytic therapy in acute occlusion of the intracranial internal carotid artery bifurcation. AJNR Am J Neuroradiol 1995;16:1977–1986
15. Zaidat OO, Suarez JI, Santillan C, et al. Response to intra-arterial and combined intravenous and intra-arterial thrombolytic therapy in patients with distal internal carotid artery occlusion. Stroke 2002;33:1821–1826
16. Sorimachi T, Fujii Y, Tsuchiya N, et al. Recanalization by mechanical embolus disruption during intra-arterial thrombolysis in the carotid territory. AJNR Am J Neuroradiol 2004;25:1391–1402
17. Fieschi C, Argentino C, Lenzi GL, Sacchetti ML, Toni D, Bozzao L. Clinical and instrumental evaluation of patients with ischemic stroke within the first six hours. J Neurol Sci 1989;91:311–321
18. Smith WS, Sung G, Starkman S, et al; MERCI Trial Investigators. Safety and efficacy of mechanical embolectomy in acute ischemic stroke: results of the MERCI trial. Stroke 2005;36:1432–1438

19. Smith WS, Sung G, Saver J, et al; Multi MERCI Investigators. Mechanical thrombectomy for acute ischemic stroke: final results of the Multi MERCI trial. Stroke 2008;39:1205–1212

20. Tomsick T, Broderick J, Carrozella J, et al; Interventional Management of Stroke II Investigators. Revascularization results in the Interventional Management of Stroke II trial. AJNR Am J Neuroradiol 2008;29:582–587

21. Rha JH, Saver JL. The impact of recanalization on ischemic stroke outcome: a meta-analysis. Stroke 2007;38:967–973

22. Hacke W, Kaste M, Bluhmki E, et al; ECASS Investigators. Thrombolysis with alteplase 3 to 4.5 hours after acute ischemic stroke. N Engl J Med 2008;359:1317–1329

23. Lansberg MG, Bluhmki E, Thijs VN. Efficacy and safety of tissue plasminogen activator 3 to 4.5 hours after acute ischemic stroke: a meta-analysis. Stroke 2009;40:2438–2441

24. Del Zoppo GJ, Saver JL, Jauch EC, Adams HP Jr; American Heart Association Stroke Council. Expansion of the time window for treatment of acute ischemic stroke with intravenous tissue plasminogen activator: a science advisory from the American Heart Association/American Stroke Association. Stroke 2009;40:2945–2948

25. Wardlaw JM, Sandercock PA, Berge E. Thrombolytic therapy with recombinant tissue plasminogen activator for acute ischemic stroke: where do we go from here? A cumulative meta-analysis. Stroke 2003; 34:1437–1442

26. del Zoppo GJ, Higashida RT, Furlan AJ, Pessin MS, Rowley HA, Gent M. PROACT: a phase II randomized trial of recombinant pro-urokinase by direct arterial delivery in acute middle cerebral artery stroke. PROACT Investigators. Prolyse in Acute Cerebral Thromboembolism. Stroke 1998; 29:4–11

27. Furlan A, Higashida R, Wechsler L, et al. Intra-arterial prourokinase for acute ischemic stroke. The PROACT II study: a randomized controlled trial. Prolyse in Acute Cerebral Thromboembolism. JAMA 1999;282: 2003–2011

28. Gobin YP, Starkman S, Duckwiler GR, et al. MERCI 1: a phase 1 study of Mechanical Embolus Removal in Cerebral Ischemia. Stroke 2004;35: 2848–2854

29. Bose A, Henkes H, Alfke K, et al; Penumbra Phase 1 Stroke Trial Investigators. The Penumbra System: a mechanical device for the treatment of acute stroke due to thromboembolism. AJNR Am J Neuroradiol 2008; 29:1409–1413

30. Hacke W, Albers G, Al-Rawi Y, et al; DIAS Study Group. The Desmoteplase in Acute Ischemic Stroke Trial (DIAS): a phase II MRI-based 9-hour window acute stroke thrombolysis trial with intravenous desmoteplase. Stroke 2005;36:66–73

31. Furlan AJ, Eyding D, Albers GW, et al; DEDAS Investigators. Dose Escalation of Desmoteplase for Acute Ischemic Stroke (DEDAS): evidence of safety and efficacy 3 to 9 hours after stroke onset. Stroke 2006;37: 1227–1231

32. Albers GW, Thijs VN, Wechsler L, et al; DEFUSE Investigators. Magnetic resonance imaging profiles predict clinical response to early reperfusion: the diffusion and perfusion imaging evaluation for understanding stroke evolution (DEFUSE) study. Ann Neurol 2006;60:508–517

33. Thomalla G, Schwark C, Sobesky J, et al; MRI in Acute Stroke Study Group of the German Competence Network Stroke. Outcome and symptomatic bleeding complications of intravenous thrombolysis within 6 hours in MRI-selected stroke patients: comparison of a German multicenter study with the pooled data of ATLANTIS, ECASS, and NINDS tPA trials. Stroke 2006;37:852–858

34. Köhrmann M, Jüttler E, Fiebach JB, et al. MRI versus CT-based thrombolysis treatment within and beyond the 3 h time window after stroke onset: a cohort study. Lancet Neurol 2006;5:661–667

35. Davis SM, Donnan GA, Parsons MW, et al; EPITHET investigators. Effects of alteplase beyond 3 h after stroke in the Echoplanar Imaging Thrombolytic Evaluation Trial (EPITHET): a placebo-controlled randomised trial. Lancet Neurol 2008;7:299–309

36. Hacke W, Furlan AJ, Al-Rawi Y, et al. Intravenous desmoteplase in patients with acute ischaemic stroke selected by MRI perfusion-diffusion weighted imaging or perfusion CT (DIAS-2): a prospective, randomised, double-blind, placebo-controlled study. Lancet Neurol 2009;8:141–150

37. Lansberg MG, Schrooten M, Bluhmki E, Thijs VN, Saver JL. Treatment time-specific number needed to treat estimates for tissue plasminogen activator therapy in acute stroke based on shifts over the entire range of the modified Rankin Scale. Stroke 2009;40:2079–2084

38. Hacke W, Donnan G, Fieschi C, et al; ATLANTIS Trials Investigators; ECASS Trials Investigators; NINDS rt-PA Study Group Investigators. Association of outcome with early stroke treatment: pooled analysis of ATLANTIS, ECASS, and NINDS rt-PA stroke trials. Lancet 2004;363: 768–774

39. Astrup J, Siesjö BK, Symon L. Thresholds in cerebral ischemia—the ischemic penumbra. Stroke 1981;12:723–725

40. Darby DG, Barber PA, Gerraty RP, et al. Pathophysiological topography of acute ischemia by combined diffusion-weighted and perfusion MRI. Stroke 1999;30:2043–2052

41. Markus R, Reutens DC, Kazui S, et al. Hypoxic tissue in ischaemic stroke: persistence and clinical consequences of spontaneous survival. Brain 2004;127(Pt 6):1427–1436

42. Esteban JM, Cervera V. Perfusion CT and angio CT in the assessment of acute stroke. Neuroradiology 2004;46:705–715

43. Kloska SP, Nabavi DG, Gaus C, et al. Acute stroke assessment with CT: do we need multimodal evaluation? Radiology 2004;233:79–86

44. Maruya J, Yamamoto K, Ozawa T, et al. Simultaneous multi-section perfusion CT and CT angiography for the assessment of acute ischemic stroke. Acta Neurochir (Wien) 2005;147:383–391, discussion 391–392

45. Muir KW, Baird-Gunning J, Walker L, Baird T, McCormick M, Coutts SB. Can the ischemic penumbra be identified on noncontrast CT of acute stroke? Stroke 2007;38:2485–2490

46. Parsons MW, Pepper EM, Bateman GA, Wang Y, Levi CR. Identification of the penumbra and infarct core on hyperacute noncontrast and perfusion CT. Neurology 2007;68:730–736

47. Klingebiel R, Siebert E, Diekmann S, et al. 4-D Imaging in cerebrovascular disorders by using 320-slice CT: feasibility and preliminary clinical experience. Acad Radiol 2009;16:123–129

48. Kudo K, Sasaki M, Ogasawara K, Terae S, Ehara S, Shirato H. Difference in tracer delay-induced effect among deconvolution algorithms in CT perfusion analysis: quantitative evaluation with digital phantoms. Radiology 2009;251:241–249

49. Wittsack HJ, Wohlschläger AM, Ritzl EK, et al. CT-perfusion imaging of the human brain: advanced deconvolution analysis using circulant singular value decomposition. Comput Med Imaging Graph 2008;32: 67–77

50. Smith WS, Roberts HC, Chuang NA, et al. Safety and feasibility of a CT protocol for acute stroke: combined CT, CT angiography, and CT perfusion imaging in 53 consecutive patients. AJNR Am J Neuroradiol 2003; 24:688–690

51. Tan JC, Dillon WP, Liu S, Adler F, Smith WS, Wintermark M. Systematic comparison of perfusion-CT and CT-angiography in acute stroke patients. Ann Neurol 2007;61:533–543

52. Wintermark M, Flanders AE, Velthuis B, et al. Perfusion-CT assessment of infarct core and penumbra: receiver operating characteristic curve analysis in 130 patients suspected of acute hemispheric stroke. Stroke 2006;37:979–985

53. Schramm P, Schellinger PD, Fiebach JB, et al. Comparison of CT and CT angiography source images with diffusion-weighted imaging in patients with acute stroke within 6 hours after onset. Stroke 2002;33: 2426–2432

54. Hellier KD, Hampton JL, Guadagno JV, et al. Perfusion CT helps decision making for thrombolysis when there is no clear time of onset. J Neurol Neurosurg Psychiatry 2006;77:417–419

55. Parsons MW, Pepper EM, Chan V, et al. Perfusion computed tomography: prediction of final infarct extent and stroke outcome. Ann Neurol 2005;58:672–679

56. Wintermark M, Meuli R, Browaeys P, et al. Comparison of CT perfusion and angiography and MRI in selecting stroke patients for acute treatment. Neurology 2007;68:694–697

57. Derex L, Hermier M, Adeleine P, et al. Clinical and imaging predictors of intracerebral haemorrhage in stroke patients treated with intravenous tissue plasminogen activator. J Neurol Neurosurg Psychiatry 2005;76: 70–75

58. Barber PA, Demchuk AM, Zhang J, Buchan AM. Validity and reliability of a quantitative computed tomography score in predicting outcome of hyperacute stroke before thrombolytic therapy. ASPECTS Study Group. Alberta Stroke Programme Early CT Score. Lancet 2000;355:1670–1674

59. Wechsler LR, Roberts R, Furlan AJ, et al; PROACT II Investigators. Factors influencing outcome and treatment effect in PROACT II. Stroke 2003; 34:1224–1229

60. Ogawa A, Mori E, Minematsu K, et al; MELT Japan Study Group. Randomized trial of intraarterial infusion of urokinase within 6 hours of middle cerebral artery stroke: the middle cerebral artery embolism local fibrinolytic intervention trial (MELT) Japan. Stroke 2007;38:2633–2639

61. Saver JL. Intra-arterial fibrinolysis for acute ischemic stroke: the message of melt. Stroke 2007;38:2627–2628

62. Fink JN, Kumar S, Horkan C, et al. The stroke patient who woke up: clinical and radiological features, including diffusion and perfusion MRI. Stroke 2002;33:988–993

63. Serena J, Dávalos A, Segura T, Mostacero E, Castillo J. Stroke on awakening: looking for a more rational management. Cerebrovasc Dis 2003; 16:128–133

64. Barreto AD, Martin-Schild S, Hallevi H, et al. Thrombolytic therapy for patients who wake-up with stroke. Stroke 2009;40:827–832
65. Adams HP Jr, Leira EC, Torner JC, et al; AbESTT-II Investigators. Treating patients with "wake-up" stroke: the experience of the AbESTT-II trial. Stroke 2008;39:3277–3282
66. Natarajan SK, Snyder KV, Siddiqui AH, Ionita CC, Hopkins LN, Levy EI. Safety and effectiveness of endovascular therapy after 8 hours of acute ischemic stroke onset and wake-up strokes. Stroke 2009;40:3269–3274
67. Zeumer H, Freitag HJ, Grzyska U, Neunzig HP. Local intraarterial fibrinolysis in acute vertebrobasilar occlusion. Technical developments and recent results. Neuroradiology 1989;31:336–340
68. Hacke W, Zeumer H, Ferbert A, Brückmann H, del Zoppo GJ. Intra-arterial thrombolytic therapy improves outcome in patients with acute vertebrobasilar occlusive disease. Stroke 1988;19:1216–1222
69. Becker KJ, Monsein LH, Ulatowski J, Mirski M, Williams M, Hanley DF. Intraarterial thrombolysis in vertebrobasilar occlusion. AJNR Am J Neuroradiol 1996;17:255–262
70. Jahan R. Hyperacute therapy of acute ischemic stroke: intraarterial thrombolysis and mechanical revascularization strategies. Tech Vasc Interv Radiol 2005;8:87–91
71. Archer CR, Horenstein S. Basilar artery occlusion: clinical and radiological correlation. Stroke 1977;8:383–390
72. Smith WS. Intra-arterial thrombolytic therapy for acute basilar occlusion: pro. Stroke 2007;38(2, Suppl)701–703
73. Lindsberg PJ, Mattle HP. Therapy of basilar artery occlusion: a systematic analysis comparing intra-arterial and intravenous thrombolysis. Stroke 2006;37:922–928
74. Levy EI, Firlik AD, Wisniewski S, et al. Factors affecting survival rates for acute vertebrobasilar artery occlusions treated with intra-arterial thrombolytic therapy: a meta-analytical approach. Neurosurgery 1999;45:539–545, discussion 545–548
75. Zeumer H, Hacke W, Ringelstein EB. Local intraarterial thrombolysis in vertebrobasilar thromboembolic disease. AJNR Am J Neuroradiol 1983;4:401–404
76. Zeumer H, Freitag HJ, Zanella F, Thie A, Arning C. Local intra-arterial fibrinolytic therapy in patients with stroke: urokinase versus recombinant tissue plasminogen activator (r-TPA). Neuroradiology 1993;35:159–162
77. Kim DJ, Kim DI, Kim SH, Lee KY, Heo JH, Han SW. Rescue localized intraarterial thrombolysis for hyperacute MCA ischemic stroke patients after early non-responsive intravenous tissue plasminogen activator therapy. Neuroradiology 2005;47:616–621
78. Pancioli AM, Broderick J, Brott T, et al; CLEAR Trial Investigators. The combined approach to lysis utilizing eptifibatide and rt-PA in acute ischemic stroke: the CLEAR stroke trial. Stroke 2008;39:3268–3276
79. Dunn B, Davis LA, Todd JW, Chalela JA, Warach S, for the ROSIE Investigators. ReoPro Retavase Reperfusion of Stroke Safety Study—Imaging Evaluation (ROSIE). Presented at the 29th International Stroke Conference February 5, 2004, San Diego, CA
80. Adams HP Jr, Effron MB, Torner J, et al; AbESTT-II Investigators. Emergency administration of abciximab for treatment of patients with acute ischemic stroke: results of an international phase III trial: Abciximab in Emergency Treatment of Stroke Trial (AbESTT-II). Stroke 2008;39:87–99
81. Investigators IMS; IMS II Trial Investigators. The Interventional Management of Stroke (IMS) II Study. Stroke 2007;38:2127–2135
82. Khatri P, Hill MD, Palesch YY, et al; Interventional Management of Stroke III Investigators. Methodology of the Interventional Management of Stroke III Trial. Int J Stroke 2008;3:130–137
83. Mattle HP, Arnold M, Georgiadis D, et al. Comparison of intraarterial and intravenous thrombolysis for ischemic stroke with hyperdense middle cerebral artery sign. Stroke 2008;39:379–383
84. Gralla J, Schroth G, Remonda L, et al. A dedicated animal model for mechanical thrombectomy in acute stroke. AJNR Am J Neuroradiol 2006;27:1357–1361
85. Gralla J, Burkhardt M, Schroth G, et al. Occlusion length is a crucial determinant of efficiency and complication rate in thrombectomy for acute ischemic stroke. AJNR Am J Neuroradiol 2008;29:247–252
86. Gralla J, Schroth G, Remonda L, Nedeltchev K, Slotboom J, Brekenfeld C. Mechanical thrombectomy for acute ischemic stroke: thrombus-device interaction, efficiency, and complications in vivo. Stroke 2006;37:3019–3024
87. McDougall CG, Clark W, Mayer T, et al, for the Penumbra Stroke Trial Investigators. The Penumbra Stroke Trial: Safety and effectiveness of a new generation of mechanical devices for clot removal in acute ischemic stroke. International Stroke Conference, February 22, 2008, New Orleans
88. Flint AC, Duckwiler GR, Budzik RF, Liebeskind DS, Smith WS; MERCI and Multi MERCI Writing Committee. Mechanical thrombectomy of intracranial internal carotid occlusion: pooled results of the MERCI and Multi MERCI Part I trials. Stroke 2007;38:1274–1280
89. Henkes H, Miloslavski E, Lowens S, Reinartz J, Liebig T, Kühne D. Treatment of intracranial atherosclerotic stenoses with balloon dilatation and self-expanding stent deployment (WingSpan). Neuroradiology 2005;47:222–228
90. Qureshi AI, Siddiqui AM, Kim SH, et al. Reocclusion of recanalized arteries during intra-arterial thrombolysis for acute ischemic stroke. AJNR Am J Neuroradiol 2004;25:322–328
91. Lubicz B, Leclerc X, Levivier M, et al. Retractable self-expandable stent for endovascular treatment of wide-necked intracranial aneurysms: preliminary experience. Neurosurgery 2006;58:451–457, discussion 451–457
92. Peluso JP, van Rooij WJ, Sluzewski M, Beute GN. A new self-expandable nitinol stent for the treatment of wide-neck aneurysms: initial clinical experience. AJNR Am J Neuroradiol 2008;29:1405–1408
93. Yavuz K, Geyik S, Pamuk AG, Koc O, Saatci I, Cekirge HS. Immediate and midterm follow-up results of using an electrodetachable, fully retrievable SOLO stent system in the endovascular coil occlusion of wide-necked cerebral aneurysms. J Neurosurg 2007;107:49–55
94. Levy EI, Mehta R, Gupta R, et al. Self-expanding stents for recanalization of acute cerebrovascular occlusions. AJNR Am J Neuroradiol 2007;28:816–822
95. Zaidat OO, Wolfe T, Hussain SI, et al. Interventional acute ischemic stroke therapy with intracranial self-expanding stent. Stroke 2008;39:2392–2395
96. Mocco J, Hanel RA, Sharma J, et al. Use of a vascular reconstruction device to salvage acute ischemic occlusions refractory to traditional endovascular recanalization methods. J Neurosurg 2010;112:557–562
97. Levy EI, Siddiqui AH, Crumlish A, et al. First Food and Drug Administration-approved prospective trial of primary intracranial stenting for acute stroke: SARIS (stent-assisted recanalization in acute ischemic stroke). Stroke 2009;40:3552–3556
98. Jovin TG, Gupta R, Uchino K, et al. Emergent stenting of extracranial internal carotid artery occlusion in acute stroke has a high revascularization rate. Stroke 2005;36:2426–2430
99. Nikas D, Reimers B, Elisabetta M, et al. Percutaneous interventions in patients with acute ischemic stroke related to obstructive atherosclerotic disease or dissection of the extracranial carotid artery. J Endovasc Ther 2007;14:279–288
100. Dabitz R, Triebe S, Leppmeier U, Ochs G, Vorwerk D. Percutaneous recanalization of acute internal carotid artery occlusions in patients with severe stroke. Cardiovasc Intervent Radiol 2007;30:34–41
101. Lavallée PC, Mazighi M, Saint-Maurice JP, et al. Stent-assisted endovascular thrombolysis versus intravenous thrombolysis in internal carotid artery dissection with tandem internal carotid and middle cerebral artery occlusion. Stroke 2007;38:2270–2274
102. Miyamoto N, Naito I, Takatama S, Shimizu T, Iwai T, Shimaguchi H. Urgent stenting for patients with acute stroke due to atherosclerotic occlusive lesions of the cervical internal carotid artery. Neurol Med Chir (Tokyo) 2008;48:49–55, discussion 55–56
103. Investigators IMS; IMS Study Investigators. Combined intravenous and intra-arterial recanalization for acute ischemic stroke: the Interventional Management of Stroke Study. Stroke 2004;35:904–911
104. Ginsberg MD. Current status of neuroprotection for cerebral ischemia: synoptic overview. Stroke 2009;40(3, Suppl)S111–S114
105. Nogueira RG, Smith WS; MERCI and Multi MERCI Writing Committee. Safety and efficacy of endovascular thrombectomy in patients with abnormal hemostasis: pooled analysis of the MERCI and multi MERCI trials. Stroke 2009;40:516–522

31

Angioplasty and Stenting for Management of Intracranial Arterial Stenosis

Andrew J. Ringer, Christopher Nichols, Shah-Naz Khan, Andrew Grande, Usman Khan, Gail Pyne-Geithman, and Todd A. Abruzzo

---

Pearls

- Although atherosclerosis of the extracranial cerebral arteries is more common and more easily treated, intracranial stenosis occurs in 20 to 40% of patients with atherosclerotic disease. Population studies show a higher incidence in blacks, Asians, and Hispanics.
- With the high risk of stroke even after the best medical therapy, endovascular surgeons may opt for angioplasty, stenting, or both to repair intracranial stenosis. Procedural risks have declined in more recent series with the use of smaller balloon dilation, acceptance of some residual stenosis, and slower balloon inflation.
- Factors affecting outcomes to consider before angioplasty include the angiographic appearance of the lesion, the severity of stenosis, and the lesion's location, length, and eccentricity.
- For a nonionic iodine-contrast preparation, an estimation of the maximum contrast volume is provided by the patient's weight in kilograms (kg) multiplied by 5 and divided by the serum creatinine level. For patients who have reacted to contrast material, prednisone, diphenhydramine, and acetaminophen should be administered before the procedure.
- Some complications of intracranial angioplasty alone, such as dissection and early restenosis, may be reduced by the use of a stent.
- Close clinical monitoring after intracranial angioplasty and stenting in an intensive care setting ensures early identification of delayed complications of angioplasty (e.g., thromboembolus, arterial dissection, restenosis, vascular perforation, or rupture). Potential complications can be reduced by careful preoperative antiplatelet loading and by being prepared to deal with these complications if necessary.
- Procedural success with reduction of stenosis to <30% without clinical complications can be achieved in 60 to 80% of patients.

The treatment of intracranial arterial stenosis as the result of arteriopathic changes in the cerebral vasculature has long been debated. Atherosclerotic disease is amenable to medical and surgical treatment in the peripheral and cardiac circulations, but poses fundamental management challenges in the intracranial vasculature. Initial management options for intracranial disease include antiplatelet medications, oral anticoagulation, and risk-factor modification, and subsequent strategies may involve surgical or endovascular treatment. Yet considering the range of treatment options, from medical management to complex surgical repair, the benefits delivered by these options remain unclear. Findings of the prospective, randomized trial that compared aspirin therapy with extracranial-intracranial (EC-IC) bypass failed to demonstrate a benefit for bypass surgery[1] and were later found to have a patient-selection bias.[2] Thus, one may reasonably surmise first that EC-IC bypass did little to reduce the thromboembolic complications of intracranial stenosis, and second that the risk of stroke with aspirin therapy remains very high. This chapter addresses the issues associated with endovascular revascularization in the treatment of patients with intracranial carotid stenosis.

◆ Indications

Natural History

The risk of stroke related to intracranial stenosis has often gone unrecognized and underreported in the past. Focus on the more easily treatable extracranial carotid and cardiac or aortic sources of stroke in fact may detract attention from coexistent intracranial disease. Although atherosclerosis of the extracranial cerebral arteries is more common, intracranial stenosis occurs in 20 to 40% of patients with atherosclerotic disease.[3,4] The most common sites of intracranial disease include the intracranial internal carotid artery (ICA), the main trunk or M1 segment of the middle cerebral artery (MCA), the distal vertebral artery or vertebrobasilar junction, and the midbasilar artery. Thus, intracranial stenosis must be considered in patients with cerebral ischemic signs and symptoms. Population studies indicate that the incidence of intracranial stenosis is higher in blacks, Asians, and Hispanics than in whites.

After intracranial stenosis is identified, estimating the risk of the lesion is difficult. Specifically, estimates of the annual risk for stroke depend on the extent of stenosis and the location of the disease. However, calculating the percent of stenosis is more reliably achieved in the extracranial ICA than in the intracranial vessels. For example, given that the diameter of certain normal intracranial arteries is 2.5 mm, stenosis of 80% is a residual lumen of only 0.5 mm—a diameter difficult to accurately measure. As most clinicians consider stenosis exceeding 50% as significant intracranial stenosis, these patients are grouped together for clinical studies. Yet, by this measure, significant intracranial stenosis poses a high risk of stroke in virtually all locations.

Intracranial ICA stenosis has a high risk of ipsilateral stroke—reported to be as high as 7.6% per year.[5] In the medical arm of the EC-IC bypass trial, the annual risk of stroke with ICA siphon or MCA stenosis was 8 to 10%.[1] Furthermore, risk of stroke with posterior circulation disease may be even higher. In the Warfarin Aspirin Symptomatic Intracranial Disease (WASID) study, patients with significant basilar artery stenosis treated with aspirin had an annual risk of stroke of >10% despite medical therapy.[6]

Although most clinicians agree that there is a high incidence of stroke with intracranial stenosis, it is often difficult to predict which patients are at highest risk and what extent of stenosis poses a clinically significant degree of risk worthy of consideration for intervention. Although most clinicians consider intracranial stenosis exceeding 50% as significant, Borozan et al[7] found that the onset of new symptoms occurred when stenosis averaged (± standard deviation) 35.4% ± 14.4%. The significance of presenting symptoms in the setting of intracranial stenosis is also unclear. In the EC-IC bypass trial, only one third of all major strokes were preceded by a transient ischemic attack.[1] Furthermore Borozan et al found no difference in stroke-free survival between symptomatic and asymptomatic patients. Collectively, these results convey the difficulty that many clinicians face in predicting which patients are at highest risk for stroke.

Medical Therapy

Appropriate medical therapy for intracranial stenosis remains a matter of debate. Several retrospective studies as well as the observational arm of the WASID trial[6] have suggested a reduced risk of stroke with warfarin therapy when compared with aspirin.[8] However, in the 1995 prospective WASID trial showing fewer strokes in patients treated with warfarin (3.6%) than with aspirin (10.4%), the incidence of major hemorrhage was 8.3% with warfarin and 3.2% with aspirin, ultimately resulting in higher mortality rates as well (9.7% versus 4.3%, respectively).

Surgical Therapy

When the EC-IC bypass trial failed to demonstrate a benefit of surgical bypass, use of this procedure all but halted. Since its publication, detractors of the EC-IC bypass trial have argued that patient selection bias may have doomed the study because the investigators made no effort to differentiate between patient symptoms resulting from either embolic events or hypoperfusion.

New imaging techniques now provide valuable data regarding brain perfusion and metabolism in specific vascular territories. These techniques include xenon computed tomography (CT), single photon emission computed tomography (SPECT), positron emission tomography (PET), and CT perfusion. Using cerebral oxygen extraction ratios to augment cerebral blood flow data, Grubb et al[9] classified cervical ICA occlusion and cerebral hypoperfusion into three stages: stage 1, vasodilatory compensation; stage 2, maximized vasodilatation with increased cerebral oxygen extraction; and stage 3, exceeding compensatory mechanisms. They reported that patients with stage 2 hypoperfusion faced a dramatically higher risk of stroke. Buoyed by these findings, a new, prospective, randomized trial for the treatment of cerebral hypoperfusion called the Carotid Occlusion Surgery Study (COSS) will examine EC-IC bypass.

Intracranial Angioplasty

Considering that the risk of stroke remains high after the best medical therapy, many endovascular surgeons opt for angioplasty, with or without stenting, to repair intracranial stenosis. Since the 1980s, angioplasty as a primary treatment of arterial atherosclerotic disease became widely accepted for coronary artery disease.[10] Its application to intracranial disease first gained popularity in the treatment of arterial vasospasm following aneurysmal subarachnoid hemorrhage.[11] Its popularity for intracranial atherosclerosis has been tempered by high procedural risks, including initial studies in which the rates of periprocedural neurologic events were as high as 33%.[12–14] However, more recent series have demonstrated complication rates of <10%,[15,16] which has been attributed to the use of smaller balloon dilation relative to the normal size of the target artery, the acceptance of some residual stenosis, and slower inflation times.

Several factors that affect angioplasty risk and success can be considered before treatment. Factors include the angiographic appearance of the lesion, the severity of stenosis, and the lesion's location, length, and eccentricity. Mori et al[17] evaluated several lesion characteristics (e.g., lesion length and eccentricity) and then assessed procedural results and angiographic follow-up. Their grading scale for intracranial stenosis was used to predict outcome after angioplasty based on lesion characteristics (**Table 31.1 and Fig. 31.1**). In their 1998 follow-up study,[15] the overall success of angioplasty, defined as uncomplicated reversal of >70% stenosis to <50%, was 79%, with clinical success in 76%. However, when lesion-specific characteristics were considered for types A, B, and C as defined in **Table 31.1**, the clinical success rates were 92%,

Table 31.1 Mori Classification of Intracranial Stenosis

	Type A	Type B	Type C
Length	Discrete <5 mm	Tubular, 5–10 mm	Diffuse >1 cm
Anatomic Features			
Concentric versus eccentric	Concentric or eccentric (70–89% diameter stenosis)	Eccentric (≥90% diameter stenosis)	
Contour	Smooth contour	Irregular contour	
Degree of occlusion	Less than totally occlusive	Total occlusion <3 months	Total occlusion ≥3 months
Calcifications	Little or no calcification	Moderate to heavy calcification	
Thrombus burden	Absence of thrombus	Some thrombus present	
Access			
Proximal vessel anatomy	Readily accessible	Moderate tortuosity of proximal segment	Excessive tortuosity of proximal segment
Segment angulation	Nonangulated segment <45 degrees	Moderate angulated segment 45–90 degrees	Extremely angulated segment ≥90 degrees
Relation to vessel branches	No major branch involvement	Bifurcation lesions requiring double guide-wires	Inability to protect major side branches

Note: Based on length of the stenosis, anatomic features of the lesion (including concentric or eccentric occlusion), degree and length of time of the occlusion, lesion contour, presence of calcification and thrombus burden, and degree of access difficulty assessed by proximal vessel tortuosity, segment angulation, and relation to side branches. Severity of lesion increases from type A to C. Lesions are classified according to the presence of any one feature found in the most severe lesion category.

86%, and 33%, respectively. For lesions of types A, B, and C, angiographic restenosis at 1 year was appreciated in 0%, 33%, and 100%, respectively, and the cumulative risk of fatal or nonfatal ipsilateral ischemic stroke was 8%, 12%, and 56%, respectively, at 1 and 2 years. The authors concluded that type A lesions were more often successfully treated with the lowest incidence of restenosis. More importantly, they demonstrated that preprocedural anatomic characteristics can be used to predict the success of angioplasty.

Accessibility of the lesion is another important factor. For example, highly tortuous proximal anatomy makes navigation of endovascular devices quite difficult and risks proximal dissection. In evaluating our success rates, we observed significant differences in the proximal anatomy. In measuring the radius of curvature of the proximal vascular loop (carotid siphon or vertebral C1 loop), we found a significantly smaller radius for unsuccessful cases (unpublished data) **(Fig. 31.2)**. Although stent devices are clearly more difficult

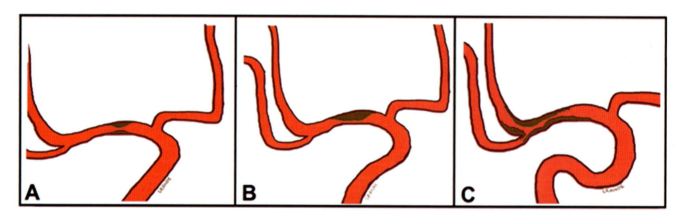

Fig. 31.1 Illustration of the Mori classification of intracranial stenosis in the middle cerebral artery. **(A)** Type A: short concentric, moderate to severe stenosis with a smooth contour in a straight segment with nontortuous proximal anatomy. **(B)** Type B: longer, <10 mm, eccentric severe stenosis with an irregular contour in a slightly angulated segment with slightly tortuous proximal anatomy. **(C)** Type C: long, >1 cm, eccentric severe stenosis with an irregular contour in a highly angulated segment that involves a major side branch with a highly tortuous proximal anatomy.

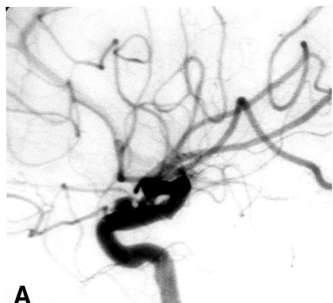

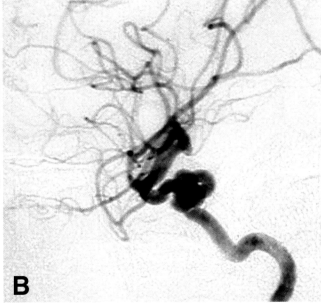

Fig. 31.2 Digital subtraction angiogram of two patients in whom intracranial carotid stent placement was attempted. **(A)** Successful attempt. Note the large radius of curvature through the carotid siphon. **(B)** Unsuccessful attempt. Note the smaller radius of curvature through the carotid siphon in a patient who suffered an asymptomatic carotid dissection during attempted stent advancement. (Courtesy of the Mayfield Clinic.)

to navigate than angioplasty balloons, greater difficulties can be encountered with virtually any device in more tortuous anatomy.

◆ Intracranial Angioplasty Technique

Perioperative Management

Preoperative preparation specific to intracranial angioplasty revolves primarily around the management of anticoagulant medication. Many patients undergo anticoagulation with warfarin when referred for treatment. Interventionalists may often rely on aggressive antiplatelet therapy to prevent perioperative complications. In our practice, we discontinue warfarin 3 days before treatment and begin combination therapy with aspirin (325 mg/day) and clopidogrel (75 mg/day) concomitantly; this practice allows adequate time for both the natural, gradual reversal of warfarin anticoagulation and the simultaneous loading of clopidogrel. For patients taking only aspirin, clopidogrel is added 3 days before treatment. For urgent cases when neither protocol can be implemented, glycoprotein IIb/IIIa inhibitors with clopidogrel are loaded postoperatively in a single 300-mg dose.

Other preoperative steps are typical of all surgical or interventional procedures. First, a complete neurologic examination is of paramount importance before the neuroendovascular procedure, not only enabling the examiner to become familiar with the patient but also aiding in rapid identification of any later neurologic compromise. In patients with preexisting neurologic deficits, documentation before the procedure can confirm later that no additional deficit accrued. Peripheral pulses should be noted, and if diminished, should be marked for easy identification during angiography. Review of any previous studies and an in-depth knowledge of the patient's history will facilitate developing an appropriate plan and complete diagnostic study tailored to the specific patient. Incomplete review of either the available studies or the history of the patient's illness may lead to the unnecessary performance of additional invasive procedures. A history of significant peripheral vascular occlusive disease or coronary artery disease should alert the practitioner to an increased risk of an arterial access complication, periprocedural myocardial infarction, or stroke. Congestive heart failure requires judicious use of periprocedural fluid intake and contrast load. Necessary laboratory work includes at least a baseline hemoglobin and hematocrit, platelet count, partial thromboplastin time, prothrombin time, blood urea nitrogen, serum creatinine, and blood glucose.

Numerous issues warrant consideration before any endovascular procedure. The maximum potential contrast load should be calculated for each patient with impaired renal function and for all spinal angiography studies. For a nonionic iodine contrast preparation, the estimation for maximum contrast volume is the patient's weight in kilograms (kg) multiplied by 5 and divided by the serum creatinine level. For example, a 90-kg patient with a 1.5 serum creatinine level could receive $90 \times 5/1.5$, or 300 cc of contrast. For longer procedures requiring large contrast loads, one can assume that a patient with adequate hydration and normal renal function excreted approximately 50% of the administered contrast load; the dosing can then be recalculated. For patients who have a history of reaction to contrast material, the administration of prednisone, diphenhydramine, and acetaminophen before the procedure will typically prevent contrast reactions and their sequelae.[12] Specifically, prednisone is administered orally 1 day before the procedure as a 10-mg dose (three times daily) and on the morning of the procedure as a single dose. Diphenhydramine (25 to 50 mg orally) and acetaminophen (10 mg) are administered 1 to 2 hours before the procedure.

The mode of sedation or anesthesia should be determined before the procedure. We generally perform all spinal angiography and interventional procedures using local anesthesia with sedative hypnotics and narcotic analgesics given intravenously before and throughout the procedure. However, the patient is maintained in a wakeful, cooperative state; during serial neurologic examinations, the angiographer is then alert to any changes in the patient's neurologic function. We reserve general anesthesia for patients who cannot remain still during the procedure, cooperate with a neurologic exam, or be recumbent for long periods.

Angioplasty Technique

Intracranial angioplasty is typically performed via the transfemoral route using the standard angiographic technique. Patients are positioned supine on the neuroangiography table; the knees can be slightly bent and supported for those with a history of low back pain. The maximum contrast load is calculated, and venous access is obtained well in advance of the procedure to permit intravenous hydration. For lengthy procedures, such as intracranial interventions, a Foley catheter is placed. Common femoral artery access is procured under sterile conditions two to three fingerbreadths below the ilioinguinal ligament using the modified Seldinger technique. We prefer the single-wall puncture technique due to the need for anticoagulation perioperatively. After placement of a 6-French sheath, anticoagulant medications are administered. Most of our patients receive heparin anticoagulation and glycoprotein (GP) IIb/IIIa blockade for antiplatelet effect. GP IIb/IIIa blockade is withheld only in patients with chronic, severe hypoperfusion or recent infarction because of the risk of hemorrhage. Selective catheterization of the appropriate vascular tree (i.e., carotid or vertebral artery) with a 6F guide catheter is performed after confirmation of appropriate anticoagulation. We target for an activated clotting time (ACT) of 220 to 250 seconds when using GP IIb/IIIa agents in conjunction with heparin or ACT >300 seconds when using heparin alone. This target can often be achieved with a heparin bolus of 40 to 50 IU/kg for use with GP IIb/IIIa or 60 to 70 IU/kg for cases with heparin alone.

After proximal access is secured, angiographic images are obtained to measure the lesion and determine the optimal view for visualization. For this purpose, the lesion is best viewed from a position perpendicular to the course of the artery. When viewed from a more acute angle, the lesion appears shorter than it really is, which may affect the surgeon's choice of balloon. The artery diameter is measured. Biplanar angiography units are typically supported by software capable of calculating the diameter, taking magnification into account **(Fig. 31.3A)**. The diameter can also be measured by comparing it to an object of known size (e.g., the diameter of

an indwelling catheter or washers affixed to either side of the patient's head) to control for magnification. The arterial diameter proximal to the lesion is used to select the appropriately sized balloon for angioplasty. This and all subsequent interventional images are performed under high magnification to improve visualization.

Access is then secured across the lesion. Access across the target lesion can be difficult in cases of severe stenosis or distal lesions, such as posterior cerebral artery (PCA) or distal MCA lesions. In our patients, the lesion is crossed with a microcatheter before insertion of the balloon catheter. Typically, a 175-cm-long, 0.014-inch-diameter wire with a soft, shapeable tip will cross with reasonable ease, allowing advancement of a small microcatheter across the lesion. With the wire removed, its position is confirmed angiographically by injecting through the microcatheter to ensure that no dissection has occurred resulting in an extraluminal catheter position. Subsequently, an exchange-length (300-cm-long, 0.014-inch-diameter) wire with a stiff proximal segment and short, soft tip is advanced to allow exchange of the balloon catheter for the microcatheter. Balloon position is confirmed angiographically before its inflation with diluted contrast/saline (2:1) using an insufflator device **(Fig. 31.3B)**. This device finely controls the pressure of inflation, permitting the interventionist to control the balloon diameter. Balloon inflation should be performed slowly so that the resulting balloon diameter is slightly less than the arterial diameter. After slow deflation, an angiogram performed through the guide catheter is used to assess the result. The balloon catheter may have to be withdrawn slightly to permit better visualization of the treated segment; however, the wire should always remain across the lesion.

Angioplasty may be repeated as necessary **(Fig. 31.3C)**. A neurologic exam is obtained before and after all balloon inflations in the conscious patient. Once a satisfactory result is attained and before withdrawal of the wire, a standard magnification angiogram visualizing the full head is obtained to rule out distal branch occlusion from emboli; maintaining wire position across the lesion during this final angiogram permits thrombolysis of distal occlusions if necessary or deemed appropriate. At completion, the balloon catheter and wire are fully withdrawn and the guide catheter is removed. The femoral artery access sheath may be left in place to be removed after reversal of anticoagulation, or the arteriotomy may be closed by one of several devices available for this purpose. We prefer closure of the arteriotomy using a sutured collagen plug (Angio-Seal Vascular Closure Device, Kensey Nash, Exton, PA) to permit early mobilization of the patient.

Strict adherence to careful technique contributes greatly to the safety of intracranial angioplasty. Nowhere is this principle more eloquently discussed than by Connors,[4] who detailed his experience from 1989 to 1998 in three periods. During the early and middle periods from 1989 to 1993, 17 patients had higher rates of complications that included angiographic evidence of dissection in 82%, stroke in 6%, and death in 6%. Since 1993, patients have experienced a 14% dissection rate, 8% neurologic event rate (of which 4% were transient ischemic attacks [TIAs]), and a 2% mortality. Two patients suffered hemorrhages (included in the strokes) in this later period. The author attributed these improvements

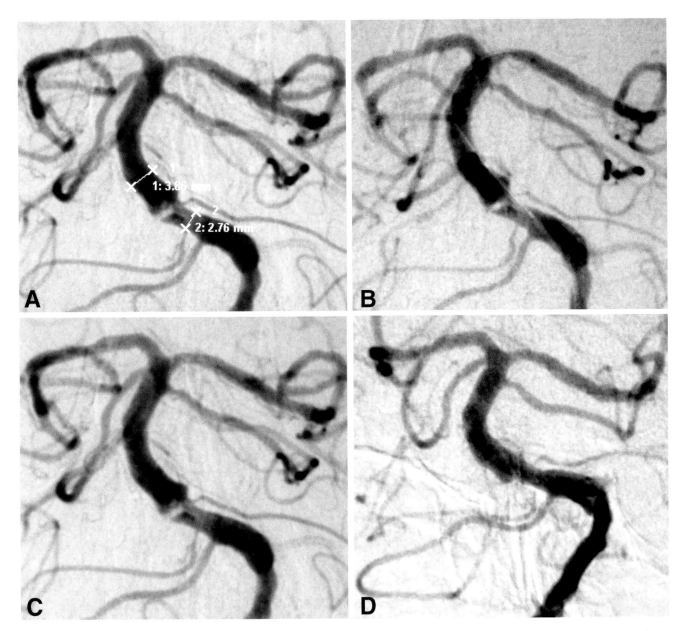

Fig. 31.3 Typical steps taken during intracranial angioplasty. **(A)** In selecting an appropriately sized balloon, the parent artery is measured to determine the size of the native lumen proximal and distal to the stenotic lesion. **(B)** Balloon position is confirmed with angiography. Even with advancement of the balloon catheter using roadmap guidance, inaccuracies can occur if the artery straightens or the patient changes position. Therefore, center the lesion on the balloon to prevent "watermelon seeding" or migration of the balloon during inflation. **(C)** After initial angioplasty attempts, angiography may show significant residual stenosis. Therefore, maintaining wire position across the lesion is paramount to prevent the need to recross the lesion, risking dissection. **(D)** Final angiography after angioplasty showing near-complete resolution of the lesion and normal filling in all distal branches. High-magnification or "coned-down" views may fail to fully evaluate these branches and may miss distal emboli. (Courtesy of the Mayfield Clinic.)

to decreasing the balloon diameter and accepting residual stenosis, very slow inflation of the balloon (2 to 5 minutes), and the routine use of GP IIb/IIIa receptor inhibitors (e.g., abciximab) during angioplasty. Connors avoided recrossing the lesion because of the increased likelihood of raising an intimal flap and vessel occlusion. In comparison with surgery, endovascular approaches offer the intrinsic advantage by allowing repair of a suboptimal result. Because the approach itself is rarely morbid, the endovascular surgeon may choose to initially treat the lesion less aggressively, knowing the result can be improved if necessary. Connors found that the use of shorter angioplasty balloons improved the ease of the procedure by preventing the straightening of the intracranial vessels with balloon inflation, thus making injury or dissection less likely.

Postoperatively, a GP IIb/IIIa blockade is maintained for 12 to 24 hours. The patient is observed in the intensive care unit by continuous blood pressure monitoring and hourly nursing evaluations. If no untoward events occur during the ensuing 24 hours, the patient can be discharged on aspirin (325 mg/day) and clopidogrel (75 mg/day).

Intracranial Stenting

Although long advocated in the treatment of coronary artery disease, stent placement after angioplasty to prevent intracranial arterial stenosis was accepted less enthusiastically because of the difficulty and risk in delivering rigid, balloon-mounted coronary stents through the tortuous intracranial anatomy. As a result, several different approaches were developed as practitioners attempted to improve the success rate of intracranial stenting. These approaches include staged stenting, primary stenting, and direct stenting (also called "sole" stenting). In staged stenting, the two procedures, angioplasty and stenting, are performed at different times, typically 1 month apart. Based on the rationale to minimize the dissection risk, the staged procedure includes a suboptimal dilatation during the first procedure, some endothelial healing, and then the attempt for full dilatation of the lesion during stent placement. In primary stenting, two steps are performed in a single procedure for angioplasty and stenting; the goal is to achieve optimal dilatation at the first procedure and eliminate the need for a second procedure. In direct stenting, stent placement during angioplasty is performed as a single step with a balloon-mounted stent, the rationale for which is to guard against dissection with the stent during the initial angioplasty.

In comparison with simple angioplasty, stent placement not only may achieve a better angiographic result but also may include the avoidance of the following: dislodgment of the plaque, plaque regrowth, elastic vessel recoil, intimal dissection, and potentially late restenosis. However, the potential stent hazards are arterial rupture, in-stent thrombosis, malpositioning of the stent, or inability to deliver the stent to the target lesion because of tortuosity of the cerebrovascular system. Severely stenotic lesions may require pre-dilatation; however, direct stenting without pre-dilatation is often feasible.

In a series of 40 patients who underwent balloon-expandable coronary stents, Jiang et al[18] reported a technical successful rate of 97.6%, total complication rate of 10%, and mortality of 2.5% (1/40 patients). During the median 10-month follow-up, no recurrence of transient ischemic attack or stroke developed in 38 available patients. In eight stented vessels in seven patients with 6-month follow-up angiography, seven had good patency and one showed restenosis.

As a multicenter, nonrandomized, prospective feasibility study, the Stenting for Symptomatic Atherosclerotic Lesions in the Vertebral or Intracranial Arteries (SSYLVIA) trial evaluated a flexible, stainless steel stent (Neurolink, Guidant Corp., Santa Clara, CA) designed for the treatment of extracranial vertebral or intracranial cerebral artery stenosis.[19] Of 61 patients with symptoms attributed to a single lesion with >50% stenosis, 43 (70.5%) had an intracranial stenosis and 18 (29.5%) had an extracranial vertebral artery stenosis. The 6-month rate for recurrence stenosis was 32.4% for intracranial vessels and 42.9% for extracranial vertebral arteries.

Stent deployment was successful in 95% of the patients; the 30-day stroke and mortality rates were 6% and 0%, respectively. During the follow-up period, 61% of patients remained asymptomatic and seven (39%) had symptomatic restenosis. Predictors of postoperative restenosis included vertebral ostial lesions, diabetes mellitus, residual stenosis of >30% after stent placement, and smaller diameter of the treated artery.

Disadvantages of Stenting

The major disadvantages of a balloon-expandable stent are its limited flexibility, which restricts navigation within the tortuous intracranial anatomy, and the risk of injury and dissection because of the high expansile force used for deployment. Unsuccessful attempts to advance a rigid stent device through tortuous diseased arteries may result in arterial or plaque dissection with distal emboli. Oversizing (i.e., expanded to greater than the nominal arterial diameter) a balloon-mounted stent can cause vessel rupture while its undersizing (i.e., expanded to <75 to 80% of nominal arterial diameter) may cause stent migration and emboli. The Wingspan stent system (Boston Scientific, Natick, MA) improves the ability to deliver a stent in the intracranial vasculature. This system uses a new concept: balloon dilatation is followed by deployment of a self-expanding nitinol microstent. The Wingspan multicenter European study enrolled 45 patients with >50% symptomatic intracranial stenosis. Technical success was achieved in 98% of patients, and the periprocedural 30-day death or ipsilateral stroke rate was 4.5%. The 6-month death or ipsilateral stroke rate was 7.1%, with an all-cause stroke rate of 9.55.

Technique

The prescribed use of the Wingspan stent is as a direct stenting technique. The stent is designed for use with the Gateway balloon. The operator should choose a balloon that dilates to approximately 75% of the normal arterial diameter to avoid overdilation. After angioplasty, the balloon is exchanged over an exchange-length (300-cm) wire (0.014-inch diameter) for the Wingspan stent, which is sized to approximately match the normal arterial diameter. The manufacturer recommends no postdilatation.

Postoperative Follow-Up

Early and continuous follow-up is paramount to ensure early identification of delayed complications of angioplasty as described later. The patient is typically seen for clinical follow-up examination 1 to 2 weeks after discharge to ensure compliance with medications and to identify any potential ischemic symptoms that may have occurred since discharge. Subsequently, clinical examinations are coupled with radiographic imaging. Typically magnetic resonance angiography is performed at 3, 6, 12, 18, and 24 months, and/or transcranial Doppler studies may be used; the latter are especially helpful if baseline studies are obtained immediately after angioplasty. Any evidence of restenosis should be evaluated angiographically. After 2 years of uneventful follow-up, annual or biannual follow-up may be sufficient.

◆ Complications and Their Management

Thromboembolus

The most feared complication of intracranial angioplasty is thromboembolism that results in downstream vascular occlusion. As with any treatment-related complication, prevention is the best management. Risk of thromboembolism can be lowered by judicious administration and monitoring of anticoagulation and antiplatelet therapy (described previously). New clot formation at the site of angioplasty can occur by several mechanisms. Local endothelial injury can cause the release of thromboxane A_2 and adenosine diphosphate, which stimulate platelet aggregation. Exposure of the subendothelium stimulates the production of thrombin through the coagulation cascade. These events may be prevented with the use of antiplatelet (aspirin and clopidogrel) and heparin. The binding of fibrin to platelets, the final common pathway in thrombus formation, is mediated by GP IIb/IIIa receptors, which are blocked by the GP IIb/IIIa inhibitors abciximab and Integrilin.

Once thromboembolism has occurred, revascularization should be attempted. In the absence of established infarction, a thrombolytic agent, such as tissue-type plasminogen activator (tPA), may be administered locally via intraarterial injection. However, use of a thrombolytic agent after cerebral ischemia is associated with intracranial hemorrhage, which increases the risk of its use for postangioplasty thrombo-embolism. Abciximab, through either intraarterial or intravenous administration, has also demonstrated thrombolytic properties and appears quite effective in the resolution of thromboembolism after angioplasty. When administered intravenously within 6 hours of acute stroke in doses typically used for acute coronary syndrome, there does not appear to be an increased risk of intracerebral hemorrhage.[20] However, fatal intracerebral hemorrhage has been reported after carotid artery angioplasty, particularly in patients with evidence of hypoperfusion before treatment.[21] Accordingly, these agents must be used cautiously and with the intent to minimize the dose administered. An alternative also includes papaverine via intraarterial injection. Acute arterial occlusion may be associated with a degree of vasospasm. In some patients, resolution of the spasm may permit reperfusion. Local thrombotic occlusion at the site of angioplasty may also be treated by any of the above-described measures. In addition, mechanical clot disruption with angioplasty or snare manipulation at the site of the thrombus has been shown to be effective in the treatment of acute intracranial occlusion resistant to thrombolysis.[22,23] Angioplasty may reestablish flow through the occluded segment, thus augmenting the delivery of thrombolytic agents and increasing the surface area of the thrombus available for binding of these agents.

Dissection

The risk of arterial dissection appears to be higher with intracranial angioplasty than in other vascular territories, including the carotid and coronary arteries **(Fig. 31.4)**. Dissection after intracranial angioplasty may affect 20% of cases,[14,24] whereas

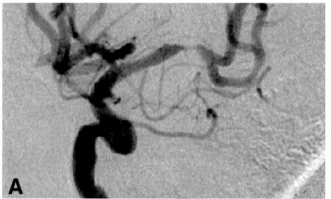

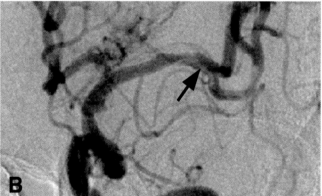

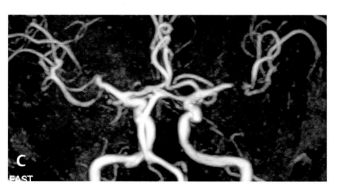

Fig. 31.4 Dissection resulting in restenosis. **(A)** Patient presented with recurrent left middle cerebral artery transient ischemic attacks (TIAs) while on warfarin. When we were unable to navigate a stent into the lesion, we resorted to angioplasty with a balloon matched to the artery size. **(B)** This resulted in dissection within the plaque *(arrow)*. Initially, the patient's symptoms resolved. Three months later, TIAs recurred and then resolved with recumbency. **(C)** Magnetic resonance angiography (MRA) revealed recurrent stenosis at the angioplasty. After confirmation of hypoperfusion on single photon emission computed tomography (SPECT) scan, patient had an extracranial to intracranial bypass and symptoms resolved. He remained symptom free 6 months later. (Courtesy of the Mayfield Clinic.)

dissection after coronary angioplasty occurs in 2 to 10% of cases.[25] The reason for this difference is unclear, but may be related to the relatively fixed position of the coronary artery in cardiac muscle as opposed to the mobile cerebral artery in the subarachnoid space. Another anatomic factor unique to the cerebral vasculature is the tortuous course of the arteries. Specifically, a highly tortuous proximal vascular anatomy or distal target location (i.e., distal MCA, PCA) increases the difficulty of reaching the target lesion with an angioplasty balloon. Therefore, dissections can occur during attempts to navigate these proximal segments. Finally, endovascular technique

influences the risk of dissection. Slow, gentle inflation and deflation without inflating beyond the normal diameter of the target artery may reduce the risk of dissection.

Restenosis

The risk of restenosis after successful intracranial angioplasty has dissuaded some clinicians from recommending this procedure for stroke prevention (**Fig. 31.3**). Yet, the reported rate varies from 0 to 50% in small series.[13,17,26] Sev-

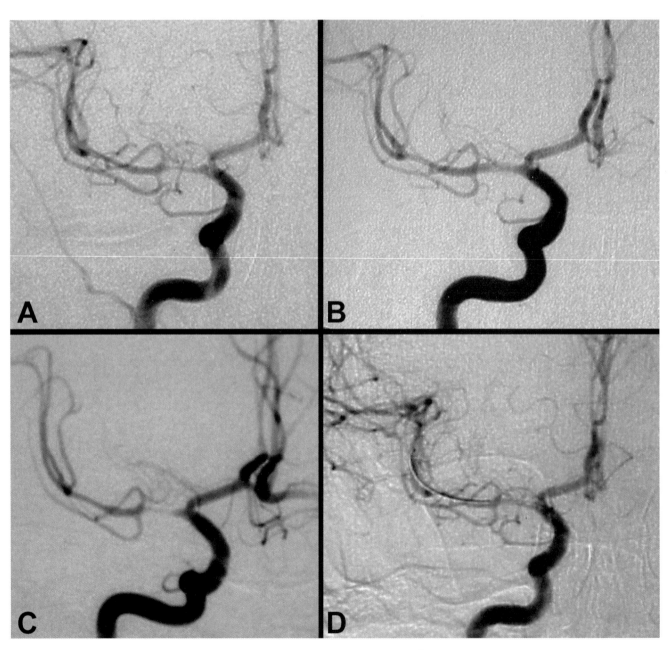

Fig. 31.5 Recurrent stenosis. **(A)** After this 65-year-old man presented with crescendo TIAs referable to this right middle cerebral artery (MCA) stenosis, he did well after angioplasty without stenting **(B).** However, 6 months later, he experienced recurrent TIAs and angiographic evidence of restenosis **(C)** and then underwent successful treatment with a second angioplasty **(D).** (Courtesy of the Mayfield Clinic.)

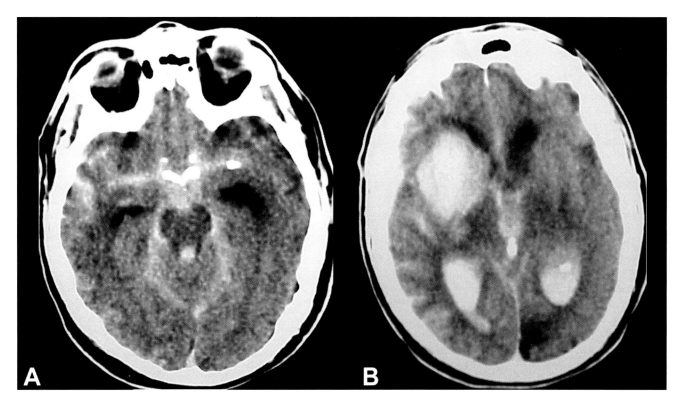

Fig. 31.6 Before **(A)** and after **(B)** reperfusion hemorrhage. After suffering a nondisabling stroke and TIAs, this patient underwent a right MCA angioplasty with abciximab antiplatelet coverage for symptomatic stenosis. The procedure was technically successful: angiographic results were good and no new neurologic signs or symptoms initially developed in the intensive care unit. Six hours after the procedure, the patient became acutely unresponsive. CT findings demonstrated the hemorrhage, which despite platelet transfusions, enlarged; the patient died as a consequence. (Courtesy of the Mayfield Clinic.)

eral factors may increase the risk of restenosis, such as long eccentric lesions[17] and procedures complicated by dissection. Accordingly, factors that increase the risk of dissection may also increase the risk of restenosis. Some authors have advocated the use of antioxidant medications to reduce the risk of restenosis. One major prospective, randomized trial demonstrated a significant reduction in restenosis after coronary angioplasty with the use of probucol and no clear benefit after the use of antioxidant vitamins alone.[27] The manufacturer discontinued production when it proved less effective than other agents for its intended use as an anticholesterolemic, and Food and Drug Administration (FDA) approval was denied because of the prolonged QT. When administered for 6 months after coronary angioplasty, Cilostazol alone and in combination with probucol has also been shown to be beneficial over placebo.[28] However, no medication has been adequately tested for prevention of intracranial restenosis.

Vascular Perforation or Rupture

Vascular perforation may occur with overzealous angioplasty that causes target artery rupture or by perforation of a more distal artery with the guidewire. Although uncommon, target artery rupture has been reported.[29] Perforation can be avoided by choosing a balloon diameter smaller than the expected normal diameter of the target artery and by avoiding overdilatation. Wire perforation of distal arteries may be less often fatal but nonetheless devastating. The use of the road-map technique to aid in wire positioning in a large distal branch and careful attention to wire stability during balloon advancement will minimize movement of the wire tip in narrow, easily perforated segments.

Complications of artery rupture and perforation are particularly troublesome when full anticoagulation with heparin and GP IIB/IIIA blockade is used. In such cases, rapid reversal of anticoagulation and transfusion of platelets is paramount. Standard procedures of emergency resuscitation are used including securing a safe airway, monitoring or providing adequate ventilation, blood pressure control, and correction of coagulopathy **(Fig. 31.5).** After emergency CT, the patient should be monitored in an intensive care unit until the coagulation status has returned to near normal. Attempts at surgical evacuation before reversal are unlikely to prove successful **(Fig. 31.6).** With appropriate reversal of pharmacologic coagulopathy and supportive care, an excellent recovery may be possible.

◆ Long-Term Results

With currently available devices, procedural success, defined as successful reduction of stenosis to less than 30%, can be achieved in up to 80% of patients.[15,16] The periprocedural neurologic complication rate is 10% in recent series. Among those successfully treated, approximately 90% remain clinically stable or improved at 6 months to 1 year follow-up.[13,30] Additional treatment is required in few patients

◆ Conclusion

Affecting 20 to 40% of patients with atherosclerotic disease, intracranial stenosis must be considered in cases of cerebral ischemic signs and symptoms, especially among some populations. In considering angioplasty or stenting for repair of intracranial stenosis, the endovascular surgeon should precisely understand the factors that influence procedural success rates, including the angiographic appearance of the lesion, severity of stenosis, and the lesion's location, length, and eccentricity. Potential complications can be reduced by careful preoperative planning and having a plan in place should they occur. Procedural success with reduction of stenosis to less than 30% can be achieved in up to 80% of patients.

References

1. The EC/IC Bypass Study Group. Failure of extracranial-intracranial arterial bypass to reduce the risk of ischemic stroke. Results of an international randomized trial. N Engl J Med 1985;313:1191–1200
2. Ausman JI, Diaz FG. Critique of the extracranial-intracranial bypass study. Surg Neurol 1986;26:218–221
3. Hass WK, Fields WS, North RR, Kircheff II, Chase NE, Bauer RB. Joint study of extracranial arterial occlusion. II. Arteriography, techniques, sites, and complications. JAMA 1968;203:961–968
4. Connors JJ III. Intracranial Angioplasty. In: Connors JJ 3rd, Wojak JC, eds. Interventional Neuroradiology: Strategies and Practical Techniques. Philadelphia: WB Saunders, 1999:500–555
5. Craig DR, Meguro K, Watridge C, Robertson JT, Barnett HJ, Fox AJ. Intracranial internal carotid artery stenosis. Stroke 1982;13:825–828
6. The Warfarin-Aspirin Symptomatic Intracranial Disease (WASID) Study Group. Prognosis of patients with symptomatic vertebral or basilar artery stenosis. Stroke 1998;29:1389–1392
7. Borozan PG, Schuler JJ, LaRosa MP, Ware MS, Flanigan DP. The natural history of isolated carotid siphon stenosis. J Vasc Surg 1984;1:744–749
8. Chimowitz MI, Kokkinos J, Strong J, et al. The Warfarin-Aspirin Symptomatic Intracranial Disease Study. Neurology 1995;45:1488–1493
9. Grubb RL Jr, Derdeyn CP, Fritsch SM, et al. Importance of hemodynamic factors in the prognosis of symptomatic carotid occlusion. JAMA 1998;280:1055–1060
10. Grüntzig A, Schneider HJ. The percutaneous dilatation of chronic coronary stenoses—experiments and morphology. Schweiz Med Wochenschr 1977;107:1588
11. Zubkov YN, Nikiforov BM, Shustin VA. Balloon catheter technique for dilatation of constricted cerebral arteries after aneurysmal SAH. Acta Neurochir (Wien) 1984;70:65–79
12. Higashida RT, Tsai FY, Halbach VV, Dowd CF, Hieshima GB. Cerebral percutaneous transluminal angioplasty. Heart Dis Stroke 1993;2:497–502
13. Terada T, Higashida RT, Halbach VV, et al. Transluminal angioplasty for arteriosclerotic disease of the distal vertebral and basilar arteries. J Neurol Neurosurg Psychiatry 1996;60:377–381
14. Takis C, Kwan ES, Pessin MS, Jacobs DH, Caplan LR. Intracranial angioplasty: experience and complications. AJNR Am J Neuroradiol 1997;18:1661–1668
15. Mori T, Fukuoka M, Kazita K, Mori K. Follow-up study after intracranial percutaneous transluminal cerebral balloon angioplasty. AJNR Am J Neuroradiol 1998;19:1525–1533
16. Nahser HC, Henkes H, Weber W, Berg-Dammer E, Yousry TA, Kühne D. Intracranial vertebrobasilar stenosis: angioplasty and follow-up. AJNR Am J Neuroradiol 2000;21:1293–1301
17. Mori T, Mori K, Fukuoka M, Arisawa M, Honda S. Percutaneous transluminal cerebral angioplasty: serial angiographic follow-up after successful dilatation. Neuroradiology 1997;39:111–116
18. Jiang WJ, Wang YJ, Du B, Wang SX, Wang GH, Jin M, Dai JP. Stenting of symptomatic M1 stenosis of middle cerebral artery: an initial experience of 40 patients. Stroke 2004;5(6):1375–1380. Epub 2004 May 6.
19. SSYLVIA Study Investigators. Stenting of Symptomatic Atherosclerotic Lesions in the Vertebral or Intracranial Arteries (SSYLVIA): study results. Stroke 2004;35:1388–1392
20. Sherman DG. Antithrombotic therapy in the acute phase: new approaches. Cerebrovasc Dis 2001;11(Suppl 1):49–54
21. Qureshi AI, Saad M, Zaidat OO, et al. Intracerebral hemorrhages associated with neurointerventional procedures using a combination of antithrombotic agents including abciximab. Stroke 2002;33:1916–1919
22. Ringer AJ, Qureshi AI, Fessler RD, Guterman LR, Hopkins LN. Angioplasty of intracranial occlusion resistant to thrombolysis in acute ischemic stroke. Neurosurgery 2001;48:1282–1288, discussion 1288–1290
23. Qureshi AI, Siddiqui AM, Suri MF, et al. Aggressive mechanical clot disruption and low-dose intra-arterial third-generation thrombolytic agent for ischemic stroke: a prospective study. Neurosurgery 2002;51:1319–1327, discussion 1327–1329
24. Alazzaz A, Thornton J, Aletich VA, Debrun GM, Ausman JI, Charbel F. Intracranial percutaneous transluminal angioplasty for arteriosclerotic stenosis. Arch Neurol 2000;57:1625–1630
25. Stauffer JC, Eeckhout E, Goy JJ, Nacht CA, Vogt P, Kappenberger L. Major dissection during coronary angioplasty: outcome using prolonged balloon inflation versus coronary stenting. J Invasive Cardiol 1995;7:221–227
26. Lee JH, Kwon SU, Lee JH, Suh DC, Kim JS. Percutaneous transluminal angioplasty for symptomatic middle cerebral artery stenosis: long-term follow-up. Cerebrovasc Dis 2003;15:90–97
27. Tardif JC, Côté G, Lespérance J, et al; Multivitamins and Probucol Study Group. Probucol and multivitamins in the prevention of restenosis after coronary angioplasty. N Engl J Med 1997;337:365–372
28. Sekiya M, Funada J, Watanabe K, Miyagawa M, Akutsu H. Effects of probucol and cilostazol alone and in combination on frequency of poststenting restenosis. Am J Cardiol 1998;82:144–147
29. Volk EE, Prayson RA, Perl J II. Autopsy findings of fatal complication of posterior cerebral circulation angioplasty. Arch Pathol Lab Med 1997;121:738–740
30. Lylyk P, Cohen JE, Ceratto R, Ferrario A, Miranda C. Angioplasty and stent placement in intracranial atherosclerotic stenoses and dissections. AJNR Am J Neuroradiol 2002;23:430–436

32

Carotid Angioplasty and Stenting

Sabareesh K. Natarajan, Adnan H. Siddiqui, Elad I. Levy, and L. Nelson Hopkins

Pearls

- Atherosclerotic disease in the carotid arteries is thought to be the cause in up to 30% of ischemic strokes. Carotid revascularization remains the principal surgical tool in the management of ischemic stroke.
- Embolic protection, rigorous training and certification, and careful patient selection are essential to keep the complications of CAS below 3% in asymptomatic patients and 6% in symptomatic patients.
- The recently published Carotid Revascularization Endarterectomy versus Stent Trial (CREST) data demonstrate that CAS and CEA are similarly effective, and therefore support CAS as a reasonable alternative to CEA.
- CEA and CAS are complementary modalities for treating patients with carotid stenosis. The choice has to be made after an individualized risk-benefit assessment for both modalities for the specific patient.

Atherosclerotic disease in the carotid arteries is thought to be the cause in up to 30% of ischemic strokes.[1] Carotid revascularization remains the principal surgical tool in the management of ischemic stroke.[1] This is corroborated by an estimated 99,000 inpatient carotid endarterectomy (CEA) procedures performed in the United States in 2006.[1] CEA, first introduced in the 1950s, was established as the gold standard for treatment of carotid stenosis by several landmark trials in the 1990s **(Table 32.1)**.[2–7]

As is the case with multiple other pathologic conditions, carotid angioplasty with stenting (also known as carotid artery stenting [CAS]) is increasingly considered an alternative to the conventional CEA procedure. The goal of CAS is restoration of a near-normal lumen. The angioplasty expands the lumen in the diseased stenotic carotid artery, and the stent prevents recoil and restrains protruding intima and plaque, thereby maintaining the restored lumen. Mathias et al[8] per-formed the first reported angioplasty of a carotid bifurcation in 1980. However, a high risk of distal embolic complications was associated with this procedure.[9,10] This led to the development of distal embolic protection devices (EPDs). The initial solutions were distal occlusion with a balloon and aspiration of debris after angioplasty, which was refined to a wire-mounted balloon for distal flow arrest. However, there was still a high rate of restenosis. The development of a stent for the carotid system shifted the balance and made CAS a promising and viable alternative for patients who were poor candidates for CEA.[11]

The major impetus for advancement of CAS came with the publication of the results of the Stenting and Angioplasty with Protection in Patients at High Risk for Endarterectomy (SAPPHIRE) trial,[12] which demonstrated effectively that patients considered high risk for CEA were less likely to have complications if treated with CAS. This resulted in Food and Drug Administration (FDA), Centers for Medicare and Medicaid Services, (CMS), and Medicare approval of CAS as a viable option in such patients. Most recently under investigation is proximal embolic protection, an entirely new method of cerebral protection achieved through flow reversal from the internal carotid artery (ICA) into the arterial guide sheath (a concept initially introduced by Parodi et al[13] and Ohki et al[14]). These technologic innovations have provided the impetus for the performance of several trials that have been conducted or are ongoing to further our understanding of the effectiveness and limitations of CAS.

With the complexity associated with risk assessment in this patient population, current standards are limited to minimizing overall surgical risk to maximize the likely benefit from surgery. The current guidelines of the American Heart Association (AHA)/American Stroke Association[15] and the Canadian Neurosurgical Society[16] establish an upper limit of 6% for perioperative risk in symptomatic patients[15] and a 3% upper limit in asymptomatic patients, assuming a life expectancy exceeding 5 years for CEA.[17]

Table 32.1 Stroke Risk in Landmark Carotid Endarterectomy (CEA) Trials

	CEA/ Medical (n)	Stenosis Severity (%)	Stroke Rate (%)		
			Medical Treatment	CEA	p Value
NASCET[2]	328/331	≥70	26	9	<.001
NASCET[6]	430/428	50–69	32.3	23.9	.026
NASCET[6]	678/690	≤50	26.2	25.7	NS
ECST[3,5]	586/389	≥70	25.9	15.8	<.001
	582/377	50–69	15.6	17.9	NS
ACAS[4]	825/834	≥60	11	5.1	.004
ACST[7]	1560/1560	≥60	11.8	6.4	.001

Abbreviation: NS, not significant.

◆ Carotid Artery Stenting Trials (Tables 32.2 and 32.3)

The first randomized trial of endovascular and surgical treatments for carotid artery stenosis was the Carotid and Vertebral Artery Transluminal Angioplasty Study (CAVATAS).[18] This trial was designed to compare balloon angioplasty alone and without embolic protection to CEA in symptomatic patients. Twenty-four centers in Europe, Australia, and Canada participated, and as in previous CEA trials, high-risk surgical patients were excluded from enrollment. For the 504 patients enrolled, no significant difference was found in the composite stroke or death rate at 30 days (10.0% endovascular group versus 9.9% CEA group) or at 3 years[19,20] (14.3% endovascular group versus 14.2% CEA group). The lack of embolic protection and low rate of stent usage (26%), which are in contrast

with current standard practice, are the main limitations of this study. The CAVATAS investigators recently reported the 5-year follow-up results.[19,20] Severe carotid restenosis (≥70%) or occlusion occurred significantly more often in patients in the endovascular arm than in patients in the endarterectomy arm (adjusted hazard ratio [HR] 3.17; p <.0001). Patients in the endovascular arm who were treated with a stent (n = 50) had a significantly lower risk of developing restenosis of ≥70%, compared with those treated with balloon angioplasty alone (n = 145; HR 0.43; p = .04).

The Wallstent trial[21,22] was the first multicenter randomized trial designed to assess CAS and CEA equivalence but was stopped early after an interim analysis revealed worse outcomes in the CAS arm, with a combined risk of stroke or death at 30 days of 12.1% in the CAS group versus 4.5% in the CEA group. Cerebral protection was not used, and this was thought to contribute in part to the high risk associated with CAS in this study.

Carotid Revascularization Using Endarterectomy or Stenting Systems (CaRESS),[23,24] a multicenter, nonrandomized, prospective study comparing CAS with embolic protection (n = 143) and CEA (n = 254) in symptomatic (32%) and asymptomatic (68%) low- and high-surgical risk patients was the first CAS versus CEA trial to use an EPD. Although this study design likely introduced selection bias, CaRESS more closely represents the real-world setting. Baseline group demographics were similar, except that patients who had previous carotid intervention more often received CAS. No statistically significant differences existed in 30-day and 1-year death or stroke rates between the CAS and CEA groups (2.1% versus 3.6% and 10.0% versus 13.6%, respectively), nor did significant differences exist for restenosis, residual stenosis, repeat angiography, and need for carotid revascularization. Overall, the morbidity and mortality in CaRESS approached North American Symptomatic Carotid Endarterectomy Trial (NASCET)[2,6] and Asymptomatic Carotid Atherosclerosis Study (ACAS)[4] standards and represented the lowest rates among contemporary CAS trials. The low stroke and death rates

Table 32.2 Summary of Completed Carotid Artery Stenting (CAS) Trials

Trial	Year	Neurologic Symptoms	CEA+ CAS (n)	30-Day Any Stroke		30-Day Stroke or Death		30-Day Stroke, Death, or MI		One-Year Death or Stroke	
				CEA %	CAS %	CEA %	CAS %	CEA %	CAS %	CEA %	CAS %
CAVATAS[18]	2001	S, AS	253+251	8.3	7.2	9.9	10	11.1	10	13.4	14.3
Wallstent[21,22]	2001	S, AS	112+107	NA	NA	4.5	12.1	4.5	12.1	3.6	12.1
CaRESS[23,24]	2003	S, AS	254+143	3.6	2.1	3.6	2.1	4.3	2.1	13.6	10.0
SAPPHIRE[12,56]	2004	S, AS	167+167	3	3.6	5.6	4.8	9.6	4.8	20.1	12.2
EVA-3S[27]	2006	S	262+265	2.7	8.7	3.9	9.6	4.6	9.8	NA	NA
SPACE[25]	2006	S	595+605	6.1	7.5	6.5	7.7	6.5	7.7	NA	NA
CRUST[98]	2010	S	653+668	3.2	5.5	3.2	6.0	5.4	6.7	NA	NA
		AS	587+594	1.4	2.5	1.4	2.5	3.6	3.5	NA	NA

Abbreviations: AS, asymptomatic; NA, data not available; S, symptomatic.

Table 32.3   Long-Term Results of Carotid Artery Stenting (CAS) Trials

Trial	Year	Neurologic Symptoms	CEA+CAS (n)	Any Stroke		Stroke or Death		Stroke, Death or MI		TLR Rate	
				CEA %	CAS %	CEA %	CAS %	CEA %	CAS %	CEA %	CAS %
EVA-3S 4 years[74]	2008	S	262+265	9.1	14.2	26.9	21.6	NA	NA	NA	NA
SAPPHIRE 3 years[56]	2008	S, AS	167+167	10.7	10.1	24.2	20.0	30.3	26.2	3.0	7.1
SPACE 2 years[73]	2009	S	595+605	10.1	10.9	15.1	17.2	NA	NA	NA	NA
CAVATAS 5 years[19,20]	2009	S,AS	253+251	15.4	21.1	23.5	29.7	NA	NA	NA	NA
CaRESS 4 years[97]	2009	S, AS	254+143	9.6	8.6	26.5	21.8	27.0	21.7	2.8	5.6
CREST 4-yr[98]	2010	S, AS	1240+1262	5.9	10.2	4.7	6.4	6.8	7.2	NA	NA

Abbreviations: AS, asymptomatic; NA, data not available; S, symptomatic; TLR, target lesion revascularization.

may be attributable to the ability of treating physicians to consider patient-specific factors and successfully assign each patient to the safest therapy.

The SAPPHIRE trial[12] was the first randomized trial to use mandatory distal EPDs. It was designed to demonstrate noninferiority of CAS in 334 patients with coexisting conditions that potentially increased the risk posed by endarterectomy and who had either a symptomatic carotid-artery stenosis of ≥50% or an asymptomatic stenosis of ≥80%. Most patients (>70%) enrolled in the trial were asymptomatic. The 30-day combined periprocedural adverse event rates were 4.8% for CAS patients and 9.8% for CEA patients ($p = .09$). At 1 year, the combined major adverse event rates were 12.2% for CAS patients and 20.1% for CEA patients ($p = .004$ for noninferiority analysis, $p = .05$ for intention-to-treat analysis). Myocardial infarction (MI) and major ipsilateral stroke rates were significantly better following CAS than following CEA (2.5% versus 8.1%, $p = .03$; 0% versus 3.5%, $p = .02$; respectively). These data strongly suggested noninferiority of CAS for high-risk, largely asymptomatic patients.

Two multicenter, randomized European trials, Stent-Protected Angioplasty versus Carotid Endarterectomy (SPACE) and Endarterectomy Versus Stenting in Patients with Symptomatic Severe Carotid Stenosis (EVA-3S) were done to establish noninferiority in standard risk, symptomatic patients. In SPACE,[25] a variety of different stents were used, and embolic protection was not mandated. The 30-day analysis in the SPACE trial comprised 1183 patients, and the primary event rates (ipsilateral stroke or death) were 6.84% in the CAS group versus 6.34% in the CEA group ($p = .09$ for noninferiority analysis). Only 27% of SPACE CAS patients were treated with embolic protection, but there were no significant differences found between those who were treated with and without an EPD. After this interim analysis, the steering committee decided to terminate the study on the basis of both futility and financial constraints, because it was revealed that 2500 patients would be needed to adequately power the study to achieve trial end points. A subsequent subgroup analysis of the 30-day results from SPACE revealed that CAS was associated with a worse outcome in older patients: the risk of ipsilateral stroke or death increased significantly with age in the CAS group ($p = .001$) but not in the CEA group ($p = .534$).[26]

Similarly, the EVA-3S trial also failed to demonstrate noninferiority of CAS in symptomatic patients.[27] The primary end point was defined as a composite of any stroke or death occurring within 30 days after treatment. A variety of different stents were used at different centers. Cerebral protection was initially not required until the safety committee instituted a protocol change as a result of a 25% 30-day rate of stroke or death in patients treated without EPDs. The study randomized 527 patients and was subsequently ended prematurely for safety reasons after an interim analysis revealed a significantly higher 30-day event rate in the CAS group (9.6%) than in the CEA group (3.9%; $p = .01$). These results persisted at 6 months, with an event rate of 11.7% in the CAS arm versus 6.1% in the CEA group ($p = .02$). A significantly higher 30-day stroke rate was observed in the CAS arm of the EVA-3S study[27] results from other studies published at that time, namely those from the SAPPHIRE trial (9.2% EVA-3S versus 3.6% in SAPPHIRE).[12] The surgeons participating in EVA-3S and performing CEA had done at least 25 endarterectomies within 1 year before trial entry, but interventionists were certified after performing less than half that number and were allowed to enroll study participants while completing their training and certification,[27] a factor that also could have, at least theoretically, increased the stroke risk in the CAS arm. Subgroup analysis based on CAS physician experience demonstrated a 12.3% stroke and death rate among endovascular physicians tutored in CAS during the trial,[27] compared with 7.1% among those tutored in CAS during their endovascular training and 10.5% among physicians with CAS experience. EVA-3S emphasizes the importance of embolic protection as well as rigorous training and credentialing for CAS physicians.

◆ Carotid Artery Stenting Registries

Carotid registries are nonrandomized outcome records for symptomatic and asymptomatic high-risk CAS patients. These registries include Arbeitsgemeinschaft Leitende Kardiologische Krankenhausarzte (ALKK), Acculink for Revascularization of Carotids in High-Risk patients (ARCHeR), Boston Scientific EPI: A Carotid Stenting Trial for High-Risk Surgical Patients (BEACH), Carotid Artery Revascularization using the Boston Scientific FilterWire EX/EZ (CABERNET), Carotid Acculink/Accunet Post Approval Trial to Uncover Unanticipated or Rare Events (CAPTURE), Carotid Artery Stenting with Emboli protection Surveillance–Post Marketing Study (CASES-PMS), and Carotid Revascularization with ev3 Arterial Technology Evolution (CREATE). Although registries do not provide direct comparison data, they do help establish true adverse event rates in high-risk CAS patients and are a crucial component in improving our understanding concerning the risks of CAS. The CABERNET collaborators found a 4.0% 30-day rate of death, stroke, and MI ($n = 446$ patients),[28] whereas the investigators of ARCHeR ($n = 581$ patients) found a 30-day stroke or death rate of 6.9% as well as a 1-year composite outcome (30-day rate of MI, stroke, or death plus the 1-year rate of ipsilateral stroke) of 9.6%.[29] CREATE ($n = 419$ patients) demonstrated a 6.2% 30-day rate of MI, stroke, and death.[30] The CAPTURE registry ($n = 3500$) determined that the post-CAS incidence of stroke, MI, and death was 6.3% for patients treated with the Acculink/Accunet CAS system (Abbott Vascular, Santa Clara, CA), and the rate of major stroke or death was 2.9%.[31,32] The BEACH investigators ($n = 747$ patients) found a 30-day MI, stroke, or death rate of 5.8%.[33] These results were similar to those in the CASES-PMS registry (5.0%), which examined the use of distal protection by endovascular carotid surgeons who either had previous experience with the EPD (Angioguard XP, Cordis Endovascular, Warren, NJ) or who underwent formal training ($n = 1493$).[34] Under these rigorous conditions, the 30-day major adverse event rate did not vary significantly between symptomatic and asymptomatic patients and among physicians with high and low volume or differing level of experience with the specific distal protection device. The German ALKK registry ($n = 1888$ patients), which included standard-risk patients, demonstrated an in-hospital death and stroke rate of 3.8%.[35] Interestingly, when this risk was stratified by time period, the investigators saw improvement from 6.3% in 1996 to 1.9% in 2004 ($p = .021$). The recently reported SAPPHIRE worldwide registry[36] is a multicenter, prospective, postapproval registry to evaluate CAS with distal protection in patients at high-risk for surgery. The registry reported results on the first 2001 patients with 30-day follow-up. The rate of adverse events was 4.4% (death 1.1%, stroke 3.2%, MI 0.7%) for the overall population. Patients with anatomic risk factors for CEA **(Table 32.4)** had a significantly lower 30-day major adverse event (MAE) rates (composite of death, MI, and stroke) than patients with physiologic risk (2.8% versus 4.9%, $p = .0306$), respectively.

Continued efforts to maintain rigorous registries like the above are critical to our eventual understanding of appropriate patient selection and procedural risks. The CABERNET investigators recently reported their 3-year results: 7.2%, all stroke; 2.8%, major stroke; 4.8%, ipsilateral stroke; 17.7%, all death; 7.1%, MI; 4.4%, target vessel revascularization.[37] Asymptomatic patients had significantly fewer major strokes than symptomatic patients (1.9% versus 5.7%, $p = .03$) and

Table 32.4 Food and Drug Administration (FDA) High-Risk Candidates for Carotid Endarterectomy (CEA)[51]

Significant medical comorbidities

- Congestive heart failure class III or IV
- Left ventricular ejection fraction <30%
- Recent myocardial infarction (>24 hour and <30 days)
- Unstable angina; Canadian Cardiovascular Society (CSS) class III or IV
- Concurrent requirement for coronary revascularization
- Abnormal stress test
- Severe pulmonary disease
- Chronic oxygen therapy
- Resting minimum arterial O_2 partial pressure (PaO_2) <60 mm Hg
- Forced expiratory volume in 1 second (FEV_1) or carbon monoxide lung

Severe pulmonary disease

- Age >80 years

Significant anatomical abnormalities

- Contralateral carotid occlusion
- Contralateral laryngeal palsy
- Previous radiation to head or neck
- Previous CEA recurrent stenosis
- Surgically difficult-to-access high cervical lesions (high cervical lesions or common carotid artery lesions below the clavicle)
- Severe tandem lesions
- Laryngectomy or tracheostomy
- Inability to extend head as a result of arthritis or other condition

patients <80 years had significantly fewer ipsilateral strokes than those ≥80 years (3.2% versus 10.7%, $p = .002$). Stroke outcomes did not differ significantly between patients with anatomic risk factors compared with those with comorbid medical risk factors.

◆ Evidence for Embolic Protection Devices

A meta-analysis by Kastrup and colleagues[38] compared 2357 patients from 26 trials who underwent carotid stenting without distal embolic protection (DEP) to 839 patients from 11 trials in which DEP was used. The primary end point of death or stroke was significantly lower in the patients treated with embolic protection (1.8 versus 5.2%, $p = .001$). There was also a significant reduction in the secondary end points of major stroke (0.3 versus 1.1%, $p = .001$) and minor stroke (0.5 versus 3.7%, $p = .001$). These results show that when distal protection is used, percutaneous carotid interventions have complication rates that are comparable to CEA. A recent meta-analysis by Garg et al[39] compared 12,263 protected CAS patients and 11,198 unprotected CAS patients. The relative risk (RR) for stroke was 0.62 (95% confidence interval [CI] 0.54–0.72) in favor of protected CAS. Subgroup analysis revealed a significant benefit for protected CAS in both symptomatic (RR 0.67; 95% CI 0.52–0.56) and asymptomatic (RR 0.61; 95% CI 0.41–0.90) patients (*p* <.05).

◆ Current Studies

The two major current, randomized trials of CAS versus CEA are the Carotid Revascularization Endarterectomy versus Stent Trial (CREST) and the International Carotid Stenting Study (ICSS; also known as CAVATAS-2).

CREST is a National Institutes of Health (NIH)-funded, multicenter, randomized trial that enrolled 2502 patients with symptomatic carotid stenosis >50% or asymptomatic carotid stenosis >70% who were considered good surgical candidates for randomization to either CEA or CAS in a 1:1 ratio. Primary end points included 30-day stroke, death, and MI, and ipsilateral stroke within 60 days and at 1 year. The trial maintained a rigorous credentialing phase for CAS providers,[40] requiring up to 20 supervised CAS procedures. During its lead-in phase, CREST demonstrated a 4.6% 30-day stroke and death rate, with stroke/death/MI rates of 3.5% for asymptomatic patients and 5.7% for symptomatic patients. There were no differences in stroke and death rates between men and women[41] or, surprisingly, between those treated with and without cerebral protection.[42] However, patients >80 years had a significantly increased stroke and death rate of 12.1%, compared with younger patients (60–69 years, 1.3%; 70–79 years, 5.3%; *p* = .0006).[43,44] The investigators have completed enrollment, analyzed the data, and presented a summary of the findings at the International Stroke Conference 2010 (W. Clark for the CREST investigators, International Stroke Conference 2010, San Antonio, TX, February 26, 2010). The salient results are as follows: For 2502 subjects with a median follow-up of 2.46 years, there was no difference in the primary end point between CEA and CAS (6.8 versus 7.2; *p* = .51); perioperatively, the primary end point was similar for CEA and CAS (4.5 versus 5.2; *p* = .38). For CEA, the rate of stroke was lower (2.3 versus 4.1%; *p* = .012) and the rate of MI was higher (2.3 versus 1.1%; *p* = .03). There were no perioperative differences in rates of stroke, MI, or death for symptomatic patients (5.4 versus 6.7%; *p* = .30) or for asymptomatic patients (3.6 versus 3.5%; *p* = .96). There were procedural differences in rates of stroke and death in symptomatic patients (3.2 versus 6.0%, *p* = .019); the differences were not significant for asymptomatic patients (1.4 versus 2.5%, *p* = .15). Thereafter, the rates of ipsilateral stroke were low for CEA and CAS (2.4 versus 2.0%; *p* = .85). The CREST data demonstrated that CAS and CEA were similarly effective and thus support CAS as a reasonable alternative for CEA.

The International Carotid Stenting Study (ICSS) is a multinational, prospective trial randomizing symptomatic, low-risk patients equally suited for CAS or CEA.[45] All CAS operators are required to attend a training course prior to enrolling

patients. Centers with limited CAS experience have been admitted to the trial on a probationary status. In addition, cerebral protection is required whenever the operator feels that an EPD can be safely deployed.

The Asymptomatic Carotid Stenosis, Stenting versus Endarterectomy Trial (ACT-I)[46] is a randomized trial of low-risk patients with asymptomatic stenosis >80% using the Xact stent and Emboshield filter cerebral protection device (Abbott Vascular, Abbott Park, IL). This trial is comparing CAS with CEA in a 3:1 ratio at multiple centers across North America. The primary end points are 30-day stroke, death, and MI rates; ipsilateral stroke at 1 year; and 5-year stroke-free survival.

The TransAtlantic Asymptomatic Carotid Intervention Trial (TACIT)[47] will randomize both standard and high-risk patients with asymptomatic carotid stenosis into one of three treatment arms: best medical therapy only (antiplatelet, antilipidemic, antihypertensive, strict diabetes control, and smoking cessation), best medical therapy plus CEA, or best medical therapy plus CAS with cerebral protection. Planned enrollment is 2400 patients with a primary end point of stroke and death at 3 years. Secondary end points include rates of transient ischemic attack (TIA) and MI, economic cost, quality-of-life analysis, neurocognitive function, and rate of carotid restenosis.

Recently, results have been made available for the Parodi flow-reversal system (Gore Flow Reversal System, W.L. Gore & Associates, Flagstaff, AZ) in the multicenter, prospective Embolic Protection with Reverse Flow (EMPiRE) trial, which demonstrated a 30-day rate of TIA, stroke, MI, and death of 4.5%.[48] Additionally, the results of the Evaluating the Use of the FiberNet Embolic Protection System in Carotid Artery Stenting (EPIC) trial demonstrated a 30-day rate of 3% for TIA, stroke, MI, and death (*n* = 237 patients) using the FiberNet DEP system (Lumen Biomedical, Plymouth, MN).[49] The ProximAl PRotection with the MO.ma device dUring caRotid stenting (ARMOUR) trial was a pivotal, prospective, multicenter, nonrandomized trial to evaluate the safety and effectiveness of cerebral protection with the MO.ma device (Invatec, Roncadelle, Italy) in high surgical risk subjects undergoing CAS. The results of this trial with 225 patients who were treated with an intention to treat in 25 United States and European centers were recently published.[50] The 30-day rate of any MI, stroke, or death was 2.7%; the stroke rate was 2.3% (major stroke rate, <1%). Continuing efforts and eventual completion of these trials or publication of the final results of these trials will improve our understanding of the relative indications and contraindications for CAS and CEA.

◆ Indications for Carotid Artery Stenting

Patients with cervical carotid artery stenosis are divided into groups according to symptoms (symptomatic or asymptomatic), age (below 80 years and 80 years and older), degree of stenosis, and surgical risk. On the basis of recent and earlier medical literature and with the exception of high surgical risk symptomatic patients, much debate remains regarding the best management of these groups, whether by medical treatment, surgical treatment, or endovascular intervention. The use of CAS in the U.S. is mainly dictated by the FDA and CMS policies.

Food and Drug Administration and Centers for Medicare and Medicaid Services Policy

Currently in the U.S., the FDA and the CMS determine the practice of CAS, directly and indirectly. The FDA's position since 2004 has "supported clinical application of CAS for carotid revascularization on symptomatic (>50% stenosis) and asymptomatic (>80%) lesions occurring on patients deemed to be high-risk candidates for CEA because of anatomical factors or severe medical comorbidities" **(Table 32.4)**.[51]

The CMS has held a position that varies from that of the FDA. Since 2005, the CMS reimburses the treatment of patients at high risk for CEA (defined as having significant comorbidities and/or anatomic risk factors—further defined in **Table 32.5**),[52] provided that they meet one of the following conditions: (1) they have symptomatic carotid artery stenosis of >70% in severity, (2) they are participating in an Investigational Device Exemption (IDE) clinical trial and are symptomatic (>50% stenosis) or asymptomatic (>80% stenosis), or (3) they are participating in an FDA-mandated postapproval study and are being treated at a study center according to the approved device indications. Hence, the CMS has increased the degree of stenosis from 50 to 70% in symptomatic patients in addition to treatment at certain approved facilities, but the CMS has made reimbursement for treatment of asymptomatic patients contingent upon trial participation, which greatly restricts the application of the procedure. The

---

Table 32.5   Centers for Medicare and Medicaid Services (CMS) Definitions of Carotid Artery Stenting (CAS)[52]

High risk is defined as having significant comorbidities and/or anatomic risk factors:

Significant comorbid conditions include:
- Congestive heart failure class III or IV
- Left ventricular ejection fraction <30%
- Unstable angina
- Contralateral carotid occlusion
- Recent myocardial infarction
- Previous CEA with recurrent stenosis
- Previous radiation treatment to the neck

Anatomic risk factors include:
- Recurrent stenosis, and/or
- Previous radical neck dissection

Symptoms of carotid artery stenosis include:
- Transient ischemic attack
- Focal cerebral ischemia producing a nondisabling stroke
- Transient monocular blindness (amaurosis fugax)

---

failure of the CMS to approve high-risk patients for reimbursement was a major setback. CMS is not convinced that CAS or CEA is indicated in asymptomatic patients. This has resulted in a dramatic decrease in the growth of CAS in the U.S. Restricting CAS to only high surgical risk symptomatic patients and only as a part of a trial results in treatment of only 7% of the potential patient base.

Symptomatic Patients

There is substantial evidence supporting the benefit of CAS for the high anatomic risk population from registry data on more than 14,000 high-risk patients.[53] Complication rates continue to show a trend toward improvement as operators gain experience.

Among randomized symptomatic patients from the SAPPHIRE trial, there was a 30-day stroke and death rate of 4.2% for CAS patients and 15.4% for CEA patients ($p = .13$).[12] Other trials had similar results for CAS: CaRESS phase I revealed no significant differences in combined death/stroke rates at 30 days (3.6% CEA versus 2.1% CAS).[24] The rate of all stroke and death in symptomatic non-octogenarians in the CREST lead-in phase was 3.9% (4.6% in the total patient population).[43]

In a review of published registries, 30-day rates of all strokes and death for symptomatic non-octogenarians in the combined Emboshield and Xact Post-Approval Carotid Stent Trial (EXACT) and CAPTURE-2 post–market surveillance studies were 7.3% and 6%, respectively.[54] With the CAPTURE, EXACT, and CAPTURE-2 studies, there were a total of 8334 patients enrolled in the largest prospective, multicenter, neurologically controlled, independently adjudicated data set for carotid intervention ever assembled.[55] In the CASES-PMS study, MAE (a composite of death, MI, and stroke) at 30 days occurred in 5.6% of symptomatic patients.[34] The overall stroke rate at 30 days was 3.8% in these high-risk patients, approaching the boundary rate of 3% put forth by the AHA guidelines for stenting outcomes in low-risk patients.[15]

Symptomatic patients have clear evidence pointing to the benefit from CAS, as the data are overwhelming in patients with >50% stenosis. Patients with >50% stenosis who are standard risk with CEA and high risk with CAS have fewer strokes if they undergo revascularization. The results are limited for standard-risk CAS for symptomatic patients. In previous studies, there was a lack of stenting (CAVATAS), lack of EPD (CAVATAS, SPACE), limited inclusion (symptomatic only in EVA-3S and SPACE), and poor trial conduct (EVA-3S). Nevertheless, except for EVA-3S, CAS appears to compare favorably to CEA in standard-risk symptomatic patients.

Asymptomatic Patients

Among asymptomatic patients in the SAPPHIRE trial, there was a 30-day stroke and death rate of 6.7% for CAS and 11.2% for CEA.[56] For the CREST lead-in phase, the rate was 3.3% for asymptomatic patients undergoing CAS.[40]

In a review of the pivotal published registries, the combined death and major stroke rate in CABERNET was 2% for patients <80 years.[28] In the large, postmarket study of high surgical risk registries, the CASES-PMS study, MAE at 30 days (a composite of death, MI, and stroke) occurred in 4.2% of all asymptomatic patients and 3.6% in asymptomatic patients <80 years.[34] EXACT and CAPTURE-2 asymptomatic 30-day outcomes showed strokes and death rates of 3.1% and 3%, respectively, in the non-octogenarians.[54]

In high surgical risk patients, stenting has achieved AHA recommendations for perioperative risk in the broad population of operators and is likely beneficial. In standard surgical risk populations, initial evidence suggests that stenting is comparable to surgery and therefore likely beneficial. CREST and the ACT-I investigational trial for patients with asymptomatic carotid stenosis will provide clearer data in this population.

Do all asymptomatic patients with severe stenosis have equal stroke risk? Clinical comorbidities, carotid stenosis severity and progression, carotid plaque morphology, and cerebrovascular characteristics reserve and "silent" infarcts/embolization are factors that raise the question of whether all asymptomatic patients are created equal. The degree of the stenosis obviously is important for lesions above or below 75%; the annual stroke rate was 1.3% in asymptomatic patients with carotid stenosis ≤75% and 3.3% in those with stenosis >75%.[57] The role of cognitive function and its improvement following CAS in asymptomatic patients likewise brings into question the categorization of symptomatic and asymptomatic patients.[58] CAS improves neurocognitive function in a considerable proportion of patients with carotid stenosis >50%. Ipsilateral anterior cerebral artery filling after CAS is associated with improved neurocognitive function, presumably due to amelioration of frontal lobe perfusion.[58] Brain perfusion deficits, observed in a majority of patients with carotid artery stenosis, tend to improve considerably by 6 months after protected CAS.[59]

◆ Procedural Technique

The processes of angioplasty and stenting create intimal injury that promotes thrombosis.[60] Therefore, patient preparation with adequate antiplatelet and anticoagulation therapy is essential. Patients receive a dual antiplatelet regimen consisting of aspirin (325 mg daily) and a thienopyridine derivative (i.e., clopidogrel, 75 mg daily, or ticlopidine, 250 mg twice daily) for at least 3 days prior to stent treatment. A loading dose of clopidogrel (300–600 mg) administered early on the day of the procedure is an alternative for patients who are already taking aspirin. An intravenous bolus dose of heparin (50–60 U/kg) is administered after catheterization of the common carotid artery (CCA). An activated coagulation time of 250 to 300 seconds is maintained throughout the procedure. The heparin infusion is usually discontinued at the conclusion of the procedure. The procedure is performed in an angiography suite with biplane digital subtraction and fluoroscopic imaging capabilities. The patient is sedated but arousable for neurologic assessment. The carotid artery is generally approached percutaneously from the common femoral artery. The operator should also be familiar with radial and brachial approaches in case femoral artery access is not possible.

An aortic arch angiogram is initially performed to define the atherosclerotic burden as well as the anatomic configuration of the great vessels, which enables the operator to predict the feasibility of carotid cannulation and select the devices needed for the procedure. Selective carotid angiography is then performed, and the degree of the stenosis is defined. The diameters of the CCA and the ICA are measured with attention paid to determining a landing zone for the EPD. A preintervention intracranial angiogram is also essential for consideration of the presence of tandem lesions in the management strategy, as well as for comparison of pre- and post-procedure intracranial angiograms to confirm the absence of any vessel dropout suggestive of embolism.

Bradycardia occurs occasionally during angioplasty, and consideration may be given to administering glycopyrrolate (0.4 mg) before performing CAS. Atropine and vasopressors (e.g., dopamine and Neo-Synephrine) should be readily available should significant bradycardia and hypotension develop. Continuous intraprocedural monitoring of heart rate, blood pressure, and neurologic status is essential. Therefore, we routinely transduce the arterial sheath in the femoral artery to maintain continuous arterial pressure monitoring.

After completion of the diagnostic angiogram and positioning of the catheter in the CCA, roadmapping of the cervical carotid artery is performed. An exchange-length 0.035-inch wire is positioned in the external carotid artery (ECA). The diagnostic catheter is exchanged over the wire for a 90-cm, 6- to 10-French (F) sheath that is then advanced into the CCA below the bifurcation. For patients who have undergone a complete diagnostic cerebral angiogram before the stenting procedure, a combination of a 6F, 90-cm shuttle over a 6.5F head-hunter 125-cm slip-catheter (Cook, Bloomington, IN) or a 5F 125-cm Vitek catheter (Cook) can be used. In these cases, the shuttle is introduced primarily in the femoral artery over a 0.035-inch wire and is parked in the descending aorta. The inner obturator and wire are removed. The 125-cm catheter is then advanced into the shuttle, and the target vessel is catheterized. The shuttle is brought over the wire and the catheter in the CCA. The size of the shuttle is usually dictated by the profile of the EPD and compatibility with the stent system. An optimal angiographic view that maximizes the opening of the bifurcation and facilitates crossing of the stenosis should be sought. The lesion is crossed with the protection device. Pre-dilation of the stenotic vessel segment is performed at the operator's discretion, but we avoid predilation whenever possible. If the lesion does require pre-dilation, we prefer to undersize the balloon to simply facilitate crossing of the stent, usually using a 2- to 3-mm diameter balloon. A 3- to 4-mm coaxial angioplasty balloon is advanced to the lesion over the 0.014-inch wire holding the protection device. On rare occasions, pre-dilation needs to be performed before the EPD is introduced.

The diameter of the stent should be sized to the caliber of the largest segment of the carotid artery to be covered (usually 1 to 2 mm more than the normal caliber of the CCA). Oversizing of the stent in the ICA does not usually result in adverse events, but a tapered stent can better conform to the vessel wall. Particular attention should be paid to the selection of a stent that is long enough to cover the entire lesion.

After removing the stent system, post-stent dilation should be performed using a balloon with a diameter matching that of the ICA distal to the stent. A coaxial balloon is usually preferred for this purpose. The EPD is then removed, using its retrieval catheter. (When a balloon occlusion catheter is used for cerebral protection, the embolic debris is aspirated before deflation and retrieval of the balloon.)

The femoral access site is then secured either through manual compression or with a local clamping device; alternatively, for faster patient mobilization and greater comfort, a device may be used for closure (e.g., Mynx, AccessClosure, Mountain View CA; Starclose, Abbott Vascular, Santa Clara, CA; Perclose, Abbott Vascular; or Angio-Seal, St. Jude Medical, Minnetonka MN), on the basis of operator preference, patient anatomy, and puncture site location.

◆ Stent Selection

Commercially available self-expanding carotid stents (**Table 32.6**) are composed of either nitinol (a nickel–titanium alloy) or stainless steel (a cobalt alloy). In general, nitinol stents are constructed from a single laser cut. The only exception is the NexStent (Boston Scientific, Natick MA), which is laser-cut from a nitinol sheet and coiled into a tube-like form. The overlap area of the coiled structure shrinks or grows as it is placed in larger or smaller diameter vessels. Once a nitinol stent is deployed in the body, the stent's thermal memory allows it to achieve a predefined shape. The only available stainless steel stent is the Carotid Wallstent (Boston Scientific), which is woven from a single piece of cobalt alloy wire into a tubular structure. The stent is delivered in a retractable sheath, and expands via a spring-like action once the sheath is withdrawn.

The stent struts engage the dilated plaque material, and the mesh design of the stent prevents dislodgment of debris through the stent interstices. Therefore, the stent's scaffolding potential (i.e., the amount of support given to the vessel wall by a stent) is of major importance in obtaining a stroke-free CAS result. The free-cell area is the best-accepted method to describe the scaffolding potential of carotid stents. In the Belgium-Italian Carotid (BIC) Registry,[61] stents with a smaller free-cell area best contained the plaque material behind the struts, resulting in significant differences in event rates, as compared with stents with large free-cell areas. The differences were more pronounced among symptomatic patients and most clear for events occurring in the postprocedural phase, during which the carotid stent alone provides protection against embolization.

Another often-used classification for stent design is the binary open- and closed-cell design, in which the differentiation is made according to the number and arrangement of bridge connectors between the ring segments. In closed-cell stents, the adjacent ring of the stent are connected at every possible junction; in the open-cell stents, not all junction points are interconnected. An open-cell design might insufficiently scaffold a plaque in, for example, tortuous anatomy because the stent cells open on the concave surface of the bend, which can cause prolapse on the open surface. Patients treated with closed-cell stents had significantly lower 30-day stroke, death, and TIA event rates than patients treated with open-cell stents, according to a retrospective study.[62] These results have been confirmed by a subanalysis of the SPACE study.[25] Nevertheless, Wholey and Finol[63] stated that this classification may be too general for comparison, and concluded that cell size and surface area coverage appear to be more important. They gave the example that a closed-cell stent with a cell diameter of 1000 μm is more likely to be responsible for plaque prolapse and embolization than an open cell stent with a cell diameter of 500 μm.

The flexibility of a stent is defined as its ability to conform to vessel tortuosity during deployment. In closed-cell stents, the adjacent ring segments are connected at every possible junction with flexible bridge connectors, and therefore only a limited degree of flexion between adjacent rings is possible. In open-cell stents, not all junction points are interconnected, and this allows more movement between adjacent ring segments and a better conformability to tortuous anatomy. The flexion benefits of an open-cell design have a cost in scaffolding uniformity, just as the scaffolding benefits of a closed-cell design have a cost in flexion and conformability.[63]

In an attempt to improve compliance with carotid anatomy, tapered stents have been developed. These are characterized by a smaller stent diameter at the distal end than at the proximal end. There are two types of tapered stents: the conical (e.g., Acculink, Xact [Abbott Vascular] and Crystallo Ideale [Invatec]) and the shouldered (e.g., Protégé [ev3]), which are the self-tapering, as mentioned in **Table 32.6**. In the first, there is a gradual decrease in diameter from the proximal to the distal end, whereas in the second, there is a short transition zone in the midsegment of the stent. The coiled nitinol sheet configuration of the NexStent (another tapered stent) allows the stent to adapt nicely to the change in diameter. The stent overlap differs from the proximal to the distal stent end. The Precise stent (Cordis Endovascular, Warren NJ) is also considered self-tapering because the different rings interact independently with the vessel wall.

In the spirit of the findings of the BIC Registry,[61] and taking into account that after stent deployment and as soon as the EPD is removed, the stent remains the only protection against brain embolization, plaque scaffolding should be the main determinant in the selection of a carotid device. Any patient presenting with a potential vulnerable lesion, that is, all symptomatic patients and patients presenting with an echogenic lesion (gray scale median >25),[64] should receive a stent that has a free-cell area that is as low as possible. If the selection of a stent with such high scaffolding capacities would potentially compromise preservation of the anatomy of the vessel (e.g., potential distal kink or significant mismatch in proximal and distal diameters), CEA should be performed.

◆ Embolic Protection Device Types

All EPD systems currently on the market can be classified into three main groups, each with its own working principle: (1) distal occlusion devices, (2) distal filtration systems, and (3) proximal occlusion devices (PODs).

Table 32.6 Specifications of Commercial Carotid Stents

Stent (Manufacturer)	Design	Cell Type	Material	Shape	Free Cell Area (mm²)	Tapering
Carotid Wallstent Monorail (Boston Scientific)	Woven	Closed	Cobalt Chromium	Tube	1.08	Self-tapering
Exponent RX (Medtronic Vascular)	Laser-cut	Open	Nitinol	Tube	6.51	Self-tapering
NexStent Monorail (Boston Scientific)	Laser-cut	Closed	Nitinol	Coiled sheet	4.7	Self-tapering
Precise (Cordis)	Laser-cut	Open	Nitinol	Tube	5.89	Self-tapering
Protégé RX (ev3)	Laser-cut	Open	Nitinol	Tube	10.71	Straight or shoulder tapered
RX Acculink (Guidant)	Laser-cut	Open	Nitinol	Tube with longitudinal spines	11.48	Straight or conical tapered
Xact (Abbott Vascular)	Laser-cut	Closed	Nitinol	Tube	2.74	Straight or conical tapered

Distal occlusion devices (distal occlusion balloons [DOBs]) work according to the principle set forth by Theron et al[65] during their first successful attempt to create cerebral protection.[66] A balloon is inflated in the ICA between the lesion and the brain to block the flow of blood toward the cerebrum. Consequently, debris cannot enter the cerebral vasculature during the procedure. The debris is aspirated and flushed, forcing it either into the ECA or out of the body, through a sheath in the CCA. The major advantages of the DOB over other types of EPDs are the low crossing profile and high flexibility, which facilitate device delivery. However, complete blockage of the distal ICA interrupts blood flow to the brain and reduces oxygen delivery to the brain in patients with insufficient cerebral collateralization. Although cerebral oxygenation can be maintained by intermittent balloon deflation, this may compromise the quality of cerebral protection. Another disadvantage of complete ICA occlusion is that angiographic assessment of the lesion is not possible during balloon infla-

tion. Additionally, the pressure needed to inflate the balloon may cause spasm and dissection at the distal ICA. The FDA-approved PercuSurge balloon (Medtronic Vascular, Santa Rosa, CA) is the commonest DOB used today.

Filtration systems (**Table 32.7 and Fig. 32.1**) function like an umbrella- or windsock-like filter hose and are deployed in between the carotid lesion and the brain to capture all debris during the CAS procedure. The distal filter (DF) and captured debris are removed at the end of the procedure. A DF can be mounted on a guidewire on which it is directly brought into place and retrieved; alternatively, it can come with a specific delivery and retrieval system. The most important features of these filters are the maintenance of cerebral perfusion during CAS and the possibility of angiographic assessment of the carotid lesion during all steps of the procedure. Thrombosis of the DF may occur during the intervention, but this can be prevented by systemic administration of heparin at the start of the procedure. In case of complete DF blockage by

Table 32.7 Food and Drug Administration (FDA)-Approved Stent and Embolic Protection Device (EPD) Combinations and Specifications

Stent	Filter	Characteristics	Pore Size (µm)	Lesion Crossing Profile (F)	Available Filter Diameters (mm)
Acculink	Accunet	Concentric	125	3.5–3.7	4.5, 5.5, 6.5, 7.5
Precise	Angioguard	Concentric	100	3.2–3.9	4, 5, 6, 7, 8
Xact	EmboShield	Concentric, bare wire	120	2.8–3.2	Small 2.5–4.8 Large 4–7
NexStent	Filterwire EZ	Eccentric	110	3.2	One size fits all
Protégé	SpiderRX	Eccentric	Variable	3.2	3, 4, 5, 6, 7
(several)	FiberNet	Occluder + filter	40	2.4–2.9	3.5–7.0

Manufacturers: Acculink and Accunet, Abbott Vascular (Santa Clara, CA); Precise and Angioguard, Cordis (Warren, NJ); Xact and EmboShield, Abbott Vascular; NexStent and EZ Filterwire, Boston Scientific (Natick, MA); Protégé and SpiderRX, ev3 (Irvine, CA); FiberNet, Lumen Biomedical (Plymouth, MN).

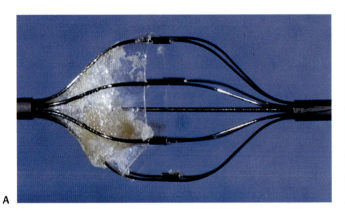

A

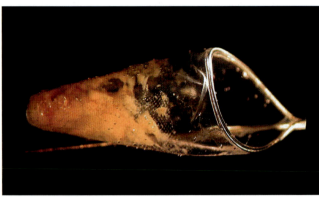

B

Fig. 32.1 **(A)** Angioguard (courtesy of Cordis, Warren NJ), and **(B)** Filterwire EX. (Courtesy of Boston Scientific, Natick, MA.) These are examples of filtration systems used for embolic protection. The

Accunet and Angioguard have a concentric profile, whereas the Filterwire EX has an eccentric profile. The Filterwire has the lowest lesion crossing profile of all these filters.

debris or thrombus, a few rescue options are available: the debris can be removed by aspiration of the filter or simply retrieved, after which the CAS procedure can be continued.

Proximal occlusion systems (**Fig. 32.2**) are characterized by two compliant balloons, of which one is inflated in the proximal CCA and one in the ECA (e.g., the MO.ma system). This double-balloon inflation creates either a no-flow or a reversed-flow pattern within the ICA that prevents debris from entering the cerebral circulation. PODs are especially attractive as complete cerebral protection is established before crossing the lesion. After the occlusion balloons have been positioned, multiple guidewires can be selected to cross highly stenotic or tortuous lesions. The procedural steps required to maneuver the POD in the carotid arteries are more laborious than those involved with other types of EPDs. Also, ICA and CCA blockage impedes blood supply to the brain in patients with insufficient intracerebral collateralization. Intraprocedural deflation of the distal balloon between the different steps of CAS may restore cerebral oxygenation but can compromise the efficacy of the protection. The concerns associated with proximal protection devices are their large size, currently requiring 9F access to the femoral artery, and the concurrent delivery of a 9F system into tortuous CCAs.

FiberNet (Lumen Biomedical, Plymouth, MN) is the first EPD that combines the features of a filter and an occlusion device in one system.[67] The system consists of a three-dimensional expandable polyethylene terephthalate fiber-based filter, which expands radially, and is mounted on a 0.014-inch wire and retrieval catheter. The system can capture particles as small as 40 μm without compromising flow. On completion of the CAS procedure, the retrieval catheter is advanced over the wire and positioned just proximal to the expanded filter. There are two focal suction steps required for this filter. The first focal suction is at the base of the filter to remove any material that may be loosely bound to the filter. The second focal suction is performed while the device is being retrieved. Contained and captured emboli are removed by focal suction through the retrieval catheter and also by retention within the filter fibers.

Selecting an Embolic Protection Device

Screening a patient to determine which EPD to use begins with assessment of the intracerebral circulation. For patients without sufficient cerebral collateralization (as documented by preoperative imaging), DFs are advisable as they preserve periprocedural oxygen delivery to the brain. DOBs and PODs should not be used because cerebral perfusion might be inadequate during the procedure. Although the protective balloons could be temporarily deflated to guarantee intracerebral circulation, we believe that this is a laborious technique that may even increase the risk of distal embolization and stroke. Next, the selected access site is evaluated. Patients with tortuous iliac access or with a type III aortic arch require low-profile, flexible protection systems because the lesion site is difficult to reach. As DOBs have crossing profiles comparable with those of guidewires, they are always steerable and flexible enough to pass tortuous anatomies. Of the DFs, only the small-profile, flexible ones are qualified in these cases. POD systems are not recommended because of their large French sizes.

The anatomy and morphology of the carotid lesion are key factors in the selection of the EPD. Highly stenotic, irregular lesions and near occlusions can be treated with any EPD. However, a DF should be carefully selected: only low-profile, soft-tipped, and flexible devices should be used to cross the lesion because they are less traumatic and their use may reduce the risk of complications. For cases with a severely angulated ICA, PODs are the most likely choice because they do not have to be navigated across the lesion site. If a DOB or DF system is chosen, the device should be highly steerable and flexible.

Because only small differences in complication rates for the different presented cases can be expected, hard data from randomized controlled trials are currently not and probably never will become available to prove the presented guidelines for selection of an EPD. In a comparison of proximal versus distal EPD during CAS, El-Koussy et al[68] found (based on diffusion-weighted magnetic resonance imaging [MRI]

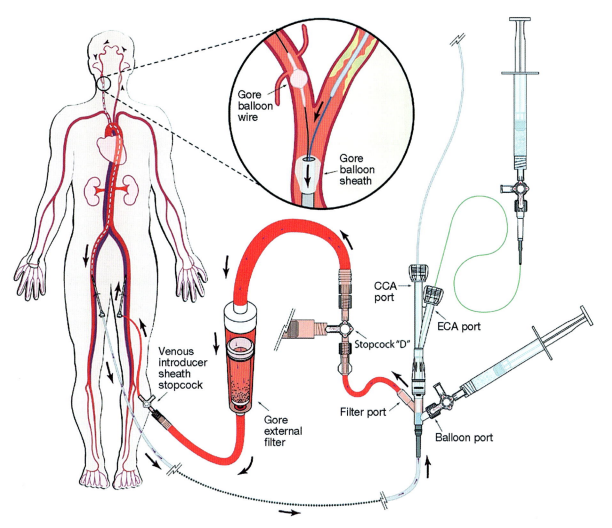

Fig. 32.2 The Gore flow reversal device causes a no-flow or a reversed-flow pattern within the internal carotid artery (ICA) that prevents debris from entering the cerebral circulation. The advantage of the Gore device is that it provides embolic protection before crossing the lesion, although it requires favorable arch anatomy and a larger access sheath is needed for delivery. CCA, common carotid artery; ECA, external carotid artery. (Courtesy of W.L. Gore & Associates, Flagstaff, AZ.)

outcome) a nonsignificant trend toward fewer embolic events after CAS with POD. These diffusion-weighted MRI differences did not result in differences in clinical outcomes relative to type of EPD used. Similarly, a subanalysis of the BIC Registry concluded that none of the observed differences in 30-day event rates between the different EPD types could be explained by EPD selection, but rather were attributable to the differences in stent types used in conjunction with the EPD.[61]

◆ Periprocedural Management

Hydration is essential before, during, and after the procedure. For patients with concurrent renal dysfunction, hydration includes alkalinization of the urine with three ampules of sodium bicarbonate added to each liter of 5% dextrose with normal saline for prophylaxis against contrast-related nephropathy. In others, 5% dextrose with normal saline (0.9% NaCl) is sufficient. Intravenous hydration should be maintained for up to 24 hours postprocedure. CAS at the carotid bulb often results in a sustained vagal bradycardia, which may be minimized by intraprocedural administration of anticholinergic agents, such as glycopyrrolate. Postprocedure hypotension should be aggressively managed with vasoconstrictors, such as Neo-Synephrine, or intravenous infusion of dopamine. The goal is to keep the patient in a normotensive condition. Frequently, carotid artery disease is associated with coronary artery disease; and sustained hypotension is a harbinger of myocardial ischemia. Conversely, sustained hypertension after CAS revascularization may be associated with a cerebral hyperperfusion syndrome and, in some cases, with breakthrough hyperperfusion hemorrhage, with disastrous consequences.[69] Hence, normotension should be continuously maintained with systolic blood pressures between 110 and 150 mm Hg. This requires postoperative observation in a continuously monitored setting. If a closure device has not been used, the arterial sheath should be removed when the activated coagulation time is <150 seconds. The patient is usually discharged on the afternoon after the procedure if hemodynamic parameters are maintained without intravenous infusions and if neurologically unchanged postprocedure. Patients require surveillance imaging to evaluate vessel patency. Duplex sonography evaluation should be obtained before discharge, at 6 weeks, 3 months, 6 months, and 1 year, and then annually thereafter. The dual antiplatelet regimen of aspirin and clopidogrel (or ticlopidine) is maintained for 12 weeks postprocedure, after which patients remain on aspirin therapy.

◆ Procedural Durability

Durability of carotid revascularization with CAS is a concern frequently expressed by the surgical community. In a retrospective study of patients undergoing stenting for de novo carotid stenosis (119 arteries) and postendarterectomy carotid stenosis (76 arteries), ≥80% stenosis was detected by follow-up Doppler imaging in 5.2% of the vessels stented.[70] Restenosis after endarterectomy was the major risk for instent restenosis. Significant (symptomatic or ≥80%) recurrent stenosis was detected by follow-up Doppler imaging in six (5%) of 112 patients in our CAS series.[71] The 3-year follow-up of the SAPPHIRE trial revealed a 4% recurrent stenosis rate following CAS.[56] This rate compares favorably with the 0.7 to 7.9% reported risk of restenosis after endarterectomy in large series.[72] Further, an increasing body of evidence is indicating a persistent benefit after CAS. It appears that the majority of the risk of the procedure is noted within the periprocedural period and up to 30 days. Thereafter, the risk falls significantly, remaining low for the duration of these studies. SAPPHIRE suggested a 6.6% ipsilateral stroke rate at 3 years as compared with 5.4% after CEA, including the periprocedural risk.[56] The 2-year data from the SPACE trial suggests a 2.2% ipsilateral stroke risk after CAS as compared with 1.9% after CEA (between postprocedure day 30 and 2 years).[73] Similarly, EVA-3S had a 1.26% stroke rate after CAS as compared with 1.97% after CEA (between postprocedure day 30 and 4 years).[74]

◆ Patient Selection

Patient selection is the most important factor in minimizing complications associated with CAS.[75,76] Categories of major risk factors for CAS include medical, neurologic, anatomic, and genetic arteriopathy. Advanced age is often listed as a risk factor, but it is the anatomic challenges and medical comorbidities that come with advanced age that increase the risk for most patients.[77–79] The major medical risk factor for patients with carotid stenosis is MI. A sudden decline in blood pressure and the onset of severe bradycardia present a major risk for MI in patients with severe left main coronary artery disease or severe triple-vessel disease. In this group, if CAS before coronary intervention is necessary, minimal or no dilation of the stent after deployment will generally avoid major hemodynamic swings, and the patient can be sent for cardiac surgery, with a plan made for follow-up evaluation and retreatment if necessary. Neurologic risk increases with recent large infarction, crescendo TIAs, and stroke in evolution. Large infarctions present a significant risk for hemorrhage.[80,81] Traditionally, patients with large infarction are allowed to "heal" the stroke for 6 weeks prior to intervention. Patients with active TIAs or stroke in evolution need to be treated but are at higher risk for neurologic injury.

Several studies have demonstrated increased rates of stroke and death among octogenarians. The CREST lead-in phase reported a 30-day stroke and death rate of 12.1% for octogenarians compared with 3.2% among non-octogenarians ($p = .0001$), prompting the study investigators to exclude patients >80 years from the study.[43] Similarly, results from Stanziale et al[82] indicated that CAS in octogenarians was associated with a statistically significant higher rate of adverse events at 30 days and at 1-year follow-up. Subgroup analysis of the SPACE trial also found that the rate of complications was significantly associated with age in the CAS group; patients in the CEA group had homogeneous event rates across all age groups.[26]

Conversely, there are reports of experienced operators performing CAS in octogenarians after careful patient and device selection with acceptable and low adverse events.[83–85] It has been suggested that adverse vascular anatomy and lesion characteristics with the potential to increase the technical complexity of CAS may account for this finding because recent studies have suggested that some of these complex anatomic features seem to be more prevalent among older patients.[86–88] Lin et al[88] found that aortic arch calcification, stenosis of the CCA and innominate artery, and tortuosity of the CCA and ICA were significantly more severe in patients >80 years. Likewise, in addition to the features mentioned earlier, others have found that unfavorable arch elongation, severe lesion stenosis (>85%), and plaque ulceration are significantly more common among patients aged ≥80 years.[86,87] Recent work has sought to determine the effect of these anatomic characteristics on outcomes after CAS. Some variables that have been associated with an increased risk of adverse events include tortuous and severe iliofemoral disease; abnormal arch anatomy[89]; proximal or distal tortuosity of the CCA or ICA[90]; long, irregular, or concentrically calcified stenotic lesions (>15 mm); pseudo-occlusion; string sign; carotid artery kinking; involvement of the internal carotid ostium[91]; intraluminal thrombus; and plaque echolucency.[64] It is important to note that although these anatomic and lesion characteristics are thought to be more common in the elderly population, younger patients may also have similar unfavorable risk factors. For example, Sayeed et al[91] reported that long stenosis and ostial involvement were associated with an increased risk of stroke that was independent of octogenarian status. Thus, the presence of certain anatomic factors that preclude safe passage or proper positioning of stents and EPDs must be considered high risk at any age, and this could possibly delineate a new group of patients who, in addition to the elderly, need proper imaging to identify these high-risk factors and appropriate therapy and device selection to decrease the risk of complications.

Creative endovascular solutions can be found even for high-risk patients when treatment is deemed necessary. For patients with intraluminal thrombus and symptomatic carotid artery disease, the traditional treatment has been heparin and warfarin therapy with reevaluation in 6 weeks to 3 months. In four patients with multiple episodes of TIAs, we used a trapping technique with proximal and distal balloon occlusion with good success.[92,93] Flow-reversal systems may prove useful in this setting and in the context of kinks that make the landing of a DEP device infeasible.[94] Not all high-risk patients can be avoided. For example, treatment should likely be delayed for 6 weeks in a patient who has a large completed infarction with territory still at risk. Conversely, treatment should promptly be undertaken in a patient in need of urgent coronary artery bypass graft (CABG) who presents with crescendo TIAs and an MI. Each case should be evaluated on an individual basis. For patients who are candidates for carotid intervention, it should be remembered that CEA remains a safe and effective operation if CAS is thought to be too risky. In fact, CEA and CAS are highly complementary procedures; in those situations for which one is high risk, the other is usually feasible with acceptable risk. It is important to remember that the surgeon's backing out of a CAS procedure is rarely a problem for the patient, whereas the surgeon's persisting in the face of technical challenges may result in an avoidable stroke.

Lower-risk patients are those with either asymptomatic or single retinal or hemispheric TIAs with no previous cardiac history.[95] Anatomically, type I aortic arches[96] with both straight proximal and distal anatomy provide the easiest anatomic substrate for CAS. Many of these patients have not been treated in the carotid stenting pool that has been reserved for "high-risk" patients. Ongoing low-risk clinical trials like ACT-I will determine how these patients fare with CAS when compared with CEA.

At our center, we use a simplified algorithm (**Table 32.8**) for the classification of patients at high risk for CAS based on patient factors, access method, lesion type, and procedural factors.

◆ Conclusion

The indications for CAS are evolving. With advances in technology, access to carotid lesions, and embolic protection, CAS is becoming increasingly safe. The SAPPHIRE trial proved that CAS is a reasonable alternative for CEA in patients at high risk for CEA. Subsequently, however, certain subgroups of patients have been identified as being at high risk for CAS. These categories need to be further defined and excluded from the CAS versus CEA trials to determine the similarity of these modalities or the superiority of one over the other. The recent CREST data support CAS as a reasonable alternative therapy to CEA for both symptomatic and asymptomatic carotid stenosis. Ultimately, it boils down to the fact that CAS and CEA should be considered as complementary therapies.

Table 32.8 A Simplified Algorithm for the Classification of Patients at High Risk for Carotid Artery Stenting

Patient-related

Recent symptoms

Age >80 years

On Coumadin therapy

Clopidogrel allergy

Access

Iliofemoral or aortic artery

1. Stenotic or occluded iliac arteries
2. Tortuous iliac or abdominal aorta
3. Occluded abdominal aorta

Arch

1. Arch type 2 or 3 anatomy
2. Bovine configuration
3. Arch disease (calcifications and plaque)

Supraaortic vessels

1. Origin disease
2. Tortuous proximal target vessels or trunk

Target vessel

1. Occluded ECA
2. Stenosis involving both ICA and ECA
3. Perilesional tortuosity

Landing zone difficulty

1. Tortuosity
2. Disease

Lesion characteristics

Severe and concentric calcification

Length >2 cm

Echolucent plaque

Intraluminal thrombus

Restenosis

Tandem intracranial lesions

Procedural

Duration of procedure >2 hours

Embolic dwell time >20 minute (the time during which the embolic protection device [EPD] is deployed)

Moreover, every patient should be evaluated for both therapies and the choice made after thorough performance of a risk-benefit analysis for the specific patient.

References

1. Lloyd-Jones D, Adams R, Carnethon M, et al; American Heart Association Statistics Committee and Stroke Statistics Subcommittee. Heart disease and stroke statistics—2009 update: a report from the American

Heart Association Statistics Committee and Stroke Statistics Subcommittee. Circulation 2009;119:e21–e181

2. North American Symptomatic Carotid Endarterectomy Trial Collaborators. Beneficial effect of carotid endarterectomy in symptomatic patients with high-grade carotid stenosis. N Engl J Med 1991;325:445–453

3. European Carotid Surgery Trialists' Collaborative Group. MRC European Carotid Surgery Trial: interim results for symptomatic patients with severe (70–99%) or with mild (0–29%) carotid stenosis. European Carotid Surgery Trialists' Collaborative Group. Lancet 1991;337:1235–1243

4. Endarterectomy for asymptomatic carotid artery stenosis. Executive Committee for the Asymptomatic Carotid Atherosclerosis Study. JAMA 1995;273:1421–1428 JAMA 1995;273:1421–1428

5. European Carotid Surgery Trialists' Collaborative Group. Randomised trial of endarterectomy for recently symptomatic carotid stenosis: final results of the MRC European Carotid Surgery Trial (ECST). Lancet 1998; 351:1379–1387

6. Barnett HJ, Taylor DW, Eliasziw M, et al. Benefit of carotid endarterectomy in patients with symptomatic moderate or severe stenosis. North American Symptomatic Carotid Endarterectomy Trial Collaborators. N Engl J Med 1998;339:1415–1425

7. Halliday A, Mansfield A, Marro J, et al; MRC Asymptomatic Carotid Surgery Trial (ACST) Collaborative Group. Prevention of disabling and fatal strokes by successful carotid endarterectomy in patients without recent neurological symptoms: randomised controlled trial. Lancet 2004; 363:1491–1502

8. Mathias K, Gospos C, Thron A, Ahmadi A, Mittermayer C. Percutaneous transluminal treatment of supraaortic artery obstruction. Ann Radiol (Paris) 1980;23:281–282

9. Diethrich EB, Ndiaye M, Reid DB. Stenting in the carotid artery: initial experience in 110 patients. J Endovasc Surg 1996;3:42–62

10. Jordan WD Jr, Voellinger DC, Fisher WS, Redden D, McDowell HA. A comparison of carotid angioplasty with stenting versus endarterectomy with regional anesthesia. J Vasc Surg 1998;28:397–402, discussion 402–403

11. Théron J, Courthéoux P, Alachkar F, Maiza D. Intravascular technics of cerebral revascularization. J Mal Vasc 1990;15:245–256

12. Yadav JS, Wholey MH, Kuntz RE, et al; Stenting and Angioplasty with Protection in Patients at High Risk for Endarterectomy Investigators. Protected carotid-artery stenting versus endarterectomy in high-risk patients. N Engl J Med 2004;351:1493–1501

13. Parodi JC, La Mura R, Ferreira LM, et al. Initial evaluation of carotid angioplasty and stenting with three different cerebral protection devices. J Vasc Surg 2000;32:1127–1136

14. Ohki T, Parodi J, Veith FJ, et al. Efficacy of a proximal occlusion catheter with reversal of flow in the prevention of embolic events during carotid artery stenting: an experimental analysis. J Vasc Surg 2001;33:504–509

15. Sacco RL, Adams R, Albers G, et al; American Heart Association; American Stroke Association Council on Stroke; Council on Cardiovascular Radiology and Intervention; American Academy of Neurology. Guidelines for prevention of stroke in patients with ischemic stroke or transient ischemic attack: a statement for healthcare professionals from the American Heart Association/American Stroke Association Council on Stroke: co-sponsored by the Council on Cardiovascular Radiology and Intervention: the American Academy of Neurology affirms the value of this guideline. Stroke 2006;37:577–617

16. Findlay JM, Tucker WS, Ferguson GG, Holness RO, Wallace MC, Wong JH. Guidelines for the use of carotid endarterectomy: current recommendations from the Canadian Neurosurgical Society. CMAJ 1997;157: 653–659

17. Moore WS, Barnett HJ, Beebe HG, et al. Guidelines for carotid endarterectomy. A multidisciplinary consensus statement from the ad hoc Committee, American Heart Association. Stroke 1995;26:188–201

18. CAVATAS Investigators. Endovascular versus surgical treatment in patients with carotid stenosis in the Carotid and Vertebral Artery Transluminal Angioplasty Study (CAVATAS): a randomised trial. Lancet 2001; 357:1729–1737

19. Bonati LH, Ederle J, McCabe DJH, et al; CAVATAS Investigators. Long-term risk of carotid restenosis in patients randomly assigned to endovascular treatment or endarterectomy in the Carotid and Vertebral Artery Transluminal Angioplasty Study (CAVATAS): long-term follow-up of a randomised trial. Lancet Neurol 2009;8:908–917

20. Ederle J, Bonati LH, Dobson J, et al; CAVATAS Investigators. Endovascular treatment with angioplasty or stenting versus endarterectomy in patients with carotid artery stenosis in the Carotid and Vertebral Artery Transluminal Angioplasty Study (CAVATAS): long-term follow-up of a randomised trial. Lancet Neurol 2009;8:898–907

21. Alberts MJ. Results of a multicenter prospective randomized trial of carotid artery stenting vs. carotid endarterectomy. (Abstract 53) Stroke 2001;32:325

22. Alberts MJ, McCann R, Smith TP, et al for the Schneider Wallstent Endoprosthesis Clinical Investigators. A randomized trial of carotid stenting vs. endarterectomy in patients with symptomatic carotid stenosis: study design. J Neurovasc Dis. 1997;2:228–234

23. CARESS Steering Committee. Carotid revascularization using endarterectomy or stenting systems (CARESS): phase I clinical trial. J Endovasc Ther 2003;10:1021–1030

24. CaRESS Steering Committee. Carotid Revascularization Using Endarterectomy or Stenting Systems (CaRESS) phase I clinical trial: 1-year results. J Vasc Surg 2005;42:213–219

25. Ringleb PA, Allenberg J, Brückmann H, et al; SPACE Collaborative Group. 30 day results from the SPACE trial of stent-protected angioplasty versus carotid endarterectomy in symptomatic patients: a randomised non-inferiority trial. Lancet 2006;368:1239–1247

26. Stingele R, Berger J, Alfke K, et al; SPACE investigators. Clinical and angiographic risk factors for stroke and death within 30 days after carotid endarterectomy and stent-protected angioplasty: a subanalysis of the SPACE study. Lancet Neurol 2008;7:216–222

27. Mas JL, Chatellier G, Beyssen B, et al; EVA-3S Investigators. Endarterectomy versus stenting in patients with symptomatic severe carotid stenosis. N Engl J Med 2006;355:1660–1671

28. Hopkins LN, Myla S, Grube E, et al. Carotid artery revascularization in high surgical risk patients with the NexStent and the Filterwire EX/EZ: 1-year results in the CABERNET trial. Catheter Cardiovasc Interv 2008; 71:950–960

29. Gray WA, Hopkins LN, Yadav S, et al; ARCHeR Trial Collaborators. Protected carotid stenting in high-surgical-risk patients: the ARCHeR results. J Vasc Surg 2006;44:258–268

30. Safian RD, Bresnahan JF, Jaff MR, et al; CREATE Pivotal Trial Investigators. Protected carotid stenting in high-risk patients with severe carotid artery stenosis. J Am Coll Cardiol 2006;47:2384–2389

31. Fairman R, Gray WA, Scicli AP, et al; for the CAPTURE Trial Collaborators. The CAPTURE registry: analysis of strokes resulting from carotid artery stenting in the post approval setting: timing, location, severity, and type. Ann Surg 2007;246:551–556, discussion 556–558

32. Gray WA, Yadav JS, Verta P, et al. The CAPTURE registry: results of carotid stenting with embolic protection in the post approval setting. Catheter Cardiovasc Interv 2007;69:341–348

33. White CJ, Iyer SS, Hopkins LN, Katzen BT, Russell ME; BEACH Trial Investigators. Carotid stenting with distal protection in high surgical risk patients: the BEACH trial 30 day results. Catheter Cardiovasc Interv 2006;67:503–512

34. Katzen BT, Criado FJ, Ramee SR, et al; CASES-PMS Investigators. Carotid artery stenting with emboli protection surveillance study: thirty-day results of the CASES-PMS study. Catheter Cardiovasc Interv 2007;70: 316–323

35. Zahn R, Roth E, Ischinger T, et al. Carotid artery stenting in clinical practice results from the Carotid Artery Stenting (CAS)-registry of the Arbeitsgemeinschaft Leitende Kardiologische Krankenhausarzte (ALKK). Z Kardiol 2005;94:163–172

36. Massop D, Dave R, Metzger C, et al; SAPPHIRE Worldwide Investigators. Stenting and angioplasty with protection in patients at high-risk for endarterectomy: SAPPHIRE Worldwide Registry first 2,001 patients. Catheter Cardiovasc Interv 2009;73:129–136

37. Hopkins LN, Myla SV, Grube E, et al. Carotid artery revascularisation in high-surgical-risk patients with the NexStent and the FilterWire EX/EZ: 3-year results from the CABERNET trial. EuroIntervention 2010;5:917–924

38. Kastrup A, Gröschel K, Krapf H, Brehm BR, Dichgans J, Schulz JB. Early outcome of carotid angioplasty and stenting with and without cerebral protection devices: a systematic review of the literature. Stroke 2003;34:813–819

39. Garg N, Karagiorgos N, Pisimisis GT, et al. Cerebral protection devices reduce periprocedural strokes during carotid angioplasty and stenting: a systematic review of the current literature. J Endovasc Ther 2009; 16:412–427

40. Hobson RW II, Howard VJ, Roubin GS, et al; CREST. Credentialing of surgeons as interventionalists for carotid artery stenting: experience from the lead-in phase of CREST. J Vasc Surg 2004;40:952–957

41. Howard VJ, Brott TG, Qureshi AI, et al for the CREST Investigators. Gender and periprocedural stroke and death following carotid artery stenting: results from the CREST lead-in phase. (Abstract P5) Stroke 2004; 35:253

42. Roubin GS, Brott TG, Hopkins LN. for the CREST Investigators. Developing embolic protection for carotid stenting in the Carotid Revascularization Endarterectomy vs Stenting Trial (CREST). (Abstract 3124) Circulation 2003;108(suppl 4):IV-687

43. Hobson RW II, Howard VJ, Roubin GS, et al; CREST Investigators. Carotid artery stenting is associated with increased complications in octoge-

narians: 30-day stroke and death rates in the CREST lead-in phase. J Vasc Surg 2004;40:1106–1111

44. Howard G, Hobson RW II, Brott TG. for the CREST Investigators. Does the stroke risk of stenting increase at older ages? thirty-day stroke death rates in the CREST lead-in phase. (Abstract 2116) Circulation 2003; 8(suppl 4):V-461

45. Featherstone RL, Brown MM, Coward LJ; ICSS Investigators. International carotid stenting study: protocol for a randomised clinical trial comparing carotid stenting with endarterectomy in symptomatic carotid artery stenosis. Cerebrovasc Dis 2004;18:69–74

46. Carotid stenting vs. surgery of severe carotid artery disease and stroke prevention in asymptomatic patients (ACT I). http://www.clinicaltrials.gov/ct/show/NCT00106938?order=1

47. Katzen B. The Transatlantic Asymptomatic Carotid Intervention Trial. Endovascular Today. 2005;1:49–50

48. Clair DG, Hopkins LN, Mehta M, et al; EMPiRE Clinical Study Investigators. Neuroprotection during carotid artery stenting using the GORE flow reversal system: 30-day outcomes in the EMPiRE Clinical Study. Catheter Cardiovasc Interv 2011;77(3):420–429

49. Myla S, Bacharach JM, Ansel GM, Dippel EJ, McCormick DJ, Popma JJ. Carotid artery stenting in high surgical risk patients using the FiberNet embolic protection system: the EPIC trial results. Catheter Cardiovasc Interv 2010;75(6):817–822

50. Ansel GM, Hopkins LN, Jaff MR, et al. Safety and effectiveness of the INVATEC HYPERLINK "http://MO.MA" \o "http://mo.ma/" MO.MA proximal cerebral protection device during carotid artery stenting: results from the ARMOUR pivotal trial. Catheter Cardiovasc Interv 2010;76: 1–8.

51. U.S. Food and Drug Administration. http://www.accessdata.fda.gov/scripts/cdrh/cfdocs/cftopic/pma/pma.cfm?num=p040012, 2004

52. Centers for Medicare & Medicaid Services. Medicare Coverage Database: Decision memo for carotid artery stenting (CAG-00085R).http://www.cms.hhs.gov/mcd/viewdecisionmemo.asp?id=157

53. White CJ, Anderson HV, Brindis RG, et al. The Carotid Artery Revascularization and Endarterectomy (CARE) registry: objectives, design, and implications. Catheter Cardiovasc Interv 2008;71:721–725

54. Gray WA, Chaturvedi S, Verta P; Investigators and the Executive Committees. Thirty-day outcomes for carotid artery stenting in 6320 patients from 2 prospective, multicenter, high-surgical-risk registries. Circ Cardiovasc Interv 2009;2:159–166

55. Jeffrey S. EXACT/CAPTURE-2: Postmarketing Carotid Stent Registry data. Medscape http://www.medscape.com/viewarticle/554613, 2007

56. Gurm HS, Yadav JS, Fayad P, et al; SAPPHIRE Investigators. Long-term results of carotid stenting versus endarterectomy in high-risk patients. N Engl J Med 2008;358:1572–1579

57. Norris JW, Zhu CZ, Bornstein NM, Chambers BR. Vascular risks of asymptomatic carotid stenosis. Stroke 1991;22:1485–1490

58. Turk AS, Chaudry I, Haughton VM, et al. Effect of carotid artery stenting on cognitive function in patients with carotid artery stenosis: preliminary results. AJNR Am J Neuroradiol 2008;29:265–268

59. Mlekusch W, Mlekusch I, Haumer M, et al. Improvement of neurocognitive function after protected carotid stenting. Catheter Cardiovasc Interv 2008;71:114–119

60. Lam JY, Chesebro JH, Steele PM, Dewanjee MK, Badimon L, Fuster V. Deep arterial injury during experimental angioplasty: relation to a positive indium-111-labeled platelet scintigram, quantitative platelet deposition and mural thrombosis. J Am Coll Cardiol 1986;8:1380–1386

61. Bosiers M, de Donato G, Deloose K, et al. Does free cell area influence the outcome in carotid artery stenting? Eur J Vasc Endovasc Surg 2007; 33:135–141, discussion 142–143

62. Hart JP, Peeters P, Verbist J, Deloose K, Bosiers M. Do device characteristics impact outcome in carotid artery stenting? J Vasc Surg 2006;44: 725–730, discussion 730–731

63. Wholey MH, Finol EA. Designing the ideal stent. Endovascular Today. 2007;6:25–34

64. Biasi GM, Froio A, Diethrich EB, et al. Carotid plaque echolucency increases the risk of stroke in carotid stenting: the Imaging in Carotid Angioplasty and Risk of Stroke (ICAROS) study. Circulation 2004;110: 756–762

65. Theron JG, Payelle GG, Coskun O, Huet HF, Guimaraens L. Carotid artery stenosis: treatment with protected balloon angioplasty and stent placement. Radiology 1996;201:627–636

66. Théron J, Cosgrove R, Melanson D, Ethier R. Embolization with temporary balloon occlusion of the internal carotid or vertebral arteries. Neuroradiology 1986;28:246–253

67. Henry M, Polydorou A, Henry I, et al. New distal embolic protection device the FiberNet 3 dimensional filter: first carotid human study. Catheter Cardiovasc Interv 2007;69:1026–1035

68. El-Koussy M, Schroth G, Do DD, et al. Periprocedural embolic events related to carotid artery stenting detected by diffusion-weighted MRI: comparison between proximal and distal embolus protection devices. J Endovasc Ther 2007;14:293–303

69. Kang HS, Han MH, Kwon OK, Kwon BJ, Kim SH, Oh CW. Intracranial hemorrhage after carotid angioplasty: a pooled analysis. J Endovasc Ther 2007;14:77–85

70. Setacci C, Pula G, Baldi I, et al. Determinants of in-stent restenosis after carotid angioplasty: a case-control study. J Endovasc Ther 2003;10: 1031–1038

71. Levy EI, Hanel RA, Lau T, et al. Frequency and management of recurrent stenosis after carotid artery stent implantation. J Neurosurg 2005;102: 29–37

72. Ecker RD, Pichelmann MA, Meissner I, Meyer FB. Durability of carotid endarterectomy. Stroke 2003;34:2941–2944

73. Eckstein HH, Ringleb P, Allenberg JR, et al. Results of the Stent-Protected Angioplasty versus Carotid Endarterectomy (SPACE) study to treat symptomatic stenoses at 2 years: a multinational, prospective, randomised trial. Lancet Neurol 2008;7:893–902

74. Mas JL, Trinquart L, Leys D, et al; EVA-3S investigators. Endarterectomy Versus Angioplasty in Patients with Symptomatic Severe Carotid Stenosis (EVA-3S) trial: results up to 4 years from a randomised, multicentre trial. Lancet Neurol 2008;7:885–892

75. Goldstein LB, McCrory DC, Landsman PB, et al. Multicenter review of preoperative risk factors for carotid endarterectomy in patients with ipsilateral symptoms. Stroke 1994;25:1116–1121

76. Ouriel K, Hertzer NR, Beven EG, et al. Preprocedural risk stratification: identifying an appropriate population for carotid stenting. J Vasc Surg 2001;33:728–732

77. Ballotta E, Renon L, Da Giau G, Barbon B, Terranova O, Baracchini C. Octogenarians with contralateral carotid artery occlusion: a cohort at higher risk for carotid endarterectomy? J Vasc Surg 2004;39:1003–1008

78. Reed AB, Gaccione P, Belkin M, et al. Preoperative risk factors for carotid endarterectomy: defining the patient at high risk. J Vasc Surg 2003;37: 1191–1199

79. Villalobos HJ, Harrigan MR, Lau T, et al. Advancements in carotid stenting leading to reductions in perioperative morbidity among patients 80 years and older. Neurosurgery 2006;58:233–240, discussion 233–240

80. Meyer FB, ed. Sundt's Occlusive Cerebrovascular Disease, 2nd ed. Philadelphia: WB Saunders, 2004

81. Pritz MB. Timing of carotid endarterectomy after stroke. Stroke 1997; 28:2563–2567

82. Stanziale SF, Marone LK, Boules TN, et al. Carotid artery stenting in octogenarians is associated with increased adverse outcomes. J Vasc Surg 2006;43:297–304

83. Chiam PT, Roubin GS, Iyer SS, et al. Carotid artery stenting in elderly patients: importance of case selection. Catheter Cardiovasc Interv 2008; 72:318–324

84. Henry M, Henry I, Polydorou A, Hugel M. Carotid angioplasty and stenting in octogenarians: is it safe? Catheter Cardiovasc Interv 2008;72:309–317

85. Velez CA, White CJ, Reilly JP, et al. Carotid artery stent placement is safe in the very elderly (> or =80 years). Catheter Cardiovasc Interv 2008; 72:303–308

86. Lam RC, Lin SC, DeRubertis B, Hynecek R, Kent KC, Faries PL. The impact of increasing age on anatomic factors affecting carotid angioplasty and stenting. J Vasc Surg 2007;45:875–880

87. Kastrup A, Gröschel K, Schnaudigel S, Nägele T, Schmidt F, Ernemann U. Target lesion ulceration and arch calcification are associated with increased incidence of carotid stenting-associated ischemic lesions in octogenarians. J Vasc Surg 2008;47:88–95

88. Lin SC, Trocciola SM, Rhee J, et al. Analysis of anatomic factors and age in patients undergoing carotid angioplasty and stenting. Ann Vasc Surg 2005;19:798–804

89. Faggioli GL, Ferri M, Freyrie A, et al. Aortic arch anomalies are associated with increased risk of neurological events in carotid stent procedures. Eur J Vasc Endovasc Surg 2007;33:436–441

90. Faggioli G, Ferri M, Gargiulo M, et al. Measurement and impact of proximal and distal tortuosity in carotid stenting procedures. J Vasc Surg 2007;46:1119–1124

91. Sayeed S, Stanziale SF, Wholey MH, Makaroun MS. Angiographic lesion characteristics can predict adverse outcomes after carotid artery stenting. J Vasc Surg 2008;47:81–87

92. Ecker RD, Tummala RP, Levy EI, Hopkins LN. "Internal cross-clamping" for symptomatic internal carotid artery thrombus. Report of two cases. J Neurosurg 2007;107:1223–1227

93. Tummala RP, Jahromi BS, Yamamoto J, Levy EI, Siddiqui AH, Hopkins LN. Carotid artery stenting under flow arrest for the management of intraluminal thrombus: technical case report. Neurosurgery 2008;63(1, Suppl 1)ONSE87-8, discussion E88

94. Parodi JC, Ferreira LM, Sicard G, La Mura R, Fernandez S. Cerebral protection during carotid stenting using flow reversal. J Vasc Surg 2005; 41:416–422

95. Goldstein LB, Samsa GP, Matchar DB, Oddone EZ. Multicenter review of preoperative risk factors for endarterectomy for asymptomatic carotid artery stenosis. Stroke 1998;29:750–753

96. Bates ER, Babb JD, Casey DE Jr, et al; American College of Cardiology Foundation; American Society of Interventional & Therapeutic Neuroradiology; Society for Cardiovascular Angiography and Interventions; Society for Vascular Medicine and Biology; Society of Interventional Radiology. ACCF/SCAI/SVMB/SIR/ASITN 2007 clinical expert consensus document on carotid stenting: a report of the American College of Cardiology Foundation Task Force on Clinical Expert Consensus Documents (ACCF/SCAI/SVMB/SIR/ASITN Clinical Expert Consensus Document Committee on Carotid Stenting). J Am Coll Cardiol 2007;49:126–170

97. Zarins CK, White RA, Diethrich EB, Shackelton RJ, Siami FS; CaRESS Steering Committee and CaRESS Investigators. Carotid revascularization using endarterectomy or stenting systems (CaRESS): 4-year outcomes. J Endovasc Ther 2009;16:397–409

98. Brott TG, Hobson RW II, Howard G, et al; CREST Investigators. Stenting versus endarterectomy for treatment of carotid-artery stenosis. N Engl J Med 2010;363(1):11–23

33

Management of Vertebral Artery Origin Stenosis

John C. Dalfino and Alan S. Boulos

Pearls

- Most posterior circulation strokes are embolic, not hemo-dynamic.
- The first-line treatment of vertebral artery stenosis is usually medical, using a combination of antiplatelet agents, statins, and risk factor reduction.
- Endovascular revascularization should be considered for symptomatic lesions with greater than 50% stenosis in patients who fail medical management.
- The use of balloon-mounted, medicated stents may help prevent restenosis after endovascular vertebral artery origin revascularization.
- Distal embolic protection during angioplasty and stenting of the vertebral artery origin may reduce the risk of embolic complications.

The vertebral artery (VA) origin is the most common site of atherosclerosis in the posterior circulation. Artery-to-artery emboli from VA-origin lesions are responsible for most posterior circulation strokes. The management of VA-origin stenosis (VAOS) is usually medical, consisting of antiplatelet agents, statins, and lifestyle modification. In patients who fail medical management, surgical revascularization procedures such as vertebral endarterectomy and transposition can help improve flow and reduce the risk of emboli to the posterior circulation, but these procedures are associated with potentially significant surgical morbidity.

Endovascular interventions such as angioplasty and stenting offer an alternative, minimally invasive way to open a stenotic vertebral artery origin. Although the long-term patency of these interventions is still being examined, the technology and techniques used to treat these lesions is continually evolving. This chapter discusses the natural history of vertebral origin stenosis, presents the available treatment options, and describes the indications and techniques used for endovascular treatment of these lesions.

◆ Epidemiology

Due to the difficulty of imaging the VA origin noninvasively, the incidence of VAOS in the general population has not been determined. In patients with vascular risk factors, approximately 2% will have VAOS and nearly 7% will have one occluded or congenitally absent VA.[1] In patients who have sustained a posterior circulation stroke or transient ischemic attack (TIA), over 30% will have a high-grade lesion of one or both VA origins. Overall, nearly 10% of all posterior circulation strokes can be attributed to VAOS.[2]

◆ Risk Factors

The New England Medical Center Posterior Circulation Registry[2] identified hypertension (75%), smoking (50%), and coronary artery disease (48%) as the most common risk factors shared among patients with VAOS. Other risk factors associated with peripheral vascular disease, such as diabetes and hyperlipidemia, were less frequently associated with VAOS.[2,3] It has been observed that VAOS is more common in Caucasian men than in other demographic groups.[4]

◆ Presentation

In greater than 90% of cases, VAOS causes posterior circulation strokes by artery-to-artery embolization. Common ischemic symptoms associated with extracranial VA disease include vertigo, diplopia, vision loss, perioral paresthesias, tinnitus, headache, and ataxia.[5] Symptoms are often vague, overlooked, or attributed to a more benign disease process. Catastrophic strokes from large emboli can result in hemiparesis, locked-in syndrome, coma, or death. Less commonly, patients with VAOS can experience posterior circulation TIA symptoms related to transient relative posterior circulation hypoperfusion. In these patients, orthostatic hypotension and anatomic obstructions may incite or exacerbate symptoms.

◆ Natural History

Isolated, asymptomatic atherosclerotic lesions of VA origin may have a benign natural history.[3] Moufarrij and colleagues[3] followed 89 patients with VAOS for an average of 4.6 years. During that time only two patients had a posterior circulation stroke. On the other hand, the 5-year survival rate of these patients was only 60% compared with 87% for age-matched controls. The increased mortality of VAOS patients in this series was attributed to a greater degree of generalized vascular disease, with most patients dying from either cardiac disease (53%) or anterior circulation hemispheric strokes (20%).

Considering the literature on symptomatic carotid lesions, it might be assumed that symptomatic lesions of VA origin might have a more aggressive course than asymptomatic lesions. There is no definitive literature, however, supporting that assumption. The Carotid and Vertebral Artery Transluminal Angioplasty Study (CAVATAS)[6] is the only randomized trial to date comparing endovascular treatment of symptomatic VA stenosis to medical treatment. In a mean follow-up of 4.7 years, not a single patient in either treatment arm had a posterior circulation stroke. The authors concluded that even symptomatic VAOS may have a benign course and that endovascular treatment was not shown to be superior to medical management.[7]

◆ Medical Treatment of Vertebral Origin Stenosis

Blood Pressure Management

There is strong evidence that even a modest reduction of systemic hypertension can substantially reduce the risk of secondary stroke. For instance, in the PROGRESS (Perindopril pROtection aGainst REcurrent Stroke Study) trial, a combination of an angiotensin-converting enzyme (ACE) inhibitor with a thiazide diuretic resulted in a decrease in the average blood pressure by 12/5 and reduced the risk of recurrent stroke by 43%.[7]

Patients with acute stroke often present with hypertension that slowly resolves over the first 24 to 48 hours. Castillo et al[8] observed that the average blood pressure during the first 24 hours of stroke has a U-shaped effect on outcome, with the best outcomes associated with a systolic blood pressure of 180 mm Hg. Patients with blood pressures 20 mm Hg higher or lower than 180 mm Hg had substantially larger stoke volumes and worse neurologic outcomes. Based on these observations, acutely lowering the systolic blood pressure below 180 mm Hg is not recommended during the first 24 hours after a stroke. However, it is important to consider lowering systolic blood pressure below 180 mm Hg in patients receiving intravenous thrombolytics, as blood pressures over 185/110 mm Hg have been associated with a significant increase in cerebral hemorrhage.[9]

Statins

There are two large trials that suggest that the use of a statin can reduce the risk of both primary and secondary stroke. In the Heart Protection Study (HPS), 20,536 patients with stroke risk factors such as hypertension, vascular disease, and diabetes were randomly assigned to receive 40 mg of simvastatin or placebo. At the end of the 5-year follow-up period, the risk of primary stroke was 25% lower in the treatment group. In the Stroke Prevention by Aggressive Reduction in Cholesterol Levels (SPARCL) trial,[10] patients with a history of stroke or TIA within 6 months were randomly assigned to treatment with either 80 mg of atorvastatin or placebo. In the 5-year follow-up period there was an 18% relative reduction in the risk of secondary stroke in patients treated with atorvastatin. Interestingly, there was an increase in the relative risk of hemorrhagic stroke among statin users that was not observed in the HPS trial.

Based on the data from these two studies, statins should be used in all patients with risk factors for ischemic stroke including VAOS. Statins, in addition to lowering total body cholesterol, may help stabilize plaque, halt or reverse atherosclerosis, and improve arterial endothelial function. In addition, statins significantly lower the risk of cardiac events in patients with vascular risk factors, a major source of morbidity and mortality in this patient population.

◆ Revascularization of Vertebral Artery Origin Stenosis

Surgical Revascularization

In experienced hands, VA revascularization can be done with acceptable risk.[11] Perioperative mortality and stroke during revascularization is uncommon (<2%).[11] Nevertheless, surgical morbidity from these procedures is common. In a recent series of 29 patients who underwent proximal VA revascularization either by transposition or endarterectomy, 48% of patients sustained some sort of surgical approach morbidity such as Horner's syndrome, recurrent laryngeal nerve injury, or chylothorax.[12] Despite its high morbidity rate, surgical revascularization is still a reasonable option in patients who fail medical management and who are poor candidates for an endovascular approach. It is also notable that surgical revascularization carries an 80% 5-year patency rate,[11] considerably better than what has been reported in most endovascular series to date.

◆ Endovascular Revascularization of Vertebral Artery Origin Stenosis

Patient Preparation

Vertebral artery origin atherosclerosis, like carotid artery disease, is often a marker of systemic vascular disease. Not surprisingly, the cause of death in most VAOS patients, even symptomatic ones, is cardiac disease. A careful history and physical examination often uncover other health issues such as congestive heart failure or angina that may require additional workup, optimization, and planning prior to an invasive procedure. Palpation of the femoral and peripheral pulses, including an Allen test, helps to identify potential problems with percutaneous access. Physiologic testing of heart function is often important in preoperative preparation before a stent is placed.

Imaging

Noninvasive Vessel Imaging

The diagnosis of VAOS is usually made on the basis of noninvasive vessel imaging. Color duplex imaging can diagnose lesions at the vertebral artery origin,[13] but does not provide the anatomic detail required for planning a revascularization procedure. Computed tomography angiography (CTA) and magnetic resonance angiography (MRA) are also capable of visualizing the VA origin. A comparison of various noninvasive imaging techniques[14] determined that contrast-enhanced MRA is more sensitive and specific than CTA in evaluating VAOS. In practice, however, noninvasive imaging is often marred by artifact from tissue and bone in the chest wall and calcifications within the atherosclerotic plaque.

Perfusion Imaging

The role of perfusion imaging in the management of VAOS remains undefined. Because most patients have redundant blood supply to the basilar artery from the contralateral VA, it is relatively uncommon for patients with VA stenosis to have a hemodynamic stroke. Rather, most posterior circulation strokes are due to artery-to-artery emboli from the plaque itself. Perfusion imaging is potentially useful in patients with a hypoplastic or stenotic contralateral VA if a hemodynamic syndrome is suspected. Nevertheless, only a handful of case reports in the literature describe the use and utility of computed tomography (CT) perfusion imaging in the posterior circulation.

Diagnostic Angiography

A complete diagnostic cerebral angiogram often yields information helpful in medical decision making. The goals of angiography include the following:

◆ Visualizing and measuring the degree of stenosis and tortuosity of the VA origin

◆ Characterizing collateral flow pathways to the posterior circulation

◆ Finding suitable donor and recipient vessels for open surgical bypass in the event that endovascular revascularization fails

◆ Identifying anatomic variants or other vascular lesions that might contribute to posterior circulation ischemia.

Antiplatelet Agents

All patients being prepared for VA stent placement require dual antiplatelet therapy, usually with aspirin and clopidogrel. In patients undergoing elective procedures the patient is started on 75 mg of clopidogrel and 325 mg of aspirin 1 week prior to the procedure. Based on the American College of Surgery (ACS) literature, patients who require more urgent treatment should be loaded with 300 mg of clopidogrel at least 8 hours prior to stenting. Alternatively, 600 mg of clopidogrel at least 3 hours prior to the procedure is effective.[15] Platelet aggregation studies may be useful in identifying patients who may be nonresponders to aspirin or clopidogrel, although they are not routinely available in all centers and their utility remains controversial.

Anesthesia

Vertebral artery origin stenting can often be performed with the patient under moderate conscious sedation. Although most patients tolerate VA-origin angioplasty and stenting under conscious sedation, it is not the best choice in all patients. General anesthesia should be considered for patients with congestive heart failure (CHF), dementia, or even severe lumbar spine disease who cannot lie flat comfortably for at least 1 hour. General anesthesia with neurophysiologic monitoring may also be a good choice for patients with poor collateral flow who may not tolerate temporary occlusion of the VA during angioplasty. If general anesthesia is selected, then somatosensory evoked potentials (SSEPs), motor evoked potentials (MEPs), and electroencephalogram (EEG) monitoring are an option to assess the presence of ischemia. A blood pressure cuff should be placed on the ipsilateral arm, so that it can be inflated during the subclavian injections to improve visualization of the VA if necessary.

Puncture

The most convenient access point is generally the common femoral artery, although radial or brachial access can be used if femoral access is impossible or the VA anatomy is not favorable for a femoral approach. Often, patients with VA stenosis have other manifestations of peripheral vascular disease (**Fig. 33.1**). A 6-French (F), 10- or 25-cm groin sheath is usually sufficient for access if a guide catheter will be used. In patients with very tortuous anatomy an 80-cm Raabe guide sheath (Cook Medical, Bloomington, IN) parked just proximal to the VA origin in the subclavian artery provides additional support.

Intravenous heparin (usually 70 units/kg) is given to all patients after arterial access is secured. The activated clotting time (ACT) is measured with a Hemochron ACT analyzer (ITC Nexus Dx, Edison, NJ) 15 minutes after heparin administration. Patients are re-bolused with intravenous heparin hourly as needed to maintain the ACT between 250 and 300 seconds.[16]

Guide Catheter Placement

A 6F guide catheter (or guide sheath) on a continuous heparinized saline flush is navigated into the subclavian artery

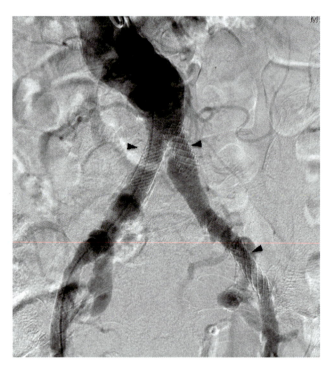

Fig. 33.1 Distal aortic runoff demonstrating extensive aortic and iliac atherosclerosis in a patient with vertebral origin stenosis. Despite the stents in the iliac and femoral arteries *(black arrowheads)*, percutaneous access was obtained via the right common femoral artery.

just proximal to the VA origin. A preprocedure angiogram of the entire length of the VA should be performed to verify balloon and stent measurements as well as to identify more distal disease. Cerebral angiography should also be performed to assess blood flow and define the baseline anatomy should an embolus occur.

On occasion, aortic arch anatomy may not provide adequate support for the guide catheter in the proximal subclavian artery. If this occurs, a "buddy wire" can provide additional support. In this technique an 0.018- or 0.014-inch wire is passed through the guide sheath and into the brachial artery. The wire is then left in place throughout the procedure to help prevent the guide catheter from slipping back into the arch **(Fig. 33.2).** A guide catheter can also be passed through a guide sheath in a coaxial arrangement to improve stability if necessary.

Measurements

Measurements of the degree and length of the stenosis, as well as the normal caliber of the artery distal to the lesion, guide the selection of the appropriate balloon(s).

Using the CAVATAS trial method as a guide, the degree of stenosis is defined by the following formula **(Fig. 33.3):**

$$\text{Percent stenosis} = 100\,(1 - A/V)$$

where A = Diameter of lumen at point of maximum stenosis
V = Diameter of VA distal to lesion where walls are parallel.

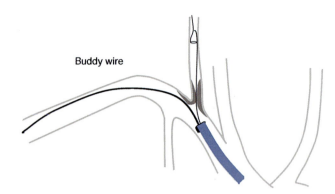

Fig. 33.2 Use of a buddy wire can help to stabilize the guide catheter in the subclavian artery. A 300-cm, 0.014- or 0.018-inch wire is generally used.

Choosing a Stent

There are no stents specifically designed for the VA origin. The well-developed muscularis layer of the VA origin requires a stent with high radial force. In many cases, balloon-mounted coronary stents are appropriate as they have adequate radial force, a low crossing profile, and track well through tortuous vessels. Most importantly, they can be placed precisely. Peripheral stents can be used in vessels that are too large for a coronary stent (generally greater than 4 mm). Both monorail and over-the-wire systems are suitable for VA-origin stenting. For the solo interventionist, a monorail system allows the use of standard-length wires, making the procedure less cumbersome. The diameter of a balloon-mounted stent should be the same size as the normal VA just distal to the lesion.

In the Stenting of Symptomatic Atherosclerotic Lesions in the Vertebral or Intracranial Arteries (SSYLVIA) study and other retrospective series, a high restenosis rate was identified after balloon-mounted stent placement. Therefore, antiproliferative drug-eluting coronary stents have been used to reduce the risk of restenosis at the VA origin.[17–19] Tacrolimus-, paclitaxel-, and sirolimus-coated stents have been successfully deployed at the VA origin.[17–21] In a series of 12 consecutive patients, Akins et al[21] showed that the restenosis rate for bare stents at the VA origin was 43% (3/7) compared with 0% (0/5) for tacrolimus-coated stents. Currently, however, there are no randomized data comparing the rate of restenosis of bare and drug-eluting stents at the VA origin. In addition, drug-eluting coronary stents only go to 4.5 mm, so vessels larger than that are not appropriate candidates for these particular stents.

Self-expanding stents can be used successfully in the VA origin, particularly when combined with a post-stent angioplasty. Self-expanding stents, which are made from memory metal alloys, are more resistant to permanent mechanical deformation than balloon expandable stents. In cases where a balloon-mounted stent has been kinked or compressed, re-stenting across the lesion with a self-expanding stent

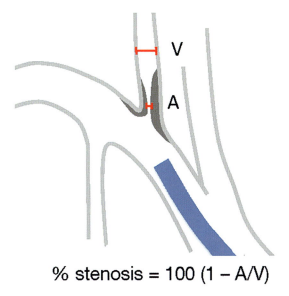

$$\% \text{ stenosis} = 100 \ (1 - A/V)$$

Fig. 33.3 The degree of stenosis was calculated in the Carotid and Vertebral Artery Transluminal Angioplasty Study (CAVATAS) trial using the formula shown at left, in which *V* is the reference diameter and *A* is the diameter of the vessel at the area of greatest stenosis. The diameter of a balloon-mounted stent should be no more than 10% larger than the reference vessel diameter. Self-expanding stents, conversely, should oversized by 1 to 2 mm to prevent the stent from migrating after deployment. A stent should be long enough to span the entire atherosclerotic lesion and protrude 2 to 3 mm into the subclavian artery to cover plaque at the vessel origin.

can help to restore the vessel lumen and provide a durable repair.

A self-expanding stent should be oversized by at least 0.5 to 1 mm to keep it snug against the vessel wall. The length of the stent should be approximately 7 to 9 mm longer than the stenotic segment to make sure the entire lesion is covered. Ideally, the stent will extend a few millimeters proximally into the subclavian artery to cover plaque around the vertebral os. Care should be taken not to let the stent extend more than 2 to 3 mm into the subclavian artery, however, as this will make reaccessing the stent in the future more difficult. Self-expanding stents are more difficult to place as precisely as balloon-expandable stents, so they should be sized longer to accommodate this potential inaccuracy. Allowing the stent to be positioned too far into the subclavian artery may also make removing the distal protection device difficult at the end of the procedure **(Fig. 33.4).**

Choosing Balloons

An appropriately sized semicompliant monorail balloon is generally sufficient for VA-origin angioplasty. The diameter of the balloon should be between 80 and 100% of the diameter of the normal vessel distal to the lesion. Using oversized balloons may result in catastrophic vessel injury and should be avoided. The balloon should generally be as long as the stent that will be used, to prevent the balloon from slipping or "watermelon seeding" out of the lesion during inflation. Compliant balloons are not recommended for angioplasty procedures because they do not generate enough outward radial force.

Unlike de novo atherosclerotic lesions, restenosis after angioplasty and stenting is due to intimal hyperplasia. These lesions are typically resistant to traditional balloon angioplasty because the thickened intimal layer causes the vessel

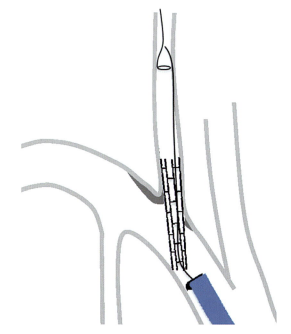

Fig. 33.4 Stenting too far into the subclavian artery makes removing the distal protection device difficult and may make reaccessing the lesion difficult.

to recoil once the balloon is deflated. Recoil can be reduced with the use of a cutting balloon, a semicompliant balloon with a series of three or four longitudinally mounted blades called atherotomes permanently mounted on its surface. During inflation, the blades score the intima (and plaque) in a controlled manner to help prevent vessel recoil after balloon deflation. The blades also reduce the balloon inflation pressure required to dilate the vessel, potentially reducing the deep vessel injury and postangioplasty inflammation that leads to neointimal proliferation and restenosis. Cutting balloon angioplasty can also be performed with care in patients with balloon-resistant de novo lesions, particularly if they have medical or anatomic contraindications to stenting.

Stepwise Stent Deployment

1. Cross the lesion. Anatomy permitting, the VA origin can usually be crossed directly with the distal protection device (**Fig. 33.5**). Careful shaping of the wire tip will aid will aid in navigating the lead wire through the vessel lumen. In patients with tortuous anatomy or a tight stenosis, consider crossing the lesion with a small microcatheter and 300-cm microwire to define a path for the filter wire through the lesion. The filter wire can then be passed through the lesion alongside the microwire. In the event that the distal protection device causes a vessel dissection or rupture, access to the true lumen is maintained by the microwire.

2. Pre-dilate the lesion (if necessary). In lesions with a lumen size <1.5 mm, pre-dilation with an undersized balloon facilitates passing a balloon-mounted or self-expanding stent through the stenotic segment. Pre-stent angioplasty also creates a more even surface for the stent to expand against during deployment, allowing the stent to be positioned more precisely. Usually a 2.0- or 2.5-mm balloon long enough to span the lesion is sufficient (**Fig. 33.6**).

3. Deploy the stent. A balloon-expandable, drug-eluting cardiac stent helps avoid restenosis. The stent should be long enough to deploy 4 to 5 mm distal to the lesion and should extend 2 to 3 mm into the subclavian artery (**Fig. 33.7**). When using a balloon-mounted stent, the balloon can be pulled back slightly and reinflated to a larger diameter to flare out the proximal tines of the stent in the subclavian artery. This facilitates reaccessing the stent in the future if necessary (**Fig. 33.8**).

4. Perform post-stent angioplasty (if necessary). The balloon diameter should be the same as the diameter of the lumen of the nondiseased VA distal to the lesion. Balloon inflation outside the stent within the VA should be avoided, as this may injure the vessel and has been associated with restenosis in the cardiac literature. In addition to enlarging the lumen of the artery, a stent often straightens out kinks that might be contributing to turbulent flow (**Fig. 33.9**).

5. Remove the distal protection device. Care must be taken not to dislodge the stent during device removal. If the retrieval catheter will not advance through the stent, the guide catheter can often be advanced through the stent to

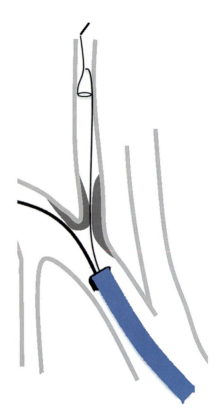

Fig. 33.5 A distal protection device can be used in vessels greater than 2.25 mm. Over-the-wire distal embolic protection devices such as the SpideRx (ev3 Endovascular, Plymouth, MN) can be deployed over any 0.014-inch microwire to help make crossing the lesion easier.

make recovering the filter easier. If advancing the guide catheter through the stent is not possible, the filter can often be retrieved using a more flexible 3.5F or 4F long diagnostic catheter.

Restenosis After Angioplasty and Stenting

Restenosis of VA-origin lesions after endovascular treatment is common. In a series of 33 patients with VAOS treated by angioplasty and stenting, Albuquerque et al[22] noted a 43% rate of in-stent restenosis after a mean follow-up period of 16 months. In-stent stenosis can be effectively treated with cutting balloon angioplasty, but reaccessing the lumen of the VA through the existing stent can be difficult. To facilitate reaccess, ending the stent on a turn or allowing the stent to protrude too far into the subclavian artery should be avoided. This is particularly important when using a closed cell design stent where wire access through the tines of the stent may be difficult or impossible.

◆ Complications Avoidance

◆ Many VAOS patients have concurrent cardiovascular and peripheral vascular disease. Consider additional medical

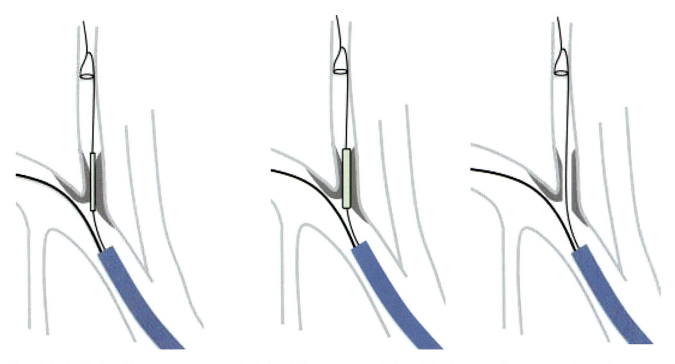

Fig. 33.6 Pre-dilation of the stenotic segment with a balloon helps to create a path through the plaque to make it easier to advance the stent. Pre-dilation also creates a smooth bed in the plaque for the stent to lie across during deployment.

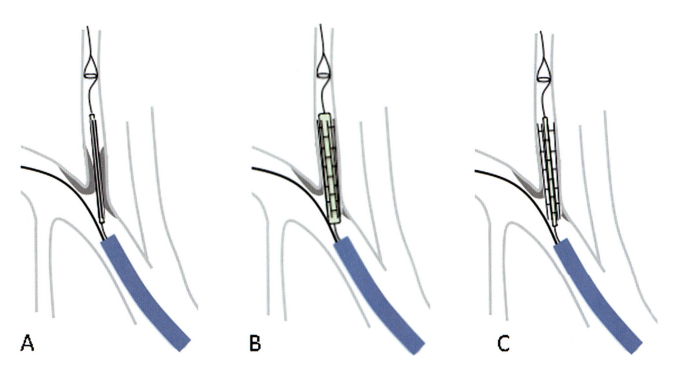

A   B   C

Fig. 33.7 Deploying a balloon-mounted stent involves the following steps: **(A)** navigating to the lesion; **(B)** inflating the balloon to deploy the stent; and **(C)** deflating the balloon and leaving the stent in place.

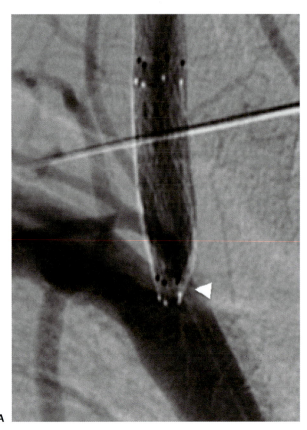
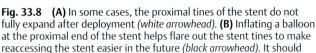

A

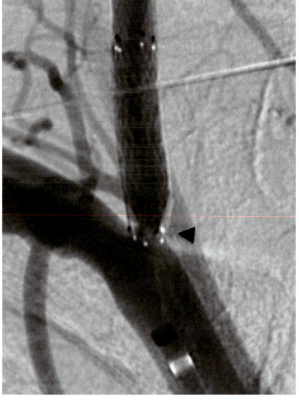

B

Fig. 33.8 **(A)** In some cases, the proximal tines of the stent do not fully expand after deployment *(white arrowhead)*. **(B)** Inflating a balloon at the proximal end of the stent helps flare out the stent tines to make reaccessing the stent easier in the future *(black arrowhead)*. It should be noted that the self-expanding stent used in this case was deployed slightly too distal in the vertebral artery (VA). This was due to the stent advancing forward during the final stage of deployment, a common problem with self-expanding stents.

screening prior to intervention to avoid perioperative myocardial infarction (MI), CHF, or renal failure.

◆ Preprocedural antiplatelet therapy, intraprocedural anticoagulation, the use of an appropriately sized distal protection device, and good catheter hygiene are critical to preventing ischemic events.

◆ Choose a balloon diameter that is 80 to 100% of the vessel lumen diameter to avoid dissection or rupture.

◆ Consider crossing the lesion with "buddy" wire in addition to a distal protection device. In addition to providing extra support during device exchanges, a second guidewire helps maintain access to the true vessel lumen if the vessel is damaged during insertion or retrieval of the distal protection device (see Case 3, below).

◆ Be prepared: protamine and an appropriately sized compliant balloon can be lifesaving in the event of vessel rupture.

◆ Case Illustrations

Case 1

A 55-year-old, right-handed man with a past medical history of treated hypertension presented to the emergency depart-ment with vertigo, nausea/vomiting, and mild left upper extremity ataxia for 2 days. A noncontrasted head CT scan revealed a subacute posterior inferior communicating artery (PICA) infarct. CTA suggested that the left VA likely ended in the PICA, but was occluded distally. A diagnostic angiogram revealed a high-grade stenosis of the right VA origin with a tandem lesion in the V4 segment just proximal to the right PICA origin. The left vertebral originated off the arch and was hypoplastic **(Fig. 33.10)**.

Because the left VA ended in the PICA and the stroke was only in the left PICA distribution, it appeared that the right VA lesions were asymptomatic. The decision was made to treat the patient medically with aspirin, clopidogrel, and simvastatin. Over 72 hours the patient's symptoms resolved and he was sent home. He was seen in follow-up 6 weeks later, complaining of intermittent vertigo and one episode of double vision. Due to his persistent symptoms on medication, endovascular revascularization of the right VA lesion was suggested, as this lesion was more severe than the more distal lesion. The proximal stenosis could be treated using a distal protection device.

Under conscious sedation a 6F, 10-cm Glidesheath (Terumo Medical, Somerset, NJ) was inserted into the right common femoral artery. A 6F angled Chaperon guide catheter (Micro-Vention, Tustin, CA) on a continuous heparinized saline flush

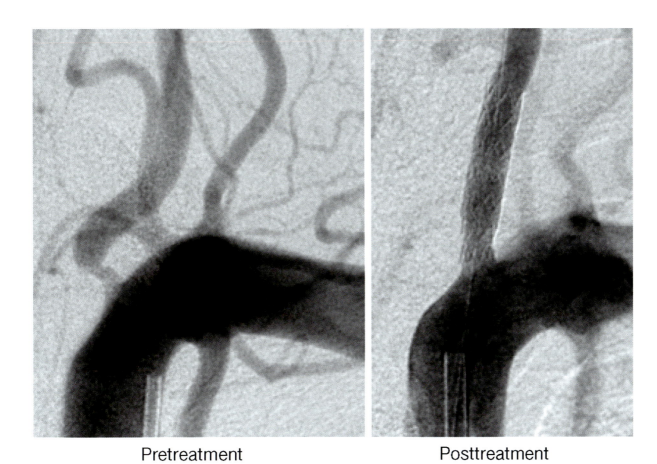

| Pretreatment | Posttreatment |

Fig. 33.9 In addition to dilating the vessel, a stent often straightens out the vessel to help reduce turbulent flow and decrease the risk of restenosis.

was advanced into the right subclavian artery over a 3.5F JB2 inner guide catheter (MicroVention). The inner guide catheter was then removed and an appropriate working angle was selected based on previous angiograms. Six thousand units of intravenous heparin was then administered, resulting in an ACT of >250 seconds. An EPI Filterwire EX (Boston Scientific, Natick, MA) with gently curved tip was navigated through the lesion under a high-definition roadmap and deployed in a straight segment of the midcervical VA. A 4 mm × 20 mm Xpert (Abbott Laboratories, Abbott Park, IL) stent was then deployed across the lesion. Control angiography revealed a small waist in the stent that was subsequently angioplastied using a 4 mm × 20 mm Maverick balloon (Boston Scientific), leaving less than 10% residual stenosis **(Fig. 33.11)**. The filter wire was then retrieved. The distal lesion was not treated. Following the procedure the patient has remained on aspirin, clopidogrel, and atorvastatin and has had no new posterior circulation ischemic events.

Case 2

A 51-year-old, right-handed man with a past medical history of treated hypertension complained of 6 months of progressive blurry vision, vertigo, and gait ataxia. During the previous month his symptoms had worsened to the extent that he was no longer able to work. CTA revealed bilateral VAOS **(Fig. 33.12)**. He was started on aspirin, clopidogrel, and atorvastatin. Within 1 week the patient returned with recurrent symptoms. Diagnostic angiography confirmed high-grade stenosis (70%) of the left VA origin. There was also 60% stenosis at the right VA origin **(Fig. 33.13)**. The decision was made to proceed with angioplasty and stenting of the left VA, as this was the dominant vessel.

With the diagnostic catheter in the left subclavian artery, a stiff 0.035-inch exchange length was passed into the left brachial artery. The diagnostic catheter and introducer were then removed. A 6F Raabe guide sheath (Cook Medical, Bloomington, IN) on a continuous heparinized saline flush was then advanced into the left subclavian artery. The exchange wire was removed and 100 units/kg of heparin was administered intravenously. Next, a 300-cm Filterwire EZ (Boston Scientific) was advanced into the left midcervical VA and deployed. A pre-stent angioplasty was performed using a 2.5 × 40 mm Maverick balloon (Boston Scientific) followed by deployment of a 3.5 mm × 18 mm Promus stent (Boston Scientific) across the lesion **(Fig. 33.14)**. The Filterwire was then recaptured and removed.

Following the procedure the patient's vertigo and ataxia resolved, but he continued to have blurry vision. He was seen

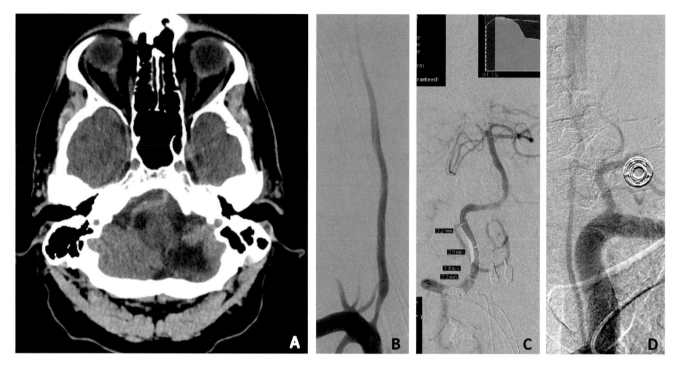

Fig. 33.10 **(A)** Computed tomography (CT) scan showing left cerebellar infarct in left posterior inferior communicating artery (PICA) distribution. **(B)** Catheter angiogram from the right subclavian artery shows high-grade (70%) stenosis of the right VA origin. **(C)** Cerebral angiogram from the right subclavian artery reveals a second stenotic segment just proximal to the PICA origin. **(D)** Catheter angiogram from the left subclavian artery reveals that the left VA is nondominant and originates directly off the aortic arch. Dynamic imaging showed delayed emptying, suggesting a distal occlusion of the left VA (not shown).

by a neuro-ophthalmologist who did not see any evidence of ischemic injury to the retina or cranial nerves. His visual acuity was 20/20 with correction. A repeat angiogram and magnetic resonance imaging (MRI) done 2 months later (not shown) did not reveal evidence of infarction, in-stent stenosis, or anterior circulation disease. He continues to complain of blurry vision, but the resolution of the vertigo and ataxia has allowed him to return to work.

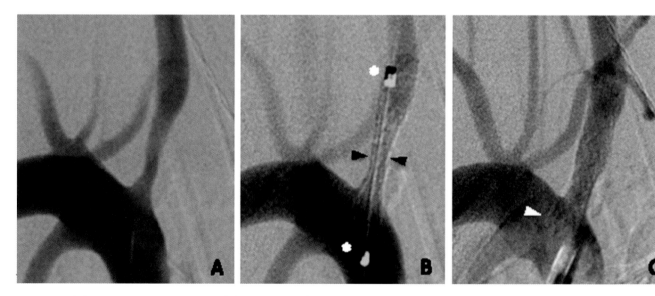

Fig. 33.11 **(A)** Pretreatment angiogram revealed 70% stenosis of the right VA origin. **(B)** A self-expanding Xpert stent (Abbott Laboratories, Abbott Park, IL) was deployed across the lesion, but left a small waist in the stent *(black arrowheads)*. A Maverick balloon (Boston Scientific, Natick, MA) was positioned across the waist in preparation for a post-stent angioplasty *(white asterisks)*. **(C)** After stenting and angioplasty there was very little residual stenosis. Note that the stent extends a few millimeters into the subclavian artery, ensuring that the entire lesion is covered *(white arrowhead)*.

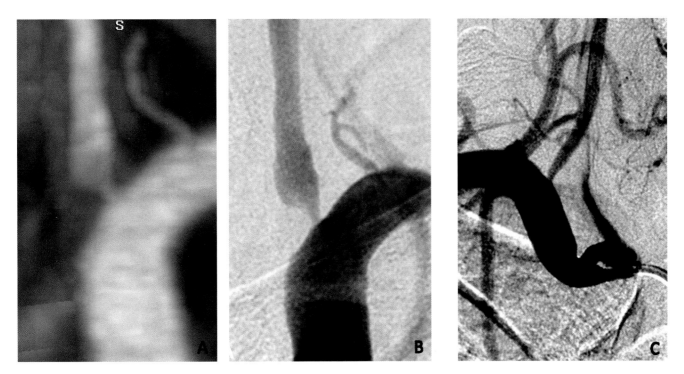

Fig. 33.12 **(A)** A CT angiogram shows a severe left (dominant) vertebral origin stenosis. **(B)** The area of stenosis was confirmed by catheter angiography. **(C)** This patient also had moderate stenosis of the right (nondominant) VA.

Case 3

A 78-year-old, right-handed man with a past medical history of peripheral vascular disease and progressive balance difficulty presented to the emergency department with slurred speech. An MRI with diffusion-weighted imaging (DWI) revealed two small embolic strokes in the posterior circulation. Attenuation of the posterior circulation on MRA suggested decreased flow in the posterior circulation, including the basilar artery. The patient recovered and was sent home on aspirin and clopidogrel but returned within 2 weeks with intermittent gait ataxia, slurred speech, and vision changes.

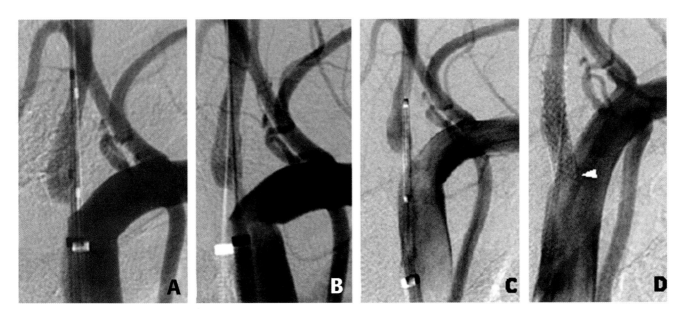

Fig. 33.13 **(A)** A 2.5-mm Maverick balloon (Boston Scientific) was positioned just distal to the lesion *(dotted rectangle)*. It was pulled back across the lesion prior to inflation. **(B)** After the pre-stent angioplasty, the stenosis improved. **(C)** A balloon-mounted Promus stent (Boston Scientific) was positioned across the lesion. **(D)** After deployment of the stent there was no significant residual stenosis. Note that the stent extends a few millimeters into the subclavian artery *(white arrowhead)*.

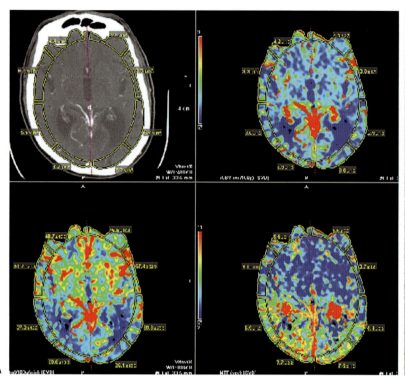
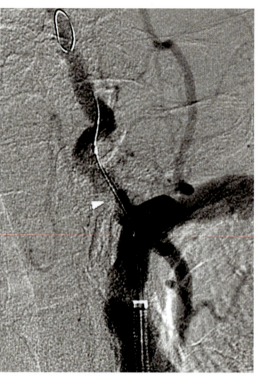

A

B

Fig. 33.14 **(A)** This patient had a history of multiple posterior circulation infarctions. A CT perfusion scan done prior to stenting shows decreased cerebral blood flow and increased mean transit time in the posterior circulation. **(B)** A preangioplasty angiogram shows high-grade stenosis at the left VA origin *(white arrowhead)*. Prior to crossing the lesion with the Filterwire, a 300-cm, 0.014-inch buddy wire was advanced through the lesion and into the distal cervical VA. In addition to providing extra support for the guide sheath, a buddy wire helps to straighten out the vessel to facilitate passing the Filterwire. In the event of vessel injury with the Filterwire, a buddy wire maintains access to the true lumen for additional rescue procedures.

A CTA and perfusion scan revealed a heavily calcified VA origin with relative hypoperfusion of the posterior circulation **(Fig. 33.14)**. The right VA was occluded at its origin, although there was some distal reconstitution via muscular branch collaterals (not shown).

A catheter angiogram under conscious sedation confirmed high-grade stenosis of the left VA origin. Due to tortuosity in the V1 segment and heavy calcification within the plaque, an angioplasty without stenting was planned. To avoid losing access to the true lumen in the event of dissection, the lesion was first crossed with a 300 cm, 0.014-inch Asahi Prowater wire (Abbott Laboratories). Once access to the true lumen was secured, a 300-cm Filterwire EZ (Boston Scientific) was passed alongside the Asahi wire and deployed in a straight segment of the VA. An angioplasty was performed with a 3.5 mm × 20 mm Maverick balloon (Boston Scientific). Due to vasospasm, retrieving the Filterwire with the relatively stiff retrieval catheter was impossible. Instead, a 4F diagnostic catheter was used to recapture the filter. A run after filter retrieval showed extravasation from the VA, so a Jostent cov-ered stent graft (Abbott Laboratories) was deployed across the lesion to stop the bleeding. Ten milligrams of intraarterial verapamil was administered to relieve the spasm and restore flow through the VA **(Fig. 33.15)**. The patient did have a small hemothorax that was visualized on subsequent chest imaging but suffered no long-term morbidity.

◆ Conclusion

Vertebral artery origin stenosis is common in patients with peripheral vascular disease. The first-line treatment of VA stenosis is medical using a combination of antiplatelet agents, statins, and risk factor reduction. Patients who fail medical management and have stenosis greater than 50% should be considered for endovascular revascularization with angioplasty and stenting. The use of balloon-mounted medicated stents at the VA origin may reduce the risk of restenosis. Distal embolic protection devices can be used safely in the VA and may reduce the risk of embolic complications.

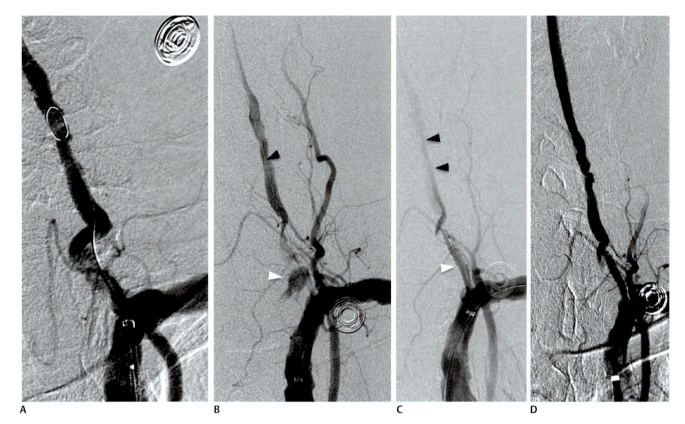

A   B   C   D

Fig. 33.15 **(A)** After angioplasty the VA origin is patent, the stenosis is improved, and there is no extravasation. No stent was planned due to the tortuosity of the V1 segment. **(B)** The retrieval catheter was difficult to advance due to vasospasm. A run after filter retrieval showed contrast extravasation from the VA *(white arrowhead)*. An 0.014-inch buddy wire is faintly seen in the true vessel lumen *(black arrowhead)*. **(C)** Contrast extravasation ceased after deployment of a covered stent *(white arrowhead)*, but little antegrade flow beyond the stent distally *(black arrowheads)*. **(D)** After 10 mg of intraarterial verapamil, antegrade flow through the VA was restored.

References

1. Hennerici M, Aulich A, Sandmann W, Freund HJ. Incidence of asymptomatic extracranial arterial disease. Stroke 1981;12:750–758
2. Wityk RJ, Chang HM, Rosengart A, et al. Proximal extracranial vertebral artery disease in the New England Medical Center Posterior Circulation Registry. Arch Neurol 1998;55:470–478
3. Moufarrij NA, Little JR, Furlan AJ, Williams G, Marzewski DJ. Vertebral artery stenosis: long-term follow-up. Stroke 1984;15:260–263
4. Caplan LR, Wityk RJ, Glass TA, et al. New England Medical Center Posterior Circulation registry. Ann Neurol 2004;56:389–398
5. Wehman JC, Hanel RA, Guidot CA, Guterman LR, Hopkins LN. Atherosclerotic occlusive extracranial vertebral artery disease: indications for intervention, endovascular techniques, short-term and long-term results. J Interv Cardiol 2004;17:219–232
6. Coward LJ, McCabe DJH, Ederle J, Featherstone RL, Clifton AC, Brown MM; CAVATAS Investigators. Long-term outcome after angioplasty and stenting for symptomatic vertebral artery stenosis compared with medical treatment in the Carotid And Vertebral Artery Transluminal Angioplasty Study (CAVATAS): a randomized trial. Stroke 2007;38:1526–1530
7. PROGRESS Collaborative Group. Randomised trial of a perindopril-based blood-pressure-lowering regimen among 6,105 individuals with previous stroke or transient ischaemic attack. Lancet 2001;358:1033–1041
8. Castillo J, Leira R, García MM, Serena J, Blanco M, Dávalos A. Blood pressure decrease during the acute phase of ischemic stroke is associated with brain injury and poor stroke outcome. Stroke 2004;35:520–526
9. Adams HP Jr, del Zoppo G, Alberts MJ, et al; American Heart Association; American Stroke Association Stroke Council; Clinical Cardiology Council; Cardiovascular Radiology and Intervention Council; Atherosclerotic Peripheral Vascular Disease and Quality of Care Outcomes in Research Interdisciplinary Working Groups. Guidelines for the early management of adults with ischemic stroke: a guideline from the American Heart Association/American Stroke Association Stroke Council, Clinical Cardiology Council, Cardiovascular Radiology and Intervention Council, and the Atherosclerotic Peripheral Vascular Disease and Quality of Care Outcomes in Research Interdisciplinary Working Groups: the American Academy of Neurology affirms the value of this guideline as an educational tool for neurologists. Stroke 2007;38:1655–1711
10. Amarenco P, Bogousslavsky J, Callahan A III, et al; Stroke Prevention by Aggressive Reduction in Cholesterol Levels (SPARCL) Investigators. High-dose atorvastatin after stroke or transient ischemic attack. N Engl J Med 2006;355:549–559
11. Berguer R, Flynn LM, Kline RA, Caplan L. Surgical reconstruction of the extracranial vertebral artery: management and outcome. J Vasc Surg 2000;31(1 Pt 1):9–18
12. Hanel RA, Brasiliense LB, Spetzler RF. Microsurgical revascularization of proximal vertebral artery: a single-center, single-operator analysis. Neurosurgery 2009;64:1043–1050, discussion 1051
13. Hua Y, Meng XF, Jia LY, et al. Color Doppler imaging evaluation of proximal vertebral artery stenosis. AJR Am J Roentgenol 2009;193:1434–1438
14. Khan S, Rich P, Clifton A, Markus HS. Noninvasive detection of vertebral artery stenosis: a comparison of contrast-enhanced MR angiography, CT angiography, and ultrasound. Stroke 2009;40:3499–3503
15. Park SJ, Lee SW. Optimal management of platelet function after coronary stenting. Curr Treat Options Cardiovasc Med 2007;9:37–45
16. Saw J, Bajzer C, Casserly IP, et al. Evaluating the optimal activated clotting time during carotid artery stenting. Am J Cardiol 2006;97:1657–1660
17. Edgell RC, Yavagal DR, Drazin D, Olivera R, Boulos AS. Treatment of vertebral artery origin stenosis with anti-proliferative drug-eluting stents. J Neuroimaging 2010;20:175–179
18. Boulos AS, Agner C, Deshaies EM. Preliminary evidence supporting the safety of drug-eluting stents in neurovascular disease. Neurol Res 2005;27(Suppl 1):S95–S102

19. Boulos AS, Levy EI, Bendok BR, et al. Evolution of neuroendovascular intervention: are view of advancement in device technology. Neurosurgery 2004;54:238–252

20. Lin YH, Hung CS, Tseng WY, et al; National Taiwan University Carotid Artery and Vertebral Artery Stenosis (NTU CAVAS) Study Group. Safety and feasibility of drug-eluting stent implantation at vertebral artery origin: the first case series in Asians. J Formos Med Assoc 2008;107: 253–258

21. Akins PT, Kerber CW, Pakbaz RS. Stenting of vertebral artery origin atherosclerosis in high-risk patients: bare or coated? A single-center consecutive case series. J Invasive Cardiol 2008;20:14–20

22. Albuquerque FC, Fiorella D, Han P, Spetzler RF, McDougall CG. A reappraisal of angioplasty and stenting for the treatment of vertebral origin stenosis. Neurosurgery 2003;53:607–614, discussion 614–616

34

Vasodilators and Angioplasty for Cerebral Vasospasm

Aditya S. Pandey, Neeraj Chaudhary, W. Christopher Fox, Byron Gregory Thompson, and Joseph J. Gemmete

Pearls

- Maximize cerebral perfusion pressure by increasing volume status, increasing mean arterial pressure, and reducing intracranial pressures.
- Obtain a computed tomography (CT) scan of the head to evaluate for cerebral infarct or hemorrhage as explanations for clinical symptoms.
- Proceed to cerebral angiography with chemical and mechanical angioplasty if medically refractory spasm persists; time is of the essence.

Cerebral vasospasm following aneurysmal subarachnoid hemorrhage (SAH) is a delayed, reversible narrowing of the intracranial vasculature that occurs most commonly 4 to 14 days after aneurysmal SAH and can lead to permanent ischemic injury. Although it has been the focus of much research and clinical effort, vasospasm remains difficult to treat and is responsible for significant morbidity and mortality in patients with ruptured cerebral aneurysms. Angiographic spasm occurs in up to 70% of SAH patients, of whom half will become symptomatic secondary to ischemic changes. In the past, mortality rates from vasospasm have been reported to range from 30 to 70%, with 10 to 20% of patients experiencing severe neurologic deficits.[1,2]

With advancements in diagnostic and interventional technology, estimates of patients suffer significant morbidity/mortality, range from 5 to 9%, with vasospasm accounting for 12 to 17% of all fatalities or cases of disability after SAH.[3,4] We have an incomplete understanding of the pathophysiology of vasospasm, and it is difficult to predict which patients will develop vasospasm after SAH. The Hunt and Hess grade, Fisher score, hypertension, smoking, cocaine use, age range of 40 to 59 years, and early rise in the middle cerebral artery blood flow on transcranial Doppler have been shown to be independent risk factors for vasospasm.[4] Cerebral salt wasting has also been associated with vasospasm. This chapter discusses the multiple medical and endovascular therapies that are utilized to prevent or treat vasospasm.

◆ Vasospasm Prophylaxis and Medical Treatment

Prophylactic treatment for cerebral vasospasm following aneurysmal SAH is controversial and varies among institutions. Calcium channel blockers, intravenous magnesium, and 3-hydroxy-3-methylglutaryl coenzyme A (HMG CoA) reductase inhibitors (statins) have all been used in attempts to prevent and treat vasospasm. In addition, triple-H (hypervolemia, hypertension, and hemodilution) therapy has been a mainstay of vasospasm treatment for years. At our institution, we initiate triple H therapy post-treatment of the cerebral aneurysm, as long as there are no medical contraindications such as congestive heart failure or severe pulmonary disease. We use prophylactic nimodipine and magnesium sulfate and are considering utilizing statins as new data emerge.

◆ Calcium Channel Antagonists

Calcium channel antagonists have been shown to decrease the overall incidence of cerebral infarction after SAH by 34% and the incidence of poor outcomes by 40%.[5] The physiologic reasoning behind the use of calcium channel blockers is that the central event in vascular smooth muscle contraction is the influx of calcium into cells, which has been shown to occur after SAH.[6] This, in turn, leads to several downstream events including free radical formation, production of vasoconstricting prostaglandins, and activation of the myosin light chain kinase that causes smooth muscle contraction. The most common calcium channel blocker used after SAH is nimodipine, which has a certain degree of specificity for the cerebral vessels. Multiple trials have shown its efficacy in improving outcomes, although it may not improve angiographic outcome.

◆ Magnesium

Obstetricians have used magnesium to treat eclampsia, as magnesium is thought to alter calcium physiology and thus alter vascular tone in the uterine circulation. Magnesium competes with calcium-binding sites, thus preventing muscular contraction and allowing vascular muscle relaxation. Level 1 evidence now exists for the usage of magnesium sulfate in the prevention of cerebral vasospasm. Westermaier et al[7] have shown that magnesium sulfate significantly reduces cerebral ischemic events after SAH.

◆ Triple-H Therapy

Hypervolemia, hypertension, and hemodilution therapy (triple-H) has long been a mainstay of medical therapy in patients with aneurysmal SAH. The rationale behind triple-H therapy is that maintenance of high circulating blood volume, increased perfusion pressures, and decreased blood viscosity will enhance cerebral blood flow in the setting of vasoconstriction. Although in healthy adults changes in cardiac output do not change the local cerebral flow, they do impact cerebral blood flow in patients suffering from cerebral vasospasm. Our goal is to maintain euvolemia as defined by the specific central venous/wedge pressure which allows for the highest cardiac output.

The vast majority of our SAH patients receive central lines so that central venous pressures can be closely monitored to achieve optimized volume expansion without causing pulmonary edema. We prefer central venous pressures in the range of 8 to 12 mm Hg, but these are highly individualized and must be closely monitored in relation to the clinical findings in each patient. Patients with cardiopulmonary disease may need to be evaluated with a Swan Ganz catheter, as the ideal venous pressure in these patients needs to be related to

the ideal cardiac output.[8] One series or 184 patients reported a 13% risk of device-related sepsis in patients with pulmonary artery catheters, as well as a 2% risk of congestive heart failure, 1.3% risk of subclavian vein thrombosis, and 1% risk of pneumothorax.[8] Most SAH patients require invasive blood pressure monitoring. In the post-clipping or -coiling vasospasm period, we often allow patients to autoregulate with systolic blood pressure in the range of 200 mm Hg. The role of red blood cell transfusion is not well studied, but transfusion could certainly increase the oxygen carrying capacity.

Endovascular Therapy

Endovascular treatment with intraarterial infusion of a vasodilator or balloon angioplasty is indicated in patients with symptomatic vasospasm refractory to medical therapy to prevent neurologic deficits referable to the vascular territory of the angiographic vasospasm. Any patient who is a candidate for cerebral angioplasty in the context of cerebral vasospasm must be evaluated with a computed tomography (CT) scan of the head to evaluate for hemorrhage as well as the presence of hypodensity within the vascular territory at question for vasospasm. A vessel diameter reduction between 25% and 50% from the initial angiographic diameter is usually treated with intraarterial infusion of vasodilators. Vessel diameter reductions greater than 50% from the initial angiographic diameter are treated with a combination of mechanical and chemical angioplasty. The timing of endovascular intervention for vasospasm is critical, and a 2-hour window from the time of symptoms may exist for restoration of blood flow to the region affected by vasospasm.[9]

Intraarterial Vasodilators (Table 34.1)

Papaverine

The most studied intraarterial pharmacologic agent to date is papaverine. It is an opium alkaloid that is thought to alter adenosine 3',5'–cyclic monophosphate levels in smooth muscles.[10] The half-life is approximately 2 hours. Hoh and Ogilvy,[11] in a review of intraarterial agents for treatment of cerebral vasospasm, reported that papaverine produced clinical improvement in only 43% of the treated patients. The effective-

Table 34.1 Intraarterial Agents for the Treatment of Vasospasm

Agent	Typical Intraarterial Dose	Half-Life (Hours)	Side Effects
Papaverine	300 mg per vascular territory at 0.3% concentration over 20 minutes.	2	Cortical necrosis, permanent neurologic deficits, raised intracranial pressure, systemic hypotension
Verapamil	1- to 2-mg bolus over 2 minutes with maximum of 10 mg per vascular territory	7	Increased intracranial pressure
Nimodipine	1 to 3 mg at 25% dilution over 10 to 30 minutes in each vascular territory; maximum dose 5 mg	9	Increased intracranial pressure
Nicardipine	0.2 to 0.5 mg/mL in 1-mL aliquots; maximum dose of 20 mg per vascular territory	16	Increased intracranial pressure

ness of treatment was short given its half-life; therefore, multiple treatments were required, which led to a variable and increased risk of complications. Platz et al[12] more recently reported a case of spontaneous hemorrhage following intraarterial use of papaverine. They hypothesized that local increased levels of infused papaverine possibly led to a blood–brain barrier (BBB) breakdown with subsequent intracranial hemorrhage. Furthermore, there has been a recent report from Pennings et al[13] that they observed an abnormal response to topical application of papaverine on the cerebral cortical microvasculature during aneurysm surgery. They noted rebound vasoconstriction in two of 14 cases. In the cases where there was some increase in vessel diameter compared with baseline, it did not reach statistical significance.

There is wide variation in the intraarterial use of papaverine in terms of dosage and duration of infusion.[13] Firlik et al[14] demonstrated no correlation with the clinical response and angiographic picture in cases of vasospasm from aneurysmal SAH treated with intraarterial papaverine. In their cohort of 15 patients they had 23 intraarterial (IA) treatments with papaverine, leading to partial angiographic reversal in 18 of the 23 IA treatments. However, major clinical improvement was seen in only six treatments and minor improvement or none in 17.

Papaverine hydrochloride is supplied as a 3% concentration, 30 mg/mL, in an acidic mixture maintained at a pH of 3.3. Papaverine may form crystal precipitates, with crystal size up to 100 μm, when mixed with human serum at 3% or 0.3% concentrations. A precipitate has also been seen when 3% papaverine solution was mixed with heparinized saline in concentrations of 2000 to 10,000 units of heparin per liter. The typical papaverine concentration infused is 0.3%, produced by diluting 300 mg of papaverine in 100 mL of normal saline. The entire dose (300 mg) is given in a vascular territory over 20 to 30 minutes. If more than one vascular territory is involved, additional infusions of 300 mg can be given. The catheter for infusion in the anterior circulation should be placed past the ophthalmic artery to prevent possible precipitate being introduced into the retina. In the posterior circulation the catheter should be positioned past the origin of the anterior inferior cerebellar artery to prevent respiratory arrest and the potential of cardiac dysfunction due to transient depression of the medullary respiratory and cardiovascular nuclei. Papaverine can cause systemic hypotension and elevation of intracranial pressure during infusion; therefore, these parameters should be monitored closely.

Side effects from intraarterial infusion of papaverine also included transient neurologic deficits such as mydriasis, transient hemiparesis, and respiratory depression. Given the short half-life, the transient effect on the local cerebral vasculature, and significant side effects, we no longer utilize papaverine for chemical angioplasty at our institution.

Calcium Channel Antagonists

With the complications associated with papaverine, use of calcium channel antagonists (verapamil, nimodipine, nicardipine) for the treatment of cerebral vasospasm has become more popular. These agents are still not approved by the Food and Drug Administration (FDA) in the United States for intraarterial use in the cerebral vasculature.

Verapamil

Verapamil is a phenylalkylamine calcium channel blocker that inhibits voltage-gated calcium channels in the arterial wall smooth muscle cells, resulting in vasodilatation. The half-life is approximately 7 hours. Feng et al[15] reported on the intraarterial use of verapamil in 29 patients who underwent 34 procedures; 52% were treated with verapamil alone, which resulted in 44% experiencing increased vessel diameters and 33% exhibiting neurologic improvements without complications or intracranial pressure (ICP) issues. The vasodilation effects of verapamil are still transient and poorly sustained, and no studies thus far have demonstrated significant patient outcome benefit.

Verapamil is usually infused in a 1- to 2-mg bolus over 2 minutes, with a total maximal dose of 10 mg administered into each vascular territory. In their small cohort of 10 patients, Keuskamp et al[16] have demonstrated the efficacy of using high doses of verapamil (total 41 ± 29 mg per procedure) without significant alteration of ICP, cerebral perfusion pressure, or other side effects. In their series, the neurologic deficits that prompted endovascular treatment of vasospasm improved in eight of 12 procedures. In a recent report of a case series of again 12 patients, Albanese et al[17] have documented the use of ultrahigh doses of verapamil for treatment of vasospasm. They used an average dose of 164.6 mg of verapamil per vessel for infiltration through an indwelling microcatheter. They have demonstrated improvement in nine of 12 patients. Only one patient had the infusion stopped due to ICP increasing beyond 20 cm H_2O.

Major complications of intravenous verapamil are hyptension and bradycardia; however, no significant changes in blood pressure or heart rate have been reported with intraarterial infusion. No prolonged or dramatic increase in intracranial pressure has been reported, as mentioned above. Intraarterial verapamil administration appears to be safe with few systemic effects in the limited number of patients studied.

Nimodipine

Nimodipine is a dihydropyridine agent that has a mechanism of action similar to that of verapamil, but it has a slightly longer half-life of 9 hours. The systemic application of nimodipine has been proven to be an effective agent on clinical outcome after SAH in several clinical trials.[18] Hänggi et al[19] recently analyzed the effect of intraarterial nimodipine in the treatment of severe cerebral vasospasm due to aneurysmal SAH. In their small cohort of 26 patients, eight (30.8%) had treatment failure with no angiographic response to intraarterial nimodipine. Seven of the 18 patients who had angiographic response went on to develop additional cerebral infarctions related to the vasospasm. Although the results do not suggest nimodipine to have sustained benefit in improving patient outcome, they do demonstrate a trend toward improved cerebral perfusion parameters that were sustained for a period of 24 hours. The authors conclude that the vasodilatory effect of intraarterial nimodipine in the treatment of vasospasm is still transient albeit better than that of papaverine. In terms of patient numbers, Hänggi et al demonstrated that of the 11 patients who were clinically assessable, seven had no change in neurologic status post-application of intraarterial nimodipine, and only two had neurologic improvement whereas two had worsening in their Glasgow Coma Scale (GCS) score. These results are in contrast to the 76% clinical improvement shown in another cohort of patients with aneurysmal SAH and vasospasm treated with IA nimodipine by Biondi et al.[20]

Nimodipine is administered by diluting 1 to 3 mg with 15 to 45 mL of normal saline to obtain a dilution of 25%. This is then infused at a slow continuous infusion over 10 to 30 minutes (approximately 0.1 mg/min). The total dose reported in the literature has not been greater than 5 mg per procedure.[21] In their recent report of 19 patients treated with IA nimodipine, Kim et al[21] demonstrated improvements in flow in 42 of 53 procedures and an improvement in clinical outcome after 23. They used nimodipine in a 10% concentration infused slowly at 0.1 mg nimodipine per minute. The main systemic complications of nimodipine include hypotension, rash, diarrhea, and bradycardia. No significant changes in heart rate, blood pressure, or intracranial pressure have been reported in the literature from intraarterial administration.

Nicardipine

Nicardipine is also a dihydropyridine agent that has an even longer half-life of almost 16 hours. It has a more selective effect on vascular smooth muscle than cardiac muscle. Several studies have demonstrated that continuous intravenous nicardipine infusion significantly decreases the incidence of symptomatic, angiographic, and transcranial Doppler (TCD) vasospasm, but the efficacy is limited by prolonged hypotension, pulmonary edema, and renal dysfunction. Badjatia et al[22] have previously demonstrated that the utilization of IA nicardipine induces more sustained reversal of vasospasm than does papaverine. They demonstrated a 42.1% neurologic improvement in patients following treatment with IA nicardipine. Although this is encouraging, the authors also highlight the incidence of increased ICP following treatment in six patients. Tejada et al[23] more recently showed that a higher dose regime of IA nicardipine is more efficacious. They used a total dose of 10 to 40 mg in each patient. GCS and Glasgow Outcome Scale (GOS) scores in 10 of 11 patients who were treated with the high-dose regimen improved. The authors also demonstrated a low complication rate and a sustained clinical outcome benefit with a GOS score of 1 or 2 in nine of 10 patients with at least 2-month follow-up.

Nicardipine is usually administered intraarterially by diluting with normal saline to a concentration of 0.2 mg/mL and infusing in 1-mL aliquots to a maximum dose between 2.5 and 20 mg per vessel.[23] The authors of this review use it in a 0.5-mg/mL dosage concentration with a maximum dosage of 20 mg per vessel.

Prolonged hypotension, pulmonary edema, and renal dysfunction have been reported following the intravenous administration of nicardipine; however, these findings have not been reported with intraarterial administration.[23] The main adverse effect reported in the literature is an increase in ICP, which usually can be controlled with ventricular drainage. Tejada et al[23] have demonstrated the safe use of a high dose of IA nicardipine in their series of 11 patients with vasospasm.[23] However, ICP monitoring was possible in only two of the 11 patients who did not demonstrate any change during IA infusion of nicardipine.

Other Agents

There are other pharmaceutical agents with various other mechanisms of vasodilatation, namely magnesium sulfate, HMG CoA reductase inhibitors, nitric oxide donors, and endothelin-1 antagonists. The neuroprotective and vasoprotective properties of magnesium sulfate have been well documented in the literature. Shah et al[24] have recently evaluated a cohort of patients in whom magnesium sulfate was used in conjunction with nicardipine for intraarterial treatment of aneurysmal SAH related vasospasm. They observed that this agent was well tolerated by the patients, with no adverse effects on ICP. They did not observe any statistically significant difference in clinical outcome improvement in comparison to other studies with cohorts treated only with nicardipine.

Transluminal Balloon Angioplasty (Table 34.2)

The mechanism of cerebral blood vessel narrowing in aneurysmal SAH is not clearly understood. Inflammatory changes mediating smooth muscle contraction, changes in the linkage of the protein matrix, and collagen deposition in the vessel wall have all been implicated as a possible cause of blood vessel narrowing in SAH related to aneurysm rupture.

Mechanical dilation of intracranial vessels was performed first in 1984 by Zubkov et al.[25] They reported their results in selected patients with large vessel spasm. Balloons for intracranial angioplasty have developed considerably since then. The most significant limitation of these angioplasty balloons remains the inability to treat spasm affecting the distal cerebral vasculature. The current thinking is that transluminal balloon angioplasty (TBA) acts by stretching the vessel wall, leading to morphologic and functional changes in the smooth muscle fibers, resulting in impairment of contractility. At a cellular level it has been shown that there is fragmentation of the collagen matrix and flattening of the endothelial cells, resulting in permanent restoration of vessel diameter. This has been demonstrated to be durable in both canine and primate models.

Eskridge et al[26] reported 50 patients with 170 treated arterial segments. They demonstrated sustained neurologic improvement in only 61% of patients within 72 hours following angioplasty. Rosenwasser et al[9] sought to identify an optimal time frame for treatment of vasospasm from aneurysmal SAH. They demonstrated that 61% of patients treated within 2 hours had an angiographic improvement leading to a sustained clinical improvement in 70% of cases; in contrast, the other 39% of cases treated more than 2 hours later achieved

Table 34.2 Balloons Utilized for Transluminal Balloon Angioplasty

Balloon Catheters	Technique	Dimensions	Manufacturer	Qualities
HyperForm	Over-the-wire balloon catheter with single lumen	Balloon diameter: 4 and 7 mm Balloon length: 7 mm	eV3	Readily conformable
HyperGlide	Over-the-wire balloon catheter with single lumen	Balloon diameter: 4 and 5 mm Balloon lengths (by diameter): 4/10, 4/15, 4/20, 4/30 5/15, 5/20	eV3	Relatively rigid and longer length
Gateway	Over-the-wire balloon catheter with separate lumen for inflation	Balloon diameter: 1.5, 2.0, 2.25, 3.0, 3.5, and 4 mm Balloon length (by diameter): 1.5/9, 2.0/9, and 15, 20 mm in the other diameters	Boston Scientific	Comparatively rigid but available in smaller diameters

88% angiographic improvement but sustained only a 40% clinical improvement.[27] Recently, the results of a phase II study that examined the role of prophylactic TBA in patients with Fisher grade III SAH demonstrated no significant difference in the primary end point (GOS score), but did demonstrate a trend toward fewer patients developing vasospasm or needing therapeutic TBA.[28] In summary, TBA has shown benefit in restoring antegrade flow in the treated cerebral vascular territory and some improvement in patient outcomes. However, there is still a lack of level 1 evidence supporting balloon angioplasty for treatment of cerebral vasospasm in the literature.

Typical locations of vessels amenable to TBA are vertebral, basilar, supraclinoid internal carotid artery (ICA), and M1 segments. Less common locations due to their small diameter are the posterior communicating, A1, M2, and P1 arteries. In general, TBA in vessels with a diameter less than 2 mm may have a higher risk of vessel rupture. Hence, the posterior inferior communicating artery (PICA), anterior inferior communicating artery (AICA), A2, M3, and P2 arterial branches are usually avoided altogether.

Two different balloon technologies have been used for treatment of vasospasm: coronary balloons and more compliant intracranial balloons. The coronary balloon catheter technology comprises a stiff balloon membrane composed of polyethylene or nylon and a double-lumen shaft, one lumen for balloon inflation and the other for passage of a range of 0.014–inch guidewires. The short Maverick coronary balloons (Boston Scientific, Natick, MA) allow greater maneuverability and cause less vessel straightening and distortion. These balloons typically have tight size to inflation pressure calibration. Typically a 2-mm-diameter balloon is used for the middle cerebral artery and 1.5 mm for A1 or M2 branches. Similar technology developed for dedicated intracranial use is the Gateway™ system (Boston Scientific), which is available in balloon sizes ranging from 1.5 to 4 mm diameter (outer diameter at nominal inflation) and 10, 15, and 20 mm in length. This system has been designed for angioplasty of intracranial stenoses.

The other more compliant balloon catheter systems utilize a softer semipermeable silicone/elastomer membrane loaded on a single-lumen, more flexible catheter shaft. These balloons are designed to navigate over a 0.010-inch X-Pedion (ev3, Irvine, CA) guidewire. There are two types of balloons: HyperForm (ev3) and HyperGlide (ev3). The HyperForm is a softer balloon (4/7 × 7 mm) than the HyperGlide, which has a longer length (4 × 10/15/20/30 mm). These balloons are both over-the-wire systems. The distal end of the catheter has a small valve at the tip, which is occluded when the 0.010-inch wire passes 10 cm past the tip of the catheter. This design allows for a smaller profile, a less dense catheter, excellent distal access, and excellent guide-catheter compatibility. In addition, by utilizing a mechanical seal for the balloon inflation, air management can be confidently and efficiently controlled. Some operators use a 0.08-inch wire such as the Mirage (EV3, Irvine, CA), claiming that it allows the balloon to decompress if overinflated, thus conferring a possible safety mechanism. The wire should not be allowed to track proximal to the balloon in vivo, as this causes blood to track into the balloon and thus makes deflation difficult or inadequate and can potentially lead to complications such as vessel rupture from overinflation of the balloon. The balloon is calibrated to the volume injected and is inflated with a highly calibrated threaded 1-mL Cadence (eV3) syringe that enables adjustments in the 0.01-mL range. The operator has to be very careful when inflating these balloons, as their maximum diameter is large; hence, inflation should cease once the soft balloon starts to conform to the vessel lumen diameter. All of the balloons mentioned above should be inflated with a 50/50 concentration of 300 mg/mL iodinated contrast and saline for optimal visualization and deflation. Higher concentrations can lead to incomplete deflation and thus vessel damage.

Transluminal balloon angioplasty itself has some potential significant risks. These include vessel rupture due to the balloon being larger than the vessel diameter. In cases of critical spasm, there may be a poor roadmap due to minimal antegrade flow with the arterial vessels. This can lead to malpositioning of the balloon, which, for example, can accidentally get lodged in the posterior communicating artery rather than the supraclinoid ICA or in a lenticulostriate vessel rather than the M1, thus resulting in rupture of that vessel. Arterial dissection can also occur from angioplasty. These balloons can be flow limiting or may cause thrombus or pseudoaneurysm formation. Furthermore, thrombus or platelet aggregates can form around the balloon or in the catheter lumen, due to the increase thrombogenic state in SAH patients. To avoid this, patients undergoing TBA typically are heparinized to an activated clotting time of 250 seconds unless contraindicated. Finally, there is the potential risk of hemorrhage or reperfusion injury by restoration of blood flow in a vascular territory with prolonged ischemia.

◆ Current Concepts in Combination Therapy

The discrepancy in the clinical correlation with large-vessel vasospasm suggests that microvascular vasospasm is more crucial to overcome to improve clinical outcome. However, flow-limiting large-vessel luminal narrowing due to spasm can compromise the concentration of IA vasodilators in the distal cerebral microvasculature. Performing TBA initially should theoretically lead to better proximal flow and thus improved delivery of IA vasodilators to distal microvasculature. It is controversial which should be performed first— TBA or IA vasodilator infusion. One argument is that initial IA vasodilator infusion may increase the proximal diameter of a target vessel to successfully place a balloon catheter in it for TBA. The durability of chemical angioplasty is unknown; however, TBA is thought to be a more durable modality than chemical angioplasty. Larger multicenter prospective randomized trials are necessary to create level 1 evidence to assess the efficacy of combination therapy with the newly available technology with compliant balloons and longer acting IA vasodilators.

◆ Future Endovascular Therapies

Our understanding of the phenomenon of vasospasm due to aneurysmal SAH is still evolving. A better understanding of the pathophysiologic insult to the brain at ictus will enable us to understand the phenomenon of vasospasm better and will enable better design in the therapy to improve patient outcome. Novel methods of production of animal vasospasm models are needed to evaluate various IA or TBA therapies to ultimately improve patient outcome. Animal models will play a key role in evaluating different variables in the understanding of cerebral vasospasm.

◆ Case Example

A 25-year-old woman was transferred to our institution with Hunt and Hess grade I SAH from a ruptured anterior communicating artery aneurysm. The patient underwent microsurgery for clip ligation without complications. On post hemorrhage day 9, she developed dense left-sided hemiparesis, which was thought to be secondary to cerebral vasospasm. After optimizing the cerebral perfusion pressure and volume status, the patient was taken to the interventional suite for

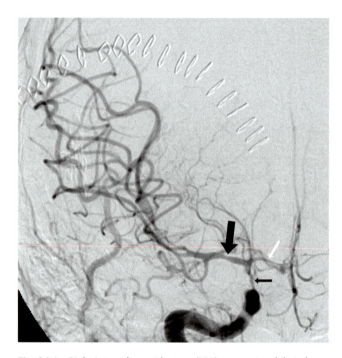

Fig. 34.1 Right internal carotid artery (ICA) conventional digital subtraction angiogram (DSA) anteroposterior (AP) projection showing vasospasm in supraclinoid ICA *(small black arrow)*, right middle cerebral artery (MCA) M1 segment *(large black arrow)*, and right anterior cerebral artery (ACA) segment *(white arrow)*.

diagnostic angiography and angioplasty. A CT scan of the head was performed, which revealed no evidence of acute hemorrhage or large territorial infarct to explain the patient's deficits. Cerebral angiography was performed revealing severe spasm involving the right middle cerebral artery (MCA), anterior cerebral artery (ACA), and intracranial ICA territories **(Fig. 34.1).** The calibre of the vessels was significantly narrower as compared with the postclipping angiography **(Fig. 34.2).** The patient was then given 10 mg of IA ni-

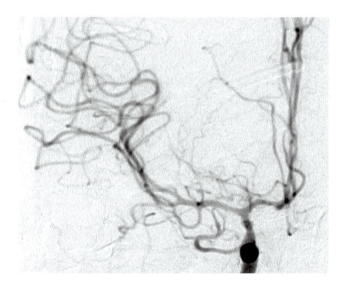

Fig. 34.2 Immediate post-clipping right ICA DSA AP projection is shown for comparison.

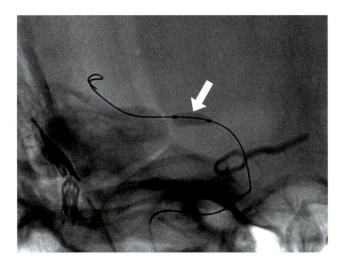

Fig. 34.3 A 4 mm × 7 mm HyperForm balloon *(white arrow)* is shown inflated in the right MCA M1 segment.

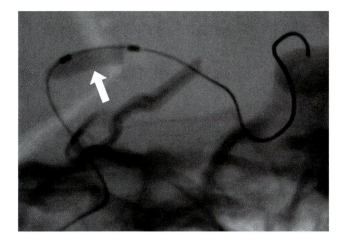

Fig. 34.4 A 2.5 mm × 9 mm Gateway balloon *(white arrow)* is shown inflated in the right A1 segment.

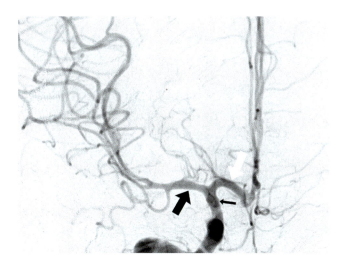

Fig. 34.5 Right ICA AP projection DSA image revealing resolution of the spasm within the ICA *(small black arrow)*, MCA *(large black arrow)*, and ACA *(white arrow)* segments.

cardipine to allow for cerebral vasodilatations. A HyperForm balloon was inflated within the MCA while a Gateway balloon was inflated within the ACA territory (**Figs. 34.3 and 34.4**). Mechanical and chemical angioplasty led to resolution of the spastic MCA, ICA, and ACA segments (**Fig. 34.5**). The patient had resolution of her symptoms and was discharged without neurologic deficits.

◆ Conclusion

The jury is still out on which pharmaceutical agent exclusively or in conjunction with TBA is the optimal treatment of cerebral vasospasm. There is a trend toward some benefit provided by the longer acting calcium channel blockers in combination with TBA. Newer agents on the horizon specifically targeting the vascular endothelium without a wide spectrum of side effects need to be tried and tested in larger prospective randomized patient cohorts. Improved animal models of vasospasm are being validated in studies. These models should form the cornerstone of optimizing treatment by helping to develop a better understanding of the phenomenon of cerebral vasospasm due to SAH from a ruptured aneurysm.

References

1. Hop JW, Rinkel GJ, Algra A, van Gijn J. Case-fatality rates and functional outcome after subarachnoid hemorrhage: a systematic review. Stroke 1997;28:660–664
2. Komotar RJ, Zacharia BE, Valhora R, Mocco J, Connolly ES Jr. Advances in vasospasm treatment and prevention. J Neurol Sci 2007;261:134–142
3. Roos YB, de Haan RJ, Beenen LF, Groen RJ, Albrecht KW, Vermeulen M. Complications and outcome in patients with aneurysmal subarachnoid haemorrhage: a prospective hospital based cohort study in the Netherlands. J Neurol Neurosurg Psychiatry 2000;68:337–341
4. Zwienenberg-Lee M, Hart5man J, Rudisill N, Muizelaar JP. Endovascular management of cerebral vasospasm. Neurosurgery 2006;59(5 Suppl 3): S139–147; discussion S3–13
5. Pickard JD, Murray GD, Illingworth R, et al. Effect of oral nimodipine on cerebral infarction and outcome after subarachnoid haemorrhage: British aneurysm nimodipine trial. BMJ 1989;298:636–642
6. Rothoerl RD, Ringel F. Molecular mechanisms of cerebral vasospasm following aneurysmal SAH. Neurol Res 2007;29:636–642
7. Westermaier T, et al. Prophylactic intravenous magnesium sulfate for treatment of aneurysmal subarachnoid hemorrhage: a randomized, placebo-controlled, clinical study. Crit Care Med 2010;38:1382–1384
8. Rosenwasser RH, Jallo JI, Getch CC, Liebman KE. Complications of Swan-Ganz catheterization for hemodynamic monitoring in patients with subarachnoid hemorrhage. Neurosurgery 1995;37:872–875, discussion 875–876
9. Rosenwasser RH, Armonda RA, Thomas JE, Benitez RP, Gannon PM, Harrop J. Therapeutic modalities for the management of cerebral vasospasm: timing of endovascular options. Neurosurgery 1999;44:975–979, discussion 979–980
10. Macdonald RL, Weir BK, Young JD, Grace MG. Cytoskeletal and extracellular matrix proteins in cerebral arteries following subarachnoid hemorrhage in monkeys. J Neurosurg 1992;76:81–90
11. Hoh BL, Ogilvy CS. Endovascular treatment of cerebral vasospasm: transluminal balloon angioplasty, intra-arterial papaverine, and intra-arterial nicardipine. Neurosurg Clin N Am 2005;16:501–516, vi vi.
12. Platz J, Baráth K, Keller E, Valavanis A. Disruption of the blood-brain barrier by intra-arterial administration of papaverine: a technical note. Neuroradiology 2008;50:1035–1039
13. Pennings FA, Albrecht KW, Muizelaar JP, Schuurman PR, Bouma GJ. Abnormal responses of the human cerebral microcirculation to papaverin during aneurysm surgery. Stroke 2009;40:317–320
14. Firlik KS, Kaufmann AM, Firlik AD, Jungreis CA, Yonas H. Intra-arterial papaverine for the treatment of cerebral vasospasm following aneurysmal subarachnoid hemorrhage. Surg Neurol 1999;51:66–74

15. Feng L, Fitzsimmons BF, Young WL, et al. Intraarterially administered verapamil as adjunct therapy for cerebral vasospasm: safety and 2-year experience. AJNR Am J Neuroradiol 2002;23:1284–1290

16. Keuskamp J, Murali R, Chao KH. High-dose intraarterial verapamil in the treatment of cerebral vasospasm after aneurysmal subarachnoid hemorrhage. J Neurosurg 2008;108:458–463

17. Albanese E, Russo A, Quiroga M, Willis RN Jr, Mericle RA, Ulm AJ. Ultra-high-dose intraarterial infusion of verapamil through an indwelling microcatheter for medically refractory severe vasospasm: initial experience. J Neurosurg 2010;113:913–922

18. Barker FG II, Ogilvy CS. Efficacy of prophylactic nimodipine for delayed ischemic deficit after subarachnoid hemorrhage: a metaanalysis. J Neurosurg 1996;84:405–414

19. Hänggi D, Beseoglu K, Turowski B, Steiger HJ. Feasibility and safety of intrathecal nimodipine on posthaemorrhagic cerebral vasospasm refractory to medical and endovascular therapy. Clin Neurol Neurosurg 2008;110:784–790

20. Biondi A, Ricciardi GK, Puybasset L, et al. Intra-arterial nimodipine for the treatment of symptomatic cerebral vasospasm after aneurysmal subarachnoid hemorrhage: preliminary results. AJNR Am J Neuroradiol 2004;25:1067–1076

21. Kim JH, Park IS, Park KB, Kang DH, Hwang SH. Intraarterial nimodipine infusion to treat symptomatic cerebral vasospasm after aneurysmal subarachnoid hemorrhage. J Korean Neurosurg Soc 2009;46:239–244

22. Badjatia N, Topcuoglu MA, Pryor JC, et al. Preliminary experience with intra-arterial nicardipine as a treatment for cerebral vasospasm. AJNR Am J Neuroradiol 2004;25:819–826

23. Tejada JG, Taylor RA, Ugurel MS, Hayakawa M, Lee SK, Chaloupka JC. Safety and feasibility of intra-arterial nicardipine for the treatment of subarachnoid hemorrhage-associated vasospasm: initial clinical experience with high-dose infusions. AJNR Am J Neuroradiol 2007;28:844–848

24. Shah QA, Memon MZ, Suri MF, et al. Super-selective intra-arterial magnesium sulfate in combination with nicardipine for the treatment of cerebral vasospasm in patients with subarachnoid hemorrhage. Neurocrit Care 2009;11:190–198

25. Zubkov YN, Nikiforov BM, Shustin VA. Balloon catheter technique for dilatation of constricted cerebral arteries after aneurysmal SAH. Acta Neurochir (Wien) 1984;70:65–79

26. Eskridge JM, McAuliffe W, Song JK, et al. Balloon angioplasty for the treatment of vasospasm: results of first 50 cases. Neurosurgery 1998;42:510–516, discussion 516–517

27. Rothoerl RD, Ringel F. Molecular mechanisms of cerebral vasospasm following aneurysmal SAH. Neurol Res 2007;29:636–642

28. Zwienenberg-Lee M, Hartman J, Rudisill N, et al; Balloon Prophylaxis for Aneurysmal Vasospasm (BPAV) Study Group. Effect of prophylactic transluminal balloon angioplasty on cerebral vasospasm and outcome in patients with Fisher grade III subarachnoid hemorrhage: results of a phase II multicenter, randomized, clinical trial. Stroke 2008;39:1759–1765

35

Aneurysm Coiling

Erol Veznedaroglu and Rashid M. Janjua

Pearls

- Master of the "push-pull" technique is essential.
- Patient selection for treatment must conform to the current literature and to clinical observations.
- The tools needed to solve intraoperative complications must be readily available before starting the treatment.
- Not every aneurysm is best treated with coiling. A low threshold for deciding to clip the aneurysm is recommended.

The treatment of intracranial aneurysms has been revolutionized over the past two decades with the advent of endovascular treatment and technologies. Although open craniotomy for clip ligation and bypass surgery are still required for certain aneurysms, technologic advancements have been decreasing the need for such invasive therapies. The prevalence of intracranial aneurysms ranges from 0.2 to 9% depending on the study, the study population, and the treatment center. Based on interpretation of the data, it is more likely that the true prevalence is closer to 1% of the adult population in young adults and 4% in the elderly.[1]

The natural history of intracranial aneurysms remains a controversial subject. The retrospective International Study of Unruptured Intracranial Aneurysms (ISUIA)[2] found that the risk of rupture of aneurysms smaller than 10 mm was much lower (by a factor of 10 to 20) than reported in previous studies or in the experience of most large centers. The prospective arm of this study reported yearly rupture rates of 1.2%, 3.1%, and 8.6% for aneurysms 7 to 12 mm, 13 to 24 mm, and greater than 25 mm, respectively.[3] This study also had significant selection bias and did not effectively combine data for aneurysms less than 7 mm. Of the 1692 patients, 534 patients were switched from observation to treatment (410 clipped and 124 coiled), and of the 193 patients who died of causes other than aneurysmal subarachnoid hemorrhage (aSAH), 52 died of intracerebral hemorrhage.[4]

Rinkel et al[4] performed a literature review between 1955 and 1996 of nine studies evaluating 3907 patients. They found an overall risk of rupture of 0.7% for aneurysms less than or equal to 10 mm and 4% for aneurysms larger than 10 mm. In a landmark study, Juvela et al[5] studied all unruptured intracranial aneurysms at their institution in Finland prior to 1979 and had 100% follow-up. In 142 patients with 181 aneurysms the cumulative rates of aSAH were 10.5% at 10 years, 23% at 20 years, and 30.3% at 30 years. Significant predictors of aSAH were aneurysm size, patient age (inverse relation), and cigarette smoking.

With a greater collecting and understanding of data, we now know that certain locations of aneurysms (posterior communicating artery aneurysms and those in the posterior circulation) have a higher risk of rupture. Irregular shape, documented growth, family history, and cigarette smoking also play a major role. With this is mind, it is generally accepted that each individual patient have a specifically tailored treatment plan.

◆ Treatment

The development of the Guglielmi detachable coil and its Food and Drug Administration (FDA) approval in 1995 introduced a potential alternative treatment for intracranial aneurysms.[6,7] Guglielmi himself must be astonished at the major paradigm shift in treatment in just the past 15 years largely based on the continual advancement of technology. The treatment paradigm for intracranial aneurysms, both ruptured and unruptured, varies wildly based on the institution and the "gatekeeper" of this patient population. At most centers the volume of clipping verses coiling is dependent on the gatekeepers' treatment expertise. Initially, aneurysms that were relegated to endovascular treatment were those in elderly patients, with high-grade aSAH or with serious medical and surgical comorbidities. The major barrier to endovascular therapy has traditionally been a wide aneurysm neck (**Fig. 35.1**), higher recurrence rates, and absent long-term data on efficacy. The release of the International Subarachnoid Aneurysm Trial (ISAT) has dramatically changed treatment practice

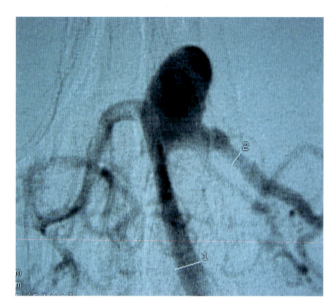

Fig. 35.1 This basilar tip aneurysm would not be able to contain a coil mass due to its wide neck. A stent placed from the basilar artery to the posterior cerebral artery acts as a buttress and contains the coil mass within the aneurysm.

for ruptured aneurysms around the world.[8,9] This prospective, randomized, international study looked at the comparison of outcomes at 1 year in ruptured aneurysms treated with either endovascular coiling or surgical clip ligation. The study found that independent survival at 1 year was superior in the endovascular cohort, and that the survival benefit continues for at least 7 years. The risk of rebleeding in the endovascular group was very low but higher than that of the surgical clipping group; long-term seizures were lower in the coiled group. Recently, the Barrow Ruptured Aneurysm Trial (BRAT) trial was completed, which eliminated the bias of experience.[10] These very experienced open and endovascular neurosurgeons replicated the ISAT study at a single center and found similar results. Interestingly, rehemorrhage was more common in the surgical clipping group.

It is important to point out that endovascular therapy is in its infancy with regard to both operator experience as well as technology. The traditional reports of "recurrence" or "coil compaction" have been as high as 14 to 34%.[11,12] These rates are often quoted but often taken out of context, as they reflect often minimal compaction with no clinical relevance and are from the pre-stent era. The ability to occlude adequately, a wide-neck aneurysm, and increased packing density with stent assistance have likely lowered this number. The pertinent question is, What amount of compaction is enough to warrant retreatment? Most experienced surgeons have many patients in both operative and endovascular treatments with small remnants at the neck that are stable and of no clinical concern. These patients must be differentiated from the ones with increased growth or any filling of the body or dome of the aneurysm. The introduction of "bioactive" coils has also shown early promise in lowering the recurrence rates.[13,14] With improved delivery and embolization techniques as well as an increase in the use of endovascular technique at most

centers, recurrence rates as well as outcomes will likely improve. With longer term follow-up it has now been well established that the risk of recurrence is also very high in cigarette smokers.[15,16] This is important in that it is one of the only truly modifiable risks, and the surgeon should play a large role in this education in addition to the primary caregiver.

Training has also reflected this paradigm shift. Most neurosurgical residency programs now have a mandatory endovascular rotation as mandated by the Residency Review Committee and the American Board of Neurological Surgery. With more physicians training and performing less invasive techniques, as in other areas of medicine, improved outcomes will follow.

◆ Patient Selection

There was little variability in patient selection prior to the ISAT trial (level 1 data), but now the widespread acceptance of endovascular treatments by the neurosurgical community and the improved technology and outcomes have increased the number of variables to consider. Thus, there is currently a wide disparity between centers in who is treated with either endovascular therapy or open craniotomy. There is a general consensus that elderly patients, patients with medical comorbidities, and most patients with high-grade subarachnoid hemorrhage (SAH) are more suitable for coiling. For dual-trained neurosurgeons, the algorithm used to be "if I can't clip them, they should be coiled"; the opposite is now true at many centers. Patients who require long-term anticoagulation are also excellent candidates in that they do not require any cessation of anticoagulation for treatment, with the caveat that anticoagulation may increase recurrence risk.

Patients should sign an informed consent form after a discussion of treatment options ideally with a surgeon who performs both coiling and clipping or who works with either a neurosurgeon or an interventionist. Too often patients are confused by the surgeon's treatment bias. In our practice, which is exclusively staffed by dual-trained neurosurgeons, we explain to the patient (or family, in cases of SAH) that there are two treatment options available and that we perform both regularly. It must be clearly stated that they both carry risks and benefits, and that the risk/benefit ratio is what should determine the choice. Treatment centers and operators have different levels of experience and different comfort levels, and this should be a large factor in the ultimate recommendation.

Our treatment algorithm is based on our experience with both open and endovascular treatments. At our center, most posterior circulation aneurysms are treated via endovascular coiling. Posterior inferior cerebellar artery (PICA) aneurysms that are distal or wide necked are often better suited for clip ligation **(Fig. 35.2).** With stent- or balloon-assisted techniques, it is very rare that a basilar artery aneurysm requires clip ligation. Most wide-necked anterior communicating artery aneurysms and middle cerebral artery aneurysms are treated via craniotomy due to the relative ease and safety of this technique. All other anterior circulation aneurysms are generally treated with endovascular methods.

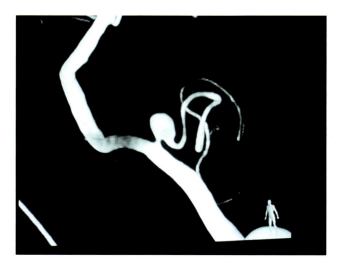

Fig. 35.2 Due to the wide neck of this posterior inferior communicating artery (PICA) aneurysm as well as the narrow lumen of the parent artery, this aneurysm may be best treated with clip ligation. If coiled this wide neck would expose a large surface of the coil mass to the parent vessel, potentially risking occlusion secondary to thrombosis.

We tell patients that the benefit of open craniotomy is the immediate cure of the aneurysm, with only one angiogram needed at 5-year follow-up. It is imperative to tell the patient that clip ligation does not guarantee a cure, but that intraoperative angiography helps reduce the risk of leaving residual aneurysm.[17] The risks of open surgery include retraction injury, wound infection, longer inpatient and outpatient recovery, and the need for antiepileptic medications postoperatively. Endovascular treatment is much less invasive, and usually entails only one night in the hospital and several days' recovery time at home. The risk of thromboembolic events, however, is greater, and the recurrence rates are higher than with open surgery, but with proper surveillance the risk of SAH is very low.[17] The patient is also counseled that they need to have at minimum one 6-month follow-up angiogram and periodic magnetic resonance angiography (MRA) thereafter.

Giant aneurysms remain a challenge to treat from an endovascular standpoint. The rate of recurrence has been reported to be as high as 50%, and surgical morbidity is higher for these aneurysms than for smaller aneurysms. The risk of recurrence and recoiling may be an acceptable trade-off for some patients. Hunterian ligation and trapping with endovascular techniques are also effective in select patients. The introduction of Onyx polymer (ev3, Irvine, CA) and closed cell stents may hold promise for this difficult aneurysm type.

◆ Technical Nuances

With the advent of endovascular treatment comes the development of new techniques and ideas, and greater understanding of the art of coil embolization. One would be hard pressed to find any two surgeons who have the exact (or even closely similar) technique and philosophy. So the following discussion reflects one surgeon's experience. However, one tenet that should be considered inviolable is to treat the patient and not the films. One should ask not "Can I do this?" but rather "Should I do this?"; when all tools are at your disposal, decision analysis is more difficult and must always play the most important role.

As already discussed, with the advent of stent technology, complex coils, and liquid embolics, outcomes continue to improve. Most wide-necked aneurysms are now readily treated with such devices **(Fig. 35.3)**. The improvement of stent delivery enables the treatment of aneurysms in distal locations as well as the ability to utilize new creative techniques. Although there have been major advances in stent design and safety, it must be cautioned that we still do not have long-term data on in-stent stenosis, durability, and safety, and the use of stents should be judicious. Indeed, there has been an increased interest in obviating the need for stent placement by using liquid polymers, complex coils, and bioactive coils **(Fig. 35.4)**.

The first goal of endovascular treatment of aneurysms is to understand the angiographic anatomy. Just as there has been a whirlwind in the evolution of devices, so too has biplane angiographic technology advanced. Three-dimensional reconstruction is available on all new biplane units, and at a minimum, biplane two-dimensional images are a must for any neurointerventional procedure **(Fig. 35.5)**. Once the anatomy is appreciated, the aneurysm must be entered via a microcatheter and microwire. Just as in angiography, the wire is used as a guide to navigate the catheter. Too stiff a wire will allow easy shaping and access to acute turns, but will inhibit the catheter from "following" over the wire around acute bends. Too soft a wire, in contrast, will not allow for navigation into these bends such as at the takeoff of the A1 segment. Catheters come in different configurations of shape, size, and stiffness. Many surgeons use a straight catheter tip and steam-shape it to fit a particular aneurysm and anatomy. In general, anywhere a wire can be navigated to, the catheter should be able to follow. Once the microwire is navigated into the aneurysm, the catheter is carefully threaded over the wire. This maneuver is one of the more common causes of difficulty and morbidity. Once the catheter is advanced, there is an immediate tension translated onto the wire, and when the wire is pulled back upon, the catheter will then automatically advance over the wire. This "push-pull" phenomenon is the hallmark of successfully and safely catheterizing an aneurysm. Once this step is mastered, most aneurysms can be entered, regardless of location.

Once the aneurysm is entered, our preference is for the catheter tip to be in midposition, which is position B in **Fig. 35.6A**. A catheter placed on the wall may increase the risk of coil protrusion, as all the kinetic force will be placed on the aneurysm wall. It is also difficult to distinguish resistance from pushing against the wall versus tension in the catheter system related to tortuous anatomy **(Fig. 35.6B)**.

Likewise, a catheter placed too close to the neck may cause prolapse of the entire catheter system into the parent vessel. Every aneurysm has different anatomic features, and placement should be adjusted accordingly. Smaller aneurysms obviously have a closer apposition of the catheter tip to the

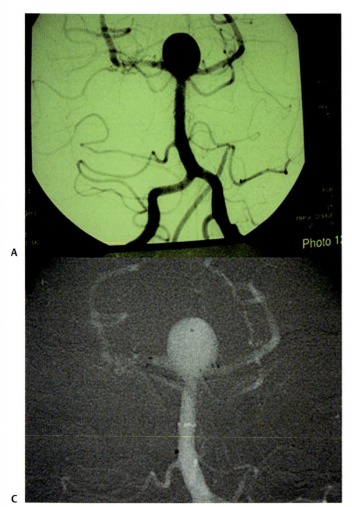

A

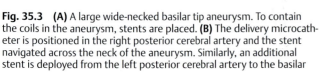

C

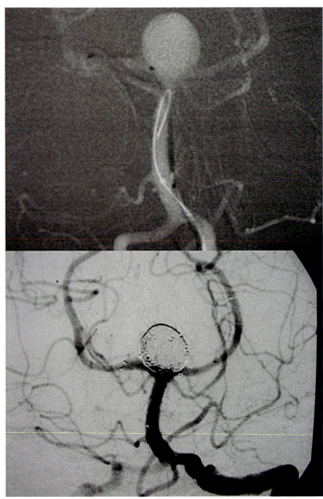

B

D

Fig. 35.3 **(A)** A large wide-necked basilar tip aneurysm. To contain the coils in the aneurysm, stents are placed. **(B)** The delivery microcatheter is positioned in the right posterior cerebral artery and the stent navigated across the neck of the aneurysm. Similarly, an additional stent is deployed from the left posterior cerebral artery to the basilar artery, resulting in a so-called Y-stenting. **(C)** The microcatheter is hereafter positioned in the dome of the aneurysm. **(D)** Several coils are deployed until satisfactory filling, and thus obliteration of the aneurysm from the circulation has been obtained.

dome, which makes them more dangerous and more prone to intraprocedural rupture. Care should be taken with irregular-shaped aneurysms in that the catheter position should be away from any excrescence, as it is the weakest point. With adequate catheter placement, the decision of what size, shape, and type of coil must be made. Nomenclature of coil size is x mm $\times$ x mm, the first number being the diameter and the second being the length **(Fig. 35.7).** The diameter should be sized according to the largest dimension of the aneurysm. The length should be correlated with the volume of the aneurysm. For example, an elongated aneurysm with a length of 7 mm may have a smaller volume than a 7-mm spherical aneurysm. This is important in that although the initial loop of coil takes excellent shape, too long a coil will cause the aneurysm to be filled, but there will be coil remaining to be placed. This scenario then mandates either "forcing" the remainder in or pulling the entire coil out, both less than ideal situations. An angiographic run or roadmap

can be done prior to detachment of the coil to ensure excellent placement and to rule out extravasation. Newer coils have been designed for giant aneurysms with much longer lengths.

A basic tenet is that the two most dangerous coil placements are the first and last, similar to the takeoff and landing of an airplane. Filling of the aneurysm is done with sequentially smaller sized coils and in general with "softer" coils towards the end. Packing of the aneurysm occurs from dome to neck. Judgment must be taken into account at this juncture. Poor filling at the neck promotes coil compaction and recurrence, but overly aggressive packing can increase the risks of rupture, prolapse of coils into the parent artery, and thromboembolism. Just as in intraprocedural rupture during open surgery, the most dreaded location of rupture is the neck, as this is much more difficult to control and repair, with significant risk to the parent arteries. A useful sign at this stage is catheter "kickback"; when the coil is advanced

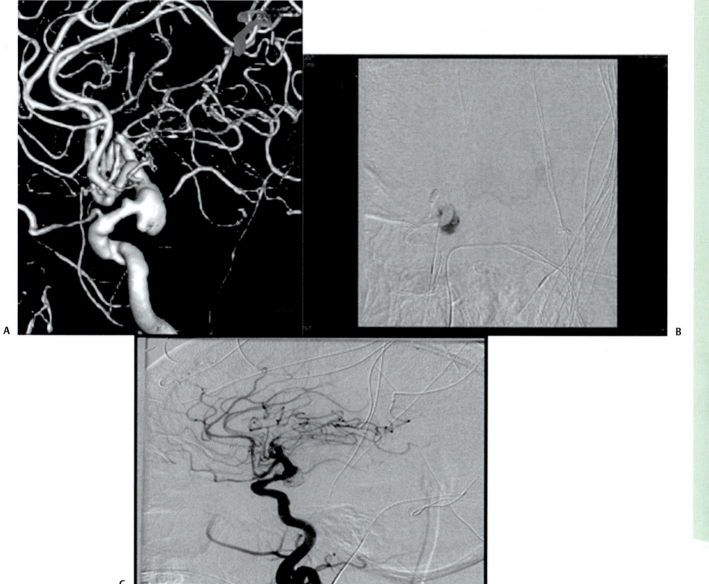

Fig. 35.4 **(A)** Three-dimensional rendition of the carotid artery with a wide-necked posterior communicating artery segment aneurysm. **(B)** The aneurysm is filled with a liquid polymer (Onyx) with temporary occlusion of the neck of the aneurysm by inflation of a balloon in the internal carotid artery. **(C)** Final result, with obliteration of the aneurysm and preservation of the parent vessel.

appropriately, the catheter should push back, as shown by arrow B in **Fig. 35.8,** during coil deployment rather than translate the force of the coil onto the neck of the aneurysm, as shown by arrow A in **Fig. 35.8.** At the completion of coiling, several views, including three-dimensional, when appropriate, can be performed to ensure complete obliteration. At this point in the mask technique the catheter should be slowly removed under direct fluoroscopic visualization to ensure no movement of coils. Once the catheter is removed from the neck, it should remain close to the neck for a final run. In case of any further filling or extravasations, the catheter can quickly be placed back in the aneurysm or be used for thrombolysis if needed.

◆ Complications

As with any surgery, the best complication management strategy is to avoid the known risks for complications but be prepared to deal with them **(Table 35.1).** One of the most common complications in endovascular therapy for aneurysms is thromboembolic. It is our preference to place high-risk patients, and patients who may potentially require a stent, on a minimum of 3 days of prophylactic antiplatelet agent. In general we avoid "loading" elective patients on the day of the procedure, as the full effect of oral agents is not in place.

Another potential cause of thromboembolic events is the length of the procedure. With stent assistance, it can be

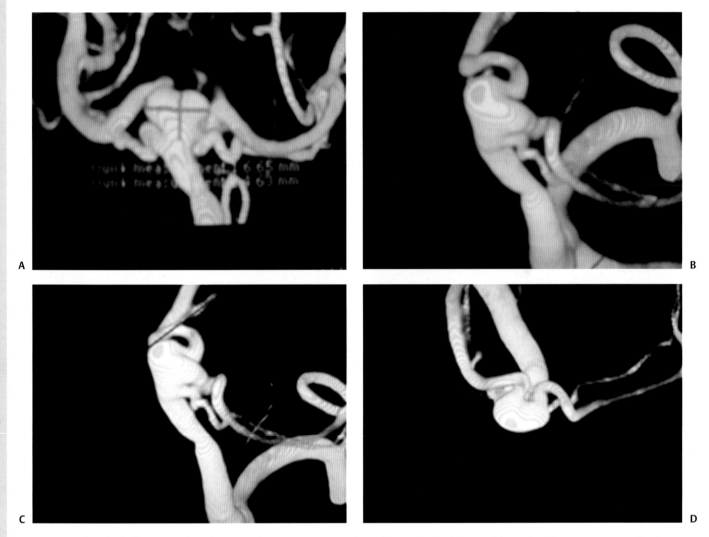

Fig. 35.5 **(A–D)** A biplane, near three-dimensional view is a must to evaluate the true size and shape of the neck of the aneurysm as well as its relationship to adjacent branches. Similar to when approached surgically, proper understanding of these anatomic features is of utmost importance. **(A)–(D)** show different views of the aneurysm as seen with the three-dimensional view.

prudent to stage the stenting and the coiling of the aneurysm when there is prolonged catheter time and difficulty with deployment of the stent. Difficult anatomy with multiple attempts at coil placement should also alert the operator that stent assistance might be required or open surgical clip ligation might need to be considered. It is standard practice at the Cerebrovascular Center of New Jersey to perform all such procedures with the patient under general anesthesia to help reduce this risk. General anesthesia also reduces the amount of movement, thereby allowing faster treatment and avoidance of untoward movement at critical junctures of the procedure. We prefer neurophysiologic monitoring in most instances. We use an experienced team with an exclusive cerebrovascular surgery focus. This team has full monitor access to the procedure to visualize what is happening during the procedure as well as to monitor the vital signs. The angiography suite is optimized for communication among the surgical team, anesthesia, nursing, and the neuromonitoring team. As an example, the anesthesia team monitors the fluoroscopic images, and the surgical team has full view of the vital signs and neurophysiologic data in real time.

All patients undergoing interventional procedures have their baseline activated clotting time (ACT) noted and are given heparin bolus to achieve an ACT twice that of baseline. Full anticoagulation does not preclude sheath placement and can be done safely in patients on Coumadin, heparin, or antiplatelet agents. The decision to continue anticoagulation is made on a case-by-case basis. An uneventful coiling usually does not mandate continuous heparin infusion; however, longer procedures or those involving stent placement may require heparin infusion for 24 hours. In addition to anticoagulation, strict blood pressure monitoring is essential, which requires a good working relationship with a dedicated anesthesiologist. Hypoperfusion should be avoided as well as hypertension during induction and prior to aneurysm treatment.

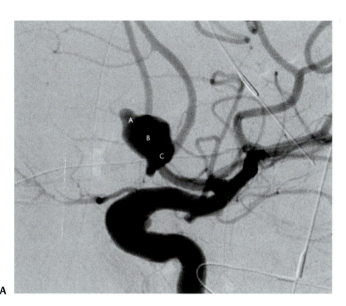

A

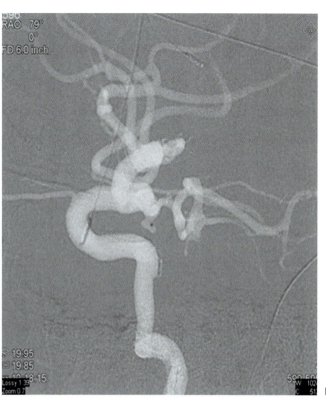

B

Fig. 35.6 **(A)** The three potential positions for microcatheter tip placement. Position A is at the top of the aneurysm. Deploying coils from this position onward enables the coils to be positioned farther away from the neck of the aneurysm; however, the trade-off is a much higher risk of perforation of the dome from the coils. Position C reverses the benefits and risks of position A, with position B allowing sufficient room away from both the neck as well as the dome. **(B)** Due to the tortuosity, tension buildup in the microcatheter can easily be translated to its tip. A tip placed too close to the dome may then result in perforation of the dome.

One of the most feared and life-threatening complications of any aneurysm treatment is intraprocedural rupture (**Fig. 35.9**). This is particularly true for endovascular procedures in that, unlike open craniotomy, direct exposure and manipulation are eliminated and most often patients are fully anti-coagulated. Once a rupture occurs, immediate action should be taken to reduce increased intracranial pressure (ICP) while *simultaneously* assessing where the rupture has occurred, and quickly developing an action plan. A ventriculostomy should be readily available in all angio suites, with nursing staff members checking the contents as they would a code cart. If the patient is anticoagulated, reversal should be done by the

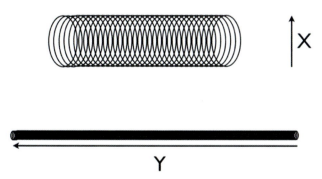

Fig. 35.7 The measurement/size of a given coil is expressed in two numbers: the diameter (X) and the length (Y). The diameter determines the "loop" that each coil segment will take when deployed within an aneurysm, with the length determined by this coil when uncoiled to a straight shape; the longer the coil, the more "loops" it contains.

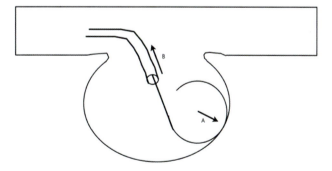

Fig. 35.8 Upon deployment, the coil experiences counterpressure from the aneurysm wall. This counterpressure is translated back to the microcatheter, which allows it to "kick back" out of the aneurysm. This potentially useful feedback alerts the surgeon to the good filling status of the aneurysm.

Table 35.1 Pearls and Pitfalls in Cerebral Angiography and Aneurysm Coiling

Complication	Avoidance
Thromboembolic	• Heparinization/antiplatelet
Aneurysm rupture	• Careful monitoring of flushes, e.g., air, turbulence
	• Limiting catheter time
	• Staging when appropriate
	• Avoiding overpacking
	• Monitoring tension on microcatheter
	• Visualization at all times of catheter and coil
	• Catheter placement
Groin	• Single vs double arterial wall puncture
• Bleeding	
• Arterial occlusion	• Sufficient local pressure
	• Proper usage of closure device
Renal	• Hydration
	• Diluted nonionic contrast
	• Radical scavengers (Mucomyst)
Wires	• Proper size/stiffness of wire
• Dissection/perforation	• Stop advancing if resistance felt
	• Avoid buckling wire against the wall
	• Avoid prolonged wire exchanges
Catheter	• Always advance over a wire
• Dissection/perforation	• Avoid buildup of tension in the catheter

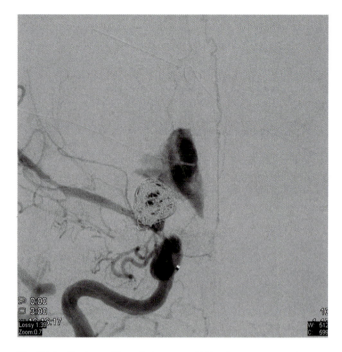

Fig. 35.9 During coiling of a large carotid body aneurysm, extravasation of contrast dye is seen above the coil mass, indicating a disruption of the wall of the aneurysm.

anesthetist, and a neurophysiologist should be notified to place the patient in burst suppression with pentobarbital.

Once the location of rupture is identified (neck, dome), it should be quickly secured with further coil placement with the smallest possible coil. The nurse or technician should have several coils of different sizes readily available. For large amounts of persistent extravasations, we have found embolization with Onyx (ev3, Irvine, CA) very useful and safe, with the ability to control the amount of injection and to perform angiographic runs to determine the cessation of extravasations (**Fig. 35.10**). Once the aneurysm appears to be secure, a second technician should slowly pull back the microcatheter while the operator is injecting puffs of contrast to ensure a secure dome. Once the catheter is removed, it is often very difficult to reach the point of extravasations safely. Temporary balloon occlusion at the neck can also be a very useful technique. If a catheter has gone through the dome, a second catheter can be used to place further coils into the aneurysm. The ICP should be monitored and managed carefully during this time. Modern biplane suites can be used to obtain computed tomography (CT) images, which can assess the extent of extravasation. A large clot may require open surgical evacuation.

◆ Follow-Up

One of the criticisms of endovascular therapy for aneurysms has been the need for long-term follow-up with invasive means such as angiography. With improved neuroimaging, noninvasive neuroradiographic surveillance has proven safe and reliable. We consider a 6-month follow-up angiogram mandatory with an MRA at the same time to establish a baseline. The Endovascular Neurosurgical Research Group recently published its multicenter experience in 2243 patients undergoing follow-up angiography after endovascular treatment of aneurysms.[18] The complication rate was 0.43% in this group, with 0.32% being temporary and minor and only 0.04% being major.[19] Once 100% obliteration has been documented on angiography and confirmed with MRA, patients are followed with MRA at 6-month intervals for 18 months and then yearly thereafter.

◆ Future Directions

With advancements in technology and technique, and with multiple options for treatment, improved outcomes are expected. The simple yet revolutionary concept of treating an aneurysm from the inside as opposed to externally has come a long way over the past several years. The proliferation of advanced technologies such as bioactive coils, liquid embolics, and covered stents has allowed us to treat many aneurysms

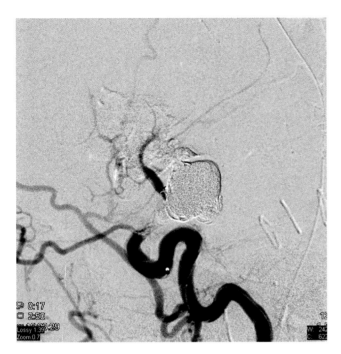

Fig. 35.10 With careful injection of Onyx into the aneurysm, the leak in the wall of the aneurysm is sealed and further hemorrhage abated.

that were not candidates for endovascular therapy just a few years ago.

Research into understanding flow dynamics has led to increased interest in determining if the best way to exclude an aneurysm from the cerebral circulation is better achieved with intraluminal parent vessel reconstruction, that is, occluding dome or interrupting flow to the aneurysm altogether. The Pipeline (Chestnut Medical, Menlo Park, CA) device is a closed cell stent that has been designed to exclude flow into the aneurysm and yet be porous enough to keep perforating arteries open. The initial series of 63 aneurysms treated with this device showed 56%, 93%, and 95% complete angiographic occlusion at 3 ($n = 42$), 6 ($n = 28$), and 12 ($n = 18$) months, respectively.[20] Although these initial results are promising, it must be taken into account that once this device is placed, the aneurysm cannot be entered with a microcatheter, thus excluding the possibility of coiling. As noted in the data, occlusion can take months, thereby eliminating its use for primary treatment in ruptured aneurysms.

The flurry of activity in device design and development and outcomes assessments is a testament to the promise of the endovascular era of cerebrovascular disease. The introduction of new technologies and devices mandates close attention to results and outcomes to determine efficacy. It is likely that the final "cure" for cerebral aneurysms has not yet been developed.

◆ Conclusion

The past decade has seen a major paradigm shift in the diagnosis and treatment of intracranial aneurysms. Along with these changes, the training and practice patterns of both academic and private physicians have also seen a major change. Aneurysms that were routinely treated in the community were referred to large academic centers solely because endovascular treatment was available. This shift was mainly due to confusion over who was a candidate, availability of interventions such as balloon angioplasty for vasospasm, and fear of litigation. With the increase in training and the need for this treatment in the community, there is an increasing shift of even the most complex cases being performed in nonacademic centers, allowing more access to this treatment. With this advance, the decision will no longer be clip versus coil but rather what is the best treatment for the specific pathology, based on outcomes data and local expertise.

References

1. Komotar RJ, Mocco J, Solomon RA. Guidelines for the surgical treatment of unruptured intracranial aneurysms: the first annual J. Lawrence Pool Memorial Research Symposium—Controversies in the Management of Cerebral Aneurysms. Neurosurgery 2008;62:183–193, discussion 193–194
2. International Study of Unruptured Intracranial Aneurysms Investigators. Unruptured intracranial aneurysms—risk of rupture and risks of surgical intervention. N Engl J Med 1998;339:1725–1733
3. Wiebers DO, Whisnant JP, Huston JP III, et al; International Study of Unruptured Intracranial Aneurysms Investigators. Unruptured intracranial aneurysms: natural history, clinical outcome, and risks of surgical and endovascular treatment. Lancet 2003;362:103–110
4. Rinkel GJ, Djibuti M, Algra A, van Gijn J. Prevalence and risk of rupture of intracranial aneurysms: a systematic review. Stroke 1998;29:251–256
5. Juvela S, Porras M, Heiskanen O. Natural history of unruptured intracranial aneurysms: a long-term follow-up study. J Neurosurg 1993;79:174–182
6. Guglielmi G, Viñuela F, Sepetka I, Macellari V. Electrothrombosis of saccular aneurysms via endovascular approach. Part 1: Electrochemical basis, technique, and experimental results. J Neurosurg 1991;75:1–7
7. Guglielmi G, Viñuela F, Duckwiler G, et al. Endovascular treatment of posterior circulation aneurysms by electrothrombosis using electrically detachable coils. J Neurosurg 1992;77:515–524
8. Molyneux AJ, Kerr RS, Yu LM, et al; International Subarachnoid Aneurysm Trial (ISAT) Collaborative Group. International subarachnoid aneurysm trial (ISAT) of neurosurgical clipping versus endovascular coiling in 2143 patients with ruptured intracranial aneurysms: a randomised comparison of effects on survival, dependency, seizures, rebleeding, subgroups, and aneurysm occlusion. Lancet 2005;366:809–817
9. Molyneux AJ, Kerr RS, Stratton I, et al; International Subarachnoid Aneurysm Trial (ISAT) Collaborative Group. International Subarachnoid Aneurysm Trial (ISAT) of neurosurgical clipping versus endovascular coiling in 2143 patients with ruptured intracranial aneurysms: a randomised trial. Lancet 2002;360:1267–1274
10. BRAT Trail Investigators. Personal communication
11. Cognard C, Weill A, Spelle L, et al. Long-term angiographic follow-up of 169 intracranial berry aneurysms occluded with detachable coils. Radiology 1999;212:348–356
12. Raymond J, Guilbert F, Weill A, et al. Long-term angiographic recurrences after selective endovascular treatment of aneurysms with detachable coils. Stroke 2003;34:1398–1403
13. Veznedaroglu E, Koebbe CJ, Siddiqui A, Rosenwasser RH. Initial experience with bioactive cerecyte detachable coils: impact on reducing recurrence rates. Neurosurgery 2008;62:799–805, discussion 805–806
14. Deshaies EM, Adamo MA, Boulos AS. A prospective single-center analysis of the safety and efficacy of the hydrocoil embolization system for the treatment of intracranial aneurysms. J Neurosurg 2007;106:226–233
15. Juvela S, Porras M, Poussa K. Natural history of unruptured intracranial aneurysms: probability of and risk factors for aneurysm rupture. J Neurosurg 2000;93:379–387
16. Ortiz R, Stefanski M, Rosenwasser R, Veznedaroglu E. Cigarette smoking as a risk factor for recurrence of aneurysms treated by endosaccular occlusion. J Neurosurg 2008;108:672–675
17. Schaafsma JD, Sprengers ME, van Rooij WJ, et al. Long-term recurrent subarachnoid hemorrhage after adequate coiling versus clipping of ruptured intracranial aneurysms. Stroke 2009;40:1758–1763

18. Ringer AJ, Lanzino G, Veznedaroglu E, et al. Does angiographic surveillance pose a risk in the management of coiled intracranial aneurysms? A multicenter study of 2243 patients. Neurosurgery 2008;63:845–849, discussion 849

19. Ringer AJ, Lanzino G, Veznedaroglu E, et al. Does angiographic surveillance pose a risk in the management of coiled intracranial aneurysms? A multicenter study of 2243 patients. Neurosurgery 2008;63:845–849, discussion 849

20. Lylyk P, Miranda C, Ceratto R, et al. Curative endovascular reconstruction of cerebral aneurysms with the pipeline embolization device: the Buenos Aires experience. Neurosurgery 2009;64:632–642, discussion 642–643, quiz N6

36

Approaches to Extracranial and Intracranial Dissection

Peter S. Amenta, Pascal M. Jabbour, and Robert H. Rosenwasser

---

Pearls

- Dissection of the intracranial and extracranial vasculature is deemed spontaneous if no evidence of preceding trauma exists.
- Extracranial carotid artery dissection represents the etiology of stroke in less than 1% of all cases.[1,2]
- Regardless of the mechanism of injury, the majority of arterial dissections will heal within 3 to 6 months of medical therapy. Luminal stenosis completely resolves in 90% of cases over this time.[3]
- Ruptured intracranial pseudoaneurysms involving the vertebrobasilar system have a high rerupture rate in the acute period.
- Intracranial dissecting pseudoaneurysms of the vertebral artery represent approximately 28% of posterior circulation aneurysms and 3.3% of all intracranial aneurysms.

Representing the etiology of stroke in less than 1% of all cases, extracranial carotid artery dissection is a relatively uncommon cause of cerebral infarction. However, dissections are a significant cause of stroke in the young, accounting for 10 to 25% of strokes in those aged 25 to 45 years.[1] The yearly incidence of spontaneous carotid dissection is approximately 2.6 per 100,000, whereas that of vertebral artery dissection is 1 to 1.5 per 100,000.[4,5] Untreated carotid artery dissections are associated with a mortality rate of 20 to 40% and a morbidity rate of approximately 40 to 80%.[6] Dissection is deemed spontaneous if no evidence of preceding trauma exists, and fibromuscular dysplasia (FMD) is present in up to 15% of these patients.[7] One percent to 5% of spontaneous dissections of the carotid or vertebral arteries are diagnosed in patients with other connective tissue diseases, such as Ehlers-Danlos syndrome type IV, Marfan's syndrome, autosomal-dominant adult polycystic kidney disease, and osteogenesis imperfecta type I.[8,9] When the cause of spontaneous dissection is unclear, the underlying etiology is usually a summation of multiple vascular risk factors, including, hypertension, diabetes mellitus, smoking, hyperlipidemia, and the use of oral contraceptives.[10-12]

In the setting of multisystem trauma, a dissection may be easily overlooked due to multiple factors contributing to a neurologic deficit on examination.[13] Traumatic dissections may be secondary to either blunt or penetrating injury to the head or neck. Blunt trauma is the more common mechanism for both carotid and vertebral dissections. Sudden impact resulting in rapid deceleration and hyperextension, such as that seen in motor vehicle accidents, may stretch the internal carotid artery over the lateral masses of the cervical vertebrae, resulting in dissection. Hyperflexion of the cervical spine has also been implicated in carotid dissection, as the artery may be compressed between the mandible and spinal column.[14] Vertebral artery dissections are associated with any mechanism that applies excessive rotational forces, distraction, or flexion-extension to the cervical spine. The vertebral arteries are placed at risk of dissection when trauma to the cervical spine results in fractures of the transverse foramina or facet dislocation. Arterial dissection may also be secondary to a relatively minor blunt force, such as that experienced in chiropractic manipulation of the neck.[15,16]

Penetrating injuries represent a less common cause of traumatic carotid and vertebral artery dissections and may be due to physical violence, such as stab and gunshot wounds to the head and neck. Additionally, iatrogenic dissections are well-known complications of neurosurgical procedures. Cerebral angiography may result in cervical or intracranial dissections, as the catheters and guidewires used to navigate the vasculature may disrupt the endothelium, leading to the formation of an intimal flap. Multiple spine procedures, including cervical lateral mass screw placement and occipital-cervical fusions, place the vertebral arteries at risk of injury and dissection.

◆ Pathophysiology and Natural History

Arterial dissections are the result of longitudinal division of the vessel wall by the entrance of blood into the tunica media. The inciting event is debatable, either being the result of an intimal tear that grants access to intraluminal blood or a direct bleed from the vasa vasorum, which forces blood into the vessel wall. Regardless of the inciting event, the expanding diameter of the vessel wall results in partial or complete occlusion of the true vessel lumen. The false lumen may remain patent and act as a conduit for continued blood flow.[17] Exposure of the subendothelial layer also brings the pro-thrombotic components of the vessel wall into contact with intraluminal blood, resulting in the formation of thrombus and a source of potential embolization[18] **(Figs. 36.1 and 36.2).**

In Sandmann et al's[19] review of 200 patients with spontaneous cervical arterial dissections, the internal carotid artery was involved in 76% of patients. Of these patients, 62% experienced unilateral dissection, whereas 14% suffered bilateral

dissections. The internal carotid and vertebral arteries were involved simultaneously in 6% of patients. Spontaneous internal carotid artery dissection most commonly occurs in the cervical segment 2 cm distal to the carotid bulb. The length of the dissected segment is variable, but the distal extent usually does not progress beyond the entry of the internal carotid into the petrous bone. The vertebral arteries most commonly dissect at the level of C1 and C2.

Cerebral infarction may occur at the time of dissection; however, approximately two thirds of strokes occur more than 24 hours after the initial injury. Stroke secondary to dissection is believed to occur for up to 1 month from the time of dissection. The majority of arterial dissections heal within 3 to 6 months, and luminal stenosis completely resolves in 90% of cases over this time. In cases of complete occlusion, 50% of the vessels recanalize within the first 2 to 3 months, resulting in the restoration of blood flow.[3]

When followed with serial imaging, dissecting aneurysms are found to be completely resolved (5–40%), decreased in

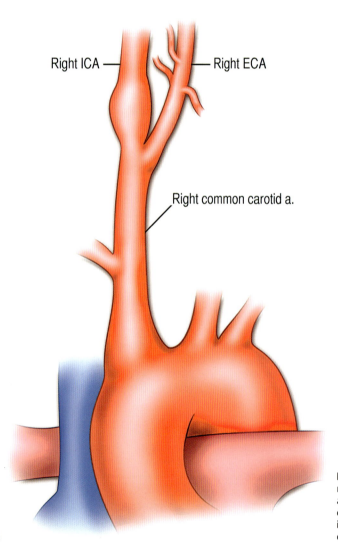

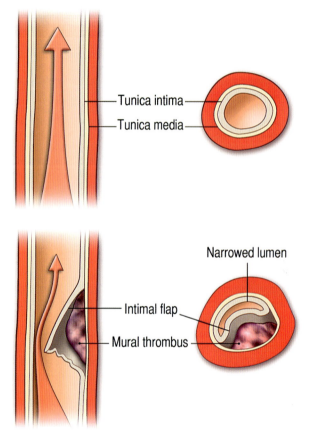

Fig. 36.1 Carotid dissection. **(A)** Illustration demonstrating the normal anatomy of the right common, external, and internal carotid arteries. **(B)** The normal carotid artery in cross section. **(C)** Schematic of a carotid dissection. Note the intimal flap and mural thrombus impinging on the vessel lumen, thereby reducing blood flow. ECA, external carotid artery; ICA, internal carotid artery.

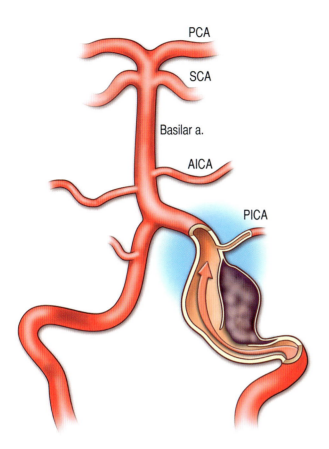

Fig. 36.2 Vertebral artery dissection. Illustration demonstrating intracranial vertebral artery dissection. Note the relationship of the origin of the posterior inferior communicating artery (PICA) to the advancing mural thrombus. Extension of a vertebral artery dissection into the PICA may result in subarachnoid hemorrhage or a clinical presentation consistent with ischemic insult to the brainstem. AICA, anterior inferior communicating artery; PCA, posterior cerebral artery; SCA, superior cerebellar artery.

size (15–30%), unchanged (50–65%), or, rarely, enlarged.[20,21] Dissecting aneurysms of the vertebral arteries are more likely to resolve than those of the carotid arteries. Persistent aneurysms are followed with imaging and are associated with a low incidence of delayed embolic events.[22]

◆ Imaging of Cervical and Vertebral Artery Dissections

Cerebral angiography remains the gold standard in the diagnosis of dissection; however, magnetic resonance imaging (MRI) and magnetic resonance angiography (MRA) offer sensitive noninvasive means by which to reliably detect cervical and intracranial dissections. T1-weighted fat saturation sequences may demonstrate a widened vessel diameter and a narrowed lumen surrounded by a hyperintense signal, representing the false lumen and intramural hematoma. The MRA may reveal a tapered or narrow vessel lumen at the site of dissection. MRI and MRA also represent the imaging mo-

dality most commonly employed in the long-term follow-up of dissections.[16,23]

Although MRI and MRA are the preferred noninvasive modalities for dissection, their lack of widespread availability in the community and the lengthy amount of time required to capture an image limit their use when dissection presents as an emergency. Computed tomography (CT) and CT angiography (CTA) are readily available in most centers and are of significant benefit when dissection presents with subarachnoid hemorrhage or ischemia due to hypoperfusion. CT is able to confirm subarachnoid hemorrhage in most instances, and in many cases is sensitive enough to detect early signs of ischemia. CTA reliably identifies changes in vessel caliber, false lumina, vessel occlusion, and pseudoaneurysms caused by dissection.[14,16]

Prior to the advent of modern imaging techniques, cerebral angiography provided the only imaging modality by which to confirm dissection. Currently, its role as a diagnostic tool has largely been supplanted by the noninvasive tools discussed above. However, angiography continues to play a critical role in the treatment of dissections, and the appearance of a dissected vessel on angiographic films bears mentioning. Dissections, both cervical and intracranial, may display one or more of the following characteristics: segmental arterial narrowing (string sign), segmental dilation (pearl sign), frank aneurysmal dilation, a double lumen representative of an intimal flap, a free-floating thrombus, and a tapered occlusion.[23]

◆ The Cervical Artery Dissection in Ischemic Stroke Patients (CADISP) Study Group: Medical Management of Dissections

In 2007, the Cervical Artery Dissection in Ischemic Stroke Patients (CADISP) Study Group published the results of a systematic meta-analysis of the existing clinical data on antithrombotic therapy for the treatment of cervical arterial dissections.[18] The study represents the most comprehensive review of the pathophysiologic and clinical considerations regarding the use of antiplatelet agents versus anticoagulation. The current medical management of dissections is largely derived from the practice guidelines put forth in this review, and an understanding of the presented data is useful in guiding clinical decision making.

The predominant risk associated with cervical arterial dissection is that of stroke, occurring as the result of either thromboembolism or hemodynamic insufficiency. The vast majority of studies support thromboembolism as the primary etiology. Transcranial Doppler of the vasculature distal to a cervical dissection of the carotid or vertebral arteries shows a high incidence of microemboli in the intracranial distribution of the involved vessels.[18,24] A review of CT and diffusion-weighted MRI imaging has revealed predominant cortical, large subcortical, or multiterritorial infarcts consistent with thromboembolic events. Multiple studies have shown an incidence of only 3 to 16% of patients with a watershed distribution infarct suggestive of hypoperfusion. Angiographic data also support thromboembolism as the predominant cause of stroke in dissection, revealing branch occlusion of intracranial vessels in the distribution of the dissected vessel.[18]

Although the evidence supports thromboembolism as the primary cause of dissection-induced stroke, making anticoagulation the intuitive option, there is currently a lack of evidence from randomized prospective studies to support its routine use.[18] Further complicating the decision-making process is a growing body of evidence that highlights the bleeding risks associated with anticoagulation. Whether the mechanism of dissection is an intimal tear or a direct bleed from the vasa vasorum, intramural blood accumulation is the common end point. When this phenomenon is taken into consideration, it is reasonable to assume that anticoagulation may lead to persistent or recurrent rehemorrhage, thereby propagating the dissection. Additionally, expansion of the mural thrombus can further narrow the true lumen, thus increasing the risk of hemodynamic compromise, delayed vessel occlusion, and possible stroke secondary to hypoperfusion. Indeed, multiple studies have shown delayed vessel occlusion in patients treated with anticoagulation, although mural thrombus rehemorrhage has not been proven.[18]

The existing data from clinical series were also found to be inconclusive, with conflicting findings of varying significance. Subarachnoid hemorrhage is believed to be a rare, yet devastating complication most commonly associated with intracranial extension of a dissection. Studies conducted with antiplatelet agents or anticoagulation failed to show a significant difference in the rate of subarachnoid hemorrhage associated with dissection, but the absolute risk of antithrombotic-associated subarachnoid hemorrhage has never been defined. Similarly, the rate of hemorrhagic conversion of an ischemic infarct is currently unknown and may represent a significant deterrent to anticoagulation. Stroke recurrence has been reported in patients treated with antiplatelets and in those treated with anticoagulation, but the literature fails to show the benefit of one intervention or define the true incidence of stroke recurrence.[18] Specific clinical scenarios, such as recurrent thromboembolic events on antiplatelets, the presence of a free-floating thrombus, and occlusion of the dissected artery, may require further consideration of anticoagulation.

The findings of the CADISP study group meta-analysis highlight the need for a large randomized controlled trial comparing anticoagulation with antiplatelet agents.[18] However, in the interim, the existing data establish a set of treatment recommendations that when paired with careful risk-benefit analysis, can be used to tailor treatment on a case-by-case basis. In all situations, the magnitude of the therapeutic benefit of long-term antithrombotic therapy must be weighed against the increased bleeding risk of anticoagulation.

◆ Surgical Intervention and the Management of Dissections

Although the vast majority of dissections may be treated with medical management, multiple scenarios, both ischemic and hemorrhagic, require the consideration of operative interven-tion. Hemodynamic insufficiency secondary to decreased luminal diameter, pseudoaneurysms, and subarachnoid hemorrhage represent commonly encountered pathology amenable to open or endovascular surgery. Traditional surgical intervention consists of craniotomy and proximal ligation of the dissected vessel, clipping or wrapping of associated pseudoaneurysms, and extracranial to intracranial bypass. Although effective in restoring blood flow and maintaining cerebral perfusion, the extended operative time required for the large exposures and delicate microsurgical technique limits the utility of these procedures in the setting of acute ischemia. Additionally, multiple studies demonstrate relatively high morbidity and mortality rates associated with such procedures, including an incidence of cranial nerve injury as high as 58% and a perioperative stroke rate of 10%.[25-27]

The limitations of these open approaches combined with advances in endovascular therapy have generated interest in stenting and stent-assisted coiling as a primary treatment modality. The relatively rapid nature of endovascular intervention dramatically reduces operative time and eliminates the need to prepare recipient and donor vessels for bypass. In contrast to open bypass procedures, which require temporary interruption of blood flow, stenting is able to reconstruct dissected vessel walls while maintaining continuous perfusion throughout the entirety of a case. In the setting of multisystem trauma, the ability to access the dissected vessel via a site remote from other injuries, such as the femoral artery, allows for effective treatment with minimal patient manipulation or positioning. Angiographic findings accurately define the collateral blood supply and determine the presence of additional vascular pathology within the same operative setting. The minimally invasive approach of endovascular intervention dramatically reduces the risk of further ischemic insult and cranial nerve injury frequently encountered in the meticulous dissections associated with open treatment.

Ischemic Presentation of Dissection and Surgical Intervention

When dissection results in acute severe stenosis or luminal occlusion, hemodynamic insufficiency and decreased perfusion, not thromboembolism, are the causative agents of cerebral infarction. Effective therapy consists of prompt recognition of hypoperfusion as the etiology of neurologic compromise and the initiation of medical therapy to stabilize the patient and optimize cerebral perfusion (see **Figure 36.3**). In the event of declining mental status or labored respiratory effort, immediate control of the airway is the first priority. Once respiratory stability has been established, and ideally in parallel, measures must be taken to maximize cerebral perfusion. High-volume fluid resuscitation and blood transfusion in the presence of anemia are utilized to at least maintain a normotensive state, with moderate hypertension most likely proving beneficial. An arterial line is useful in providing continuous monitoring of the mean arterial pressure. Likewise, routine insertion of a Foley catheter allows for strict monitoring of urinary output, with the goal of achieving a

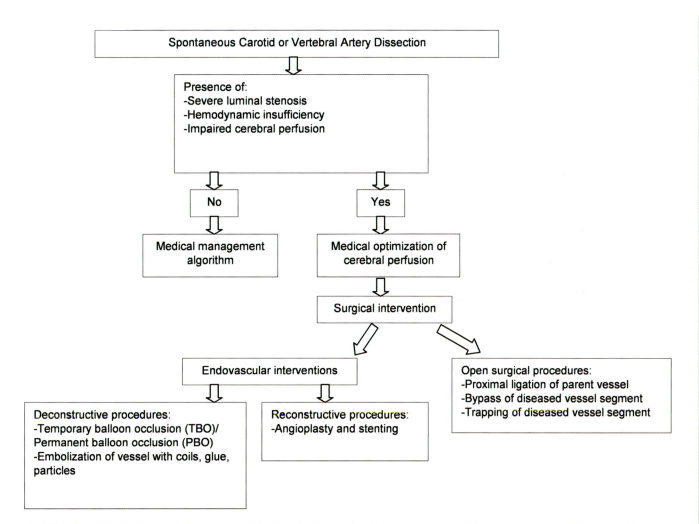

Fig. 36.3 Algorithm for the surgical management of ischemic disease related to spontaneous carotid and vertebral artery dissections. (From Redekop GJ. Extracranial carotid and vertebral artery dissection: a review. Can J Neurol Sci 2008;35:146–152.)

euvolemic to slightly hypervolemic goal. When stable, surgical intervention, either open or endovascular, should be considered to restore normal luminal diameter and cerebral blood flow.

At our institution, acute hemodynamically significant cervical and intracranial dissections are routinely evaluated for possible angioplasty and stenting. Current stent technology enables reconstruction of the vessel wall, while maintaining cerebral perfusion throughout the entirety of the case. Stenting supports the true vessel lumen, reapproximates the edges of the intimal tear, and traps the intramural hematoma within the vessel wall, thereby restoring the original anatomy and decreasing the risk of thromboembolic events. As the dissection heals, the stent is incorporated into the vessel wall via endothelialization and the underlying hematoma is resorbed (**Fig. 36.4**).

Stenting has also found utility in the management of subacute and chronic symptomatic dissections refractory to medical therapy and in patients with contraindications to anticoagulation. Additionally, patients with asymptomatic dissections but persistent severe stenosis may also be considered for surgical intervention, as the incidence of thromboembolism is more than doubled (0.7% versus 0.3%) in this population. In these situations, stenting is usually the preferred modality, yet no guidelines exist to indicate the appropriate time interval over which to initiate treatment. Multiple studies cite the North American Symptomatic Carotid Endarterectomy Trial (NASCET) criteria, referring to the benefit of surgical intervention over medical therapy in symptomatic patients with 50 to 70% stenosis secondary to atherosclerotic disease.[27] Clearly, prospective randomized studies are needed to better define the role of surgical management in this population.

Delivery of a stent to the extracranial or intracranial vasculature introduces a foreign body into the vessel lumen and further disrupts the antithrombogenic endothelial surface. Thus, in the acute setting, placement of an intravascular stent creates a prothrombotic environment, induces local platelet aggregation, and promotes thromboembolism. As a result, antiplatelet therapy is routinely initiated at the time of stenting and continued until re-endothelialization of the vessel wall is complete. Protocols differ between institutions, but

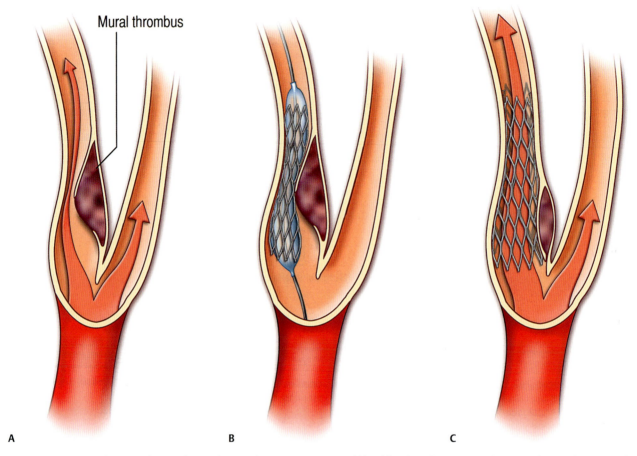

Mural thrombus

A   B   C

Fig. 36.4 Stenting of a cervical internal carotid artery dissection. **(A)** Mural thrombus beneath intimal flap causing hemodynamically significant stenosis. **(B)** Inflation of balloon-assisted stent over guidewire. **(C)** Stent in position across dissection. Luminal diameter and blood flow have been returned to normal. Note the intimal flap and mural thrombus pinned to the vessel wall, thereby reducing the risk of thromboembolism.

most consist of a 600-mg load of clopidogrel with or without aspirin followed by daily dual therapy. Due to the need for antiplatelet therapy, intracranial hemorrhage, primarily subarachnoid hemorrhage due to intracranial extension of a cervical dissection, should be ruled out via head CT prior to stenting. The presence of subarachnoid hemorrhage may alter treatment protocols or entirely exclude stenting as a treatment option. In these situations, temporary balloon occlusion and sacrifice of the vessel with or without bypass may be the preferred intervention.

Close follow-up with angiographic or noninvasive imaging modalities is critical in patients who have been stented for cervical or intracranial dissections. Myointimal hyperplasia represents the chronic response of the vessel to the presence of a foreign body and results in the gradual thickening of the vessel wall. Over time, significant in-stent stenosis or occlusion may occur, resulting in delayed infarction remote from the original event. When discovered prior to additional neurologic insult, significant narrowing or occlusion may require further treatment with angioplasty, stenting, or open bypass.

Clinical Cases

Case 1 demonstrates endovascular stenting of a carotid dissection presenting with hemodynamic insufficiency **(Figs. 36.5 and 36.6).** Case 2 demonstrates dissection and complete occlusion of the cavernous carotid presenting with an acute stroke **(Figs. 36.7 and 36.8).**

Posterior Circulation Dissections and Surgical Treatment Options

Despite the ever-growing role of endovascular therapy in the treatment of dissections, instances remain where open surgical intervention may provide the superior treatment option. More often than not, these complex circumstances arise with intracranial dissections of the posterior circulation. Intracranial vertebral artery dissections may occur anywhere from the piercing of the dura to the termination of the vessel at the origin of the basilar artery. This segment of vessel is rich in small brainstem perforators that arise as proximal as 14 mm to the confluence of the vertebral arteries and are

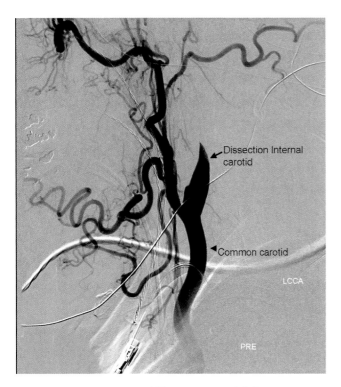

Fig. 36.5 Case 1: A 60-year-old hypertensive and diabetic woman experienced the acute onset of right hemiplegia and aphasia 2 hours prior to admission. Computed tomography (CT) of the head was unremarkable. Cerebral angiogram revealed a left carotid dissection and complete occlusion just above the bifurcation.

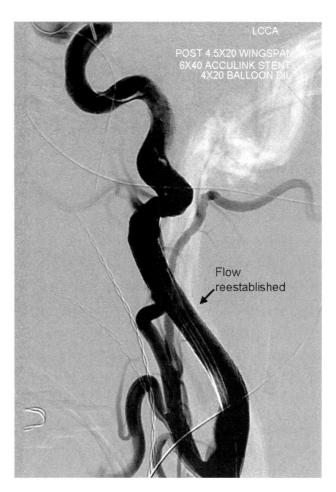

Fig. 36.6 Case 1, continued: A cerebral angiogram post-deployment of stents in the cervical carotid artery and intracranial stent deployment in the cavernous portion of the carotid are performed.

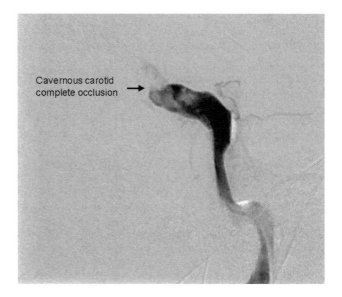

Fig. 36.7 Case 2: A 70-year-old patient presented with an acute onset of a left hemiplegia. The angiogram showed dissection and complete occlusion of the cavernous carotid artery.

present up to 16 mm distal to their union. Endovascular sacrifice of a dissected vertebral artery risks occlusion of these perforators, with the risk increasing as the dissection approaches the vertebrobasilar junction. In contrast to endovascular techniques, open surgical approaches provide direct visualization of these perforators and allow for their preservation, thereby avoiding brainstem infarction.

Dissection of the posterior inferior communicating artery (PICA), whether in isolation or in association with a vertebral artery dissection, presents a particularly challenging problem and one in which open surgical intervention may prove to be the preferable option. PICA dissections commonly present with ischemic symptoms referable to the brainstem or subarachnoid hemorrhage. In the event of ischemic disease, consideration should be given to surgical trapping or endovascular occlusion, yet most cases are treated with antiplatelet agents and close follow-up. When subarachnoid hemorrhage is the presenting pathology, exclusion of the dissection from the circulation is mandatory. In hemodynamically and neurologically stable patients, temporary balloon occlusion is advantageous in determining whether or not the vessel may be sacrificed without further neurologic compromise. If the patient fails the occlusion test, open surgical intervention with trapping of the dissected segment and a bypass procedure is the preferred treatment option. Open intervention allows for meticulous surgical dissection, precise placement of vascular clips, preservation of critical perforators, and the

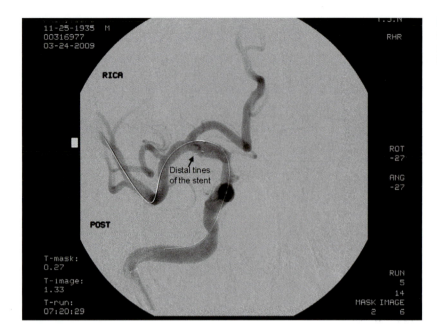

Fig. 36.8 Case 2, continued: A wingspan stent was deployed across the dissection with immediate flow restoration, the patient was discharged on day 4 neurologically intact.

utilization of intraoperative Doppler to confirm preserved flow. The two most commonly performed bypasses in this region are the PICA-to-PICA and occipital artery-to-PICA anastomoses.

Pseudoaneurysms and Subarachnoid Hemorrhage

Intracranial dissections may extend into the subadventitia, resulting in subarachnoid hemorrhage or the formation of a pseudoaneurysm. Subarachnoid hemorrhage classically presents with the acute onset of "the worst headache of my life," photophobia, neck pain, and intractable nausea and vomiting. CT of the head is usually sufficient to identify blood in the subarachnoid space; however, in the presence of a normal CT and high clinical suspicion, a lumbar puncture should be performed to rule out the diagnosis. Unruptured pseudoaneurysms commonly present with headache, neck pain, and, particularly in the posterior circulation, compressive symptoms such as cranial neuropathies.

In cases of subarachnoid hemorrhage, the goal of surgical management is complete exclusion of the dissection and associated pseudoaneurysms from the circulation. Failure to achieve this final result, poses a significant risk of rehemorrhage, usually with catastrophic results. Surgical intervention at most institutions begins with a diagnostic angiogram to evaluate the collateral blood flow, length of the dissected segment, the presence of pseudoaneurysms, and, in the posterior circulation, vertebral dominance.

In the anterior circulation, subarachnoid hemorrhage resulting from intracranial carotid dissection is rare and is often the result of a penetrating or iatrogenic injury. These scenarios are true surgical emergencies, and treatment options have been traditionally limited. In the event that temporary balloon occlusion establishes the presence of adequate collat-

eral blood flow, the dissected carotid may be occluded via coil embolization. Postoperative signs and symptoms of hypoperfusion are treated with hypertensive and hypervolemic therapy, and, rarely, emergent bypass. In the setting of poor collateral circulation, treatment was previously restricted to clip ligation of the carotid and bypass. The emergence of new stenting techniques has provided additional options in the management of this complex clinical scenario. Multiple authors have reported success with "artery-saving procedures" to treat complex dissections of the anterior and posterior circulations. Stents are used to reconstruct the vessel wall, and multiple stents can be layered via a stent-in-stent technique to decrease the diameter of the stent interstices. The vessel is thereby preserved while blood flow is diverted away from the friable dissected wall.[28]

Intracranial dissections of the posterior circulation presenting with subarachnoid hemorrhage represent the class of dissections associated with the highest morbidity and mortality. Intracranial dissecting pseudoaneurysms of the vertebral artery represent approximately 28% of posterior circulation aneurysms and 3.3% of all intracranial aneurysms. Although rupture of these aneurysms accounts for less than 10% of all nontraumatic subarachnoid hemorrhage, the mortality rate has been reported as high as 83%. Once ruptured, intracranial vertebrobasilar dissections and associated pseudoaneurysms have a rerupture rate of approximately 70% within the first 24 hours of presentation, rendering prompt diagnosis and surgical treatment emergent.[23]

Occlusion of the entire dissected segment of the vertebral artery is the treatment option associated with the lowest risk of rehemorrhage following subarachnoid hemorrhage. In many instances, this outcome can be achieved through proximal occlusion of the dissected vertebral artery. However, in the presence of retrograde filling of the dissected segment from the contralateral vertebral artery, the dissection is not completely removed from the circulation and the risk of rehemorrhage persists. In these situations, trapping of the dissected segment with or without bypass may be the superior option. Endovascular trapping of dissected segments is possible and may be used effectively in certain situations. However, the direct visualization provided by open surgery and trapping will also assist in identification and preservation of the PICA and brainstem perforators.[23,29]

Ruptured vertebral artery dissections that extend into the basilar artery remain among the most difficult lesions to treat. Proximal occlusion of the vertebral artery does not sufficiently exclude the basilar dissection from the circulation. Temporary balloon occlusion may be used to determine if the patient can tolerate proximal occlusion of the basilar artery and sufficiently supply the posterior circulation via the posterior communicating arteries. If the balloon occlusion test is tolerated, bilateral vertebral artery occlusions or permanent occlusion of the proximal basilar may be performed. Endovascular coiling of bilateral vertebral arteries is preferred over open techniques, and basilar occlusion may be performed via open or endovascular procedures. In the setting of inadequate collateral circulation, treatment of a ruptured basilar dissection was previously limited to open surgery and wrapping of the vessel to provide additional structural support. Currently, the stent-in-stent technique has provided an additional option for these rare clinical circumstances. Fusiform and saccular pseudoaneurysms may then be coiled through the stents.[23,29]

Nevertheless, a risk of rehemorrhage following stent-assisted coiling remains. Multiple factors have been linked to rehemorrhage, including recanalization of an endovascularly occluded vessel, incomplete coiling of the pseudoaneurysm, and postoperative antiplatelet therapy. Additionally, there are case reports of rehemorrhage associated with the administration of intraventricular and intrathecal thrombolytics to clear the cerebrospinal fluid of blood.[23,29]

Clinical Case

Case 3 demonstrates a stent-in-stent reconstruction of a dissected carotid artery presenting with subarachnoid hemorrhage (**Figs. 36.9 and 36.10**).

◆ Technical Nuances of Endovascular Stenting and Stent-Assisted Coiling

As with all surgical procedures, preoperative preparation is crucial in determining the success or failure of an endovascular intervention. Prior to entering the interventional suite, all pertinent noninvasive imaging should be reviewed, with attention paid to the length of the dissected segment, the likelihood of small perforators originating from that segment, and the presence of pseudoaneurysms. CT and MRI must be evaluated for signs of ischemia or intracranial hemorrhage, as these variables may influence the decision of whether or not postoperative antiplatelet agents will be a practical treat-

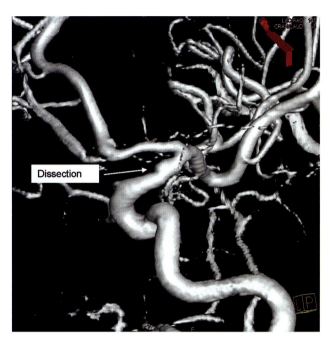

Fig. 36.9 Case 3: A 52-year-old hypertensive man presented with the acute onset of "the worst headache of my life," nausea, and vomiting. On exam, the patient was nonfocal but confused, and CT scan of the head confirmed subarachnoid hemorrhage. The ensuing cerebral angiogram revealed a right internal carotid artery dissecting aneurysm involving the anterior wall of the intracranial carotid artery proximal to the bifurcation.

ment option. At our institution, neuromonitoring is utilized in all endovascular interventions to continuously evaluate the stability of brainstem auditory evoked responses (BAERs), somatosensory evoked potentials (SSEPs), and motor potentials. Preferably, a neuroanesthesiologist is present, as a continuous dialogue is necessary among the surgeon, neuromonitoring team, and anesthetist.

Iatrogenic thromboembolism remains the most common and devastating complication of endovascular intervention. Comorbid atherosclerotic disease, excessive maneuvering through the vasculature, and prolonged exposure of the catheters and guidewires to blood flow all increase the risk of a thromboembolic event. Preexisting vascular disease is obviously beyond the control of the surgeon; however, there are several steps that may be taken to decrease the incidence of iatrogenic ischemic insults. The catheters and guidewires are prothrombotic, and the risk of thromboembolism increases with prolonged exposure to the blood flow. As a result, it is of significant benefit to treat the lesion in a timely and efficient manner. Additionally, heparinization of the entire system should extend throughout the intervention with only minimal interruption for the injection of contrast. Prior to the start of the procedure, all tubing and catheters are flushed free of air to decrease the risk of air embolization. Finally, surgeon experience with the chosen guidewires, catheters, stents, and coils cannot be underestimated, with greater surgeon experience translating into shorter operative time and less manipulation of the vessels.

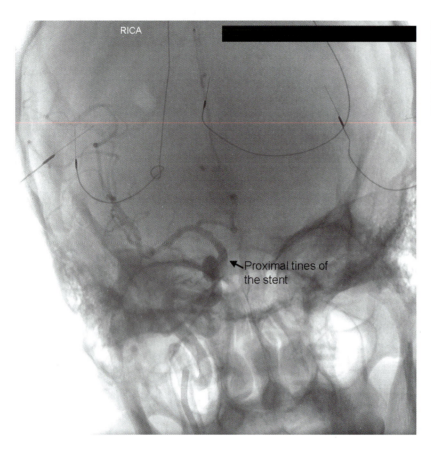

RICA

Proximal tines of the stent

Fig. 36.10 Case 3, continued: Endovascular intervention consisted of deployment of three Enterprise stents (Cordis, Miami Lakes, FL) via the stent-in-stent technique with resultant diversion of flow. The patient was placed on antiplatelet therapy to reduce the risk of stent-induced thromboembolic complications and was discharged neurologically intact.

A comprehensive review of the stents currently available to the treating surgeon is beyond the scope of this chapter, yet it is important to understand the basic characteristics of the stents routinely used in the treatment of dissections. Balloon-expandable and self-expanding stents provide multiple options when attempting to reconstruct the vessel lumen, and each has its own advantages and limitations. The extracranial carotid and vertebral arteries represent larger caliber vessels that maintain a relatively regular and linear course throughout the neck. In dissections of the cervical segments of these arteries, the use of balloon-expanding coronary stents has been shown to be advantageous. These stents possess an increased metal-to-artery wall surface area and exert a greater radial force to the dissected wall, thereby reestablishing and maintaining patency of the true vessel lumen.[30] Both of these properties have also been implicated in initiating an intimal response and promoting endothelialization and incorporation of the stent into the vessel wall. In dissections associated with free-floating thrombus, balloon-expanding stents may tack the clot to the vessel wall, thereby preventing thromboembolic events. Aneurysms associated with cervical dissections of the carotid and vertebral arteries have also been effectively treated with these stents via the "stent-within-a-stent" technique.[28,30] The stents promote thrombosis of the aneurysm by decreasing inflow secondary to the overlapping interstices of the stent walls and a summation of the radial forces applied to the vessel wall from each individual stent.

Although effective in treating extracranial dissections, balloon-expanding stents have multiple limitations and are restricted in their use within the distal carotid and vertebral arteries and intracranial vasculature. Due to a lack of flexibility, balloon-expanding stents are difficult to guide into position through the tortuous vascular anatomy. The relative rigidity of the stent design also limits their use at the skull base, where flexion and extension of the neck may result in kinking and stent occlusion.[30] Additionally, the smaller caliber vessels of the distal vasculature are less likely to tolerate the large radial force that these stents exert on the vessel wall. As a result, delivery of a balloon-expanding stent to a distal or intracranial dissected vessel could promote further dissection or induce rupture.

Self-expanding stents offer a more flexible design and apply a lesser radial force to the dissected vessel wall. These properties allow the stents to be more easily advanced into the distal vasculature, while simultaneously reexpanding the vessel lumen with minimal additional trauma.[27,30] Multiple self-expanding stents currently exist on the market, each with its own specifications, advantages, and limitations **(Table 36.1).**

◆ Conclusion

Cervical and intracranial dissections represent an uncommon etiology of cerebral infarction, yet are a prominent causative

Table 36.1 Balloon-Assisted Versus Self-Expanding Stents

	Balloon-Assisted Stents	Self-Expanding Stents
Preferred target vessel	Larger caliber cervical vessels	Distal cervical and intracranial vasculature
Radial force	Increased metal-to-artery wall surface area increases radial force	Less radial force ideal for delicate intracranial vessels
Postoperative antiplatelet therapy required?	Yes	Yes
Specific uses	1. Tacking of free floating thrombus to vessel wall 2. Stent-in-stent vessel reconstruction for cervical dissecting pseudoaneurysms 3. Stent-assisted coiling of cervical pseudoaneurysms	1. Stent-in-stent vessel reconstruction for fusiform intracranial dissections 2. Stent-assisted coiling of intracranial pseudoaneurysms

agent of stroke in the young. The morbidity and mortality associated with dissection is most commonly the result of a thromboembolic event, whereas acute hemodynamic insufficiency and hypoperfusion account for a far smaller number of strokes. Spontaneous dissections of the extracranial and intracranial vasculature have no association with a preceding traumatic event, and 1 to 5% are diagnosed in patients with connective tissue disorders. When trauma results in dissection, blunt mechanisms are the predominant underlying cause, with penetrating injuries being largely limited to iatrogenesis or the consequence of interpersonal violence.

Arterial dissections heal over 3 to 6 months, with the vast majority of patients achieving complete resolution of luminal stenosis. Dissecting aneurysms usually remain unchanged and may be folllowed with serial imaging in most cases. Although the existing data are limited, the literature supports medical therapy with antiplatelet agents or anticoagulation as the primary treatment modality in the treatment of most dissections. Distinct clinical scenarios, including acute hypoperfusion, patients with contraindications to antithrombotic therapy, patients who have failed medical treatment, and dissections resulting in subarachnoid hemorrhage or pseudoaneurysm formation, must be evaluated for surgical intervention. Traditionally, these patients were candidates for open surgical procedures; however, advances in the field of endovascular surgery have revolutionized the approach to this patient population.

References

1. Ducrocq XLJ, Lacour JC, Debouverie M, Bracard S, Girard F, Weber M. Cerebral ischemic accidents in young subjects. A prospective study of 296 patients aged 16 to 45 years. Rev Neurol (Paris) 1999;155:575–582
2. Hart RGEJ, Easton JD. Dissections. Stroke 1985;16:925–927
3. Kremer CMM, Mosso M, Georgiadis D, et al. Carotid dissection with permanent and transient occlusion or severe stenosis: Long-term outcome. Neurology 2003;60:271–275
4. Bogousslavsky J, Regli F. Ischemic stroke in adults younger than 30 years of age. Cause and prognosis. Arch Neurol 1987;44:479–482
5. Davis JWHT, Holbrook TL, Hoyt DB, Mackersie RC, Field TO Jr, Shackford SR. Blunt carotid artery dissection: incidence, associated injuries, screening, and treatment. J Trauma 1990;30:1514–1517
6. Krajewski LPHN, Hertzer NR. Blunt carotid artery trauma: report of two cases and review of the literature. Ann Surg 1980;191:341–346
7. Mas JLBM, Bousser MG, Hasboun D, Laplane D. Extracranial vertebral artery dissections: a review of 13 cases. Stroke 1987;18:1037–1047
8. Schievink WIMV, Michels VV, Piepgras DG. Neurovascular manifestations of heritable connective tissue disorders. A review. Stroke 1994;25:889–903
9. Schievink WIBJ, Björnsson J, Piepgras DG. Coexistence of fibromuscular dysplasia and cystic medial necrosis in a patient with Marfan's syndrome and bilateral carotid artery dissections. Stroke 1994;25:2492–2496
10. Ast GWF, Woimant F, Georges B, Laurian C, Haguenau M. Spontaneous dissection of the internal carotid artery in 68 patients. Eur J Med 1993;2:466–472
11. Mokri B, Schievink WI, Olsen KD, Piepgras DG. Spontaneous dissection of the cervical internal carotid artery. Presentation with lower cranial nerve palsies. Arch Otolaryngol Head Neck Surg 1992;118:431–435
12. Provenzale JM, Morgenlander JC, Gress D. Spontaneous vertebral dissection: clinical, conventional angiographic, CT, and MR findings. J Comput Assist Tomogr 1996;20:185–193
13. Cohen JEB-HT, Ben-Hur T, Rajz G, Umansky F, Gomori JM. Endovascular stent-assisted angioplasty in the management of traumatic internal carotid artery dissections. Stroke 2005;36:e45–e47
14. Kraus RRBJ, Bergstein JM, DeBord JR. Diagnosis, treatment, and outcome of blunt carotid arterial injuries. Am J Surg 1999;178:190–193
15. Mokri B. Traumatic and spontaneous extracranial internal carotid artery dissections. J Neurol 1990;237:356–361
16. Provenzale JMBD, Barboriak DP, Taveras JM. Exercise-related dissection of craniocervical arteries: CT, MR, and angiographic findings. J Comput Assist Tomogr 1995;19:268–276
17. Anson JCR, Crowell RM. Cervicocranial arterial dissection. Neurosurgery 1991;29:89–96
18. Engelter STBT, Brandt T, Debette S, et al; for the Cervical Artery Dissection in Ischemic Stroke Patients (CADISP) Study Group. Antiplatelets versus anticoagulation in cervical artery dissection. Stroke 2007;38:2605–2611
19. Sandmann WHM, Hennerici M, Aulich A, Kniemeyer H, Kremer KW. Progress in carotid artery surgery at the base of the skull. J Vasc Surg 1984;1:734–743
20. Benninger DHGJ, Gandjour J, Georgiadis D, Stöckli E, Arnold M, Baumgartner RW. Benign long-term outcome of conservatively treated cervical aneurysms due to carotid dissection. Neurology 2007;69:486–487
21. Guillon BBL, Brunereau L, Biousse V, Djouhri H, Lévy C, Bousser MG. Long-term follow-up of aneurysms developed during extracranial internal carotid artery dissection. Neurology 1999;53:117–122
22. Redekop GJ. Extracranial carotid and vertebral artery dissection: a review. Can J Neurol Sci 2008;35:146–152
23. Boet RWH, Wong HT, Yu SC, Poon WS. Vertebrobasilar artery dissections: current practice. Hong Kong Med J 2002;8:33–38
24. Srinivasan JND, Newell DW, Sturzenegger M, Mayberg MR, Winn HR. Transcranial Doppler in the evaluation of internal carotid artery dissection. Stroke 1996;27:1226–1230
25. Müller BTLB, Luther B, Hort W, Neumann-Haefelin T, Aulich A, Sandmann W. Surgical treatment of 50 carotid dissections: indications and results. J Vasc Surg 2000;31:980–988
26. Schievink WIPD, Piepgras DG, McCaffrey TV, Mokri B. Surgical treatment of extracranial internal carotid artery dissecting aneurysms. Neurosurgery 1994;35:809–815, discussion 815–816

27. Surdell DLBR, Bernstein RA, Hage ZA, Batjer HH, Bendok BR. Symptomatic spontaneous intracranial carotid artery dissection treated with a self-expanding intracranial nitinol stent: a case report. Surg Neurol 2009;71:604–609

28. Benndorf GHU, Herbon U, Sollmann WP, Campi A. Treatment of a ruptured dissecting vertebral artery aneurysm with double stent placement: case report. AJNR Am J Neuroradiol 2001;22:1844–1848

29. Taha MMSH, Sakaida H, Asakura F, et al. Endovascular management of vertebral artery dissecting aneurysms: review of 25 patients. Turk Neurosurg 2010;20:126–135

30. Ansari SATB, Thompson BG, Gemmete JJ, Gandhi D. Endovascular treatment of distal cervical and intracranial dissections with the neuroform stent. Neurosurgery 2008;62:636–646, discussion 636–646

37

Cranial Arteriovenous Malformation Embolization

Yin C. Hu, C. Benjamin Newman, Cameron G. McDougall, and Felipe C. Albuquerque

Pearls

◆ Cranial arteriovenous malformations (AVMs) are a heterogeneous group of intracranial vascular lesions that require a multidisciplinary team that includes neurosurgical, endovascular, and radiosurgical expertise to optimize the risk-to-benefit ratio of treatment.

◆ The function of endovascular therapy in AVM treatment can be divided into the following categories: presurgical embolization, preradiosurgical embolization, targeted embolization (i.e., securing an associated aneurysm), curative embolization, and palliative embolization.

◆ Superselective angiographic imaging must be reviewed diligently to identify the following characteristics of the AVM angioarchitecture: (1) *en passage* feeders into normal neural tissue from the pedicle, (2) the first appearance of venous drainage, (3) potential proximal vessels that may be compromised by reflux, and (4) the rate of contrast opacification through the nidus.

◆ The advantage of Onyx over *n*-butyl cyanoacrylate (nBCA) is that the injection can be stopped periodically to evaluate its progression, the patency of the venous drainage, and the remaining nidal angioarchitecture.

◆ The "plug-and-push" technique can cast additional new areas of nidus, and several milliliters of Onyx are often used for a single pedicle injection. However, the procedure is stopped when adequate Onyx casting is achieved or if retrograde reflux threatens to occlude proximal *en passage* branches.

Brain arteriovenous malformations (AVMs) are highly complex vascular lesions that account for approximately 2% of all hemorrhagic strokes.[1] Although they are relatively rare, AVMs can cause significant long-term morbidity and mortality because most patients are healthy and young. The angioarchitecture of AVMs consists of arterial feeders directly connected to the venous system without an intervening capillary bed, creating high-flow arteriovenous (AV) shunts (**Fig. 37.1**). AVMs are considered congenital pathologies that occur sporadically, but they can be associated with several hereditary syndromes, such as Rendu-Osler-Weber syndrome and Wyburn-Mason syndrome, and with Sturge-Weber disease. Reports of familial cases are extremely rare.[2]

Most AVMs are discovered after patients experience an intracranial hemorrhage. Other presentations include headaches, seizures, or a focal neurologic deficit. The natural history of these lesions is poorly understood because most studies are retrospective and biased (i.e., relatively uncommon and heterogeneous lesions are included, and there is a selection bias toward untreatable AVMs). Many investigators estimate an annual risk of hemorrhage for an AVM to be 2 to 4%, with an increased risk of hemorrhage in the first few years after a ruptured presentation of 6 to 18%.[3,4] The risk then gradually returns to baseline.

The treatment paradigms for cerebral AVMs have evolved into a multidisciplinary strategy with the goal of optimizing the risk-to-benefit ratio after a thorough evaluation of the angioarchitecture of the lesion. The current armamentarium includes microvascular neurosurgery, radiosurgery, and endovascular embolization. Based on prospective studies, the Spetzler and Martin grading system (**Table 37.1**) reasonably predicts the surgical morbidity and mortality rates associated with cerebral AVMs.[5] Multiple investigators have reported low rates of surgical morbidity and mortality for grade I through III AVMs. The risk of hemorrhage associated with grade I and II AVMs typically outweighs that of microsurgical resection. Smaller AVMs are more prone to rupture than larger ones. The inverse relationship between AVM size and feeding artery pressure suggests that smaller AVMs have a significantly higher rate of hemorrhage. Usually, the risk associated with preoperative embolization of grade I AVMs may exceed the surgical risk. Grade II AVMs in highly eloquent regions may be

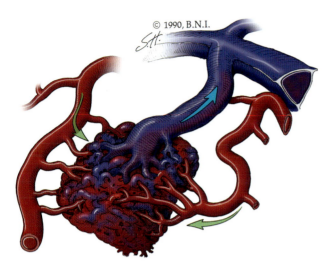

© 1990, B.N.I.

Fig. 37.1 Illustration showing two main arterial feeding pedicles *(green arrows)* branching into the nidus of an arteriovenous malformation (AVM). Note the large vein *(blue arrow)* draining into the dural sinus. (Courtesy of the Barrow Neurological Institute.)

Table 37.1 Spetzler-Martin Grading System of Arteriovenous Malformations

Description	Points
Size of AVM (cm)	
Small (<3)	1
Medium (3–6)	2
Large (>6)	3
Eloquence of adjacent brain	
Noneloquent	0
Eloquent	1
Deep venous drainage[†]	
Superficial only	0
Deep	1

Eloquent cortex defined as primary motor or sensory cortex, visual cortex, language cortex, internal capsule, hypothalamus, thalamus, cerebellar peduncles, brainstem, or deep cerebellar nuclei

[†] Deep veins are defined as internal cerebral veins, basal vein of Rosenthal, or the precentral cerebellar vein.

Source: Spetzler RF, Martin NA. A proposed grading system for arteriovenous malformations. J Neurosurg 1986;65:476–483. Reprinted by permission from the Journal of Neurosurgery.

treated with stereotactic radiosurgery rather than surgical resection.

Grade III AVMs are the most complex and heterogeneous group. Lawton[6] subcategorized grade III lesions into four types based on size (S), venous drainage (V), and eloquent location (E), and determined the relative risks of surgical morbidity and mortality. The surgical risk for small AVMs (S1, V1, E1), medium and deep AVMs (S2, V1, E0), and medium/eloquent AVMs (S2, V0, E1) was 2.9%, 7.1%, and 14.8%, respectively. Presurgical embolization is often required to occlude deep arterial feeders that can be difficult to visualize during microsurgery, thus minimizing intraoperative blood loss. Furthermore, embolized arterial vessels can be used as surgical landmarks.

The surgical excision of grade IV and V AVMs is associated with a high rate of major and minor perioperative deficits, which reach 31% and 50%, respectively. Han et al[7] examined the outcomes of 73 consecutive patients with grade IV and V AVMs and found that the risk of hemorrhage (1% per year) in these two subgroups was lower than the risk of surgical complications. They recommended observing these lesions rather than intervening. Other publications have reported that partial treatment may increase the risk of future hemorrhage.[7,8] Current recommendations reserve treatment of these high-grade AVMs for patients with progressive or disabling neurologic symptoms such as repeated hemorrhage, intractable seizures, venous hypertension, or vascular steal syndromes **(Fig. 37.2)**. These data suggest the need for judicious selection of patients for the appropriate treatment algorithm to maximize the risk-to-benefit ratio.

◆ Endovascular Therapies

The treatment goals for cerebral AVMs dictate the role of endovascular interventions. The function of endovascular therapy in AVM treatment can be divided into the following categories: presurgical embolization, preradiosugical embolization, curative embolization, targeted embolization (i.e., securing an associated aneurysm), and palliative embolization. We discuss the first two categories in the following subsections.

Presurgical Embolization

At many medical centers, microvascular surgery remains the treatment of choice for cerebral AVMs. Preoperative embolization often has little or no role in the therapeutic management of superficial grade I or II cerebral AVMs because the additional risks of embolization may be unwarranted. An exception is the presence of deep arterial feeders that are surgically inaccessible. Grade III or higher cerebral AVMs are often embolized before microsurgical resection **(Figs. 37.3 and 37.4)**. By occluding deep or surgically inaccessible arterial feeders, embolization can improve surgical outcomes. Surgery for a cerebral AVM with deep or surgically inaccessible feeders, which was once considered perilous, can be made a safer operation with preoperative embolization. Furthermore, embolization can decrease the size of the nidus and the amount of blood flow, which minimizes blood loss and decreases operative time. Embolized vessels can be identified easily during surgery, thereby helping to delineate a surgical plane and preventing resection of *en passage* vessels to adjacent eloquent cortex. Grade IV and V AVMs considered for surgical resection often require staged embolization because of their size and the additional risk of normal perfusion

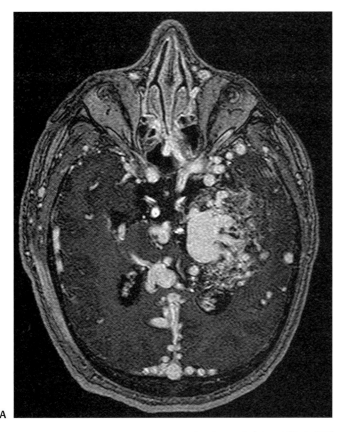

A

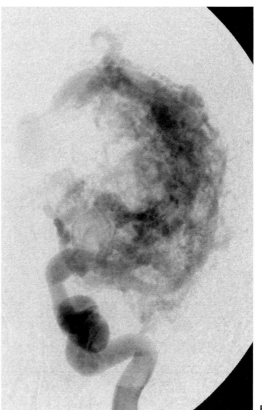

B

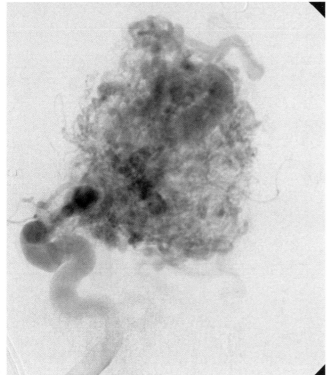

C

Fig. 37.2 Grade V AVM in a patient with progressive neurologic deficits who underwent palliative endovascular treatments. **(A)** T1-weighted magnetic resonance imaging with gadolinium enhancement shows the complex AVM in the left medial temporal lobe. Anteroposterior (AP) **(B)** and lateral **(C)** angiographic views before embolization showing multiple arterial feeders from the left middle cerebral artery. (*continued on next page*)

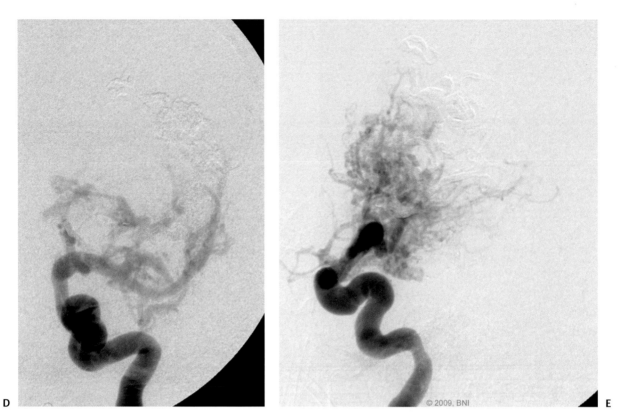

Fig. 37.2 (*continued*) AP **(D)** and lateral **(E)** angiographic views showing postembolization in stages with nBCA and Onyx. (Courtesy of the Barrow Neurological Institute.)

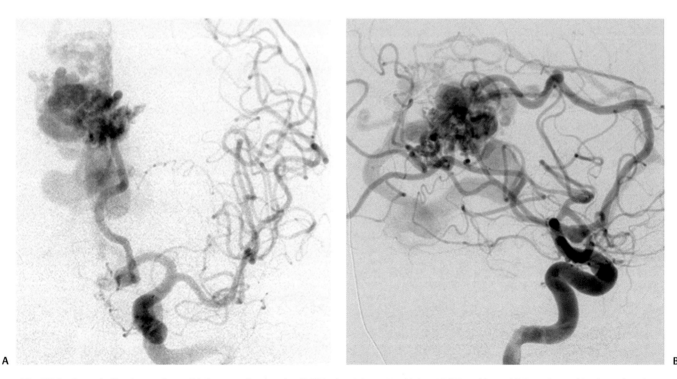

Fig. 37.3 Preembolization angiographic images of a complex AVM in the right parietal lobe. AP **(A)** and lateral **(B)** angiographic views showing arterial feeders from the left anterior cerebral artery.

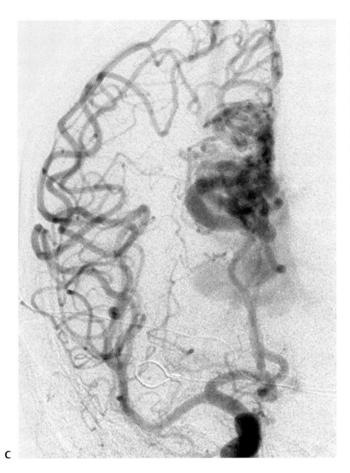

C

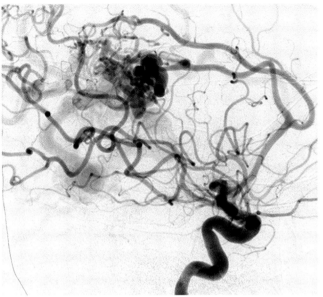

D

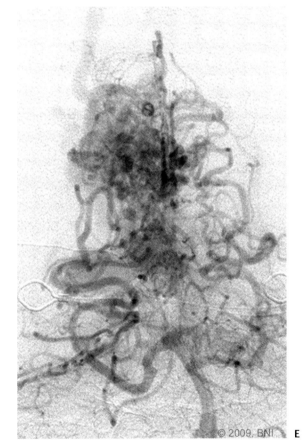

© 2009. BNI   E

Fig. 37.3 (*continued*) AP (**C**) and lateral (**D**) angiographic views showing arterial feeders from right anterior cerebral artery and middle cerebral artery. (**E**) AP angiographic view showing arterial feeders from bilateral posterior cerebral arteries. (Courtesy of the Barrow Neurological Institute.)

pressure breakthrough (NPPB) from the hemodynamic changes that occur within the lesion. Embolization of high-risk angioarchitectural features, such as the feeding vessel and intranidal aneurysms, may stabilize the nidus before surgery and decrease the risk of intraoperative hemorrhage.[9]

Preradiosurgical Embolization

Stereotactic radiosurgery is a common therapeutic option for AVMs that are not appropriate for surgical resection, such as those located in eloquent or deep-seated regions. The radio-

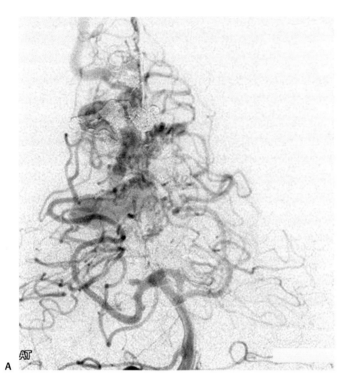

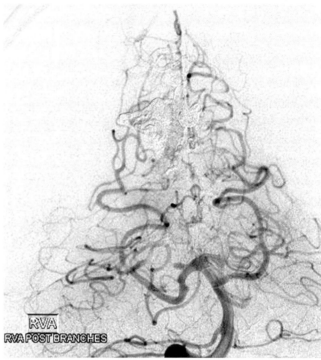

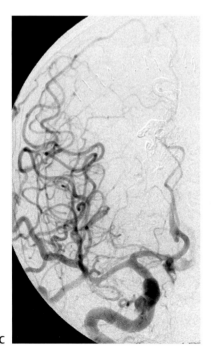

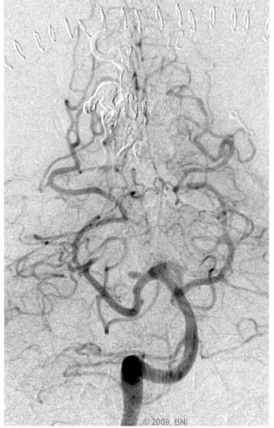

Fig. 37.4 Preoperative angiographic images before endovascular treatment in three stages: coils, *n*-butyl cyanoacrylate (nBCA), and Onyx. **(A)** Preembolization AP angiographic projection of posterior circulation. **(B)** Angiographic image of posterior circulation after all three stages of embolization; AP angiographic views of the right internal carotid artery circulation **(C)** and posterior circulation **(D)** showing complete resection of the right parietal AVM after embolization. (Courtesy of the Barrow Neurological Institute.)

surgical obliteration response of an AVM is highly dependent on dose and volume. Small cerebral AVMs that are less than 3 cm in diameter can be cured in 3 years with radiosurgery, with a documented rate of success in the range of 70 to 95% after a single session.[10,11] One role of endovascular embolization is to shrink a large AVM to a smaller single target that is amenable to stereotactic radiosurgery. This strategy allows the delivery of a higher dose of radiation, thus minimizing the side effects of radiation to surrounding tissues and improving the rate of radiosurgical cure. In some cases, high-dose radiation is not possible. Staged volume radiosurgery can be an option when two or more distinct regions of residual nidus are present after embolization.[12] Other high-risk AVM features such as intranidal or feeding vessel aneurysms can be embolized before radiotherapy (**Fig. 37.5**). High-flow arteriovenous (AV) fistulas are often refractory to radiosurgery and are treated by endovascular embolization. Persistent residual AVMs after radiosurgery are also potential lesions that can be embolized or removed surgically, depending on their angioarchitecture.[13,14]

◆ Technical Nuances

Whether patients should undergo general anesthesia for AVM embolization has been debated extensively. Some argue that provocative testing with a short-acting barbiturate (amobarbital) while the patient undergoes a continuous neurologic examination helps avoid ischemic complications.[15] Proponents of general anesthesia suggest that complete suppression of patient motion during embolization[16] is a safer option and eliminates the need for the continuous neurologic evaluation. This group argues that thorough examination of the angioarchitecture and microcatheter position may be more reliable for avoiding ischemic complications than provocative testing.

In our practice, all patients undergo general anesthesia with neurophysiologic monitoring (both somatosensory evoked potentials and electroencephalography). A 6-French (F) sheath is placed into the common femoral artery, regardless of the agent used. A baseline activated coagulation time (ACT) is obtained, and heparin is administered to patients to achieve a targeted ACT of 200 to 250 seconds throughout the procedure. We believe that the risk of rebleeding with periprocedural anticoagulation therapy is low compared with the risks of embolic complications. A 6F guide catheter, either an Envoy (Codman, Miami Lakes, FL) or a Neuron (Penumbra, Alameda, CA) depending on the tortuosity of the vessel, is placed in the distal primary targeted vessel.

Arterial pedicles are identified on initial angiographic images. Flow-directed microcatheters are often used based on their preferential selectivity toward the vessel with the higher flow, which is usually a feeder into the AVM. The microwire is usually confined within the microcatheter to provide proximal structural support. Occasionally, the microwire is needed to redirect the microcatheter if it repeatedly flows toward a nontargeted vessel or if it must be maneuvered through tortuous feeding vessels. When the microcatheter has reached its pre-nidal or perianeurysmal position, it is confirmed with a gentle contrast injection on a blank roadmap. If the pedicle is a potential vessel for embolization, a superselective angiogram is obtained.

In the presence of high-flow AV shunting, adaptive changes occur in vessels in adjacent neural tissues. As the pedicles supplying the AVM become more exclusively dedicated to the lesion, collateral pathways are opened to supply blood to the surrounding parenchyma. Over an extended period, these collateral vessels can undergo "angiomatous change" that results in markedly dilated and abnormal vessels in the immediate vicinity of the AVM.[17] When significant AV shunting is present, high frame rates (5 to 6/sec) may improve delineation of the angioarchitecture.

Superselective angiographic imaging must be reviewed diligently to identify the following characteristics: (1) *en passage* feeders into normal neural tissue from the pedicle, (2) the first appearance of venous drainage, (3) potential proximal vessels that may be compromised by reflux, and (4) the rate of contrast opacification through the nidus.

Typically, pedicles that contain arterial feeders to normal parenchyma are not embolized. To protect normal parenchyma, coils can be deployed distally in branches that supply the nidus over a long segment and then continue to normal tissue. The branches can be occluded proximally with liquid embolysates. This approach requires the presence of retrograde flow within the distal aspect of the branch, presumably from leptomeningeal contribution, to the normal neural tissue.

The position of the microcatheter in relation to the orientation of the pedicle and nidus is a crucial factor for success. The microcatheter should not overlap with either the nidus or draining veins in at least one image intensifier. This configuration allows early visualization of embolysate reflux to minimize the risk of gluing the microcatheter with *n*-butyl cyanoacrylate (nBCA) or occluding proximal feeders into normal tissues.

Contrast transit time through a nidus provides an estimate of the rate of AV shunting. This information translates into formulating the optimal composition of the nBCA-to-Ethiodol mixtures and initial injection rate. The transit time also determines which Onyx (ev3, Plymouth, MN) concentration should be used. Typically, Onyx-18 (6%) is used for most embolizations, whereas Onyx-34 (8%) is used for the high-flow fistulous portions of AVMs.

Before infusing liquid embolics, interventionists must be aware of the location of the venous drainage. The venous structures should be clearly delineated on both image intensifiers to identify the first sign of embolysates passing through the nidus and approaching the draining veins. It is helpful to use the angiographic image that demonstrates the pedicle and the first visualization of venous drainage on an in-suite monitor as a reference image to guide the injection periodically. It also can be helpful to outline the nidus and draining vein of complicated angioarchitecture during infusion.

Infusion of nBCA requires two experienced operators working in tandem. Before the nBCA is infused, it is appropriate for the neuroanesthesiologist to readminister paralytics if necessary and to reduce the mean arterial pressure by 20 to

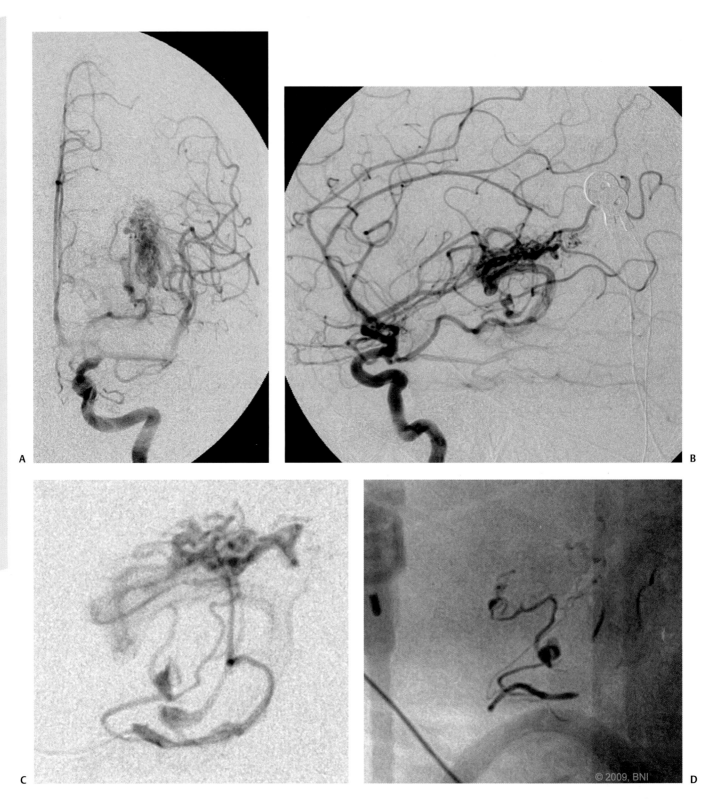

Fig. 37.5 Anteroposterior **(A)** and lateral **(B)** angiographic views of an AVM in the left basal ganglia before radiosurgical embolization. **(C)** Superselective microinjection shows a high-risk feature, an intra-nidal aneurysm. **(D)** Angiographic image after embolization with nBCA confirms elimination of the intranidal aneurysm. (Courtesy of the Barrow Neurological Institute.)

30% to slow the AV shunting. The microcatheter is cleared with 5% dextrose in water to flush all ionic catalysts from the lumen. In a wedged catheter position without arterial contamination, the forward flow is controlled by the rate of injection. This procedure allows a slow, more controlled injection of a dilute nBCA-to-Ethiodol mixture.

Under continuous subtracted fluoroscopic roadmap, the nBCA mixture is then injected slowly into the nidus to obtain a solid cast. The injection is paused for several seconds if a drop of nBCA is observed in the draining vein. The infusion is continued if additional casting of the nidus is noted.

The procedure is terminated when one of three observations is noted: (1) the desired nidal filling is achieved, (2) proximal reflux occurs, or (3) the nBCA penetrates into the draining vein. The microcatheter is gently aspirated and briskly pulled from the patient. A postembolization angiogram is obtained to evaluate the status of the nidus and remaining arterial feeders, the patency of draining veins, and the presence of any complications (e.g., parent vessel injuries, thromboembolic events, extravasation).

In a nonwedged position, a lower concentration of nBCA-to-Ethiodol mixture is used because it flows more rapidly. The injection rate is faster, and the total period of injection is shorter compared with when the microcatheter is in a wedge position. In the setting of extremely high-flow fistulas, coil deployment is used as a strategy to impede the flow rate and to provide a structural lattice for nBCA adherence. A higher concentration of nBCA mixture is also infused to achieve the desired polymerization and casting within the fistulas.

The technique of infusing Onyx is completely different from that of injecting nBCA. Before it is used, the Onyx solution must be shaken vigorously for 20 minutes to fully suspend the tantalum powder. Otherwise, sedimentation of the tantalum causes inadequate opacification during infusion. Once the microcatheter is in satisfactory position as described previously, the dead space of the microcatheter is slowly purged with dimethylsulfoxide (DMSO, 0.25 mL/90 s). The Onyx is drawn into a DMSO-compatible 1-mL syringe and connected to the microcatheter. Next, the Onyx is injected slowly over 120 seconds to displace the DMSO, and subtracted fluoroscopic roadmap is initiated just before the injection is completed. The slow, steady injection should be approximately 0.1 mL/min and usually should not exceed 0.25 mL/min to avoid the angiotoxicity of the solvent.

The advantage of Onyx over nBCA is that the injection can be stopped periodically to evaluate its progression, the patency of the venous drainage, and the remaining nidal angioarchitecture. When reflux occurs proximally, the infusion is stopped for as long as 2 minutes to allow the Onyx to solidify around the catheter. This strategy allows a plug to form at the catheter tip, thereby increasing the probability of antegrade flow. Each time, a subtracted fluoroscopic roadmap is refreshed to prevent confusion about the progression of the Onyx. This process may need to be repeated multiple times. The goal is to establish forward flow into the AVM nidus.

If there is antegrade infusion into the draining veins, the infusion is also halted to allow the Onyx to solidify to prevent venous occlusion. This "plug-and-push" technique can cast additional new areas of nidus, and several milliliters of Onyx

are often used for a single pedicle injection. However, the procedure is stopped when adequate Onyx casting is achieved or if retrograde reflux threatens to occlude proximal *en passage* branches.

Retrieving the microcatheter after Onyx injection requires patience, gentle aspiration, and constant tension. Deflection of the Onyx cast is common, and gentle traction should be maintained as tension is slowly increased over several minutes. If the microcatheter cannot be removed, it is cut at the groin sheath. Breakaway tip microcatheters are in the research and development phase and currently in use outside the United States. In the future, their use should facilitate removal and help avoid potential complications.

◆ Available Agents

Endovascular embolic agents can be broadly categorized as solid occlusive devices, particulates, or liquid embolysates. Solid occlusive devices such as coils and balloons are mainly used to occlude direct AV fistulas. More developed materials such as polyvinyl alcohol (PVA) and microspheres have replaced earlier particulates, including silk sutures and microfibrillar collagen materials. Most centers using liquid embolic agents have also replaced particulates, as evidence has shown that embolization with liquid agents, such as ethanol, cyanoacrylates, and Onyx, is more effective.

Solid Occlusive Devices

Balloons

Balloons can be excellent devices for occluding an artery that supplies an AVM; however, they are ineffective in treating the AVM nidus. Balloons can migrate antegrade into the veins or retrograde into the parent vessels leading to hemorrhagic or ischemic complications, respectively. With the emergence of liquid embolics, balloons have become obsolete.

Coils

Both detachable and injectable coils are useful and complementary components for occluding AV fistulas within the AVM nidus. When using detachable coils, we have a mixture of nBCA-to-Ethiodol prepared before pedicle catheterization while we position the microcatheter by an over-the-wire technique. The over-the-wire technique has the potential to perforate the friable, abnormal arterial feeders. The availability of prepared nBCA mixture minimizes wasting precious moments if a vessel is perforated. Choosing an appropriate coil dimension is important because undersized coils can migrate through the fistula and into the venous system. Based on the vessel size, we typically use a complex three-dimensional geometry or fibrous 0.018-inch detachable coil. The initial coil is usually oversized by 1 to 2 mm.

The coil is formed within the desired artery under fluoroscopic imaging to achieve optimal configuration and position and subsequently deployed. A second coil of similar vessel diameter is then introduced immediately. After several coils have created a stable arrangement, liquid coils can be deployed. Once antegrade flow through the fistula has been reduced substantially, the vessel can be occluded with an nBCA injection. In small fistulas, pushable or injectable coils may be placed primarily via flow-directed microcatheters, eliminating the need for over-the-wire catheterization. Once the flow rate has been decreased, nBCA is injected. Medically induced hypotension is helpful and may be necessary to prevent the migration of nBCA through the fistula into the venous drainage.

Particulates

The particulates initially used for embolization were composed of silk sutures and microfibrillar collagen materials. With technologic advances these materials fell into disuse. Before liquid agents were introduced, PVA particles (50 to 1000 μm) were commonly used to embolize cerebral AVMs. Because PVA is nonradiopaque, iodinated contrast was needed for fluoroscopic delivery.

There are fundamental differences between using PVA particles and liquid agents. For PVA the inner diameter of the delivery microcatheter must be bigger than the particles to prevent clumping and clogging. Typically, larger over-the-wire microcatheters, with their disadvantages of a large profile and less flexibility compared with smaller flow-directed microcatheters, are required for PVA. Superselective catheterization of pedicles feeding the nidus with the larger microcatheters is more labor intensive and entails a greater risk of vessel perforation. The diameter and shunting of vessels coursing into the nidus often vary, making it difficult to select the optimal particle size. Although iodinated contrast is mixed with the PVA particles, it is not possible to identify where they are deposited, unlike with liquid embolic agents. PVA can often accumulate in proximal arterial feeders rather than in the nidus and may contribute to a higher rate of recanalization. Significantly high recanalization rates have been reported on follow-up angiography for cerebral AVMs embolized with PVA particles.[18]

The lack of durable occlusion with PVA particles makes it highly undesirable as a preradiosurgical treatment because the embolized regions are excluded from the radiation field. This lack of permanency is not as important when PVA is used as a presurgical adjunct. In a large prospective trial, the efficacy, surgical resection time, degree of nidal reduction, and Glasgow Outcome Scale scores of PVA and nBCA were similar.[9]

Liquid Agents

Alcohol

Ethanol dehydrates and denudes the endothelial cells from the vascular wall. This process leads the vessel walls to fracture to the level of internal elastic lamina. As a result, acute thrombosis occurs. Although cures have been obtained when ethanol is used to embolize cerebral AVMs, myriad complications are associated with its use.[19] Alcohol can cause cerebral

edema, necessitating treatment with high-dose steroids before and after the procedure. Mannitol may be required in patients with elevated intracranial pressure, which can be difficult to detect when a patient is under general anesthesia. A Cushing triad may be the only indicator of a life-threatening level of increased intracranial pressure. When ethanol is used in high concentrations as an embolic agent to treat peripheral AVMs, it can cause pulmonary precapillary vasospasm leading to cardiopulmonary collapse.[20] The relative lack of inexperience with using ethanol combined with the prevalent and familiar use of cyanoacrylate embolysates for cerebral AVMs has limited the use of ethanol as a routine embolic agent.

nBCA

In 2000 the Food and Drug Administration (FDA) approved the use of nBCA (Trufill, Johnson and Johnson, Miami Lakes, FL) for embolization of cerebral AVMs. These liquid embolysates offered several advantages compared with particulates. nBCA can be injected through small, flow-directed microcatheters positioned just proximal to the nidus. The nidus is penetrated deeply, maximizing permanent occlusion of the lesion.

The nBCA embolysate is a mixture of nBCA, Ethiodol, and tantalum powder. When polymerized, it forms an adhesive, nonbiodegradable solid. The tantalum powder further increases the radiopacity of the Ethiodol-nBCA mixture. The correct ratio is that which matches the angioarchitecture and hemodynamics of the AVM. During superselective angiography, the rate of contrast opacification provides a rough estimate of the mixture required. For most applications, we typically use a mixture of 1.5:1 to 3:1 (Ethiodol to nBCA). The slowing of polymerization by Ethiodol permits better penetration of the nidus. A small quantity of glacial acetic acid may be added to increase the polymerization time without increasing the viscosity of the mixture.[21] After nBCA solidifies, recanalization rarely occurs after an adequate embolization.

Ethylene-Vinyl Alcohol Copolymer-Dimethylsulfoxide Solvent (Onyx)

In 2005 the FDA approved the ethylene-vinyl alcohol (EVOH) copolymer-DMSO solvent for use in preoperative embolization of brain AVMs. The compound is a mixture of EVOH, tantalum powder, and DMSO. It is sold in the United States as Onyx. Onyx is as effective as nBCA in reducing the volume of a cerebral AVM by more than 50% before surgery.[22]

Although Onyx does not adhere to the endothelium, it can adhere to the microcatheter, making withdrawal of the catheter precarious. The DMSO solvent prevents polymerization of Onyx. When Onyx is injected and contacts the aqueous solution, the DMSO diffuses away rapidly. The copolymer precipitates into a soft, spongy solid. The angiotoxicity of DMSO in humans is well established.[23] These detrimental qualities are directly related to the volume of DMSO infused and its length of contact with the endothelium. Limiting the DMSO infusion rate (less than 0.25 mL/90 s) eliminates these undesirable side effects. An inadequate mixture of the solution before infusion can lead to sedimentation of the tantalum powder, producing suboptimal opacification and visualization.

The long-term findings regarding the permanency of Onyx are unclear, and its role as a curative agent or as an adjunct for radiosurgery has not yet been established definitively. Several short-term angiographic follow-up studies have found no recanalization associated with its use.[22] Further evaluation is needed to delineate the significance of Onyx in a neurointerventionist's armamentarium.

◆ Outcome of Endovascular Treatment of Arteriovenous Malformations and Complication Avoidance

Embolization of cerebral AVMs with the goal of complete cure (**Fig. 37.6**) or as an adjunct before microsurgery or radiosurgery is an accepted treatment modality. The cure rates for embolization alone varies widely (0 to 80%) with the type of embolysate used. Several recent case series have reported cure rates between 20% and 50% for all AVMs treated with embolization alone.[24] Preoperative embolization for higher grade AVMs (i.e., greater than Spetzler-Martin grade II) significantly improves outcomes compared with surgical resection alone.[25,26]

No objective, randomized comparisons of nBCA and Onyx as preoperative treatments have been reported. However, noninferiority data for Onyx compared with nBCA have emerged.[25] Many neurointerventionists believe that the handling characteristics of Onyx allow safer, more controlled embolization, and enable a wider variety of AVMs to be treated compared with nBCA. Anecdotal evidence suggests the superior handling of an AVM nidus that has been cast with Onyx at surgery, in which case vessels are less friable and the border between AVM and normal brain is more clearly delineated.

Radiosurgery is often used to treat small residual AVMs or recanalized AVMs after embolization. The role of preradiosurgery embolization of AVMs is less clear. The chief benefit of radiosurgery is to reduce the threat of spontaneous intracranial hemorrhage by gradually eliminating the nidus over several years. The optimal time between embolization and radiosurgery is unclear and requires further investigation. The primary rationale for the use of embolization before radiosurgery is to reduce the volume of the nidus, which theoretically should increase the efficacy of the radiation treatment. At the moment, there are no authoritative guidelines for the role of preradiosurgery embolization of AVMs.

Complications

Despite meticulous attention and cautious techniques, complications can never be avoided completely during embolization of cerebral AVMs. Advances in fluoroscopy and superselective microcatheter technology have widened the scope of AVMs that can be treated by endovascular means. Hemorrhage, antegrade and retrograde thrombosis, and migration of embolic materials into vessels supplying normal brain parenchyma remain major complications.

The overall complication rate for endovascular embolization of cerebral AVMs is approximately 10% for temporary morbidity and 8% for permanent morbidity, whereas the mortality rate is 1%.[16,25] Death or major morbidity is usually related to hemorrhage or ischemia, either venous or arterial. Considerable variability exists in the prediction of hemorrhage from an AVM because these lesions are rare, and randomized trials comparing treatment strategies are lacking.

Intraprocedural or postprocedural hemorrhage is a major concern, but other complications (occlusion of *en passage* arteries supplying functional brain, venous outflow obstruction, venous infarction, cerebral edema, seizures, steal phenomenon,

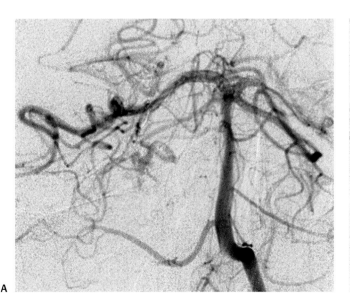
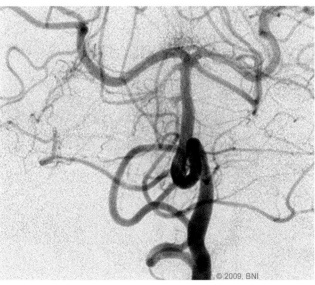

A

B

Fig. 37.6 **(A)** Anteroposterior angiographic view of a small AVM involving the right superior cerebellar artery before embolization. **(B)** AP angiographic image showing curative embolization of the AVM with nBCA. (Courtesy of the Barrow Neurological Institute.)

mass effect) have the potential to inflict substantial morbidity on patients, despite recent advances in microcatheters and liquid embolic agents. The factors contributing to procedure-related complications are incompletely understood and the subject of intense investigation. Patient age, anatomic AVM characteristics (size, location, associated aneurysms, vessel architecture, etc.), hemodynamic disruptions, and many other factors have been postulated to contribute to the risk profile of AVM rupture.

Haw et al[17] observed that intraprocedural complications tend to be related to arterial occlusion, whereas postprocedural complications tend to be related to venous occlusion. They also identified three risk factors that were associated with embolization-related complications: a nidus located in eloquent brain, a pure fistula or nidus with a fistulous component, and venous penetration of the embolysate. Increasing patient age, absence of a pretreatment neurologic deficit, a greater number of embolization sessions, infused volume of nBCA >1 mL, venous embolization, and venous stasis in or around the nidus after embolization also appear to correlate with new postembolization deficits.[27] Antegrade or retrograde reflux of embolysates can result in ischemic complications. Embolic strokes can occur during withdrawal of the microcatheter if nBCA droplets from the tip shower distally. Many neurointerventionists believe that even under the best possible embolization circumstances, perforating arteries that feed normal brain and that are too small to be seen on angiography are occluded, thus providing yet another possible source of complications.

Overestimation of the volume of the nidus can result in overembolization and mismanagement at surgery, or it can cause a falsely large target for radiotherapy. It also can produce NPPB hemorrhage. NPPB hemorrhage is thought to arise from the repressurization of previously hypoperfused regions of brain parenchyma adjacent to the lesion. The cerebral vasculature in these regions displays impaired autoregulation and is unable to tolerate the reestablishment of normal cerebral perfusion pressure after abrupt closure of the fistula or AVM shunt. Hyperemia, cerebral edema, hemorrhage, and even death can result. Therefore, NPPB hemorrhage is a serious consideration in any AVM embolization.

Avoidance of Complications

Following fundamental surgical tenets can minimize complications. We use fastidious outside-the-body technique during the peri-embolization period. Fresh, sterile towels are laid over the patient's legs to create a working area isolated from extracorporeal blood and contrast. The gloves of the physician performing the liquid embolic injection are replaced. Careful handling of the embolic agent may prevent unintended or premature precipitation of embolysate. Vessel perforation is a common complication of embolization because the arterial pedicles are friable, but many authors believe it primarily reflects technical errors that decrease with patience and experience.

Improved fluoroscopic software and detectors have drastically enhanced the visualization of the angioarchitecture of AVMs. Angiomatous changes in perilesional vessels can be difficult to distinguish from an AVM nidus. By increasing the rate of image acquisition from the standard 3 frames per second (fps) to 4 or even 6 fps can help differentiate between a true nidus and adaptive changes in the perilesional vasculature.

The need for a clear understanding of the angioarchitecture of the AVM from a microcatheter injection cannot be overemphasized. In particular, the locations of venous drainage and branching vessels that supply normal parenchyma must be noted. Absence of early venous opacification implies that the selected vessel is a vessel in transit with angiomatous changes. Occasionally, retrograde filling of the nidus from injections of the perilesional adaptive vessels complicates the task of delineating the nidus and feeding vessels. In such cases, the timing of opacification of the nidus or draining veins in relationship to the surrounding vasculature should provide a clue about whether the flow pattern is retrograde or antegrade.

Venous outflow from the nidus must not be compromised until the arterial supply has been eliminated. Failure to do so may result in catastrophic hemorrhage as the arterial blood causes the remaining nidus or venous channels to rupture. Regardless of the embolysate used, meticulous care must be taken to ensure that venous outflow channels are preserved during embolization. Venous infarcts have been associated with delayed venous thrombosis. Any evidence of embolysate migrating into venous outflow pathways typically terminates embolization from the current microcatheter position, if not the entire embolization session.

Suspected antegrade or retrograde migration of embolysate into the arterial tree warrants expeditious angiography to investigate the distal branches. Showering of nBCA emboli as the microcatheter is removed also produces ischemic events. Tearing of the vessel when the catheter is removed can produce devastating hemorrhages, especially since patients receive anticoagulation therapy. If intracranial hemorrhage is suspected, anticoagulation must be reversed immediately. Careful attention to superselective angiography and thorough embolization techniques can minimize ischemic and hemorrhagic events.

Pulmonary emboli have been associated with the use of PVA and liquid embolysates.[28,29] Most patients are asymptomatic, but in some patients it can lead to respiratory distress and death. These incidents are more common in the setting of high-flow fistulas. Nonflow arrest techniques or slowing polymerization with more diluted nBCA-to-Ethiodol mixture or the addition of glacial acetic acid increases the risk.

Occasionally, removing the microcatheter can be problematic, if not impossible, as previously described. If microcatheter removal is deemed impossible, we advocate cutting the microcatheter where it exits the groin sheath. In such cases, patients are placed on aspirin and glycoprotein IIa/IIIb inhibitor, if not contraindicated, to minimize embolic events. The implanted catheter can be resected and removed from the patient at the time of surgery.

Postoperative care is as important as meticulous periprocedural techniques. We typically embolize an AVM aggressively in anticipation of resection the next day. Large lesions are staged over several days before they are resected to minimize the probability of NPPB hemorrhage. We routinely do not reverse heparinization after the procedure unless intraprocedural hemorrhage is a concern. Occasionally, a heparin drip is continued if there is evidence of sluggish venous flow or occlusion.

NPPB hemorrhage is a potential source of complications, particularly if large AV shunts or a large volume of nidus has been embolized. Multiple staged embolization of large high-flow AVMs with gradual reduction of shunting reduces the risk of NPPB hemorrhage. We prefer aggressive maintenance of lower systolic blood pressure after a procedure. Each patient is treated on an individual basis, depending on baseline blood pressure or the presence of other abnormalities (e.g., stenoses). If neurologic deficits are detected, patients undergo immediate computed tomography of the head. Patients may require emergent evacuation of a hematoma. Such patients usually improve significantly after a hematoma is removed, and, if possible, the AVM is resected.

◆ Strategies

Each patient with a cerebral AVM is evaluated on an individual basis. Many factors, including rupture status, high-risk angioarchitecture features, AVM location in relation to eloquent cortex, size, and venous drainage, are thoroughly considered and studied before treatment is selected (**Fig. 37.7**).

There are no authoritative guidelines for the number of embolization sessions needed to obtain optimal endovascular treatment. Furthermore, there is no consensus on the timing between sessions or the time between the final session and surgical resection. Practically speaking, the number of embolizations that can be performed safely in a single session is determined primarily by the anatomy of the lesion and the treatment preferences of the neurointerventionist.

Because AVMs are so highly variable, clear clinical guidelines for determining how much embolization is safe in a single session are lacking. Mounayer et al[30] advocate staging any embolization for AVMs larger than 2 cm to minimize the risk of NPPB. Anecdotally, Katsaridis et al[24] reported that adherence to this strategy prevented NPPB in their series, whereas deviation from this protocol resulted in new neurologic deficits in several patients. We have found that AVMs as large as 3 cm can be embolized safely in a single session. If a lesion is supplied by multiple vascular distributions and multiple sessions are anticipated, our preference is to embolize within one vascular distribution per session.

◆ Conclusion

Cerebral AVMs are rare, heterogeneous intracranial vascular lesions associated with significant morbidity and mortality rates. Treatment of these lesions requires a multidisciplinary team that includes cerebrovascular neurosurgeons, neurointerventionists, and radiosurgeons. Endovascular technologic advances and innovations have significantly improved the understanding of the angioarchitecture of these complex lesions and have extended the capability of achieving poten-

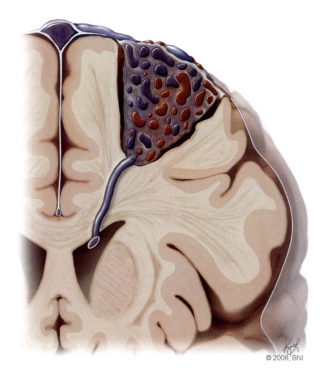

Fig. 37.7 Illustration showing a left frontal arteriovenous malformation with superficial and deep venous drainages. Note the absence of neural tissue within the nidus of the arteriovenous malformation. (© 2008, Courtesy of the Barrow Neurological Institute.)

tial endovascular cures. Despite these revolutionary steps, the treatment of cerebral AVMs requires a well-designed, rational plan that maximizes the benefit-to-risk ratio.

References

1. Choi JH, Mohr JP. Brain arteriovenous malformations in adults. Lancet Neurol 2005;4:299–308
2. Amin-Hanjani S, Robertson R, Arginteanu MS, Scott RM. Familial intracranial arteriovenous malformations. Case report and review of the literature. Pediatr Neurosurg 1998;29:208–213
3. Hernesniemi JA, Dashti R, Juvela S, Väärt K, Niemelä M, Laakso A. Natural history of brain arteriovenous malformations: a long-term follow-up study of risk of hemorrhage in 238 patients. Neurosurgery 2008; 63:823–829, discussion 829–831
4. Fults D, Kelly DL Jr. Natural history of arteriovenous malformations of the brain: a clinical study. Neurosurgery 1984;15:658–662
5. Spetzler RF, Martin NA. A proposed grading system for arteriovenous malformations. J Neurosurg 1986;65:476–483
6. Lawton MT; UCSF Brain Arteriovenous Malformation Study Project. Spetzler-Martin Grade III arteriovenous malformations: surgical results and a modification of the grading scale. Neurosurgery 2003;52: 740–748, discussion 748–749
7. Han PP, Ponce FA, Spetzler RF. Intention-to-treat analysis of Spetzler-Martin grades IV and V arteriovenous malformations: natural history and treatment paradigm. J Neurosurg 2003;98:3–7
8. Wikholm G, Lundqvist C, Svendsen P. The Göteborg cohort of embolized cerebral arteriovenous malformations: a 6-year follow-up. Neurosurgery 2001;49:799–805, discussion 805–806
9. n-BCA Trail Investigators. N-butyl cyanoacrylate embolization of cerebral arteriovenous malformations: results of a prospective, randomized, multi-center trial. AJNR Am J Neuroradiol 2002;23:748–755
10. Chang TC, Shirato H, Aoyama H, et al. Stereotactic irradiation for intracranial arteriovenous malformation using stereotactic radiosurgery or hypofractionated stereotactic radiotherapy. Int J Radiat Oncol Biol Phys 2004;60:861–870

11. Lunsford LD, Kondziolka D, Flickinger JC, et al. Stereotactic radiosurgery for arteriovenous malformations of the brain. J Neurosurg 1991;75:512–524
12. Sirin S, Kondziolka D, Niranjan A, Flickinger JC, Maitz AH, Lunsford LD. Prospective staged volume radiosurgery for large arteriovenous malformations: indications and outcomes in otherwise untreatable patients. Neurosurgery 2006;58:17–27, discussion 17–27
13. Marks MP, Lane B, Steinberg GK, et al. Endovascular treatment of cerebral arteriovenous malformations following radiosurgery. AJNR Am J Neuroradiol 1993;14:297–303, discussion 304–305
14. Steinberg GK, Chang SD, Levy RP, Marks MP, Frankel K, Marcellus M. Surgical resection of large incompletely treated intracranial arteriovenous malformations following stereotactic radiosurgery. J Neurosurg 1996;84:920–928
15. Moo LR, Murphy KJ, Gailloud P, Tesoro M, Hart J. Tailored cognitive testing with provocative amobarbital injection preceding AVM embolization. AJNR Am J Neuroradiol 2002;23:416–421
16. Fiorella D, Albuquerque FC, Woo HH, McDougall CG, Rasmussen PA. The role of neuroendovascular therapy for the treatment of brain arteriovenous malformations. Neurosurgery 2006;59(5, Suppl 3)S163–S177, discussion S3–S13
17. Haw CS, terBrugge K, Willinsky R, Tomlinson G. Complications of embolization of arteriovenous malformations of the brain. J Neurosurg 2006;104:226–232
18. Sorimachi T, Koike T, Takeuchi S, et al. Embolization of cerebral arteriovenous malformations achieved with polyvinyl alcohol particles: angiographic reappearance and complications. AJNR Am J Neuroradiol 1999;20:1323–1328
19. Yakes WF, Rossi P, Odink H. How I do it. Arteriovenous malformation management. Cardiovasc Intervent Radiol 1996;19:65–71
20. Hiraki T, Mimura H, Gobara H, et al. Pulmonary edema as a complication of transcatheter embolization of renal angiomyolipoma in a patient with pulmonary lymphangioleiomyomatosis due to tuberous sclerosis complex. J Vasc Interv Radiol 2009;20:819–823
21. Gounis MJ, Lieber BB, Wakhloo AK, Siekmann R, Hopkins LN. Effect of glacial acetic acid and ethiodized oil concentration on embolization with N-butyl 2-cyanoacrylate: an in vivo investigation. AJNR Am J Neuroradiol 2002;23:938–944
22. Jahan R, Murayama Y, Gobin YP, Duckwiler GR, Vinters HV, Viñuela F. Embolization of arteriovenous malformations with Onyx: clinicopathological experience in 23 patients. Neurosurgery 2001;48:984–995, discussion 995–997
23. Chaloupka JC, Viñuela F, Vinters HV, Robert J. Technical feasibility and histopathologic studies of ethylene vinyl copolymer (EVAL) using a swine endovascular embolization model. AJNR Am J Neuroradiol 1994;15:1107–1115
24. Katsaridis V, Papagiannaki C, Aimar E. Curative embolization of cerebral arteriovenous malformations (AVMs) with Onyx in 101 patients. Neuroradiology 2008;50:589–597
25. Hartmann A, Mast H, Mohr JP, et al. Determinants of staged endovascular and surgical treatment outcome of brain arteriovenous malformations. Stroke 2005;36:2431–2435
26. DeMeritt JS, Pile-Spellman J, Mast H, et al. Outcome analysis of preoperative embolization with N-butyl cyanoacrylate in cerebral arteriovenous malformations. AJNR Am J Neuroradiol 1995;16:1801–1807
27. Hartmann A, Pile-Spellman J, Stapf C, et al. Risk of endovascular treatment of brain arteriovenous malformations. Stroke 2002;33:1816–1820
28. Kjellin IB, Boechat MI, Vinuela F, Westra SJ, Duckwiler GR. Pulmonary emboli following therapeutic embolization of cerebral arteriovenous malformations in children. Pediatr Radiol 2000;30:279–283
29. Pelz DM, Lownie SP, Fox AJ, Hutton LC. Symptomatic pulmonary complications from liquid acrylate embolization of brain arteriovenous malformations. AJNR Am J Neuroradiol 1995;16:19–26
30. Mounayer C, Hammami N, Piotin M, et al. Nidal embolization of brain arteriovenous malformations using Onyx in 94 patients. AJNR Am J Neuroradiol 2007;28:518–523

38

Endovascular Management of Intracranial Dural Arteriovenous Fistulas

Michael C. Hurley, Guilherme Dabus, Ali Shaibani, Eric J. Russell, and Bernard R. Bendok

Pearls

◆ Dural arteriovenous fistulas (DAVFs) are both a result and a cause of dural sinus thrombosis.
◆ The pattern of venous drainage determines lesion grade, and cortical venous drainage heralds an extremely aggressive course.
◆ Transvenous occlusion of the common draining vein requires careful mapping of cerebral venous drainage to avoid inadvertent venous infarcts and hemorrhage.
◆ Transarterial occlusion is now more feasible using the liquid embolic agent Onyx but requires a detailed understanding of dural arterial anatomy to avoid eloquent collaterals and cranial nerve injury.

Dural arteriovenous fistulas (DAVFs) account for 15% of all high-flow intracranial vascular lesions.[1] Evaluation of the prognosis of a lesion and its potential therapies requires a detailed angiographic workup combined with a sound knowledge of dural arterial and venous anatomy. After reviewing this vital basis, we shall discuss the main transvenous and transarterial endovascular approaches to endovascular therapy as well as modified/combined techniques.

◆ Applied Dural Arterial Anatomy

Dural fistulas tend to recruit regional supply from adjacent arterial pedicles in a predictable fashion. Large shunts can eventually draw in supply from contralateral arterial pedicles (**Fig. 38.1**). Understanding the dural arterial anatomy and potential direct cranial nerve supply or anastomotic supply to the brain and orbit is of increased importance due to the increased application of transarterial liquid embolization

since the availability of ethylene vinyl alcohol (Onyx, ev3, Irvine, CA) in 2005.[2]

The dura mater is supplied almost exclusively by extra-dural branches of the external carotid (ECA), internal carotid (ICA), and vertebral arteries (VA). A notable exception is the artery of Davidoff and Schechter, a dural branch arising from the posterior cerebral artery (PCA) that supplies the tentorial dura (**Fig. 38.2**).[3] Normal intraaxial cerebral and posterior fossa brainstem/cerebellar arteries are delimited peripherally by the pia-arachnoid (leptomeninges) and subject to the blood–brain barrier. However, if there is a large and chronic shunt, these arteries may be recruited by a "sump effect" to supply the dural lesion (**Fig. 38.3**).

A brief account of pertinent dural arterial anatomy follows. The locations of potentially dangerous anastomoses among the ECA, ICA, and VA are summarized in **Figs. 38.4 and 38.5**.

The middle meningeal artery (MMA) arises from the proximal internal maxillary artery (IMaxA) and takes a characteristic hairpin bend as it traverses the foramen spinosum. After becoming intracranial it gives off immediate branches to the dura of the cavernous sinus and petrous ridge (the latter constituting an important supply to the geniculate portion of the facial nerve, along with the stylomastoid branch of the posterior auricular artery). It then gives off the main squamosal and frontoparietal branches, which course posteriorly across the calvaria in a smooth anteriorly convex arc. The latter are distinguished from the overlapping superficial temporal artery (STA) on lateral angiograms by the marked tortuosity of the latter's subcutaneous branches.

The accessory middle meningeal artery (aMMA) may arise from a common trunk with the MMA or arise independently and more distally along the IMaxA. After traversing the skull either with the mandibular nerve through the foramen ovale or the adjacent foramen of Vesalius, it gives off branches to

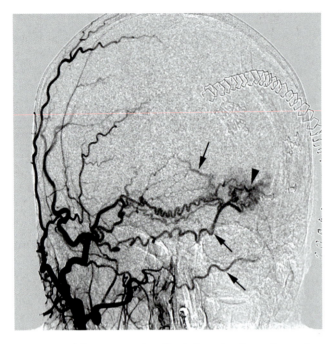

Fig. 38.1 A left transverse sinus fistula *(arrowhead)* recruits supply from the contralateral occipital territory *(arrows)*.

the cavernous dura and can anastomose with the corresponding branches of the inferolateral trunk (ILT) of the ipsilateral cavernous ICA.

The most distal IMaxA supply arises from the artery of the foramen rotundum, which has a characteristic sawtooth pattern on a lateral angiogram as it travels superiorly

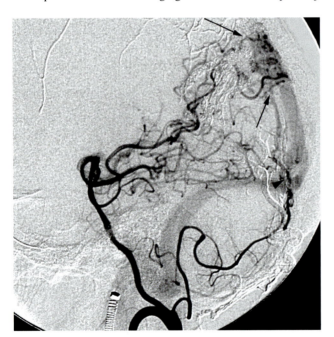

Fig. 38.3 After transarterial embolization of its dural supply, this dural arteriovenous fistula (DAVF) of the posterior falx/superior sagittal sinus (SSS) retains pial collateral supply from the parieto-occipital posterior cerebral arteries *(arrows)*. A satellite DAVF supplied by calcarine feeders drains superiorly via a falcine sinus *(arrowhead)*.

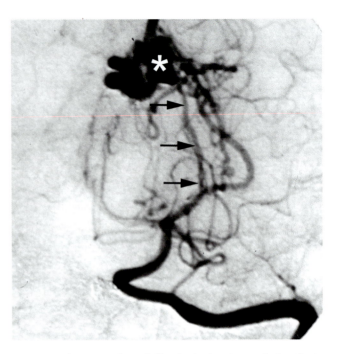

Fig. 38.2 The artery of Davidoff and Schechter is a rarely described dural branch arising from the proximal posterior cerebral artery (PCA) and courses along the tentorial margin, seen here on the left *(arrows)* supplying a pineal region arteriovenous malformation (AVM).

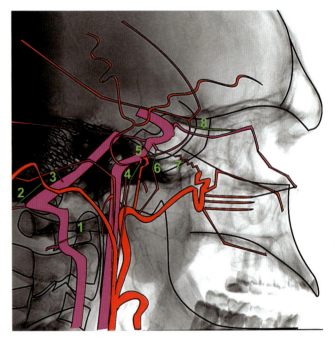

Fig. 38.4 Potentially dangerous external carotid artery (ECA) to internal carotid artery (ICA) and vertebral artery (VA) anastomoses: 1, ascending pharyngeal artery (APA) to the muscular branch of VA C2 segment; 2, occipital artery to VA C1 segment; 3, posterior meningeal branches of APA and VA; 4, carotid branch of APA to lateral ICA segment; 5, middle meningeal artery (MMA) to meningohypophyseal trunk (MHT) of cavernous ICA; 6, accessory middle meningeal artery to inferolateral trunk (ILT) of cavernous ICA; 7, artery of foramen of rotundum to the ILT; 8, MMA to ophthalmic artery.

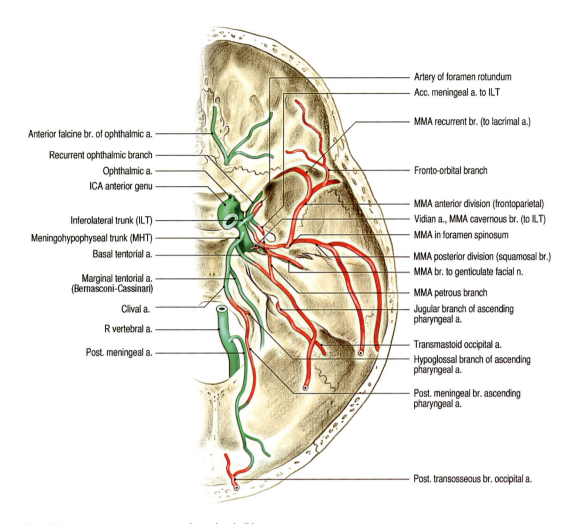

Fig. 38.5 Important anastomoses along the skull base.

Labels (clockwise from top right):
- Artery of foramen rotundum
- Acc. meningeal a. to ILT
- MMA recurrent br. (to lacrimal a.)
- Fronto-orbital branch
- MMA anterior division (frontoparietal)
- Vidian a., MMA cavernous br. (to ILT)
- MMA in foramen spinosum
- MMA posterior division (squamosal br.)
- MMA br. to genticulate facial n.
- MMA petrous branch
- Jugular branch of ascending pharyngeal a.
- Transmastoid occipital a.
- Hypoglossal branch of ascending pharyngeal a.
- Post. meningeal br. ascending pharyngeal a.
- Post. transosseous br. occipital a.
- Post. meningeal a.
- R vertebral a.
- Clival a.
- Marginal tentorial a. (Bernasconi-Cassinari)
- Basal tentorial a.
- Meningohypophyseal trunk (MHT)
- Inferolateral trunk (ILT)
- ICA anterior genu
- Ophthalmic a.
- Recurrent ophthalmic branch
- Anterior falcine br. of ophthalmic a.

and posteriorly along with the maxillary nerve to supply the cavernous dura **(Fig. 38.6)**. The terminal IMaxA can anastomose with the ophthalmic artery via sphenopalatine to ethmoidal networks and with the accessory meningeal via the pterygovaginal artery, which supplies the roof of the pharynx and eustachian orifice. The vidian artery provides an extremely diminutive connection between the IMaxA and the lateral carotid segment, but can be enlarged in chronic collateralization states **(Fig. 38.6)**.

The STA gives off a small transosseous supply to the dura, particularly over the vertex close to the superior sagittal sinus. A palpebral branch may anastomose with the ophthalmic artery at the lateral orbital margin.

The occipital artery (OccA) gives off transmastoid and transoccipital transosseous branches. As with the superficial

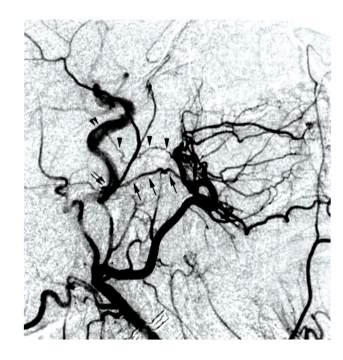

Fig. 38.6 Lateral projection ECA angiogram demonstrates a grossly enlarged vidian artery *(arrows)* and artery of the foramen of rotundum *(arrowheads)* giving collateral supply to the lateral segment *(double arrows)* and cavernous segment *(double arrowheads)* of the ICA, respectively. This patient had a critical stenosis of the ICA origin.

temporal artery, these can be difficult to traverse, and necrosis of the scalp is a risk if the OccA or STA is embolized with liquid embolic agents.

The ascending pharyngeal artery (APA) gives off neuromeningeal branches that traverse the hypoglossal and jugular foramina with a variable meningeal supply that is balanced with the posterior meningeal branch of the vertebral artery. It gives an important supply to the cranial nerves IX to XII. A branch to the periodontoid arcade can anastomose with the C3 vertebral segmental artery. The superior pharyngeal branch gives off a carotid branch that traverses the foramen lacerum to anastomose with the ICA.

The meningohypophyseal trunk (MHT) of the posterior cavernous ICA gives off the marginal tentorial branch of Bernasconi-Cassinari (**Fig. 38.5**) and also supplies the cavernous dura along with branches of the ILT, which arises from the anterior cavernous ICA. The latter may anastomose with the artery of foramen rotundum and the ophthalmic artery via a recurrent branch. Medial and lateral clival branches course inferiorly from the MHT and ILT, respectively, where they anastomose with corresponding hypoglossal and neuromeningeal branches of the ascending pharyngeal artery. There are no normal dural branches arising from the intradural ICA. In extreme cases of high-flow shunting, the dural territory may recruit supply from the adjacent pial branches of the cerebral arterial territories (**Fig. 38.7**).

The ethmoidal branches of the ophthalmic artery (OA) traverse the floor of the anterior cranial fossa at the foramen cecum and give off an anterior falcine branch. They are almost always the main supply to fistulas in this region, often with the bilateral OAs involved.[4] The MMA may also contribute to their supply but is usually secondary.

◆ Applied Dural and Cortical Venous Anatomy

Dural arteriovenous fistulas are defined and graded by their means of dural or cortical venous drainage (see below). Dural sinuses are venous channels within the dura itself and tend to have a triangular cross-sectional profile with flattened sides. Cortical veins and the perimedullary veins around the brainstem traverse the subarachnoid space and are rounded in cross sections and more tortuous as they pass over adjacent anatomy such as cortical gyri. **Figures 38.8 and 38.9** demonstrate the lateral projection venous phases, from ICA and VA injections, respectively, superimposed on the same patient's sagittal magnetic resonance (MR) anatomy.

Dural Venous Anatomy

The superior sagittal sinus (SSS) has a variable size anteriorly and gradually enlarges as it passes posteriorly to accommodate the draining paramedian medial and lateral convexity hemispheric (frontal, parietal, and occipital) cortical veins. Due to the small size of the SSS anteriorly, DAVFs of the floor of the anterior cranial fossa tend to drain into a cortical vein before reaching the SSS (**Fig. 38.10**).[5] The anatomic arrangement of the torcular herophili varies widely but it usually receives the SSS and the straight and occipital sinuses, and divides into the left and dominant right transverse sinuses (TSs). In addition to the deep venous drainage though the vein of Galen, the straight sinus receives the inferior sagittal sinus, which is normally a tiny structure in the inferior margin of the falx cerebri. A vestigial embryonic posterior falcine sinus can be recanalized in pathologic states and extends from the vein of Galen to the SSS several centimeters above the torcular (**Fig. 38.11**).[5] The transverse sinuses receive the adjacent occipital and temporal cortical veins, either directly or via inconstant tentorial sinuses. A midline occipital sinus usually drains up into the torcular but may drain inferiorly around the foramen magnum via a marginal sinus into the jugular or condylar-suboccipital vein. The sigmoid sinus is applied to the inner surface of the petrous bone as it descends from the TS to the jugular fossa, and turbulent flow may be audible to the patient in this location even in the absence of an arteriovenous malformation (essential vascular tinnitus).[6] It is also prone to involvement by inflammatory diseases of the middle ear and mastoid sinus.

The paired cavernous sinuses are located directly behind the superior orbital fissures on each side. They receive drainage from the superficial middle cerebral vein, sphenoparietal sinus, and superior and inferior ophthalmic veins, the latter often joining before draining into the sinus. Drainage is usually predominantly via the superior and inferior petrosal sinuses into the transverse sinus and jugular bulb, respectively, and with variable drainage via the basilar plexus and transforaminal emissary veins mainly through the foramen ovale to the pterygoid plexus. As with other large dural sinuses, the cavernous sinus may be compartmentalized by fibrous trabeculae (Willis cords) complicating transvenous treatment. Further confusion is added by the inconstant presence of a laterocavernous sinus, a separate entity in the lateral wall of the cavernous sinus that commonly drains the superficial middle cerebral vein (SMCV) to the pterygoid veins or petrosal sinus, but which only communicates with the cavernous sinus in about a third of cases.[7] Intercavernous sinuses communicate between the two cavernous sinuses under the diaphragma sella, together creating a "circular sinus" around the pituitary infundibulum. There may also be intercavernous communication through part of the clival plexus over the back of the dorsum sellae.

Superficial Intradural Veins

The sylvian vein (superficial middle cerebral vein) receives the superficial perisylvian cortical venous drainage and passes anteriorly and medially over the lesser sphenoidal wing to drain into either the cavernous sinus or the laterocavernous sinus, directly via emissary veins through the foramen ovale into the pterygoid plexus, or extending back over the floor of the middle cranial fossa to the transverse sinus. The term *sphenoparietal sinus* is often used as a synonym for the sylvian vein, but anatomic studies have shown that the former is a separate structure, paralleling the sylvian vein at the lesser sphenoidal wing, and it receives dural venous drainage alone.[8] Perisylvian drainage may also pass to the posterior

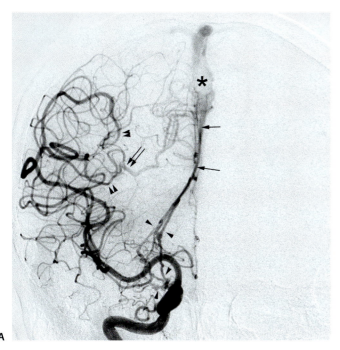

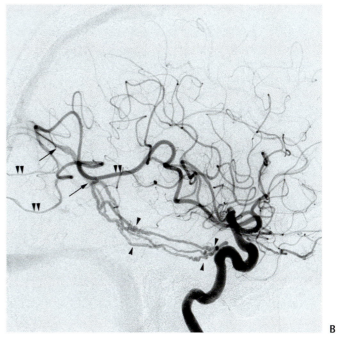

A   B

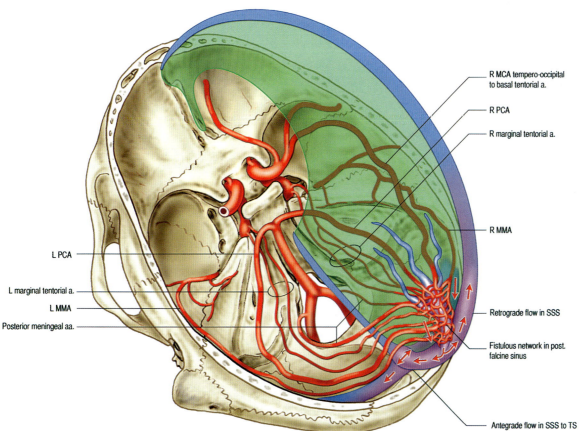

- R MCA tempero-occipital to basal tentorial a.
- R PCA
- R marginal tentorial a.
- R MMA
- Retrograde flow in SSS
- Fistulous network in post. falcine sinus
- Antegrade flow in SSS to TS

L PCA
L marginal tentorial a.
L MMA
Posterior meningeal aa.

C

Fig. 38.7 Anteroposterior (AP) **(A)** and lateral **(B)** projections of the right ICA territory show grossly enlarged marginal tentorial branches *(arrowheads)* that demarcate the right incisural margin and converge on a common channel in the posterior falx *(arrows)* to supply a grade 2a posterior falcine sinus fistula (*) with retrograde flow in the superior sagittal sinus. As in Fig. 38.3 (same patient), there are pial to dural feeders, in this case from the distal angular branches of the right middle cerebral artery (MCA) *(double arrowheads)* converging on a channel in the right tentorial leaflet *(double arrows)*. **(C)** The multiple vertebral, external, and internal carotid dural and pial supplies to this chronic posterior falcine fistula.

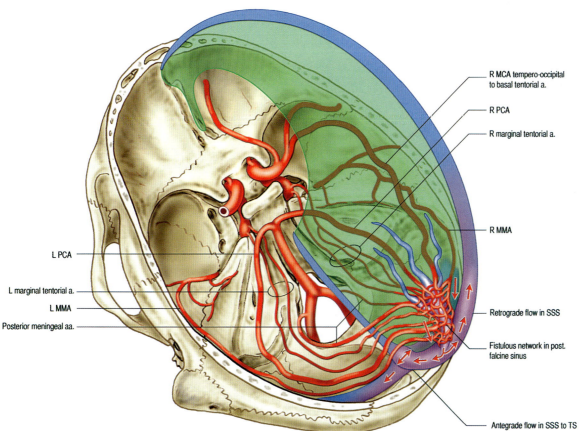

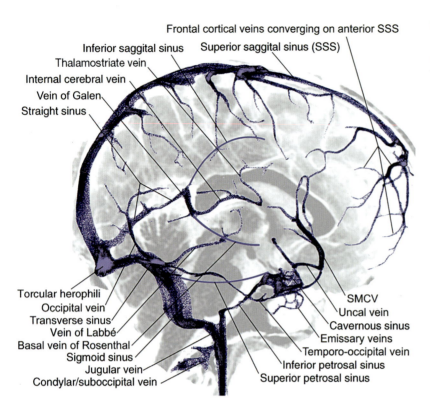

Frontal cortical veins converging on anterior SSS
Inferior saggital sinus
Superior saggital sinus (SSS)
Thalamostriate vein
Internal cerebral vein
Vein of Galen
Straight sinus

Torcular herophili
Occipital vein
Transverse sinus
Vein of Labbé
Basal vein of Rosenthal
Sigmoid sinus
Jugular vein
Condylar/suboccipital vein

SMCV
Uncal vein
Cavernous sinus
Emissary veins
Temporo-occipital vein
Inferior petrosal sinus
Superior petrosal sinus

Fig. 38.8 Lateral projection ICA venous phase angiogram superimposed on the patient's midline sagittal magnetic resonance imaging (MRI) anatomy for reference. SMCV, superficial middle cerebral vein.

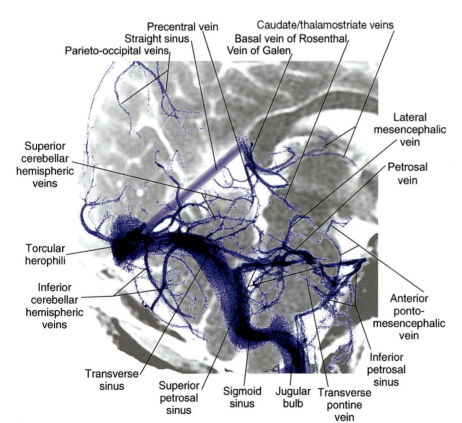

Precentral vein
Straight sinus
Parieto-occipital veins
Caudate/thalamostriate veins
Basal vein of Rosenthal
Vein of Galen

Superior cerebellar hemispheric veins

Lateral mesencephalic vein

Petrosal vein

Torcular herophili

Inferior cerebellar hemispheric veins

Anterior ponto-mesencephalic vein

Inferior petrosal sinus

Transverse sinus
Superior petrosal sinus
Sigmoid sinus
Jugular bulb
Transverse pontine vein

Fig. 38.9 Lateral projection VA venous phase angiogram superimposed on the patient's midline sagittal MRI anatomy for reference.

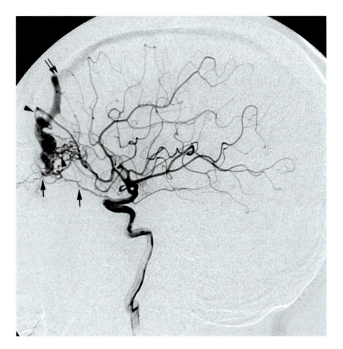

Fig. 38.10 Anterior cranial fossa DAVF supplied by the ethmoidal branches of the ophthalmic artery *(arrows)* and pial to dural supply from the orbitofrontal and frontopolar branches of the anterior cerebral artery (ACA) *(arrowheads)*. An ectatic frontal cortical vein drains superiorly to enter the SSS *(double arrows)*.

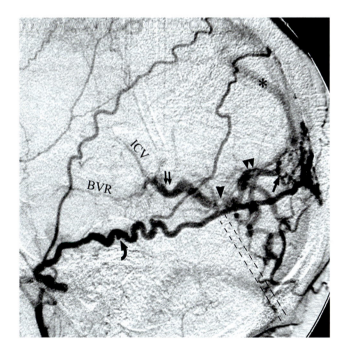

Fig. 38.11 An enlarged MMA *(curved arrow)* supplies a complex fistulous network centered on the posterior SSS *(arrow)* and which drains retrogradely via a posterior falcine sinus *(double arrowhead)*, through a stenosis *(arrowhead)*, SSS, vein of Galen *(double arrows)*, internal cerebral vein (ICV), and basal vein of Rosenthal (BVR). Drainage also occurs via parieto-occipital vein to the SSS (*). The inferior segment of the straight sinus is occluded *(dashed lines)*.

transverse sinus and the superior sagittal sinus via the anastomotic veins of Labbé and Trolard, respectively. Any of these three perisylvian routes can dominate over the others. Although the remaining superficial cortical veins drain relatively directly into the nearest sinus, they do so at an angle **(Fig. 38.8)** and can run a variable distance adjacent and parallel to the sinus before joining it. The junction between the cortical vein and sinus is relatively inelastic and can appear focally (pseudo)-stenosed if receiving a pathologically dilated vein.

Posterior and lateral cerebellar hemispheric cortical veins drain either directly into the torcular and transverse sinuses, or enter them via sinuses in the tentorium. The vermian veins and more anterior cerebellar hemispheric veins drain into the galenic or petrosal routes.

Deep Intradural Veins

The deep system drains the periventricular medullary/transependymal, septal, caudate, thalamostriate and thalamic veins via the paired internal cerebral veins, vein of Galen, and straight sinus. The bilateral basal veins of Rosenthal traverse the ambient cisterns above the posterior cerebral arteries and receive a variable contribution from the deep middle cerebral, orbitofrontal, inferior thalamic, and lateral mesencephalic veins.

The perimedullary veins of the brainstem run longitudinally (anterior pontomesencephalic, anterior medullary, lateral mesencephalic, and lateral pontomesencephalic) and transversely (posterior mesencephalic, pontomesencephalic sulcal, transverse pontine, and pontomedullary sulcal veins). They are closely applied to the surface of the brainstem **(Fig. 38.9)**. Drainage can predominate superiorly via the basal vein of Rosenthal, superiorly via the precentral vein to the vein of Galen, laterally via the petrosal vein to the superior petrosal sinus, or inferiorly to the spinal venous system.[9,10]

◆ Pathogenesis

Although simple, direct arteriovenous fistulas are often seen incidentally on angiograms performed soon after severe head trauma or surgical craniotomy, these are usually small, self-limiting, and not clinically significant. In cases of trauma and intracranial hemorrhage where there is uncertainty whether the trauma may have occurred secondary to collapse after an initial hemorrhagic event, traumatic fistulas may be recognized by their proximity to skull fractures or extradural hematomas, the clean appearance of a single irregular artery and parallel draining dural vein, the lack of recruitment, and the dilatation of feeding vessels **(Fig. 38.12)**. In contrast, the "idiopathic acquired" DAVFs that constitute the subject matter of this chapter usually have established multiple feeders with a "leash" or network centered on the fistula itself **(Fig. 38.13)**.

As many DAVFs recruit a prominent leash of dural vessels, it is not surprising that until about 30 years ago these were mistakenly considered to be congenital dural-based arteriovenous malformations (AVMs), analogous to pial AVMs. The realization of their acquired nature gained momentum after

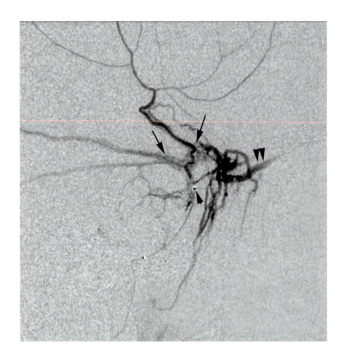

Fig. 38.12 Traumatic DAVF. This 35-year-old man collapsed at work and struck his head on a photocopy machine. Computed tomography (CT) demonstrated multiple cerebral contusions, and extraaxial and subarachnoid hemorrhage without skull fracture. The findings seemed out of keeping with the degree of trauma, so he underwent cerebral angiography, on which the only abnormal finding was a direct MMA to the adjacent dural vein DAVF located close to the pterion. Microcatheter tip *(arrowhead)*; tramtrack dural venous specification paralleling the artery *(arrows)*; sphenoparietal sinus *(double arrowhead)*.

several case series demonstrated the de-novo angiographic evolution of complex fistulas after previous sinus thrombosis[11] or trauma.[12] Terada et al[13] were later able to generate a DAVF by inducing venous hypertension in a rat model. The finer details of normal dural vascularization, which are grossly underappreciated by clinical angiography, were elucidated by histologic analysis, which can distinguish normal arteries and veins in the wall of the dura.[14] These same networks (vasa venorum) are responsible for the "empty delta sign" of enhancement evident in the wall of a thrombosed sinus on contrast-enhanced computed tomography (CT) or magnetic resonance imaging (MRI) **(Fig. 38.14)**.[15] Small dural arteries (<200 μm) and veins are intimately related in the dural subintima, concentrated at points of dural fusion along the margins of the sinuses as well as at junctions between the sinus and cortical veins[14]—the latter arrangement explaining the prevalence of high-grade lesions draining primarily into cortical veins (see below). Direct pathologic communication between these vessels has been documented histopathologically in cases of DAVF. These arterialized veins then traverse the intima to empty into the sinus. Sinus thrombosis, usually occult, is considered to be the initial insult leading to the genesis of a DAVF in the majority of cases. During the period of sinus occlusion, fistulas are created due to elevated back pressure leading to dilatation of preexisting microscopic anastomoses (which explains the frequent finding of "satellite" DAVFs), local ischemia leading to neovascularization by pathologic vessels, or inflammatory injury to the intervening capillary network during the period of thrombosis with subsequent fibrinolysis. To add confusion, sinus thrombosis may itself be a result of a preexisting DAVF due to turbulent flow and an occlusive venopathy that can occur due to intimal hyperplasia and intimal swelling consequent to the dilated vasa venorum. The potential for subsequent occlusion or recanalization of venous drainage explains the possible spontaneous evolution of a fistula that can upgrade due to thrombosis of a previously benign drainage route. However, as described in the following section, low-grade fistulas tend to have a benign natural history. Venous thrombosis can also lead to spontaneous improvement and even complete obliteration of a fistula.[16,17]

◆ Grading

The two established grading systems were published in quick succession by Borden et al[18] and then Cognard et al[19] in 1995. The Cognard classification is illustrated in **Fig. 38.15**. Both systems relate the pattern of venous drainage of a DAVF to the risk of having an aggressive outcome, such as intracranial hemorrhage or nonhemorrhagic neurologic deficit (NHND) due to venous hypertension.

Cognard's data were based on a retrospective single center experience of 205 patients over an 18-year period. As an example of the difficulty in subanalyzing such rare disorders, there were only 10 patients in the CG2b group. Also, of the 205 patients, only 120 received follow-up with a range of 6 months to 23 years (mean 52 months), and, apart from the CG1 lesions, Cognard's data do not distinguish between symptoms occurring at presentation versus during follow-up. However their data remain the benchmark for estimating the risk of a particular lesion having an adverse outcome. In brief, in patients without any cortical drainage (CG1 and 2a) there were no cases of intracranial hemorrhage, whereas hemorrhage occurred in 10% of CG2b, 6% of CG2a+b, 40% of CG3, and 65% of CG4. Nonhemorrhagic aggressive symptoms were found in less than 2% of CG1, 37% of CG2a, 10% of CG2b, 61% of CG2a+b, 36% of CG3, and 31% of CG4. Intracranial hemorrhage is usually parenchymal, in the territory of an involved cortical vein, with possible subarachnoid breakthrough or subdural hematoma. Cognard found that fisulas in the anterior fossa, tentorium, and torcular had higher rates of aggressive symptoms (88%, 92%, and 100%, respectively), but this correlated with the likelihood of cortical venous drainage and, allowing for this, location itself was not an independent arbiter of risk. Of 12 patients with CG5 lesions draining from an intracranial fistula into perimedullary spinal veins, six suffered a progressive myelopathy, five had subarachnoid hemorrhage, and one had a focal neurologic deficit.

Borden's classification is as follows: BG1, drainage into a sinus only (antegrade or retrograde); BG2, reflux from a sinus into a cortical vein; and BG3, drainage into a cortical/subarachnoid vein only. Borden et al illustrated their system with cases but did not publish data to quantify the outcomes

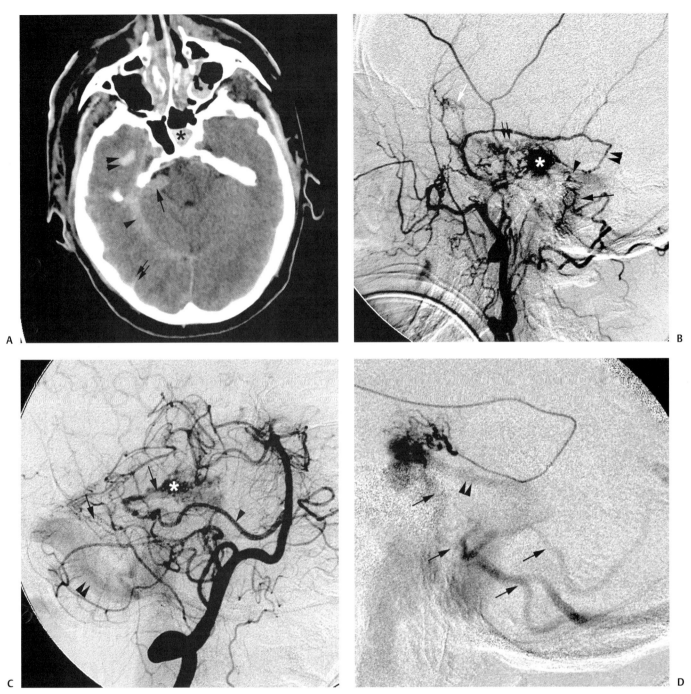

Fig. 38.13 "Chicken and egg" dilemma—distinguishing whether a fistula is the cause of or the result of trauma. This 40-year-old workman fell off a roof with loss of consciousness and multiple injuries including **(A)** cerebral contusions *(double arrowheads)*, subdural hematoma over the tentorium *(arrowhead)*, subarachnoid hemorrhage *(double arrows)*, and air-fluid level in the sphenoid sinus (*) indicative of a skull fracture. An unusual rounded lesion in the right cerebellopontine angle *(arrow)* was initially considered to be loculated subarachnoid blood. **(B)** Right ECA angiogram shows a dense leash of vessels and varix (*) centered on the anterior right superior petrosal sinus (SPS, *arrowhead*) and supplied by a recurrent branch of the right squamosal MMA *(double arrowheads)* and a transmastoid occipital artery branch *(arrow)*. This

high-grade lesion also drains by tortuous perimesencephalic veins *(double arrows)*. Note the separate traumatic dural fistula *(white arrow)*, which is acute, low-grade, and unrelated to the high-grade SPS lesion. **(C)** Right VA injection shows the right anterior inferior communicating artery (AICA) *(arrowhead)* also supplies the fistulous leash (*) centered on the anterior SPS *(arrows)*, which drains into the transverse sinus *(double arrowheads)*. **(D)** Magnified lateral view of a microcatheter angiogram via the MMA feeder shows drainage not only via the SPS *(double arrowheads)*, but also via the subarachnoid petrosal vein into inferior cerebellar hemispheric veins *(arrows)*, which empty into the transverse sinus. *(continued on next page)*

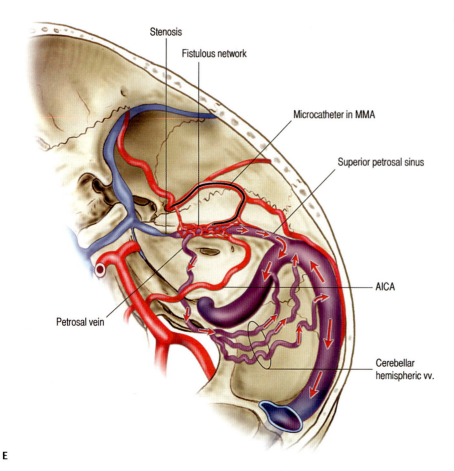

E

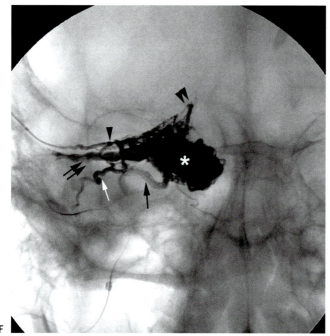

F

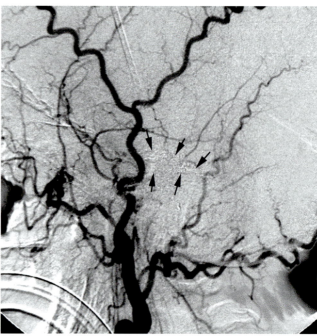

G

Fig. 38.13 (*continued*) (**E**) The anatomy of the fistula. The varix (not shown) is located at the junction of the petrosal vein and SPS. (**F**) AP projection post–Onyx injection via microcatheter in the MMA feeder. Onyx cast extends from the catheter tip *(arrowhead)* through a leash of vessels in the tentorium to the incisura *(double arrowheads)*, to fill the varix (*) and a segment of the SPS *(double arrows)*. Note some reflux into the AICA *(arrow)* and occipital artery *(white arrow)* feeders. (**G**) Final right ECA angiogram shows complete obliteration of the fistula. The Onyx cast is outlined *(arrows)*.

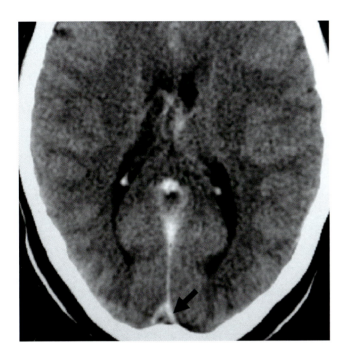

Fig. 38.14 The "empty delta sign" on a postcontrast CT of the head in a case of SSS thrombosis *(arrow)*. The mural enhancement is caused by engorgement of the vasa venorum in the wall of the sinus.

associated with their different grades, as did Cognard et al. Instead, they had two subclassifications: type a, single fistulas; and type b, multiple fistulas. They considered the spinal epidural veins to be equivalent to intracranial sinuses and classified the majority of spinal DAVFs as type 3 (dural lesion draining directly into the subarachnoid coronal venous plexus).

As mentioned, apart from CG1 lesions, neither analysis quantifies the risk of a future adverse event from the time a patient has been diagnosed with a DAVF. Most high-grade lesions are treated and cured urgently. The Toronto group followed over a mean of 4.3 years 20 patients with DAVF and cortical venous reflux (CVR) who had either failed or refused treatment. This cohort had an annual event rate of 15% (8.1% intracranial hemorrhage and 6.9% NHND) and a 10.4% annual mortality rate.[20] However, it appears that not all patients with cortical venous reflux are at such a high risk; Strom et al[21] analyzed a cohort of DAVFs with CVD in 17 patients presenting with aggressive symptoms versus 11 patients without aggressive symptoms, and found respective annual rates of hemorrhage or NHND of 19% versus 1.4%.

Barrow et al[22] devised a classification of cavernous sinus fistulas in 1985 that includes the type A, direct ICA to cavernous fistula, usually due to a traumatic tear of the ICA or a ruptured aneurysm; and types B to D, which are dural fistulas subclassified by their arterial supply.[22] Type B receives dural supply from the cavernous branches (ILT and MHT) of the ICA alone, type C is supplied only by dural branches of the ECA, and type D is supplied by both the ICA and ECA branches.

◆ Presentation

Symptoms can be categorized as nonaggressive or aggressive, the latter relating to hemorrhage or cerebral venous congestion. Nonaggressive symptoms include tinnitus, isolated headaches, and ocular symptoms (diplopia, reduced visual acuity, chemosis, etc.), the latter relating to the local effects of cavernous sinus fistulas rather than elevated intracranial pressure (ICP). Tinnitus is a common complaint in the general population, most commonly a ringing in the ear that is associated with hearing loss of various causes.[23] Pulsatile tinnitus suggests a vascular etiology, particularly if it is objective (audible on auscultation). However, the most common vascular etiology, essential pulsatile tinnitus, is simply turbulent flow in an otherwise normal petrous carotid or jugular vein, occasionally associated with variations such as a high jugular bulb or a stenosed vein (the latter causing a "venous hum"). DAVFs and other high-flow lesions such as glomus tumors are rare causes. If nonaggressive symptoms are tolerable and the lesion is low grade without cortical venous reflux, then observation without treatment is a good option. As mentioned above, high-grade lesions presenting with nonaggressive symptoms have a much lower incidence of adverse outcome, 1.4% compared with 19% per year for those presenting with aggressive symptoms,[21] and in these cases one can consider options such as radiation treatment, which is otherwise usually avoided in emergent cases due to its delayed effect, taking 1 to 3 years to result in a cure.[24]

Aggressive symptoms are associated with CVR, may be hemorrhagic or nonhemorrhagic (venous congestion) in etiology, and can vary from acute stroke syndromes to prolonged dementing processes. Although the latter syndromes are nonspecific, if caused by a DAVF they are usually associated with headaches.[25] NHND may be caused by intracranial hypertension (nausea, vomiting, headache, papilledema, and visual deterioration) or cerebral venous congestion causing nonhemorrhagic infarction or edema **(Fig. 38.16)**. Note that NHND occurred in over a third of Cognard's patients graded as 2a (sinus reflux but no CVR).[19]

◆ Patient Selection and Treatment Strategy

Patients who have DAVFs without cortical venous reflux or aggressive symptoms may not require treatment if their benign symptoms are tolerable. Ocular symptoms due to cavernous fistulas usually warrant treatment as does disabling tinnitus or headache. Radiation therapy may be an option in these cases. Endovascular treatment, even if not curative, may reduce the flow enough to sufficiently ameliorate the symptoms while radiotherapy is taking time to have its effect.

Lesions presenting with cortical venous reflux in general require early treatment with particular urgency required in those presenting with aggressive symptoms. Endovascular treatment is the first treatment of choice if there is a viable means of safely accessing the lesion by a transvenous or transarterial route. Open surgical treatment is usually reserved for cases of failed endovascular treatment or inaccessible

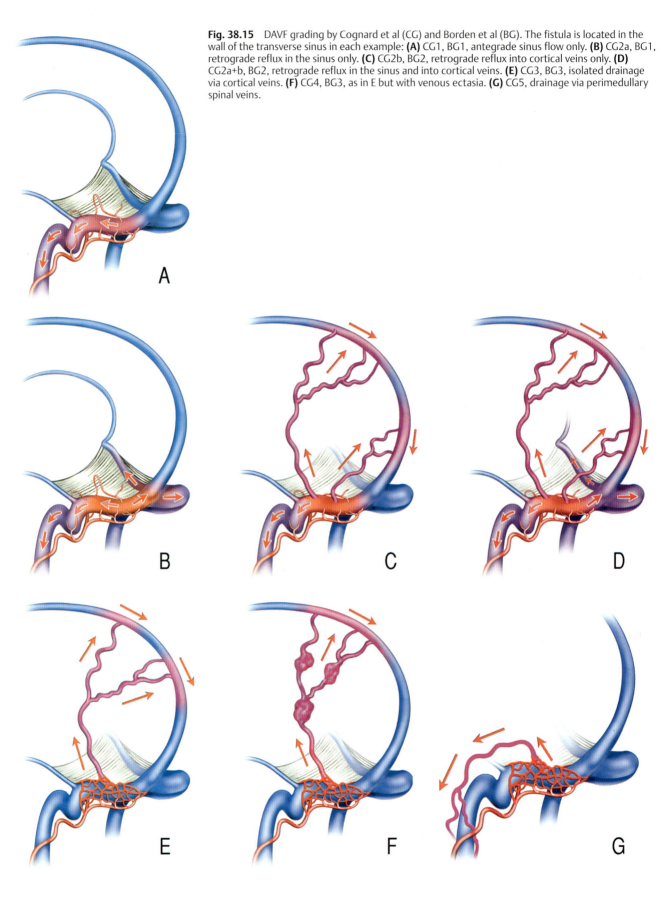

Fig. 38.15 DAVF grading by Cognard et al (CG) and Borden et al (BG). The fistula is located in the wall of the transverse sinus in each example: **(A)** CG1, BG1, antegrade sinus flow only. **(B)** CG2a, BG1, retrograde reflux in the sinus only. **(C)** CG2b, BG2, retrograde reflux into cortical veins only. **(D)** CG2a+b, BG2, retrograde reflux in the sinus and into cortical veins. **(E)** CG3, BG3, isolated drainage via cortical veins. **(F)** CG4, BG3, as in E but with venous ectasia. **(G)** CG5, drainage via perimedullary spinal veins.

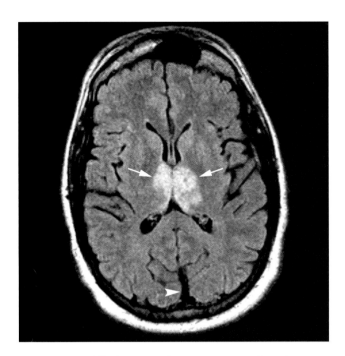

Fig. 38.16 Axial fluid-attenuated inversion recovery (FLAIR) MRI brain demonstrates confluent edema largely restricted to the bilateral thalami *(arrows)* in a patient presenting with a subacute onset of severe short-term memory loss similar to a Korsakoff's syndrome. Note the prominent flow void between the occipital lobes, which was caused by a DAVF shunting into a persistent posterior falcine sinus *(arrowhead)* (same case as in Fig. 38.11). The patient made a full recovery after transarterial embolization of the fistula with Onyx.

lesions. Radiation treatment can be curative for smaller lesions but takes several years to have its effect, so it is not a good stand-alone treatment in these cases.[24]

◆ Imaging Workup

Computed Tomography

In the absence of hemorrhage, noncontrast CT head is usually normal but may reveal subtle signs such as enlargement of foramina around ectatic dural arteries such as the foramen spinosum or transcalvarial channels for emissary vens.[26] If grossly enlarged, fistulized intracranial veins and varices may be evident without contrast. Hemorrhagic complications are well demonstrated. Cerebral edema and hydrocephalus may also be evident as aggressive signs of high-grade lesions. Contrast-enhanced CT may demonstrate distended cortical veins, but a formal CT angiogram (CTA) is usually necessary to determine the presence of abnormal vascularity **(Fig. 38.17).** Even on CTA, a DAVF without significant vascular ectasia may be occult apart from subtle focal dural enhancement related to the dural arterial leash at the site of the fistula. CTA does have particular utility in pinpointing the anatomic location of a known DAVF and can be combined with CT venography in one session to perform a three-dimensional assessment of the lesion and its surroundings.[27]

Magnetic Resonance Imaging

Standard T1, T2, and postgadolinium T1 spin-echo imaging may demonstrate the sequelae of a DAVF, including dilated cortical or ophthalmic veins, parenchymal hemorrhage, or hydrocephalus.[28] Although there are some reports of a modest detection rate for the arterial nidus itself, these published assessments were performed in retrospect and the findings were very subtle.[29] Time-of-flight (TOF) magnetic resonance angiography (MRA) without intravenous contrast relies on arterial high-flow rates to generate a "slice entry phenomenon" vascular signal, whereas the relatively slow normal venous flow is subjected to "radiofrequency saturation" along with the surrounding tissue and will appear dark. Thus, although the spatial resolution is low, bright arterialized venous drainage from a DAVF usually stands out clearly enough to suggest the diagnosis **(Fig. 38.18),** although the nidus and important features such as sinus stenosis or occlusion are only variably depicted.[29,30] Time-resolved MRA (TRMRA) exploits shortcuts in image acquisition including partial filling of K-space, sliding window sampling of K-space, and parallel imaging to give ultrafast imaging of approximately 2 frames per second on commercially available time-resolved imaging of contrast kinetics (TRICKS) protocols,[31,32] whereas frame rates of up to 6 per second have been reported for experimental sequences.[33] These allow for imaging of a contrast bolus transit through the vascular territories, with the trade-off being diminished spatial resolution. Several reports have demonstrated at least 90% accuracy in grading DAVFs by TRMRA compared with digital subtraction angiography (DSA).[31,34] However, current standard practice would still be to perform DSA in the workup of a DAVF. Susceptibility-

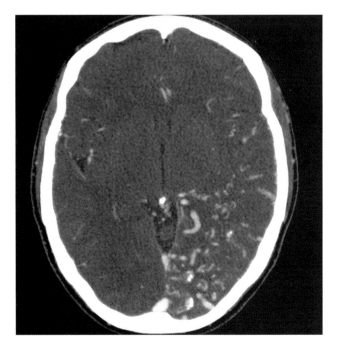

Fig. 38.17 Left hemispheric cortical venous congestion is well demonstrated on this axial CT angiogram.

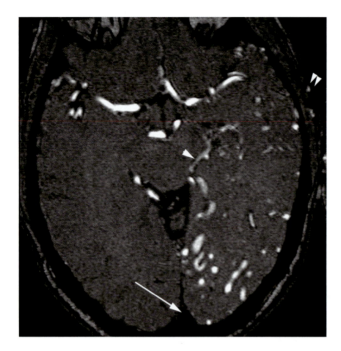

Fig. 38.18 Noncontrast time-of-flight (TOF) magnetic resonance angiography (MRA) shows cortical venous congestion. Note the lack of signal in the SSS *(arrow)*, indicating normal venous flow (whereas on the computed tomography angiography [CTA] in Fig. 38.17, the sinus is opacified regardless of normal or increased flow). Also note abnormal signal in the arterialized BVR *(arrowhead)* and enlarged superficial temporal artery (STA) branches in the scalp, indicating their recruitment by the shunt.

weighted imaging (SWI) combines a three-dimensional (3D) gradient echo with a phase contrast mask, resulting in exquisite sensitivity for blood products, including hemorrhage, thrombus, and deoxyhemoglobin (in normal venous blood) depicted as signal void.[35] Arterialized veins demonstrate nulled or high signal, whereas engorged veins due to venous hypertension are of low signal.

Digital Subtraction Angiography

Conventional DSA remains the gold standard for diagnosis, assessment of grade, and treatment options. Diagnostic angiography is described in detail elsewhere in this book. Every craniodural and intracranial cerebral territory should be included due to the propensity for recruitment from multiple sources. Often, a nondominant supply from a contralateral or other neighboring territory better localizes the site of the fistula, as the multiple rapidly enhancing enlarged vessels from the main ipsilateral pedicle may overwhelmingly obscure the image. In addition to grading a lesion by its early venous drainage, it is important to closely scrutinize the normal venous phase of the brain parenchyma. Any normal venous drainage through a sinus precludes its sacrifice **(Fig. 38.19).** Because of the time and contrast volume necessary for a detailed angiogram, in nonemergent situations we recommend performing separate diagnostic studies prior to an initial intervention. A radiographic frame rate of 6 frames per second

is usually adequate to image the shunt. If further clarification is required, the 4- or 5-French (F) diagnostic catheter placed in the ECA can suffice as a guide for a microcatheter to perform superselective diagnostic angiography. Although poorly understood, there have been reports of unexpected spontaneous DAVF thrombosis and cure occurring in the period after diagnostic angiography.[36]

◆ Therapeutic Options

The first decision to be made is whether a DAVF should be treated at all. A low-grade lesion without cortical venous reflux may be observed without treatment if any symptoms are tolerable to the patient. For low-grade lesions, the patient can also be instructed on performing regular manual compression of the ipsilateral carotid artery; in a series of cavernous DAVFs, this was reported to lead to a thrombosis of the sinus in 30% of cases, though others have found it to be less efficacious.[37,38] Radiation treatment is a viable option if there is no imminent risk of aggressive symptoms, but it takes up to 2 to 3 years to cure a lesion. Most lesions with any cortical venous reflux undergo endovascular treatment if this is possible. If no safe venous or arterial access is available, then a direct surgical approach may be necessary. If there is purely cortical venous drainage, then disconnection of a common draining vein should result in a cure, whereas fistulas of the dural sinus may require direct surgical sinus packing (coils, fat, or muscle) or stripping the sinus wall (skeletonization of the sinus) if there are multiple inputs.[39] Particular risks of surgery are operative blood loss[40] or cranial nerve injury in locations such as the cavernous sinus.[38]

◆ Endovascular Treatment Options

The endovascular technique depends on the accessibility of the lesion to transarterial or transvenous navigation. The goal in most cases is complete obliteration of the shunt, as partially treated lesions can rapidly recruit new supply. Also, incomplete venous embolization can risk diverting flow into cortical veins with potentially grave consequences. However, in extreme cases the secondary goal may be to downgrade a lesion enough to relieve symptoms or buy time for radiation therapy to have its effect. Embolization may not be the only means of downgrading a lesion; several authors have reported stenting to open a venous sinus stenosis and relieve intracranial hypertension or cortical venous reflux.[41] Finally, multiple innovative combined surgical-endovascular approaches have been described to access difficult lesions.

◆ Transvenous Versus Transarterial Approach

The main considerations are accessibility, safety, and likelihood of cure. Many high-grade fistulas are associated with sinus occlusion and reversed flow. Therefore, more complex transvenous routes may be required as described below, and

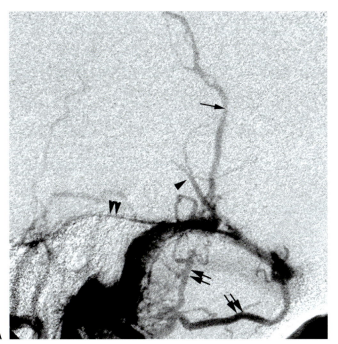

A

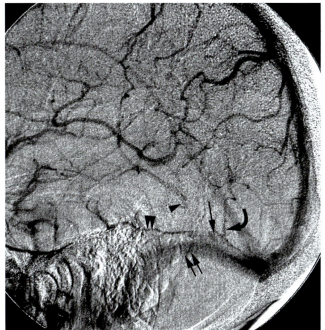

B

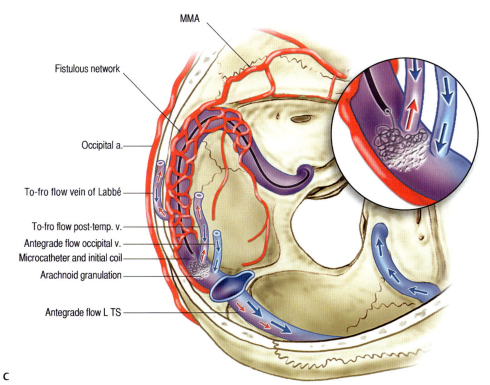

MMA

Fistulous network

Occipital a.

To-fro flow vein of Labbé

To-fro flow post-temp. v.

Antegrade flow occipital v.

Microcatheter and initial coil

Arachnoid granulation

Antegrade flow L TS

C

Fig. 38.19 Avoiding sacrifice of a normal cortical vein represents the importance of the normal cerebral venous phase. **(A)** Occipital branches *(double arrows)* and MMA supply a CG2a+b DAVF of the left transverse sinus with reflux into the vein of Labbé *(arrowhead)*, a posterior temporal vein *(double arrowhead)*, and a parietal diploic vein *(arrow)*. **(B)** On injection of the ipsilateral ICA, the normal venous phase demonstrates sluggish "to-and-fro" flow in the vein of Labbé *(arrow-* *head)* and posterior temporal vein *(double arrowheads)* into the posterior segment of the right transverse sinus (TS) *(arrow)*, which also receives a normally draining occipital vein *(curved arrow)*. The arterialized anterior TS is not opacified, as the normal venous drainage is reversed across the torcular and through the left TS *(double arrows)*. This arrangement is illustrated **(C).** *(continued on next page)*

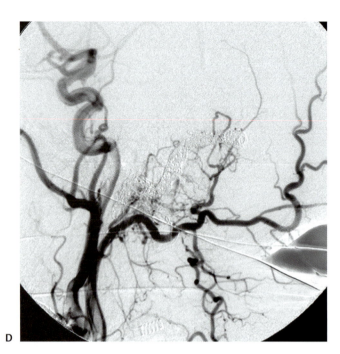

D

Fig. 38.19 (*continued*)   In this case, we were able to use an arachnoid granulation located anterior to the occipital vein as a landmark for the posterior limit of a safe coil sacrifice of the TS that resulted in an uneventful cure (**D**).

in certain cases there may be no transvenous option. The safety of transarterial access depends on the territory requiring embolization and its proximity to and potential anastomosis with eloquent vessels (see Applied Dural Arterial Anatomy, above). If there is balanced choice between the two approaches, much depends on the experience of the operator. If venous access is straightforward, coiling a single draining venous channel is a relatively controlled and less complex procedure. Transarterial treatment has a longer learning curve, and each anatomic region has its particular dangers as outlined below.

◆ Transvenous Embolization

Considerations

If the primary drainage site of a single-input DAVF is accessible by transvenous access, then its complete occlusion should lead to total obliteration of the fistula.[42] In contradistinction to pial AVMs, the risk of a dural fistula nidus rupturing consequent to the sudden occlusion of its outflow is negligible. The transvenous approach in general carries a lower risk profile and is still usually the first endovascular consideration. Multiple inputs along a sinus segment can be treated together by coiling the entire segment. As the treated vein is permanently occluded, it is paramount that the operator ensures that it does not drain brain parenchyma in addition to the fistula (**Fig. 38.19**). Otherwise, cerebral edema, venous infarction, and hemorrhage are potential con-

sequences. Fistulas may drain primarily via a channel in the wall of a sinus, which is difficult to discern due to overlap with the sinus itself but which, if identified, may be sacrificed to close the fistula while preserving the sinus.[43] If a fistula drains into a cortical vein that communicates with the sinus, as is frequently seen in the anterior cranial fossa, it may be possible to reach this vein with standard femoral or transjugular venous access.[44] High-grade fistulas with only retrograde cortical venous drainage are usually inaccessible transvenously unless there are large cortical collaterals (**Fig. 38.20**) or combined surgical-transvenous approaches are employed (**Fig. 38.21**).

Technique

The femoral vein is easily accessed by advancing a micropuncture needle 1 to 2 cm medial to the femoral pulse while gently aspirating. Bright red blood and pulsatile flow indicates a misdirected arterial puncture, although the latter may not be appreciated through a standard 21-gauge micropuncture needle. Sheath/guide combinations vary depending on the anticipated level of complexity and manipulation anticipated, and therefore the amount of proximal support required. When accessing the superior sagittal sinus or contralateral transverse sinus, insufficient catheter length can be an issue, and redundant lengths of guide catheter or the guide catheter remaining external to the puncture site should be minimized. An 80-cm sheath (e.g., 6F or 7F Shuttle, Cook, Bloomington, IN, or Brite-tip, Cordis, Miami, FL) will usually reach the mid–internal jugular level on the right, and a 90-cm length may be preferable on the left. This gives excellent support in the neck and, if necessary, allows for more distal intracranial placement of recently developed flexible guide catheters such as the Neuron (Penumbra, Alameda, CA).[45] We prefer to navigate long sheaths coaxially over a long diagnostic catheter such as a 125-cm vertebral catheter. Alternatively, a short sheath can be combined with a guide catheter such as the Envoy (Codman Neurovascular, Raynham, MA) or Neuropath (Micrus Endovascular, San Jose, CA), which with the multipurpose 20-degree angle tip can be navigated directly over a guidewire.

At least one venous valve is usually encountered in the brachiocephalic, subclavian, and jugular venous system. These can be difficult to traverse even with a hydrophilic guidewire, and undue force can risk damaging the valve. Sometimes the catheter passes more easily without a leading wire. The valve is more likely to be open during respiratory inspiration.

The internal jugular vein is usually easily selected and navigated. If there is difficulty selecting the correct vein, a roadmap subtraction can be achieved by injecting the arterial territory supplying the DAVF, due to the rapid opacification of the arterialized vein that is the target of the embolization. By delaying the fluoroscopic mask until immediately after the arterial bolus has been delivered, it may be possible to avoid having the cervical arteries cluttering the roadmap. This is particularly useful in the more challenging catheterizations of the external jugular, facial, ophthalmic, and pterygoid systems. An arterial catheter is mandatory in any case to local-

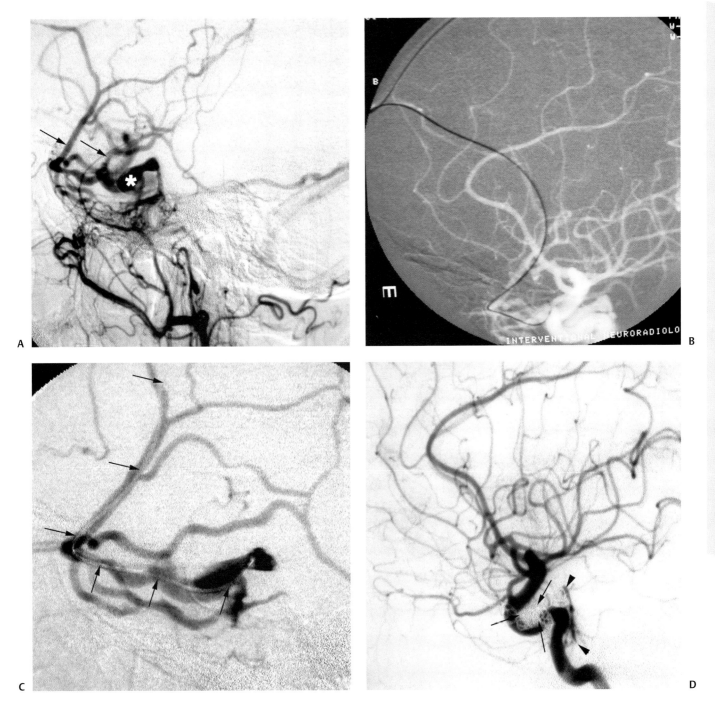

Fig. 38.20 **(A)** This high-grade cavernous fistula (*) drains only via cortical veins, predominantly the superficial middle cerebral vein *(arrows)*. **(B)** It was possible to use a transfemoral route to navigate a microcatheter through the SSS and a dilated frontal cortical branch of the SMCV. **(C)** A contrast injection in the cavernous sinus (CS) demonstrates the venous anatomy; catheter is outlined by *arrows*. **(D)** Final right ICA angiogram demonstrates the coil-occluded CS *(arrows)* with staining in the redundant ICA feeders *(arrowheads)*.

ize the fistula and the monitor the progress of the venous embolization during the procedure.

If femoral venous access is unsatisfactory due to unnavigable anatomy or insufficient catheter length to reach the target, then direct percutaneous puncture of the internal jugular vein can be performed relatively easily. Other cervical veins may be targeted by ultrasound. Direct transorbital puncture of the cavernous sinus has been described by advancing a needle over the orbital floor toward the superior orbital fissure using fluoroscopic landmarks.[46] Alternatively, direct puncture of the superior ophthalmic vein is performed via surgical cut-down, as a failed uncontrolled catheterization of the arterialized vein could result in catastrophic orbital hemorrhage.[47]

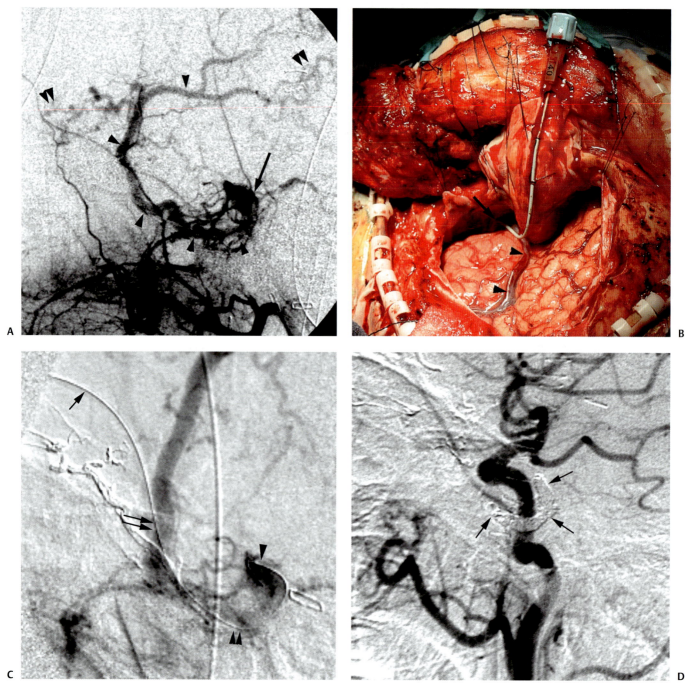

Fig. 38.21 **(A)** Combined surgical-endovascular approach to a high-grade cavernous fistula *(arrow)* draining via the SMCV *(arrowheads)* to opacify dilated cortical veins *(double arrowheads)*. Unlike the example in Fig. 38.18, the venous drainage lacked a collateral communication to another major sinus. An attempt at transarterial embolization was abandoned due to dangerous collaterals to the ophthalmic territory (see Fig. 38.25). **(B)** After frontozygomatic craniotomy, retraction of the temporal lobe was avoided by cannulating the arterialized SMCV *(arrowheads)* at its junction with the sphenoidal dura *(arrow)*. **(C)** Intraoperative venography via a microcatheter *(arrow)* navigated through the SMCV *(double arrows)* over the greater sphenoidal wing *(double arrowhead)* into the CS *(arrowhead)*. **(D)** Final angiography demonstrates coil occlusion of the sinus and fistula *(arrows)*.

We fully heparinize patients for elective procedures (activated coagulation time [ACT] >250 seconds) to reduce the risk of catheter thromboembolism. If there has been recent hemorrhage, we start either without heparin or at a reduced dose.

The venous drainage through the segment to be embolized must be scrutinized to ensure that it does not receive eloquent drainage from any source. In the example in **Fig. 38.19**, temporo-occipital and occipital veins drain into the transverse sinus posterior to the segment involved by the CG2a+b DAVF (to-and-fro flow was present in the vein of Labbé). Care was taken to occlude the sinus, fistula, and the vein of Labbé while sparing the normal drainage routes. One should also appreciate the possibility of compartmentalization within a venous sinus. In this situation, a visible channel is created by the fistula in the wall of the sinus, postthrombotic septations create a separate intraluminal channel for arterialized flow while the true lumen can accommodate normal venous drainage, or there is an accessory sinus paralleling the main sinus.[43] The implication is that, if selectively catheterized, the fistulized channel can be occluded while sparing normal venous drainage in the true lumen of the sinus. Conversely, embolizing the true lumen alone not only may be detrimental to the patient but also may fail to result in a cure of the fistula.

Venous sacrifice also carries the risk of upgrading a lesion if there is incomplete obliteration of the fistula. This usually results from a treatment that occludes a relatively benign drainage route and diverts the fistula into retrograde sinus or cortical pathways. If possible, it is prudent to deliberately select and occlude the eloquent pathways first before embolizing the main draining structure. Lee et al[48] illustrate the potential consequence of partial treatment where diversion into the superior petrosal sinus (SPS) resulted in cerebellopontine hemorrhage and infarction.

Embolic materials may comprise coils or liquids (n-butyl-2-cyanoacrylate [nBCA] and Onyx). Detachable balloons were also used in the past but are no longer being manufactured. Most venous sacrifices are performed with coils. To reduce the risk of the coil mass migrating and embolizing to the pulmonary circulation, we recommend starting with detachable coils to build the initial coil mass before moving onto less expensive pushable/injectable coils (note that it can take more than 50 coils to sacrifice a sinus, and each detachable coil can cost at least $1000). Liquid embolic agents (nBCA and Onyx) have been used transvenously, particularly in the cavernous sinus, usually after first slowing the flow with coils **(Fig. 38.22)**. Liquid embolic agents are less likely to push the catheter out of the desired position; however, they do carry a higher risk of pulmonary emboli.

The draining vein is packed to complete occlusion as determined by concurrent angiography from the arterial side. A small amount of residual drainage through a coiled sinus may undergo complete thrombosis after the procedural heparinization has worn off. However, if a fistula does remain patent, it is likely to recruit more arterial pedicles and can enlarge rapidly or gradually. As mentioned above, partial transvenous treatment also risks diversion of venous drainage to another route with potential adverse consequences.

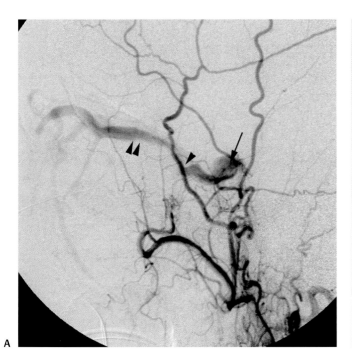
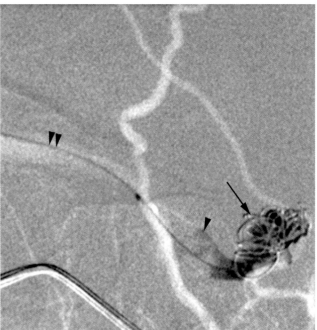

A   B

Fig. 38.22 This 52-year-old woman presented with bilateral orbital chemosis and proptosis. **(A)** Angiography demonstrated a cavernous sinus fistula (*arrow*, Barrow type D) draining only via an ectatic superior ophthalmic vein *(double arrowhead)*, with a focal venous stenosis *(arrowhead)*. There was a mirror image fistula of the contralateral sinus (not shown). A transfemoral approach was used to navigate the external jugular, angular, and superior ophthalmic veins into the cavernous sinus **(B)**. After several coils were placed to slow the flow down, 3 cc of Onyx-34 was injected to fill the CS back into the posterior ophthalmic vein. *(continued on next page)*

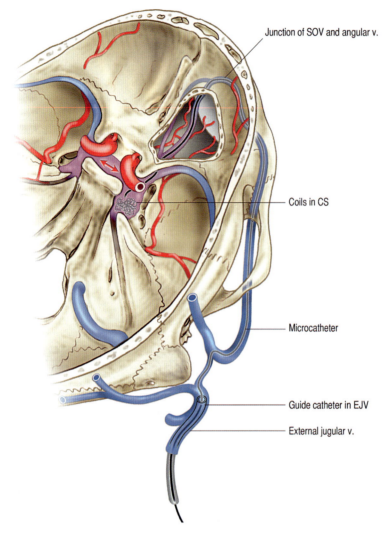

Junction of SOV and angular v.

Coils in CS

Microcatheter

Guide catheter in EJV

External jugular v.

C

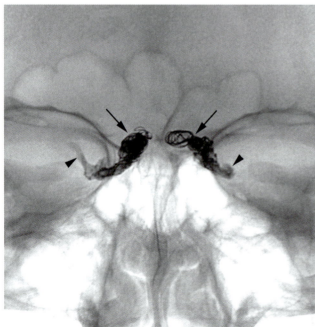

D

Fig. 38.22 (*continued*) **(C)** The technique is illustrated. CS, cavernous sinus; EJV, external jugular vein; SOV, superior ophthalmic vein. Both sides were treated over two elective procedures and the final appearance of the coils and Onyx is shown (**D**). The patient's symptoms completely resolved. Coils in bilateral cavernous sinus *(arrows)*; Onyx extending from the cavernous sinuses to the superior ophthalmic veins *(arrowheads)*.

◆ Venous Recanalization

The rationale behind venous recanalization as a therapy is to rapidly downgrade a dural fistula by opening up a more benign drainage route, as has been described in cases of TS occlusion associated with DAVF.[41] In one of these cases, bare metal stent placement across the fistulized sinus also resulted in complete obliteration of the fistula, presumably due to compression of the fistulous channels in the wall of the sinus.

◆ Transarterial Treatment

Enthusiasm for transarterial treatment has come full circle from the early days of limited success with ethanol[49] and particles such as polyvinyl alcohol,[50] through the establishment of transvenous embolization as a safe and effective treatment, and now with the renewed interest in transarterial occlusion for difficult transvenous cases after reports of good success with polymerizing acrylic, nBCA (Trufill, Codman, Miami, FL),[51] and now with the availability of the more user friendly nonpolymerizing liquid embolic, ethylene vinyl alcohol (Onyx, ev3, Irvine, CA).[52]

As described above, most DAVFs recruit several surrounding arterial pedicles with ramifying vasa venorum creating a leash in the wall of the arterialized sinus. To achieve a cure, ideally the liquid embolic will be pushed through the entire pathologic network with, at least, penetration and casting of the venous side of the fistula.

n-Butyl-2-cyanoacrylate (nBCA; Trufill) is a clear polymerizing glue, one of the cyanoacrylates (same family as commercial Super Glue). Cyanoacrylates are activated by the presence of water, and nBCA rapidly forms an adhesive and brittle mass on contact with blood, accelerated by the presence of anions.[53] As most injected agents including saline and contrast agents are water based, adequate opacification of the nBCA is usually provided by combination with the oil-based iodinated contrast lipiodol. The polymerization time can be manipulated by altering the ratio of nBCA to lipiodol or by the addition of several microdrops of glacial acetic acid.[54] It can be injected through any standard microcatheter after pre-flushing with (nonionic) 5% dextrose to reduce the risk of catheter occlusion. The injection is short, usually several seconds to minutes, as the feeding vessel is rapidly casted. Longer injections and deeper penetration may be achieved by more diluted solutions of 20% or less, combination with acetic acid or concomitant perfusion of the territory with dextrose through the guide catheter. Once the nBCA refluxes back to the catheter tip, the operator applies suction and the catheter is rapidly withdrawn to prevent its being permanently glued in position. nBCA in higher concentrations can be used to ligate larger vessels but will be less radiopaque (tantalum powder can be added to increase opacity). If one is concerned about the lack of radiopacity of a mixture, it may be prudent to check it by passing the syringe directly through the fluoroscopic beam. The advantages of nBCA over Onyx are reduced fluoroscope time,[55] freedom to use any microcatheter type, more distal penetration before reflux occurs, and the ability to use concentrated mixtures to ligate large

shunts. Its main disadvantages are the reduced control during the more rapid injections; its brittle cast that can break up and embolize distally before flow arrest is achieved; and the higher risk of catheter retention, which can occur if it is not removed rapidly after any reflux.

Onyx solidifies by precipitating out of solution as the dimethylsulfoxide (DMSO) rapidly diffuses into the bloodstream. DMSO trapped within the enlarging mass of Onyx takes longer to diffuse, and this results in the core of the injected Onyx remaining in liquid form while the surface forms an elastic crust. This enables prolonged injection of Onyx to push the leading edge distally. Onyx comes in two concentrations approved for embolization of AVMs—18 and 34 cP (centipoise). Retrograde Onyx migration around the catheter tip can be tolerated to a certain degree depending on vascular tortuosity as the Onyx is nonadhesive, and prolonged retraction of the catheter with straightening and spasm of the dural and external carotid branches is less of an issue than with the cerebral vasculature. Whenever reflux is observed, the injection is paused for about 30 seconds and restarted. Usually there will be eventual further antegrade penetration, although it can take 10 to 15 minutes before the Onyx cast "breaks" favorably. Of course, if there is continued reflux, the operator will have to terminate the embolization, remove the catheter, and consider another pedicle. Although the extended arterial penetration of Onyx is a major advantage, one must be vigilant to observe dangerous penetration of side branches, which can travel to anastomose with eloquent territories (see Applied Dural Arterial Anatomy, above). Intermittent angiograms to check the arterial supply to the fistula in addition to the adjacent eloquent territory is advisable. The main advantages of Onyx are better penetration and greater control over the injection, as the operator can pause to reassess the progress and then continue with the injection. Onyx comes in a vial, already mixed with tantalum and is more reliably visualized than nBCA preparations. Onyx must be shaken for 20 minutes prior to use (machine provided) and delays between shaking and injection should be minimized to avoid the tantalum gravitating in the syringe. The recommended injection rate is less than 0.3 mL/min to avoid possible vasospasm or angionecrosis caused by DMSO.

Strategy

As with transvenous embolization, meticulous angiographic assessment is paramount to success and safety. The artery chosen for embolization should be the least eloquent and most distant from potentially dangerous anastomoses (**Figs. 38.4 and 38.5**). In certain locations such as the cavernous region and around the foramen magnum, proximity to such anastomoses is unavoidable. In these cases, the margin for error is tight, and vascular landmarks must be memorized or mapped onto the monitor; nonpermanent markers can be used to draw important boundaries directly onto the monitor. For external carotid territory embolizations, a check angiogram can usually be adequately performed through the guide catheter positioned in the common carotid artery, particular exceptions being embolization through the occipital, posterior auricular, and ascending pharyngeal arteries, where a second catheter should be placed in the ipsilateral vertebral artery. In general, the best chance of success is achieved by positioning the microcatheter as close to the fistula as possible, bearing in mind that the catheter may have to be retracted through Onyx or glue at the end of the procedure.

After choosing the optimal working angle that lays out the fistulous anatomy and, it is hoped, separates it from eloquent and potentially anastomosed vessels, landmarks are referenced and a blank roadmap performed. Onyx is injected at <0.3 mL/min and should be visible in the catheter before entering the artery. If there is a large shunt, the Onyx or nBCA can potentially break off and pass through the fistula, risking occlusion of an eloquent vein downstream or pulmonary embolism (usually the latter are tiny and well tolerated). Placing the microcatheter tip up against the vessel wall helps Onyx to solidify and settle; however, in extreme cases it may be necessary to slow down the flow first with a few coils before the liquid embolic is injected. Balloon assistance has also been described using a HyperForm balloon (ev3, Irvine, CA) placed either in the more proximal arterial pedicle to slow down flow or within the recipient venous sinus to prevent its filling with Onyx.[56] As the Onyx is injected, it may start to reflux back around the catheter tip. As it is nonadhesive, this can be permitted for several centimeters without permanently fixing the catheter in position. With reflux, the injection is paused for about 30 seconds and then a tiny repeat injection is made; if this causes the Onyx to break in the desired direction, then it is continued, otherwise it is paused again for another 30 seconds and so forth—the so-called the reflux-hold-reinjection technique. In a worst-case scenario, the Onyx may persistently reflux on each injection, and at some point the operator must decide when to abandon that pedicle and remove the catheter. Notably, reflux in the MMA to the foramen spinosum may risk facial nerve ischemia. Some operators attempt to get some early reflux around the catheter tip to form a plug that will subsequently force the remaining injection forward. CG 3 and 4 lesions usually converge on a common draining leptomeningeal vein, and if the liquid embolic penetrates the fistula point, it is usual to try and cast this arterialized segment of vein just distal to the fistula, as this gives the best chance of a robust cure (**Figs. 38.23 and 38.24**).

When withdrawing the catheter after Onyx injection, it is best to wait a minute for the last injected Onyx to become less liquid, then aspiration is performed on the microcatheter and it is slowly retracted. If resistance prevents immediate catheter removal, it can be stretched back by approximately 3 cm and locked in that position by the Tuohy valve for about a minute to allow the applied tension to gradually work the tip back. This gradual process usually enables catheter removal even after considerable reflux. Overstretching the catheter can result in catheter fracture and partial retention, usually not a significant problem if a short fragment lies entirely within a noneloquent vessel, such as the ECA. Snare catheters can be used to help retract a catheter[57] or to remove catheter fragments. As the occluded dural artery is relatively forgiving, it is rare to have to leave an entire catheter in situ, though if necessary (more often after using nBCA glue) this can be performed by stretching it through the skin by a few centimeters,

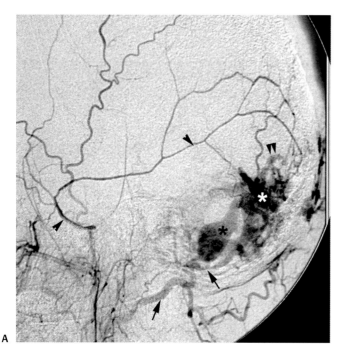

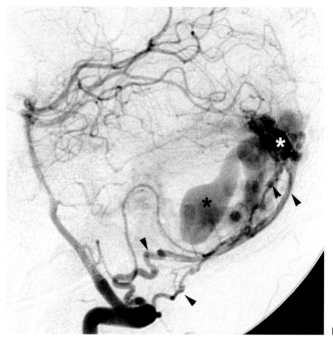

A   B

Fig. 38.23 A 32-year-old man presenting with headaches and large posterior fossa varix visible on CT. **(A)** Right ECA angiogram shows MMA *(arrowheads)* and occipital artery *(arrows)* supply to a CG4 fistula centered on the torcular *(white asterisk)* draining predominantly into cerebellar cortical veins with a large interhemispheric varix *(black asterisk)* and less prominent drainage via occipital cortical veins *(double arrowhead)*. The fistula is also supplied by posterior meningeal branches *(arrowheads* [**B**]).

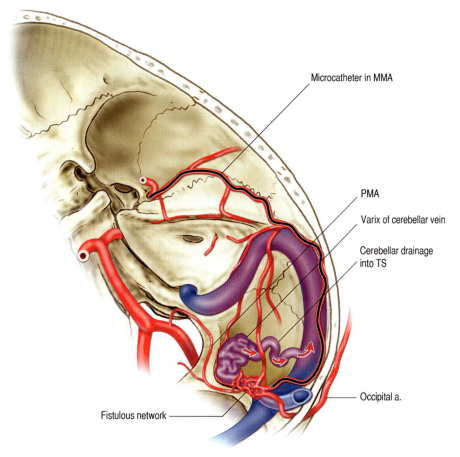

Microcatheter in MMA

PMA

Varix of cerebellar vein

Cerebellar drainage into TS

Occipital a.

Fistulous network

C

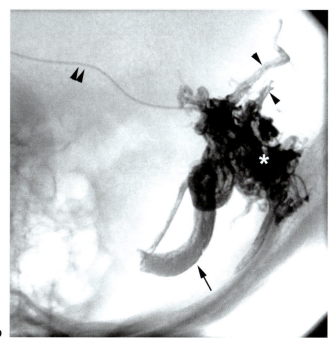

D

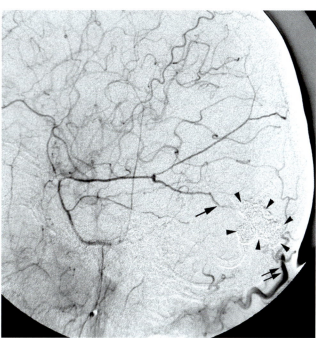

E

Fig. 38.23 (*continued*)   **(C)** The MMA feeder was chosen as the safest transarterial access. PMA, posterior meningeal artery; TS, transverse sinus. **(D)** Lateral view post–6-cc Onyx-18 embolization of the fistula demonstrates the microcatheter prior to extraction *(double arrowheads)*, with complete casting of the fistulous network (*) and the ectatic vein leading to the varix *(arrow)* as well as the involved occipital veins *(arrowheads)*. **(E)** Posttreatment ECA angiogram shows occlusion of the MMA *(arrow)* and occipital *(double arrows)* arterial feeders. The Onyx cast is outlined by the arrowheads.

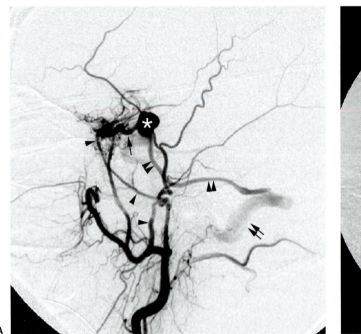

A

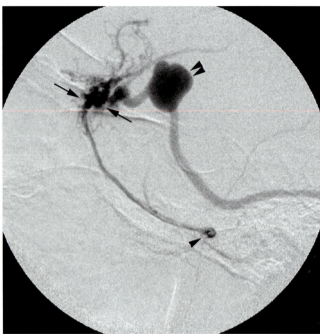

B

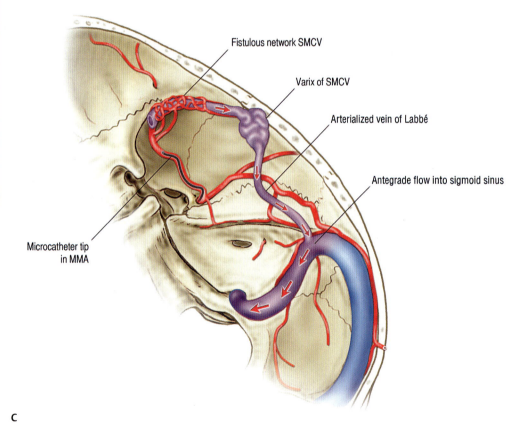

Fistulous network SMCV

Varix of SMCV

Arterialized vein of Labbé

Antegrade flow into sigmoid sinus

Microcatheter tip in MMA

C

Fig. 38.24 This 27-year-old man complained of headache accompanied by double vision. The double vision resolved but the headaches persisted. An MRI of the brain showed prominent flow voids close to the lesser sphenoid wing, leading to further workup. **(A)** Right ECA injection shows an enlarged MMA *(arrowheads)* feeding a leash of fistulized vessels centered at the lateral aspect of the lesser sphenoid wing and draining solely via the SMCV *(arrow)*, which becomes varicose *(*)* before emptying via the vein of Labbé *(double arrowheads)* into the transverse sinus *(double arrows)*. **(B)** Selective MMA injection shows the microcatheter tip close to the foramen spinosum *(arrowhead)*. The complex leash of vessels *(arrows)* is better appreciated as is the prominent varicosity *(double arrowheads)*. The arrangement is illustrated **(C)**.

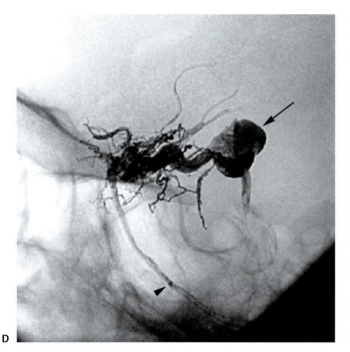

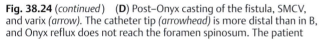

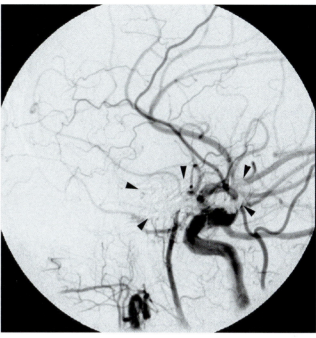

D

E

Fig. 38.24 (*continued*) (**D**) Post–Onyx casting of the fistula, SMCV, and varix *(arrow).* The catheter tip *(arrowhead)* is more distal than in B, and Onyx reflux does not reach the foramen spinosum. The patient suffered no new symptoms and his headaches resolved. (**E**) Final right common carotid artery (CCA) angiography shows no residual fistula. The Onyx cast is outlined *(arrowheads).*

cutting it at the skin level and allowing the proximal end to recoil back into the femoral artery, preferably back into the nonmobile iliac segment to avoid chronic irritation. Parts of the catheter are eventually incorporated into the arterial endothelium,[58] and with the patient on aspirin, the risk of thromboembolic complication from a retained catheter is remarkably low. A novel microcatheter, the Sonic (Balt, Montmerci, France) is flow directable, Onyx compatible, and has an engineered weak zone 1.5 or 2.5 cm from its tip, enabling detachment with moderate traction (not yet available in the United States).[59]

Barrow's type D carotid-cavernous fistulas (CCFs) and paracavernous and clival fistulas present a major challenge due to the proximity of short feeders arising from the ILT and MHT branches of the cavernous ICA (**Fig. 38.5**). We have utilized a HyperGlide (ev3) balloon temporarily inflated across the cavernous ICA during Onyx embolization of the ECA feeder(s). This provides a landmark for the ICA position; any backfilling of the ICA is easily detected as a linear opacity along the balloon, and distal migration should be prevented by the balloon. This occurred in the case illustrated in **Fig. 38.25,** and after allowing the Onyx to set over several minutes, we deflated the balloon and delivered a stent across the cavernous segment to prevent any delayed migration of the Onyx. The combined use of a covered stent placed in the cavernous ICA to occlude the ICA feeders, followed by Onyx embolization of the ECA supply, has been reported.[60] Another case demonstrates unexpected penetration of Onyx into the lacrimal territory of the ophthalmic artery during attempted CCF embolization via a sphenoid branch of the MMA (**Fig. 38.26).**

◆ Conclusion

There are now a multitude of endovascular options available in the treatment of DAVFs. A sound understanding of the complex dural arterial and venous anatomy is important in first choosing the most suitable therapy and then performing it safely. Our understanding of the natural history of DAVFs continues to evolve but at a slow pace due to the low number of cases, making subanalysis difficult.

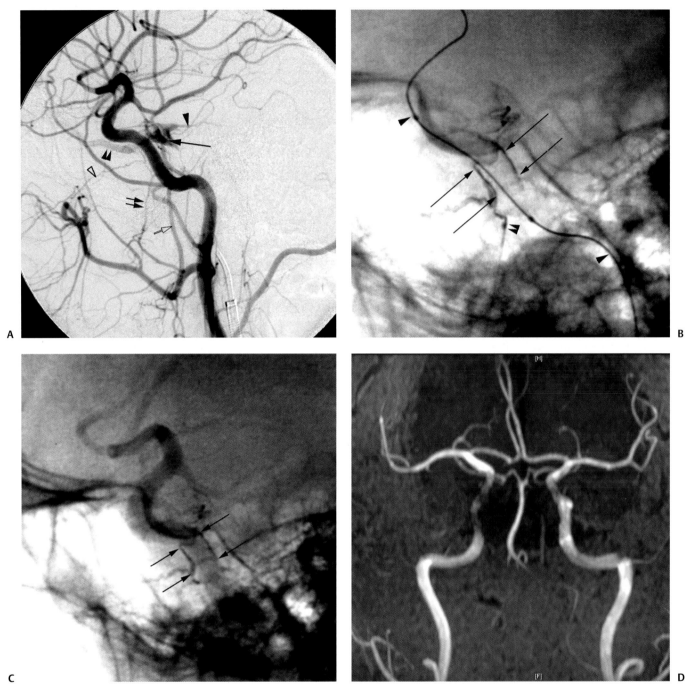

A

B

C

D

Fig. 38.25 A 62-year-old woman complained of progressive orbital proptosis and chemosis, initially attributed to her known Graves' disease. **(A)** A right common carotid injection shows a cavernous fistula *(arrow)* draining via the superior ophthalmic vein *(double arrowhead)* and an uncal vein *(arrowhead)*. Feeders arise from the MMA *(open arrow)*, accessory MMA *(double arrows)*, and the artery of foramen rotundum *(open arrowhead)*. There were also short feeders arising from the cavernous ICA. During embolization of the accessory MMA, Onyx-18 migrated through the cavernous feeder to marginate between a protective HyperGlide balloon and the wall of the ICA lumen. **(B)** Post-embolization lateral image demonstrates the microcatheter tip *(double arrowhead)*, deflated balloon microcatheter *(arrowheads)*, and linear Onyx cast outlining the wall of the cavernous ICA *(arrows)*. **(C)** ICA injection confirms the Onyx cast along the carotid wall *(arrows)*. An Enterprise stent was delivered across the cavernous ICA to fix the endoluminal Onyx in place. The patient's proptosis gradually resolved with no new symptoms. **(D)** Follow-up magnetic resonance angiography (MRA) at 6 months shows no evidence of residual fistula. Attenuated signal of the right cavernous ICA is due to artifact from the nitinol stent.

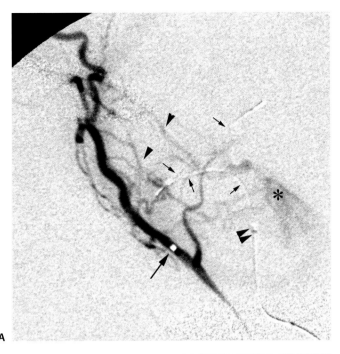

A

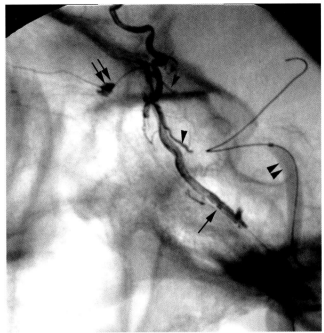

B

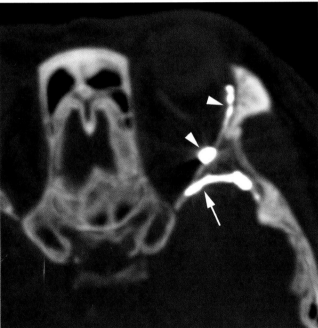

C

Fig. 38.26 A failed attempt to treat a left Barrow type D, CG3 cavernous fistula by transarterial Onyx embolization of the cavernous MMA supply. **(A)** A microcatheter tip *(arrow)* injecting the MMA at the floor of the middle cranial fossa. Cavernous branches *(arrowheads)* supply the cavernous fistula (*). Note protective balloon catheter *(double arrowheads)* and wire *(small arrows)* outlining the course of the ICA. **(B)** Onyx cast extends from the catheter tip *(arrow)* into the origins of the cavernous feeders *(arrowheads)*, some distance from the cavernous sinus; note inflated balloon in the posterior cavernous carotid *(double arrowheads)*. The injection was abandoned after Onyx penetrated a tiny recurrent lacrimal connection to the MMA to opacify the lacrimal branch of the ophthalmic artery *(double arrows)*. There was no penetration of the main ophthalmic artery, and the patient's vision was unaffected. **(C)** CT shows the Onyx in the MMA over the greater sphenoid wing *(arrow)* and within the lacrimal artery *(arrowheads)*. The recurrent lacrimal branch traverses the foramen of Hyrtl.

References

1. Newton TH, Cronqvist S. Involvement of dural arteries in intracranial arteriovenous malformations. Radiology 1969;93:1071–1078
2. Geibprasert S, Pongpech S, Armstrong D, Krings T. Dangerous extracranial-intracranial anastomoses and supply to the cranial nerves: vessels the neurointerventionalist needs to know. AJNR Am J Neuroradiol 2009;30: 1459–1468
3. Wollschlaeger PB, Wollschlaeger G. An infratentorial meningeal artery. Radiologe 1965;5:451–452
4. Agid R, Terbrugge K, Rodesch G, Andersson T, Söderman M. Management strategies for anterior cranial fossa (ethmoidal) dural arteriovenous fistulas with an emphasis on endovascular treatment. J Neurosurg 2009;110:79–84
5. Kesava PP. Recanalization of the falcine sinus after venous sinus thrombosis. AJNR Am J Neuroradiol 1996;17:1646–1648
6. Russell EJ, Wiet R, Meyer J. Objective pulse-synchronous "essential" tinnitus due to narrowing of the transverse dural venous sinus. Int Tinnitus J 1995;1:127–137
7. Gailloud P, San Millán Ruíz D, Muster M, Murphy KJ, Fasel JH, Rüfenacht DA. Angiographic anatomy of the laterocavernous sinus. AJNR Am J Neuroradiol 2000;21:1923–1929
8. San Millán Ruíz D, Fasel JH, Rüfenacht DA, Gailloud P. The sphenoparietal sinus of Breschet: does it exist? An anatomic study. AJNR Am J Neuroradiol 2004;25:112–120
9. Huang YP, Wolf BS. The veins of the posterior fossa—superior or galenic draining group. Am J Roentgenol Radium Ther Nucl Med 1965;95: 808–821
10. Huang YP, Wolf BS, Antin SP, Okudera T. The veins of the posterior fossa—anterior or petrosal draining group. Am J Roentgenol Radium Ther Nucl Med 1968;104:36–56
11. Houser OW, Campbell JK, Campbell RJ, Sundt TM Jr. Arteriovenous malformation affecting the transverse dural venous sinus—an acquired lesion. Mayo Clin Proc 1979;54:651–661
12. Chaudhary MY, Sachdev VP, Cho SH, Weitzner I Jr, Puljic S, Huang YP. Dural arteriovenous malformation of the major venous sinuses: an acquired lesion. AJNR Am J Neuroradiol 1982;3:13–19
13. Terada T, Higashida RT, Halbach VV, et al. Development of acquired arteriovenous fistulas in rats due to venous hypertension. J Neurosurg 1994;80:884–889
14. Nishijima M, Takaku A, Endo S, et al. Etiological evaluation of dural arteriovenous malformations of the lateral and sigmoid sinuses based on histopathological examinations. J Neurosurg 1992;76:600–606
15. Buonanno FS, Moody DM, Ball MR, Laster DW. Computed cranial tomographic findings in cerebral sinovenous occlusion. J Comput Assist Tomogr 1978;2:281–290
16. Luciani A, Houdart E, Mounayer C, Saint Maurice JP, Merland JJ. Spontaneous closure of dural arteriovenous fistulas: report of three cases and review of the literature. AJNR Am J Neuroradiol 2001;22:992–996
17. Magidson MA, Weinberg PE. Spontaneous closure of a dural arteriovenous malformation. Surg Neurol 1976;6:107–110
18. Borden JA, Wu JK, Shucart WA. A proposed classification for spinal and cranial dural arteriovenous fistulous malformations and implications for treatment. J Neurosurg 1995;82:166–179
19. Cognard C, Gobin YP, Pierot L, et al. Cerebral dural arteriovenous fistulas: clinical and angiographic correlation with a revised classification of venous drainage. Radiology 1995;194:671–680
20. van Dijk JM, terBrugge KG, Willinsky RA, Wallace MC. Clinical course of cranial dural arteriovenous fistulas with long-term persistent cortical venous reflux. Stroke 2002;33:1233–1236
21. Strom RG, Botros JA, Refai D, et al. Cranial dural arteriovenous fistulae: asymptomatic cortical venous drainage portends less aggressive clinical course. Neurosurgery 2009;64:241–247, discussion 247–248
22. Barrow DL, Spector RH, Braun IF, Landman JA, Tindall SC, Tindall GT. Classification and treatment of spontaneous carotid-cavernous sinus fistulas. J Neurosurg 1985;62:248–256
23. Crummer RW, Hassan GA. Diagnostic approach to tinnitus. Am Fam Physician 2004;69:120–126
24. Wu HM, Pan DH, Chung WY, et al. Gamma knife surgery for the management of intracranial dural arteriovenous fistulas. J Neurosurg 2006; 105(Suppl):43–51
25. Hurst RW, Bagley LJ, Galetta S, et al. Dementia resulting from dural arteriovenous fistulas: the pathologic findings of venous hypertensive encephalopathy. AJNR Am J Neuroradiol 1998;19:1267–1273
26. Alatakis S, Koulouris G, Stuckey S. CT-demonstrated transcalvarial channels diagnostic of dural arteriovenous fistula. AJNR Am J Neuroradiol 2005;26:2393–2396
27. Nakagawa M, Sugiu K, Tokunaga K, et al. Usefulness of 3-dimensional CT angiograms obtained by 64-section multidetector row CT scanner for dural arteriovenous fistula. J Neuroimaging 2009;19:179–182
28. De Marco JK, Dillon WP, Halback VV, Tsuruda JS. Dural arteriovenous fistulas: evaluation with MR imaging. Radiology 1990;175:193–199
29. Kwon BJ, Han MH, Kang HS, Chang KH. MR imaging findings of intracranial dural arteriovenous fistulas: relations with venous drainage patterns. AJNR Am J Neuroradiol 2005;26:2500–2507
30. Chen JC, Tsuruda JS, Halbach VV. Suspected dural arteriovenous fistula: results with screening MR angiography in seven patients. Radiology 1992;183:265–271
31. Farb RI, Agid R, Willinsky RA, Johnstone DM, Terbrugge KG. Cranial dural arteriovenous fistula: diagnosis and classification with time-resolved MR angiography at 3T. AJNR Am J Neuroradiol 2009;30:1546–1551
32. Meckel S, Maier M, Ruiz DS, et al. MR angiography of dural arteriovenous fistulas: diagnosis and follow-up after treatment using a time-resolved 3D contrast-enhanced technique. AJNR Am J Neuroradiol 2007; 28:877–884
33. Eddleman CS, Jeong HJ, Hurley MC, et al. 4D radial acquisition contrast-enhanced MR angiography and intracranial arteriovenous malformations: quickly approaching digital subtraction angiography. Stroke 2009;40:2749–2753
34. Nishimura S, Hirai T, Sasao A, et al. Evaluation of dural arteriovenous fistulas with 4D contrast-enhanced MR angiography at 3T. AJNR Am J Neuroradiol 2010;31:80–85
35. Tsui YK, Tsai FY, Hasso AN, Greensite F, Nguyen BV. Susceptibility-weighted imaging for differential diagnosis of cerebral vascular pathology: a pictorial review. J Neurol Sci 2009;287:7–16
36. Moriya M, Itokawa H, Fujimoto M, et al. Spontaneous closure of dural arteriovenous fistula after performing diagnostic angiography. No Shinkei Geka 2007;35:65–70
37. Higashida RT, Hieshima GB, Halbach VV, Bentson JR, Goto K. Closure of carotid cavernous sinus fistulae by external compression of the carotid artery and jugular vein. Acta Radiol Suppl 1986;369:580–583
38. Tu YK, Liu HM, Hu SC. Direct surgery of carotid cavernous fistulae and dural arteriovenous malformations of the cavernous sinus. Neurosurgery 1997;41:798–805, discussion 805–806
39. Ushikoshi S, Houkin K, Kuroda S, et al. Surgical treatment of intracranial dural arteriovenous fistulas. Surg Neurol 2002;57:253–261
40. Sundt TM Jr, Piepgras DG. The surgical approach to arteriovenous malformations of the lateral and sigmoid dural sinuses. J Neurosurg 1983; 59:32–39
41. Murphy KJ, Gailloud P, Venbrux A, Deramond H, Hanley D, Rigamonti D. Endovascular treatment of a grade IV transverse sinus dural arteriovenous fistula by sinus recanalization, angioplasty, and stent placement: technical case report. Neurosurgery 2000;46:497–500, discussion 500–501
42. Dawson RC III, Joseph GJ, Owens DS, Barrow DL. Transvenous embolization as the primary therapy for arteriovenous fistulas of the lateral and sigmoid sinuses. AJNR Am J Neuroradiol 1998;19:571–576
43. Piske RL, Campos CM, Chaves JB, et al. Dural sinus compartment in dural arteriovenous shunts: a new angioarchitectural feature allowing superselective transvenous dural sinus occlusion treatment. AJNR Am J Neuroradiol 2005;26:1715–1722
44. Defreyne L, Vanlangenhove P, Vandekerckhove T, et al. Transvenous embolization of a dural arteriovenous fistula of the anterior cranial fossa: preliminary results. AJNR Am J Neuroradiol 2000;21:761–765
45. Hurley MC, Sherma AK, Surdell D, Shaibani A, Bendok BR. A novel guide catheter enabling intracranial placement. Catheter Cardiovasc Interv 2009;74:920–924
46. Narayanan S, Murchison AP, Wojno TH, Dion JE. Percutaneous trans-superior orbital fissure embolization of carotid-cavernous fistulas: technique and preliminary results. Ophthal Plast Reconstr Surg 2009; 25:309–313
47. Tress BM, Thomson KR, Klug GL, Mee RR, Crawford B. Management of carotid-cavernous fistulas by surgery combined with interventional radiology. Report of two cases. J Neurosurg 1983;59:1076–1081
48. Lee RJ, Chen CF, Hsu SW, Lui CC, Kuo YL. Cerebellar hemorrhage and subsequent venous infarction followed by incomplete transvenous embolization of dural carotid cavernous fistulas: a rare complication: case report. J Neurosurg 2008;108:1245–1248
49. Barbier C, Legeais M, Cottier JP, Bibi R, Herbreteau D. Failure of transverse sinus dural fistula embolization using ethanol injection. J Neuroradiol 2008;35:230–235
50. Nichols DA, Rufenacht DA, Jack CR Jr, Forbes GS. Embolization of spinal dural arteriovenous fistula with polyvinyl alcohol particles: experience in 14 patients. AJNR Am J Neuroradiol 1992;13:933–940
51. Nelson PK, Russell SM, Woo HH, Alastra AJ, Vidovich DV. Use of a wedged microcatheter for curative transarterial embolization of complex intracranial dural arteriovenous fistulas: indications, endovascular technique, and outcome in 21 patients. J Neurosurg 2003;98:498–506
52. Nogueira RG, Dabus G, Rabinov JD, et al. Preliminary experience with onyx embolization for the treatment of intracranial dural arteriovenous fistulas. AJNR Am J Neuroradiol 2008;29:91–97

53. Coover HW, McIntire JM. Cyanoacrylate adhesives. In: Skeist I, ed. Handbook of Adhesives. New York: Van Nostrand Reinhold, 1977:569–591

54. Gounis MJ, Lieber BB, Wakhloo AK, Siekmann R, Hopkins LN. Effect of glacial acetic acid and ethiodized oil concentration on embolization with N-butyl 2-cyanoacrylate: an in vivo investigation. AJNR Am J Neuroradiol 2002;23:938–944

55. Velat GJ, Reavey-Cantwell JF, Sistrom C, et al. Comparison of N-butyl cyanoacrylate and onyx for the embolization of intracranial arteriovenous malformations: analysis of fluoroscopy and procedure times. Neurosurgery 2008;63(1, Suppl 1)ONS73–ONS78, discussion ONS78–ONS80

56. Shi ZS, Loh Y, Duckwiler GR, Jahan R, Viñuela F. Balloon-assisted transarterial embolization of intracranial dural arteriovenous fistulas. J Neurosurg 2009;110:921–928

57. Kelly ME, Turner R IV, Gonugunta V, Rasmussen PA, Woo HH, Fiorella D. Monorail snare technique for the retrieval of an adherent microcatheter from an onyx cast: technical case report. Neurosurgery 2008;63(1, Suppl 1)E89, discussion E89

58. Zoarski GH, Lilly MP, Sperling JS, Mathis JM. Surgically confirmed incorporation of a chronically retained neurointerventional microcatheter in the carotid artery. AJNR Am J Neuroradiol 1999;20:177–178

59. Tahon F, Salkine F, Amsalem Y, Aguettaz P, Lamy B, Turjman F. Dural arteriovenous fistula of the anterior fossa treated with the Onyx liquid embolic system and the Sonic microcatheter. Neuroradiology 2008;50:429–432

60. Shi ZS, Qi TW, Gonzalez NR, Ziegler J, Huang ZS. Combined covered stent and onyx treatment for complex dural arteriovenous fistula involving the clivus and cavernous sinus. Surg Neurol 2009;72:169–174

39

Spinal Arteriovenous Malformation and Dural Fistula Embolization

Timothy Uschold, Richard Lochhead, Felipe C. Albuquerque, and Cameron G. McDougall

---

Pearls

- General strategies for optimal visualization and complication avoidance include (1) reconfirmation of index levels using multiple techniques, (2) angiographic visualization of pathologic and adjacent normal anatomy, (3) maximized image quality and prolonged venous phase imaging, and (4) minimized neurologic compromise via intraoperative monitoring (IOM) and provocative infusion testing (when necessary).
- A primary role for polyvinyl alcohol (PVA) particles in spinal arteriovenous fistula (AVF)/arteriovenous malformation (AVM) embolization is no longer supported. Cyanoacrylate glue is appropriate for many AVFs and some AVMs, but Onyx has gained wider interest due to its technical advantages.
- Lesion classification is best achieved by the Spetzler nomenclature, differentiating lesions by anatomic location and pathophysiology. This scheme serves as a useful starting point for understanding shunting patterns and developing embolization strategies.
- For spinal AVFs of all types, catheter proximity immediately adjacent to the fistulous point is essential to achieve AVF obliteration, minimize recurrence risk, and maximize safety.
- Preoperative angiography and in many cases embolization are mainstays of multimodal spinal AVM treatment (for all types). Patient selection, identification of risk features (e.g., nidal aneurysms, location of the anterior spinal artery), and provocative infusion testing help guide subsequent embolization and surgical decisions.

Spinal arteriovenous lesions, by virtue of their varied pathophysiology and complex angioarchitecture, present unique neurosurgical challenges in diagnosis and management. As a progressively nuanced understanding of spinal arteriovenous fistulas (AVFs) and arteriovenous malformations (AVMs) has developed, classification schemes and treatment strategies have become more coherent. Within this emerging paradigm, percutaneous catheter-based approaches increasingly play a crucial role in multimodal treatment strategies, and in some instances represent a first-line option for cure. This chapter focuses on the technical aspects of endovascular spinal AVM and AVF embolization. The review of the literature presented here emphasizes trends in endovascular innovation, capabilities, decision making, and outcomes.

◆ Spinal Vascular Anatomy

Thorough understanding of normal spinal vascular anatomy and its common variations is essential to the endovascular diagnosis and treatment of spinal arteriovenous lesions. The spinal cord receives its blood supply from the singular anterior spinal artery (ASA) found in the anterior median sulcus, as well as from the paired posterior spinal arteries (PSAs) running along the dorsolateral surface of the cord (**Fig. 39.1**). The intrinsic vascular supply of centrifugal and centripetal perforators to the cord is only rarely angiographically apparent.

Segmental contributions to the spinal arteries are highly variable. The ASA begins as a paired derivative of the intracranial vertebral arteries, and ultimately receives contributions from only six to eight radiculomedullary arteries throughout the length of the cord.[1] In the cervical region, inconstant anastomoses may derive from the vertebral arteries, costocervical trunk, thyrocervical trunk, and ascending pharyngeal arteries. The relatively constant artery of the cervical enlargement (usually found at C5–6 from the vertebral arteries) and the eponymous artery of Adamkiewicz (commonly found on the left between T9 and T12 depending upon reports) help demarcate the intervening anterior cord into watershed regions. These regions, and in particular the upper-middle thoracic cord, are theoretically more prone to ischemic injury during aggressive embolization or hypotension. The PSA typically derives bilaterally from the vertebrals

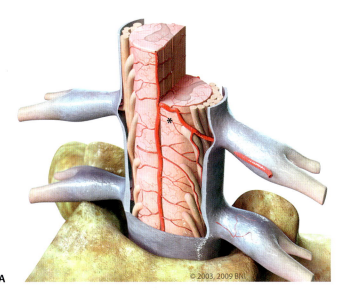

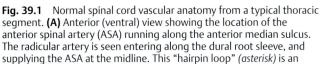

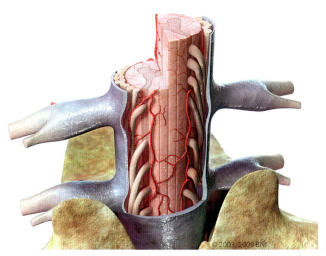

A

B

Fig. 39.1 Normal spinal cord vascular anatomy from a typical thoracic segment. **(A)** Anterior (ventral) view showing the location of the anterior spinal artery (ASA) running along the anterior median sulcus. The radicular artery is seen entering along the dural root sleeve, and supplying the ASA at the midline. This "hairpin loop" *(asterisk)* is an important angiographic sign. **(B)** The paired posterior spinal arteries (PSAs) are seen in this posterior (dorsal) view. They are inconstantly supplied from radiculopial feeding vessels. (Used with permission from Barrow Neurological Institute.)

and is maintained by 10 to 20 inconstant radiculopial branches from the segmental arteries.[1] The two PSAs and the ASA are directly anastomotic only at the conus, which bears particular relevance to AVMs and fistulas in that region. Below the termination of the cord and the spinal arteries, vascular supply may derive from the aorta (lower lumbar or median sacral arteries) as well as the internal iliacs (iliolumbar or lateral sacral arteries).

In contrast to the inconstant segmental contributions to cord perfusion, nerve roots are more predictably supplied by paired segmental arteries emerging from the thoracolumbar aorta. Radicular arteries are derived from the dorsospinal trunk of each segmental artery, and branch anatomically to supply the dorsal and ventral nerve roots. Complete endovascular investigation of the spine, including adjacent segmental arteries as well as extrasegmental vessels, is an essential component of complication avoidance.[1,2]

◆ Spinal Angiography and Embolization: Technical Considerations

Small-caliber vasculature, anatomic variability, relative rarity of the lesions, complex angioarchitecture, and highly eloquent surrounding parenchyma are the principal factors that make spinal angiography and embolization uniquely demanding. Despite these challenges inherent to spinal arteriovenous lesions, angiographic investigation can safely be performed in the majority of cases. General technical strategies for optimal visualization and complication avoidance include the following[2]:

1. Correct identification of the index level: A combination of methods such as counting ribs, numbering vertebrae, and the use of a reference landmark such as a radiopaque ruler are most helpful. Misidentification of levels due to parallax can be minimized when biplanar angiography is adjusted to account for deformity, kyphosis, and lordosis.

2. Visualization of the lesion and adjacent normal vasculature in entirety: Preprocedure planning to narrow the region of interest based on noninvasive imaging modalities (magnetic resonance imaging [MRI]/magnetic resonance angiography [MRA]) and clinical findings is essential to minimize contrast loads and fluoroscopy exposure. Given the relative futility of aortography in these cases, staged angiography or treatment may be a consideration. At our institution, we typically explore the thoracolumbar region with a Cobra or Mickelson catheter designed to selectively engage the segmental ostia. This should proceed bilaterally for several levels, centered at the level of the lesion to identify major ASA (e.g., artery of Adamkiewicz) and PSA feeding vessels. Nonsegmental vessels contributing to cervical or lumbosacral perfusion (detailed above) should be injected when necessary. We prefer hand injections of relatively smaller contrast boluses (approximately 3 cc).

3. Maximized image quality: General anesthesia with apnea during contrast runs helps minimize motion artifact and is routinely employed for all interventional cases and for diagnostic cases that are likely to require interrogation of more than a few levels. Higher sampling rates and longer venous phase imaging times (up to 20 to 30 seconds for some fistulas displaying sluggish venous flow) are commonly necessary to detect the full spectrum of pathology. Administration of 0.5 to 1.0 mg of systemic glucagon has been reported to limit motion artifact due to gastrointestinal (GI) motility and is occasionally helpful in this regard.[3]

4. Minimized risks of vascular compromise: The amount of tolerable embolysate reflux, the degree of anterograde embolus, the proximity of the microcatheter relative to the target site, and the lesional anatomy are the most important determinants of safety during embolization. Provocative infusion testing with Amytal and Lidocaine, or the so-called spinal Wada test, has been reported as a useful pretest for potential deficits associated with embolization via a particular vascular pedicle. Given the relative lack of specificity and technical requirements associated with this procedure, however, clinical acumen based on the factors above is often a more useful guide for AVFs. Provocative testing is of greater predictive utility for AVMs compared with AVFs. For the latter class of lesions, a single fistulous point may represent a more anatomically predictable target for embolization. Intraoperative electrophysiologic monitoring (IOM) with somatosensory (SSEP) and motor (MEP) evoked potentials is employed during all embolizations. Most procedures are performed under systemic anticoagulation using heparin, and periprocedural steroids are used judiciously when swelling or ischemic injury are potential concerns.[4]

◆ Embolic Agents

Polyvinyl alcohol (PVA) foam particles are selected by size, presuming that this characteristic determines distal penetration. For example, particles chosen for spinal AVM embolization are smaller than the anterior spinal artery (340 to 1100 µm) but larger than the normal central spinal arteries (60 to 72 µm). After delivery, the particles expand to occlude the arterial lumen, causing a transient inflammatory reaction. Subsequent fibroblast ingrowth is thought to stabilize long-term vessel occlusion, but clinical studies from a variety of spinal applications have consistently demonstrated comparatively higher rates of recanalization following PVA embolization than with other materials. Although of historical interest, there is largely no supported first-line role for particulate embolization of spinal AVFs and AVMs due to this fact.

Cyanoacrylate glues are composed of either isobutyl-2-cyanoacrylate (IBCA) or n-butyl-cyanoacrylate (nBCA); nBCA is a newer, softer isomer of IBCA. These agents are useful for high-flow fistulas and larger caliber vessels because they rapidly polymerize after injection upon contact with ionized blood or vessel intima. Cyanoacrylate is not resorbable, and therefore theoretically not associated with vessel recanalization. Hardening time is somewhat controllable by mixing the glue with different amounts of contrast solution or dextrose. Considerable skill is required to use this agent. Catheters may be inadvertently "glued in" during slow injections. Unexpected proximal reflux may result from rapid injections. A dilute mixture of cyanoacrylate of inadequate viscosity may migrate too distally, causing venous thrombosis and possible hemorrhage.

Onyx (ev3, Irvine, CA) is an ethylene vinyl alcohol copolymer dissolved in dimethylsulfoxide (DMSO). When Onyx is injected, the DMSO rapidly diffuses away, causing the polymer to precipitate into a spongy, soft, nonadherent embolus.

Onyx applications to the spine remain relatively new, but several theoretical advantages have been reported. First, there is a high degree of angiographic control with Onyx compared with glue. It can be injected over several minutes with minimal risk of catheter adhesion. This allows for deep penetration into the nidus with a decreased chance of unwanted proximal reflux. Onyx tends to stay cohesive, and is less likely to penetrate distally into the veins, causing venous thrombosis and possible hemorrhage. Although not always advisable in the spine, some authors describe wedging the microcatheter within a proximal Onyx plug to arrest blood flow. This allows for embolic material to be pushed strictly anterograde for optimal nidal penetration and decreased chance of reflux. The most cited disadvantage of Onyx remains the potential vascular toxicity from DMSO. Animal experiments demonstrate that vascular toxicity is primarily related to the speed of injection. Vascular recanalization and excessive venous penetration with Onyx, although less common, have been noted.[5]

◆ Classification of Spinal Vascular Lesions

The ideal nomenclature for spinal vascular lesions must organize similar entities by both anatomic location and pathophysiology inclusive of all lesion types. In such a scenario, it follows suit that each named category would share general likenesses in terms of neuroimaging, arteriovenous shunting, operative findings, natural history, and associated treatment strategies.[6] This is most effectively accomplished by the Spetzler et al (2002) classification scheme. AVM and AVF are broadly distinguished by the presence of a nidus, with more specific anatomic relationships defining specific pathologies. A detailed review of the pathophysiology, angiographic diagnosis, and endovascular decision making for each lesion type is organized accordingly in the following discussion (**Tables 39.1 and 39.2; Figs. 39.2 and 39.3**). Treatment of vascular lesions without arteriovenous (AV) shunting (e.g., cavernous malformations, spinal artery aneurysms) is reviewed elsewhere.

Spinal Arteriovenous Fistulas

Intradural Dorsal Spinal Fistulas

These lesions may be encountered in the older literature as spinal dural AVFs, long dorsal AVMs, angioma racemosum, dorsal extramedullary AVMs, and angioma racemosum venosum. Such names are derived from the typical pathologic (and subsequent angiographic) appearance of these lesions. The observed arterialization and dilation of the intradural coronal venous plexus situated on the dorsal surface of the cord can only be understood in the context of an intradural lesion. As a rule, dilated epidural veins are not encountered. The AV shunt is universally found at the intradural interface of the radicular artery and dural root sleeve. Further recruitment of additional arterial feeders from nearby levels has been reported. Such lesions are denoted as type B, as in the

Table 39.1 Spinal Arteriovenous Fistula Classification

	Extradural	Intradural Dorsal	Intradural Ventral
Pathophysiology	Compression, myelopathy, steal, congestion	Vascular congestion	Mass effect, steal, hemorrhage progressive with grade
Flow characteristics	High	Low	Progressive with grade
Symptoms	Progressive myeloradiculopathy	Progressive myelopathy	Progressive myelopathy
Treatment options	Primarily endovascular	Surgical versus endovascular	Higher grade may favor endovascular

Note: Lesions are demarcated primarily by anatomic location. Pathophysiology, flow characteristics, and symptoms follow suit. The classification scheme is not intended as a strict guideline to determine mode of therapy (e.g., embolization versus open surgical), but serves as a useful starting point to guide decision making.

Source: Modified from Spetzler RF, Detwiler PW, Riina HA, Porter RW. Modified classification of spinal cord vascular lesions. J Neurosurg 2002;96(Spine 2):145–156.

Anson and Spetzler (1992) classification system.[7] Of key importance, despite the presence of multiple arterial feeding vessels, there remains a single fistulous point in all cases **(Fig. 39.2A,B).** Frustrated arterial collateralization observed with angiography at the level of the root sleeve must not be incorrectly interpreted as a nidus or a multiplicity of feeding pedicles.

Because the slow-flow, elevated-pressure arterialized veins also drain functional spinal cord, neurologic deterioration results from venous congestion or hypertension. Progressive myelopathy, dominated by lower extremity weakness, gait changes, paresthesias, and sphincter dysfunction, ensues. Although periods of more acute or discrete decline are not infrequently observed, symptomatic progression typically follows a slow but malignantly progressive course.[8] The protean natural history of intradural dorsal AVFs typically results in significant diagnostic delay, as long as 27 months as reported by Gilbertson et al[9] between symptom onset and angiographic confirmation. Intradural dorsal AVFs comprise nearly 60 to 80% of spinal vascular anomalies, most commonly affecting men of ages 40 to 60, and display a predilection for the thoracolumbar spine. Intradural dorsal AVFs are believed to be acquired lesions, presumably the result of a cascade of impairments in distal venous outflow. Noninvasive

imaging such as MRI has drawn increasing attention as a diagnostic tool for intradural dorsal AVF. T2-signal hyperintensity (in the absence of primary compressive pathology) found in combination with prominent dorsal flow voids should be interpreted as essentially pathognomonic in the appropriate clinical setting. This has been largely corroborated in the literature, and extended to include MRA as a useful adjunct. MRI/MRA has shown considerable promise in defining AVF anatomy, locating feeding pedicles, identifying recurrence, and even in assessing the adequacy of embolization.[9,10] Digital subtraction angiography (DSA), however, remains the imaging modality of choice for initial diagnosis as well as follow-up. All patients suspected of intradural dorsal AVF should have a DSA investigation. It has been our practice to obtain confirmatory or reassuring posttreatment MRI/MRA images at intervals to verify improvement in spinal cord edema following resolution of venous hypertension.

Absolute contraindications to first-line endovascular treatment are strictly anatomic. Microsurgical clipping remains the treatment of choice for all intradural dorsal fistulas sharing an ASA-feeding vascular pedicle. This is due to the inability to tolerate any unwanted anterograde embolization or reflux. A small subset of fistulas identified by noninvasive imaging and symptomatology remain angiographically occult due

Table 39.2 Spinal Arteriovenous Malformation Classification

	Extradural-Intradural	Intramedullary	Conus Medullaris
Pathophysiology	Compression, myelopathy, steal, hemorrhage	Hemorrhage, compression, steal	Venous hypertension, compression, hemorrhage
Flow characteristics	High	High	High
Symptoms	Pain, progressive myelopathy	Acute or progressive myelopathy, pain	Progressive myelopathy, radiculopathy
Treatment options	Palliative embolization or surgery to decrease mass effect, vascular steal, venous hypertension	Surgery for superficial or midline lesions with dorsal-feeding vessels. Endovascular for deep lesions and preoperative embolization for complex lesions and ventral-feeding vessels	Preoperative embolization with surgical decompression of large veins from nerve roots and spinal cord

Note: Lesions are demarcated primarily by anatomic location. Pathophysiology, flow characteristics, and symptoms follow suit. The classification scheme is not intended as a strict guideline to determine mode of therapy but serves as general guidelines for decision making.

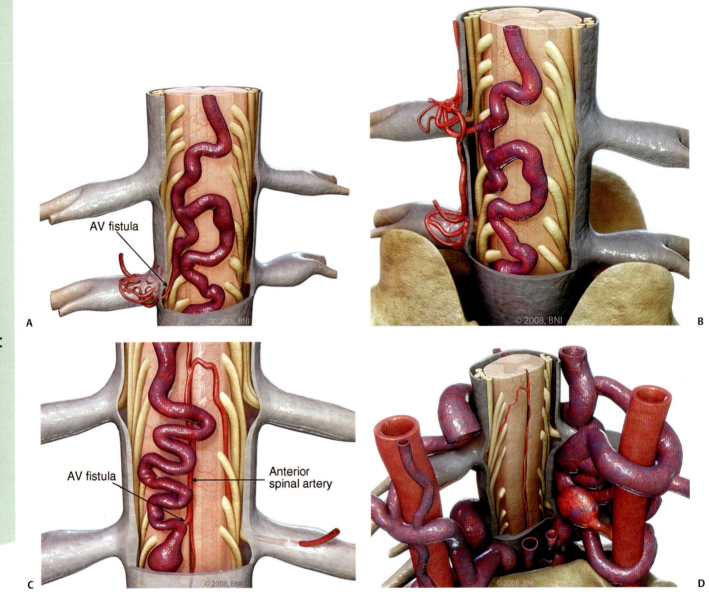

Fig. 39.2 Spinal arteriovenous fistulas (AVFs). **(A)** Dorsal view of an intradural dorsal (type a) spinal AVF. Note that the fistulous point between the radicular feeder and the dilated coronal venous plexus is intradural. Frustrated vascular recruitment at the root sleeve should not be interpreted as nidus. **(B)** Dorsal view of an intradural dorsal (type b) spinal AVF. Radicular feeders are identified at multiple levels. However, there remains a single fistulous point. **(C)** Ventral view of an intradural ventral spinal AVF. Note the dilated venous plexus, fistulous connection to the ASA, and venous varix immediately adjacent to fistulous point. **(D)** Ventral view of a cervical extradural spinal fistula. Note the venous epidural venous engorgement, and lack of intradural involvement. (Used with permission from Barrow Neurological Institute.)

to aberrant anatomy, atherosclerosis limiting endovascular access, or presumably even sluggish venous filling.[11] All such cases warrant open surgical exploration. The majority of fistulas, reported as high as 94% by Niimi et al,[12] remain amenable to attempted first-line embolization strictly by anatomic criteria. The decision to proceed with endovascular treatment follows with frank consideration of recurrence risks compared with those of surgery.

In a meta-analysis spanning over 40 years of the literature, Steinmetz et al[13] reported favorable results for 98% of intra-dural dorsal AVFs treated surgically compared with 48% of cases treated endovascularly. Recent endovascular publications and experience, however, have highlighted improving results facilitated by advances in technology and technique. Embolization with PVA particles has been abandoned, due to an unacceptably high incidence of recurrence (often over 80%) among limited older case series.[14] Results with nBCA glue have shown considerable improvement, with definitive single-treatment success rates approaching 75%, according to Song et al,[15] and only 39% of patients subsequently re-

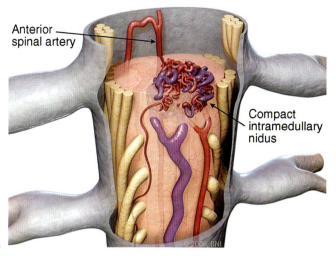

Anterior spinal artery

Compact intramedullary nidus

A

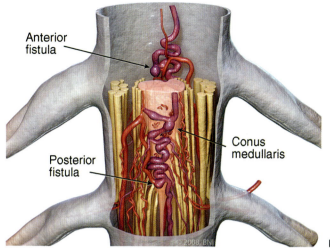

Anterior fistula

Posterior fistula

Conus medullaris

B

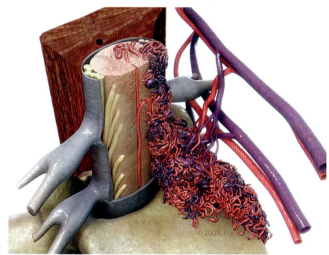

C

Fig. 39.3 Spinal arteriovenous malformations (AVMs). **(A)** Dorsal view of an intramedullary spinal AVM. Note the intramedullary location of the nidus, more compact nature of the nidus in this case, and feeding pedicles (at least one from the ASA is commonly noted). **(B)** Conus medullaris type spinal AVM. At the conus level, the ASA and PSA are directly anastomotic in normal patients. The AVM itself has been described as "glomus" in this subtype. Multiple fistulas and a highly complex angioarchitecture are commonly noted. **(C)** Extradural-intradural AVM. The size of the nidus may be extensive, and involves intradural as well as extradural tissues as the name implies. Symptoms may result from parenchymal involvement, steal, hemorrhage, or compression. (Used with permission from Barrow Neurological Institute.)

quired definitive surgical treatment, according to Eskandar et al.[16] Similarly, flexible microcatheter technology has improved successful embolization rates. The growing use of ethylene vinyl alcohol (Onyx) may herald further improvements in the precision of delivery based on observed benefits in opacity, viscosity, tolerance for slow injection rates, and microcatheter compatibility.

In terms of outcomes, the literature has generally shown comparable neurologic improvements in Aminoff-Logue scores among adequately treated surgical and endovascular patients.[17] Narvid et al[18] reported significant differences in length of hospital stay favoring an observed trend toward lower morbidity among endovascular patients. Considering these trends and our own institutional experience, we concur with several recent studies favoring the inclusion of embolization as a first-line option for cure in anatomically favorable cases.

Defining the goals, strategies, and end points of adequate embolization is crucial to achieving ideal treatment and to complication avoidance. Niimi et al[12] defined "adequate embolization" as (1) use of liquid embolic agent, (2) embolic occlusion of the proximal vein and fistulous point, (3) preserved venous drainage and angioarchitecture, and (4) angiographic disappearance of the AVF on bilateral injections extending two segments above and below the index level. Selective microcatheter navigation within the feeding pedicle immediate to the fistulous point is essential **(Fig. 39.4)**. Proximal arterial embolization may obscure angiographic visualization of the fistula, but distal collateralization may lead to subsequent recurrence. Palliative attempts at partial treatment for flow reduction are similarly unsuccessful. As the dilated coronal venous plexus remains responsible for venous drainage of functional cord tissue, overly aggressive distal venous embolization may exacerbate symptomatic edema due to further obstructions in outflow.

Intradural Ventral Spinal Fistulas

Intradural ventral spinal fistulas have been previously described as perimedullary, intradural extramedullary, and Anson and Spetzler type IV lesions. In contrast to intradural dorsal lesions, ventral AVFs are higher flow fistulas due to a

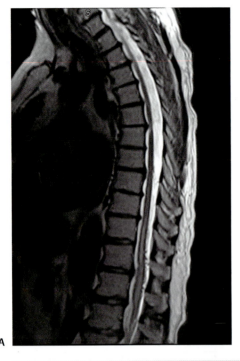

A

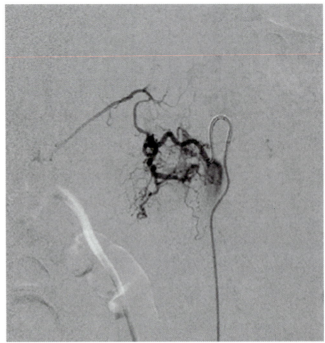

B

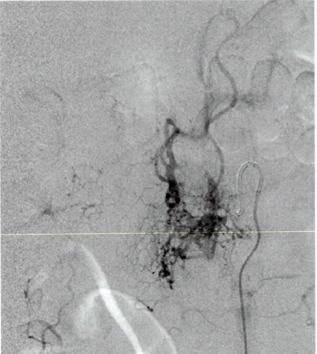

C

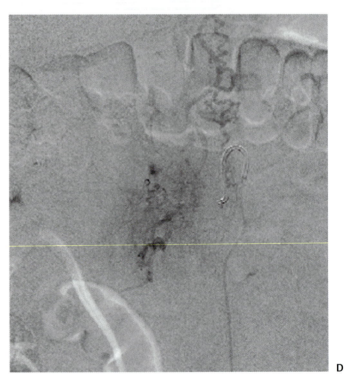

D

Fig. 39.4 A 62-year-old man with progressive bilateral leg weakness worsening over 10 months. He previously walked 4 miles a day. Lower extremity paresthesias worsened on the day prior to admission. The patient subsequently progressed to paresis and incontinence over 24 hours. **(A)** A T2-weighted sagittal magnetic resonance imaging (MRI) showing hyperintense cord signal near the conus and dorsal flow voids. The patient was subsequently taken for urgent spinal angiography for presumed spinal AVF. Anteroposterior (AP) preembolization runs are seen here **(B–D)**. **(B)** Early arterial phase injection at right L1 showed frustrated collateralization at the root sleeve. **(C)** Middle arterial phase injection displays the dilated coronal venous plexus. **(D)** Late arterial phase injection showing extensively arterialized coronal venous plexus and sluggish venous outflow.

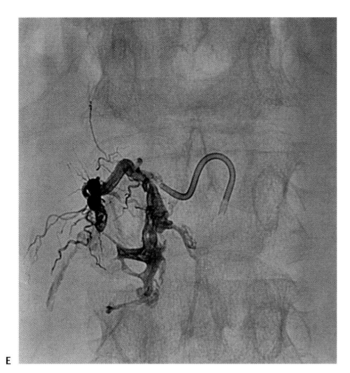

E

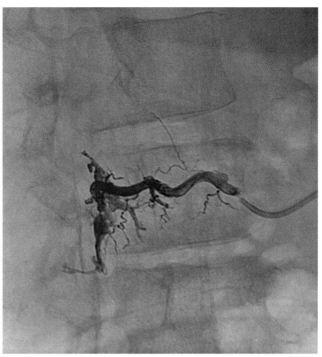

F

Fig. 39.4 (*continued*) (**E**) Postembolization Onyx cast seen on AP projection showing fistula obliteration, with cast penetration to the fistulous point. (**F**) Lateral projection. The patient ultimately returned to full strength and was discharged on postprocedure day 3. Although the extent of recovery is atypical, the case highlights the urgent nature of diagnosis and treatment. (Used with permission from Barrow Neurological Institute.)

direct connection with the ASA. Intradural ventral AVFs are recognized angiographically by a variable degree of variceal venous dilation immediately distal to the fistulous point, association with the ASA, as well as their ventral and midline location (**Fig. 39.2C**).[2] Left-to-right shift of the ASA and fistula from the midline, presumably due to associated arteriovenous pathology, has been reported in a significant percentage of patients and should not be allowed to confound the diagnosis.[19] Varix formation should not be misinterpreted as evidence of a coexistent mass lesion or AVM on MRI/MRA. These lesions are further subdivided into types A, B, and C, which may be differentiated by the degree of variceal dilation, multiplicity of arterial feeding pedicles, complexity of the associated angioarchitecture, and flow rate. Symptoms due to cord compression, steal, and subarachnoid hemorrhage predominate over venous congestion with progression of grade.[6,7] Patients are typically younger compared with intradural dorsal lesions, and most commonly present with locations near the conus (**Fig. 39.5**).

The relative rarity of intradural ventral AVFs has resulted in a more limited experience and literature. Nonetheless, careful examination of the following trends in the literature supports a growing role for the endovascular specialist in the management of these lesions beyond preoperative diagnostic angiography alone:

1. Selected series representative of the earlier literature utilizing awake anesthesia, detachable balloons, and PVA particles fail to reflect current abilities, outcomes, and technology. General anesthesia with electrophysiologic monitoring and liquid embolic agents reflect the current standard of care.

2. Endovascular candidate selection is governed largely by class and anatomy. Type A lesions possess the ideal anatomy for embolization given their more straightforward anatomy and single arterial feeding pedicle. Narrow-caliber feeding vessels, however, may limit microcatheter access to the fistulous point. The caliber of multiple thin feeders in type B lesions may present similar challenges. Type C lesions are generally considered most favorable to endovascular embolization given their complex angioarchitecture, larger caliber vessels, and high flow rates. Anterior or anterolateral surgical access may be problematic for particularly complex type C lesions situated high above the conus. Embolization of class a, b, and c lesions has been reported with varying success.

3. Partial embolization for flow reduction fails to result in ultimate cure or symptomatic improvement. The goal of embolization remains microcatheter navigation to the fistulous point, complete obliteration of the fistulous point and proximal-most vein, and strict intolerance of reflux.

4. Pre- and intraoperative angiography has shown additional value for surgical localization, preoperative classification and diagnosis, as well as verification of treatment. Nonetheless, some authors prefer surgical resection given high rates of gross total resection (up to 92%), generally favorable outcomes associated with surgery, and the possibility of direct visualization (and presumably therefore preservation) of the ASA.[6]

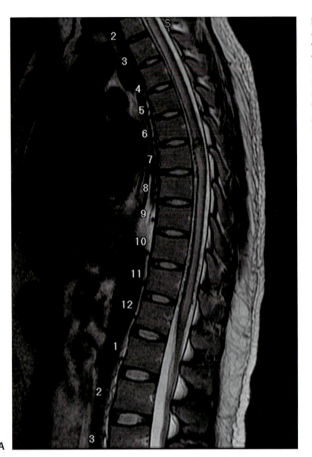

A

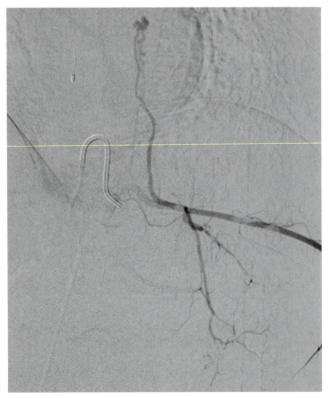

B

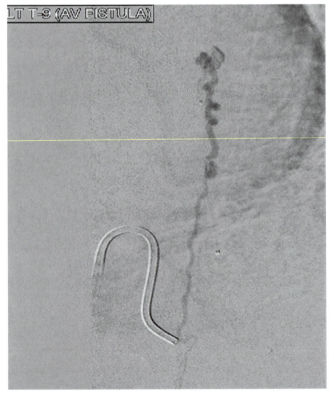

C

Fig. 39.5 A 20-year-old man with 2 weeks of radiating abdominal pain. Five days prior to admission he developed onset of bilateral lower extremity weakness, progressing to left leg paresis and hemisensory loss. **(A)** A T2-weighted sagittal MRI sequence showing presumed intramedullary mass/hemorrhage at T6/7 with scant ventral flow voids. Presumed diagnosis of spinal AVM. **(B)** Early arterial phase of left selective T9 injection via Mickelson catheter. Intradural ventral spinal (type a) AVF noted with small associated venous varix, relatively moderate flow rate, and direct association with the ASA. **(C)** Later arterial phase (subtracted) view showing ventral venous arterialization.

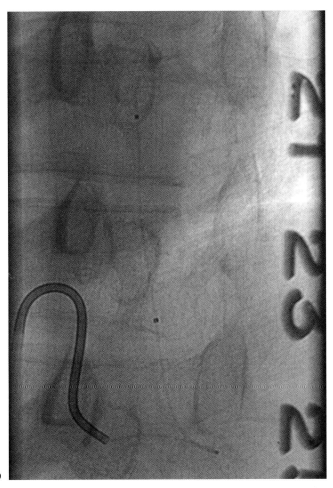
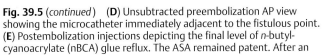
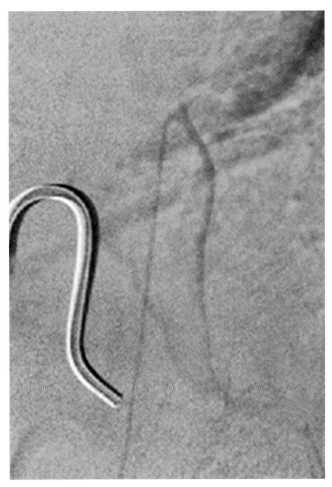

D   E

Fig. 39.5 (*continued*) (**D**) Unsubtracted preembolization AP view showing the microcatheter immediately adjacent to the fistulous point. (**E**) Postembolization injections depicting the final level of *n*-butyl-cyanoacrylate (nBCA) glue reflux. The ASA remained patent. After an initial deterioration, the patient improved dramatically to 4/5 strength on the left and was ambulatory approximately 1 month postprocedure. (Used with permission from Barrow Neurological Institute.)

Ultimately, selection of endovascular candidates requires a case-by-case consideration of the factors enumerated above, and the management of such lesions typically mandates a multimodal approach.[20,21]

Extradural Spinal Fistulas

Extradural spinal fistulas are characteristically high flow in nature due to large vessel, segmental, dural, or radicular arterial shunting to the epidural venous network (**Fig. 39.2D**). Although defined solely by epidural venous engorgement, fistulas with intradural as well as extradural involvement have been described. Although many reports are confounded by a lack of consistent nomenclature predating the current classification scheme, such cases are presumably due to venous valvular incompetence. Multiple feeding arterial pedicles may be identified, especially in the case of traumatic fistulas. The majority of cases remain idiopathic in nature. Congenital and syndromic associations (e.g., neurofibromatosis type 1 [NF1]) as well as traumatic etiologies have been reported. The largest review to date reported by Zhang et al[22] highlighted a female predominance with a widely separated bimodal age distribution. Neurologic symptoms typically result from thecal compression, subarachnoid hemorrhage, and less commonly steal or bruit.[2] Extradural fistulas are uniquely well suited to endovascular treatment due to the potential for extensive venous hemorrhage during surgery, high flow rates, and larger caliber feeding arterial pedicles (**Fig. 39.6**). The latter two characteristics generally limit the utility of particulate agents, and in instances of especially high flow, can favor the more controlled deployment of detachable coils with or without liquid embolic agents. Larger delivery catheters and coil deployment, however, may limit distal or superselective navigation.[2] Transvenous routes for embolization have also been reported. The goals of embolization remain angiographic obliteration of the fistulous point (often requiring treatment of the distal-most feeding arterial segment) as well as a small segment of the proximal arterialized vein. Surgical intervention is typically reserved for the setting of neurologic decline, which may occur secondary to extrinsic compression, for example, by enlarged draining veins.

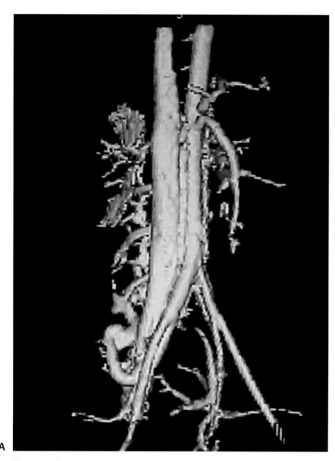

A

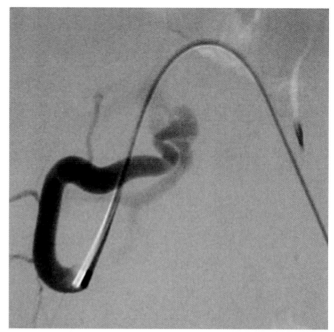

B

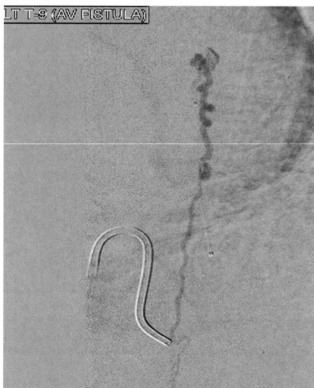

LT T-9 (AV FISTULA)

C

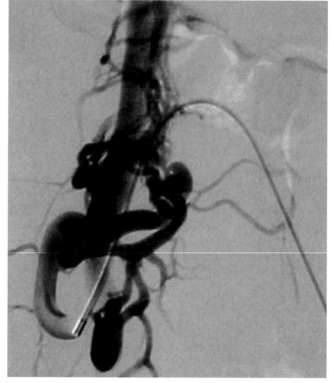

D

Fig. 39.6 A 2-year-old child presented with failure to reach lower extremity milestones. A bruit was auscultated in the right groin. **(A)** Screening magnetic resonance angiography (MRA) revealed an extradural high-flow AVF fed by the internal iliac artery. Early **(B)**, middle **(C)**, and late **(D)** arterial phase injections. Note the lack of intradural pathology.

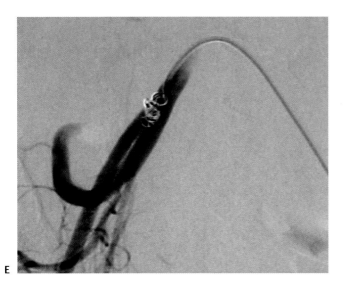

E

Fig. 39.6 (continued) (**E**) Post–coil embolization injection. (Actual distal location of the coil-pack is obscured by the AP projection). The child recovered nicely with motor improvement and ambulation at latest follow-up. (Used with permission from Barrow Neurological Institute.)

Spinal Arteriovenous Malformations

Extradural-Intradural Arteriovenous Malformations

Extradural-intradural AVMs have been previously termed juvenile, metameric, or type III spinal AVMs. They represent a class of large, rare lesions that typically present with pain and progressive myelopathy in childhood or adolescence. These are high-flow lesions with multiple arterial feeders that do not respect tissue boundaries and often involve paraspinal bone, muscle, skin, subcutaneous tissues, the spinal canal, spinal cord, and nerve roots (**Fig. 39.3C**). Neurologic deficits may result from a combination of spinal cord compression, venous congestion, vascular steal phenomena, and hemorrhage.

Most previous endovascular studies have employed PVA particles for treatment, and thus may not demonstrate current endovascular abilities.[23,24] Bondi et al[23] embolized 15 metameric lesions within their larger spinal AVM cohort, requiring a total of 158 embolization procedures due to recanalization. The authors reported an 8% rate of postprocedure clinical decline. The literature has supported the value of particulate embolization for the reduction of hemorrhage risk, improved clinical symptoms, and limited progression with a relatively low complication rate. Higher recanalization rates requiring follow-up DSA and possible retreatment have eliminated PVA embolization as a first-line option for extradural-intradural AVMs.

Corkill et al[25] reported their results with Onyx for the treatment of six extradural-intradural AVMs. Complete obliteration was obtained in one patient, but later recurrence was noted. Three of six patients had clinical improvement, two with stabilization of symptoms, and one developed persistent neurologic decline. Short- and long-term clinical outcome data of greater sample size and significance is highly antici-

pated, but general experience with Onyx suggests considerable promise.

Extradural-intradural AVMs are in general surgically and endovascularly formidable lesions and typically carry a poor prognosis (**Fig. 39.7**). Complex angioarchitecture, flow rate, size, and local involvement typically obscure surgical or angiographic visualization of the normal spinal vasculature. Complete obliteration is often not possible without significant neurologic injury. Spetzler et al[26] reported complete resection of a metameric AVM with clinical improvement using staged resection with preoperative and intraoperative embolization. Such results are generally atypical, however, and most realistic goals for treatment are palliative. In large unresectable lesions, embolization is used to ameliorate neurologic deficits caused by mass effect, vascular steal, or venous hypertension. Surgery is typically reserved for decompression of mass effect along the nerve roots and spinal cord. In potentially resectable lesions, preoperative angiography and embolization are an essential part of any multimodality treatment strategy.

Intramedullary Arteriovenous Malformations

Intramedullary AVMs, also known as glomus-type or type II AVMs, are more common than intramedullary-extramedullary AVMs and usually present relatively early in life. As with in tracranial AVMs, the nidus may be compact or diffuse. Symptoms are often acute secondary to hemorrhage, although progressive or fluctuating myelopathy and pain are not outside the norm. Angiography typically reveals a high-pressure and high-flow lesion that fills rapidly with early venous drainage. Venous drainage may be bidirectional into the coronal venous plexus that surrounds the spinal cord. The arterialized plexus can be tortuous and distended for a variable distance from the nidus, and should not be misinterpreted as evidence of a metameric lesion or AVF (**Fig. 39.3A**). The identification of high-risk features (such as aneurysms) remains a key role in preintervention angiography.

Treatment strategies can be surgical, endovascular, or multimodal. Although complete cure is always the ideal goal, it is critical to identify those lesions in which an attempt at cure would likely cause neurologic decline. This is accomplished by examination of the anatomic margins, nidus location, and preembolization provocative infusion testing. At our institution, all spinal AVMs are deemed to warrant preintervention DSA to identify the feeding vessels, characterize the pattern of venous drainage, determine the presence of high-risk features, and establish relationships to the normal cord vasculature. Superselective angiography is most essential to identify peri- and intramedullary anastomosis and collateral recruitment, and to achieve images uncontaminated by adjacent vessels (**Fig. 39.8**). Treatment plans must be individualized based on lesion characteristics, angioarchitecture, location, patient age, lifetime risk of hemorrhage, and history of recent hemorrhage or recovery.

There is sufficient literature to justify embolization primarily or prior to surgical resection in appropriately selected cases. In general, AVMs with a diffuse intraparenchymal nidus or those located anterolaterally are not easily treated with

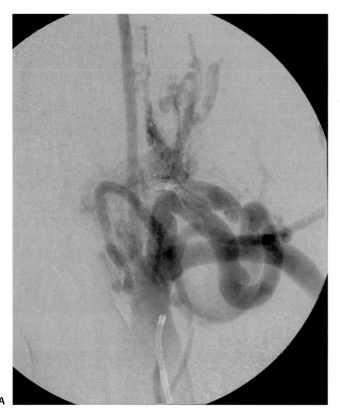

A

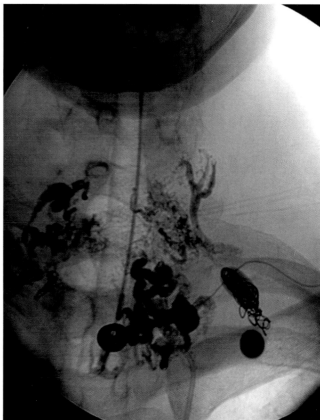

B

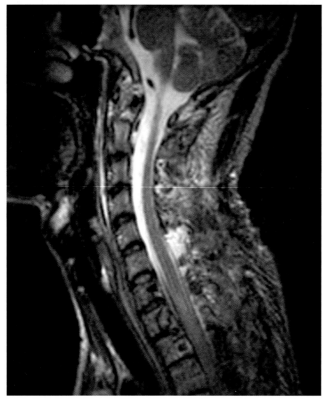

C

Fig. 39.7 A 29-year-old man with worsening left (4-/5), more so than right (4/5) lower extremity strength over 3 months. The patient reported a general decrease in sensation below T4. **(A)** Left subclavian injection reveals the typical "metameric" configuration of this spinal AVM. There is early venous drainage, and high-risk features are identified (not seen). Treatment consisted of staged embolization in combination with surgical resection for palliation. **(B)** Unsubtracted view depicts the multiple techniques used to achieve flow reduction prior to subtotal resection. **(C)** Post–multimodal treatment midsagittal T2-weighted MRI. Good epidural venous decompression was achieved along with extensive resection. Scant T2-hyperintense cord signal was still apparent. Postoperatively, the patient's weakness was improved. (Used with permission from Barrow Neurological Institute.)

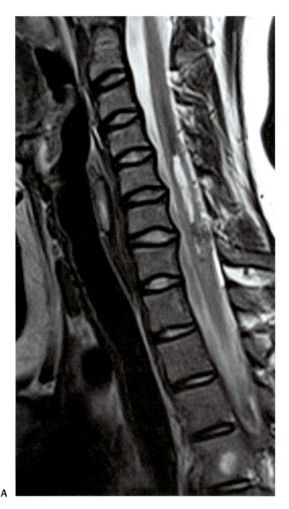

A

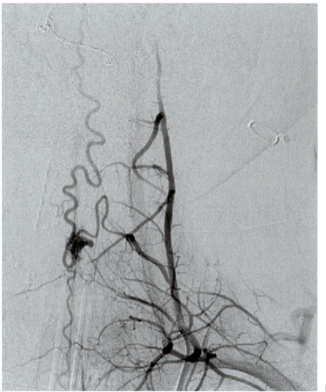

B

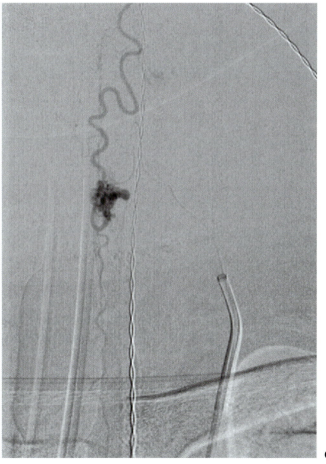

C

Fig. 39.8 A 15-year-old girl with a remote history of surgical exploration for presumed tumor after sudden onset of left-sided weakness. In the interval, the patient had returned to baseline. **(A)** A T2-weighted sagittal MRI revealing evidence of flow voids, myelomalacia, and old hemorrhage. **(B)** Left thyrocervical injection seen here in the AP plane reveals an intramedullary spinal AVM with perimedullary venous drainage. The ASA is not clearly seen due to preferential shunting. **(C)** AP superselective catheterization with the catheter tip lodged at the AVM nidus. *(continued on next page)*

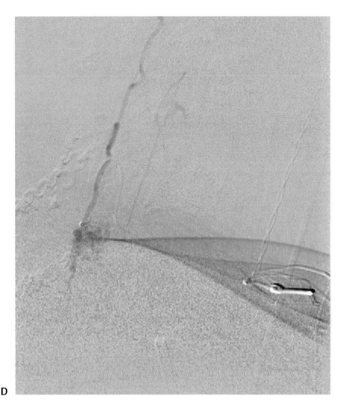

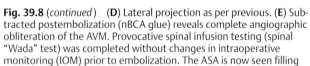

D

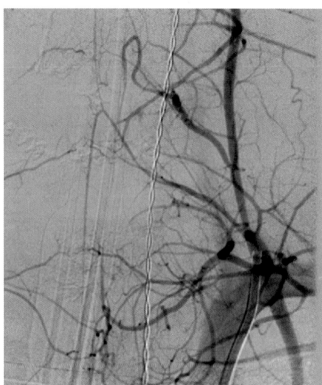

E

Fig. 39.8 (*continued*) (**D**) Lateral projection as per previous. (**E**) Subtracted postembolization (nBCA glue) reveals complete angiographic obliteration of the AVM. Provocative spinal infusion testing (spinal "Wada" test) was completed without changes in intraoperative monitoring (IOM) prior to embolization. The ASA is now seen filling

from an adjacent pedicle off the thyrocervical trunk. The patient underwent subsequent surgical resection, and was discharged at her neurologic baseline. (Used with permission from Barrow Neurological Institute.)

surgery. The results of partial embolization alone with regard to reduction of hemorrhage risk are not known, but subtotal embolization likely confers nominal benefit unless high risk features like nidal aneurysms are selectively targeted. Further data on the durability of clinical or functional improvement correlated with decreased blood flow, mass effect, and vascular steal will be useful. Given the relatively low complication rate associated with endovascular intervention, repeated embolization attempts represents an alternative strategy if surgery is less desirable.

Endovascular management is particularly appropriate for deep lesions, ventrally located lesions, and poor surgical candidates. Identification of the ASA is a crucial first step during angiography, as nearly all intramedullary AVMs possess a main feeding pedicle related to this vessel. PSA contributions are common, but typically more variable. In some cases, the ASA remains angiographically occult due to preferential shunting to the AVM. During embolization and progressive obliteration of the shunt, the normal spinal arteries may subsequently opacify. Serial and frequent runs, initially cautious embolization, and preembolization Wada testing are important components of complication avoidance.

The incidence of neurologic deficit following embolization of intramedullary spinal AVMs may range as high as 10%, but this may in fact be underestimated if the anterior spinal artery requires catheterization. This usually occurs from inadvertent occlusion of normal feeding arteries as described above. The common causes for this include unwanted reflux

of embolic material, failure to recognize normal vasculature, displacement of catheter during embolization, and choice of embolic material. As a general rule for complication avoidance, the safest and most effective embolizations deliver material as close to the nidus as possible. This helps to achieve more robust embolization with reduced risk for reflux and inadvertent embolization of normal arteries.

As previously described, many of the early embolization studies using PVA particles showed initial promise, but suffered from similar criticisms of unacceptably high rates of recanalization necessitating retreatment.[23,24] Acrylic glue, however, is also less desirable for intramedullary AVMs due to its technical demands and unpredictability in even the most experienced hands. Complications include unwanted proximal reflux, distal penetration with venous occlusion, and catheter gluing from slow injections. Onyx has shown promise in this regard, allowing injection over several minutes to provide more predictable and controllable nidal embolization. It can also allow angiography or repeat provocative spinal Wada testing through the guide catheter during a pause of injection. Some find this characteristic very helpful when embolizing tiny feeding pedicles from the anterior spinal axis, when absolute injection control is critical.[25] As previously highlighted, animal studies have suggested that vessel toxicity may be related to injection rate, necessitating frequent stops for 1 to 2 minutes during embolization procedures. A useful strategy is to coordinate angiographic runs via the guide catheter during these injection pauses or when Onyx reflux is noticed. Embolization can then be resumed after a few minutes, ultimately allowing for deep nidus penetration and occlusion.[25] Corkill et al[25] reported a 37.5% rate of angiographic occlusion among their series of 17 patients with spinal AVMs treated with Onyx embolization (six intradural-extradural, 11 intramedullary). Onyx has almost completely replaced cyanoacrylate glue and PVA particles and is widely considered the embolic agent of choice for intramedullary spinal AVMs. Further advances in catheter technology, novel embolic agents, and further development of the literature will likely expand the role of the endovascular surgeon in intramedullary spinal AVMs.

Nonetheless, surgical resection remains the gold standard and well-supported treatment modality for many spinal intramedullary AVMs. Surgery is especially well suited for simple, midline, and superficial lesions that have dorsally located feeding vessels. Spetzler et al[6] achieved gross total resection in 92% of 27 treated intramedullary AVMs. In this study 67% of patients had clinical improvement, and only 8% had neurologic decline. In this study, however, an unspecified number of AVMs likely underwent preoperative embolization. The authors suggested that complex, multipedicled lesions are in general most appropriately managed with preoperative embolization before surgical resection is attempted. Similar results have been supported by Yasargil et al,[27] Rosenblum et al,[28] and Connolly et al[29] with clinical improvement in 33 to 48% of patients in roughly 3 to 8.5 years of follow-up.

Conus Medullaris Arteriovenous Malformations

Conus medullaris AVMs are a relatively new category of spinal AVMs[6] that warrant specific attention given their unique characteristics. These AVMs by definition are always located at the conus medullaris and cauda equina but can extend along the entire filum terminale. They have glomus-type niduses that are usually extramedullary and pial-based, but almost always have an intramedullary component. They typically have multiple feeding arteries, multiple niduses, and complex patterns of venous drainage. The complex angioarchitecture seen in these lesions is typically composed of multiple feeding pedicles with direct arteriovenous shunts and large dilated veins (**Fig. 39.3C**). Angiographic and surgical interpretation is further complicated by the direct anastomoses of anterior and posterior spinal circulations at the level of the conus.

Clinically these patients can present with myelopathy, radiculopathy, or myeloradiculopathy. Symptoms are usually secondary to hemorrhage or venous hypertension, ischemia, and mass effect from large veins. Radiculopathy, in particular, may significantly improve with time after successful treatment.

These lesions are treated with combined endovascular and microsurgical approach (**Fig. 39.9**). Angiographic identification of the ASA and PSA as well as the possible sites of anastomosis is crucial. Endovascular embolization followed

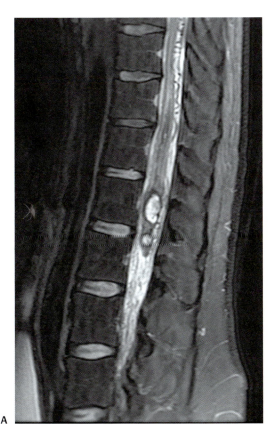
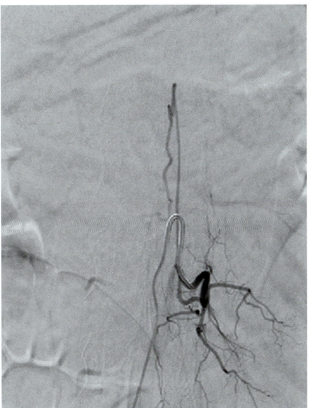

A   **B**

Fig. 39.9 A 40-year-old man with a prior history of hemorrhage, lower extremity dysfunction, and three attempted embolizations. **(A)** Sagittal T2-weighted MRI scan revealing the sequelae of hemorrhage, extensive flow voids, and myelomalacia at the conus. Presumed diagnosis of partially treated conus AVM. Selective left L2 injection early **(B)**, *(continued on next page)*

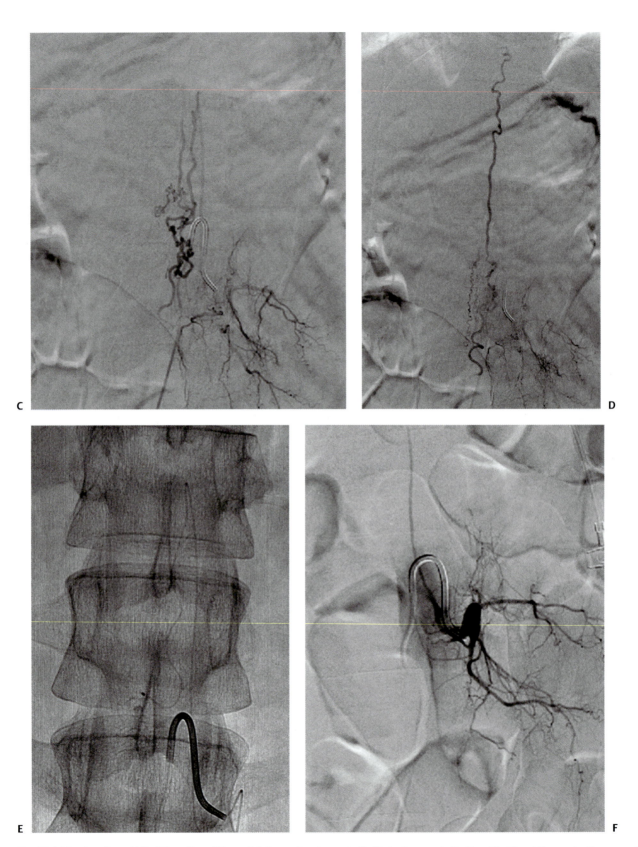

C

D

E

F

Fig. 39.9 (*Continued*)   middle **(C)**, and late **(D)** arterial phases showing early venous drainage, diffuse shunting pattern, and complex anastomoses between the anterior and posterior spinal circulation. **(E)** Unsubtracted view showing superselective catheterization of the conus AVM to facilitate Onyx embolization. Significant flow reduction was achieved prior to surgery. **(F)** Postsurgical left L2 injection revealing obliteration of AV shunting after multimodality treatment. (Used with permission from Barrow Neurological Institute.)

by surgical resection to ultimately facilitate the decompression of large dilated veins from the spinal cord and nerve roots can cause dramatic relief of neurologic symptoms. Aggressive multimodal treatment for these lesions is most appropriate.[6]

◆ Conclusion

Arteriovenous lesions of the spinal neuroaxis represent a complex spectrum of pathologies most appropriately demarcated by anatomic location, shunting patterns, and clinical symptoms. AVFs and AVMs warrant angiographic investigation, and in many cases endovascular intervention can be safely offered in the same setting as a means to preoperative treatment or cure. The growing range of endovascular materials and techniques are certain to foster further innovation in the catheter-based treatment of these lesions.

References

1. Wells-Roth D, Zonenshayn M. Vascular anatomy of the spine. Operatives Techniques in Neurosurgery. 2003;6:116–121
2. McDougall CG, Deshmukh VR, Fiorella DJ, Albuquerque FC, Spetzler RF. Endovascular techniques for vascular malformations of the spinal axis. Neurosurg Clin N Am 2005;16:395–410, x–xi
3. Rabe FE, Yune HY, Klatte EC, Miller RE. Efficacy of glucagon for abdominal digital angiography. AJR Am J Roentgenol 1982;139:618–619
4. Britz GW, Eskridge J. Endovascular treatment of spinal cord arteriovenous malformations. In: Winn HR, Youmans JR, eds. Youmans' Neurological Surgery, 5th ed. Philadelphia: WB Saunders, 2004:2363–2373
5. Chaloupka JC, Huddle DC, Alderman J, Fink S, Hammond R, Vinters HV. A reexamination of the angiotoxicity of superselective injection of DMSO in the swine rete embolization model. AJNR Am J Neuroradiol 1999;20:401–410
6. Spetzler RF, Detwiler PW, Riina HA, Porter RW. Modified classification of spinal cord vascular lesions. J Neurosurg 2002;96(2, Suppl)145–156
7. Anson JA, Spetzler RF. Classification of spinal arteriovenous malformations and implications for treatment. BNI Q 1992;8:2–8
8. Niimi Y, Berenstein A. Endovascular treatment of spinal vascular malformations. Neurosurg Clin N Am 1999;10:47–71
9. Gilbertson JR, Miller GM, Goldman MS, Marsh WR. Spinal dural arteriovenous fistulas: MR and myelographic findings. AJNR Am J Neuroradiol 1995;16:2049–2057
10. Eddleman CS, Jeong H, Cashen TA, et al. Advanced noninvasive imaging of spinal vascular malformations. Neurosurg Focus 2009;26:E9
11. Oldfield EH, Bennett A III, Chen MY, Doppman JL. Successful management of spinal dural arteriovenous fistulas undetected by arteriography. Report of three cases. J Neurosurg 2002;96(2, Suppl)220–229
12. Niimi Y, Berenstein A, Setton A, Neophytides A. Embolization of spinal dural arteriovenous fistulae: results and follow-up. Neurosurgery 1997;40:675–682, discussion 682–683
13. Steinmetz MP, Chow MM, Krishnaney AA, et al. Outcome after the treatment of spinal dural arteriovenous fistulae: a contemporary single-institution series and meta-analysis. Neurosurgery 2004;55:77–87, discussion 87–88
14. Morgan MK, Marsh WR. Management of spinal dural arteriovenous malformations. J Neurosurg 1989;70:832–836
15. Song JK, Gobin YP, Duckwiler GR, et al. N-butyl 2-cyanoacrylate embolization of spinal dural arteriovenous fistulae. AJNR Am J Neuroradiol 2001;22:40–47
16. Eskandar EN, Borges LF, Budzik RF Jr, Putman CM, Ogilvy CS. Spinal dural arteriovenous fistulas: experience with endovascular and surgical therapy. J Neurosurg 2002;96(2, Suppl)162–167
17. Cenzato M, Versari P, Righi C, Simionato F, Casali C, Giovanelli M. Spinal dural arteriovenous fistulae: analysis of outcome in relation to pretreatment indicators. Neurosurgery 2004;55:815–822, discussion 822–823
18. Narvid J, Hetts SW, Larsen D, et al. Spinal dural arteriovenous fistulae: clinical features and long-term results. Neurosurgery 2008;62:159–166, discussion 166–167
19. Hida K, Iwasaki Y, Goto K, Miyasaka K, Abe H. Results of the surgical treatment of perimedullary arteriovenous fistulas with special reference to embolization. J Neurosurg 1999;90(2, Suppl)198–205
20. Barrow DL, Colohan ART, Dawson R. Intradural perimedullary arteriovenous fistulas (type IV spinal cord arteriovenous malformations). J Neurosurg 1994;81:221–229
21. Cho KT, Lee DY, Chung CK, Han MH, Kim HJ. Treatment of spinal cord perimedullary arteriovenous fistula: embolization versus surgery. Neurosurgery 2005;56:232–241, discussion 232–241
22. Zhang H, He M, Mao B. Thoracic spine extradural arteriovenous fistula: case report and review of the literature. Surg Neurol 2006;66(Suppl 1):S18–S23, discussion S23–S24
23. Biondi A, Merland JJ, Reizine D, et al. Embolization with particles in thoracic intramedullary arteriovenous malformations: long-term angiographic and clinical results. Radiology 1990;177:651–658
24. Touho H, Karasawa J, Ohnishi H, Yamada K, Ito M, Kinoshita A. Intravascular treatment of spinal arteriovenous malformations using a microcatheter—with special reference to serial xylocaine tests and intravascular pressure monitoring. Surg Neurol 1994;42:148–156
25. Corkill RA, Mitsos AP, Molyneux AJ. Embolization of spinal intramedullary arteriovenous malformations using the liquid embolic agent, Onyx: a single-center experience in a series of 17 patients. J Neurosurg Spine 2007;7:478–485
26. Spetzler RF, Zabramski JM, Flom RA. Management of juvenile spinal AVM's by embolization and operative excision. Case report. J Neurosurg 1989;70:628–632
27. Yaşargil MG, Symon L, Teddy PJ. Arteriovenous malformations of the spinal cord. Adv Tech Stand Neurosurg 1984;11:61–102
28. Rosenblum B, Oldfield EH, Doppman JL, Di Chiro G. Spinal arteriovenous malformations: a comparison of dural arteriovenous fistulas and intradural AVM's in 81 patients. J Neurosurg 1987;67:795–802
29. Connolly ES Jr, Zubay GP, McCormick PC, Stein BM. The posterior approach to a series of glomus (type II) intramedullary spinal cord arteriovenous malformations. Neurosurgery 1998;42:774–785, discussion 785–786

40

Promising Advances and Innovations in Neurointerventional Surgery

Omar M. Arnaout, Rudy J. Rahme, Salah G. Aoun, Christopher S. Eddleman, Anitha Nimmagadda, Michael C. Hurley, Guilherme Dabus, Jeffery Miller, Sameer A. Ansari, Ali Shaibani, and Bernard R. Bendok

---

Pearls

- Recent neurointerventional advances include better mechanical devices for stroke treatment, improved liquid embolic agents, and enhanced access devices.
- Future advances may include nanotechnologies and interventional MRI.
- Local delivery of stem cells and pharmacotherapy may be on the horizon.

The past two decades have witnessed tremendous strides in interventional therapeutic options for the treatment of cerebrovascular diseases. These advances include new management strategies for hemorrhagic disease and ischemic stroke. Notably, the introduction of detachable platinum coils in the early 1990s offered an additional tool for the treatment of intracranial aneurysms. More recently, advances in device-assisted coiling techniques, complex coil shapes, and gel-coated and bioactive-coil technology have further evolved the interventional capabilities.[1] Similarly, the management of intracranial stenosis has shifted from angioplasty or stenting with cardiac devices to new flexible systems specifically designed for the cerebral circulation.[2] In addition, the 2000s have seen the birth of the first mechanical clot retrieval devices for the treatment of acute ischemic stroke. As our experience continues to grow in this rather novel area, these devices will continue to be perfected and tailored to the needs of the neurointerventionist, for optimal patient outcomes. From an imaging standpoint, interventional work has benefited from exciting advances in biplane angiography, computed tomography (CT), and magnetic resonance imaging (MRI) modalities.[3] Finally, from a basic science perspective, vascular biology studies of the underlying molecular and genetic basis of cerebrovascular diseases are rapidly expanding with exciting discoveries[4] and the promising development of cell-mediated therapies.[5] Moreover, sophisticated genetic epidemiologic studies are laying the foundation for future rational screening protocols. This chapter reviews promising advances and future directions for the endovascular treatment of neurovascular diseases and tumors.

◆ Ischemic Stroke

Time Is Brain

Each year, 600,000 individuals in the United States suffer a new stroke, and an additional 180,000 experience recurrent attacks[6]; ischemic stroke accounts for 87% of all strokes, whereas hemorrhagic stroke accounts for the other 13%.[6] The treatment and outcome of acute ischemic stroke is time dependent in that there exists a very brief period after the onset of stroke during which ischemic brain tissue may be salvageable. Intravenous tissue-type plasminogen activator (tPA) has been shown to improve outcome if given up to 3 hours after acute ischemic stroke.[7] Recently the time window has extended to 4.5 hours in select patients.[8] Not surprisingly, earlier recanalization has been associated with better outcomes within this time window.[9] Despite our understanding of time-sensitivity and of the potential reversible nature of the disease, it is estimated that fewer than 5% of patients receive Food and Drug Administration (FDA)-approved thrombolytic therapy.[10] This can be partially explained by multiple causes, which are more often than not related to the narrow time window and patients' comorbidities that preclude treatment.[11] Therefore, it becomes evident that the logistics of care delivery as well as treatment options must be improved so that more patients are properly and promptly transferred to, and evaluated at, appropriate treatment centers.

Logistics of Care

Improved stroke care begins at the prehospital stage; the California Acute Stroke Prototype Registry (CASPR) investigators estimate more than a 10-fold increase in the number of patients receiving appropriate treatment if the hospital arrival time is within 1 hour of symptom onset,[12] highlighting the importance of public education and emergency medical services response time. Future first responders to the scene of a suspected stroke may be able to perform real-time neuroimaging rapidly with subsequent transmission of images to the receiving medical center such that the time to diagnosis, triage, and catheterization (if deemed necessary) is optimized. Real-time neuroimaging using transcranial ultrasonography, especially with the concurrent use of ultrasound contrast agents, may prove beneficial in providing such rapid assessment of occluded cerebral vessels in the field.[13] Color-coded duplex ultrasonography has been shown to correctly differentiate hemorrhagic stroke from ischemic stroke in 95% of cases when compared with CT scanning.[14] Furthermore, the use of cerebroprotective agents, again possibly administered in the field or early in the provision of stroke care, may further contribute to improved outcomes.

With our current knowledge, patients arriving at a stroke treatment center outside of the defined windows for thrombolysis have few options outside of future stroke prevention and rehabilitation; therefore, extension of the therapeutic window is critical for enabling more patients to benefit from acute stroke treatment. The replacement of the traditional "stopwatch" approach to stroke with a more dynamic and functional time window is likely to take place, with growing evidence in clinical trials with the usefulness of MRI-based patient selection for thrombolysis (Desmoteplase in Acute Ischemic Stroke [DIAS], Diffusion-weighted imaging Evaluation For Understanding Stroke Evolution [DEFUSE], and Dose Escalation of Desmoteplase for Acute Ischemic Stroke [DEDAS] trials).[15] The ongoing Third International Stroke Trial (IST-3) and the Magnetic Resonance and REcanalization of Stroke Clots Using Embolectomy (MR RESCUE) trial will also likely impact whether patients in the future are offered thrombolysis outside the conventional window.

Technologic Advances

The incorporation of interventional approaches as an adjunct or alternative to intravenous thrombolysis in the setting of acute stroke is a rapidly growing field with a recent explosion in the number of devices available to the interventionist. The Prolyse in Acute Cerebral Thromboembolism (PROACT) trial was one of the first large multicenter trials to investigate the use of intravenous thrombolytic agents for the treatment of acute stroke; the study was followed by several other randomized trials including the Interventional Management of Stroke (IMS) study, which described the use of intravenous tPA as a bridge toward catheter directed arterial infusion of the thrombolytic. IMS-II introduced data regarding the use of low-energy sonography in addition to local thrombolysis. Subsequent studies have evaluated mechanical clot retrieval devices including the Mechanical Embolus Removal in Cerebral Ischemia (MERCI) and Penumbra (San Leandro, CA) trials.[15] Investigations and breakthroughs are likely to continue in both pharmacologic and mechanical thrombolysis, with the future generation of devices likely to include a combination of the two modalities to achieve increased recanalization rates.[16,17] Future devices are also likely to address the issue of distal emboli during clot manipulation.[18]

In addition to clot removal and microinfusion devices, the use of retrievable stents for the acute revascularization of thromboembolic stroke is a topic of great interest that is currently being evaluated.[19,20] Stenting may prove useful as an adjunct to thrombolysis for immediate re-reperfusion with subsequent retrieval, or alternatively left in place for permanent deployment.

Pharmacologic Advances

Promising pharmacologic options for the treatment of acute ischemic stroke can be categorized as follows:

1. *Novel thromboembolytic agents and adjuvants* (including antiplatelet and anticoagulation agents). Microplasmin, a recombinant form of human plasmin may have a reduced propensity to cause bleeding compared with tPA and has been shown to be tolerable in human volunteers and efficacious in animal models of stroke. Microplasmin is currently under investigation to determine the clinical efficacy in human acute ischemic stroke patients.[21]

2. *Neuroprotective agents,* which have been an attractive but so far elusive target. At the time of this writing, over 160 trials for ischemic stroke neuroprotective agents have been initiated.[22] Unfortunately, few have produced positive results. However, notable recent exceptions include high-dose human albumin therapy, which showed promising results in the original Albumin in Acute Stroke (ALIAS) trial.[23] A larger randomized multicenter placebo-controlled efficacy trial is now underway.[15] Additionally, magnesium, which has been shown so far to be a rather weak neuroprotectant,[24] continues to be under investigation, as it is a safe and relatively inexpensive agent that may be administered in the hyperacute prehospital setting or during interventional procedures.[15]

3. Agents that contribute to the *recovery of lost or dormant neuronal function.* Although currently in their infancy, future interventional approaches may include local administration of neurorestorative agents, such as stem cells of both exogenous and endogenous origins, or neurotrophic molecules that promote and direct endogenous neurogenesis.[25,26]

◆ Intracranial Atherosclerotic Disease

Intracranial atherosclerotic disease (ICAD) accounts for 8 to 10% of all strokes.[27] Furthermore, the degree of stenosis is known to directly correlate with the risk of stroke; although the 1-year rate of stroke in patients with history of stroke or transient ischemic attack (TIA) and ≥70% stenosis is 18%, this risk falls to 6% in individuals with the same clinical history but <70% stenosis.[28]

Despite the significant stroke risk, the interventional management of ICAD remains controversial. Although significant technical progress has been made in the endovascular treatment of ICAD over the past decade, including staged angioplasty and stenting[29,30] and more recently self-expanding nitinol stents, clear benefit of stenting over maximal medical management (antiplatelet, statins, overall risk factor modification) has not yet been shown clearly.[31] Furthermore, there appears to be a high degree of restenosis after stenting, although efforts are underway to address this issue with various strategies.[32] Although a significant amount of data has been generated regarding the interventional approaches to ICAD, it has been partially plagued by a lack of standardization; a standardized protocol will likely allow direct comparison of outcome data in the future.[33]

Technologic Advances

The deployment of drug-eluting stents, a common place practice in interventional cardiology, is a promising venue[34] but one that is currently marked with concerns regarding delayed restenosis and thrombosis. Ideally, a stent will undergo early and stable endothelialization, which reduces the risk of thrombosis. This may be achieved in the new generation of intracranial stents by including bioactive coating that attracts or stimulates endothelial cells, or circulating growth factors.[34] Conversely, biodegradable stents, which are currently under investigation in the realm of interventional cardiology, may prove a useful addition to the endovascular armamentarium as they perform their function and subsequently dissolve, theoretically eliminating the risk of future complications.[35]

◆ Intracranial Aneurysms

The approval of detachable platinum coils by the FDA more than a decade ago revolutionized the treatment of both ruptured and unruptured intracranial aneurysms. The International Subarachnoid Aneurysm Trial (ISAT),[36] which compared the safety and efficacy of endovascular coiling to those of microsurgical clipping of ruptured intracranial aneurysms, produced some controversy regarding patient selection and randomization with subsequent concerns regarding the results. Nevertheless, endovascular embolization emerged as a suitable option for select aneurysms. Although the definition of "suitable aneurysm" is constantly evolving, some lesions have so far eluded simple coiling, for example, giant aneurysms,[37,38] complex bifurcation aneurysms, and fusiform aneurysms.[39–41] Furthermore, in an environment that is growing more cost-conscious, the potential high cost of endovascular therapy compared with open surgery will need to be addressed to ensure the continued expansion of the field.[42]

Technologic Advances

Advances in the materials and methods employed in the endovascular embolization of intracranial aneurysms are chiefly driven by the need for improved outcome and durability. To that end, several promising technologies are currently under development and testing[43] **(Fig. 40.1).** Although intracranial stenting has been primarily employed as an adjunct to coiling,[39,44,45] by which the presence of a stent in the parent vessel acts as a "buttress," preventing coil extrusion into the parent vessel, novel uses for intracranial and extracranial[46,47] stenting are becoming available as the technology advances. Perhaps generating the most interest is the use of flow-diverting intracranial stents as the primary treatment for aneurysms, where the stent in the parent vessel diverts flow from the aneurysm and promotes thrombosis. This technology holds promise of improved obliteration rates as well as decreased recanalization rates with possible applications to giant aneurysms.[48] Adequate data demonstrating those benefits are pending at this time. On the other hand, the use of stenting in the setting of aneurysmal rupture has been discouraged primarily due to the need for adequate antiplatelet therapy, which is likely detrimental in that setting.[49] Advances in stent materials may soon overcome this limitation, however. In addition to using traditional stents, the development of stents customized for use in low- and high-perforator density vessels are likely to further improve occlusion rates while preserving flow to critical vessels.[50]

Bifurcation lesions such as middle cerebral artery (MCA) aneurysms have predominantly remained in the surgical domain due to largely unfavorable anatomy and concerns about long-term recurrences.[51] The endovascular treatment of such lesions, in addition to benefiting from more durable embolization materials, is likely to benefit from the development of specialized bifurcation or Y-stents, which are now available for coronary stenting. Similarly, flow-reversal stents, such as the Pipeline braided stent (ev3 Neurovascular, Irvine, CA), are being designed to reduce the impact of fluid momentum on the aneurysm wall while providing a scaffold to induce "aneurysm healing" and remodeling.[52] These devices may have a significant impact on the treatment of such lesions as well as others, as aneurysms can be precluded from the circulation without coil deposition.

In addition to coil embolization materials, liquid embolics such as Onyx (ev3 Neurovascular) may witness more frequent use, especially in the treatment of complex lesions.[53,54] On the other hand, bioactive coil materials have recently garnered significant interest, although preliminary results have been marginal at best.[55] The materials used to impregnate coils fall into three categories: (1) substances meant to induce aneurysmal sac healing (such as polyglycolic acid)[56]; (2) coils such as the Hydrogel coil (MicroVention, Tustin, CA),

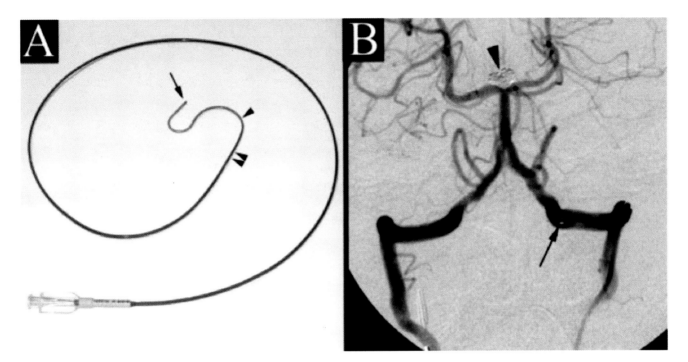

Fig. 40.1 The Neuron guide-catheter (Penumbra, San Leandro, CA) has a distal flexible tip of 6 or 12 cm, and can be placed at or above the skull base. **(A)** The *double-arrowheads* indicate the transition zone from 6 to 5 French. Also note the distal flexible segment *(single arrowhead)* and the radiopaque tip marker *(arrow)*. **(B)** Distal placement at the V3-V4 junction. Arrow indicates coiled and partially coiled aneurysms.

which undergoes volume expansion upon deployment with subsequent theoretical improved sac occlusion[57]; these Hydogel coils may be more durable than plain platinum coils,[58] and although there were initially some concerns about coil stiffness, recent technologic advances have successfully addressed this issue; and (3) embolization materials that may directly impact the local aneurysm biology either by locally delivering growth factors (such as vascular endothelial growth factor [VEGF], transforming growth factor-β [TGF-β], and fibroblast growth factor [FGF]) or containing genetic vectors that induce and promote aneurysm healing.[59] The development of the latter category of embolization materials will depend on advances in our understanding of the biology and genetics of intracranial aneurysms, which is an area of active research.

Pharmacologic Advancements

Although the majority of research and interest has focused on the development and testing of novel endovascular devices and embolic agents, the development of pharmacologic adjuvants will likely contribute to improved outcomes in the future. The role of preoperative antiplatelet or anticoagulation therapy, for instance, has yet to be fully elucidated, and guidelines for the use of such agents are yet to be established. Furthermore, active trials are ongoing to investigate the use of cerebral neuroprotection agents during an endovascular intervention to reduce the frequency and impact of post-intervention diffusion "hits."[15] Similarly, agents that reduce the incidence and severity of post–subarachnoid hemorrhage

vasospasm are highly sought after, and may reduce dependence on pharmacologic and mechanical (balloon) angioplasty for this patient population.[60,61]

Genetics, Pathophysiology, and Screening

Our fundamental understanding of the pathophysiology and the underlying genetic factors predisposing to aneurysm formation and aneurysm rupture is limited. Future expansion of our knowledge on the biology of these lesions will undoubtedly have a major impact on the whole approach to aneurysms and on outcomes. For instance, although the overall initial results from bioactive endovascular coils has been underwhelming, there is a suggestion of the presence of responders and nonresponders in the population.[55] The evolution of bioactive coils may also incorporate genetic or pharmacologic therapy addressing the underlying individualized pathology of each patient. Furthermore, a more complete understanding of the populations at risk for the development of cerebral aneurysms will afford targeted screening protocols with resultant earlier treatment of lesions before they acquire complex anatomic configurations. For instance, Deka et al[62] identified single nucleotide polymorphisms associated with intracranial aneurysms and the increased risk of developing aneurysms in individuals with those variants who are cigarette smokers. Similarly, the identification of patient populations with known aneurysms who are at increased risk for rupture, such as radiographic evidence or with serum markers of intraaneurysmal inflammation, will help direct appropriate therapy.

◆ Arteriovenous Malformations

Arteriovenous malformations (AVMs) are a heterogeneous group of vascular malformations, some of which are amenable to endovascular treatment. Fewer than 15% of AVMs of the brain and spine can be cured with endovascular treatment.[16] Although vein of Galen malformations and carotid-cavernous fistulas (CCFs) are often amenable to endovascular treatment and rarely require open surgical intervention, most other complex lesions require multimodality approaches that often include embolization in the earlier stages of management.

Technologic Advances

The main recent advance in the interventional approaches to AVMs is the advent of Onyx (ethylene-vinyl alcohol). Subsequent advances are likely to focus on novel and improved embolization agents and delivery catheters. Calcium alginate has recently generated interest as a potential novel embolic agent, and preliminary outcomes data are highly anticipated.[63]

Considering the frequency of multimodality treatment of complex AVMs that often incorporates endovascular embolization and radiosurgery, future embolization agents, in addition to improved penetration and safety, would ideally improve radiosensitivity. Furthermore, an ideal agent would not pose the risk of thromboembolism and retain the potential for dissolution in the event of unintended vessel embolization. Finally, with our ever-improving understanding of the biology of arteriovenous malformation, particularly on the role of angiogenic factors in the formation and expansion of AVMs, the introduction of bioactive embolization materials with antiangiogenic attributes may contribute to the healing or involution of the malformation as well as to their occlusion.

◆ Dural Arteriovenous Fistulas

Dural arteriovenous fistulas (DAVFs) are acquired intracranial arteriovenous shunts, with an incompletely understood etiology, which represent approximately 15% of all intracranial AVMs. The clinical manifestations, management options, and prognosis of DAVF are largely determined by venous drainage patterns.

Prior to the introduction of Onyx, the armamentarium of the neurointerventionist consisted of polyvinyl alcohol (PVA), n-butyl-2-cyanoacrylate (nBCA), and detachable coils, and the aims of transarterial embolization depended on the individual case and did not always include curative occlusion of the fistula. Since the introduction of onyx, curative occlusion of many fistulas has become more feasible as the overall angiographic occlusion rates have more than doubled compared with treatment using other materials.[64] Similar to the treatment of AVMs at large, future advances are likely to include novel embolic agents including bioactive materials and improved catheters.

◆ Carotid Disease

The treatment of carotid stenosis, first described in the mid-1950s, continues to be a topic of debate and intense study. Although carotid endarterectomy (CEA) continues to be the treatment of choice for patients with significant (>50%) symptomatic stenosis, the decision to offer CEA to patients with low-grade or asymptomatic stenosis remains controversial. Over the past decade the debate regarding medical versus surgical management of carotid artery disease has expanded to include the interventional techniques of carotid angioplasty and stenting (CAS).

As the general trend toward the use of minimally invasive approaches has increased, interest has intensified in the use of CAS for the treatment of carotid stenosis. In addition to vessel dilation or stenting, recent devices include a distal embolic protection component to reduce the risk of intraoperative stroke. Generally, distal protection devices function by deploying a semipermeable membrane downstream from the stenotic segment prior to angioplasty; alternatively, proximal flow arrest may also offer similar protection while avoiding the risk of maneuvering a device past vulnerable plaque. A number of trials[65–67] have compared carotid endarterectomy and carotid artery stenting, and perhaps the most significant study to date to compare CEA and CAS has been the Carotid Revascularization Endarterectomy versus Stenting Trial (CREST),[68] which emphasized rigorous trial methods in an attempt to produce the most reliable evidence regarding the roles of CEA and CAS in the management of CAS. The final analysis of over 2000 randomized patients, in centers that met strict qualification criteria, revealed no difference in the primary outcomes of the study, namely periprocedural stroke, myocardial infarction (MI), or death or ipsilateral stroke within 4 years. Interestingly, subgroup analysis was notable for stroke occurring more frequently with CAS then CEA (4.1% and 2.3% respectively, $p = .01$), whereas perioperative MI was reported to be more prevalent in the CEA group (1.1% during CAS and 2.3% during CEA; $p = .03$). The results of the trial suggest that both techniques are complementary, and that the variables, including the practitioner's personal experience and the patient's comorbidities, age, and anatomic features, should be carefully considered in the decision making.

Stenting of the external carotid artery (ECA), often in the setting of symptomatic ipsilateral internal carotid artery occlusion, has also been reported, as the ECA may be an important source of collateral circulation.[46,69] Initial results from a multicenter retrospective analysis is promising, with five of 12 patients demonstrating resolution of neurologic symptoms at 2-year follow-up, although large-scale studies are necessary to fully elucidate the clinical indications for ECA stenting.

Technologic Advances

Currently available distal protection filter devices have the potential for embolization during introduction, and may not be able to successfully trap small emboli after deployment.[70]

Furthermore, most require a relatively long and straight segment of vessel distal to the stenosis, which may not always be available. Flow-reversal devices also exist, whereby flow through the internal cerebral artery is reversed prior to the introduction of a wire past the stenotic segment.[71]

As stent technology continues to improve, the prospect of intraprocedural imaging with subsequent patient-specific stent choice has become more attractive. The use of optical coherence tomography (OCT) has recently been reported in case reports,[72] and may represent the first modality of delineating the intraluminal characteristics of plaque and perhaps identify patients at risk for long-term embolic events and those who may benefit from coated or fine mesh stents.

Additional improvements in the outcomes of CAS are expected with the next generation of distal protection devices and stents.

◆ Microdevices, Endovascular Navigation, and Endovascular Access

The notion of deploying untethered microdevices and nanorobots for the purpose of conducting endovascular diagnostic and therapeutic interventions has been the subject of recent interest and research (**Fig. 40.2**). In fact, nanorobotics research groups have recently published reports of real-time control over a ferromagnetic object in a living animal model under simulated human anatomic conditions using a standard MRI system.[73] Ferromagnetic components built into intravascular catheters are also under investigation and represent a novel method of navigating interventional devices that may increase the precision and speed of procedures. Additionally, intraluminal tracking devices, for instance ultrasonic

devices, have been demonstrated to be feasible and accurate when used to track devices within vessels.[74]

The introduction of endovascular devices into the endovascular space is not without risk, including the recently well-documented risk of MRI-confirmed silent cerebral ischemic lesions in as many as one in four patients.[75] This observation highlights the importance of future efforts aimed at reducing the rate of intra- and immediate postprocedure stroke risks.

As for achieving endovascular access, the transfemoral approach remains the preferred route in the majority of patients. In select subpopulations, however, alternative access may be necessary. Although transbrachial,[76] transaortic,[77] and transcarotid[78] approaches have been previously described, each is not without significant risk and limitations. Bendok at al[79] reported the first case series of successful intracranial endovascular procedures performed through a transradial approach (**Fig. 40.3**), and note that as devices continue to become smaller such an approach may become increasingly preferred in select patients.[79]

◆ Neurointerventional Imaging

Imaging of the central nervous system is a fast-growing technologic field. With respect to the neurointerventionist, the two main categories of advances are those that relate to preoperative planning and patient selection, and those that are used intraprocedurally.

Although conventional catheter angiography remains the gold standard for the diagnosis of many cerebrovascular lesions, time-resolved magnetic resonance angiography (TR-MRA) is a promising diagnostic modality that provides

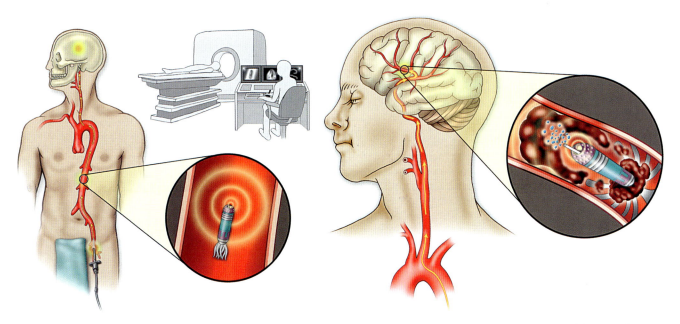

Fig. 40.2 Concept illustration of a micro-robot inserted through the femoral artery and navigated wirelessly with an magnetic resonance imaging (MRI)-guided system to distal cerebral arteries for various therapeutic options such as ultrasound, local drug delivery, and mechanical clot removal.

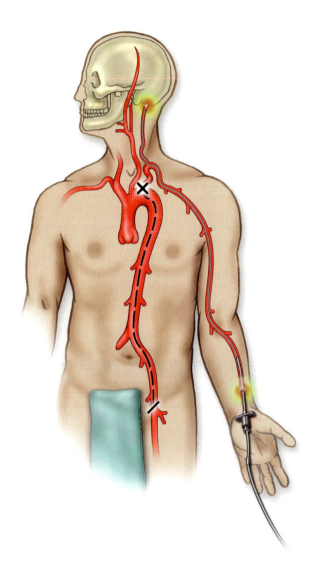

targets. As the technology moves from qualitative and semi-qualitative imaging toward quantitative imaging, it is likely that new guidelines will emerge providing superior diagnostic and prognostic utility as well as improved patient selection criteria for intervention.[81] Furthermore, qualitative MR perfusion imaging may provide similarly improved utility in pathologic conditions of brain hypoperfusion, including occlusive cerebrovascular disease and post–subarachnoid hemorrhage vasospasm.

Magnetic resonance imaging also holds most of the future promise for intraoperative imaging. Already introduced to the neurosurgical operating room, intraprocedural MRI navigation systems are starting to emerge for the neurointerventional suite. Additionally, the preoperative MR images may be fused with real-time MR-guided catheter navigational data to provide enhanced three-dimensional images with better extravascular anatomic context for navigation and treatment.[82] Similarly, holographic angiography techniques may allow the clinician to visualize data acquired by conventional angiography while eliminating the need for scrolling through multiple sequences.

◆ Conclusion

Neurointerventional surgery is a rapidly expanding field with constantly improving tools and ever-evolving indications for treatment of spinal, head and neck, cerebral, and cerebrovascular diseases. As data continues to accumulate regarding new treatment modalities and technologies, neurosurgeons, radiologists, and neurologists should continue to push the field forward in an evidence-based and creative manner. Exciting developments are around the corner in all aspects of the field, including imaging, nanotechnology, custom neuroendovascular devices and implants, and basic science investigation into the pathophysiologic targets of disease.

Fig. 40.3 Illustration of the transradial access route to the posterior cerebral circulation in neuroendovascular procedures. This constitutes a useful technical alternative to the transfemoral approach.

high temporal as well as spatial resolution allowing for the identification of the vascular architecture of lesions such as DAVFs.[80] Similarly, computed tomography angiography (CTA) continues to gain widespread popularity for cerebrovascular imaging by providing ever-improving spatial resolution, three-dimensional reconstructions, and short image-acquisition time, as well as by taking advantage of an established framework of CT scanners; it is often the modality of choice in more critical patients, such as those in whom an emergent noncontrasted CT study raises the concern that a vascular lesion is present, and may be the only modality necessary for interventional decision making and planning. Perfusion-weighed MRI techniques are becoming increasingly important to the neurointerventionist as they may be able to identify areas of salvageable hypoperfused parenchyma in addition to areas of acute stroke, therefore identifying therapeutic

References

1. Boulos AS, Levy EI, Bendok BR, et al. Evolution of neuroendovascular intervention: a review of advancement in device technology. Neurosurgery 2004;54:438–452, discussion 452–453
2. Bendok BR, Hopkins LN. Cutting balloon angioplasty to treat carotid in-stent restenosis. J Invasive Cardiol 2004;16:A16, discussion A16
3. Bendok BR, Sherma AK, Hage ZA, et al. Periprocedural MRI perfusion imaging to assess and monitor the hemodynamic impact of intracranial angioplasty and stenting for symptomatic atherosclerotic stenosis. J Clin Neurosci 2010;17:54–58
4. Rahme RJ, Bendok BR. Beyond opening a closed vessel. Neurosurgery 2010;66:N11–N12
5. Koebbe CJ, Pandey A, Veznedaroglu E, Rosenwasser RH. The evolution and future directions of endovascular therapy. Clin Neurosurg 2006; 53:191–195
6. Rosamond W, Flegal K, Furie K, et al; American Heart Association Statistics Committee and Stroke Statistics Subcommittee. Heart disease and stroke statistics–2008 update: A report from the American Heart Association Statistics Committee and Stroke Statistics Subcommittee. Circulation 2008;117:e25–e146
7. Marler JR, Tilley BC, Lu M, et al. Early stroke treatment associated with better outcome: the NINDS rt-PA stroke study. Neurology 2000;55: 1649–1655
8. Hacke W, Kaste M, Bluhmki E, et al; ECASS Investigators. Thrombolysis with alteplase 3 to 4.5 hours after acute ischemic stroke. N Engl J Med 2008;359:1317–1329

9. Rha JH, Saver JL. The impact of recanalization on ischemic stroke outcome: a meta-analysis. Stroke 2007;38:967–973

10. Katzan IL, Hammer MD, Furlan AJ, Hixson ED, Nadzam DM; Cleveland Clinic Health System Stroke Quality Improvement Team. Quality improvement and tissue-type plasminogen activator for acute ischemic stroke: a Cleveland update. Stroke 2003;34:799–800

11. Part 9: Adult stroke. Circulation 2005;112:IV-111–IV-120

12. California Acute Stroke Pilot Registry (CASPR) Investigators. Prioritizing interventions to improve rates of thrombolysis for ischemic stroke. Neurology 2005;64:654–659

13. Seidel G, Meairs S. Ultrasound contrast agents in ischemic stroke. Cerebrovasc Dis 2009;27(Suppl 2):25–39

14. Mäurer M, Shambal S, Berg D, et al. Differentiation between intracerebral hemorrhage and ischemic stroke by transcranial color-coded duplex-sonography. Stroke 1998;29:2563–2567

15. Goldberg M. Stroke trials registry. 2010 http://www.strokecenter.org/trials/

16. Hopkins LN, Ecker RD. Cerebral endovascular neurosurgery. Neurosurgery 2008;62(6, Suppl 3)1483–1501, discussion 1501–1502

17. Sugrue PA, Hage ZA, Surdell DL, Foroohar M, Liu J, Bendok BR. Basilar artery occlusion following C1 lateral mass fracture managed by mechanical and pharmacological thrombolysis. Neurocrit Care 2009;11:255–260

18. Liebig T, Reinartz J, Hannes R, Miloslavski E, Henkes H. Comparative in vitro study of five mechanical embolectomy systems: effectiveness of clot removal and risk of distal embolization. Neuroradiology 2008;50:43–52

19. Wakhloo AK, Gounis MJ. Retrievable closed cell intracranial stent for foreign body and clot removal. Neurosurgery 2008;62(5, Suppl 2)ONS390–ONS393, discussion ONS393–ONS394

20. Zaidat OO, Wolfe T, Hussain SI, et al. Interventional acute ischemic stroke therapy with intracranial self-expanding stent. Stroke 2008;39:2392–2395

21. Thijs VN, Peeters A, Vosko M, et al. Randomized, placebo-controlled, dose-ranging clinical trial of intravenous microplasmin in patients with acute ischemic stroke. Stroke 2009;40:3789–3795

22. Internet Stroke Center WU. Stroke trials registry. 2010

23. Palesch YY, Hill MD, Ryckborst KJ, Tamariz D, Ginsberg MD. The ALIAS Pilot Trial: a dose-escalation and safety study of albumin therapy for acute ischemic stroke—II: neurologic outcome and efficacy analysis. Stroke 2006;37:2107–2114

24. Muir KW, Lees KR, Ford I, Davis S; Intravenous Magnesium Efficacy in Stroke (IMAGES) Study Investigators. Magnesium for acute stroke (Intravenous Magnesium Efficacy in Stroke trial): randomised controlled trial. Lancet 2004;363:439–445

25. Burns TC, Verfaillie CM, Low WC. Stem cells for ischemic brain injury: a critical review. J Comp Neurol 2009;515:125–144

26. Chen J, Sanberg PR, Li Y, et al. Intravenous administration of human umbilical cord blood reduces behavioral deficits after stroke in rats. Stroke 2001;32:2682–2688

27. Wityk RJ, Lehman D, Klag M, Coresh J, Ahn H, Litt B. Race and sex differences in the distribution of cerebral atherosclerosis. Stroke 1996;27:1974–1980

28. Derdeyn CP, Chimowitz MI. Angioplasty and stenting for atherosclerotic intracranial stenosis: rationale for a randomized clinical trial. Neuroimaging Clin N Am 2007;17:355–363, viii–ix

29. Levy EI, Hanel RA, Boulos AS, et al. Comparison of periprocedure complications resulting from direct stent placement compared with those due to conventional and staged stent placement in the basilar artery. J Neurosurg 2003;99:653–660

30. Gross BA, Hurley MC, Bernstein R, Shaibani A, Batjer HH, Bendok BR. Endovascular recanalization for subacute symptomatic intracranial arterial occlusion: a report of two cases. Clin Neurol Neurosurg 2008;110:1058–1063

31. Samaniego EA, Hetzel S, Thirunarayanan S, Aagaard-Kienitz B, Turk AS, Levine R. Outcome of symptomatic intracranial atherosclerotic disease. Stroke 2009;40:2983–2987

32. Fiorella DJ, Levy EI, Turk AS, et al. Target lesion revascularization after wingspan: assessment of safety and durability. Stroke 2009;40:106–110

33. Schumacher HC, Meyers PM, Higashida RT, et al. Reporting standards for angioplasty and stent-assisted angioplasty for intracranial atherosclerosis. Stroke 2009;40:e348–e365

34. Parkinson RJ, Demers CP, Adel JG, et al. Use of heparin-coated stents in neurovascular interventional procedures: preliminary experience with 10 patients. Neurosurgery 2006;59:812–821, discussion 821

35. Tamai H, Igaki K, Kyo E, et al. Initial and 6-month results of biodegradable poly-l-lactic acid coronary stents in humans. Circulation 2000;102:399–404

36. Molyneux A, Kerr R, Stratton I, et al; International Subarachnoid Aneurysm Trial (ISAT) Collaborative Group. International Subarachnoid Aneurysm Trial (ISAT) of neurosurgical clipping versus endovascular coiling in 2143 patients with ruptured intracranial aneurysms: a randomised trial. Lancet 2002;360:1267–1274

37. Parkinson RJ, Eddleman CS, Batjer HH, Bendok BR. Giant intracranial aneurysms: endovascular challenges. Neurosurgery 2008;62(6, Suppl 3)1336–1345

38. Parkinson RJ, Eddleman CS, Batjer HH, Bendok BR. Giant intracranial aneurysms: endovascular challenges. Neurosurgery 2006;59(5, Suppl 3)S103–S112, discussion S3–S13

39. O'Shaughnessy BA, Getch CC, Bendok BR, Batjer HH. Late morphological progression of a dissecting basilar artery aneurysm after staged bilateral vertebral artery occlusion: case report. Surg Neurol 2005;63:236–243, discussion 243

40. Parkinson RJ, Bendok BR, Getch CC, et al. Retrograde suction decompression of giant paraclinoid aneurysms using a No. 7 French balloon-containing guide catheter. Technical note. J Neurosurg 2006;105:479–481

41. Surdell DL, Hage ZA, Eddleman CS, Gupta DK, Bendok BR, Batjer HH. Revascularization for complex intracranial aneurysms. Neurosurg Focus 2008;24:E21

42. Hoh BL, Chi YY, Dermott MA, Lipori PJ, Lewis SB. The effect of coiling versus clipping of ruptured and unruptured cerebral aneurysms on length of stay, hospital cost, hospital reimbursement, and surgeon reimbursement at the university of Florida. Neurosurgery 2009;64:614–619, discussion 619–621

43. Hurley MC, Sherma AK, Surdell D, Shaibani A, Bendok BR. A novel guide catheter enabling intracranial placement. Catheter Cardiovasc Interv 2009;74:920–924

44. Adel JG, Sherma AK, Bendok BR. CT angiography for assessment of intracranial basilar apex aneurysm neck diameter reduction poststenting for treatment planning. Catheter Cardiovasc Interv 2010;75:644–647

45. Bendok BR, Parkinson RJ, Hage ZA, Adel JG, Gounis MJ. The effect of vascular reconstruction device-assisted coiling on packing density, effective neck coverage, and angiographic outcome: an in vitro study. Neurosurgery 2007;61:835–840, discussion 840–841

46. Xu DS, Abruzzo TA, Albuquerque FC, et al. External carotid artery stenting to treat patients with symptomatic ipsilateral internal carotid artery occlusion: a multicenter case series. Neurosurgery 2010;67:314–321

47. Adel JG, Bendok BR, Hage ZA, Naidech AM, Miller JW, Batjer HH. External carotid artery angioplasty and stenting to augment cerebral perfusion in the setting of subacute symptomatic ipsilateral internal carotid artery occlusion. Case report. J Neurosurg 2007;107:1217–1222

48. Lubicz B, Bandeira A, Bruneau M, Dewindt A, Balériaux D, De Witte O. Stenting is improving and stabilizing anatomical results of coiled intracranial aneurysms. Neuroradiology 2009;51:419–425

49. Kessler IM, Mounayer C, Piotin M, Spelle L, Vanzin JR, Moret J. The use of balloon-expandable stents in the management of intracranial arterial diseases: a 5-year single-center experience. AJNR Am J Neuroradiol 2005;26:2342–2348

50. Levy EI, Chaturvedi S. Perforator stroke following intracranial stenting: a sacrifice for the greater good? Neurology 2006;66:1803–1804

51. Suzuki S, Tateshima S, Jahan R, et al. Endovascular treatment of middle cerebral artery aneurysms with detachable coils: angiographic and clinical outcomes in 115 consecutive patients. Neurosurgery 2009;64:876–888, discussion 888–889

52. Fiorella D, Woo HH, Albuquerque FC, Nelson PK. Definitive reconstruction of circumferential, fusiform intracranial aneurysms with the pipeline embolization device. Neurosurgery 2008;62:1115–1120, discussion 1120–1121

53. Cekirge HS, Saatci I, Ozturk MH, et al. Late angiographic and clinical follow-up results of 100 consecutive aneurysms treated with Onyx reconstruction: largest single-center experience. Neuroradiology 2006;48:113–126

54. Hurley MC, Gross BA, Surdell D, et al. Preoperative Onyx embolization of aggressive vertebral hemangiomas. AJNR Am J Neuroradiol 2008;29:1095–1097

55. Fiorella D, Albuquerque FC, McDougall CG. Durability of aneurysm embolization with matrix detachable coils. Neurosurgery 2006;58:51–59, discussion 51–59

56. Murayama Y, Tateshima S, Gonzalez NR, Vinuela F. Matrix and bioabsorbable polymeric coils accelerate healing of intracranial aneurysms: long-term experimental study. Stroke 2003;34:2031–2037

57. Kallmes DF, Fujiwara NH. New expandable hydrogel-platinum coil hybrid device for aneurysm embolization. AJNR Am J Neuroradiol 2002;23:1580–1588

58. O'Hare AM, Fanning NF, Ti JP, Dunne R, Brennan PR, Thornton JM. HydroCoils, occlusion rates, and outcomes: a large single-center study. AJNR Am J Neuroradiol 2010;31:1917–1922

59. Abrahams JM, Forman MS, Grady MS, Diamond SL. Delivery of human vascular endothelial growth factor with platinum coils enhances wall thickening and coil impregnation in a rat aneurysm model. AJNR Am J Neuroradiol 2001;22:1410–1417

60. Eddleman CS, Hurley MC, Naidech AM, Batjer HH, Bendok BR. Endovascular options in the treatment of delayed ischemic neurological deficits due to cerebral vasospasm. Neurosurg Focus 2009;26:E6

61. Mindea SA, Yang BP, Bendok BR, Miller JW, Batjer HH. Endovascular treatment strategies for cerebral vasospasm. Neurosurg Focus 2006;21:E13

62. Deka R, Koller DL, Lai D, et al; FIA Study Investigators. The relationship between smoking and replicated sequence variants on chromosomes 8 and 9 with familial intracranial aneurysm. Stroke 2010;41:1132–1137

63. Becker TA, Preul MC, Bichard WD, Kipke DR, McDougall CG. Preliminary investigation of calcium alginate gel as a biocompatible material for endovascular aneurysm embolization in vivo. Neurosurgery 2007;60:1119–1127, discussion 1127–1128

64. Macdonald JH, Millar JS, Barker CS. Endovascular treatment of cranial dural arteriovenous fistulae: a single-centre, 14-year experience and the impact of Onyx on local practise. Neuroradiology 2010;52:387–395

65. Endovascular versus surgical treatment in patients with carotid stenosis in the Carotid and Vertebral Artery Transluminal Angioplasty Study (CAVATAS): a randomised trial. Lancet 2001;357:1729–1737

66. Ringleb PA, Allenberg J, Brückmann H, et al; SPACE Collaborative Group. 30 day results from the SPACE trial of stent-protected angioplasty versus carotid endarterectomy in symptomatic patients: a randomised non-inferiority trial. Lancet 2006;368:1239–1247

67. Yadav JS, Wholey MH, Kuntz RE, et al; Stenting and Angioplasty with Protection in Patients at High Risk for Endarterectomy Investigators. Protected carotid-artery stenting versus endarterectomy in high-risk patients. N Engl J Med 2004;351:1493–1501

68. Brott TG, Hobson RW II, Howard G, et al; CREST Investigators. Stenting versus endarterectomy for treatment of carotid-artery stenosis. N Engl J Med 2010;363:11–23

69. Xu DS, Abruzzo TA, Albuquerque FC, et al. External carotid artery stenting to treat patients with symptomatic ipsilateral internal carotid artery occlusion: a multicenter case series. Neurosurgery 2010;67:314–321

70. Clair DG. Carotid stenting: new devices on the horizon and beyond. Semin Vasc Surg 2008;21:88–94

71. Rabe K, Sugita J, Gödel H, Sievert H. Flow-reversal device for cerebral protection during carotid artery stenting—acute and long-term results. J Interv Cardiol 2006;19:55–62

72. Yoshimura S, Kawasaki M, Hattori A, Nishigaki K, Minatoguchi S, Iwama T. Demonstration of intraluminal thrombus in the carotid artery by optical coherence tomography: technical case report. Neurosurgery 2010;67(3, Suppl Operative)E305, discussion E305

73. Martel S, Mathieu JB, Felfoul O, et al. A computer-assisted protocol for endovascular target interventions using a clinical MRI system for controlling untethered microdevices and future nanorobots. Comput Aided Surg 2008;13:340–352

74. Bond AE, Weaver FA, Mung J, Han S, Fullerton D, Yen J. The influence of stents on the performance of an ultrasonic navigation system for endovascular procedures. J Vasc Surg 2009;50:1143–1148

75. Bendszus M, Koltzenburg M, Burger R, Warmuth-Metz M, Hofmann E, Solymosi L. Silent embolism in diagnostic cerebral angiography and neurointerventional procedures: a prospective study. Lancet 1999;354:1594–1597

76. Gritter KJ, Laidlaw WW, Peterson NT. Complications of outpatient transbrachial intraarterial digital subtraction angiography. Work in progress. Radiology 1987;162(1 Pt 1):125–127

77. Glower DD, Clements FM, Debruijn NP, et al. Comparison of direct aortic and femoral cannulation for port-access cardiac operations. Ann Thorac Surg 1999;68:1529–1531

78. Berkmen T, Troffkin N, Wakhloo AK. Direct percutaneous puncture of a cervical internal carotid artery aneurysm for coil placement after previous incomplete stent-assisted endovascular treatment. AJNR Am J Neuroradiol 2003;24:1230–1233

79. Bendok BR, Przybylo JH, Parkinson R, Hu Y, Awad IA, Batjer HH. Neuroendovascular interventions for intracranial posterior circulation disease via the transradial approach: technical case report. Neurosurgery 2005;56:E626, discussion E626

80. Meckel S, Maier M, Ruiz DS, et al. MR angiography of dural arteriovenous fistulas: diagnosis and follow-up after treatment using a time-resolved 3D contrast-enhanced technique. AJNR Am J Neuroradiol 2007;28:877–884

81. Schellinger PD, Bryan RN, Caplan LR, et al; Therapeutics and Technology Assessment Subcommittee of the American Academy of Neurology. Evidence-based guideline: The role of diffusion and perfusion MRI for the diagnosis of acute ischemic stroke: report of the Therapeutics and Technology Assessment Subcommittee of the American Academy of Neurology. Neurology 2010;75:177–185

82. Saybasili H, Faranesh AZ, Saikus CE, Ozturk C, Lederman RJ, Guttman MA. Interventional MRI using multiple 3D angiography roadmaps with real-time imaging. J Magn Reson Imaging 2010;31:1015–1019

Index

Note: Page references followed by *f* indicate figures; page references followed by *t* indicate tables.

Index

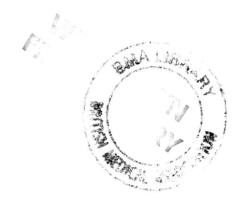